The GALE ENCYCLOPEDIA of CANCER

A GUIDE TO CANCER AND ITS TREATMENTS

THIRD EDITION

Barnes & Noble 2/9/12 $456.00

The GALE ENCYCLOPEDIA *of* CANCER

A GUIDE TO CANCER AND ITS TREATMENTS

THIRD EDITION

VOLUME

2

L–Z

JACQUELINE L. LONGE, EDITOR

GALE
CENGAGE Learning™

Detroit • New York • San Francisco • New Haven, Conn • Waterville, Maine • London

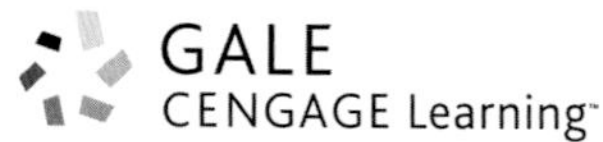

Gale Encyclopedia of Cancer: A Guide To Cancer And Its Treatments

Project Editors: Jacqueline L. Longe

Editorial: Kristin Key

Product Manager: Kate Hanley

Editorial Support Services: Andrea Lopeman

Indexing Services: Factiva, a Dow Jones Company

Rights Acquisition and Management: Margaret Abendroth, Dean Dauphinais, and Savannah Gignac

Composition: Evi Abou-El-Seoud

Manufacturing: Wendy Blurton

Imaging: John Watkins

Product Design: Pam Galbreath

For product information and technology assistance, contact us at
Gale Customer Support, 1-800-877-4253.
For permission to use material from this text or product,
submit all requests online at **www.cengage.com/permissions.**
Further permissions questions can be emailed to
permissionrequest@cengage.com

Library of Congress Cataloging-in-Publication Data

The Gale encyclopedia of cancer : a guide to cancer and its treatments. -- 3rd ed. / Jacqueline L. Longe, editor.
p. ; cm.
Other title: Encyclopedia of cancer
Includes bibliographical references and index.
ISBN-13: 978-1-4144-7598-1 (set)
ISBN-13: 978-1-4144-7599-8 (vol. 1)
ISBN-13: 978-1-4144-7600-1 (vol. 2)
ISBN-10: 1-4144-7598-5 (set)
[etc.]
1. Cancer--Encyclopedias. 2. Oncology--Encyclopedias. I. Longe, Jacqueline L. II. Title: Encyclopedia of cancer.
[DNLM: 1. Neoplasms--Encyclopedias--English. 2. Medical Oncology--Encyclopedias--English. QZ 13 G151 2010]

RC254.5.G353 2010
616.99'4003--dc22 2010002075

Gale
27500 Drake Rd.
Farmington Hills, MI, 48331-3535

ISBN-13: 978-1-4144-7598-1 (set)
ISBN-13: 978-1-4144-7599-8 (vol. 1)
ISBN-13: 978-1-4144-7600-1 (vol. 2)

ISBN-10: 1-4144-7598-5 (set)
ISBN-10: 1-4144-7599-3 (vol. 1)
ISBN-10: 1-4144-7600-0 (vol. 2)

This title is also available as an e-book.
ISBN-13: 978-1-4144-7601-8 ISBN-10: 1-4144-7601-9
Contact your Gale, a part of Cengage Learning sales representative for ordering information.

Printed in China by China Translation & Printing Services Limited
1 2 3 4 5 6 7 11 10

CONTENTS

LIST OF ENTRIES

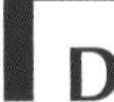

D

E

F

G

H

I

K

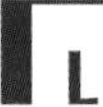

L

M

N

O

P

Q

R

S

T

U

V

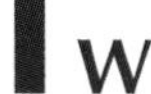

W

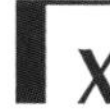

X

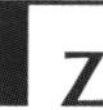

Z

PLEASE READ—IMPORTANT INFORMATION

The *Gale Encyclopedia of Cancer: A Guide To Cancer And Its Treatments* is a health reference product designed to inform and educate readers about a wide variety of cancers, diseases and conditions related to cancers, nutrition and dietary practices beneficial to cancer patients, and various cancer treatments including drug treatments. Cengage Learning believes the product to be comprehensive, but not necessarily definitive. It is intended to supplement, not replace, consultation with a physician or other healthcare practitioners. While Cengage Learning has made substantial efforts to provide information that is accurate, comprehensive, and up-to-date, Cengage Learning makes no representations or warranties of any kind, including without limitation, warranties of merchantability or fitness for a particular purpose, nor does it guarantee the accuracy, comprehensiveness, or timeliness of the information contained in this product. Readers should be aware that the universe of medical knowledge is constantly growing and changing, and that differences of opinion exist among authorities. Readers are also advised to seek professional diagnosis and treatment for any medical condition, and to discuss information obtained from this book with their healthcare provider.

INTRODUCTION

The *Gale Encyclopedia of Cancer: A Guide to Cancer and Its Treatments* is a unique and invaluable source of information for anyone touched by cancer. This collection of over 450 entries provides in-depth coverage of specific cancer types, diagnostic procedures, treatments, cancer side effects, and cancer drugs. In addition, entries have been included to facilitate understanding of common cancer-related concepts, such as cancer biology, carcinogenesis, and cancer genetics, as well as cancer issues such as clinical trials, home health care, fertility issues, and cancer prevention. This encyclopedia minimizes medical jargon and uses language that laypersons can understand, while still providing thorough coverage that will benefit health science students as well.

Scope

Entries follow a standardized format that provides information at a glance. Rubrics include:

Cancer types

- Definition
- Description
- Demographics
- Causes and symptoms
- Diagnosis
- Treatment team
- Clincial staging, treatments, and prognosis
- Coping with cancer treatment
- Clinical trials
- Prevention
- Special concerns
- Resources
- Key terms

Cancer drugs

- Definition
- Purpose
- Description
- Recommended dosage
- Precautions
- Side effects
- Interactions

Drugs, herbs, vitamins

- Definition
- Description
- Recommended dosage
- Precautions
- Side effects
- Interactions
- Caregiver concerns
- "Questions to ask the doctor"
- Resources
- Key Terms

Inclusion criteria

A preliminary list of cancers and related topics was compiled from a wide variety of sources, including professional medical guides and textbooks, as well as consumer guides and encyclopedias. The advisory board, made up of medical doctors and oncology pharmacists, evaluated the topics and made suggestions for inclusion. Final selection of topics to include was made by the advisory board in conjunction with the Gale editor.

About the contributors

The essays were compiled by experienced medical writers, including physicians, pharmacists, nurses, and other health care professionals. The advisors reviewed the completed essays to ensure that they are appropriate, up-to-date, and medically accurate.

How to use this book

The *Gale Encyclopedia of Cancer* has been designed with ready reference in mind.

- Straight **alphabetical arrangement** of topics allows users to locate information quickly.
- **Bold-faced terms** within entries direct the reader to related articles.
- **Cross-references** placed throughout the encyclopedia direct readers from alternate names and related topics to entries.
- A list of **key terms** is provided where appropriate to define unfamiliar terms or concepts.
- A list of **questions to ask the doctor** is provided whevever appropriate to help facilitate discussion with the patient's physician.
- The **Resources** section for non-drug entries directs readers to additional sources of medical information on a topic.
- Valuable **contact information** for organizations and support groups is included with each cancer type entry. Appendix II at the back of Volume 2 contains an extensive list of organizations arranged in alphabetical order.
- A comprehensive **general index** guides readers to all topics mentioned in the text.
- A note about **drug entries**: Drug entries are listed in alphabetical order by common **generic names**. However, because many oncology drugs have more than one common generic name, and because in many cases, the brand name is also often used interchangeably with a generic name, drugs can be located in one of three ways. The reader can: find the generic drug name in alphabetical order, be directed to the entry from an alternate name cross-reference, or the reader can use the **index** to look up a **brand name**, which will direct the reader to the equivalent generic name entry. If the reader would like more information about oncology drugs than these entries provide, the reader is encouraged to consult with a physician, pharmacist, or the reader may find helpful any one of a number of books about cancer drugs. Two that may be helpful are: D. Solimando's *Drug Information Handbook for Oncology*, or R. Ellerby's *Quick Reference Handbook of Oncology Drugs*.

Graphics

The *Gale Encyclopedia of Cancer* is also enhanced by color photographs,illustrations, and tables.

FOREWORD

Unfortunately, humans must suffer disease. Some diseases are totally reversible and can be effectively treated. Moreover, some diseases with proper treatment have been virtually annihilated, such as polio, rheumatic fever, smallpox, and, to some extent, tuberculosis. Other diseases seem to target one organ, such as the heart, and there has been great progress in either fixing defects, adding blood flow, or giving medications to strengthen the diseased pump. Cancer, however, continues to frustrate even the cleverest of doctors or the most fastidious of health conscious individuals. Why?

By its very nature, cancer is a survivor. It has only one purpose: to proliferate. After all, that is the definition of cancer: unregulated growth of cells that fail to heed the message to stop growing. Normal cells go through a cycle of division, aging, and then selection for death. Cancer cells are able to circumvent this normal cycle, and escape recognition to be eliminated.

There are many mechanisms that can contribute to this unregulated cell growth. One of these mechanisms is inheritance. Unfortunately, some individuals can be programmed for cancer due to inherited disorders in their genetic makeup. In its simplest terms, one can inherit a faulty gene or a missing gene whose role is to eliminate damaged cells or to prevent imperfect cells from growing. Without this natural braking system, the damaged cells can divide and lead to more damaged cells with the same abnormal genetic makeup as the parent cells. Given enough time, and our inability to detect them, these groups of cells can grow to a size that will cause discomfort or other symptoms.

Inherited genetics are obviously not the only source of abnormalities in cells. Humans do not live in a sterile world devoid of environmental attacks or pathogens. Humans must work, and working environments can be dangerous. Danger can come in the form of radiation, chemicals, or fibers to which we may be chronically exposed with or without our knowledge. Moreover, man must eat, and if our food is contaminated with these environmental hazards, or if we prepare our food in a way that may change the chemical nature of the food to hazardous molecules, then chronic exposure to these toxins could damage cells. Finally, man is social. He has found certain habits which are pleasing to him because they either relax him or release his inhibitions. Such habits, including smoking and alcohol consumption, can have a myriad of influences on the genetic makeup of cells.

Why the emphasis on genes in the new century? Because they are potentially the reason as well as the answer for cancer. Genes regulate our micro- and macrosopic events by eventually coding for proteins that control our structure and function. If the abovementioned environmental events cause errors in those genes that control growth, then imperfect cells can start to take root. For the majority of cases, a whole cascade of genetic events must occur before a cell is able to outlive its normal predecessors. This cascade of events could take years to occur, in a silent, undetected manner until the telltale signs and symptoms of advanced cancer are seen, including pain, lack of appetite, cough, loss of blood, or the detection of a lump. How did these cells get to this state where they are now dictating the everyday physical, psychological, and economic events for the person afflicted?

At this time, the sequence of genetic catastrophes is much too complex to comprehend or summarize because, it is only in the past year that we have even been able to map what genes we have and where they are located in our chromosomes. We have learned, however, that cancer cells are equipped with a series of self-protection mechanisms. Some of the altered genes are actually able to express themselves more than in the normal situation. These genes could then code for more growth factors for the transforming cell, or they could make proteins that could keep our own immune system from eliminating these interlopers. Finally, these cells are chameleons: if we treat them with drugs to try to kill them, they can "change their colors" by mutation, and then be resistant to the drugs that may have harmed them before.

Then what do we do for treatment? Man has always had a fascination with grooming, and grooming involves removal—dirt, hair, waste. The ultimate removal involves cutting away the spoiled or imperfect portion. An abnormal growth? Remove it by surgery ... make sure the edges are clean. Unfortunately, the painful reality of cancer surgery is that it is highly effective when performed in the early stages of the disease. "Early stages of the disease" implies that there is no spread, or, hopefully, before there are symptoms. In the majority of cases, however, surgery cannot eradicate all the disease because the cancer is not only at the primary site of the lump, but has spread to other organs. Cancer is not just a process of growth, but also a metastasizing process that allows for invasion and spread. The growing cells need nourishment so they secrete proteins that allow for the growth of blood vessels (angiogenesis); once the blood vessels are established from other blood vessels, the tumor cells can make proteins that will dissolve the imprisoning matrix surrounding them. Once this matrix is dissolved, it is only a matter of time before thecancer cells will migrate to other places making the use of surgery fruitless.

Since cancer cells have a propensity to leave home and pay a visit to other organs, therapies must be geared to treat the whole body and not just the site of origin. The problem with these chemotherapies is that they are not selective and wreak havoc on tissues that are not affected by the cancer. These therapies are not natural to the human host, and result in nausea, loss of appetite, fatigue, as well as a depletion in our cells that protect us from infection and those that carry oxygen. Doctors who prescribe such medications walk a fine line between helping the patient (causing a "response" in the cancer by making it smaller) or causing "toxicity" which, due to effects on normal organs, causes the patient problems. Although these drugs are far from perfect, we are fortunate to have them because when they work, their results can be remarkable.

But that's the problem—"when they work." We cannot predict who is going to benefit from our therapies, and doctors must inform the patient and his/her family about countless studies that have been done to validate the use of these potentially beneficial/potentially harmful agents. Patients must suffer the frustration that oncologists have because each individual afflicted with cancer is different, and indeed, each cancer is different. This makes it virtually impossible to personalize an individual's treatment expectations and life expectancy. Cancer, after all, is a very impersonal disease, and does not respect sex, race, wealth, age, or any other "human" characteristics.

Cancer treatment is in search of "smart" options. Like modern-day instruments of war, successful cancer treatment will necessitate the construction of therapies which can do three basic tasks: search out the enemy, recognize the enemy, and kill the enemy without causing "friendly fire." The successful therapies of the future will involve the use of "living components," "manufactured components," or a combination of both. Living components, white blood cells, will be educated to recognize where the cancer is, and help our own immune system fight the foreign cells. These lymphocytes can be educated to recognize signals on the cancer cell which make them unique. Therapies in the future will be able to manufacture molecules with these signature, unique signals which are linked to other molecules specifically for killing the cells. Only the cancer cells are eliminated in this way, hopefully sparing the individual from toxicity.

Why use these unique signals as delivery mechanisms? If they are unique and are important for growth of the cancer cell, why not target them directly? This describes the ambitious mission of gene therapy, whose goal is to supplement a deficient, necessary genetic pool or diminish the number of abnormally expressed genes fortifying the cancer cells. If a protein is not being made that slows the growth of cells, gene therapy would theoretically supply the gene for this protein to replenish it and cause the cells to slow down. If the cells can make their own growth factors that sustain them selectively over normal cells, then the goal is to block the production of this growth factor. There is no doubt that gene therapy is the wave of the future and is under intense investigation and scrutiny at present. The problem, however, is that there is no way to tell when this future promise will be fulfilled.

No book can describe the medical, psychological, social, and economic burden of cancer, and if this is your first confrontation with the enemy, you may find yourself overwhelmed with its magnitude. Books are only part of the solution. Newly enlisted recruits in this war must seek proper counsel from educated physicians who will inform the family and the patient of the risks and benefits of a treatment course in a way that can be understood. Advocacy groups of dedicated volunteers, many of whom are cancer survivors, can guide and advise. The most important component, however, is an intensely personal one. The afflicted individual must realize that he/she is responsible for charting the course of his/her disease, and this requires the above described knowledge as well as great personal intuition. Cancer comes as a series of shocks: the symptoms, the diagnosis, and the treatment. These shocks can be followed by cautious optimism or profound disappointment. Each one of these shocks either reinforces or chips away at one's resolve, and how an individual reacts to these issues is as unique as the cancer that is being dealt with.

While cancer is still life-threatening, strides have been made in the fight against the disease. Thirty years ago, a young adult diagnosed with testicular cancer had few options for treatment that could result in cure. Now, chemotherapy for good risk Stage II and III testicular cancer can result in a complete response of the tumor in 98% of the cases and a durable response in 92%. Sixty years ago, there were no regimens that could cause a complete remission for a child diagnosed with leukemia; but now, using combination chemotherapy, complete remissions are possible in 96% of these cases. Progress has been made, but more progress is needed. The first real triumph in cancer care will be when cancer is no longer thought of as a life-ending disease, but as a chronic disease whose symptoms can be managed. Anyone who has been touched by cancer or who has been involved in the fight against it lives in hope that that day will arrive.

Helen A. Pass, M.D., F.A.C.S.
Director, Breast Care Center
William Beaumont Hospital
Royal Oak, Michigan

ADVISORS

A number of experts in the medical community provided invaluable assistance in the formulation of this encyclopedia. Our advisory board performed a myriad of duties, from defining the scope of coverage to reviewing individual entries for accuracy and accessibility. The editor would like to express her appreciation to them.

Melinda Granger Oberleitner, R.N., D.N.S.
Acting Department Head and Associate Professor
Department of Nursing
University of Louisiana at Lafayette
Lafayette, Louisiana

Helen A. Pass, M.D., F.A.C.S.
Director, Breast Care Center
William Beaumont Hospital
Royal Oak, Michigan

Marianne Vahey, M.D.
Clinical Instructor in Medicine
Yale University School of Medicine
New Haven, Connecticut

James E. Waun, M.D., M.A., R. Ph..
Associate Clinical Professor
Department of Family Practice
Faculty
Center for Ethics and the Humanities
Michigan State University
Adjunct Assistant Professor of Clinical Pharmacy
Ferris State University
East Lansing, Michigan

CONTRIBUTORS

Margaret Alic, Ph.D.
Science Writer
Eastsound, Washington

Lisa Andres, M.S., C.G.C.
Certified Genetic Counselor and Medical Writer
San Jose, California

Racquel Baert, M.Sc.
Medical Writer
Winnipeg, Canada

Julia R. Barrett
Science Writer
Madison, Wisconsin

Maria Basile, PhD
Neuropharmacologist
Neward, New Jersey

Nancy J. Beaulieu, RPh., B.C.O.P.
Oncology Pharmacist
New Haven, Connecticut

Linda K. Bennington, C.N.S., M.S.N.
Clinical Nurse Specialist
Department of Nursing
Old Dominion University
Norfolk, Virginia

Kenneth J. Berniker, M.D.
Attending Physician
Emergency Department
Kaiser Permanente Medical Center
Vallejo, California

Olga Bessmertny, Pharm.D.
Clinical Pharmacy Manager
Pediatric Hematology/Oncology/Bone Marrow Transplant
Children's Hospital of New York
Columbia Presbyterian Medical Center
New York, New York

Patricia L. Bounds, Ph.D.
Science Writer
Zürich, Switzerland

Cheryl Branche, M.D.
Retired General Practitioner
Jackson, Mississippi

Tamara Brown, R.N.
Medical Writer
Boston, Massachusetts

Diane M. Calabrese
Medical Sciences and Technology Writer
Silver Spring, Maryland

Rosalyn Carson-DeWitt, M.D.
Durham, North Carolina

Lata Cherath, Ph.D.
Science Writer
Franklin Park, New York

Lisa Christenson, Ph.D.
Science Writer
Hamden, Connecticut

Rhonda Cloos, R.N.
Medical Writer
Austin, Texas

David Cramer, M.D.
Medical Writer
Chicago, Illinois

Tish Davidson, A.M.
Medical Writer
Fremont, California

Dominic DeBellis, Ph.D.
Medical Writer and Editor
Mahopac, New York

Tiffani A. DeMarco, M.S.
Genetic Counselor
Cancer Control
Georgetown University
Washington, DC

Lori DeMilto
Medical Writer
Sicklerville, New York

Stefanie B. N. Dugan, M.S.
Genetic Counselor
Milwaukee, Wisconsin

Janis O. Flores
Medical Writer
Sebastopol, California

Paula Ford-Martin
Medical Writer
Chaplin, Minnesota

Rebecca J. Frey, Ph.D.
Research and Administrative Associate
East Rock Institute
New Haven, Connecticut

Jason Fryer
Medical Writer
Lubbock, Texas

Jill Granger, M.S.
Senior Research Associate
University of Michigan
Ann Arbor, Michigan

David E. Greenberg, M.D.
Medicine Resident
Baylor College of Medicine
Houston, Texas

Maureen Haggerty
Medical Writer
Ambler, Pennsylvania

Kevin Hwang, M.D.
Medical Writer
Morristown, New Jersey

Michelle L. Johnson, M.S., J.D.
Patent Attorney and Medical Writer
Portland, Oregon

Paul A. Johnson, Ed.M.
Medical Writer
San Diego, California

Cindy L. A. Jones, Ph.D.
Biomedical Writer
Sagescript Communications
Lakewood, Colorado

Crystal H. Kaczkowski, M.Sc.
Medical Writer
Montreal, Canada

David S. Kaminstein, M.D.
Medical Writer
Westchester, Pennsylvania

Beth Kapes
Medical Writer
Bay Village, Ohio

Bob Kirsch
Medical Writer
Ossining, New York

Melissa Knopper
Medical Writer
Chicago, Illinois

Monique Laberge, Ph.D.
Research Associate
Department of Biochemistry and Biophysics
University of Pennsylvania
Philadelphia, Pennsylvania

Jill S. Lasker
Medical Writer
Midlothian, Virginia

G. Victor Leipzig, Ph.D.
Biological Consultant
Huntington Beach, California

Lorraine Lica, Ph.D.
Medical Writer
San Diego, California

John T. Lohr, Ph.D.
Utah State University
Logan, Utah

Warren Maltzman, Ph.D.
Consultant, Molecular Pathology
Demarest, New Jersey

Richard A. McCartney M.D.
Fellow, American College of Surgeons
Diplomat, American Board of Surgery
Richland, Washington

Sally C. McFarlane-Parrott
Medical Writer
Mason, Michigan

Monica McGee, M.S.
Science Writer
Wilmington, North Carolina

Alison McTavish, M.Sc.
Medical Writer and Editor
Montreal, Quebec

Molly Metzler, R.N., B.S.N.
Registered Nurse and Medical Writer
Seaford, Delaware

Beverly G. Miller
MT(ASCP), Technical Writer
Charlotte, North Carolina

Mark A. Mitchell, M.D.
Medical Writer
Seattle, Washington

Laura J. Ninger
Medical Writer
Weehawken, New Jersey

Nancy J. Nordenson
Medical Writer
Minneapolis, Minnesota

Teresa G. Odle
Medical Writer
Albuquerque, New Mexico

Melinda Granger Oberleitner
Acting Department Head and Associate Professor
Department of Nursing
University of Louisiana at Lafayette
Lafayette, Louisiana

Lee Ann Paradise
Science Writer
Lubbock, Texas

J. Ricker Polsdorfer, M.D.
Medical Writer
Phoenix, Arizona

Elizabeth J. Pulcini, M.S.
Medical Writer
Phoenix, Arizona

Kulbir Rangi, D.O.
Medical Doctor and Writer
New York, New York

Esther Csapo Rastegari, Ed.M., R.N., B.S.N.
Registered Nurse, Medical Writer
Holbrook, Masachusetts

Toni Rizzo
Medical Writer
Salt Lake City, Utah

Martha Floberg Robbins
Medical Writer
Evanston, Illinois

Richard Robinson
Medical Writer
Tucson, Arizona

Edward R. Rosick, D.O., M.P.H., M.S.
University Physician, Clinical Assistant Professor
Student Health Services
The Pennsylvania State University
University Park, Pennsylvania

Nancy Ross-Flanigan
Science Writer
Belleville, Michigan

Belinda Rowland, Ph.D.
Medical Writer
Voorheesville, New York

Andrea Ruskin, M.D.
Whittingham Cancer Center
Norwalk, Connecticut

Laura Ruth, Ph.D.
Medical, Science, & Technology Writer
Los Angeles, California

Kausalya Santhanam, Ph.D.
Technical Writer
Branford, Connecticut

Marc Scanio
Doctoral Candidate in Chemistry
Stanford University
Stanford, California

Joan Schonbeck, R.N.
Medical Writer
Nursing
Massachusetts Department of Mental Health
Marlborough, Massachusetts

Kristen Mahoney Shannon, M.S., C.G.C.
Genetic Counselor
Center for Cancer Risk Analysis
Massachusetts General Hospital
Boston, Massachusetts

Judith Sims, MS
Science Writer
Logan, Utah

Genevieve Slomski, Ph.D.
Medical Writer
New Britain, Connecticut

Anna Rovid Spickler, D.V.M., Ph.D.
Medical Writer
Salisbury, Maryland

Laura L. Stein, M.S.
Certified Genetic Counselor
Familial Cancer Program-Department of Hematology/Oncology
Dartmouth Hitchcock Medical Center
Lebanon, New Hampshire

Phyllis M. Stein, B.S., C.C.R.P.
Affiliate Coordinator
Grand Rapids Clinical Oncology Program
Grand Rapids, Michigan

Kurt Sternlof
Science Writer
New Rochelle, New York

Deanna M. Swartout-Corbeil
Registered Nurse, Freelance Writer
Thompsons Station, Tennessee

Jane M. Taylor-Jones, M.S.
Research Associate
Donald W. Reynolds Department of Geriatrics
University of Arkansas for Medical Sciences
Little Rock, Arkansas

Carol Turkington
Medical Writer
Lancaster, Pennsylvania

Samuel Uretsky, PharmD
Medical Writer
Wantagh, New York

Marianne Vahey, M.D.
Clinical Instructor
Medicine
Yale University School of Medicine
New Haven, Connecticut

Malini Vashishtha, Ph.D.
Medical Writer
Irvine, California

Ellen S. Weber, M.S.N.
Medical Writer
Fort Wayne, Indiana

Ken R. Wells
Freelance Writer
Laguna Hills, California

Barbara Wexler, M.P.H.
Medical Writer
Chatsworth, California

Wendy Wippel, M.Sc.
Medical Writer and Adjunct Professor of Biology
Northwest Community College
Hernando, Mississippi

Debra Wood, R.N.
Medical Writer
Orlando, Florida

Kathleen D. Wright, R.N.
Medical Writer
Delmar, Delaware

Jon Zonderman
Medical Writer
Orange, California

Michael V. Zuck, Ph.D.
Writer
Boulder, Colorado

ILLUSTRATIONS OF BODY SYSTEMS

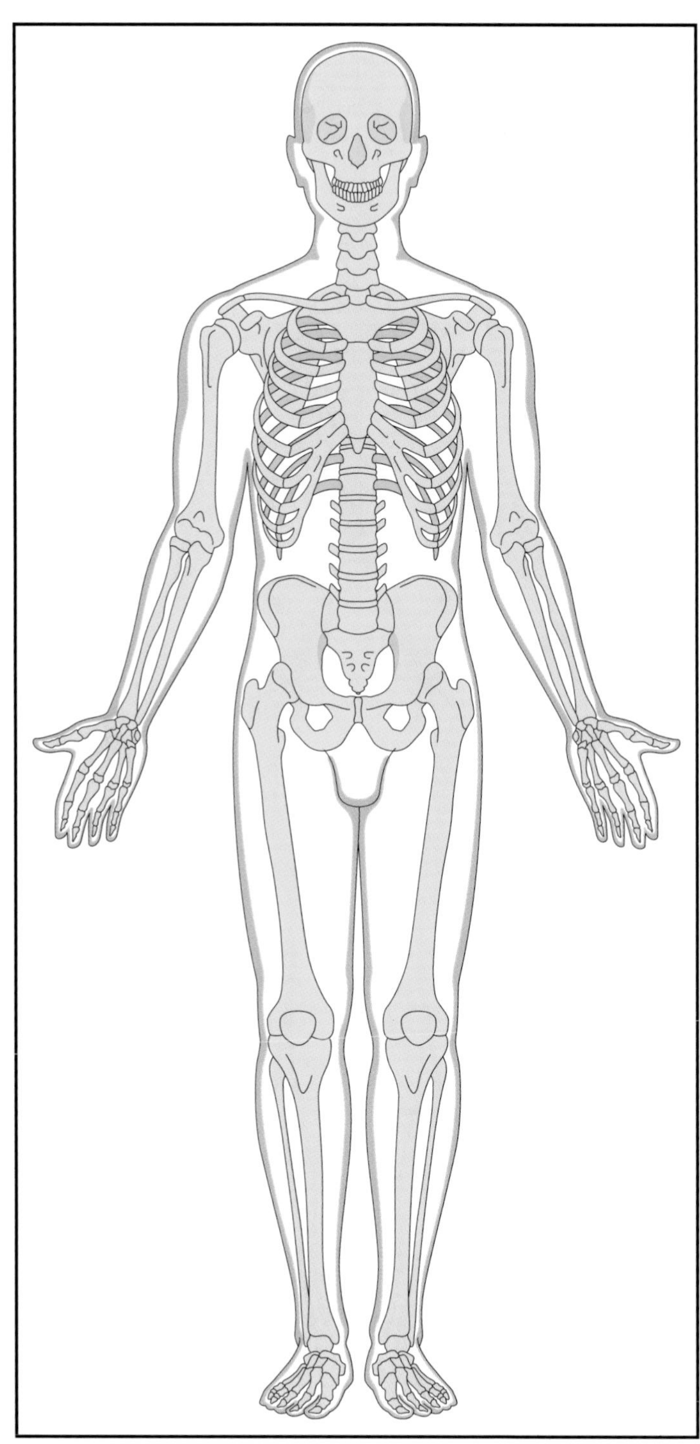

HUMAN SKELETON and SKIN. Some cancers that affect the skeleton are: Osteosarcoma; **Ewing's sarcoma**; **Fibrosarcoma** (can also be found in soft tissues like muscle, fat, connective tissues, etc.). Some cancers that affect tissue near bones: **Chondrosarcoma** (affects joints near bones); **Rhabdomyosarcoma** (formed from cells of muscles attached to bones); **Malignant fibrous histiocytoma** (common in soft tissues, rare in bones). SKIN CANCERS: **Basal cell carcinoma**; **Melanoma**; **Merkel cell carcinoma**; **Squamous cell carcinoma of the skin**; and **Trichilemmal carcinoma**. Precancerous skin condition: **Bowen's disease**. Lymphomas that affect the skin: **Mycosis fungoides**; **Sézary syndrome**. *(Illustration by Argosy Publishing Argosy Publishing. Cengage Learning, Gale.)*

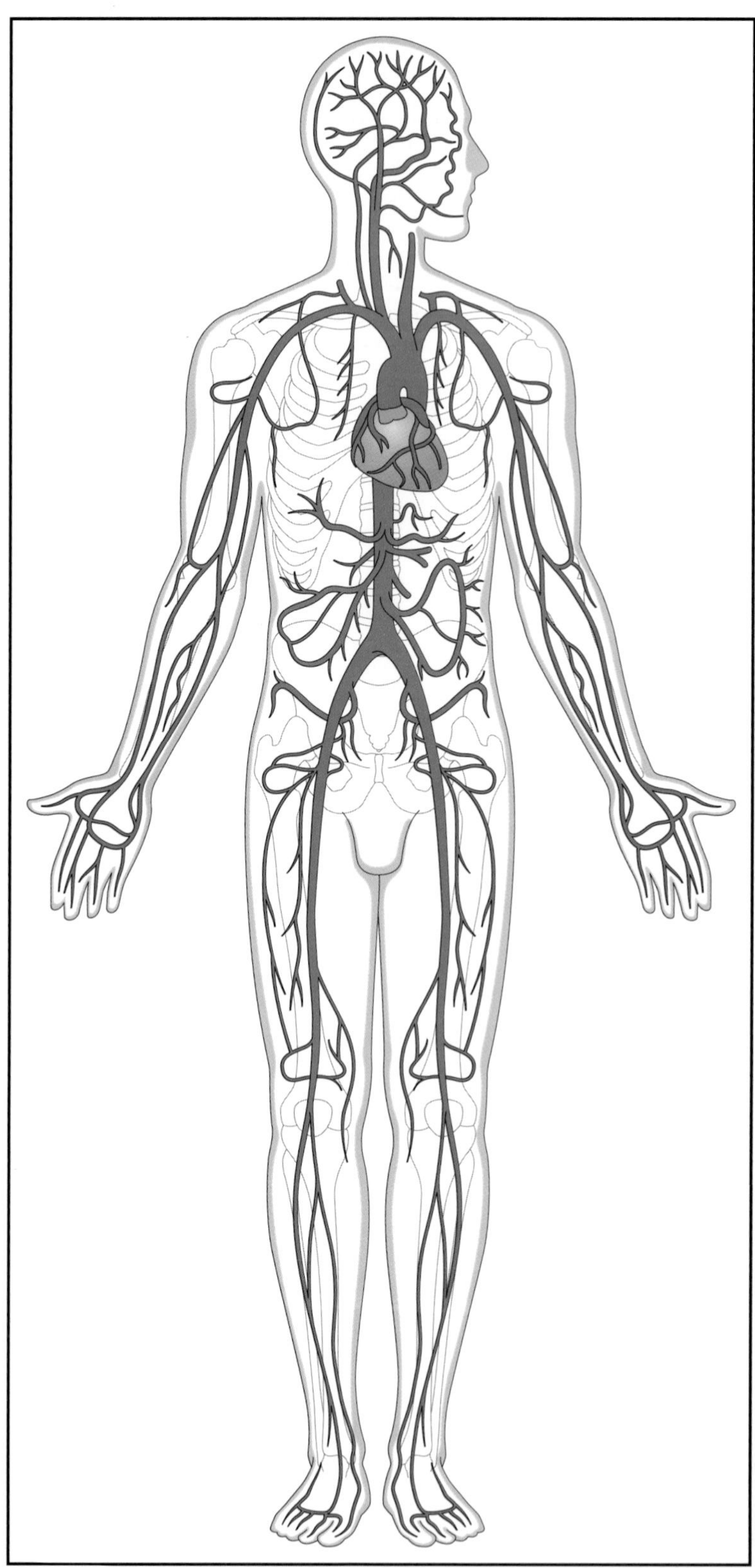

HUMAN CIRCULATORY SYSTEM. Some cancers of the blood cells are: Acute erythroblastic leukemia; **Acute lymphocytic leukemia**; **Acute myelocytic leukemia**; **Chronic lymphocytic leukemia**; **Chronic myelocytic leukemia**; **Hairy cell leukemia**; and **Multiple myeloma**. One condition associated with various cancers that affects blood is called **Myelofibrosis**. *(Illustration by Argosy Publishing Argosy Publishing. Cengage Learning, Gale.)*

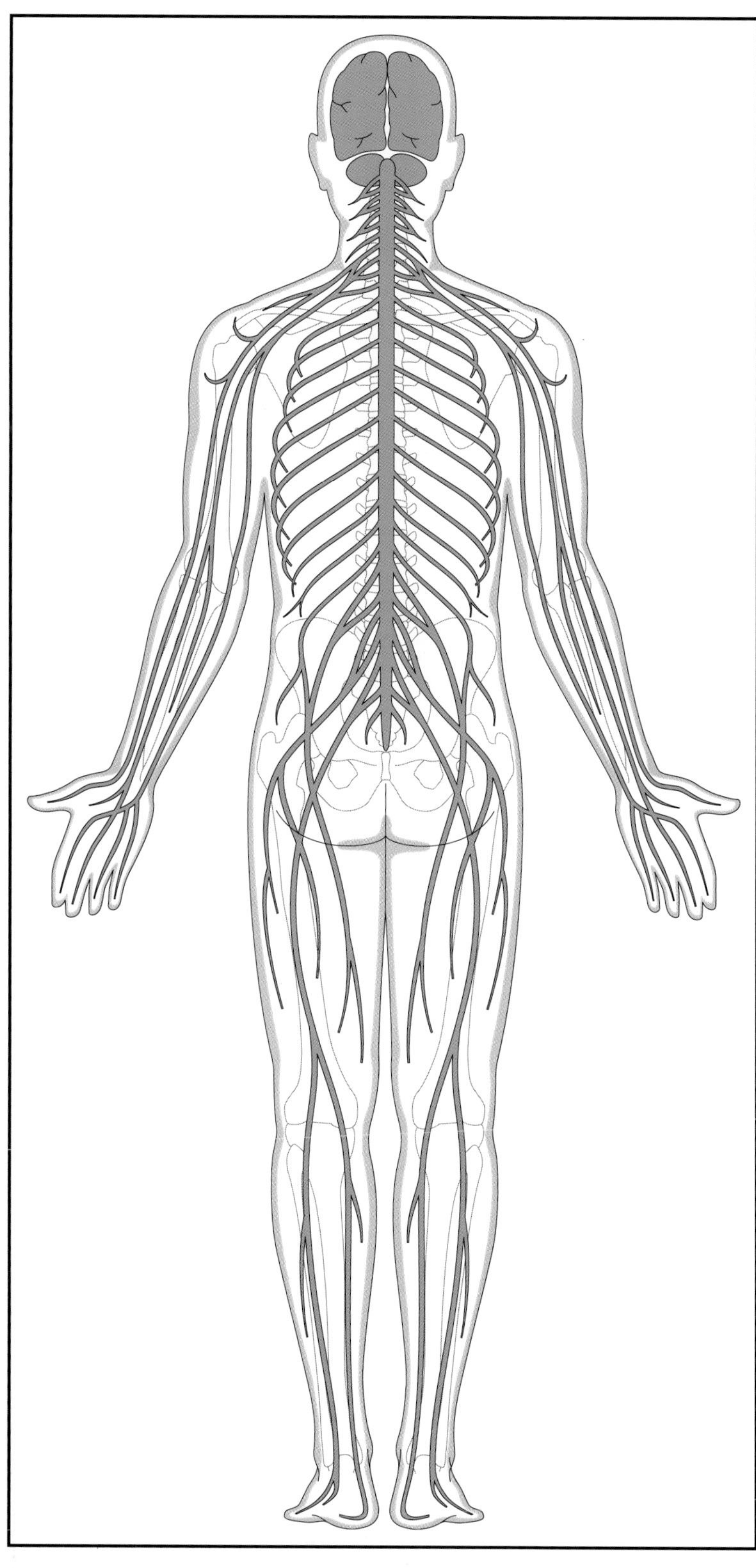

HUMAN NERVOUS SYSTEM. Some brain and central nervous system tumors are: **Astrocytoma**; **Carcinomatous meningitis**; **Central nervous system carcinoma**; **Central nervous system lymphoma**; **Chordoma**; **Choroid plexus tumors**; **Craniopharyngioma**; **Ependymoma**; **Medulloblastoma**; **Meningioma**; **Oligodendroglioma**; and **Spinal axis tumors**. One kind of noncancerous growth in the brain: **Acoustic neuroma**. *(Illustration by Argosy Publishing Argosy Publishing. Cengage Learning, Gale.)*

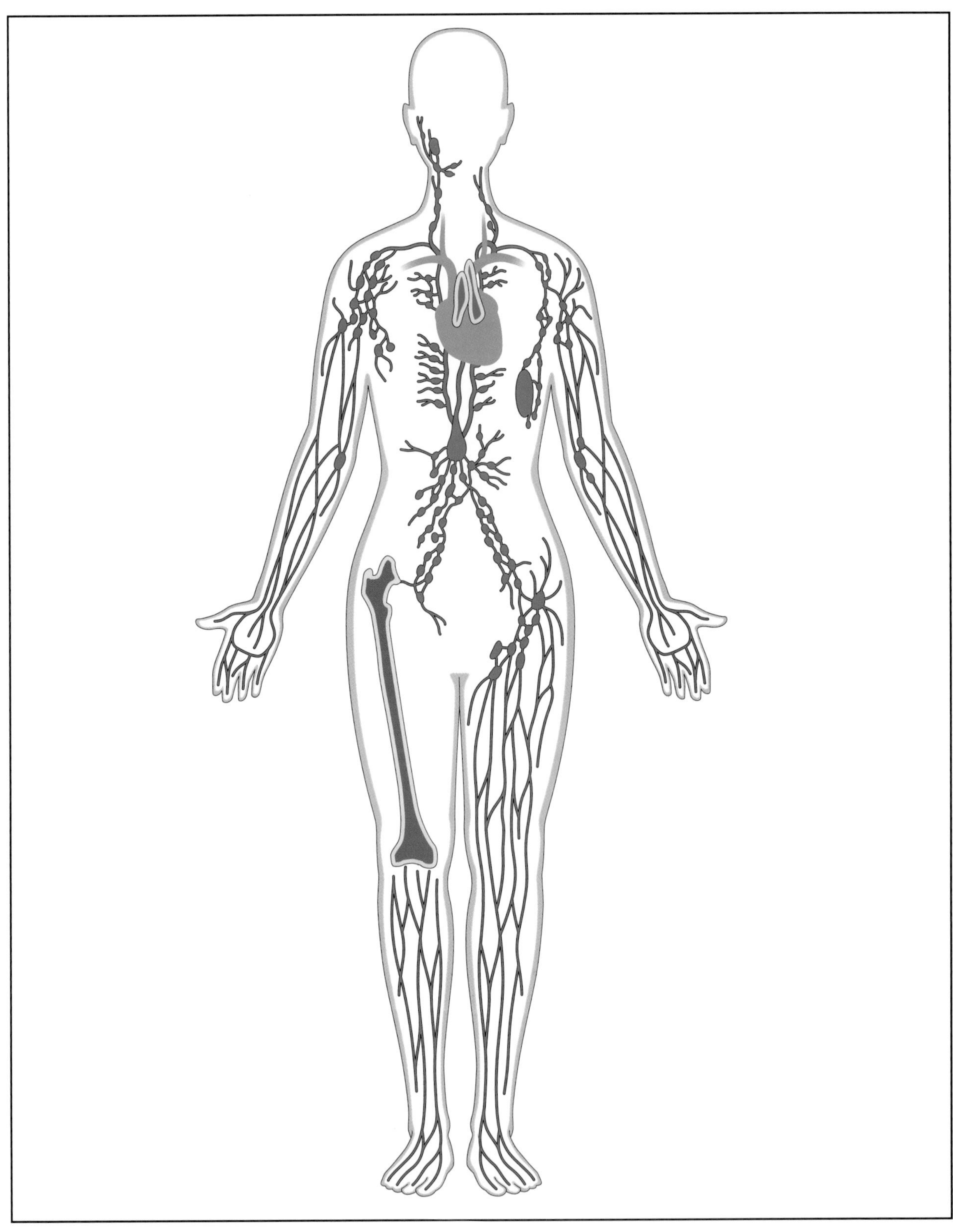

HUMAN LYMPHATIC SYSTEM. The lymphatic system and lymph nodes are shown here in pale green, the thymus in deep blue, and one of the bones rich in bone marrow (the femur) is shown here in purple. Some cancers of the lymphatic system are: Burkitt's lymphoma; **Cutaneous T-cell lymphoma**; **Hodgkin's disease**; **MALT lymphoma**; **Mantle cell lymphoma**; **Sézary syndrome**; and **Waldenström's macroglobulinemia**. *(Illustration by Argosy Publishing. Cengage Learning, Gale.)*

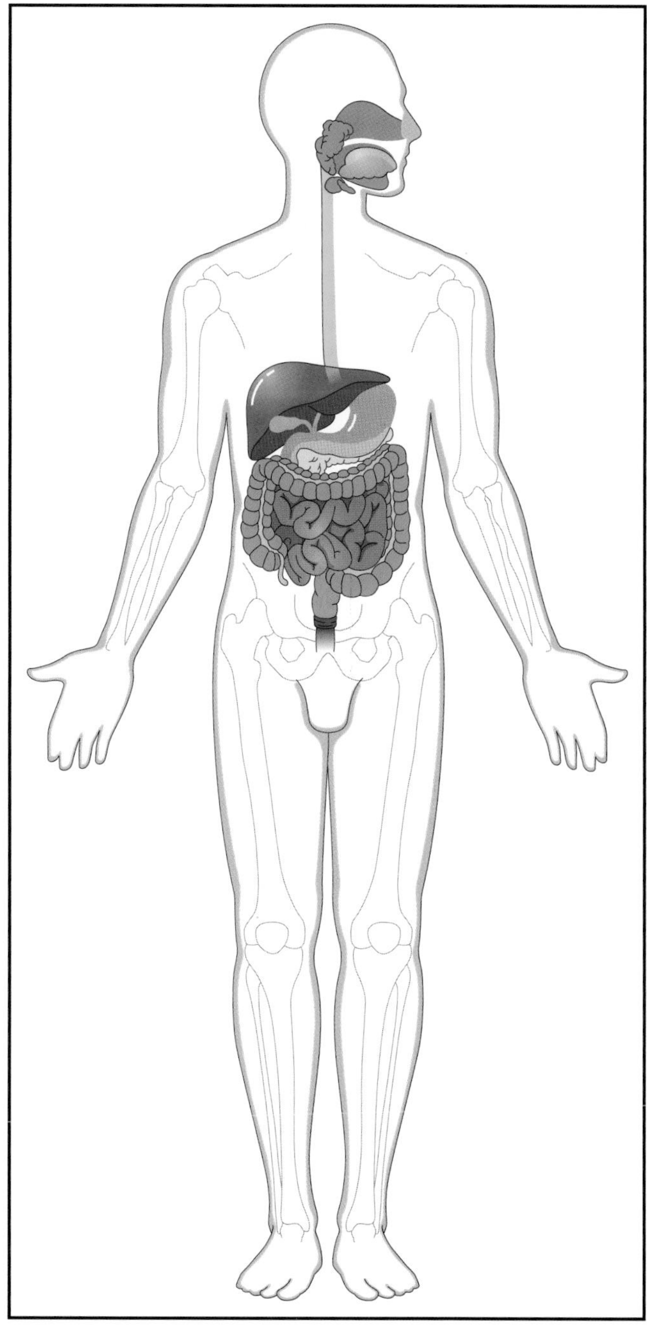

HUMAN DIGESTIVE SYSTEM. Organs and cancers of the digestive system include: Salivary glands (shown in turquoise): Salivary gland tumors. Esophagus (shown in bright yellow): **Esophageal cancer**. Liver (shown in bright red): **Bile duct cancer**; **Liver cancer**. Stomach (pale gray-blue): **Stomach cancer**. Gallbladder (bright orange against the red liver): **Gallbladder cancer**. Colon (green): **Colon cancer**. Small intestine (purple): **Small intestinal cancer**; can have malignant tumors associated with **Zollinger-Ellison syndrome**. Rectum (shown in pink, continuing the colon): **Rectal cancer**. Anus (dark blue): **Anal cancer**. *(Illustration by Argosy Publishing. Cengage Learning, Gale.)*

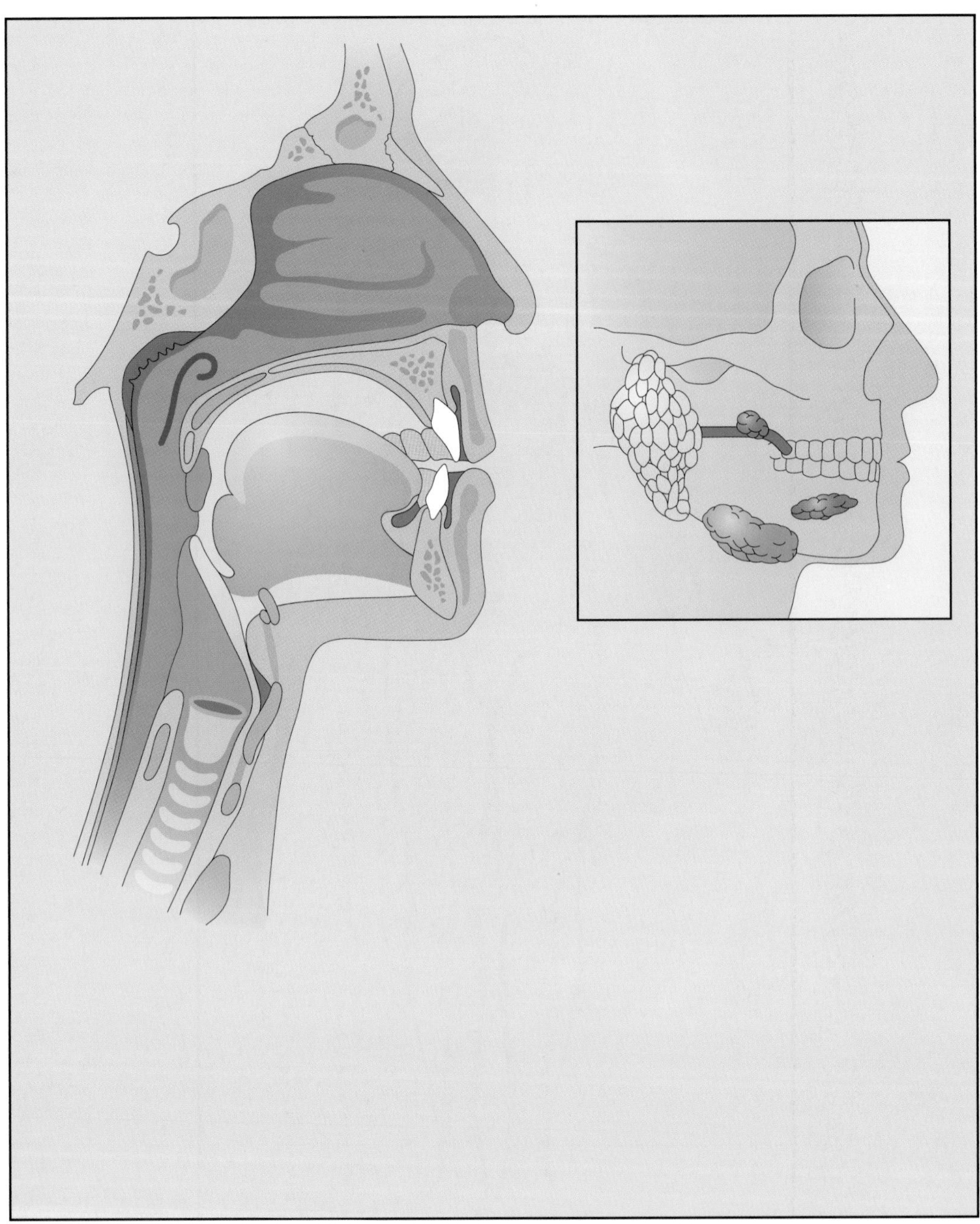

HEAD AND NECK. The pharynx, the passage that leads from the nostrils down through the neck is shown in orange. This passage is broken into several divisions. The area posterior to (behind) the nose is the nasopharynx. The area posterior to the mouth is the oropharynx. The oropharynx leads into the laryngopharynx, which opens into the esophagus (still in orange) and the larynx (shown in the large image in medium blue). Each of these regions may be affected by cancer, and the cancers include: Nasopharyngeal cancer; **Oropharyngeal cancer**; **Esophageal cancer**; and **Laryngeal cancer**. **Oral cancers** can affect the lips, gums, and tongue (pink). Referring to the smaller, inset picture of the salivary glands, **salivary gland tumors** can affect the parotid glands (shown here in yellow), the submandibular glands (inset picture, turquoise), and the sublingual glands (purple). *(Illustration by Argosy Publishing. Cengage Learning, Gale.)*

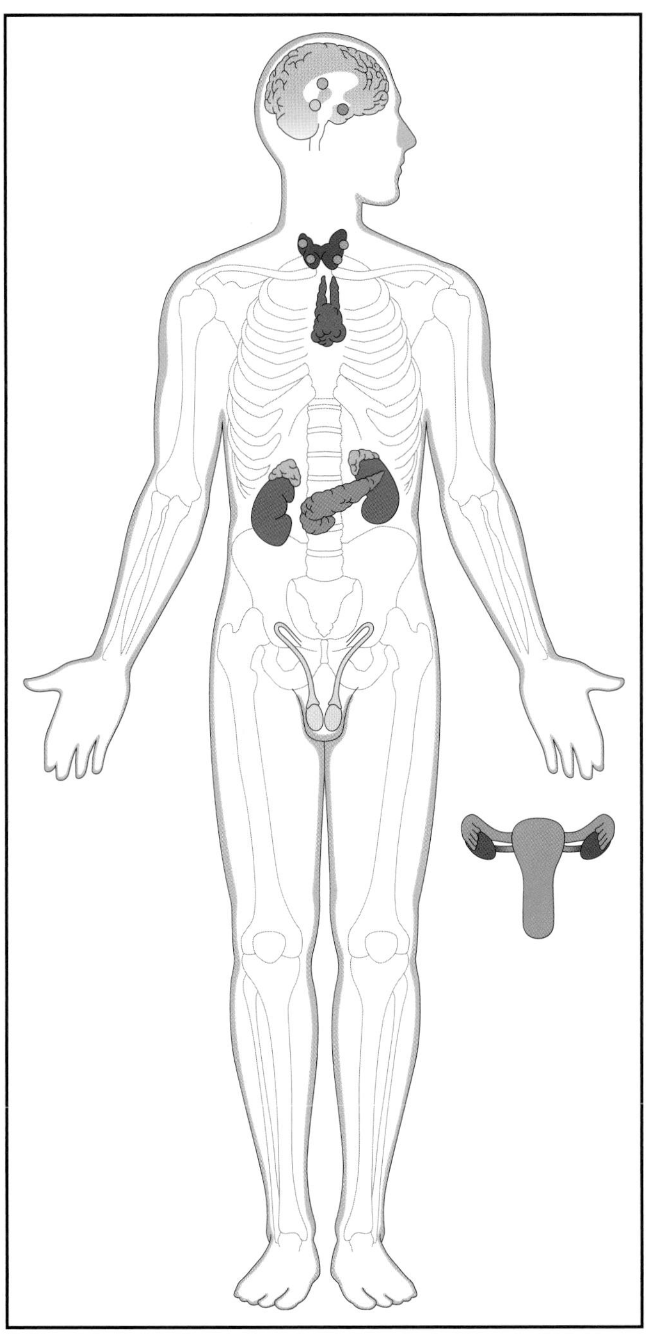

HUMAN ENDOCRINE SYSTEM. The glands and cancers of the endocrine system include: In the brain: the pituitary gland shown in blue (pituitary tumors), the hypothalamus in pale green, and the pineal gland in bright yellow. Throughout the rest of the body: Thyroid (shown in dark blue): **Thyroid cancer**. Parathyroid glands, four of them adjacent to the thyroid: **Parathyroid cancer**. Thymus (green): **Thymic cancer**; **Thymoma**. Pancreas (turquoise): **Pancreatic cancer, endocrine**; **Pancreatic cancer, exocrine**; **Zollinger-Ellison syndrome** tumors can be malignant and can be found in the pancreas. Adrenal glands (shown in apricot, above the kidneys): **Neuroblastoma** often originates in these glands; **Pheochromocytoma** tumors are often found in adrenal glands. Testes (in males, shown in yellow): **Testicular cancer**. Ovaries (in females, shown in dark blue in inset image): **Ovarian cancer**. *(Illustration by Argosy Publishing. Cengage Learning, Gale.)*

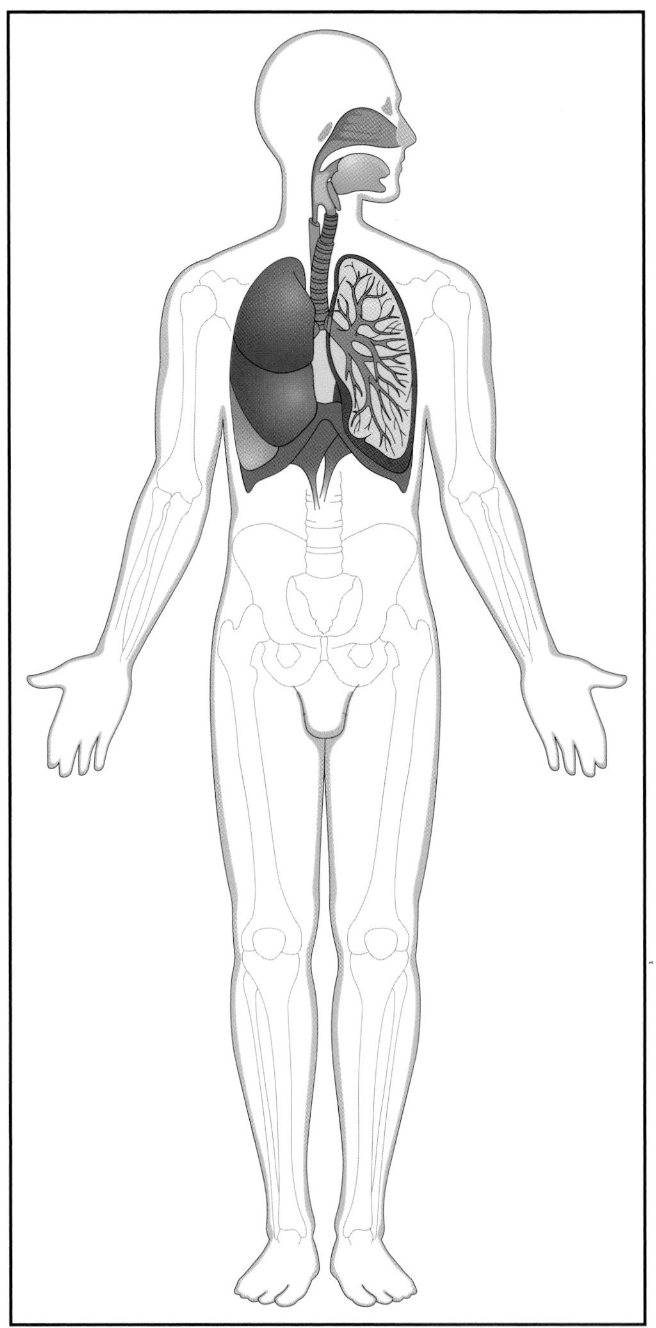

HUMAN RESPIRATORY SYSTEM. Air is breathed in through nose or mouth, enters the pharynx, shown here in orange, and passes through the larynx, shown here as a green tube with a ridged texture. (The smooth green tube shown is the esophagus, which is posterior to the larynx and which is involved in digestion instead of breathing.) The air then passes into the trachea (purple), a tube that divides into two tubes called bronchi. One bronchus passes into each lung, and continues to branch within the lung. These branches are called bronchioles and each bronchiole leads to a tiny cluster of air sacs called alveoli, where the exchange of gases occurs, so that the air and gases breathed in get diffused to the blood. The lungs (deep blue) are spongy and have lobes and can be affected by Lung cancer, both the non-small cell and small-cell types. *(Illustration by Argosy Publishing. Cengage Learning, Gale.)*

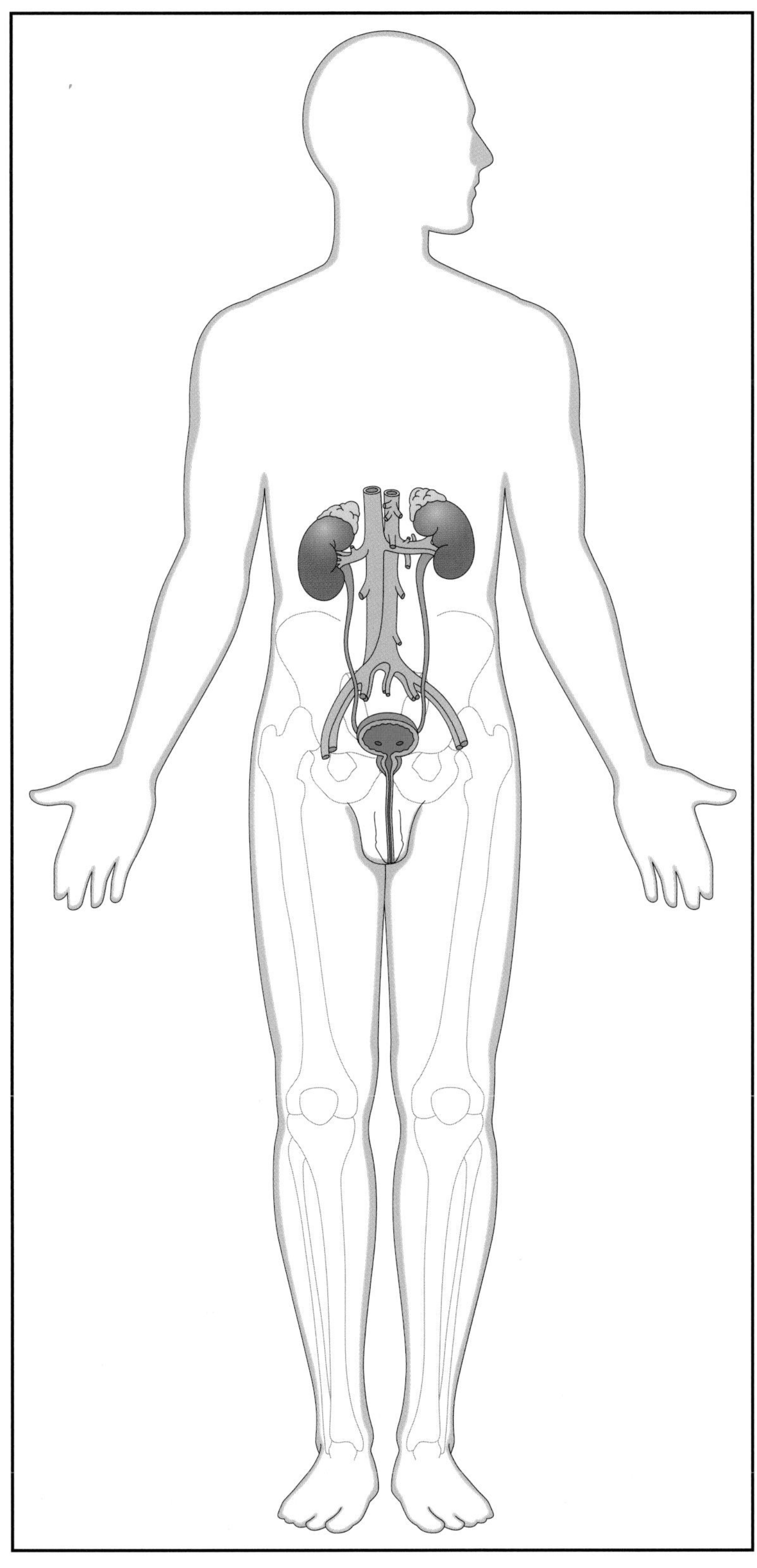

HUMAN URINARY SYSTEM. Organs and cancers of the urinary system include: Kidneys (shown in purple): Kidney cancer; **Renal pelvis tumors**; **Wilms' tumor.** Ureters are shown in green. Bladder (blue-green): **Bladder cancer**. The kidneys, bladder, or ureters can be affected by a cancer type called **Transitional cell carcinoma**. *(Illustration by Argosy Publishing. Cengage Learning, Gale.)*

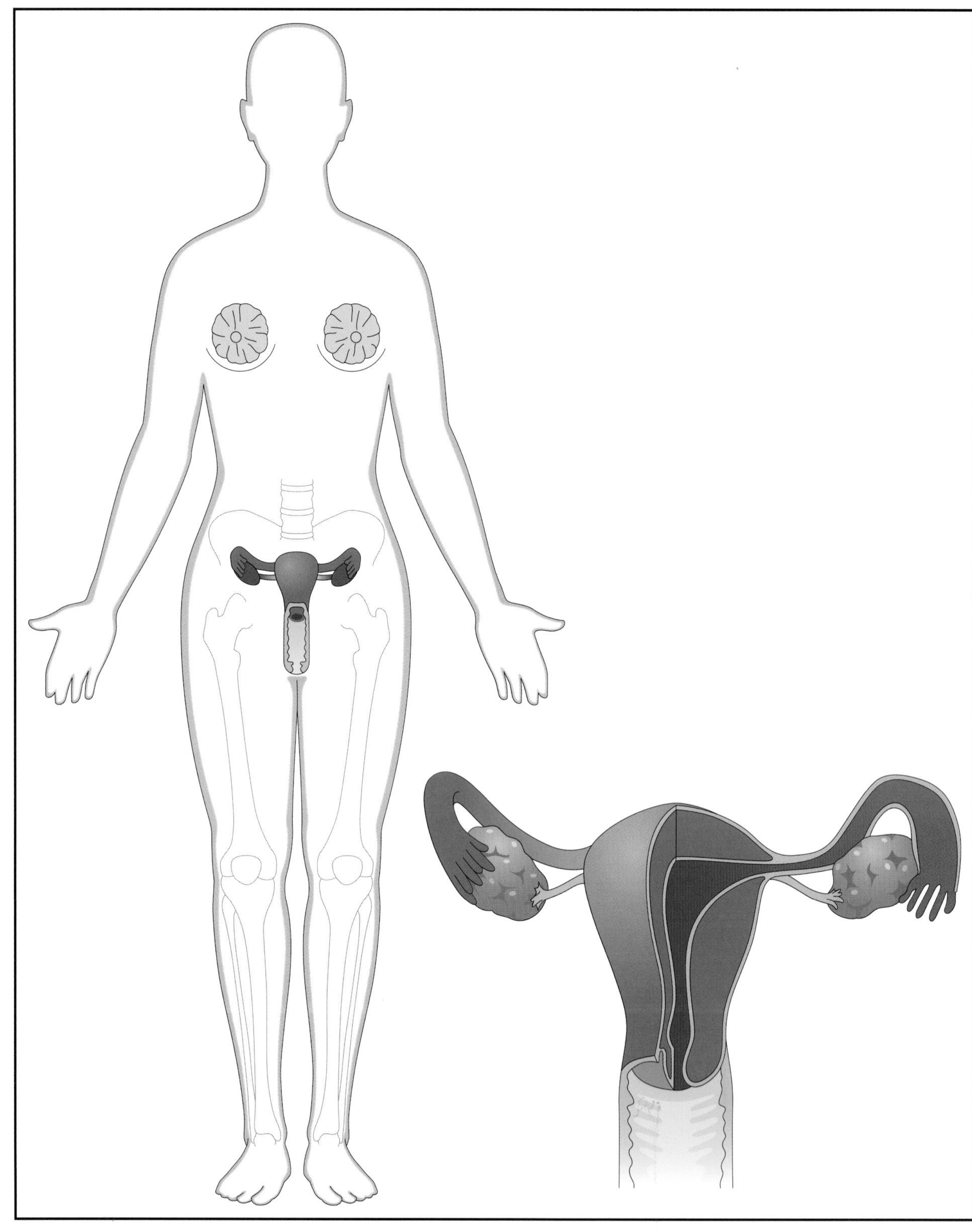

FEMALE REPRODUCTIVE SYSTEM. Organs and cancers of the female reproductive system include: Uterus, shown in red with the uterine or Fallopian tubes: Endometrial cancer. Ovaries (blue): **Ovarian cancer**. Vagina (shown in pink with a yellow interior or lining): **Vaginal cancer**. Breasts: **Breast cancer**; **Paget's disease of the breast**. Shown in detailed inset only in turquoise, Cervix: **Cervical cancer**. *(Illustration by Argosy Publishing. Cengage Learning, Gale.)*

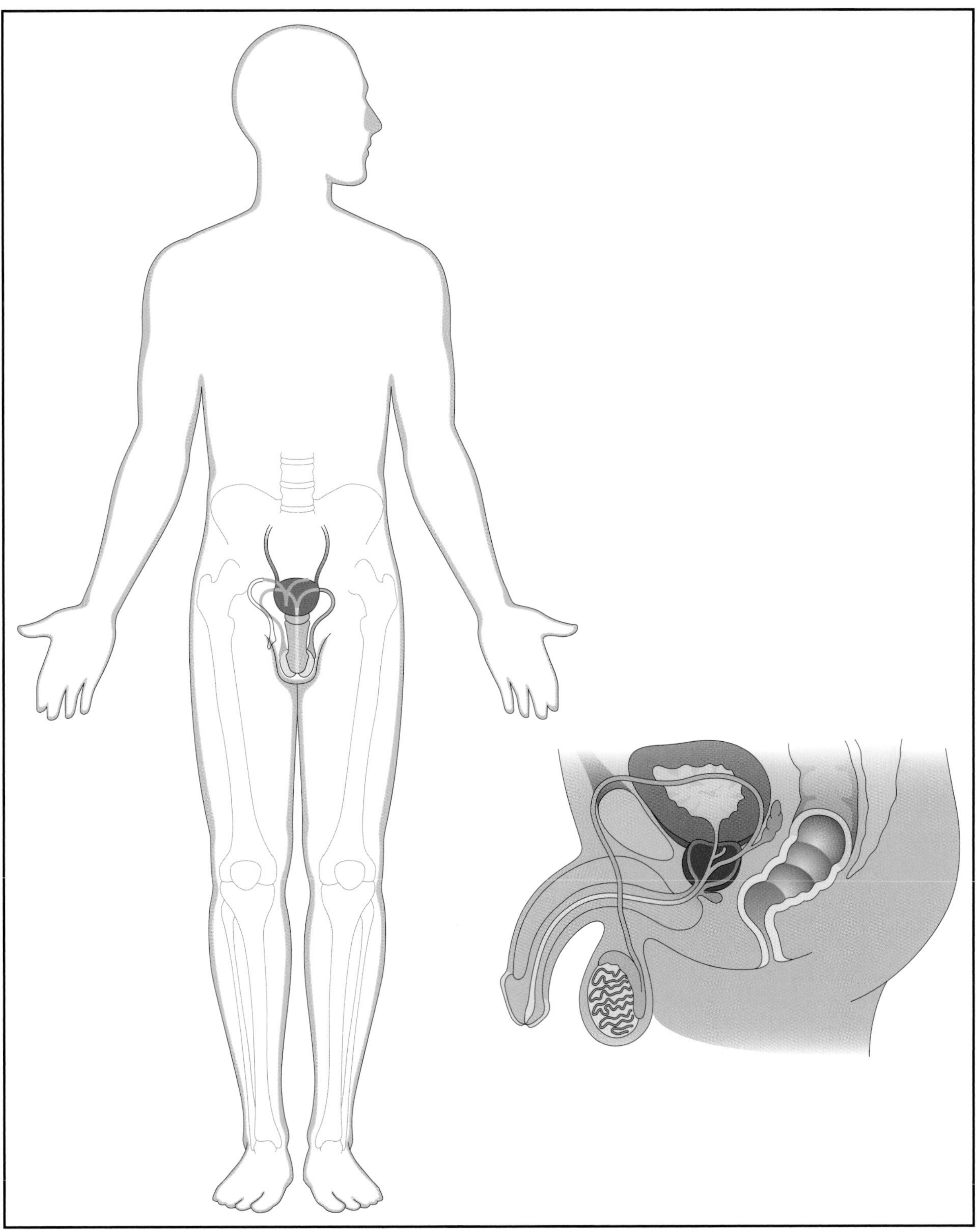

MALE REPRODCTIVE SYSTEM. Organs, glands, and cancers of the male reproductive system include: Penis (shown in pink): Penile cancer. Testes (shown in yellow): **Testicular cancer**. Prostate gland (shown in full-body illustration in a peach/ apricot color, and in the inset as the dark blue gland between the bladder and the penis): **Prostate cancer**. *(Illustration by Argosy Publishing. Cengage Learning, Gale.)*

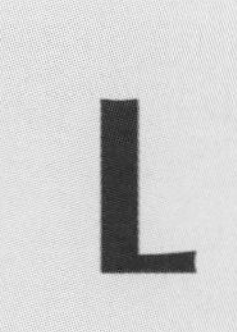

Lactulose *see* **Laxatives**

Lambert-Eaton myasthenic syndrome

Definition

Lambert-Eaton myasthenic syndrome (LEMS), sometimes called Eaton-Lambert syndrome, is a rare disorder affecting the muscles and nerves. LEMS is known to be associated with small-cell lung **cancer**. It may also be associated with such cancers as **lymphoma**, **non-Hodgkin's lymphoma**, T-cell leukemia, non-small-cell lung cancer, **prostate cancer**, and **thymoma**. LEMS was first identified in 1956 by a team of three American neurologists, Lee Eaton, Edward Lambert, and Edward Rooke.

Demographics

LEMS is a rare disorder; the number of people affected by it is at best an estimate. Various figures that have been given are that 400 people in the United States have the disorder at any one time. This figure does not include patients with LEMS who do not have cancer. About half of patients diagnosed with LEMS do not have cancer; this form of LEMS is called idiopathic LEMS, which means that its origin is unknown.

Another estimate is that LEMS affects 3% of patients with small-cell lung cancer (SCLC), or about 4 people in every million. Between 50% and 70% of patients diagnosed with LEMS have an identifiable cancer of some type, the vast majority having SCLC. LEMS has also been associated with non-SCLC, lymphosarcoma, malignant thymoma, or **carcinoma** of the breast, stomach, colon, prostate, bladder, kidney, or gallbladder.

Description

LEMS is a disorder characterized by muscular weakness and **fatigue** caused by a disruption of electrical impulses between the nerves and muscle cells. The disruption in turn results from an autoimmune process.

About half of all cases of LEMS are associated with cancer, particularly small-cell lung cancer (SCLC). The other half of cases have no known cause and are called idiopathic LEMS. The disorder is typically slow in onset; it usually begins with a dry mouth and some weakness or aching in the legs, progressing to difficulty swallowing or holding up the head, problems in focusing the eyes, and general fatigue. LEMS chiefly affects the patient's quality of life and ability to carry out everyday activities; patients with cancer-associated LEMS usually die from the cancer, not the muscle syndrome.

Risk factors

Risk factors for LEMS include:

- Being diagnosed with SCLC or another type of cancer.
- Age. LEMS is more common in middle-aged and older adults than in children and adolescents. The average age at diagnosis is 60 years.
- Sex. LEMS is slightly more common in men than in women. It is most likely to be diagnosed in men over 40.
- Having another autoimmune disorder.
- Smoking. All patients with SCLC diagnosed with LEMS have been found to be heavy smokers.

Causes and symptoms

Causes

The symptoms of LEMS are the result of an insufficient release of a neurotransmitter called acetylcholine at the junctions between the nerves and muscle cells. Acetylcholine is a chemical that passes signals from the nerve cells to the muscles in order for the muscles to move. The decreased level of acetylcholine causes a muscle reaction to the nerve signal that is lower than normal. The underlying cause of the lower-than-normal neurotransmitter release seen in LEMS patients is believed to be related to a disorder of the immune system (an autoimmune reaction). This autoimmune reaction is caused by antibodies produced by the patient in response to small-cell lung cancer or one of the other cancers associated with LEMS.

Since continued use of the muscles may lead to a buildup of acetylcholine to normal levels, symptoms of LEMS can often be lessened or alleviated by using the affected muscles. **Myasthenia gravis** (MG), another disorder that has symptoms similar to LEMS, is caused by a blockage of neurotransmitters by antibodies. Symptoms of myasthenia gravis do not improve with continued muscle use. The improvement in symptoms that is observable in LEMS patients often helps to differentiate LEMS from myasthenia gravis. In contrast to MG, the symptoms of LEMS tend to be worse in the morning and improve toward evening with exercise and nerve stimulation. In addition, LEMS usually does not affect the muscles that control breathing as severely as MG does.

LEMS is made worse by neuromuscular blocking agents used during surgery; certain **antibiotics**, such as the aminoglycosides and fluoroquinolones; magnesium; calcium channel blockers; and iodinated intravenous contrast agents used in medical imaging.

Symptoms

The symptoms of LEMS in cancer patients typically begin 2–4 years before the cancer is diagnosed. The primary symptom is muscular weakness or paralysis that varies in intensity and location throughout the body. Other symptoms of LEMS include tingling sensations on the skin, double vision, difficulty maintaining a steady gaze, and dry mouth or difficulty in swallowing.

The first signs of LEMS tend to be a dry mouth and weakness or soreness in the legs. Some patients also complain of a metallic taste in the mouth as well as dryness. Later symptoms of LEMS include:

- changes in vision
- decreased posture and muscle tone
- difficulty in chewing or swallowing
- difficulty in climbing stairs
- difficulty in lifting simple objects
- speech impairment
- impotence in men
- a drooping head
- fatigue
- and/or a need to use the hands to get up from a sitting or lying position

Diagnosis

LEMS is often misdiagnosed as myasthenia gravis because of the similarities between the symptoms of these two disorders. The diagnosis is usually made by a combination of chest x-rays (to detect lung cancer), blood tests for antibodies to the calcium channels at the ends of nerve fibers, and electrical stimulation tests. An increased response of muscle fibers to very high frequencies of electrical stimulation indicates LEMS rather than MS.

If the doctor does not find a tumor within the first two years after the onset of the patient's symptoms, the patient probably has idiopathic LEMS.

Examination

The doctor may notice drooping eyelids, a dry mouth, and weakness when the patient is asked to stand up. The patient's reflexes will be weaker than normal, and the muscles may appear smaller than usual or wasted.

Treatment

Traditional

The goal of treatment for LEMS patients is to improve muscle strength while also treating the cancer or other underlying disorder that is causing LEMS.

When possible, patients affected with LEMS should undergo a physical therapy program that is tailored to their health status and abilities. This may include stretching and flexibility manuevers as well as light strength and cardiovascular exercises. Symptoms of LEMS tend to be aggravated by prolonged exercise, so any physical therapy undertaken should be relatively short in duration.

Some LEMS patients are not able to undergo physical therapy because of their current state of health. In these cases, plasmapheresis (also called plasma exchange), a procedure in which blood plasma is removed from the patient and replaced, may be recommended. This procedure can be effective in a majority of LEMS patients.

Heat appears to worsen the symptoms of LEMS; patients typically feel much worse in hot weather and when they are running a **fever**. The doctor will usually advise the patient to take lukewarm rather than hot showers or baths.

Drugs

Medications that suppress the **immune response** or that suppress the antibodies responsible for the

QUESTIONS TO ASK YOUR DOCTOR

- Should I be tested for LEMS if I have an autoimmune disorder?
- What are the differences between LEMS and myasthenia gravis?
- What are my chances of developing LEMS after I have been diagnosed with cancer?
- Have you ever treated anyone with LEMS?

muscle weakness have also been shown to improve LEMS symptoms in some patients. These medications include high-dose intravenous immunoglobulin, **azathioprine**, and steroid drugs like prednisone. Another type of drug that has been shown to be beneficial is drugs that improve the transmission of nerve impulses to the muscles. These drugs include di-amino pyridine (DAP) and pyridostigmine bromide (Mestinon).

Alternative and complementary therapies

Yoga and other stretching exercises may be effective treatments for alleviating the physical symptoms of LEMS patients. Some LEMS patients also report improvement of symptoms after deep body massage or hydrotherapy.

Prognosis

The most important prognostic factor for LEMS patients diagnosed with cancer is the prognosis of the cancer. People with idiopathic LEMS have a better prognosis than those with cancer; however, recovery of muscle strength varies from patient to patient. In general, patients whose symptoms progress more rapidly have a worse prognosis.

Prevention

There is no way to prevent LEMS as of 2009 because its underlying cause is presently unknown.

Resources

BOOKS

Benatar, Michael. *Neuromuscular Disease: Evidence and Analysis in Clinical Neurology*. Totowa, NJ: Humana Press, 2006.

Kalman, Bernadette, and Thomas H. Brannagan III. *Neuroimmunology in Clinical Practice*. Malden, MA: Blackwell Publishing, 2008.

PERIODICALS

Titulaer, M. J., et al. "Screening for Small-cell Lung Cancer: A Follow-up Study of Patients with Lambert-Eaton Myasthenic Syndrome." *Journal of Clinical Oncology* 26 (September 10, 2008): 4276–81.

Ueda, T., et al. "Dropped Head Syndrome Caused by Lambert-Eaton Myasthenic Syndrome." *Muscle and Nerve* 40 (July 2009): 134–36.

Weimer, M. B., and J. Wong. "Lambert-Eaton Myasthenic Syndrome." *Current Treatment Options in Neurology* 11 (March 2009): 77–84.

Wirtz, P.W., et al. " Efficacy of 3,4-diaminopyridine and Pyridostigmine in the Treatment of Lambert-Eaton Myasthenic Syndrome: A Randomized, Double-blind, Placebo-controlled, Crossover Study." *Clinical Pharmacology and Therapeutics* 86 (July 2009): 44–48.

OTHER

Kleinschmidt, Paul. "Lambert-Eaton Myasthenic Syndrome." *eMedicine*, February 15, 2007.http://emedicine.medscape.com/article/792803-overview

Medline Plus Medical Encyclopedia. *Lambert-Eaton Syndrome*. http://www.nlm.nih.gov/medlineplus/ency/article/000710.htm.

National Institute of Neurological Disorders and Stroke (NINDS). *Lambert-Eaton Myasthenic Syndrome Information Page*. http://www.ninds.nih.gov/disorders/lambert_eaton/lambert_eaton.htm.

Stickler, David E., and Donald B. Sanders. "Lambert-Eaton Myasthenic Syndrome." *eMedicine*, January 20, 2009. http://emedicine.medscape.com/article/1170810-overview.

ORGANIZATIONS

American Academy of Neurology (AAN), 1080 Montreal Avenue, Saint Paul, MN, 55116, 651-695-2717, 800-879-1960, 651-695-2791, http://www.aan.com/.

American Physical Therapy Association (APTA), 1111 North Fairfax Street, Alexandria, VA, 22314-1488, 703-684-APTA (2782), 800-999-APTA (2782), 703-684-7343, http://www.apta.org//AM/Template.cfm?Section=Home.

National Institute of Neurological Disorders and Stroke (NINDS), P.O. Box 5801, Bethesda, MD, 20824, 800-352-9424, 301-496-5751, http://www.ninds.nih.gov/index.htm.

National Organization for Rare Disorders (NORD), P.O. Box 1968, Danbury, CT, 06813-1968, 203-744-0100, 800-999-NORD, 203-798-2291, http://www.rarediseases.org.

Paul A. Johnson, Ed.M.
Rebecca J. Frey, PhD

Langerhans cell histiocytosis *see* **Histiocytosis X**

Laparoscopy

Definition

Laparoscopy is a type of surgical procedure in which a small incision is made, usually in the navel, through which a viewing tube (laparoscope) is inserted. The viewing tube has a small camera on the eyepiece. This allows the doctor to examine the abdominal and pelvic organs on a video monitor connected to the tube. Other small incisions can be made to insert instruments to perform procedures. Laparoscopy can be done to diagnose conditions or to perform certain types of operations. It is less invasive than regular open abdominal surgery (laparotomy).

Purpose

Since the late 1980s, laparoscopy has been a popular diagnostic and treatment tool. The technique dates back to 1901, when it was reportedly first used in a gynecologic procedure performed in Russia. In fact, gynecologists were the first to use laparoscopy to diagnose and treat conditions relating to the female reproductive organs: uterus, fallopian tubes, and ovaries.

Laparoscopy was first used with **cancer** patients in 1973. In these first cases, the procedure was used to observe and **biopsy** the liver. Laparoscopy plays a role in the diagnosis, staging, and treatment for a variety of cancers.

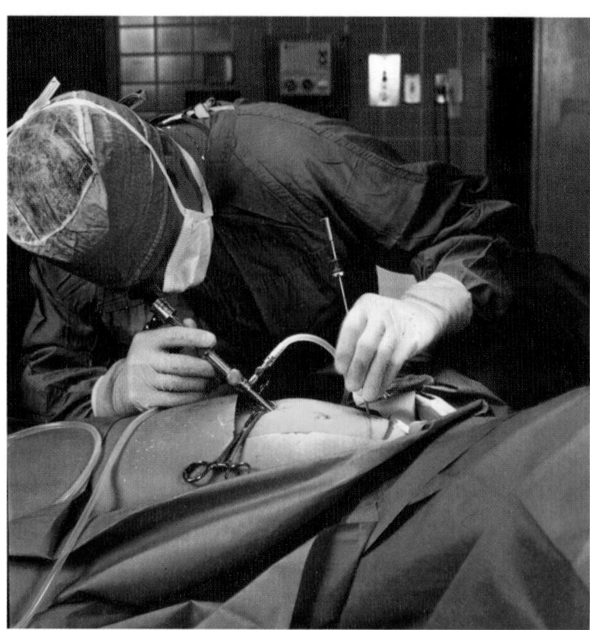

This surgeon is performing a laparoscopic procedure on a patient. *(Photo Researchers, Inc. Reproduced by permission.)*

As of 2009, the use of laparoscopy to completely remove cancerous growths and surrounding tissues (in place of open surgery) is still debated. The procedure is being studied to determine if it is as effective as open surgery in complex operations. Laparoscopy is also being investigated as a screening tool for **ovarian cancer**.

Laparoscopy is widely used in procedures for noncancerous conditions that in the past required open surgery, such as removal of the appendix (appendectomy) and gallbladder removal (cholecystectomy).

Diagnostic procedure

As a diagnostic procedure, laparoscopy is useful in taking biopsies of abdominal or pelvic growths, as well as lymph nodes. It allows the doctor to examine the abdominal area, including the female organs, appendix, gallbladder, stomach, and the liver.

Laparoscopy is used to determine the cause of pelvic pain or gynecological symptoms that cannot be confirmed by a physical exam or ultrasound. For example, ovarian cysts, endometriosis, ectopic pregnancy, or blocked fallopian tubes can be diagnosed using this procedure. It is an important tool when trying to determine the cause of infertility.

Operative procedure

While laparoscopic surgery to completely remove cancerous tumors, surrounding tissues, and lymph nodes is used on a limited basis, this type of operation is widely used in noncancerous conditions that once required open surgery. These conditions include:

- Tubal ligation. In this procedure, the fallopian tubes are sealed or cut to prevent subsequent pregnancies.
- Ectopic pregnancy. If a fertilized egg becomes embedded outside the uterus, usually in the fallopian tube, an operation must be performed to remove the developing embryo. This often can be done with laparoscopy.
- Endometriosis. This is a condition in which tissue from inside the uterus is found outside the uterus in other parts of (or on organs within) the pelvic cavity. This can cause cysts to form. Endometriosis is diagnosed with laparoscopy, and in some cases the cysts and other tissue can be removed during laparoscopy.
- Hysterectomy. This procedure to remove the uterus can, in some cases, be performed using laparoscopy. The uterus is cut away with the aid of the laparoscopic

QUESTIONS TO ASK THE DOCTOR

- Whate is your complication rate?
- What is the purpose of this procedure?
- How often do you do laparoscopies?
- What type of anesthesia will be used?
- Will a biopsy be taken during the laparoscopy if anything abnormal is seen?
- If more surgery is needed, can it be done with a laparoscope?
- What area will be examined with the laparoscope?
- What are the risks?
- How long is the recovery time?

instruments and then the uterus is removed through the vagina.

- Ovarian masses. Tumors or cysts in the ovaries can be removed using laparoscopy.
- Appendectomy. This surgery to remove an inflamed appendix required open surgery in the past. It is now routinely performed with laparoscopy.
- Cholecystectomy. Like appendectomy, this procedure to remove the gallbladder used to require open surgery. Now it can be performed with laparoscopy, in some cases.

In contrast to open abdominal surgery, laparoscopy usually involves less pain, less risk, less scarring, and faster recovery. Because laparoscopy is so much less invasive than traditional abdominal surgery, patients can leave the hospital sooner.

Cancer staging

Laparoscopy can be used in determining the spread of certain cancers. Sometimes it is combined with ultrasound. Although laparoscopy is a useful staging tool, its use depends on a variety of factors, which are considered for each patient. Types of cancers where laparoscopy may be used to determine the spread of the disease include:

- Liver cancer. Laparoscopy is an important tool for determining if cancer is present in the liver. When a patient has non-liver cancer, the liver is often checked to see if the cancer has spread there. Laparoscopy can identify up to 90% of malignant lesions that have spread to that organ from a cancer located elsewhere in the body. While computed tomography (CT) can find cancerous lesions that are 0.4 in (10 mm) in size, laparoscopy is capable of locating lesions that are as small as 0.04 in (1 millimeter).
- Pancreatic cancer. Laparoscopy has been used to evaluate pancreatic cancer for years. In fact, the first reported use of laparoscopy in the United States was in a case involving pancreatic cancer.
- Esophageal and stomach cancers. Laparoscopy has been found to be more effective than magnetic resonance imaging (MRI) or computed tomography (CT) in diagnosing the spread of cancer from these organs.
- Hodgkin's disease. Some patients with Hodgkin's disease have surgical procedures to evaluate lymph nodes for cancer. Laparoscopy is sometimes selected over laparotomy for this procedure. In addition, the spleen may be removed in patients with Hodgkin's disease. Laparoscopy is the standard surgical technique for this procedure, which is called a splenectomy.
- Prostate cancer. Patients with prostate cancer may have the nearby lymph nodes examined. Laparoscopy is an important tool in this procedure.

Cancer treatment

Laparoscopy is sometimes used as part of a palliative cancer treatment. This type of treatment is not a cure, but can often lessen the symptoms. An example is the feeding tube, which cancer patients may have if they are unable to take in food by mouth. The feeding tube provides nutrition directly into the stomach. Inserting the tube with a laparoscopy saves the patient the ordeal of open surgery.

Precautions

As with any surgery, patients should notify their physicians of any medications they are taking (prescription, over-the-counter, or herbal) and of any allergies. Precautions vary due to the several different purposes for laparoscopy. Patients should expect to rest for several days after the procedure, and should set up a comfortable environment in their homes (with items such as pain medication, heating pads, feminine products, comfortable clothing, and food readily accessible) prior to surgery.

Description

Laparoscopy is a surgical procedure that is done in the hospital under anesthesia. For diagnosis and biopsy, local anesthesia is sometimes used. In operative procedures, such as abdominal surgery, general anesthesia is required. Before starting the procedure, a

KEY TERMS

Biopsy—Microscopic evaluation of a tissue sample. The tissue is closely examined for the presence of abnormal cells.

Cancer staging—Determining the course and spread of cancer.

Cyst—An abnormal lump or swelling that is filled with fluid or other material.

Palliative treatment—A type of treatment that does not provide a cure, but eases the symptoms.

Tumor—A growth of tissue, benign or malignant, often referred to as a mass.

catheter is inserted through the urethra to empty the bladder, and the skin of the abdomen is cleaned.

After the patient is anesthetized, a hollow needle is inserted into the abdomen in or near the navel, and carbon dioxide gas is pumped through the needle to expand the abdomen. This allows the surgeon a better view of the internal organs. The laparoscope is then inserted through this incision to look at the internal organs. The image from the camera attached to the end of the laparoscope is seen on a video monitor.

Sometimes, additional small incisions are made to insert other instruments that are used to lift the tubes and ovaries for examination or to perform surgical procedures.

Preparation

Patients should not eat or drink after midnight on the night before the procedure.

Aftercare

After the operation, nurses will check the vital signs of patients who had general anesthesia. If there are no complications, the patient may leave the hospital within four to eight hours. (Traditional abdominal surgery requires a hospital stay of several days).

There may be some slight pain or throbbing at the incision sites in the first day or so after the procedure. The gas that is used to expand the abdomen may cause discomfort under the ribs or in the shoulder for a few days. Depending on the reason for the laparoscopy in gynecological procedures, some women may experience some vaginal bleeding. Many patients can return to work within a week of surgery and most are back to work within two weeks.

Risks

Laparoscopy is a relatively safe procedure, especially if the physician is experienced in the technique. The risk of complication is approximately 1%.

The procedure carries a slight risk of puncturing a blood vessel or organ, which could cause blood to seep into the abdominal cavity. Puncturing the intestines could allow intestinal contents to seep into the cavity. These are serious complications and major surgery may be required to correct the problem. For operative procedures, there is the possibility that it may become apparent that open surgery is required. Serious complications occur at a rate of only 0.2%.

Rare complications include:

- hemorrhage
- inflammation of the abdominal cavity lining
- abscess
- problems related to general anesthesia

Laparoscopy is generally not used in patients with certain heart or lung conditions, or in those who have some intestinal disorders, such as bowel obstruction.

Normal results

In diagnostic procedures, normal results would indicate no abnormalities or disease of the organs or lymph nodes that were examined.

Abnormal results

A diagnostic laparoscopy may reveal cancerous or benign masses or lesions. Abnormal findings include tumors or cysts, infections (such as pelvic inflammatory disease), cirrhosis, endometriosis, fibroid tumors, or an accumulation of fluid in the cavity. If a doctor is checking for the spread of cancer, the presence of malignant lesions in areas other than the original site of malignancy is an abnormal finding.

See also Endoscopic retrograde cholangiopancreatography; Gynecologic cancers; Liver biopsy; Lymph node biopsy; Nutritional support; Tumor grading; Tumor staging; Ultrasonography.

Resources

BOOKS

Kurtz, Robert C., and Robert J. Ginsberg. "Cancer Diagnosis: Endoscopy." In *Cancer: Principles & Practice of Oncology*, edited by Vincent T. DeVita, Jr. Philadelphia: Lippincott, Williams & Wilkins, 2004, 725-27.

Lefor, Alan T. "Specialized Techniques in Cancer Management." In *Cancer: Principles & Practice of Oncology*, edited by Vincent T. DeVita Jr., et al., 6th ed. Philadelphia: Lippincott, Williams & Wilkins, 2004, 739-57.

OTHER

Iannitti, David A. "The Role of Laparoscopy in the Management of Pancreatic Cancer." *Home Journal Library Index*. [cited June 27, 2009]. http://bioscience.org/1998/v3/e/iannitti/e181-185.htm.

Carol A. Turkington
Rhonda Cloos, R.N.

Lapatinib

Definition

Lapatinib is an anti-cancer drug designed to treat **cancer** of the breast. Lapatinib inhibits tumor cellular signaling by antagonizing a signaling pathway effecting tumor cell development. The tumor cells lapatinib is used against have a receptor on their cell surface called the human epidermal growth factor receptor type 2 (HER2).

Purpose

Lapatinib is used to treat advanced or metastatic **breast cancer** that has high levels of the growth factor receptor HER2 on the tumor cell surface. Lapatinib is used in patients who have received prior therapy including drugs that are an anthracycline, a taxane, and **trastuzumab** and now need a new agent to treat their cancer.

Description

Lapatinib is an anticancer drug that acts on receptor tyrosine kinases to inhibit the growth of tumors. Receptor tyrosine kinases are receptors for growth factors that are a natural part of cell development and necessary for normal cell growth. When tyrosine kinase receptors are activated, they initiate chemical signals that tell the cell how to grow and develop. Normal tyrosine kinase receptors turn on and off as needed for usual amounts of growth. However, when cells have constantly activated tyrosine kinase receptors, it can lead to abnormal growth and cancer. Drugs in the class of lapatinib inhibit these overly active tyrosine kinase receptors.

Lapatinib is an inhibitor of two growth factor receptors, HER2 and epidermal growth factor receptor (EGFR). Both receptors are tyrosine kinases. Lapatinib is used in combination with the drug **capecitabine** for the treatment of advanced or metastatic HER2 breast cancer. The combination of capecitabine and lapatinib has an additive anti-cancer effect.

KEY TERMS

Cytochrome P450— Enzymes present in the liver that metabolize drugs.

Epilepsy—Neurological disorder characterized by recurrent seizures.

Metastasize—The process by which cancer spreads from its original site to other parts of the body.

QT prolongation—Potentially dangerous heart condition that affects the rhythm of the heart beat and alters the ECG reading of the heart.

Receptor tyrosine kinase—Cell surface receptors that interact with growth factors and hormones to affect the normal life cycle of a cell.

Tuberculosis—Potentially fatal infectious disease that commonly affects the lungs, is highly contagious, and is caused by an organism known as mycobacterium.

Lapatinib is manufactured by GlaxoSmithKline under the trade name Tykerb. Studies have shown that lapatinib is an effective drug, affecting both time to tumor progression and progression-free survival. The term time to tumor progression describes a period of time from when disease is diagnosed (or treated) until the disease starts to get worse. Progression-free survival describes the length of time during and after treatment in which a patient is living with a disease that does not get worse. Both time to tumor progression and progression-free survival may be used in a clinical study or trial to help find out how well a new treatment works. In studies done on lapatinib, patients receiving lapatinib in combination with capecitabine had a longer median time to tumor progression and a longer median progression-free survival than those receiving placebo or capecitabine alone.

Recommended dosage

Lapatinib is taken as an oral medication once a day. Lapatinib should not be taken with food and needs to be administered at least one hour apart from meals (one hour before or after meals). Lapatinib may be given in combination with the drug capecitabine. The usual adult dose of lapatinib is 1.25 g per day. If a dose is missed the patient should seek the advice of their physician and not double their next dose. It is important that the medication not be taken more than once daily. In patients with severe liver impairment the dose of lapatinib may need to be reduced to 750 mg a day. Treatment with lapatinib is continued until disease progression occurs or until unacceptable levels of toxicity occur, whichever comes first.

Precautions

Lapatinib is not recommended for use in pregnant women. Birth control is recommended while using this drug. Lapatinib is a pregnancy Category D drug. Category D describes drugs in which there is evidence of potential human fetal risk based on adverse reaction data from investigational or marketing experience or studies in humans, but potential benefits may warrant use of the drug in pregnant women despite potential risks. For Category D drugs, medical necessity must be great enough to warrant risking harm to the fetus. Lapatinib is both a teratogen and lethal to fetuses in animal studies. Lapatinib is contraindicated for use in breast feeding women. Lapatinib is only used in adults as the safety for use in patients less than 18 years of age has not been established. Lapatinib is absorbed through the skin and lungs if breathed in powder form. Women who are pregnant or who may become pregnant should not handle lapatinib or breathe the dust from the tablets.

Lapatinib may cause a heart condition that affects the rhythm of the heartbeat known as QT prolongation. Sometimes QT prolongation can cause a serious cardiac condition that includes a fast and irregular heartbeat, with severe dizziness and fainting. The risk of developing QT prolongation syndrome may be increased if the patient is taking other drugs that also affect the rhythm of the heart, or if the patient has cardiac problems. Low blood levels of potassium or magnesium may also increase risk of QT prolongation. Lapatinib toxicity may cause other adverse side effects affecting heart function, and multiple other medical heart conditions may result from use of lapatinib.

Lapatinib may not be suitable for patients with a history of certain types of heart failure. Caution must be used for lapatinib treatment in patients with liver disease or impairment. The liver is responsible for metabolizing lapatinib into inactive compounds. If this metabolism is impaired, higher levels of lapatinib in the bloodstream may cause toxicity. Patients with liver impairment may need a lower dose for treatment. Caution may be needed in patients with kidney impairment as safety and effectiveness has not been fully established in this group of patients.

Side effects

Lapatinib is used when the medical benefit is judged to be greater than the risk of side effects. The most frequent side effects of lapatinib treatment are **diarrhea**, dry skin, rash, upset stomach, **fatigue**, diarrhea, **nausea**, and **vomiting**. Lapatinib also commonly causes hand foot syndrome, caused by leakage of lapatinib out of small blood vessels in the hands and feet. During some types of **chemotherapy**, small amounts of medication in the blood stream leak out of capillaries in the palms of the hands and the soles of the feet. Drug leakage is increased by heat exposure or friction. The result is redness, tenderness, and sometimes peeling of the skin of the palms and soles. The appearance of sunburn, numbness, and tingling may develop, and may interfere with the activity level of the patient.

Less commonly, lapatinib therapy may cause insomnia, body aches, and inflammation of the tissue lining the inside of the mouth. Lapatinib may cause abnormal liver function tests, liver disease, difficulty breathing, lung disease and inflammation, heart failure, and the heart condition called prolonged QT interval.

Interactions

Patients should make their doctor aware of any and all medications or supplements they are taking before using lapatinib. Lapatinib interacts with many other drugs. Some drug interactions may make lapatinib unsuitable for use, while others may be monitored and attempted.

Lapatinib may have dangerous additive effects with other drugs that also cause QT prolongation. Drugs that interact with lapatinib in this way include amiodarone, dofetilide, pimozide, procainamide, quinidine, sotalol, and macrolide **antibiotics** such as erythromycin.

Lapatinib is metabolized by a set of liver enzymes known as cytochrome P450 (CYP-450) subtype 3A4.

QUESTIONS TO ASK YOUR PHARMACIST

- How long will I need to take this drug before you can tell if it helps for me?
- How often do I have to have blood work and other laboratory tests done to check the effect the drug is having?
- Is this drug safe to take with the other drugs that I am currently taking?
- What side effects should I watch for? When should I call the doctor about them?
- Are there any clinical trials of this drug combined with other therapies that might benefit me?

Drugs that induce, or activate these enzymes increase the metabolism of lapatinib. This results in lower levels of therapeutic lapatinib, thereby negatively affecting treatment of cancer. For this reason drugs that induce CYP-450 subtype 3A4 may not be used with lapatinib. This includes some anti-epileptic drugs such as **carbamazepine**, some anti-inflammatory drugs such as **dexamethasone**, anti-tuberculosis drugs such as rifampin, and the herb St. John's Wort.

Drugs that act to inhibit the action of CYP-450 subtype 3A4 may cause undesired increased levels of lapatinib in the body. This could lead to toxic doses. Some examples are antibiotics such as clarithromycin, antifungal drugs such as ketoconazole, antiviral drugs such as indinavir, antidepressants such as fluoxetine, and some cardiac agents such as verapamil. Grapefruit juice may also increase the amount of lapatinib in the body. Patients should avoid drinking grapefruit juice or eating grapefruit while taking lapatinib.

Resources

BOOKS

Goodman and Gilman's The Pharmacological Basis of Therapeutics, Eleventh Edition. McGraw Hill Medical Publishing Division, 2006.

Tarascon Pharmacopoeia Library Edition. Jones and Bartlett Publishers, 2009.

OTHER

Epocrates. *Lapatinib.* http://www.epocrates.com.

Medscape. *Lapatinib.* http://www.medscape.com.

RxList. *Lapatinib.* http://www.rxlist.com.

ORGANIZATIONS

FDA U.S. Food and Drug Administration. 10903 New Hampshire Ave, Silver Spring, MD 20993. (888)INFO-FDA. http://www.fda.gov.

National Cancer Institute. 6116 Executive Boulevard, Room 3036A, Bethesda, MD 20892-8322. (800)4-CANCER. http://www.cancer.gov.

Maria Basile, Ph.D.

Laryngeal cancer

Definition

Laryngeal **cancer** is cancer of the larynx or voice box.

Description

The larynx is located where the throat divides into the esophagus and the trachea. The esophagus is the tube that takes food to the stomach. The trachea, or windpipe, takes air to the lungs. The area where the larynx is located is sometimes called the Adam's apple.

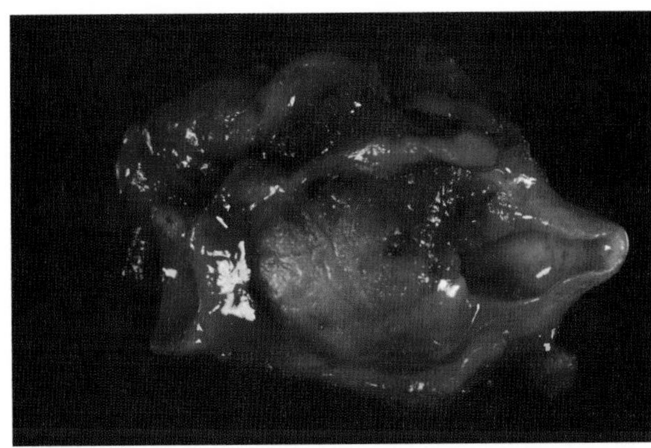

A pathology photograph of an extracted tumor found on the larynx. *(Photograph by William Gage. Custom Medical Stock Photo. Reproduced by permission.)*

The larynx has two main functions. It contains the vocal cords, cartilage, and small muscles that make up the voice box. When a person speaks, small muscles tighten the vocal cords, narrowing the distance between them. As air is exhaled past the tightened vocal cords, it creates sounds that are formed into speech by the mouth, lips, and tongue.

The second function of the larynx is to allow air to enter the trachea and to keep food, saliva, and foreign material from entering the lungs. A flap of tissue called the epiglottis covers the trachea each time a person swallows. This blocks foreign material from entering the lungs. When not swallowing, the epiglottis retracts, and air flows into the trachea. During treatment for cancer of the larynx, both of these functions may be lost.

Cancers of the larynx develop slowly. About 95% of these cancers develop from thin, flat cells similar to skin cells called squamous epithelial cells. These cells line the larynx. Gradually, the squamous epithelial cells begin to change and are replaced with abnormal cells. These abnormal cells are not cancerous but are pre-malignant cells that have the potential to develop into cancer. This condition is called dysplasia. Most people with dysplasia never develop cancer. The condition simply goes away without any treatment, especially if the person with dysplasia stops smoking or drinking alcohol.

The larynx is made up of three parts, the glottis, the supraglottis, and the subglottis. Cancer can start in

KEY TERMS

Dysplasia—The abnormal change in size, shape or organization of adult cells.

Lymph—Clear, slightly yellow fluid carried by a network of thin tubes to every part of the body. Cells that fight infection are carried in the lymph.

Lymphatic system—Primary defense against infection in the body. The lymphatic system consists of tissues, organs, and channels (similar to veins) that produce, store, and transport lymph and white blood cells to fight infection.

Lymph nodes—Small, bean-shaped collections of tissue found in a lymph vessel. They produce cells and proteins that fight infection, and also filter lymph. Nodes are sometimes called lymph glands.

Malignant—Cancerous. Cells tend to reproduce without normal controls on growth and form tumors or invade other tissues.

Metastasize—Spread of cells from the original site of the cancer to other parts of the body where secondary tumors are formed.

QUESTIONS TO ASK THE DOCTOR

- What stage is my cancer, and what exactly does that mean?
- What are possible treatments for my cancer?
- How long will my treatment last?
- What are some of the changes in my activities that will occur because of my treatment?
- What is daily life like after a laryngectomy?
- How will I speak?
- I've heard about clinical trials using radiation and drugs to treat cancer of the larynx. Where can I find out more about these trials?
- What changes in my lifestyle can I make to help improve my chances of beating this cancer?
- How often will I have to have check-ups?
- What is the likelihood that I will survive this cancer?
- Can you suggest any support groups that would be helpful to me or my family?

any of these regions. Treatment and survival rates depend on which parts of the larynx are affected and whether the cancer has spread to neighboring areas of the neck or distant parts of the body.

The glottis is the middle part of the larynx. It contains the vocal cords. Cancers that develop on the vocal cords are often diagnosed very early because even small vocal cord tumors cause hoarseness. In addition, the vocal cords have no connection to the lymphatic system. This means that cancers on the vocal cord do not spread easily. When confined to the vocal cords without any involvement of other parts of the larynx, the cure rate for this cancer is 75–95%.

The supraglottis is the area above the vocal cords. It contains the epiglottis, which protects the trachea from foreign materials. Cancers that develop in this region are usually not found as early as cancers of the glottis because the symptoms are less distinct. The supraglottis region has many connections to the lymphatic system, so cancers in this region tend to spread easily to the lymph nodes and may spread to other parts of the body (lymph nodes are small bean-shaped structures that are found throughout the body; they produce and store infection-fighting cells). In 25–50% of people with cancer in the supraglottal region, the cancer has already spread to the lymph nodes by the time they are diagnosed. Because of this, survival rates are lower than for cancers that involve only the glottis.

The subglottis is the region below the vocal cords. Cancer starting in the subglottis region is rare. When it does, it is usually detected only after it has spread to the vocal cords, where it causes obvious symptoms such as hoarseness. Because the cancer has already begun to spread by the time it is detected, survival rates are generally lower than for cancers in other parts of the larynx.

Demographics

About 12,000 new cases of cancer of the larynx develop in the United States each year. Each year, about 3,600 die of the disease. Laryngeal cancer is between four and five times more common in men than in women. Almost all men who develop laryngeal cancer are over age 55. Laryngeal cancer is about 50% more common among African-American men than among other Americans.

It is thought that older men are more likely to develop laryngeal cancer than women because the two main risk factors for acquiring the disease are lifetime habits of smoking and alcohol abuse. More men smoke and drink more than women, and more African-American men are heavy smokers than other men in the United States. However, as smoking becomes more prevalent among women, it seems likely that more cases of laryngeal cancer in females will be seen.

Causes and symptoms

Laryngeal cancer develops when the normal cells lining the larynx are replaced with abnormal cells (dysplasia) that become malignant and reproduce to form tumors. The development of dysplasia is strongly linked to life-long habits of smoking and heavy use of alcohol. The more a person smokes, the greater the risk of developing laryngeal cancer. It is unusual for someone who does not smoke or drink to develop cancer of the larynx. Occasionally, however, people who inhale asbestos particles, wood dust, paint or industrial chemical fumes over a long period of time develop the disease.

The symptoms of laryngeal cancer depend on the location of the tumor. Tumors on the vocal cords are rarely painful, but cause hoarseness. Anyone who is continually hoarse for more than two weeks or who has a cough that does not go away should be checked by a doctor.

Tumors in the supraglottal region above the vocal cords often cause more, but less distinct symptoms. These include:

- persistent sore throat
- pain when swallowing
- difficulty swallowing or frequent choking on food
- bad breath
- lumps in the neck
- persistent ear pain (called referred pain; the source of the pain is not the ear)
- change in voice quality

Tumors that begin below the vocal cords are rare, but may cause noisy or difficult breathing. All the symptoms above can also be caused other cancers as well as by less serious illnesses. However, if these symptoms persist, it is important to see a doctor and find their cause, because the earlier cancer treatment begins, the more successful it is.

Diagnosis

On the first visit to a doctor for symptoms that suggest laryngeal cancer, the doctor first takes a complete medical history, including family history of cancer and lifestyle information about smoking and alcohol use. The doctor also does a physical examination, paying special attention to the neck region for lumps, tenderness, or swelling.

The next step is examination by an otolaryngologist, or ear, nose, and throat (ENT) specialist. This doctor also performs a physical examination, but in addition will also want to look inside the throat at the larynx. Initially, the doctor may spray a local anesthetic on the back of the throat to prevent gagging, then use a long-handled mirror to look at the larynx and vocal cords. This examination is done in the doctor's office. It may cause gagging but is usually painless.

A more extensive examination involves a **laryngoscopy**. In a laryngoscopy, a lighted fiberoptic tube called a laryngoscope that contains a tiny camera is inserted through the patient's nose and mouth and snaked down the throat so that the doctor can see the larynx and surrounding area. This procedure can be done with a sedative and local anesthetic in a doctor's office. More often, the procedure is done in an outpatient surgery clinic or hospital under general anesthesia. This allows the doctor to use tiny clips on the end of the laryngoscope to take biopsies (tissue samples) of any abnormal-looking areas.

Laryngoscopies are normally painless and take about one hour. Some people find their throat feels scratchy after the procedure. Since laryngoscopies are done under sedation, patients should not drive immediately after the procedure, and should have someone available to take them home. Laryngoscopy is a standard procedure that is covered by insurance.

The locations of the samples taken during the laryngoscopy are recorded, and the samples are then sent to the laboratory where they are examined under the microscope by a pathologist who specializes in diagnosing diseases through cell samples and laboratory tests. It may take several days to get the results. Based on the findings of the pathologist, cancer can be diagnosed and staged.

Once cancer is diagnosed, other tests will probably be done to help determine the exact size and location of the tumors. This information is helpful in determining which treatments are most appropriate. These tests may include:

- Endoscopy. Similar to a laryngoscopy, this test is done when it appears that cancer may have spread to other areas, such as the esophagus or trachea.
- Computed tomography (CT or CAT) scan. Using x-ray images taken from several angles and computer modeling, CT scans allow parts of the body to be seen as a cross section. This helps locate and size the

tumors, and provides information on whether they can be surgically removed.

- Magnetic resonance imaging (MRI). MRI uses magnets and radio waves to create more detailed cross-sectional scans than computed tomography. This detailed information is needed if surgery on the larynx area is planned.
- Barium swallow. Barium is a substance that, unlike soft tissue, shows up on x rays. Swallowed barium coats the throat and allows x-ray pictures to be made of the tissues lining the throat.
- Chest x ray. Done to determine if cancer has spread to the lungs. Since most people with laryngeal cancer are smokers, the risk of also having lung cancer or emphysema is high.
- Fine needle aspiration (FNA) biopsy. If any lumps on the neck are found, a thin needle is inserted into the lump, and some cells are removed for analysis by the pathologist.
- Additional blood and urine tests. These tests do not diagnose cancer, but help to determine the patient's general health and provide information to determine which cancer treatments are most appropriate.

Treatment team

An otolaryngologist and an oncologist (cancer specialist) generally lead the treatment team. They are supported by radiologists to interpret CT and MRI scans, a head and neck surgeon, and nurses with special training in assisting cancer patients.

A speech pathologist is often involved in treatment, both before surgery to discuss various options for communication if the larynx is removed, and after surgery to teach alternate forms of voice communication. A social worker, psychologist, or family counselor may help both the patient and the family meet the changes and challenges that living with laryngeal cancer brings.

At any point in the process, the patient may want to get a second opinion from another doctor in the same specialty. This is a common practice and does not indicate a lack of faith in the original doctor, but simply a desire for more information. Some insurance companies require a second opinion before surgery is done.

Clinical staging, treatments, and prognosis

Staging

Once cancer of the larynx is found, more tests will be done to find out if cancer cells have spread to other parts of the body. This is called staging. A doctor needs to know the stage of the disease to plan treatment. In cancer of the larynx, the definitions of the early stages depend on where the cancer started.

STAGE I. The cancer is only in the area where it started and has not spread to lymph nodes in the area or to other parts of the body. The exact definition of stage I depends on where the cancer started, as follows:

- Supraglottis: The cancer is only in one area of the supraglottis and the vocal cords can move normally.
- Glottis: The cancer is only in the vocal cords and the vocal cords can move normally.
- Subglottis: The cancer has not spread outside of the subglottis.

STAGE II. The cancer is only in the larynx and has not spread to lymph nodes in the area or to other parts of the body. The exact definition of stage II depends on where the cancer started, as follows:

- Supraglottis: The cancer is in more than one area of the supraglottis, but the vocal cords can move normally.
- Glottis: The cancer has spread to the supraglottis or the subglottis or both. The vocal cords may or may not be able to move normally.
- Subglottis: The cancer has spread to the vocal cords, which may or may not be able to move normally.

STAGE III. Either of the following may be true:

- The cancer has not spread outside of the larynx, but the vocal cords cannot move normally, or the cancer has spread to tissues next to the larynx.
- The cancer has spread to one lymph node on the same side of the neck as the cancer, and the lymph node measures no more than 3 centimeters (just over 1 inch).

STAGE IV. Any of the following may be true:

- The cancer has spread to tissues around the larynx, such as the pharynx or the tissues in the neck. The lymph nodes in the area may or may not contain cancer.
- The cancer has spread to more than one lymph node on the same side of the neck as the cancer, to lymph nodes on one or both sides of the neck, or to any lymph node that measures more than 6 centimeters (over 2 inches).
- The cancer has spread to other parts of the body.

RECURRENT. Recurrent disease means that the cancer has come back (recurred) after it has been treated. It may come back in the larynx or in another part of the body.

Treatment

Treatment is based on the stage of the cancer as well as its location and the health of the individual. Generally, there are three types of treatments for cancer of the larynx. These are surgery, radiation, and **chemotherapy**. They can be used alone or in combination based in the stage of the caner. Getting a second opinion after the cancer has been staged can be very helpful in sorting out treatment options and should always be considered.

SURGERY. The goal of surgery is to cut out the tissue that contains malignant cells. There are several common surgeries to treat laryngeal cancer.

Stage III and stage IV cancers are usually treated with total **laryngectomy**. This is an operation to remove the entire larynx. Sometimes other tissues around the larynx are also removed. Total laryngectomy removes the vocal cords. Alternate methods of voice communication must be learned with the help of a speech pathologist.

Smaller tumors are sometimes treated by partial laryngectomy. The goal is to remove the cancer but save as much of the larynx (and corresponding speech capability) as possible. Very small tumors or cancer in situ are sometimes successfully treated with laser excision surgery. In this type of surgery, a narrowly targeted beam of light from a laser is used to remove the cancer.

Advanced cancer (Stages III and IV) that has spread to the lymph nodes often requires an operation called a neck dissection. The goal of a neck dissection is to remove the lymph nodes and prevent the cancer from spreading. There are several forms of neck dissection. A **radical neck dissection** is the operation that removes the most tissue.

Several other operations are sometimes performed because of laryngeal cancer. A tracheotomy is a surgical procedure in which an artificial opening is made in the trachea (windpipe) to allow air into the lungs. This operation is necessary if the larynx is totally removed. A **gastrectomy** tube is a feeding tube placed through skin and directly into the stomach. It is used to give nutrition to people who cannot swallow or whose esophagus is blocked by a tumor. People who have a total laryngectomy usually do not need a gastrectomy tube if their esophagus remains intact.

RADIATION. **Radiation therapy** uses high-energy rays, such as **x rays** or gamma rays, to kill cancer cells. The advantage of radiation therapy is that it preserves the larynx and the ability to speak. The disadvantage is that it may not kill all the cancer cells. Radiation therapy can be used alone in early stage cancers or in combination with surgery. Sometimes it is tried first with the plan that if it fails to cure the cancer, surgery still remains an option. Often, radiation therapy is used after surgery for advanced cancers to kill any cells the surgeon might not have removed.

There are two types of radiation therapy. External beam radiation therapy focuses rays from outside the body on the cancerous tissue. This is the most common type of radiation therapy used to treat laryngeal cancer. With internal radiation therapy, also called brachytherapy, radioactive materials are placed directly on the cancerous tissue. This type of radiation therapy is a much less common treatment for laryngeal cancer.

External radiation therapy is given in doses called fractions. A common treatment involves giving fractions five days a week for seven weeks. **Clinical trials** are underway to determine the benefits of accelerating the delivery of fractions (accelerated fractionation) or dividing fractions into smaller doses given more than once a day (hyperfractionation). Side effects of radiation therapy include dry mouth, sore throat, hoarseness, skin problems, trouble swallowing, and diminished ability to taste.

CHEMOTHERAPY. Chemotherapy is the use of drugs to kill cancer cells. Unlike radiation therapy, which is targeted to a specific tissue, chemotherapy drugs are either taken by mouth or intravenously (through a vein) and circulate throughout the whole body. They are used mainly to treat advanced laryngeal cancer that is inoperable or that has metastasized to a distant site. Chemotherapy is often used after surgery or in combination with radiation therapy. Clinical trials are underway to determine the best combination of treatments for advanced cancer.

The two most common chemotherapy drugs used to treat laryngeal cancer are **cisplatin** and 5-fluorouracil (5-FU or **fluorouracil**). There are many side effects associated with chemotherapy drugs, including **nausea and vomiting**, loss of appetite (**anorexia**), hair loss (**alopecia**), **diarrhea**, and mouth sores. Chemotherapy can also damage the blood-producing cells of the bone marrow, which can result in low blood cell counts, increased chance of **infection**, and abnormal bleeding or bruising.

Prognosis

Cure rates and survival rates can predict group outcomes, but can never precisely predict the outcome for a single individual. However, the earlier laryngeal cancer is discovered and treated, the more likely it will be cured.

Cancers found in stage 0 and stage 1 have a 75–95% cure rate depending on the site. Late stage cancers that have metastasized have a very poor survival rate, with intermediate stages falling somewhere in between. People who have had laryngeal cancer are at greatest risk for recurrence (having cancer come back), especially in the head and neck, during the first two to three years after treatment. Check-ups during the first year are needed every other month, and four times a year during the second year. It is rare for laryngeal cancer to recur after five years of being cancer-free.

Alternative and complementary therapies

Alternative and complementary therapies range from herbal remedies, vitamin supplements, and special diets to spiritual practices, acupuncture, massage, and similar treatments. When these therapies are used in addition to conventional medicine, they are called complementary therapies. When they are used instead of conventional medicine, they are called alternative therapies.

Complementary or alternative therapies are widely used by people with cancer. One large study published in the *Journal of Clinical Oncology* in July 2000, found that 83% of all cancer patients studied used some form of complementary or alternative medicine as part of their cancer treatment. No specific alternative therapies have been directed toward laryngeal cancer. However, good nutrition and activities that reduce stress and promote a positive view of life have no unwanted side effects and appear to be beneficial in boosting the immune system in fighting cancer.

Unlike traditional pharmaceuticals, complementary and alternative therapies are not evaluated by the United States Food and Drug Administration (FDA) for either safety or effectiveness. These therapies may have interactions with traditional pharmaceuticals. Patients should be wary of "miracle cures" and notify their doctors if they are using herbal remedies, vitamin supplements or other unprescribed treatments. Alternative and experimental treatments normally are not covered by insurance.

Coping with cancer treatment

Cancer treatment, even when successful, has many unwanted side effects. In laryngeal cancer, the biggest side effects are the loss of speech due to total laryngectomy and the need to breathe through a hole in the neck called a stoma. Several alternative methods of sound production, both mechanical and learned, are available, and should be discussed with a speech pathologist. Support groups also exist for people who have had their larynx removed. Coping with speech loss and care of the stoma is discussed more extensively in the laryngectomy entry.

Chemotherapy brings with it a host of unwanted side effects, many of which disappear after the chemotherapy stops. For example, hair will re-grow, and until it does, a wig can be used. Medications are available to treat **nausea** and **vomiting**. Side effects such as dry skin are treated symptomatically.

Clinical trials

Clinical trials are government-regulated studies of new treatments and techniques that may prove beneficial in diagnosing or treating a disease. Participation is always voluntary and at no cost to the participant. Clinical trials are conducted in three phases. Phase 1 tests the safety of the treatment and looks for harmful side effects. Phase 2 tests the effectiveness of the treatment. Phase 3 compares the treatment to other treatments available for the same condition.

The selection of clinical trials underway changes frequently. Clinical trials for laryngeal cancer currently focus treating advanced cancers by combining radiation and surgical therapy, radiation and chemotherapy, and different combinations of chemotherapy drugs. Other studies are examining the most effective timing and duration of radiation therapy.

Current information on what clinical trials are available and where they are being held is available by entering the search term "laryngeal cancer" at the following web sites:

- National Cancer Institute: http://cancertrials.nci.nih.gov or (800) 4-CANCER
- National Institutes of Health Clinical Trials: http://clinicaltrials.gov
- Center Watch: A Clinical Trials Listing: http://www.centerwatch.com

Prevention

By far, the most effective way to prevent laryngeal cancer is not to smoke. Smokers who quit smoking also significantly decrease their risk of developing the disease. Other ways to prevent laryngeal cancer include limiting the use of alcohol, eating a well-balanced diet, seeking treatment for prolonged heartburn, and avoiding inhaling asbestos and chemical fumes.

Special concerns

Being diagnosed with cancer is a traumatic event. Not only is one's health affected, one's whole life suddenly revolves around trips to the doctor for cancer treatment and adjusting to the side effects of these treatments. This is stressful for both the cancer patient and his or her family members. It is not unusual for family members to feel resentful of the changes that occur in the family, and then feel guilty about feeling resentful.

The loss of voice because of laryngeal surgery may be the most traumatic effect of laryngeal cancer. Losing the ability to communicate easily with others can be isolating. Support groups and psychological counseling is helpful for both the cancer patient and family members. Many national organizations that support cancer education can provide information on in-person or on-line support and education groups.

See also Alcohol consumption; Cigarettes; Smoking cessation.

Resources

PERIODICALS

Ahmad, I., B. N. Kumar, K. Radford, J. O'Connell, and A. J. Batch. "Surgical Voice Restoration Following Ablative Surgery for Laryngeal and Hypopharyngeal Carcinoma." *Journal or Laryngology and Otolaryngology* 114 (July 2000): 522–5.

OTHER

"Laryngeal Cancer." *CancerNet*. [cited July 19, 2009]. http://www.graylab.ac.uk/cancernet/201519.html#3_STAGE EXPLANATION.

"What you Need to Know About Cancer of the Larynx." *CancerNet* November 2000. [cited July 19, 2009]. http://www.cancernet.nci.nih.gov.

ORGANIZATIONS

American Cancer Society. National Headquarters, 1599 Clifton Rd. NE, Atlanta, GA 30329. 800 (ACS)-2345. http://www.cancer.org.

National Cancer Institute. Cancer Information Service. Bldg. 31, Room 10A19, 9000 Rockville Pike, Bethesda, MD 20892. (800) 4-CANCER. http://www.nci.nih.gov/cancerinfo/index.html.

National Cancer Institute Office of Cancer Complementary and Alternative Medicine. <http://occam.nci.nih.gov>.

National Center for Complementary and Alternative Medicine. P. O. Box 8218, Silver Spring, MD 20907-8281. (888) 644-6226. <http://nccam.nih.gov>.

Tish Davidson, A.M.

Laryngeal nerve palsy

Description

Laryngeal nerve palsy is damage to the recurrent laryngeal nerve (or less commonly the vagus nerve) that results in paralysis of the larynx (voice box). Paralysis may be temporary or permanent. Damage to the recurrent laryngeal nerve is most likely to occur during surgery on the thyroid gland to treat **cancer** of the thyroid. Laryngeal nerve palsy is also called recurrent laryngeal nerve damage.

The vagus nerve is one of 12 cranial nerves that connect the brain to other organs in the body. It runs from the brain to the large intestine. In the neck, the vagus nerve gives off a paired branch nerve called the recurrent laryngeal nerve. The recurrent laryngeal nerves lie in grooves along either side of the trachea (windpipe) between the trachea and the thyroid gland.

The recurrent laryngeal nerve controls movement of the larynx. The larynx is located where the throat divides into the esophagus, a tube that takes food to the stomach, and the trachea (windpipe) that takes air to the lungs. The larynx contains the apparatus for voice production: the vocal cords, and the muscles and ligaments that move the vocal cords. It also controls the flow of air into the lungs. When the recurrent laryngeal nerve is damaged, the movements of the larynx are reduced. This causes voice weakness, hoarseness, or sometimes the complete loss of voice. The changes may be temporary or permanent. In rare life-threatening cases of damage, the larynx is paralyzed to the extent that air cannot enter the lungs.

Causes

Laryngeal nerve palsy is an uncommon side effect of surgery to remove the thyroid gland (thyroidectomy). It occurs in 1–2% of operations for total thyroidectomy to treat cancer, and less often when only part of the thyroid is removed. Damage can occur to either one or both branches of the nerve, and it can be temporary or permanent. Most people experience only transient laryngeal nerve palsy and recover their normal voice within a few weeks.

Laryngeal nerve palsy can also occur from causes unrelated to thyroid surgery. These include damage to either the vagus nerve or the laryngeal nerve, due to tumors in the neck and chest or diseases in the chest such as aortic aneurysms. Both tumors and aneurysms press on the nerve, and the pressure causes damage.

Treatments

Once the recurrent laryngeal nerve is damaged, there is no specific treatment to heal it. With time, most cases of recurrent laryngeal palsy improve on their own. In the event of severe damage, the larynx may be so paralyzed that air cannot flow past it into the lungs. When this happens, an emergency tracheotomy must be performed to save the patient's life. A tracheotomy is a surgical procedure to make an artificial opening in the trachea (windpipe) to allow air to bypass the larynx and enter the lungs. If paralysis of the larynx is temporary, the tracheotomy hole can be surgically closed when it is no longer needed.

Some normal variation in the location of the recurrent laryngeal nerve occurs among individuals. Occasionally the nerves are not located exactly where the surgeon expects to find them. Choosing a board certified head and neck surgeon who has had a lot of experience with thyroid operations is the best way to prevent laryngeal nerve palsy.

Alternative and complementary therapies

There are no alternative or complementary therapies to heal laryngeal nerve palsy. The passage of time alone restores speech to most people. Some alternatives for artificial speech exist for people whose loss of speech is permanent.

See also Laryngectomy.

Resources

PERIODICALS

Harti, Dana M., and Daniel F. Brasnu. "Recurrent laryngeal nerve paralysis:Current concepts and treatment." *Ear, Nose and Throat Journal* 79, no. 12 (December 2000): 918.

OTHER

Grebe, Werner, M.D. "Thyroid Operations." *EndocrineWeb.com.* [cited July 19, 2009]. http://www.endocrineweb.com/surthyroid.html.

University of Virginia Health System. "Surgical Tutorial: Surgical Approach for a Thyroid Mass." *University of Virginia Health System, Department of Surgery.* [cited July 19, 2009]. http://hsc.virginia.edu/surgery/tutorialsurgthyroid.html.

Tish Davidson, A.M.

Laryngectomy

Definition

Laryngectomy is the partial or complete surgical removal of the larynx, usually as a treatment for **cancer** of the larynx.

Purpose

Normally a laryngectomy is performed to remove tumors or cancerous tissue. In rare cases, it may be done when the larynx is badly damaged by gunshot, automobile injuries, or similar violent accidents. Laryngectomies can be total or partial. Total laryngectomies are done when cancer is advanced. The entire larynx is removed. Often if the cancer has spread, other surrounding structures in the neck, such as lymph nodes, are removed at the same time. Partial laryngectomies are done when cancer is limited to one spot. Only the area with the tumor is removed. Laryngectomies may also be performed when other cancer treatment options, such as **radiation therapy** or **chemotherapy**, fail.

Precautions

Laryngectomy is done only after cancer of the larynx has been diagnosed by a series of tests that allow the otolaryngologist (a specialist often called an ear, nose, and throat doctor) to look into the throat and take tissue samples (biopsies) to confirm and stage the cancer. People need to be in good general health to undergo a laryngectomy, and will have standard preoperative blood work and tests to make sure they are able to safely withstand the operation.

Description

The larynx is located slightly below the point where the throat divides into the esophagus, which takes food to the stomach, and the trachea (windpipe), which takes air to the lungs. Because of its location, the larynx plays a critical role in normal breathing, swallowing, and speaking. Within the larynx, vocal folds (often called vocal cords) vibrate as air is exhaled past, thus creating speech. The epiglottis protects the trachea, making sure that only air gets into the lungs. When the larynx is removed, these functions are lost.

Once the larynx is removed, air can no longer flow into the lungs. During this operation, the surgeon removes the larynx through an incision in the neck. The surgeon also performs a tracheotomy. He makes an artificial opening called a stoma in the front of the neck. The upper portion of the trachea is brought to

KEY TERMS

Larynx—Also known as the voice box, the larynx is composed of cartilage that contains the apparatus for voice production. This includes the vocal cords and the muscles and ligaments that move the cords.

Lymph nodes—Accumulations of tissue along a lymph channel, which produce cells called lymphocytes that fight infection.

Tracheostomy—A surgical procedure in which an artificial opening is made in the trachea (windpipe) to allow air into the lungs.

QUESTIONS TO ASK THE DOCTOR

- Is laryngectomy my only viable treatment option?
- What specific lifestyle changes will I have to make?
- Is there a support group in the area that can assist me post-surgery?
- How long will it be until I can verbally communicate? What are my options?
- How sizable is the risk of recurring cancer?

the stoma and secured, making a permanent alternate way for air to get to the lungs. The connection between the throat and the esophagus is not normally affected, so after healing, the person whose larynx has been removed (called a laryngectomee) can eat normally. However, normal speech is no longer possible. Several alternate means of vocal communication can be learned with the help of a speech pathologist.

Preparation

As with any surgical procedure, the patient will be required to sign a consent form after the procedure is thoroughly explained. Many patients prefer a second opinion, and some insurers require it. Blood and urine studies, along with chest x ray and EKG may be ordered as the doctor deems necessary. The patient also has a pre-operative meeting with an anesthesiologist. If a complete laryngectomy is planned, it may be helpful to meet with a speech pathologist and/or an established laryngectomee for discussion of post-operative expectations and support.

Aftercare

A person undergoing a laryngectomy spends several days in intensive care (ICU) and receives intravenous (IV) fluids and medication. As with any major surgery, the blood pressure, pulse, and respirations are monitored regularly. The patient is encouraged to turn, cough, and deep breathe to help mobilize secretions in the lungs. One or more drains are usually inserted in the neck to remove any fluids that collect. These drains are removed after several days.

It takes two to three weeks for the tissues of the throat to heal. During this time, the laryngectomee cannot swallow food and must receive nutrition through a tube inserted through the nose and down the throat into the stomach. During this time, even people with partial laryngectomies are unable to speak.

When air is drawn in normally through the nose, it is warmed and moistened before it reaches the lungs. When air is drawn in through the stoma, it does not have the opportunity to be warmed and humidified. In order to keep the stoma from drying out and becoming crusty, laryngectomees are encouraged to breathe artificially humidified air. The stoma is usually covered with a light cloth to keep it clean and to keep unwanted particles from accidentally entering the lungs. Care of the stoma is extremely important, since it is the person's only way to get air to the lungs. After a laryngectomy, a healthcare professional will teach the laryngectomee and his or her caregivers how to care for the stoma.

Immediately after a laryngectomy, an alternate method of communication such as writing notes, gesturing, or pointing must be used. A partial laryngectomy patient will gradually regain some speech several weeks after the operation, but the voice may be hoarse, weak, and strained. A speech pathologist will work with a complete laryngectomee to establish new ways of communicating.

There are three main methods of vocalizing after a total laryngectomy. In esophageal speech the laryngectomee learns how to "swallow" air down into the esophagus and creates sounds by releasing the air. This method requires quite a bit of coordination and learning, and produces short bursts (7 or 8 syllables) of low-volume sound.

Tracheoesophageal speech diverts air through a hole in the trachea made by the surgeon. The air then passes through an implanted artificial voice prosthesis (a small tube that makes a sound when air goes through it). Recent advances have been made in implanting voice prostheses that produce good voice quality.

The third method of artificial sound communication involves using a hand-held electronic device that translates vibrations into sounds. There are several different styles of these devices, but all require the use of at least one hand to hold the device to the throat. The choice of which method to use depends on many things including the age and health of the laryngectomee, and whether other parts of the mouth, such as the tongue, have also been removed.

Many patients resume daily activities after surgery. Special precautions must be taken during showering or shaving. Special instruction and equipment is also required for those who wish to swim or water ski, as it is dangerous for water to enter the windpipe and lungs through the stoma.

Regular follow-up visits are important following treatment for cancer of the larynx because there is a higher-than-average risk of developing a new cancer in the mouth, throat, or other regions of the head or neck. Many self-help and support groups are available to help patients meet others who face similar problems.

Risks

Laryngectomy is often successful in curing early stage cancers. However it does cause lifestyle changes. Laryngectomees must learn new ways of speaking. They must be continually concerned about the care of their stoma. Serious infections can occur if water or other foreign material enters the lungs through an unprotected stoma. Also, women who undergo partial laryngectomy or who learn some types of artificial speech will have a deep voice similar to that of a man. For some women this presents psychological challenges.

Normal results

Ideally, removal of the larynx will remove all cancerous material. The person will recover from the operation, make lifestyle adjustments, and return to an active life.

Abnormal results

Sometimes cancer has spread to surrounding tissues and it is necessary to remove lymph nodes, parts of the tongue, or other cancerous tissues. As with any major operation, post-surgical **infection** is possible. Infection is of particular concern to laryngectomees who have chosen to have a voice prosthesis implanted, and is one of the major reasons for having to remove the device.

Resources

ORGANIZATIONS

American Cancer Society. National Headquarters, 1599 Clifton Road NE, Atlanta, GA 30329. (800) ACS - 2345.http://www.cancer.org.

Cancer Information Service. National Cancer Institute, Building 31, Room 10A19, 9000 Rockville Pike, Bethesda, MD 20892. (800)4-CANCER. http://www.nci.nih.gov/cancerinfo/index.html.

International Association of Laryngectomees(IAL). http://www.larynxlink.com/.

National Institute on Deafness and Other Communication Disorders. National Institutes of Health, 31 Center Drive, MSC 2320, Bethesda, MD 20892-2320. http://www.nidcd.nih.gov.

The Voice Center at Eastern Virginia Medical School. Norfolk, VA 23507 http://www.voice-center.com.

Kathleen Dredge Wright
Tish Davidson, A.M.

Laryngoscopy

Definition

Laryngoscopy refers to a procedure used to view the inside of the larynx (the voice box).

Description

The purpose and advantage of seeing inside the larynx is to detect tumors, foreign bodies, nerve or structural injury, or other abnormalities. Two methods allow the larynx to be seen directly during the examination. In one, a flexible tube with a fiber-optic device is threaded through the nasal passage and down into the throat. The other method uses a rigid viewing tube passed directly from the mouth, through the throat, into the larynx. A light and lens affixed to the endoscope are used in both methods. The endoscopic tube may also be equipped to suction debris or remove material for **biopsy**. **Bronchoscopy** is a similar, but more extensive procedure in which the tube is continued through the larynx, down into the trachea and bronchi.

Preparation

Laryngoscopy is done in the hospital with a local anesthetic spray to minimize discomfort and suppress the gag reflex. Patients are requested not to eat for several hours before the examination.

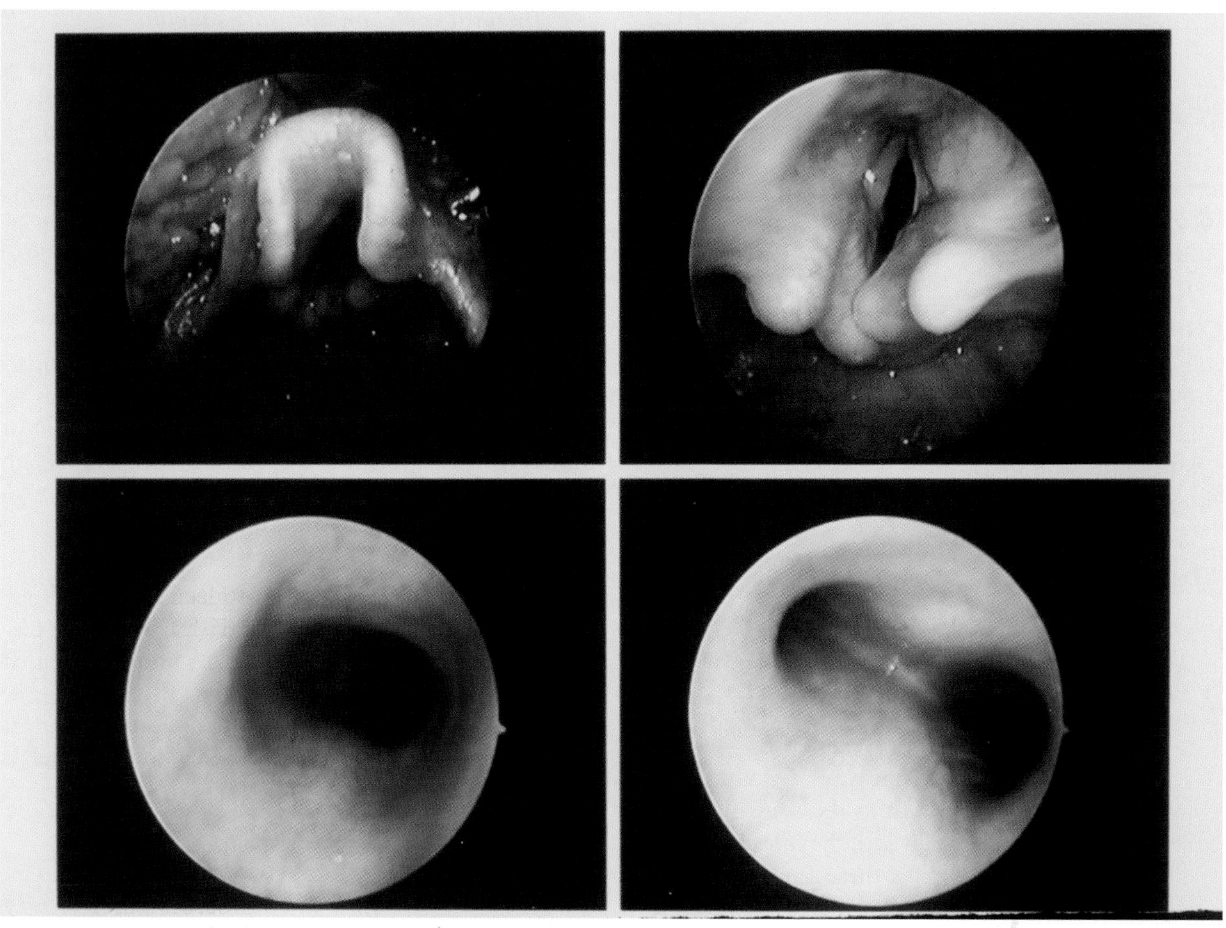

Laryngoscopy. Multiple images of epiglottis, vocal cords, and interior of trachea and bronchus. *(Custom Medical Stock Photo. Reproduced by permission.)*

KEY TERMS

Endoscopic tube—A tube that is inserted into a hollow organ permitting a physician to see the inside it.

Aftercare

If the throat is sore, soothing liquids or lozenges will probably relieve any temporary discomfort.

Risks

This procedure carries no serious risks, although the patient may experience soreness of the throat or cough up small amounts of blood until the irritation subsides.

Normal results

A normal result would be the absence of signs of disease or damage.

Abnormal results

An abnormal finding, such as a tumor or an object lodged in the tissue, would either be removed or described for further medical attention.

Jill S. Lasker

Laxatives

Definition

A laxative is a drug that helps relieve constipation.

Purpose

Laxatives are used to prevent or treat constipation. They are also used to prepare the bowel for an examination or surgical procedure.

KEY TERMS

Cathartic—A general term for any agent that causes the bowel to empty. Cathartics are also known as purgatives.

Constipation—Difficult or infrequent bowel movements.

Diarrhea—Frequent, watery stools.

Electrolyte levels—In the bloodstream, electrolyte levels are the amounts of certain acids, bases, and salts. Abnormal levels of certain electrolyes can be life-threatening.

Encephalopathy—A brain disease.

Peristalsis—Wave-like movement of the colon to pass feces along.

Tetany—Muscle spasms that can be life-threatening.

Description

Laxatives work in different ways, by stimulating colon movement, adding bulk to the contents of the colon, or drawing fluid or fat into the intestine. Some laxatives work by combining these functions. Most primary care physicians recommend that patients try the bulk-producing laxatives first before taking saline or stimulant laxatives.

Bisacodyl

Bisacodyl is a non-prescription stimulant laxative. It reduces short-term constipation and is also used to prepare the colon or rectum for an examination or surgical procedure. The drug works by stimulating colon movement (peristalsis); constipation is usually relieved within 15 minutes to one hour after administration of a suppository form and in 6 to 12 hours after taking the drug orally.

Calcium polycarbophil

Calcium polycarbophil is a non-prescription bulk-forming laxative that is used to reduce both constipation and **diarrhea**. It draws water to the intestine, enlarging the size of the colon and thereby stimulating movement. It reduces diarrhea by taking extra water away from the stool. This drug should relieve constipation in 12 to 24 hours and have maximum effect in three days. Colitis patients should see a reduction in diarrhea within one week.

Docusate calcium/docusate sodium

Docusate, a non-prescription laxative, helps a patient avoid constipation by softening the stool. It works by increasing the penetration of fluids into the stool by emulsifying feces, water and fat. Docusate prevents constipation and softens bowel movements and fecal impactions. This laxative should relieve constipation within one to three days.

Lactulose

Lactulose, a prescription laxative, reduces constipation and lowers blood ammonia levels. It works by drawing fluid into the intestine, raising the amount of water in the stool, and preventing the colon from absorbing ammonia. It is used to help people who suffer from chronic constipation.

Psyllium

Psyllium is a non-prescription bulk-forming laxative that reduces both constipation and diarrhea. It mixes with water to form a gel-like mass that can be easily passed through the colon. Constipation is relieved in 12 to 24 hours and maximum relief is achieved after several days.

Senna/senokot

Senna/senokot is a non-prescription laxative that reduces constipation by promoting colon movement. It is used to treat bouts of constipation and to prepare the colon for an examination or surgical procedure. This laxative reduces constipation in eight to 10 hours.

New and investigational treatments for constipation

Some newer options for the treatment of chronic constipation are being developed by various groups of researchers. These include such alternative therapies as biofeedback; newer drugs like tegaserod (Zelnorm) and prucalopride, which stimulate peristalsis; a nerve growth factor known as neurotrophin-3; and electrical stimulation of the colon.

Recommended dosage

Laxatives may be taken by mouth or rectally (suppository or enema).

Bisacodyl

- Adults or children over 12 years: 5–15 mg taken by mouth in morning or afternoon (up to 30 mg for surgical or exam preparation).

- Adult (rectal): 10 mg.
- Children age 2 to 11 years: 10 mg rectally as single dose.
- Children over three years: 5–10 mg by mouth as single dose.
- Children under two years: 5 mg rectally as single dose.

Calcium polycarbophil

- Adult: 1 g by mouth every day, up to four times a day as needed (not to exceed 6 g by mouth in a 24-hour time period).
- Children age 6 to 12 years: 500 mg by mouth twice a day as needed (not to exceed 3 g in a 24-hour time period).
- Children age 3 to 6 years: 500 mg twice a day by mouth, as needed (not to exceed 1.5 g in a 24-hour time period).

Docusate

- Adult (docusate sodium): 50–300 mg by mouth per day.
- Adult (docusate calcium or docusate potassium): 240 mg by mouth as needed.
- Adult (docusate sodium enema): 5 ml.
- Children over 12 years (docusate sodium enema): 2 ml.
- Children age 6 to 12 years (docusate sodium): 40–120 mg by mouth per day.
- Children age 3 to 6 years (docusate sodium): 20–60 mg by mouth per day.
- Children under 3 years (docusate sodium): 10–40 mg by mouth every day.

Lactulose

FOR CONSTIPATION:.

- Adult: 15–60 ml by mouth every day.
- Children: 7.5 ml by mouth every day.

FOR ENCEPHALOPATHY:.

- Adult: 20–30 g three or four times a day until stools become soft. Retention enema: 30–45 ml in 100 ml of fluid.
- Infants and children: Parents should follow physician's directions for infants and children with encephalopathy.

Psyllium

- Adult: 1–2 teaspoons mixed in 8 ounces of water two or three times a day by mouth, followed by 8 ounces water; or one packet in 8 ounces water two or three times a day, followed by 8 ounces of water.
- Children over 6 years: 1 teaspoon mixed in 4 ounces of water at bedtime.

Senna/senokot

- Adult (Senokot): 1 to 8 tablets taken by mouth per day or 1/2–4 teaspoons of granules mixed in water or juice.
- Adult (rectal suppository): 1 to 2 at bedtime.
- Adult (syrup): 1–4 teaspoons at bedtime.
- Adult (Black Draught): 3/4 ounce dissolved in 2.5 ounces liquid given between 2 P.M. and 4 P.M. on the day prior to a medical exam or procedure.
- Children: Parents should ask their doctor as dosage is based on weight. Black Draught is not to be used by children.
- Children age 1 month to 1 year (Senokot): 1.25–2.5 ml of syrup at bedtime.

Precautions

The doctor should be informed of any prior allergic drug reaction, especially prior reactions to any laxatives. Pregnancy is also a concern. Animal studies have shown laxatives to have adverse effects on pregnancy, but no human studies regarding pregnancy are currently available. These drugs are only given in pregnancy after the risks to the fetus have been taken under consideration. Nursing mothers should use caution and consult their doctors before receiving these drugs.

Bisacodyl should not be administered to patients with rectal fissures, abdominal pain, **nausea**, **vomiting**, appendicitis, abdominal surgery, ulcerated hemorrhoids, acute hepatitis, fecal impaction, or blockage in the biliary tract. Calcium polycarbophil should not be given to anyone with a gastrointestinal blockage (obstruction).

Both psyllium and docusate calcium/docusate sodium should be avoided by patients with intestinal blockage, fecal impaction, or **nausea and vomiting**. Lactulose should be avoided by patients who are elderly, have diabetes mellitus, eat a low galactose diet, or whose general health is poor.

Senna/senokot is inadvisable for patients with congestive heart failure, gastrointestinal bleeding, intestinal blockage, abdominal pain, nausea and vomiting, appendicitis, or prior abdominal surgery.

The American College of Toxicology states that cathartics should *not* be used as a means of clearing poisons from the digestive tract of a poisoning victim. Although some physicians have administered these laxatives along with activated charcoal in order to reduce the body's absorption of the poison, this treatment is no longer recommended.

Side effects

Laxatives may have side effects. Some, such as nausea and vomiting, are more common than others. Side effects related to specific laxatives are described in this section. With repeated use, people may become dependent on laxatives. All side effects should be reported to a doctor.

Bisacodyl

Common side effects:

- nausea
- vomiting
- loss of appetite (anorexia)
- cramps

Less common side effects:

- muscle weakness
- diarrhea
- electrolyte changes
- rectal burning (when suppositories are used).

Life-threatening:

- severe muscle spasms (tetany)

Calcium polycarbophil

Side effects may include:

- abdominal bloating (distention)
- gas
- laxative dependency

Life-threatening:

- gastrointestinal obstruction

Docusate calcium/docusate sodium

Side effects include:

- bitter taste in the mouth
- irritated throat
- nausea
- cramps
- diarrhea
- loss of appetite
- rash

Lactulose

Common side effects include:

- nausea
- vomiting
- loss of appetite
- abdominal cramping
- bloating
- belching
- diarrhea

Psyllium

Common side effects include:

- nausea
- vomiting
- loss of appetite
- diarrhea

Less common side effects include:

- abdominal cramping
- blockage of the esophagus or intestine

Senna/senokot

Common side effects include:

- nausea
- vomiting
- loss of appetite
- abdominal cramping

Less common side effects include:

- diarrhea
- gas
- urine that is pink-red or brown-black in color
- abnormal electrolyte levels

Life-threatening:

- Severe muscle spasms (tetany)

Interactions

Laxatives may interact with other drugs. Sometimes, the laxative can interfere with proper absorption of another drug. A patient must notify their doctor or pharmacist if he or she is already taking any medications so that the proper laxative can be selected or prescribed. Specific drug interactions are:

- Bisacodyl: Antacids, H2 blockers, and some herbal remedies (lily of the valley, pheasant's eye, squill).
- Calcium polycarbophil: (lowers the absorption of) tetracycline.
- Docusate calcium/docusate sodium: Unknown.

- Lactulose: Neomycin and other laxatives.
- Psyllium: Cardiac glycosides, oral anticoagulants, and salicylates.
- Senna/senokot: Disulfiram should never be taken with this drug. Also, senna/senokot lowers the absorption of other drugs taken by mouth.

Resources

BOOKS

Beers, Mark H., MD, and Robert Berkow, MD, editors. "Diarrhea and Constipation." In *The Merck Manual of Diagnosis and Therapy*. Whitehouse Station, NJ: Merck Research Laboratories, 2007.

Karch, A. M. *Lippincott's Nursing Drug Guide*. Springhouse, PA: Lippincott Williams & Wilkins, 2003.

PERIODICALS

DiPalma, J. A. "Current Treatment Options for Chronic Constipation." *Reviews in Gastroenterological Disorders* 4, Supplement 2 (2004): S34–S42.

Newton, G. D., W. S. Pray, and N. G. Popovich. "New OTC Drugs and Devices 2003: A Selective Review." *Journal of the American Pharmaceutical Association* 44 (March-April 2004): 211–225.

"Position Paper: Cathartics." *Journal of Toxicology: Clinical Toxicology* 42 (March 2004): 243–253.

Schiller, L. R. "New and Emerging Treatment Options for Chronic Constipation." *Reviews in Gastroenterological Disorders* 4, Supplement 2 (2004): S43–S51.

Talley, N. J. "Management of Chronic Constipation." *Reviews in Gastroenterological Disorders* 4 (Winter 2004): 18–24.

ORGANIZATIONS

American Society of Health-System Pharmacists (ASHP). 7272 Wisconsin Avenue, Bethesda, MD 20814. (301) 657-3000. www.ashp.org.

National Digestive Diseases Information Clearinghouse. 2 Information Way, Bethesda, MD 20892-3570. nddic@aerie.com. http://www.niddk.nih.gov/Brochures/NDDIC.htm.

United States Food and Drug Administration (FDA). 5600 Fishers Lane, Rockville, MD 20857-0001. (888) INFO-FDA. www.fda.gov.

Rhonda Cloos, R.N.
Rebecca J. Frey, Ph.D.

Leiomyosarcoma

Definition

Leiomyosarcoma is **cancer** that consists of smooth muscle cells and small cell **sarcoma** tumor. The cancer begins in smooth muscle cells that grow uncontrollably and form tumors.

Description

Leiomyosarcomas can start in any organ that contains smooth muscle, but can be found in the walls of the stomach, large and small intestines, esophagus, uterus, or deep within the abdomen (retroperitoneal). But for perspective, smooth muscle cancers are quite rare: Less than 1% of all cancers are leiomyosarcomas. Very rarely, leiomyosarcomas begin in blood vessels or in the skin.

Most leiomyosarcomas are in the stomach. The second most common site is the small bowel, followed by the colon, rectum, and esophagus.

Demographics

Leiomyosarcomas do occur in the breast and uterus, but they are very rare. Uterine sarcomas comprise less than 1% of gynecological malignancies and 2–5% of all uterine malignancies. Of these numbers, leiomyosarcomas are found in only 0.1% of women of childbearing age who have tumors of the uterus. Less than 2% of tumors in women over age 60 who are undergoing hysterectomy are leiomyosarcomas.

Causes and symptoms

The exact causes of leiomyosarcoma are not known, but there are genetic and environmental risk factors associated with it. Certain inherited conditions that run in families may increase the risk of developing leiomyosarcoma. High-dose radiation exposure, such as radiotherapy used to treat other types of cancer, has also been linked to leiomyosarcoma. It is possible that exposure to certain chemical herbicides may increase the risk of developing sarcomas, but this association has not been proven.

Since leiomyosarcoma can occur in any location, the symptoms are different and depend on the site of the tumor. When leiomyosarcoma begins in an organ in the abdomen, such as the stomach or small bowel, the physician may be able to feel a large lump or mass when he examines the abdomen. When leiomyosarcoma affects a blood vessel, it may block the flow of blood to the body part supplied by the artery. Commonly occurring symptoms include:

- painless lump or mass
- painful swelling
- abdominal pain
- weight loss
- nausea and vomiting

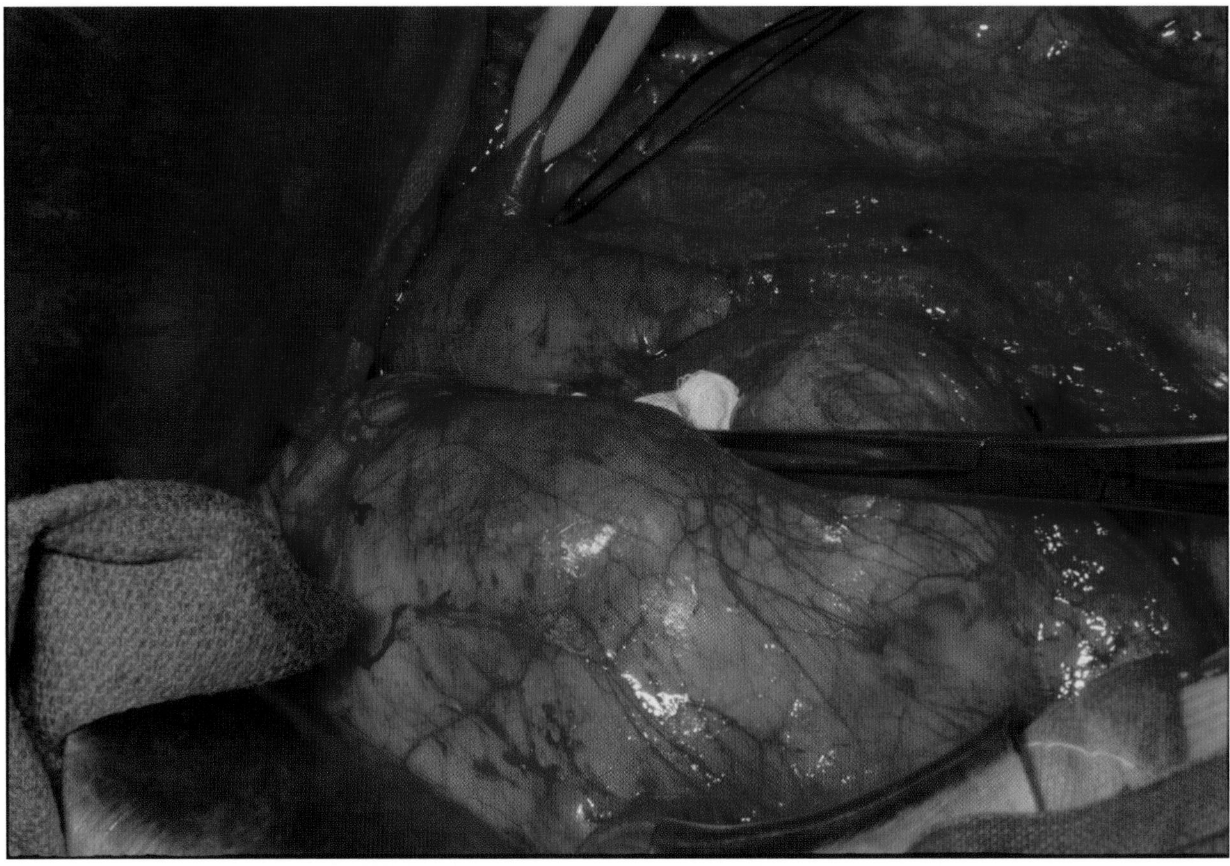

Surgery to remove a leiomyosarcoma in the tissue near a kidney. *(Custom Medical Stock Photo. Reproduced by permission.)*

Diagnosis

Some patients who have leiomyosarcomas may be visiting the doctor because they have discovered a lump or mass or swelling on a body part. Others have symptoms related to the internal organ that is affected by the leiomyosarcoma. For example, a tumor in the stomach may cause **nausea**, feelings of fullness, internal bleeding, and **weight loss**. The patient's doctor will take a detailed medical history to find out about the symptoms. The history is followed by a complete physical examination with special attention to the suspicious symptom or body part.

Depending on the location of the tumor, the doctor may order **imaging studies** such as x ray, **computed tomography** (CT) scan, and **magnetic resonance imaging** (MRI) to help determine the size, shape, and exact location of the tumor. A **biopsy** of the tumor is necessary to make the definitive diagnosis of leiomyosarcoma. The tissue sample is examined by a pathologist (specialist in the study of diseased tissue).

Types of biopsy

The type of biopsy done depends on the location of the tumor. For some small tumors, the doctor may perform an excisional biopsy, removing the entire tumor and a margin of surrounding normal tissue. Most often, the doctor will perform an incisional biopsy, a procedure that involves cutting out only a piece of the tumor that is used to determine its type and grade.

Treatment team

Patients with leiomyosarcoma are usually cared for by a multidisciplinary team of health professionals. The patient's family or primary care doctor may refer the patient to other specialists, such as surgeons and oncologists (specialists in cancer medicine), radiologic technicians, nurses, and laboratory technicians. Depending on the tumor location and treatment plan, patients may benefit from rehabilitation therapy with physical therapists and nutritional counseling from dieticians.

KEY TERMS

Biopsy—The surgical removal and microscopic examination of living tissue for diagnostic purposes.

Chemotherapy—Treatment of cancer with synthetic drugs that destroy the tumor either by inhibiting the growth of cancerous cells or by killing them.

Oncologist—A doctor who specializes in cancer medicine.

Pathologist—A doctor who specializes in the diagnosis of disease by studying cells and tissues under a microscope.

Radiation therapy—Treatment using high energy radiation from x-ray machines, cobalt, radium, or other sources.

Stage—A term used to describe the size and extent of spread of cancer.

Clinical staging, treatments, and prognosis

Staging

The purpose of staging a tumor is to determine how far it has advanced. This is important because treatment varies depending on the stage. Stage is determined by the size of the tumor, whether the tumor has spread to nearby lymph nodes, whether the tumor has spread elsewhere in the body, and what the cells look like under the microscope.

Examining the tissue sample under the microscope, using special chemical stains, the pathologist is able to classify tumors as high grade or low grade. High-grade tumors have the more rapidly growing cells and so are considered more serious.

Tumors are staged using numbers I through IV. The higher the number, the more the tumor has advanced. Stage IV leiomyosarcomas have involved either lymph nodes or have spread to distant parts of the body.

Treatment

Treatment for leiomyosarcoma varies depending on the location of the tumor, its size and grade, and the extent of its spread. Treatment planning also takes into account the patient's age, medical history, and general health.

QUESTIONS TO ASK THE DOCTOR

- What stage is the leiomyosarcoma?
- What are the recommended treatments?
- What are the side effects of the recommended treatment?
- Is treatment expected to cure the disease or only to prolong life?

Leiomyosarcomas on the arms and legs may be treated by **amputation** (removal of the affected limb) or by limb-sparing surgery to remove the tumor. These tumors may also be treated with **radiation therapy**, **chemotherapy**, or a combination of both.

Generally, tumors inside the abdomen are surgically removed. The site, size, and extent of the tumor determine the type of surgery performed. Leiomyosarcomas of organs in the abdomen may also be treated with radiation and chemotherapy.

Side effects

The surgical treatment of leiomyosarcoma carries risks related to the surgical site, such as loss of function resulting from amputation or from nerve and/or muscle loss. There also are risks associated with any surgical procedure, such as reactions to general anesthesia or **infection** after surgery.

The side effects of radiation therapy depend on the site being radiated. Radiation therapy can produce side effects such as **fatigue**, skin rashes, nausea, and **diarrhea**. Most of the side effects lessen or disappear completely after the radiation therapy has been completed.

The side effects of chemotherapy vary depending on the medication, or combination of **anticancer drugs**, used. Nausea, **vomiting**, **anemia**, lower resistance to infection, and hair loss (**alopecia**) are common side effects. Medication may be given to reduce the unpleasant side effects of chemotherapy.

Alternative and complementary therapies

Many patients explore alternative and complementary therapies to help to reduce the stress associated with illness, improve immune function, and feel better. While there is no evidence that these therapies specifically combat disease, activities such as biofeedback, relaxation, therapeutic touch, massage therapy, and guided imagery have been reported to enhance well-being.

Prognosis

The outlook for patients with leiomyosarcoma varies. It depends on the location and size of the tumor and its type and extent of spread. Some patients, such as those who have had small tumors located in or near the skin surgically removed, have excellent prognoses. Their 5-year survival is greater than 90%. Among patients with leiomyosarcomas in organs in the abdomen, survival is best when the tumor has been completely removed. In general, high-grade tumors that have spread widely throughout the body are not associated with favorable survival rates.

Coping with cancer treatment

Fatigue is one of the most common complaints during cancer treatment and recovery. Many patients benefit from learning energy-conserving approaches to accomplish their daily activities. They should be encouraged to rest when tired and take breaks from strenuous activities. Planning activities around times of day when energy is highest is often helpful. Mild exercise, small, frequent nutritious snacks, and limiting physical and emotional stress also help to combat fatigue.

Depression, emotional distress, and anxiety associated with the disease and its treatment may respond to counseling from a mental health professional. Many cancer patients and their families find participation in mutual aid and group support programs helps to relieve feelings of isolation and loneliness. By sharing problems with others who have lived through similar difficulties, patients and families can exchange ideas and coping strategies.

Clinical trials

Several clinical studies were underway as of 2001. For example, doctors at Memorial Sloan-Kettering Cancer Center were using specific chemotherapeutic drugs to treat patients with leiomyosarcoma that cannot be removed by surgery or has recurred. These drugs, **gemcitabine**, **docetaxel**, and **filgrastim** (G-CSF), work by stopping tumor cells from dividing, so they cannot grow. To learn more about this clinical trial and the availability of others, patients and families may wish to contact Memorial Sloan-Kettering Cancer Center at (212) 639-6555, or visit the National Cancer Institute (NCI) website at http://cancertrials.nci.nih.gov.

Prevention

Since the causes of leiomyosarcoma are not known, there are no recommendations about how to prevent its development. It is linked to radiation exposure; however, much of this excess radiation exposure is the result of therapy to treat other forms of cancer. Among families with an inherited tendency to develop soft tissue sarcomas, careful monitoring may help to ensure early diagnosis and treatment of the disease.

Special concerns

Leiomyosarcoma, like other cancer diagnoses, may produce a range of emotional responses. Education, counseling, and participation in support group programs may help to reduce feelings of fear, anxiety and hopelessness. For many patients suffering from spiritual distress, visits with clergy members and participation in organized prayer may offer comfort.

Resources

BOOKS

Pelletier, Kenneth R. *The Best of Alternative Medicine.* New York: Simon & Schuster, 2000.

PERIODICALS

Ishida, J., et al. "Primary Leiomyosarcoma of the Greater Omentum." *Journal Of Clinical Gastroenterology* 28, no. 2 (March 1999): 167-170.

OTHER

National Cancer Institute Clinical Cancer Trials. <http://cancertrials.nci.nih.gov>.

ORGANIZATIONS

American Cancer Society. 1599 Clifton Road, N.E., Atlanta, GA 30329. (800) 227-2345.

Cancer Research Institute. 681 Fifth Avenue, New York, NY 10022. (800) 992-2623.

National Cancer Institute (National Institutes of Health). 9000 Rockville Pike, Bethesda, MD 20892. (800) 422-6237.

Barbara Wexler, M.P.H.

Letrozole *see* **Aromatase inhibitors**

Leucovorin

Definition

Leucovorin (also known as Wellcovorin and citrovorum factor or folinic acid) is a drug that can be used either to protect healthy cells from

chemotherapy or to enhance the anti-cancer effect of chemotherapy.

Purpose

Leucovorin is most often used in **cancer** patients undergoing either **methotrexate** or **fluorouracil** chemotherapy. Methotrexate is used to treat a wide range of cancers including **breast cancer**, **head and neck cancers**, **acute leukemias**, and Burkitt's **lymphoma**. Fluorouracil is used in combination with leucovorin to treat colorectal cancer. When leucovorin and methotrexate are used together, this therapy often is called leucovorin rescue because leucovorin rescues healthy cells from the toxic effects of methotrexate. In patients with colorectal cancer, however, leucovorin increases the anti-cancer effect of fluorouracil.

Leucovorin also is used to treat megaloblastic **anemia**, a blood disorder in which red blood cells become larger than normal, and to treat accidental overdoses of drugs such as methotrexate.

Description

Leucovorin is a faster acting and stronger form of **folic acid**, and has been used for several decades. Folic acid also is known as vitamin B_9, and is needed for the normal development of red blood cells. In humans, dietary folic acid must be reduced metabolically to tetrahydrofilic acid (THFA) to exert its vital biochemical functions. The coenzyme THFA and its subsequent other cofactors participate in many important reactions including DNA synthesis.

Leucovorin rescue

Some chemotherapy drugs, such as methotrexate (Mexate, Folex), work by preventing cells from using folic acid. Methotrexate therapy causes cancer cells to develop a folic acid deficiency and die. However, normal cells also are affected by folic acid deficiency. As a result, patients treated with drugs such as methotrexate often develop blood disorders and other toxic side effects. When these patients are given leucovorin, it goes into normal cells and rescues them from the toxic effects of the methotrexate. Leucovorin cannot enter cancer cells, however, and they continue to be killed by methotrexate. Leucovorin also works by rescuing healthy cells in patients who take an accidental overdose of drugs similar to methotrexate.

Combination therapy

Patients with colorectal cancer frequently are treated with fluorouracil (Adrusil). Fluorouracil, commonly called 5-FU, is effective, but only works for a short time once it is in the body. Leucovorin enhances the effect of fluorouracil by increasing the time that it stays active. As a result, the combination of the two drugs produces a greater anti-cancer effect than fluorouracil alone.

KEY TERMS

Folic acid—Vitamin B_9.

Leucovorin rescue—A cancer therapy where the drug leucovorin protects healthy cells from toxic chemotherapy.

Recommended dosage

Leucovorin can be given as an injection, intravenously, or as oral tablets. For rescue therapy, leucovorin usually is given intravenously or orally within 24 hours of methotrexate treatment. Dosage varies from patient to patient. When used in combination with fluorouracil, leucovorin is given to the patient intravenously first, followed by fluorouracil treatment. To treat unintentional folic acid antagonist overdose, leucovorin is usually given intravenously as soon as possible after the overdose. Patients with megaloblastic anemia receive oral leucovorin.

Precautions

Patients with anemia, or any type of blood disorder, should tell their doctors. Leucovorin can treat only anemia caused by folic acid deficiency. Patients with other types of anemia should not take leucovorin. The effect of leucovorin on the fetus is not known, and it is not known if the drug is found in breast milk. Leucovorin should therefore be used with caution during pregnancy. Elderly patients treated with leucovorin and fluorouracil for advanced colorectal cancer are at greater risk for developing severe side effects.

Side effects

The vast majority of patients do not experience side effects from leucovorin therapy. Side effects are usually caused by the patient's chemotherapy, not by leucovorin. In rare cases, however, some patients can develop allergic reactions to the drug. These include skin rash, hives, and **itching**. In 2004, Swiss researchers found that oral desensitization may work in cases of severe allergic reaction to leucovorin.

Interactions

Although there are no listed drug interactions for leucovorin, patients should tell their doctors about any over the counter or prescription medication they are taking, particularly medication that can cause seizures.

Resources

PERIODICALS

"Oral Desensitization May Work in Some Cases of Allergy to Leucovorin." *Drug Week* November 14, 2003: 128.

Alison McTavish, M.Sc.
Teresa G. Odle

Leukapheresis *see* **Pheresis**

Leukemia *see* **Acute erythroblastic leukemia; Acute lymphocytic leukemia; Acute myelocytic leukemia; Chronic lymphocytic Leukemia; Leukemia, Acute; leukemia, chronic**

Leukemias, acute

Definition

Acute leukemia is a type of **cancer** in which excessive quantities of abnormal white blood cells are produced.

Demographics

Leukemias account for 2% of all cancers. Because leukemia is the most common form of childhood cancer, it is often regarded as a disease of childhood. However, leukemias affect far more adults than children. Half of the cases adult leukemia occur in people who are 60 years of age or older. Chronic leukemia is diagnosed slightly more often than acute leukemia in adults. According to the estimates of the American Cancer Society (ACS), approximately 45,000 new cases of leukemia are diagnosed each year in the United States. An estimated 22,000 people will die from leukemia in 2009.

In adults, the most common types of leukemia are acute myeloid leukemia (AML) and **chronic lymphocytic leukemia** (CLL). Leukemia accounts for about one-third of cancer cases in children. The most commonly diagnosed type of leukemia in children is **acute lymphocytic leukemia** (ALL) which is more prevalent in early childhood with a peak incidence between the ages of 2 and 4 years of age. Chronic leukemia is rare in children.

Description

Medical science classifies acute leukemia by the type of white blood cell that undergoes mutation. The most common of these are:

- Acute lymphoblastic leukemia (ALL), in which excessive quantities of lymphoblasts, or immature lymphocyte white blood cells, are produced. ALL is also referred to as acute lymphocytic leukemia.
- Acute myeloblastic leukemia (AML), also known as acute myeloid leukemia and acute nonlymphocytic leukemia (ANLL), in which excessive quantities of other types of immature white blood cells are produced.

Acute leukemias progress rapidly, while the **chronic leukemias** progress more slowly.

The cells that make up blood are produced in the bone marrow and the lymphatic system. Bone marrow is the spongy tissue found in the large bones of the body. The lymphatic system includes the spleen (an organ in the upper abdomen), the thymus (a small gland beneath the breastbone), and the tonsils (a mass of lymphatic tissue located in the throat). In addition, the lymphatic vessels (tiny tubes that branch like blood vessels into all parts of the body) and lymph nodes (pea-shaped organs that are found along the network of lymphatic vessels) are also part of the lymphatic system. Lymph is a milky fluid that contains cells. Clusters of lymph nodes are found in the neck, underarm, pelvis, abdomen, and chest.

The cells found in the blood include red blood cells (RBCs) that carry oxygen and other materials to all tissues of the body; white blood cells (WBCs) that fight **infection**; and platelets, which play an important role in the clotting of the blood. White blood cells can be further subdivided into three main types: granulocytes, monocytes, and lymphocytes.

The granulocytes, as their name suggests, have particles (granules) inside them. These granules contain special proteins (enzymes) and several other substances that can break down chemicals and destroy microorganisms, such as bacteria. Monocytes are the second type of white blood cell. They are also important in defending the body against pathogens.

Lymphocytes are the third type of white blood cell. There are two primary types of lymphocytes—T lymphocytes and B lymphocytes—with different functions in the immune system. B cells protect the body by making antibodies. Antibodies are proteins that can attach to the surfaces of bacteria and viruses. This "attachment" sends signals to many other cell types to come and destroy the antibody-coated organism. T cells protect the body against viruses. When a virus enters a cell, it produces certain proteins that are projected onto the surface of the infected cell. T cells recognize these proteins and make certain chemicals that are capable of destroying the virus-infected cells. In addition, T cells can destroy some types of cancer cells.

Bone marrow makes stem cells, which are the precursors of the different blood cells. These stem cells mature through stages into RBCs, WBCs, or platelets. In acute leukemias, the maturation process of the white blood cells is interrupted. The immature cells (or "blasts") proliferate rapidly and begin to accumulate in various organs and tissues, thereby affecting their normal function. This uncontrolled proliferation of the immature cells in the bone marrow affects the production of the normal red blood cells and platelets as well.

As noted, there are two types of acute leukemias—acute lymphocytic leukemia and acute myelogenous leukemia. Different types of white blood cells are involved in the two leukemias. In acute lymphocytic leukemia (ALL), it is the T or the B lymphocytes that are involved. The B cell leukemias are more common than T cell leukemias. Acute myelogenous leukemia, also known as acute nonlymphocytic leukemia (ANLL), is a cancer of the monocytes and/or granulocytes.

Risk factors

Several risk factors have been identified as playing a role in the development of acute leukemia including:

- exposure to ionizing radiation
- exposure to medical radiation such as the radiation used to treat cancer patients
- previous treatment with certain types of chemotherapy agents
- history of Down syndrome and other genetic factors
- history of cigarette smoking
- exposure to certain chemicals such as benezene

Causes and symptoms

The cause of most leukemias is not known. Leukemia occurs in both sexes and all ages. The human T-cell leukemia virus (HTLV-I), a virus with similarities to the human immunodeficiency virus (HIV), is believed to be the causative agent for a rare form of ALL. The Epstein Barr virus, which causes mononucleosis, has also been linked to a form of ALL.

The number of treatment-related cases of AML (individuals previously treated for cancer with **chemotherapy** and/or **radiation therapy**) is increasing particularly in survivors of childhood and adolescent cancers such as Hodgkin disease, **lymphoma**, **sarcoma**, **testicular cancer** and **breast cancer**.

ALL is more common among Caucasians than among African-Americans, while acute myeloid leukemia (AML) affects both races equally. The incidence of acute leukemia is slightly higher among men than women. People with Jewish ancestry have a higher likelihood of getting leukemia. A higher incidence of leukemia has also been observed among persons with Down syndrome and some other genetic abnormalities.

Exposure to ionizing radiation, such as occurred in Japan after the atomic bomb explosions, has been shown to increase the risk of getting leukemia. Electromagnetic fields are suspected of being a possible cause, as are certain organic chemicals, such as benzene. Having a history of diseases that damage the bone marrow, such as aplastic **anemia**, or a history of cancers of the lymphatic system puts people at a high risk for developing acute leukemias. Similarly, the use of anticancer medications, immunosuppressants, and the antibiotic chloramphenicol are also considered risk factors for developing acute leukemias.

The symptoms of leukemia are generally vague and non-specific. A patient may experience all or some of the following symptoms:

- weakness or chronic fatigue
- fever of unknown origin, chills and flu-like symptoms
- weight loss that is not due to dieting or exercise
- frequent bacterial or viral infections
- headaches
- skin rash
- non-specific bone pain
- easy bruising
- bleeding from gums or nose
- blood in urine or stools
- swollen and tender lymph nodes and/or spleen
- abdominal fullness
- night sweats
- petechiae, or tiny red spots under the skin
- more rarely, sores in the eyes or on the skin

Diagnosis

Examination

For a successful outcome, treatment for acute leukemia must begin as soon as possible, but there are no screening tests available. If the doctor has reason to suspect leukemia, he or she will conduct a very thorough physical examination to look for enlarged lymph nodes in the neck, underarm, and pelvic region. Swollen gums, enlarged liver or spleen, bruises, or pinpoint red rashes all over the body are some of the signs of leukemia.

Tests

Urine and blood tests may be ordered to check for microscopic amounts of blood in the urine and to obtain a complete differential blood count. This count will give the numbers and percentages of the different cells found in the blood. An abnormal blood test might suggest leukemia; however, the diagnosis must be confirmed by more specific tests.

Standard imaging tests, such as **x rays**, **computed tomography** scans (CT scans), and **magnetic resonance imaging** (MRI) may be used to check whether the leukemic cells have invaded other areas of the body, such as the bones, chest, kidneys, abdomen, or brain.

Sophisticated cytogenetic studies, which examine the number and shape of chromosomes in the DNA of individual blast (immature) cells, should be conducted in addition to the immunophenotyping of cells of the bone marrow. This procedure involves applying various stains to the marrow cells. These stains help doctors identify some of the proteins lying on the surface of the cells.

Procedures

The doctor may perform a **bone marrow biopsy** to confirm the diagnosis of leukemia. During the **biopsy**, a cylindrical piece of bone and marrow is removed. The tissue is generally taken out of the hipbone. These samples are sent to the laboratory where they are examined under a microscope by a hematologist, oncologist, or pathologist. In addition to the diagnostic biopsy, another biopsy will also be performed during the treatment phase of the disease to see if the leukemia is responding to therapy.

A spinal tap (**lumbar puncture**) is another procedure that the doctor may order to diagnose leukemia. In this procedure, a small needle is inserted into the spinal cavity in the lower back to withdraw some cerebrospinal fluid and to look for leukemic cells.

Treatment

As noted, treatment must be begun as soon as possible. The goal of treatment is remission, or an arresting of the disease process of the leukemia. There are two phases of treatment for leukemia. The first phase is called induction therapy. As the name suggests, during this phase, the primary aim of the treatment is to reduce the number of leukemic cells as much as possible and induce a remission in the patient. Once the patient shows no obvious signs of leukemia (no leukemic cells are detected in blood tests and bone marrow biopsies), the patient is said to be in remission.

The second phase of treatment is then initiated. This is called consoliation or maintenance therapy, and the goal is to kill any remaining cancer cells and to maintain the remission for as long as possible.

Chemotherapy

Chemotherapy is the use of drugs to kill cancer cells. It is usually the treatment of choice in leukemia, and is used to relieve symptoms and achieve long-term remission of the disease. Generally, combination chemotherapy, in which multiple drugs are used, is more efficient than using a single drug for the treatment. Some drugs may be administered intravenously through a vein in the arm; others may be given by mouth in the form of pills. If the cancer cells have invaded the brain, then chemotherapeutic drugs may be put into the fluid that surrounds the brain through a needle in the brain or back. This is known as **intrathecal chemotherapy**. Because leukemia cells can spread to all the organs via the blood stream and the lymphatic vessels, surgery is not considered an option for treating leukemias.

Radiation

Radiation therapy, which involves the use of x rays or other high-energy rays to kill cancer cells and shrink tumors, may be used in some cases. For acute leukemias, the source of radiation is usually outside the body (external radiation therapy). If the leukemic cells have spread to the brain, radiation therapy can be given to the brain.

Targeted therapies and other biologic therapies, such as the use of **monoclonal antibodies**, are increasingly being utilized in the treatment of acute leukemia. For example, the monoclonal antibody, **rituximab** (Rituxan) may be used to treat adult ALL patients whose leukemic cells are positive for the CD20

QUESTIONS TO ASK YOUR DOCTOR

- What type of acute leukemia do I or does my child have?
- How common is this particular type of acute leukemia?
- How is this type of leukemia treated?
- Can this type be treated in my community or should I be referred to a treatment center that specializes in my particular type of acute leukemia?
- How rigorous will my treatment be? What kind of side effects can I expect from treatment?
- How long will my treatments last?
- What is the long-term prognosis for my type of leukemia?

antigen. Some patients with Philadelphia chromosome positive ALL may receive the targeted therapy agents imatinib (Gleevec) or **dasatinib** (Sprycel) to treat their leukemia.

Prognosis

Like all cancers, the prognosis for leukemia depends on the patient's age and general health. According to statistics, more than 60% of patients with leukemia survive for at least a year after diagnosis. Acute myelocytic leukemia (AML), with a five year overall survival rate of only 22%, has a poorer prognosis rate than acute lymphocytic leukemias (ALL) and the chronic leukemias. In the last 20 years, the five-year survival rate for patients with ALL has increased from 42–66%.

Interestingly enough, since most childhood leukemias are of the ALL type, chemotherapy has been highly successful in their treatment. This is because chemotherapeutic drugs are most effective against actively growing cells. Due to the new combinations of **anticancer drugs** being used, the survival rates among children with ALL have improved dramatically. Ninety-five percent of all childhood ALL patients will enter remission, and 60–88% will remain in remission after five years, depending upon the type. T-cell ALL is considered curable in half of all cases, while B-cell ALL is rarely, if ever curable.

Prevention

Many cancers can be prevented by changes in lifestyle or diet, which will reduce the risk factors. However, in leukemias, there are no such known risk factors. Therefore, at the present time, no way is known to prevent leukemias from developing. People who are at an increased risk for developing leukemia because of proven exposure to ionizing radiation or exposure to the toxic liquid benzene, and people with Down syndrome, should undergo periodic medical checkups.

Resources

PERIODICALS

Belson, M., Kingsley, B., & Holmes, A."Risk Factors for Acute Leukemia in Children: A Review." *Environ Health Perspect* 115 (2007):138–45.

Brown, P., Hunger, S.P., Smith, F.O., Carroll, W.L., & Reaman, G.H."Novel Targeted Drug Therapies for the Treatment of Childhood Acute Leukemia"*Expert Rev Hematol* 2 (2009):145–58.

Pui, CH., Robinson, L.L., & Look, A.T."Acute Lymphoblastic Leukemia" *Lancet* 371 no.9617 (March 22, 2008): 166–78.

Stock, W."Clinical Trials in Adult AML"*Clin Adv Hematol Oncol* 7 (2009):8–10.

OTHER

National Comprehensive Cancer Network. *NCCN Practice Guidelines in Oncology Acute Myeloid Leukemia* [cited October 2, 2009] https://www.nccn.org/professionals/physician_gls/PDF/aml.pdf.

University of Pennsylvania Cancer Center. Oncolink. http://cancer.med.upenn.edu.

ORGANIZATIONS

American Cancer Society. 1599 Clifton Road, N.E., Atlanta, Georgia 30329. (800) 227-2345. http://www.cancer.org.

Cancer Research Institute. 681 Fifth Avenue, New York, N.Y. 10022. (800) 992-2623. http://www.cancerresearch.org.

The Leukemia & Lymphoma Society. 1311 Mamaroneck Ave., Suite 310 White Plains, NY 10605. (800) 955-4572. www.leukemia-lymphoma.org.

Melinda Granger Oberleitner, R.N., D.N.S., A.P.R.N., C.N.S.

Leukemias, chronic

Definition

Chronic leukemia is a type of **cancer** in which excessive quantities of abnormal white blood cells are produced, usually slowly, often over a period of years.

The most common types of chronic leukemia are **chronic lymphocytic leukemia** (CLL) and **chronic myelocytic leukemia** (CML).

Demographics

Leukemias account for about 2% of all cancers. Because leukemia is the most common form of childhood cancer, it is often regarded as a disease of childhood. However, leukemias affect far more adults than children. Half of the cases of adult leukemia occur in people who are 60 years of age or older. Chronic leukemia is diagnosed slightly more often than acute leukemia in adults. According to the estimates of the American Cancer Society (ACS), approximately 45,000 new cases of leukemia are diagnosed each year in the United States. An estimated 22,000 people will die from leukemia in 2009.

In adults, the most common types of leukemia are acute myeloid leukemia (AML) and chronic lymphocytic leukemia (CLL). Leukemia accounts for about one-third of cancer cases in children. The most commonly diagnosed type of leukemia in children is **acute lymphocytic leukemia** (ALL) which is more prevalent in early childhood with a peak incidence between the ages of 2 and 4 years of age. Chronic leukemia is rare in children.

Eighty percent of cases of CLL are observed in patients who are 60 years or older, with an average age at diagnosis of 72 years. Rarely is CLL diagnosed in a patient who is less than 40 years of age. CLL almost never occurs in children. The incidence of this disease increases with age. According to estimates of the American Cancer Society, approximately 15,000 new cases of CLL will be diagnosed in 2009. About 4,000 Americans will die of CLL in 2009. Average lifetime risk of developing CLL is one-half of 1% or about 1 in 200. CLL affects both sexes. Among patients younger than 65, the disease is slightly more common in men. However, among patients older than 75 years of age, CLL appears almost equally among men and women. Over the past 50 years, the incidence rate of CLL has increased significantly. However, many scientists think this increase is not necessarily due to the disease being more common than in the past, but instead due to the fact that the disease is now more likely to be accurately diagnosed when it does occur. Fifty years ago, only one of ten CLL patients was diagnosed during early stages. Today, half of all CLL patients are diagnosed in the early stage of the disease.

CML accounts for about 15% of all leukemias. The average lifetime risk of developing CML is about 1 in 500. Slightly more men than women are affected by CML. The average age at diagnosis is 67 years. CML can affect people of any age although it very rarely appears in children. The American Cancer Society estimates about 5,000 new cases of CML will be diagnosed in the United States in 2009 and 450 deaths will occur from the disease in that year. Between 1973 and 1991, the rate at which CML appeared in the United States decreased slightly.

Description

Medical science classifies chronic leukemia by the type of white blood cell that undergoes mutation. The most common of these are:

- Chronic lymphocytic leukemia (CLL), in which mature-appearing white blood cells called lymphocytes are produced.
- Chronic myeloid (or myelogenous) leukemia (CML), also known as chronic granulocytic leukemia (CGL), is the result of uncontrolled proliferation of white blood cells called granulocytes.

Chronic leukemias are typically much less rapid-growing than acute leukemia, and affect adults far more often than children. In fact, nearly all the people who develop CLL are over 50 years of age. CML is also a disease primarily of middle-aged to elderly people.

The cells that make up blood are produced in the bone marrow and the lymph system. The bone marrow is the spongy tissue found in the large bones of the body. The lymph system includes the spleen (an organ in the upper abdomen), the thymus (a small organ beneath the breastbone), and the tonsils (an organ in the throat). The lymph vessels (tiny tubes that branch like blood vessels into all parts of the body) and lymph nodes (small pea-shaped organs that are found along the network of lymph vessels) are also part of the lymph system. The lymph itself is a milky fluid that contains cells. Clusters of lymph nodes are found in the neck, underarm, pelvis, abdomen, and chest.

The cells found in the blood are the red blood cells (RBCs), which carry oxygen and other materials to all tissues of the body; white blood cells (WBCs), which fight **infection**; and the platelets, which play an important role in the clotting of the blood. The white blood cells can be further subdivided into three main types: granulocytes, monocytes, and lymphocytes.

The granulocytes have particles (granules) inside them that contain special proteins (enzymes) and several other substances that can break down chemicals and destroy microorganisms such as bacteria.

Monocytes are the second type of white blood cell. They are also important in defending the body against pathogens.

The lymphocytes form the third type of white blood cell. The two primary types of lymphocytes, T lymphocytes and B lymphocytes, have different functions within the immune system. The B cells protect the body by making antibodies, which are proteins that can attach to the surfaces of bacteria and viruses. This attachment sends signals to many other cell types to destroy the antibody-coated organism. The T cells protect the body against viruses. When a virus enters a cell, it produces certain proteins that are projected onto the surface of the infected cell. The T cells recognize these proteins and make certain chemicals that are capable of destroying the virus-infected cells. In addition, the T cells can destroy some types of cancer cells.

The bone marrow makes stem cells, which are the precursors of the different blood cells. Stem cells mature into RBCs, WBCs, or platelets. In chronic leukemias, blood cells suddenly begin to proliferate rapidly and begin to accumulate in various organs and tissues, thereby affecting their normal function. This uncontrolled proliferation of the immature cells in the bone marrow affects the production of the normal red blood cells and platelets as well.

Different types of white blood cells are involved in chronic lymphocytic leukemia and chronic myeloid leukemia. Although some blasts, or immature cells (the hallmark of acute leukemia), are also present in chronic leukemia, it is the T or B lymphocytes that gradually mutate and become cancerous. The scenario is similar for chronic myelogenous leukemia, also known as chronic granulocytic leukemia (CGL), which occurs when unusually large numbers of granulocytes begin to appear in the bloodstream.

Risk factors

There are very few established risk factors related to the development of CLL. Results of some research studies related to the link between chemical exposure and the development of CLL implicate exposure to Agent Orange, an herbicide used in the Vietnam War, and long-term exposure to pesticides as possible causes of CLL. Family history also appears to be a risk factor for CLL. First-degree relatives (parents, siblings, and children) of CLL patients are two to four times more likely to be diagnosed with CLL as people who have no family history of CLL.

As with CLL there are very few established risk factors related to the development of CML. The only known risk factor for the development of CML is exposure to high-dose radiation such as radiation from an atomic blast or from a nuclear reactor accident.

Causes and symptoms

Leukemia occurs in both sexes and in all ages. The human T-cell leukemia virus (HTLV-I), a virus with similarities to the human immunovirus (HIV), is believed to be the causative agent for some kinds of leukemias. To date, the cause of most leukemias is not known. Lymphoid leukemias are more common among Caucasians than among African-Americans, while myeloid leukemias affects both races equally. The incidence of leukemia is slightly higher among men than women. A higher incidence of leukemia has also been observed among persons with Down syndrome and some other genetic abnormalities. Patients with chronic myeloid leukemia often show a chromosome abnormality called the Philadelphia chromosome that occurs when one chromosome attaches to another.

Exposure to ionizing radiation, such as occurred in Japan after the atomic bomb explosions, has been shown to increase the risk of getting leukemia. Electromagnetic fields are suspected of being a possible cause, as are certain organic chemicals such as benzene. Having a history of diseases that damage the bone marrow, such as aplastic **anemia**, or a history of cancers of the lymphatic system puts people at a high risk for developing leukemias. Similarly, the use of anticancer medications, immunosuppressants, and the antibiotic chloramphenicol are also considered risk factors for developing leukemias.

In 2003, the Institute of Medicine (IOM) released a report based upon scientific studies that found “sufficient evidence of an association” between CLL and exposure to herbicides during the Vietnam War. This report came from a Veterans Administration (VA) request to IOM to explore some similarities between CLL and **non-Hodgkin's lymphoma**. Non-Hodgkin's **lymphoma** has already been linked to Agent Orange exposure and is recognized by VA as a presumptive condition.

The symptoms of chronic leukemia are generally vague and non-specific, and are frequently overlooked until they are noticed on routine physical examination, especially when a routine blood test such as a complete blood count (CBC) is performed. A CBC may show unusually large numbers of a certain type of lymphocyte in the blood. Chronic leukemias may go for years without manifesting any symptoms at all, but also can develop symptoms similar to **acute leukemias**.

Chronic myeloid leukemia, in particular, has a two- or three-stage progression, a chronic phase that can last for several years, an accelerated phase, and a terminal blastic phase, a malignant phase in which immature granulocytes are suddenly generated in huge numbers, producing similar symptoms to acute leukemia. In such cases, a patient may experience all or some of the following symptoms:

- weakness or chronic fatigue
- fever of unknown origin, chills, and flu-like symptoms
- unexplained weight loss
- frequent bacterial or viral infections
- viscous (sticky) blood (which slows down the supply to various organs)
- headache
- non-specific bone pain
- easy bruising
- bleeding from gums or nose
- blood in urine or stools
- swollen and tender lymph nodes and/or spleen
- abdominal fullness
- night sweats
- petechiae, or tiny red spots under the skin
- priapism, or persistent, painful erection of the penis
- rarely, sores in the eyes or on the skin

Diagnosis

Examination

There are often no symptoms present for chronic leukemia, and there are no screening tests available. If the physician has reason to suspect leukemia, a very thorough physical examination will be conducted to look for enlarged lymph nodes in the neck, underarm, and pelvic region. Swollen gums, enlarged liver or spleen, bruises, or pinpoint red rashes all over the body are some of the signs of leukemia.

Tests

Urine and blood tests may be ordered to check for microscopic amounts of blood in the urine and to obtain a complete differential blood count, which gives the numbers and percentages of the different cells found in the blood. An abnormal blood test might suggest leukemia. However, the diagnosis has to be confirmed by more specific tests.

The presence of the Philadelphia (Ph) chromosome is a crucial factor in the diagnosis of CML. People who have CML have an unusually high number of white blood cells. Somewhat less than half of CML patients will also have high numbers of blood platelets. Most CML patients have mild anemia. The composition of the bone marrow in CML patients also differs from that of a healthy person. The marrow is described as being hypercellular. This means that the number of cells present in the bone marrow is unusually great.

Laboratory findings indicate when a CML patient enters the accelerated phase from the chronic phase of CML. In the chronic phase, there are less than 10% blasts or immature cells in the blood or the bone marrow. Once there are more than 10% but less than 20% blasts detected in the blood or bone marrow of the patient with CML, the patient is said to be in the accelerated phase of the disease. When greater than 20% blasts are detected in the blood or the bone marrow the CML patient is said to be in the blast phase. Other names for this phase are the acute phase or blast crisis. In this phase, the CML acts more like an aggressive acute form of leukemia.

Some CLL patients will have a condition called hypogammaglobulinemia which can be detected by blood tests. Immunoglobulins are normal parts of the body's immune system, the system used to fight off infections. Patients with hypogammaglobulinemia have very low levels of all of the various types of immunoglobulins. The physician may also order immunophenotyping tests. This involves taking a sample of the blood and looking at what types of cells of the immune system are being affected by the CLL. Approximately 19 out of 20 CLL patients have the B-cell type of CLL. In addition, the doctor may look for abnormalities in the chromosomes of affected cells. Patients exhibiting no chromosomal abnormalities have a better prognosis than those who do have such abnormalities.

Standard imaging tests such as **x rays**, **computed tomography** (CT) scans, and **magnetic resonance imaging** (MRI) may be used to check whether the leukemic cells have invaded other areas of the body, such as the bones, chest, kidneys, abdomen, or brain.

Procedures

The physician may perform a **bone marrow biopsy**, during which a small piece of bone and marrow is removed, generally taken from hipbone. A spinal tap (**lumbar puncture**) is another procedure that may be ordered. In this procedure, a small needle is inserted into the spinal cavity in the lower back to withdraw some cerebrospinal fluid and to look for leukemic cells.

Treatment

Treatment for CML

In recent years, targeted therapy, specifically the tyrosine kinase inhibitors, have become the standard treatment of choice for CML and have revolutionized the treatment of CML. These drugs seem to work best for those in the chronic phase of the disease although they may also be effective for patients with more advanced disease. In 2009, National Comprehensive Cancer Center (NCCN) practice guidelines for the treatment of CML recommend primary treatment with the tyrosine kinase inhibitor, **imatinib mesylate** (Gleevec), for newly diagnosed patients with Philadelphia chromosome or BCR-ABL positive chronic phase CML. Gleevec targets the one special protein almost all CML cells possess. Nearly all CML patients respond to Gleevec with responses often lasting for many years. Follow-up clinical studies indicate most patients who received the drug and who were followed for five years or more years are experiencing a high response rate without relapse of the disease. Gleevec is given in pill form and is usually taken once per day with food. Some side effects include **diarrhea**, **nausea**, **fatigue**, muscle pain, and skin rashes. Another side effect is edema around the eyes, feet, or abdomen.

Chemotherapy use in CML is now reserved for patients as part of treatment preceding stem cell transplants. **Radiation therapy** is used only sparingly in the treatment of CML. It may be used to shrink an enlarged spleen, to treat pain caused by an increase in leukemia cells in the bone marrow or in low doses as pre-treatment for stem cell transplant.

Because of the apparent long-term effectiveness of Gleevec in sustaining remission in most CML patients, the role of stem cell transplant in the treatment of CML is being re-examined. Currently, NCCN guidelines recommend allogeneic stem cell transplant in CML as an alternative treatment option for patients who are not able to achieve remission after 3 months of Gleevec or other targeted therapy, for those patients who achieve no response or for those who relapse 6, 12, or 18 months after achieving initial remission on Gleevec therapy and finally, for those patients who are already on Gleevec yet who progress from the chronic phase to the accelerated phase or the blast crisis phase of CML.

The current treatment recommendation by phase of CML are: chronic phase - treatment with Gleevec; accelerated phase—Gleevec has brought about remission in this phase but remission may not be long-term. Chemotherapy may be used to induce remission prior to undergoing stem cell transplant; blast phase - high dose Gleevec may be effective for patients who haven't been treated previously. Newer tyrosine kinase inhibitors **dasatinib** and **nilotinib** may be more effective in this phase but that has not yet been conclusively determined. Patients who do not respond to Gleevec or to the newer agents may be offered stem cell transplants. The transplant is more likely to be effective if the CML can be brought into remission prior to the transplant.

Treatment for CLL

Because the long-term prognosis for many patients with CLL is excellent, many patients (about 1/3) receive no treatment at all at first. Many patients (1/3) go for years before developing aggressive disease that requires treatment. Another 1/3 will require immediate treatment intervention at the time of diagnosis.

Treatment for CLL is typically initiated in a stepwise progression from the least invasive method of monitoring blood work and symptoms at regular intervals, known as watchful waiting, to treatment with chemotherapy and/or stem cell transplantation. Decisions to initiate treatment are based on stage of disease, presence of symptoms, and activity of the disease. At this time, in 2009, patients with limited stage disease should not be treated until they become symptomatic.

Treatment for early stage CLL should be started only when one of the following conditions appears:

- Symptoms of the disease are growing worse, for example, there is a greater degree of fever, weight loss, night sweats, and so forth.
- The spleen is enlarging or enlargement of the spleen has become painful.
- Disease of the lymph nodes has become more severe.
- The condition of the bone marrow has deteriorated and there is anemia and a marked reduction in the number of blood platelets for reasons not specifically related to the condition of the bone marrow.
- The population of lymphocytes is rapidly growing.
- The patient is experiencing numerous infections caused by bacteria.

Therapy for CLL usually starts with chemotherapy. Depending on the stage of the disease, single or multiple drugs may be given. Drugs commonly prescribed include **fludarabine**, **cladribine**, **chlorambucil** and **cyclophosphamide**. The standard first-line therapy in 2009 is fludarabine and cyclophosphamide used in combination. Another combination is a regimen consisting of the monoclonal antibody **rituximab** and/or cyclophosphamide. Another monoclonal antibody, **alemtuzumab**, may be used when patients are refractory to fludarabine-based regimens. Close

QUESTIONS TO ASK YOUR DOCTOR

- What type of chronic leukemia do I have?
- How will the leukemia be treated?
- Can I receive treatment in my community or should I consider receiving treatment in a specialized treatment center?
- How long will my treatment last?
- What side effects can I expect from the treatment?
- What is my long-term prognosis?

monitoring for life-threatening infections is important when the patient is receiving alemtuzumab.

Another option for CLL patients is allogenic stem cell transplantation. This option is typically reserved for patients less than 65 years old because of the intensity of the conditioning regimen and due to the considerable risk for mortality.

Clinical trials are ongoing to evaluate the effectiveness of newer agents to treat CLL including flavopiridol and lenalidomide.

Prognosis

The newer, more effective drugs now used to treat CML first became available in 2001. Currently, there are no long term data to predict how long patients treated with these drugs will survive. However, one large study conducted with patients who were treated with Gleevec revealed that 90% of patients were still alive and in remission with no evidence of leukemia after 5 years of treatment. Longer follow-up of these patients is still needed and is ongoing.

For many CLL patients, the prognosis is based on stage at diagnosis. Using the Binet and Rai staging systems criteria, patients staged as low risk usually survive more than 10 years. Patients staged as intermediate risk usually survive about 7 years. Patients staged as high risk usually survive about 2 to 5 years. The average patient survives 9 or more years after diagnosis.

Prevention

There is no known way to prevent chronic leukemia. People who are at an increased risk for developing chronic leukemia because of proven exposure to radiation, Agent Orange or long-term exposure to pesticides and people with a family history of chronic leukemia should be encouraged to undergo periodic medical evaluations.

Resources

BOOKS

Caligaris-Cappio, Federico, and Riccardo Dalla Favera *Chronic Lymphocytic Leukemia* New York: Springer, 2005.

PERIODICALS

Maddocks, K.J.,& Lin, T.S."Update in the Management of Chronic Lymphocytic Leukemia."*J Hematol Oncol* 2 (2009):29.

Jabbour, E., Cortes, J.E., et al."Current and Emerging Treatment Options in Chronic Myeloid Leukemia." *Cancer* 109 (2007):2171–81.

Hochhaus, A., Druker, B., Sawyers, C., et al. "Favorable Long-term Follow-up Results Over 6 Years for Response, Survival, and Safety with Imatinib Mesylate Therapy in Chronic-phase Chronic Myeloid Leukemia after Failure with Interferon-alpha Treatment." *Blood* 111 (2008):1039–43.

Robak, T."Novel Drugs for Chronic Lymphoid Leukemias: Mechanism of Action and Therapeutic Activity."*Curr Med Chem* 16 (2009):2212–34.

Schiffer, C.A."BCR-ABL Tyrosine Kinase Inhibitors for Chronic Myelogenous Leukemia"*N Engl J Med* 357 (2007):258–65.

OTHER

National Comprehensive Cancer Network. *NCCN Practice Guidelines in Oncology* v.2. 2010 *Chronic Myelogenous Leukemia* [cited October 2, 2009] http://www.nccn.org/professionals/physician_gls/PDF/cml.pdf

Oncolink. University of Pennsylvania Cancer Center. http://cancer.med.upenn.edu.

ORGANIZATIONS

American Cancer Society. 1599 Clifton Road, N.E., Atlanta, Georgia 30329. (800) 227-2345. http://www.cancer.org.

Cancer Research Institute. One Exchange Place, 55 Broadway, Suite 1802 New York, N.Y. 10006. (800) 992-2623. http://www.cancerresearch.org.

The Leukemia & Lymphoma Society. 1311 Mamaroneck Ave., White Plains, NY 10605. (800) 955-4572. http://www.leukemia-lymphoma.org

Melinda Granger Oberleitner, R.N., D.N.S., A.P.R.N., C.N.S.

Leukoencephalopathy

Description

Leukoencephalopathy is a disease occurring primarily in the white matter of the brain that involves defects in either the formation or the maintenance of the myelin sheath, a fatty coating that protects nerve cells. Leukoencephalopathy has several different forms and causes.

The symptoms of leukoencephalopathy reflect the mental deterioration that occurs as, at multiple sites within the brain, the myelin cover of nerve cells is eroded, leaving nerve cells exposed and with no protective insulation. Patients may exhibit problems with speech and vision, loss of mental function, uncoordinated movements, and extreme weakness and **fatigue**. Patients may have no desire to eat. The disease is usually progressive; patients continue to lose mental function, may have seizures, and finally lapse into a coma before death. Some patients stabilize, however, although loss of neurologic function is usually irreversible.

Leukoencephalopathy as it relates to **cancer** patients is primarily associated with **methotrexate-chemotherapy**, which is used in treatment of many different types of cancer. Some other medications, including **cytarabine**, **fludarabine**, **carmustine** and **fluorouracil** in conjunction with **levamisole**. The disease may appear years after the administration of methotrexate. Although rare, the incidence of leukoencephalopathy is increasing, as stronger drugs are developed and increased survival times allow time for the side effects of the treatments to appear.

A devastating type of leukoencephalopathy, called multifocal, or disseminated, necrotizing leukoencephalopathy, has been shown to occur primarily when methotrexate or cytarabine therapy is used in conjunction with a large cumulative dose of whole head irradiation. This disease is characterized by multiple sites of necrosis of the nerve cells in the white matter of the brain, involving both the myelin coating and the nerve cells themselves. Although some patients may stabilize, the course is usually progressive, with patients experiencing relentless mental deterioration and, finally, death.

Although leukoencephalopathy is primarily associated with methotrexate therapy, this disease has also been observed in association with other chemotherapeutic drugs (like intrathecal cytarabine) and occasionally been reported in association with cancers that have not yet been treated.

Another, particularly lethal, type of leukoencephalopathy called progressive multifocal leukoencephalopathy (PML) is an opportunistic **infection** that occurs in cancer patients who experience long-term immunosuppression as a result of the cancer (as in leukemia or **lymphoma**) or as a result of chemotherapy or immunosuppressive drugs. PML results when, due to chronic immunosuppression, the JC virus, widely found in the kidneys of healthy people, becomes capable of entering the brain. The virus infects the cells that produce myelin and causes multiple sites in the brain of nerve cells without the protective fatting coating. For reasons that are not completely clear, PML has a rapid and devastating clinical course, with death occurring typically less than six months after diagnosis.

Causes

It is only relatively recently that longer survival times for cancer patients have enabled scientists to identify an association of leukoencephalopathy with intensive chemotherapy (particularly methotrexate), especially when combined with large doses of whole head radiation. The causes of the neural degeneration observed are still not completely understood.

Most cases of leukoencephalopathy observed have occurred in patients who received methotrexate (either directly into the brain, through a tube in the skull, or intravenously) or who have received large doses of radiation to the head. Up to 50% of children who have received both treatments have developed necrotizing leukoencephalopathy, which differs from regular leukoencephalopathy in that the multiple sites of demyelinization also involve necrosis (the death of cells due to the degradative action of enzymes). Deterioration of the nerve tissue in necrotizing leukoencephalopathy appears to begin with the nerve and then spread into the myelin coating.

The method of action in PML is also not well understood. Long-term immunosuppression somehow appears to create an environment where the JC virus that inhabits most healthy human kidneys can mutate into a form that gains access to the brain. When in the brain, the virus infects and kills the cells that produce the myelin that forms a protective coating around the nerve.

Treatments

Unfortunately, there is no cure for any form of leukoencephalopathy, and no treatments approved. Although some medications have shown some effect against the deterioration involved in this disease, those identified have been highly toxic themselves, and none so far have been effective enough to justify use. The treatment of people with this disorder, therefore, tends to concentrate on alleviating discomfort.

Since there are no effective treatments, prevention must be emphasized. As the risks of certain treatment choices have become more defined, physicians must pursue careful treatment planning to produce optimal chance of tumor eradication while avoiding increased risk of the onset of a fatal and incurable side effect. This is especially true in children. The cases observed have largely been in children, which implies that the developing brain is at higher risk of developing treatment-associated leukoencephalopathy.

Alternative and complementary therapies

There are no commonly used alternative treatments, although since the disease is incurable, there is little risk involved in trying nontraditional medications. Complementary therapies (yoga, t'ai chi, etc.) that improve patient wellbeing are appropriate if the patient finds them helpful.

Resources

BOOKS

Abeloff, Martin. *Clinical Oncology*. 2nd ed. Camden Town: Churchhill Livingstone, Inc., 2004.

Mandell, Gerald. *Principles and Practice of Infectious Diseases*. 5th ed. St. Louis: Harcourt Health Sciences Group, 2000.

OTHER

"Progressive Multifocal Leukoencephalopathy." *A Healthy Me*. [cited July 5, 2009]. http://www.ahealthyme.com/article/gale/100083914.

Wendy Wippel, M.Sc.

Leukotriene inhibitors

Definition

Leukotriene inhibitors are drugs used to treat asthma and allergy symptoms. Leukotrienes are fatty compounds that function as part of the immune system, and cause inflammation and constriction of the airways. Leukotriene inhibitors act to prevent this mechanism and open the airways to facilitate breathing. The three main leukotriene inhibitors are the drugs montelukast, zafirlukast, and zileuton.

Purpose

Leukotriene inhibitors are mainly used to treat chronic asthma as part of maintenance therapy. Maintenance therapy helps keep acute asthma attacks from happening and maintains a baseline of open airways. Leukotriene inhibitors are not used to treat acute asthma attacks, only prevent them from happening.

KEY TERMS

Asthma—Disorder involving chronic inflammation in which the airways are narrowed in a reversible manner making it difficult to breathe normally, especially during acute exacerbations known as asthma attacks.

Bronchi—Airway passage in the respiratory system that conducts air into the lungs.

Bronchospasm—Spasm of the smooth muscles surrounding the bronchi causing constriction and obstructed airways.

Cytochrome P450—Enzymes present in the liver that metabolize drugs.

Phenylketonuria—Disorder of metabolism involving a deficiency in liver enzymes that metabolize the amino acid phenylalanine, causing it to accumulate and resulting in severe medical problems.

QT prolongation—Potentially dangerous heart condition that affects the rhythm of the heart beat and alters the ECG reading of the heart.

Asthma induced by exercise may also be treated by leukotriene inhibitors. Allergy symptoms of sneezing, runny nose, and wheezing may be treated by leukotriene inhibitors.

Description

Leukotriene inhibitors are used to treat respiratory conditions that are caused by obstruction of the airways. Breathing involves the passage of air through the nose or mouth, down the trachea within the throat and into air passages called bronchi that lead into the lungs. Obstruction of the airways may be due to the constriction of the smooth muscle that lines the bronchi, causing a condition known as bronchospasm (spasm of the smooth muscle). Relaxation of the smooth muscle allows opening of the airway, thereby facilitating the breathing process. Leukotrienes are released by the body during an allergic reaction or in patients with asthma, and cause contraction of the bronchial airway smooth muscle, as well as inflammation and mucous production. All of these effects disrupt breathing and are ameliorated by leukotriene inhibitors.

Multiple leukotriene inhibitors are available, including the drugs montelukast, zafirlukast, and zileuton. Montelukast is manufactured by Merck under the trade name Singulair. Zafirlukast is manufactured by AstraZeneca Pharmaceuticals under the trade name Accolate. Zileuton is manufactured by Cornerstone Therapeutics under the trade name Zyflo. Leukotriene inhibitors specifically target the receptor for leukotrienes (body chemicals that induce inflammation) present on cell surfaces in the respiratory tract. Leukotriene inhibitors are a type of chemical receptor that sits on the outer membrane of cells present in the respiratory system. These receptors activate a sequence of cellular events known as a chemical cascade or signaling pathway. It is these signaling pathways that are responsible for many normal body functions. Drugs or natural chemicals that bind to and activate the receptor signaling pathway are known as receptor agonists. Drugs or natural chemicals that bind to the receptor and block them from creating a signaling pathway are known as receptor antagonists, because they antagonize the effects of that receptor. Leukotriene receptors bind leukotriene agonists to create signaling cascades that are a natural part of the **immune response** and create inflammation of the airways. In patients with asthma and allergies this natural inflammatory process is excessive and creates uncomfortable symptoms. Leukotriene inhibitors antagonize the leukotriene receptor by binding and prevent the signaling pathway for inflammation from happening, restoring a normal balance.

Recommended dosage

The dose of montelukast used for asthma maintenance therapy or allergy symptoms is 10 mg taken orally in the evening. For asthma induced by exercise in patients who are not already on montelukast maintenance therapy, the dose is 10 mg given at least two hours before exercise with a maximum dose of 10 mg per day. The same dose is used for both adults and children greater than 15 years of age. For children from 6 to 14 years of age a dose of 5 mg a day is used. For children from 1 to 5 years of age a dose of 4 mg a day is used, available as a chewable tablet or as powder that may be mixed with food. Montelukast is not appropriate for use in children less than 1 year of age.

The dose of zafirlukast used for asthma maintenance therapy is 20 mg taken orally twice a day. The maximum dose used is 40 mg per day. The same dose is used for both adults and children greater than 12 years of age. For children from 5 to 11 years of age a dose of 10 mg twice a day is used. Doses are taken 1 hour before or 2 hours after meals. Zafirlukast is not appropriate for use in children less than 5 years of age.

The dose of zileuton used for asthma maintenance therapy is 1,200 mg taken orally twice a day. The maximum dose used is 2,400 mg per day. The same dose is used for both adults and children greater than 12 years of age. Doses are taken within an hour of meals. Zafirlukast is not appropriate for use in children less than 12 years of age.

Precautions

Leukotriene inhibitors are used as a part of asthma maintenance and are not effective for acute asthma attacks. However, treatment with leukotriene inhibitors is not stopped during acute asthma exacerbations when other drugs are necessary for the acute attack. Leukotriene inhibitors may not be appropriate for use in patients with existing liver disease, anxiety, **depression**, dream disorders, hallucinations, alcoholism, mood swings, or tremors. Use of leukotriene inhibitors during breastfeeding is not recommended.

Montelukast and zafirlukast are pregnancy category B drugs. Pregnancy category B drugs are drugs in which there is no evidence of fetal risk in studies done on animals and there are no studies done in pregnant women, or drugs in which there is evidence of fetal harm in animal studies but studies done in pregnant women have not shown risk. These drugs may be used during pregnancy as fetal harm is possible but unlikely. Zafirlukast is not approved for use in children less than five years of age. Montelukast is not approved for use in children less than 1 year of age. The chewable form of montelukast may not be appropriate for use in children with the metabolic disorder phenylketonuria.

Zafirlukast may cause a heart condition that affects the rhythm of the heartbeat known as QT prolongation. Sometimes QT prolongation can cause a serious cardiac condition that includes a fast and irregular heartbeat, with severe dizziness and fainting. The risk of developing QT prolongation syndrome may be increased if the patient is taking other drugs that also affect the rhythm of the heart, or if the patient has cardiac problems. Low blood levels of potassium or magnesium may also increase risk of QT prolongation.

Zileuton is a pregnancy category C drug, and is used during pregnancy only when medically necessary. A pregnancy category C drug is one for which studies done in animals have shown potential harm to a fetus but there is not sufficient data in humans. If the potential benefits for the patient outweigh the potential risks to the fetus, the drug may be used during pregnancy. Zileuton is not approved for use in children less than 12 years of age. Use of zileuton in children may cause mood changes, patients in this age range should be

QUESTIONS TO ASK YOUR PHARMACIST

- How long will I need to take this drug before you can tell if it helps for me?
- How often do I have to have blood work and other laboratory tests done to check the effect the drug is having?
- Is this drug safe to take with the other drugs that I am currently taking?
- What side effects should I watch for? When should I call the doctor about them?
- Are there any clinical trials of this drug combined with other therapies that might benefit me?

monitored cautiously. Use of zileuton in females greater than 65 years of age may cause alterations in liver enzymes that need to be monitored.

Side effects

Leukotriene inhibitors generally have very few side effects and are well tolerated. Headaches are the most common symptom. Leukotriene inhibitors may be associated with the side effects of upset stomach, irritation of the nasal passages, dizziness, **nausea**, inflammation of the sinuses, sore throat, abdominal pain and cramping, **vomiting**, **diarrhea**, liver disease, muscle pain, rash, upper respiratory infections. Very rarely leukotriene inhibitors may cause aggressive behavior, anxiety, depression, dream disorders, hallucinations, insomnia, suicidal thoughts, and tremors. Montelukast and zafirlukast have been associated with the severe side effects of liver failure, alterations of the immune system, and inflammation of the blood vessels. Montelukast has been associated with bronchitis, weakness, and vision disturbances.

Interactions

Leukotriene inhibitors are metabolized by a set of liver enzymes known as cytochrome P450 (CYP450). Multiple subtypes of CYP450 metabolize leukotriene inhibitors, with subtype 3A4 as the main metabolizer. Drugs that induce, or activate these enzymes increase the metabolism of leukotriene inhibitors. This results in lower levels of therapeutic leukotriene inhibitors, thereby negatively affecting treatment. For this reason drugs that induce CYP450 subtype 3A4 may not be used with leukotriene inhibitors. This includes some anti-epileptic drugs such as **carbamazepine**, some anti-inflammatory drugs such as **dexamethasone**, anti-tuberculosis drugs such as rifampin, and the herb St. John's Wort.

Drugs that act to inhibit the action of CYP450 subtype 3A4 may cause undesired increased levels of leukotriene inhibitors in the body. This could lead to toxic doses. Some examples are **antibiotics** such as clarithromycin, antifungal drugs such as ketoconazole, antiviral drugs such as indinavir, antidepressants such as fluoxetine, and some cardiac agents such as verapamil. Grapefruit juice may also increase the amount of leukotriene inhibitors in the body. Patients should avoid drinking grapefruit juice or eating grapefruit while taking leukotriene inhibitors.

Zafirlukast may have dangerous additive effects with other drugs that also cause QT prolongation. Drugs that interact with zafirlukast in this way include cisapride, amiodarone, dofetilide, pimozide, procainamide, quinidine, sotalol, and macrolide antibiotics such as erythromycin. Interactions with the blood thinning drug **warfarin** may increase risk of bleeding.

Leukotriene inhibitors may also interact with other drugs to increase their toxicity. Interactions with the blood thinning drug warfarin may increase risk of bleeding. The dose of the bronchodilator theophylline needs to be reduced when initiating leukotriene inhibitor therapy to prevent toxicity. The blood pressure and cardiac drug propranolol and related compounds may cause toxicity when used with leukotriene inhibitors.

Resources

BOOKS

*Goodman and Gilman's The Pharmacological Basis of Therapeutics, Eleventh Edition*McGraw Hill Medical Publishing Division, 2006.

*Tarascon Pharmacopoeia Library Edition*Jones and Bartlett Publishers, 2009.

OTHER

Epocrates. *Montelukast.* http://www.epocrates.com.

Epocrates. *Zafirlukast.* http://www.epocrates.com.

Epocrates. *Zileuton.* http://www.epocrates.com.

Medscape. *Montelukast.* http://www.medscape.com.

Medscape. *Zafirlukast.* http://www.medscape.com.

Medscape. *Zileuton.* http://www.medscape.com.

RxList. *Montelukast.* http://www.rxlist.com.

RxList. *Zafirlukast.* http://www.rxlist.com.

RxList. *Zileuton.* http://www.rxlist.com.

ORGANIZATIONS

American Academy of Allergy, Asthma, and Immunology. 611 East Wells St., Milwaukee, WI 53202. (800) 822-2762. http://www.aaaai.org.

Asthma and Allergy Foundation of America. 1233 20th Street, NW, Suite 402, Washington, DC 20036. (800) 727-8462. http://www.aafa.org.

FDA U.S. Food and Drug Administration. 10903 New Hampshire Ave, Silver Spring, MD 20993. (888)INFO-FDA. http://www.fda.gov.

National Heart, Lung and Blood Institute. P.O. Box 30105, Bethesda, MD 20824-0105. (301) 251-1222. http://www.nhlbi.nih.gov.

Maria Basile, Ph.D.

Leuprolide acetate

Definition

Leuprolide acetate is a synthetic (man-made) hormone that acts similarly to the naturally occurring gonadotropin releasing hormone (GnRH). It is available under the tradename Lupron.

Purpose

Leuprolide acetate is used primarily to counter the symptoms of advanced **prostate cancer** in men when surgery to remove the testes or estrogen therapy is not an option or is unacceptable to the patient. It is often used to ease the pain and discomfort of women suffering from endometrosis, advanced **breast cancer**, or advanced **ovarian cancer**.

Two less common uses of this drug are the treatment of **anemia** caused by bleeding uterine fibroids, and the treatment of early onset (precocious) puberty.

Description

Leuprolide acetate is a man-made protein that mimics many of the actions of gonadotropin releasing hormone. In men, it decreases blood levels of the male hormone **testosterone**. In women, it decreases blood levels of the female hormone estrogen.

Recommended dosage for prostate cancer

In men, there are three methods of dosing: daily injections, a monthly injection, or an annual implanted capsule. In the case of daily injections, 1 mg of leuprolide acetate is injected under the skin (subcutaneously). In the case of monthly injections, an implanted capsule that contains 7.5 mg of leuprolide acetate is injected into a muscle. In the case of an annual implanted capsule, the capsule contains 72 mg of leuprolide acetate. Both the monthly and the annual capsules are specially designed to slowly release the drug into the patient's bloodstream over the specified time. The monthly capsule dissolves completely over the course of the month. The annual capsule must be removed after 12 months.

In the case of self-administered daily injections, a patient who misses a dose should take that dose as soon as it is noticed. However, if he or she does not remember until the next day, the missed dose should be skipped. Dosages should not be doubled.

Precautions

People taking leuprolide acetate should not drive a car, cook, or engage in any activity that requires alertness until they have been taking the medication long enough to be sure how it affects them.

Leuprolide acetate may cause birth defects if taken during pregnancy, and may be passed to an infant via breast milk. Therefore, women who are pregnant or nursing should not take leuprolide acetate without first consulting their doctors.

Leuprolide acetate will also interfere with the chemical actions of birth control pills. For this reason, sexually active women who do not wish to become pregnant should use some form of birth control other than birth control pills.

Side effects

In patients of both sexes, common side effects of leuprolide acetate include:

- tumor flare, which is exhibited as bone pain (due to a temporary initial increase in testosterone/estrogen before its production is finally decreased)

KEY TERMS

Endometrial tissue—The tissue lining the uterus that is sloughed off during a woman's menstrual period.

Fibroid—A benign smooth muscle tumor of the uterus.

Gonadotropin releasing hormone (GnRH)—A hormone produced in the brain that controls the release of other hormones that are responsible for reproductive function.

Prostate gland—A small gland in the male genitals that contributes to the production of seminal fluid.

- sweating accompanied by feelings of warmth (hot flashes)
- lack of energy (lethargy)
- depression, or other mood changes
- headache
- enlargement of the breasts
- decreased sex drive

Other common side effects in women include:

- light, irregular vaginal bleeding
- no menstrual period
- pelvic pain
- vaginal dryness and/or itching
- emotional instability
- increase in facial or body hair
- deepening of the voice

Less common side effects, in patients of either sex, include:

- burning or itching at the site of the injection
- nausea and vomiting
- insomnia
- weight gain
- swollen feet or lower legs
- constipation

Other side effects in men can include impotence and decreased testicle size.

A doctor should be consulted immediately if the patient experiences any of the above symptoms.

Interactions

There are no known interactions of leuprolide acetate with any food or beverage. People taking leuprolide acetate should consult their physician before taking any other prescription drug, over-the-counter drug, or herbal remedy. People currently taking any other hormone or steroid-based medications should not take leuprolide acetate without first consulting their physician.

See also Endometrial cancer.

Paul A. Johnson, Ed.M.

Levamisole

Definition

Levamisole is used to treat **colon cancer**, specifically stage III colon **cancer**. Levamisole takes the full name of levamisole hydrochloride, and it is also known by the brand name Ergamisol.

Purpose

Levamisole is used to treat patients with stage III colon cancer after they have had surgery to remove the tumor, or as much of the tumor as possible. In stage III colon cancer, the cancer has spread to nearby lymph nodes. Levamisole is approved for use with **fluorouracil** (specifically, 5-fluorouracil), a drug that is thought to prevent cells from replicating, or making more of themselves, by interfering with the manufacture of the hereditary material the cells carry. The use of levamisole with fluorouracil makes it an adjuvant therapy, or one that when used in conjunction with another drug seems to increase the defenses of the patient.

Description

Levamisole was first made (by laboratory synthesis) in 1966, and since then it has been used in veterinary medicine to eliminate intestinal, or lower gut, parasites in domestic animals. It was found to be immunostimulant in 1972 and approved for use for colon cancer in 1990.

The drug seems to have a number of benefits for the patient. It increases the response of T cells, or cells belonging to the lymphatic system that can fight cancer cells. It also seems to increase the activity of cells that attack and destroy invading or cancer cells, including both monocytes and macrophages.

Because of the response levamisole brings from T cells, causing them to be more active, it falls into the category of drugs known as **biological response modifiers**.

Recommended dosage

The drug is given orally in tablet form. Tablets contain 50 milligrams of levamisole hydrochloride, and a standard dose is one tablet every eight hours for three days. Thereafter, the patient takes the same three-day course every two weeks for about a year.

Dosage must be adjusted according to the count of white blood cells and platelets in a patient's blood. In some cases, levamisole can be continued, even when fluorouracil must be stopped.

KEY TERMS

Adjuvant therapy—Addition of a drug to another course of drug therapy to increase or enhance the immune response of a patient.

Macrophage—Large cell-eating cell.

Monocyte—A specialized type of white blood cell that attacks other cells, and acts as a phagocyte.

Neutrophil—A specialized type of white blood cell that attacks other cells, and acts as a phagocyte.

Parasite—An organism that lives by taking its nourishment from another organism.

Phagocyte—Cell-eating cell.

T cell—A cell in the lymphatic system that contributes to immunity by attacking foreign bodies, such as bacteria and viruses, directly.

Precautions

The drug can cause changes in the composition of the blood, which can be fatal. For example, agranulocytosis, also known as **neutropenia**, may develop. The condition refers to a drop in a kind of white blood cells known as neutrophils that are important in the defense against bacteria and fungus. Thus, the patient becomes more likely to get a bacterial or fungal **infection**.

Side effects

Nausea and vomiting, **diarrhea**, hair loss (**alopecia**), and changes in the composition of the white blood cells, such as neutropenia, are among the most common side effects.

Interactions

Levamisole often interacts with alcohol in the same way that the drug disulfiram, which is used to discourage **alcohol consumption** in alcoholics (alcohol deterrent), does. The reaction is extremely unpleasant, and alcohol use is best avoided when levamisole is being taken.

The drug also interacts with **warfarin**, which is often given to heart patients to reduce the chance of blood clots forming. Levamisole can interfere with the action of warfarin, allowing blood clots to form; therefore, adjustments in the amount of warfarin heart patients take may be necessary if they are also taking levamisole.

Diane M. Calabrese

Li-Fraumeni syndrome

Definition

Li-Fraumeni syndrome (LFS) is a genetic disorder caused by a hereditary mutation in a **cancer** susceptibility gene. Individuals with LFS have an increased risk for developing certain types of cancer, often at younger ages than is typically observed in the general population.

Description

Li-Fraumeni syndrome (LFS) was first described by Dr. Frederick Li and Dr. Joseph Fraumeni in 1969. It is caused by mutations in the TP53 gene, located on chromosome 17. The types of mutations that cause LFS are known as hereditary mutations, and therefore can be inherited, or passed from a parent to a child.

Cancer risks

The TP53 gene is a tumor suppressor gene. When an individual inherits a mutation in this type of gene from one of his or her parents, there is an increased risk for developing certain kinds of cancer. The most common kinds of cancer associated with LFS are sarcomas, or tumors that arise in connective tissue, like bone or cartilage.

Females with LFS have an increased risk for developing **breast cancer**. Males and females may also be at risk for developing leukemia, **melanoma**, colon, pancreatic, and brain cancer. They may also develop adrenalcorticoid tumors, which develop on the outer surface of the adrenal glands. These cancers often occur at younger ages than are typically observed in the general population, often before age 45.

Some individuals with LFS may develop certain cancers, such as **brain tumors**, sarcomas, or adrenalcorticoid tumors in childhood. In addition, individuals

Age of onset for cancers associated with Li-Fraumeni syndrome

Age of onset	Type of cancer
Infancy	Development of adrenocortical carcinoma
Under five years of age	Development of soft-tissue sarcomas
Childhood and young adulthood	Acute leukemias and brain tumors
Adolescence	Osteosarcomas
Twenties to thirties	Premenopausal breast cancer is common

(Table by GGS Creative Resources. Cengage Learning, Gale.)

KEY TERMS

Adrenalcorticoid tumors—Cancer that arises on the outer surface of the adrenal glands.

Adrenal glands—Structures located on top of the kidneys that secrete hormones.

Cancer—The process by which cells grow out of control and subsequently invade nearby cells and tissue.

Cancer susceptibility gene—The type of genes involved in cancer. If a mutation is identified in this type of gene it does not reveal whether or not a person has cancer, but rather whether an individual has an increased risk (is susceptible) to develop cancer (or develop cancer again) in the future.

Chromosome—Structures found in the center of a human cell on which genes are located.

Gene—Packages of DNA that control the growth, development and normal function of the body.

Genetic counselor—A specially trained health care provider who helps individuals understand if a disease (such as cancer) is running in their family and their risk for inheriting this disease. Genetic counselors also discuss the benefits, risks and limitations of genetic testing with patients.

Leukemia—Cancer that arises in blood cells.

Mammogram—A screening test that uses x rays to look at a woman's breasts for any abnormalities, such as cancer.

Mutation—An alteration in the number or order of the DNA sequence of a gene.

Penetrance—The likelihood that a person will develop a disease (such as cancer), if he or she has a mutation in a gene that increases the risk for developing that disorder.

Sarcoma—Cancer that occurs in connective tissue, such as cartilage or bone.

Sequencing—A method of performing genetic testing where the chemical order of a patient's DNA is compared to that of normal DNA.

Tumor suppressor gene—Genes that typically prevent cells from growing out of control and forming tumors that may be cancerous.

Ultrasound—A test that uses sound waves to examine organs in the body

with a mutation in the TP53 gene have a higher risk for developing multiple primary cancers. For example, a person with LFS who develops a **sarcoma** at a young age and survives that cancer has an increased risk for developing a second, or possibly even a third different kind of cancer.

Genetic counseling and testing

Genetic testing for mutations in the TP53 gene is usually performed on a blood sample from the relative in the family who has had one of the cancers associated with LFS at a young age. One of the most effective ways to test for mutations in the TP53 gene is by sequencing, a process whereby the chemical components of a patient's DNA is compared to that of DNA that is known to be normal. If the entire DNA code of the TP53 gene is sequenced, it is believed that the majority (98%) of the (mutations) that are responsible for Li-Fraumeni syndrome can be identified. However, as the process of sequencing is a difficult and often time-consuming process, it is not always performed for every patient. Often, only specific areas of the TP53 gene, where there is most likely to be a mutation associated with LFS, are analyzed. The length of time to receive results depends on the extent of testing that is performed and the laboratory that is used.

Due to the fact that some of the cancers associated with LFS can occur at very young ages, there is a question as to whether genetic testing should be an option for at-risk children. Typically, genetic testing is not offered to anyone under the age of 18. However, because there are some screening options available for children with LFS, it is thought that the option of testing could not be denied if a parent feels that it is important for his or her son or daughter's future health. Groups such as the National Society of Genetic Counselors are beginning to explore the issue of genetic testing in minors (those under age 18) for mutations in cancer susceptibility gene, especially if these minors would be at risk for developing **childhood cancers**.

It is important to understand the various categories of results that are associated with undergoing genetic testing for mutations in the TP53 gene. A positive result indicates the presence of a genetic mutation that is known to be associated with an increased risk for developing the types of cancer associated with

QUESTIONS TO ASK THE DOCTOR

- What is the likelihood that the cancer in my family is due to a mutation in a cancer susceptibility gene, particularly the TP53 gene?
- If my family is found to have Li-Fraumeni syndrome, what is the chance that I carry a mutation in the TP53 gene?
- What are the benefits, limitations and risks of undergoing genetic testing?
- What is the cost of genetic testing and how long will it take to obtain results?
- If I undergo genetic testing, will my insurance company pay for testing? If so, will I want to share my results with them?
- What does a positive test result mean for me?
- What does a negative test result mean for me?
- If I test positive for a mutation in a cancer susceptibility gene, what are the best options available for screening and prevention? What research studies may I be eligible to participate in?
- What legislation is in effect to protect me against discrimination by my insurer or employer?

LFS. Once this kind of mutation has been found in an individual, it is possible to test this person's relatives, such as the children, for the presence or absence of that particular mutation. Individuals who have a mutation in the TP53 gene have a 50% chance of passing on this mutation to their children.

Even if a patient has a mutation in the TP53 gene, it does not mean that he or she will definitely develop one of the cancers that are associated with Li-Fraumeni. However, the risk for those with the mutation is much higher than for someone in the general population. The likelihood that a person will develop cancer if they have a mutation in a cancer susceptibility gene like TP53 is called penetrance.

If the first person tested within a family is not found to have an alteration in the TP53 gene, his or her result is negative. Often this result is called indeterminate, because a negative test result cannot completely rule out the possibility of hereditary cancer being present within a family. The interpretation of this type of result can be very complex. For example, a negative result may mean that the method used to detect mutations in the TP53 gene may not be sensitive enough to identify all mutations. Additionally, the mutation might be located in a part of the gene that is difficult to analyze. It may also mean that a person has a mutation in another cancer susceptibility gene that has not yet been discovered or is very rare. Finally, a negative result could mean that the person tested does not have an increased risk for developing cancer because of a mutation in a single cancer susceptibility gene.

Screening and prevention options

With the exception of screening for breast cancer, there are no effective means to screen for and/or prevent the cancers that are associated with Li-Fraumeni syndrome. However, researchers have developed some screening guidelines for those with LFS. For men and women, it is recommended that they undergo a thorough physical exam with their doctor every year. This should include skin and **colon cancer** screening along with a complete exam of the nervous system. Women should also undergo breast cancer screening, which consists of annual mammograms, self-breast exams, and breast exams by a physician or health care provider. Individuals with Li-Fraumeni syndrome may choose to undergo screening more often and at an earlier age then people in the general population.

For children with a TP53 mutation, it is recommended that they also undergo a complete physical exam once a year by their physician. This should include an analysis of their urine and blood and an abdominal ultrasound.

See also Genetic testing.

Resources

OTHER

"Li-Fraumeni Support Group." *Oncolink*. 5 April 2001. [cited June 27, 2009]. http://cancer.med.upenn.edu/disease/misc/.

"Li-Fraumeni Syndrome." *GeneClinics*. 16 Dec. 1998. [cited June 27, 2009]. http://www.geneclinics.com.

ORGANIZATIONS

American Cancer Society. 1599 Clifton Rd. NE, Atlanta, GA 30329. (800)ACS-2345. http://www.cancer.org.

National Cancer Institute. 31 Center Dr., MSC 2580, Bethesda, MD 20892-2580. (800) 4-CANCER. http://www.nci.nih.gov.

National Society of Genetic Counselors. 233 Canterbury Dr., Wallingord, PA 19086-6617. (610) 872-7608. http://www.nsgc.org.

Tiffani A. DeMarco, M.S.

Limb salvage

Definition

Limb salvage is a type of surgery that removes a cancerous tumor or lesion while preserving the nearby muscles, tendons, and blood vessels.

Purpose

Doctors perform limb salvage to remove **cancer** and avoid **amputation**, while preserving the patient's appearance and the greatest possible degree of function in the affected limb. The procedure is most commonly performed for bone tumors and bone sarcomas, but is also commonly performed for soft tissue sarcomas affecting the extremities.

This complex alternative to amputation is used to cure cancers that are slow to spread from the limb where they originate to other parts of the body, or that have not invaded soft tissue.

Precautions

Limb salvage should only be performed by experienced surgeons with specialized expertise. It should also be limited to cases in which the surgery would restore more and longer-lasting function than could be achieved by amputating the affected limb and fitting the patient with an artificial replacement (prosthesis).

If the cancer's location makes it impossible to remove the malignancy without damaging or removing vital organs, essential nerves, key blood vessels, or if it is impossible to reconstruct a limb that will function satisfactorily, salvage surgery may not be an appropriate treatment.

Biopsy is a critical component of limb-salvage surgery. A poorly planned or improperly performed biopsy can limit the patient's surgical options and make amputation unavoidable.

Description

Also called limb-sparing surgery, limb salvage involves removing the cancer and about an inch of healthy tissue surrounding it, and, if bone was removed, replacing the removed bone. The replacement can take the form of synthetic metal rods or plates (prostheses), pieces of bone (grafts) taken from the patient's own body (autologous transplant), or pieces of bone removed from a donor body (cadaver) and frozen until needed for transplant (allograft). In time, transplanted bone grows into the patient's remaining bone. **Chemotherapy**, radiation, or a combination of both treatments may be used to shrink the tumor before surgery is performed.

QUESTIONS TO ASK THE DOCTOR

- Why do you think limb salvage will be successful in my case?
- How will I look and feel after the operation?
- Will I be able to enjoy my favorite sports and other activities after the operation?

Stages of surgery

Limb salvage is performed in three parts. Doctors remove the cancer and a margin of healthy tissue, implant a prosthesis or bone graft (when necessary), and close the wound by transferring soft tissue and muscle from other parts of the patient's body to the surgical site. This treatment cures some cancers as successfully as amputation.

Surgical techniques

BONE TUMORS. Doctors remove the malignant lesion and a cuff of normal tissue (wide excision) to cure low-grade tumors of bone or its components. To cure high-grade tumors, they also remove muscle, bone, and other tissues affected by the tumor (radical resection).

SOFT TISSUE SARCOMAS. Doctors use limb-sparing surgery to treat about 80% of soft tissue sarcomas affecting extremities. The surgery removes the tumor, lymph nodes or tissues to which the cancer has spread, and at least one inch of healthy tissue on all sides of the tumor.

Radiation and/or chemotherapy may be administered before or after the operation. Radiation may also be administered during the operation by placing a special applicator against the surface from which the tumor has just been removed, and inserting tubes containing radioactive pellets at the site of the tumor. These tubes remain in place during the operation and are removed several days later.

To treat a **soft tissue sarcoma** that has spread to the patient's lung, the doctor may remove the original tumor, administer radiation or chemotherapy treatments to shrink the lung tumor, and surgically remove the lung tumor.

Limb salvage for children

Doctors use expandable prostheses to perform limb-salvage surgery on children who have not stopped growing (skeletal immaturity). These children may need as many as four additional operations, at intervals of six to 12 months, to expand the prostheses as their limbs lengthen.

Because expandable prostheses have been available only since the 1980s, the long-term effects of using them are unknown.

Preparation

Before deciding that limb salvage is appropriate for a particular patient, the doctor considers what type of cancer the patient has, the size and location of the tumor, how the illness has progressed, and the patient's age and general health.

After determining that limb salvage is appropriate for a particular patient, the doctor makes sure that the patient understands what the outcome of surgery is likely to be, that the implant may fail, and that additional surgery—even amputation—may be necessary.

Preoperative rehabilitation

Physical and occupational therapists help prepare the patient for surgery by introducing the muscle-strengthening, ambulation, and range of motion (ROM) exercises the patient will begin performing right after the operation.

Aftercare

During the five to ten days the patient remains in the hospital following surgery, nurses monitor sensation and blood flow in the affected extremity and watch for signs that the patient may be developing **pneumonia**, pulmonary embolism, or deep-vein thrombosis.

The doctor prescribes broad-spectrum **antibiotics** for at least the first 48 hours after the operation and often prescribes medication (prophylactic anticoagulants) and antiembolism stockings to prevent blood clots. A drainage tube placed in the wound for the first 24–48 hours prevents blood (hematoma) and fluid (seroma) from accumulating at the surgical site. As postoperative pain becomes less intense, mild narcotics or anti-inflammatory medications replace the epidural catheter or patient-controlled analgesic pump used to relieve pain immediately after the operation.

Exercise intervention

Limb salvage requires extensive surgical incisions, and patients who have these operations need extensive rehabilitation. The amount of bone removed and the type of reconstruction performed dictate how soon and how much the patient can exercise, but most patients begin muscle-strengthening, continuous passive motion (CPM), and ROM exercises the day after the operation and continue them for the next 12 months.

A patient who has had upper-limb surgery can use the opposite side of the body to perform hand and shoulder exercises. Patients should not do active elbow or shoulder exercises for two to eight weeks after having surgery involving the bone between the shoulder and elbow (humerus). Rehabilitation following lower-extremity limb salvage focuses on strengthening the muscles that straighten the legs (quadriceps), maintaining muscle tone, and gradually increasing weight-bearing so that the patient is able to stand on the affected limb within three months of the operation. A patient who has had lower-extremity surgery may have to learn a new way of walking (gait retraining) or wear a lift in one shoe.

Goals of rehabilitation

Physical and occupational therapy regimens are designed to help the patient move freely, function independently, and accept changes in **body image**. Even patients who look the way they did before surgery are likely to feel that the operation has altered their appearance.

Before a patient goes home from the hospital or rehabilitation center, the doctor decides whether the patient needs a walker, brace, cane, or other device, and should make sure that the patient can climb stairs. Also, the doctor should emphasize the life-long importance of preventing **infection** and give the patient written instructions about how to prevent infection and what to do if infection does develop.

Risks

The major risks associated with limb salvage include superficial or deep infection at the site of the surgery; loosening, shifting, or breakage of implants; rapid loss of blood flow or sensation in the affected limb; and severe blood loss and **anemia** from the surgery.

Postoperative infection is a serious problem. Chemotherapy or radiation can weaken the immune system, and extensive bone damage can occur before the infection is identified. Tissue may die (necrosis) if the surgeon used a large piece of tissue (flap) to close the wound. This is most likely to occur if the surgical site was treated with radiation before the operation. Treatment for postoperative infection involves removing the graft or implant, inserting drains at the infected site, and giving the patient oral or intravenous antibiotic therapy for as long as 12 months. Doctors may have to amputate the affected limb.

Normal results

A patient who has had limb-sparing surgery will remain disease-free as long as a patient whose affected extremity has been amputated.

Salvaged limbs always function better than artificial ones. However, it takes a year for patients to learn to walk again following lower-extremity limb salvage, and patients who have undergone upper-extremity salvage must master new ways of using the affected arm or hand.

Successful surgery reduces the frequency and severity of patient falls and of the fractures that often result from disease-related changes in bone. Although successful surgery results in limbs that look and function very much like normal, healthy limbs, it is not unusual for patients to feel that their appearance has changed.

Abnormal results

Some patients will need additional surgery within five years of the first operation. Some will eventually require amputation.

Post-operation directives from the patient's physician may include the following items:

- Patients may be told that they should never jog, lift heavy objects, or play racquet sports.
- Wearing a splint or cast can damage nerves and veins in the affected limb.
- Implants can loosen, shift to a new position, or break.

See also Chondrosarcoma; Ewing's sarcoma; Osteosarcoma.

Resources

BOOKS

Ignatavicius, Donna D., et al. *Medical-Surgical Nursing Across the Health Care Continuum*. 3rd ed. Philadelphia: W. B. Saunders Company, 1999.

OTHER

"Adult Soft Tissue Sarcoma." "Bone Cancer." *CancerNet*. 2000. [cited July 11, 2009]. http://www.cancernet.nci.nih.gov.

"Bone Cancer." *ACS Cancer Resource Center* American Cancer Society. 2000. [cited July 11, 2009]. http://www3.cancer.org.

"Sarcoma." *ACS Cancer Resource Center*. American Cancer Society. March 22, 2000. [cited July 11, 2009]. http://www3.cancer.org.

"Soft-Tissue Sarcoma." *Memorial Sloan-Kettering Cancer Center*. 2001. [cited July 11, 2009]. http://www.mskcc.org/.

Maureen Haggerty

Lip cancers

Definition

Lip **cancer** is a malignant tumor, or neoplasm, that originates in the surface layer cells of the epithelial tissue in the upper or lower lip.

Description

The upper and lower lips are the well-defined red (often called vermilion) areas that surround the opening to the mouth. They contain muscles and special cells (receptors) that are sensitive to heat and cold and feeling. Largely taken for granted, the lips are important in identifying types of food to the brain and in getting food into the mouth. Lips also play a crucial role in speech.

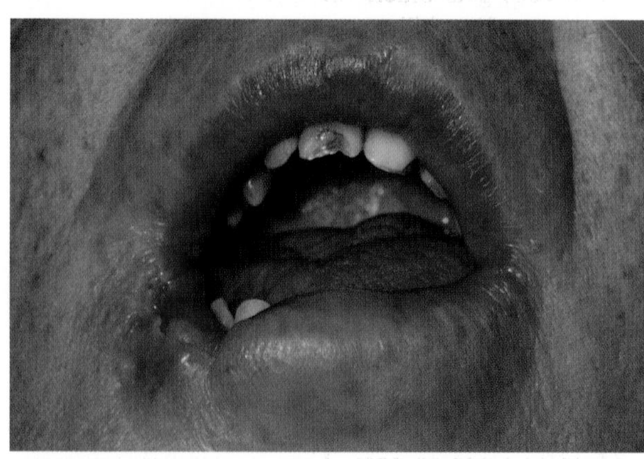

Squamous cell carcinoma on lip. *(Custom Medical Stock Photo. Reproduced by permission.)*

KEY TERMS

Biopsy—A procedure in which a tissue sample is taken from the body for examination.

Epithelial tissue—The collection of cells that form coverings for the surfaces of the body.

Immunity—Ability to resist the effects of agents, such as bacteria and viruses, that cause disease.

Lymph node—A concentration of lymphatic tissue and part of the lymphatic system that collects fluid from around the cells and returns it to the blood vessels, and helps with the immune response.

Squamous cells—Flat epithelial cells, which usually make up the outer layer of epithelial tissue, the layer farthest away from the surface the epithelium covers.

QUESTIONS TO ASK THE DOCTOR

- Is this cancer curable?
- What is the stage of the cancer?
- What is the likelihood the cancer will recur?
- Is there a clinical trial in which I should participate?

A malignant tumor, or neoplasm, that originates in the cells of one of the lips is a cancer of the lip. Lip cancer almost always begins in the flat, or squamous, epithelial cells. Epithelial cells form coverings (tissues) for the surfaces of the body. Skin, for example, has an outer layer of epithelial tissue.

If a part of the lip is affected by cancer and must be removed by surgery, there will be significant changes in eating ability and speech function. The more lip tissue removed, the greater the disturbances to the normal patterns of talking and eating.

Demographics

Nine out of 10 cases of lip cancer are diagnosed in people over the age of 45. Age, or the aging process, may contribute to the way the cancer develops. As a line of cells gets older, the genetic material in a cell loses some of its ability to repair itself. When the repair system is operating normally, damage to the genetic material, or DNA, caused by ultraviolet light from the sun is quickly weeded out. When the system fails, changes in the genetic material are kept, and they multiply when a cell divides.

If the genetic material cannot repair itself, damage caused by exposure to environmental factors such as sunlight and chemicals can quickly set in motion the uncontrolled growth of cells.

The effects of factors that are known to cause lip cancer, such as smoking and exposure to sunlight, also add up as a person ages. Thus, the combination of a breakdown in the repair system in the genetic material and the considerable periods of time (decades) over which a person is exposed to cancer agents probably causes lip cancers. However, researchers are still investigating how lip cancers start.

Men are at greater risk for lip cancer than women. Depending on where they live, men are two or three times more likely to be diagnosed than women. Fair-skinned people are more likely to get lip cancer than those with dark skin. For reasons not yet understood, people in Asia have a much lower risk of lip cancer than those living on other continents. In many parts of Asia, lip cancer is extremely rare. In North America, nearly 13 out of 100,000 men will be diagnosed with lip cancer during their lifetime. In Australia, about 13.5 men per 100,000 will be diagnosed.

The frequency of lip cancer is often lumped together with oral cancer, although lip cancer is probably much more like **skin cancer** in origin. There are about 30,000 new diagnoses of mouth and lip cancer in the United States each year. About 38% percent of all cancers of the mouth begin in the lower lip; on the other hand, cancers of the upper lip are more aggressive than those of the lower lip.

In some places, such as South Australia, women are experiencing a striking increase in lip cancer diagnoses. There are several theories to explain the trend. Among them, perhaps fewer women regularly wear hats, which offer protection from the sun. Women might also be forgoing lipstick, which serves as another barrier to sunlight.

Causes and symptoms

Exposure to sunlight and smoking, particularly pipe smoking, increases the risk of developing lip cancer. However, the way they do so is not understood. **Alcohol consumption** is tied to **oral cancers** and may contribute to lip cancer as well.

Much of the evidence about the link between time spent in the sun and lip cancer comes from a look at those who are most likely to be diagnosed. Among them are farmers, golfers, and others who spend long periods of time outdoors.

Lip cancer seems to share some properties with skin cancer in the way it originates. Yet several studies suggest that it takes more than exposure to sun to increase the risk of lip cancer. Viral **infection** is a risk factor, as is reduced immunity, which is a condition that may be caused by viral infection. A team of researchers in the Netherlands recently reported a link between liver transplants and a higher risk of lip and skin cancer following the transplant. The results are not unexpected. In this procedure, drugs are used to suppress, or lower, the activity of a recipient's immune system so that a donor organ will be accepted. Thus, the immunity of the organ recipient is low, and lower immunity is linked to lip cancer.

Individuals with acquired immunodeficiency syndrome (AIDS) are at a greater risk for lip cancer. People infected with **herpes simplex** viruses, papilloma viruses and other viruses may also be at greater risk.

Vitamin deficiency may also be a factor that contributes to lip cancer. The sorts of **vitamins** found in fruits and vegetables, particularly carotene, the substance the body uses to form vitamins A and C, seem to be important in preventing lip cancer.

Particular symptoms of this cancer include white spots, sores, or lumps on the lip. Pain can also be a symptom, particularly pain in a lymph node near the affected part of the lip. This is a troubling symptom, since it indicates that the cancer has metastasized (spread) beyond the lip.

Diagnosis

Dentists frequently identify a suspicious spot, sore, or lump on the lip. A good dental exam includes an examination of the lips and the mouth. X ray and **biopsy**, the taking of a tissue sample for analysis, can be used to determine whether or not cancer is present.

Because spots and sores on the lips can be short-lived, people should not be alarmed by every change that appears. However, when there is a change that occurs and stays, it should be investigated. If the next scheduled dental visit is several months away, a special appointment with the dentist or a physician should be made. Dentists should tell their patients, particularly older ones, how to undertake a regular self-exam of the lips between check-ups.

Treatment team

A physician who specializes in oncology, the study and treatment of cancer, will probably take the lead on treatment. A surgeon will remove the cancer. Not all oncologists are surgeons, so it is likely that the team will include a medical oncologist, who coordinates treatment, as well as a surgical oncologist, who performs the surgery.

Because surgery on the lip can interfere with eating and talking, most teams include a nutritionist and a speech pathologist. Scars and alterations of facial features can produce changes in **body image**, and a psychiatrist or social worker may participate in the team to help a patient cope with such changes. It is possible that a dentist or oral surgeon will also play a role. Nurses who administer **chemotherapy** and monitor the status of patients will be involved, as will radiation technicians and a radiation oncologist. If reconstruction of a lip is necessary because of the amount of tissue removed or the size of a scar, a plastic surgeon will be added to the team.

Clinical staging, treatments, and prognosis

The ability to see a suspicious area on the lips and to detect lip cancer early combine to form the staging process. (One inch equals 2.5 cm.)

- Stage I: The cancer is less than one inch in diameter and has not spread.
- Stage II: The cancer is up to approximately two inches in diameter and has not spread.
- Stage III: The cancer is either larger than two inches or has spread to a lymph node on the side of the neck that matches the primary location of the lip cancer. The lymph node is enlarged, but not much more than an inch.
- Stage IV: One or more of several things can occur. There may be a spread of cancer to the mouth or to the areas around the lip, more than one lymph node with cancer, or metastasis (spread) to other parts of the body.

The outlook for recovery from lip cancer is very good if it is diagnosed early. For stage I and stage II cancers, surgery to remove the cancer or radiation treatment of the affected area is sometimes all that is required to produce a cure. Decisions about which method to use depend on many factors, but the size of the tumor and the tolerance a patient has for radiation or chemotherapy are particularly important. The larger the tumor, the more urgent is its removal. Smaller tumors can be treated with radiation or other methods in an effort to shrink them before surgery. In some cases, surgery might be avoided. For stage III cancer with lymph node involvement, the cancerous lymph nodes are also removed.

Chemotherapy may be used at any stage, but it is particularly important for stage IV cancer. In some cases, chemotherapy is used before surgery, just as radiation is, to try to eliminate the cancer without cutting, or at least to make it smaller before it is cut out (excised). After surgery, **radiation therapy** and chemotherapy are both used to treat patients with stage IV lip cancer, sometimes in combination.

There are many new and promising types of treatment for lip cancer. For example, heat kills some cancer cells, and a treatment known as **hyperthermia** uses heat to eliminate cancer in some patients.

Because lip cancers are well-studied and often successfully treated, the best practices for dealing with the cancer, or a suspected cancer, are specific. In the case of how to extract and study tissue to determine whether a suspicious growth is malignant (biopsy), size is an extremely useful guide.

It is possible to take tissue from a suspected lip cancer for examination, or biopsy, by simply piercing and extracting tissue with a large, hollow needle. The technique is called a punch biopsy. However, the method is not recommended for any tumor that is thicker than about one-sixteenth of an inch. For thicker tumors, a tissue sample is better taken by cutting into the tumor, that is, making an incision.

The success with identifying lip cancer early and eliminating it means that it is not a big killer. Only four in 2.5 million people die from lip cancer each year, or about 112 individuals in the entire United States population. In contrast, cancers in the oral cavity, including on the tongue, cause more than 8,000 deaths in the United States each year.

Alternative and complementary therapies

Because there seems to be some link between a chronic absence of vitamins A and C in the diet and lip cancer, some complementary therapies promote taking massive amounts of the vitamins, or megavitamins. The value of such therapy has not been demonstrated. In order to avoid possible side effects or harmful interactions with standard cancer treatment, patients should always notify their treatment team of any over-the-counter or herbal remedies that they are taking.

Coping with cancer treatment

The doctor and patient should discuss the need for a way to communicate if speech is impaired after surgery. A pad and pencil may be all that is needed for a short interval. If there will be a long period of speech difficulty, patients should be ready with additional means, such as TYY phone service.

A change in appearance after the removal of a lip cancer can lead to concerns about body image, and social interaction may suffer. A support group can help. Discussions with a social worker, loved ones, or other patients who have undergone similar treatment can be of major benefit.

If a significant portion of lip is removed, speech therapy may be necessary to relearn how to make certain sounds. Scars and alterations of the lips usually can be reduced or hidden entirely with the techniques available from plastic surgery, so any alteration in appearance because of lip cancer is typically transient.

Reconstruction of the lip will help with appearance, but it might not make it easier to talk, especially if muscle tissue is removed during the surgery to eliminate the cancer. In many cases, the reconstruction process actually damages more muscle and sensory tissue. New methods of **reconstructive surgery** are being developed to avoid such an outcome. Some of these newer methods involve grafts of skin and muscle taken from the forearm or the area of the cheek near the angle of the jawbone. In general, reconstruction of the lower lip is more difficult than reconstruction of the upper lip.

Appetite may be affected before, during and after treatment. Before treatment, the presence of a tumor can interfere with the tasting of food, and food might not seem as appealing as it once did. During treatment, particularly radiation treatment, the area of the lips and mouth might be sore and make eating difficult. After treatment, a loss of sensation in the part of the lip affected can reduce appetite. A nutritionist can help with supplements for those who experience significant **weight loss** and who do not have an appetite.

Clinical trials

The Cancer Information Service at the National Institutes of Health offers information about **clinical trials** that are looking for volunteers. The service can be reached at http://cancertrials.nci.nih.gov or (800) 422-6237.

Prevention

The best preventive measures are minimizing sun exposure and avoiding tobacco and alcohol. Eating plenty of fruits and vegetables is a good measure. Even though the importance of fruits and vegetables is not proven to prevent lip cancer, overall fruits and vegetables are demonstrated cancer-fighters. Any precaution that is taken against contracting human immunodeficiency virus (HIV), which causes AIDS, is also likely to reduce the chance of developing lip cancer.

Special concerns

Certain diseases can mimic a possible lip cancer. They must be ruled out if a suspicious spot is found. This is particularly true in areas where diseases that cause lesions, or sores, on the lips are found. One such disease is *histoplasmosis capsulatum*, which is caused by a fungus. It sometimes produces an ulcer, or lesion, on the lip that leads to suspicion of lip cancer.

Sometimes lip cancer cannot be cured. It may keep recurring. It may also metastasize, particularly to the lungs. But overall, lip cancer is considered highly curable. Talking openly with the physician in charge of care is important in order for the patient to understand the course of the disease and be prepared to make decisions.

See also Oropharyngeal cancer.

Resources

BOOKS

Beers, Mark H., MD, and Robert Berkow, MD, editors. "Disorders of the Oral Region: Neoplasms." Section 9, In *The Merck Manual of Diagnosis and Therapy*. Whitehouse Station, NJ: Merck Research Laboratories, 2007.

PERIODICALS

Adler, N., A. Amir, and D. Hauben. "Modified von Bruns' Technique for Total Lower Lip Reconstruction." *Dermatologic Surgery* 30 (March 2004): 433–437.

Brennan, P., et al. "Secondary Primary Neoplasms Following Non-Hodgkin's Lymphoma in New South Wales, Australia." *British Journal of Cancer* 82 (April 2000): 1344–7.

Bucur, A., and L. Stefanescu. "Management of Patients with Squamous Cell Carcinoma of the Lower Lip and Neck." *Journal of Craniomaxillofacial Surgery* 32 (February 2004): 16–18.

Dupin, C., S. Metzinger, and R. Rizzuto. "Lip Reconstruction after Ablation for Skin Malignancies." *Clinics in Plastic Surgery* 31 (January 2004): 69–85.

Gardetto, A., K. Erdinger, and C. Papp. "The Zygomatic Flap: A Further Possibility in Reconstructing Soft-Tissue Defects of the Nose and Upper Lip." *Plastic and Reconstructive Surgery* 113 (February 2004): 485–490.

Haagsma, E.B., et al. "Increased Cancer Risk After Liver Transplantation: A Population-Based Study." *Journal of Hepatology* 34 (January 2001): 84–91.

ORGANIZATIONS

American Academy of Facial Plastic and Reconstructive Surgery (AAFPRS). 310 South Henry Street, Alexandria, VA 22314. (703) 299-9291. http://www.facemd.org.

American Society of Plastic Surgeons (ASPS). 444 East Algonquin Road, Arlington Heights, IL 60005. (847) 228-9900. http://www.plasticsurgery.org.

Support for People with Oral and Head and Neck Cancer (SPOHNC). P.O. Box 53, Locust Valley, NY 11560-0053. (800) 377-0928. http://www.spohnc.org.

Diane M. Calabrese, Ph.D.
Rebecca J. Frey, Ph.D.

Liver biopsy

Definition

A liver **biopsy** is a medical procedure performed to obtain a small piece of liver tissue for diagnostic testing. Liver biopsies are sometimes called percutaneous liver biopsies, because the tissue sample is obtained by going through the patient's skin.

Purpose

A liver biopsy is usually done to diagnose a tumor, or to evaluate the extent of damage that has occurred to the liver because of chronic disease. Biopsies are often performed to identify abnormalities in liver tissues after **imaging studies** have failed to yield clear results.

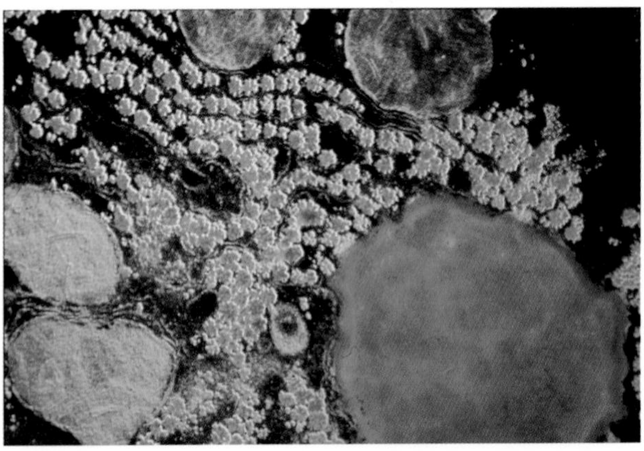

A false-color scanning electron micrograph (SEM) of hepatocyte cells of the liver that secrete bile. *(Photograph by John Bavosi. Custom Medical Stock Photo. Reproduced by permission.)*

QUESTIONS TO ASK THE DOCTOR

- Which medications should I stop taking before the biopsy?
- How soon can I return to my normal activities after the biopsy?
- How soon will I get my results?

KEY TERMS

Biopsy—A procedure where a piece of tissue is removed from a patient for diagnostic testing.

Menghini needle—A special needle used to obtain a sample of liver tissue.

Percutaneous biopsy—A biopsy in which a needle is inserted and a tissue sample removed through the skin.

Prothrombin time—A blood test that determines how quickly a person's blood will clot.

Vital signs—A person's essential body functions, usually defined as the pulse, body temperature, and breathing rate.

A liver biopsy may be ordered to evaluate any of the following conditions or disorders:

- jaundice
- cirrhosis
- hemochromatosis, which is a condition of excess iron in the liver
- repeated abnormal results from liver function tests
- unexplained swelling or enlargement of the liver
- primary cancers of the liver, such as hepatomas, cholangiocarcinomas, and angiosarcomas
- metastatic cancers of the liver

Precautions

Some patients should not have percutaneous liver biopsies. They include patients with any of the following conditions:

- a platelet count below 60,000
- a longer-than-normal prothrombin time
- a liver tumor that contains a large number of blood vessels
- a history of unexplained bleeding
- a watery (hydatid) cyst
- an infection in either the cavity around the lungs, or the diaphragm

Description

Percutaneous liver biopsy is done with a special hollow needle, called a Menghini needle, attached to a suction syringe. Doctors who specialize in the digestive system or liver will sometimes perform liver biopsies. But in most cases, a radiologist (a doctor who specializes in **x rays** and imaging studies) performs the biopsy. The radiologist will use **computed tomography** scan (CT scan) or ultrasound to guide the choice of the site for the biopsy.

An hour or so before the biopsy, the patient may be given a sedative to help relaxation. He or she is then asked to lie on the back with the right elbow to the side and the right hand under the head. The patient is instructed to lie as still as possible during the procedure. He or she is warned to expect a sensation resembling a punch in the right shoulder, but to hold still in spite of the momentary feeling.

The doctor marks a spot on the skin where the needle will be inserted and thoroughly cleanses the right side of the upper abdomen with an antiseptic solution. The patient is then given an anesthetic at the biopsy site.

The needle with attached syringe is inserted into the patient's chest wall. The doctor then draws the plunger of the syringe back to create a vacuum. At this point the patient is asked to take a deep breath, exhale the air and hold their breath at the point of complete exhalation. The needle is inserted into the liver and withdrawn quickly, usually within two seconds or less. The negative pressure in the syringe draws or pulls a sample of liver tissue into the biopsy needle. As soon as the needle is withdrawn, the patient can breathe normally. Pressure is applied at the biopsy site to stop any bleeding, and a bandage will be placed over it. The entire procedure takes 10 to 15 minutes. Test results are usually available within a day.

Preparation

Aspirin and **non-steroidal anti-inflammatory drugs** (NSAIDs) such as ibuprofen are known to thin the blood and interfere with clotting. These medications should be avoided for at least a week before the biopsy. Four to eight hours before the biopsy, patients should stop eating and drinking.

The patient's blood will be tested prior to the biopsy to make sure that it is clotting normally. Tests will include a platelet count and a prothrombin time. Doctors will also ensure that the patient is not taking any other medications, such as blood thinners like Coumadin, that might affect blood clotting.

Aftercare

Liver biopsies are outpatient procedures in most hospitals. After the biopsy, patients are usually instructed to lie on their right side for about two hours. This provides pressure to the biopsy site and helps prevent bleeding. A nurse will check the patient's vital signs at regular intervals. If there are no complications, the patient is sent home within about four to eight hours.

Patients should arrange to have a friend or relative take them home after discharge. Bed rest for a day is recommended, followed by a week of avoiding heavy work or strenuous exercise. The patient can resume eating a normal diet.

Some mild soreness in the area of the biopsy is normal after the anesthetic wears off. Irritation of the muscle that lies over the liver can also cause mild discomfort in the shoulder for some patients. Tylenol can be taken for minor soreness, but aspirin and NSAIDs are best avoided. Patients should call their doctor if they have severe pain in the abdomen, chest or shoulder, difficulty breathing, or persistent bleeding. These signs may indicate that there has been leakage of bile into the abdominal cavity, or that air has been introduced into the cavity around the lungs.

Risks

The risks of a liver biopsy are usually very small. When complications do occur, over 90% are apparent within 24 hours after the biopsy. The most significant risk is internal bleeding. Bleeding is most likely to occur in elderly patients, in patients with cirrhosis, or in patients with a tumor that has many blood vessels. Other complications from percutaneous liver biopsies include the leakage of bile or the introduction of air into the chest cavity (pneumothorax). There is also a small chance that an **infection** may occur, or an internal organ such as the lung, gallbladder, or kidney could be punctured.

Normal results

After the biopsy, the liver sample is sent to the pathology laboratory for study under a microscope. A normal (negative) result would find no evidence of **cancer** or other disease in the tissue sample.

Abnormal results

Changes in liver tissue that are visible under the microscope indicate abnormal results. Possible causes for the abnormality include the presence of a tumor, or a disease such as hepatitis.

Resources

BOOKS

Brown, Kyle E., et al. "Liver Biopsy: Indications, Technique, Complications and Interpretation" In *Liver Disease. Diagnosis and Management*, edited by Bacon, Bruce R., and Adrian M. Di Bisceglie. Philadelphia, PA: Churchill Livingstone, 2000.

Reddy, K. Rajender, and Lennox J. Jeffers. "Evaluation of the Liver. Liver Biopsy and Laparoscopy." In *Schiff's Diseases of the Liver*, edited by Eugene R. Schiff, et al. Philadelphia, PA: Lippincott-Raven, 1999.

PERIODICALS

Bravo, Arturo A., et al. "Liver Biopsy" *New England Journal of Medicine* 344, no. 7 (February 15, 2001): 495-500.

Lata Cherath, Ph.D.

Liver cancer

Definition

Liver **cancer** is a relatively rare form of cancer but has a high mortality rate. Liver cancers can be classified into two types. They are either primary, when the cancer starts in the liver itself, or metastatic, when the cancer has spread to the liver from some other part of the body.

Description and demographics

Primary liver cancer

Primary liver cancer is a relatively rare disease in the United States, representing about 2% of all malignancies and 4% of newly diagnosed cancers. Hepatocellular **carcinoma** (HCC) is the fifth most common cancer in the world as of 2004. It is much more common outside the United States, representing 10% to 50% of malignancies in Africa and parts of Asia. Rates of HCC in men are at least two to three times higher than for women. In high-risk areas (East and Southeast Asia, sub-Saharan Africa), men are even more likely to have HCC than women.

According to the American Cancer Society, 22,620 people in the United States will be diagnosed with primary liver cancer in 2009, and 18,160 persons will die from the disease. The incidence of primary

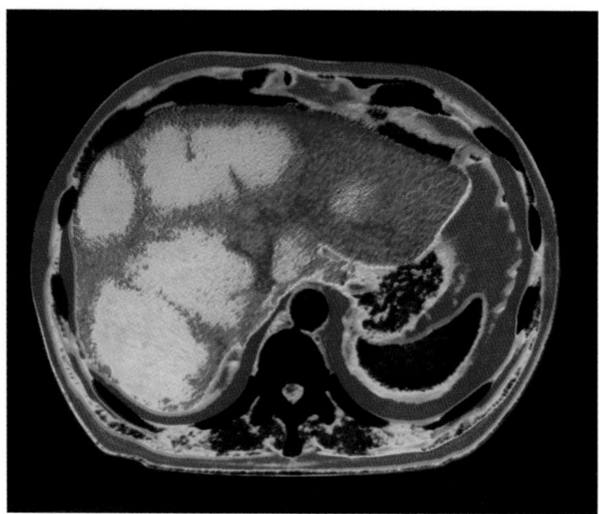

Colored computed tomography (CT) scan of axial section through the abdomen showing liver cancer. The vertebra appears dark blue, the liver is large and appears light blue, and the light patches on the liver are the cancerous tumors. *(Copyright Department of Clinical Radiology, Salisbury District Hospital, Science Source/Photo Researchers, Inc. Photo reproduced by permission.)*

liver cancer has been rising in the United States and Canada since the mid-1990s, most likely as a result of the rising rate of hepatitis C infections.

TYPES OF PRIMARY LIVER CANCER. In adults, most primary liver cancers belong to one of two types: hepatomas, or hepatocellular carcinomas (HCC), which start in the liver tissue itself; and cholangiomas, or cholangiocarcinomas, which are cancers that develop in the bile ducts inside the liver. About 80–90% of primary liver cancers are hepatomas. In the United States, about five persons in every 200,000 will develop a hepatoma (70–75% of cases of primary liver cancers are HCC). In Africa and Asia, over 40 persons in 200,000 will develop this form of cancer (more than 90% of cases of primary liver are HCC). Two rare types of primary liver cancer are mixed-cell tumors and Kupffer cell sarcomas.

One type of primary liver cancer, called a hepatoblastoma, usually occurs in children younger than four years of age and between the ages of 12 and 15. Unlike liver cancers in adults, hepatoblastomas have a good chance of being treated successfully. Approximately 70% of children with hepatoblastomas experience complete cures. If the tumor is detected early, the survival rate is over 90%.

Metastatic liver cancer

The second major category of liver cancer, metastatic liver cancer, is about 20 times more common in

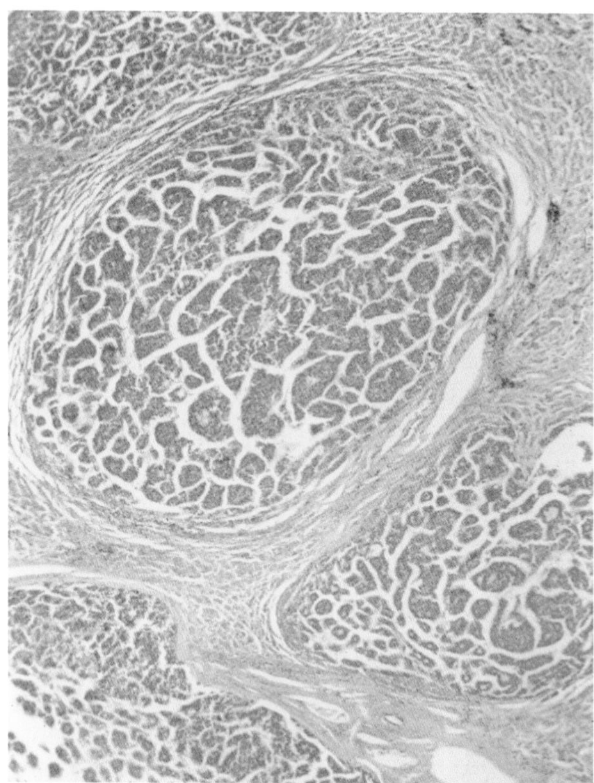

Light micrograph of a section through a primary carcinoma from a human liver. Healthy liver cells are normally arranged in roughly hexagonal structures called lobules. In this cancerous liver, the lobules are disintegrating, and abnormal fibrous tissue has proliferated around them. *(Copyright John Burbridge, Science Source/Photo Researchers, Inc. Reproduced by permission.)*

the United States than primary liver cancer. Because blood from all parts of the body must pass through the liver for filtration, cancer cells from other organs and tissues easily reach the liver, where they can lodge and grow into secondary tumors. Primary cancers in the colon, stomach, pancreas, rectum, esophagus, breast, lung, or skin are the most likely to metastasize (spread) to the liver. It is not unusual for the metastatic cancer in the liver to be the first noticeable sign of a cancer that started in another organ. After cirrhosis, metastatic liver cancer is the most common cause of fatal liver disease.

Causes and symptoms

Risk factors

The exact cause of primary liver cancer is still unknown. In adults, however, certain factors are known to place some individuals at higher risk of developing liver cancer. These factors include:

QUESTIONS TO ASK THE DOCTOR

- What type of liver cancer do I have?
- What is the stage of the disease?
- What are the treatment choices? Which do you recommend? Why?
- What are the risks and possible side effects of each treatment?
- What are the chances that the treatment will be successful?
- What new treatments are being studied in clinical trials?
- How long will treatment last?
- Will I have to stay in the hospital?
- Will treatment affect my normal activities? If so, for how long?
- What is the treatment likely to cost?

- Male sex.
- Age over 60 years.
- Ethnicity. Asian Americans with cirrhosis have four times as great a chance of developing liver cancer as Caucasians with cirrhosis, and African Americans have twice the risk of Caucasians. In addition, Asians often develop liver cancer at much younger ages than either African Americans or Caucasians.
- Exposure to substances in the environment that tend to cause cancer (carcinogens). These include: a substance produced by a mold that grows on rice and peanuts (aflatoxin); thorium dioxide, which was once used as a contrast dye for x rays of the liver; vinyl chloride, used in manufacturing plastics; and cigarette smoking.
- Use of oral estrogens for birth control.
- Hereditary hemochromatosis. This is a disorder characterized by abnormally high levels of iron storage in the body. It often develops into cirrhosis.
- Cirrhosis. Hepatomas appear to be a frequent complication of cirrhosis of the liver. Between 30% and 70% of hepatoma patients also have cirrhosis. It is estimated that a patient with cirrhosis has 40 times the chance of developing a hepatoma than a person with a healthy liver.
- Exposure to hepatitis viruses: Hepatitis B (HBV), Hepatitis C (HCV), Hepatitis D (HDV), or Hepatitis G (HGV). It is estimated that 80% of worldwide HCC is associated with chronic HBV infection. In Africa and most of Asia, exposure to hepatitis B is an important factor; in Japan and some Western countries, exposure to hepatitis C is connected with a higher risk of developing liver cancer. In the United States, nearly 25% of patients with liver cancer show evidence of HBV infection. Hepatitis is commonly found among intravenous drug abusers. The increase in HCC incidence in the United States is thought to be due to increasing rates of HBV and HCV infections due to increased sexual promiscuity and illicit drug needle sharing. The association between HDV and HGV and HCC is unclear as of the early 2000s.

Symptoms of liver cancer

The early symptoms of primary, as well as metastatic, liver cancer are often vague and not unique to liver disorders. The long period between the beginning of the tumor's growth and the first signs of illness is the major reason why the disease has a high mortality rate. At the time of diagnosis, patients are often fatigued, with **fever**, abdominal pain, and loss of appetite (**anorexia**). They may look emaciated and generally ill. As the tumor enlarges, it stretches the membrane surrounding the liver (the capsule), causing pain in the upper abdomen on the right side. The pain may extend into the back and shoulder. Some patients develop a collection of fluid, known as **ascites**, in the abdominal cavity. Others may show signs of bleeding into the digestive tract. In addition, the tumor may block the ducts of the liver or the gall bladder, leading to jaundice. In patients with jaundice, the whites of the eyes and the skin may turn yellow, and the urine becomes dark–colored.

Diagnosis

Physical examination

If the doctor suspects a diagnosis of liver cancer, he or she will check the patient's history for risk factors and pay close attention to the condition of the patient's abdomen during the physical examination. Masses or lumps in the liver and ascites can often be felt while the patient is lying flat on the examination table. The liver is usually swollen and hard in patients with liver cancer; it may be sore when the doctor presses on it. In some cases, the patient's spleen is also enlarged. The doctor may be able to hear an abnormal sound (bruit) or rubbing noise (friction rub) if he or she uses a stethoscope to listen to the blood vessels that lie near the liver. The noises are caused by the pressure of the tumor on the blood vessels.

Laboratory tests

Blood tests may be used to test liver function or to evaluate risk factors in the patient's history. Between 50% and 75% of primary liver cancer patients have abnormally high blood serum levels of a particular protein (alpha-fetoprotein or AFP). The AFP test, however, cannot be used by itself to confirm a diagnosis of liver cancer, because cirrhosis or chronic hepatitis can also produce high alpha–fetoprotein levels. Tests for alkaline phosphatase, bilirubin, lactic dehydrogenase, and other chemicals indicate that the liver is not functioning normally. About 75% of patients with liver cancer show evidence of hepatitis **infection**. Again, however, abnormal liver function test results are not specific for liver cancer.

Imaging studies

Imaging studies are useful in locating specific areas of abnormal tissue in the liver. Liver tumors as small as an inch across can now be detected by ultrasound or computed tomography scan (CT scan). Imaging studies, however, cannot tell the difference between a hepatoma and other abnormal masses or lumps of tissue (nodules) in the liver. A sample of liver tissue for **biopsy** is needed to make the definitive diagnosis of a primary liver cancer. CT or ultrasound can be used to guide the doctor in selecting the best location for obtaining the biopsy sample.

Chest **x rays** may be used to see whether the liver tumor is primary or has metastasized from a primary tumor in the lungs.

Liver biopsy

Liver biopsy is considered to provide the definite diagnosis of liver cancer. A sample of the liver or tissue fluid is removed with a fine needle and is checked under a microscope for the presence of cancer cells. In about 70% of cases, the biopsy is positive for cancer. In most cases, there is little risk to the patient from the biopsy procedure. In about 0.4% of cases, however, the patient develops a fatal hemorrhage from the biopsy because some tumors are supplied with a large number of blood vessels and bleed very easily.

Laparoscopy

The doctor may also perform a **laparoscopy** to help in the diagnosis of liver cancer. First, the doctor makes a small cut in the patient's abdomen and inserts a small, lighted tube called a laparoscope to view the area. A small piece of liver tissue is removed and examined under a microscope for the presence of cancer cells.

Clinical staging

Currently, the pathogenesis of HCC is not well understood. It is not clear how the different risk factors for HCC affect each other. In addition, the environmental factors vary from region to region.

Treatment

Treatment of liver cancer is based on several factors, including the type of cancer (primary or metastatic); stage (early or advanced); the location of other primary cancers or metastases in the patient's body; the patient's age; and other coexisting diseases, including cirrhosis. For many patients, treatment of liver cancer is primarily intended to relieve the pain caused by the cancer but cannot cure it.

Surgery

Few liver cancers in adults can be cured by surgery because they are usually too advanced by the time they are discovered. If the cancer is contained within one lobe of the liver, and if the patient does not have either cirrhosis, jaundice, or ascites, surgery is the best treatment option. Patients who can have their entire tumor removed have the best chance for survival. Unfortunately, only about 5% of patients with metastatic cancer (from primary tumors in the colon or rectum) fall into this group. If the entire visible tumor can be removed, about 25% of patients will be cured. The operation that is performed is called a partial hepatectomy, or partial removal of the liver. The surgeon will remove either an entire lobe of the liver (a **lobectomy**) or cut out the area around the tumor (a wedge resection).

A newer technique that is reported to be safe and effective is laparoscopic **radiofrequency ablation** (RFA). RFA is a technique in which the surgeon places a special needle electrode in the tumor under guidance from MRI or CT scanning. When the electrode has been properly placed, a radiofrequency current is passed through it, heating the tumor and killing the cancer cells. RFA can be used to treat tumors that are too small or too inaccessible for removal by conventional open surgery.

Chemotherapy

Some patients with metastatic cancer of the liver can have their lives prolonged for a few months by **chemotherapy**, although cure is not possible. If the tumor cannot be removed by surgery, a tube (catheter) can be placed in the main artery of the liver and an implantable infusion pump can be installed. The pump allows much higher concentrations of the cancer drug to be carried to the tumor than is possible with chemotherapy carried through the bloodstream. The drug that is used for infusion pump therapy is usually **floxuridine** (FUDR), given for 14-day periods alternating with 14-day rests. Systemic chemotherapy can also be used to treat liver cancer. The medications usually used are 5-fluorouracil (Adrucil, Efudex) or **methotrexate** (MTX, Mexate). Systemic chemotherapy does not, however, significantly lengthen the patient's survival time.

Radiation therapy

Radiation therapy is the use of high-energy rays or x rays to kill cancer cells or to shrink tumors. Its use in liver cancer, however, is only to give short-term relief from some of the symptoms. Liver cancers are not sensitive to radiation, and radiation therapy will not prolong the patient's life.

Liver transplantation

Removal of the entire liver (total hepatectomy) and liver transplantation can be used to treat liver cancer. However, there is a high risk of tumor recurrence and metastases after transplantation. In addition, most patients have cancer that is too far advanced at the time of diagnosis to benefit from liver transplantation.

Other therapies

Other therapeutic approaches include:

- Hepatic artery embolization with chemotherapy (chemoembolization).
- Alcohol ablation via ultrasound-guided percutaneous injection.
- Ultrasound-guided cryoablation.
- Immunotherapy with monoclonal antibodies tagged with cytotoxic agents.
- Gene therapy with retroviral vectors containing genes expressing cytotoxic agents.

Alternative and complementary therapies

Many patients find that alternative and complementary therapies help to reduce the stress associated with illness, improve immune function, and boost spirits. While there is no clinical evidence that these therapies specifically combat disease, such activities as biofeedback, relaxation, therapeutic touch, massage therapy and guided imagery have no side effects and have been reported to enhance well-being.

Several other healing therapies are sometimes used as supplemental or replacement cancer treatments, such as antineoplastons, cancell, cartilage (bovine and shark), laetrile, and **mistletoe**. Many of these therapies have not been the subject of safety and efficacy trials by the National Cancer Institute (NCI). The NCI has conducted trials on cancell, laetrile, and some other alternative therapies and found no anticancer activity. These treatments have varying effectiveness and safety considerations. Patients using any alternative remedy should first consult their doctors in order to prevent harmful side effects or interactions with traditional cancer treatment.

Prognosis

Liver cancer has a very poor prognosis because it is often not diagnosed until it has metastasized. Fewer than 10% of patients survive three years after the initial diagnosis; the overall five-year survival rate for patients with hepatomas is around 4%. Most patients with primary liver cancer die within six months of diagnosis, usually from liver failure; fewer than 5% are cured of the disease. Patients with liver cancers that metastasized from cancers in the colon live slightly longer than those whose cancers spread from cancers in the stomach or pancreas.

As of 2004, African American and Hispanic patients have much lower 5-year survival rates than Caucasian patients. It is not yet known, however, whether cultural differences as well as biological factors may be partly responsible for the variation in survival rates.

Coping with cancer treatment

Side effects of treatment, nutrition, emotional well-being, and other issues are all parts of coping with cancer. There are many possible side effects for a cancer treatment that include:

- constipation
- delirium
- fatigue
- fever, chills, sweats
- nausea and vomiting
- mouth sores, dry mouth, bleeding gums
- pruritus (itching)
- affected sexuality
- sleep disorders

Anxiety, **depression**, feelings of loss, post-traumatic stress disorder, affected **sexuality**, and **substance abuse** are all possible emotional side-effects. Patients should seek out a support network to help them through treatment. Loss of appetite before, during, and after a treatment can also be of concern. Other complications of coping with cancer treatment include fever and pain.

Clinical trials

As of 2004, the National Cancer Institute is sponsoring 55 **clinical trials** of treatments for primary liver cancer in adults and 13 trials for treatments of primary liver cancer in children. These trials allow researchers to investigate new types of radiation therapy and chemotherapy, new drugs and drug combinations, biological therapies, ways of combining various types of treatment for liver cancer, side effect reduction, and quality of life. Information on clinical trials can be acquired from the National Cancer Institute at http://www.nci.nih.gov or (800) 4-CANCER.

Prevention

There are no useful strategies at present for preventing metastatic cancers of the liver. Primary liver cancers, however, are 75–80% preventable. Current strategies focus on widespread vaccination for hepatitis B, early treatment of hereditary hemochromatosis (a metabolic disorder), and screening of high-risk patients with alpha-fetoprotein testing and ultrasound examinations.

Lifestyle factors that can be modified in order to prevent liver cancer include avoidance of exposure to toxic chemicals and foods harboring molds that produce aflatoxin. Most important, however, is avoidance of alcohol and drug abuse. Alcohol abuse is responsible for 60–75% of cases of cirrhosis, which is a major risk factor for eventual development of primary liver cancer. Hepatitis is a widespread disease among persons who abuse intravenous drugs.

See also Alcohol consumption; CT-guided biopsy; Hepatic arterial infusion; Immunologic therapy.

Resources

BOOKS

Beers, Mark H., MD, and Robert Berkow, MD, editors. "Primary Liver Cancer." In *The Merck Manual of Diagnosis and Therapy*. Whitehouse Station, NJ: Merck Research Laboratories, 2007.

PERIODICALS

Berber, E., A. Senagore, F. Remzi, et al. "Laparoscopic Radiofrequency Ablation of Liver Tumors Combined with Colorectal Procedures." *Surgical Laparoscopy, Endoscopy and Percutaneous Techniques* 14 (August 2004): 186–190.

Cahill, B. A., and D. Braccia. "Current Treatment for Hepatocellular Carcinoma." *Clinical Journal of Oncology Nursing* 8 (August 2004): 393–399.

Decadt, B., and A. K. Siriwardena. "Radiofrequency Ablation of Liver Tumours: Systematic Review." *Lancet Oncology* 5 (September 2004): 550–560.

Harrison, L. E., T. Reichman, B. Koneru, et al. "Racial Discrepancies in the Outcome of Patients with Hepatocellular Carcinoma." *Archives of Surgery* 139 (September 2004): 992–996.

Nguyen, M. H., A. S. Whittemore, R. T. Garcia, et al. "Role of Ethnicity in Risk for Hepatocellular Carcinoma in Patients with Chronic Hepatitis C and Cirrhosis." *Clinical Gastroenterology and Hepatology* 2 (September 2004): 820–824.

Stuart, Keith E., MD. "Hepatic Carcinoma, Primary." *eMedicine* July 20, 2004. http://www.emedicine.com/med/topic2664.htm.

OTHER

American Cancer Society (ACS). *Cancer Facts & Figures 2004*.http://www.cancer.org/downloads/STT/CAFF_finalPWSecured.pdf.

ORGANIZATIONS

American Cancer Society. 1599 Clifton Rd. NE, Atlanta, GA 30329. (800) 227-2345. http://www.cancer.org.

American Institute for Cancer Research (AICR). 1759 R St. NW, Washington, DC 20009. (800) 843-8114. http://www.aicr.org.

American Liver Foundation. 908 Pompton Ave., Cedar Grove, NJ 07009. (800) 223-0179.

Cancer Care, Inc. 275 Seventh Ave., New York, NY 10001.(800) 813-HOPE. http://www.cancercare.org.

Cancer Hope Network. Suite A., Two North Rd., Chester, NJ 07930. (877) HOPENET. http://www.cancerhopenetwork.org.

Hospicelink. Hospice Education Institute, 190 Westbrook Rd., Essex, CT, 06426-1510. (800) 331-1620. http://www.hospiceworld.com.

National Cancer Institute (National Institutes of Health). 9000 Rockville Pike, Bethesda, MD 20892. (800) 422-6237. http://www.nci.nih.gov.

The Wellness Community. Suite 412, 35 E. Seventh St., Cincinnati, OH 45202. (888) 793-9355. http://www.wellness-community.org.

Rebecca J. Frey, Ph.D.
Laura Ruth, Ph.D.

Liver cancer, secondary *see* **Metastasis**

Liver scan *see* **Nuclear medicine scans**

Lobectomy

Definition

A lobectomy is the removal of a lobe of one of the organs, usually referring to the brain, the lung, or the liver.

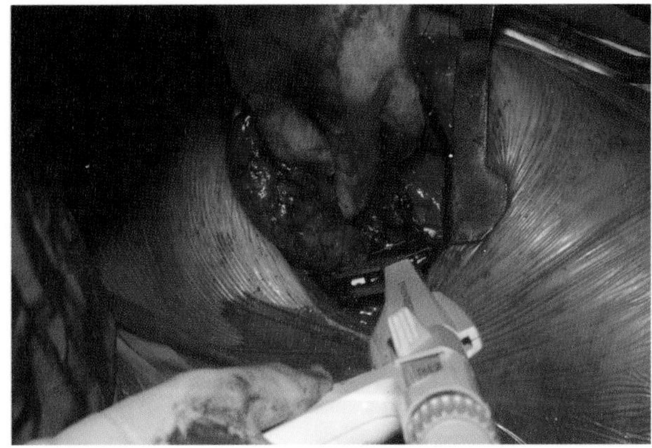

Left upper lobectomy. A surgeon is using a stapling device to ligate (tie or bind) the left upper bronchus. The lobar veins and arteries have already been ligated. *(Custom Medical Stock Photo. Reproduced by permission.)*

Purpose

Lobectomies are usually performed to prevent the spread of **cancer** from one part of an organ to other parts or to other parts of the body. Lobectomies also are performed on patients with severe seizure disorders (such as some forms of epilepsy) to prevent further seizures. However, there are differences in each of the three organs on which lobectomies may be performed.

Description

The brain

Each lobe of the brain performs a different function, and when part of the brain is removed, it does not grow back. However, other parts of the brain can take over some, or all, of the function of the missing part of the brain. Depending on the part of the brain removed, the effects may be quite severe, or nearly nonexistent.

Left upper lobectomy. A surgeon is using a stapling device to ligate (tie or bind) the left upper bronchus. The lobar veins and arteries have already been ligated.

The most commonly referenced brain lobectomy in the medical literature is the removal of the temporal lobe. Temporal lobectomy usually is performed to prevent debilitating seizures. Seizures are commonly caused by temporal lobe epilepsy, but can also be caused by **brain tumors** in the temporal lobe. Thus, lobectomy of the temporal lobe in patients with a temporal lobe tumor reduces or eliminates seizures, and has the beneficial side effect of removing the tumor mass.

QUESTIONS TO ASK THE DOCTOR

- What benefits can I expect from this operation?
- What are the risks of this operation?
- What are the normal results of this operation?
- What happens if this operation doesn't go as planned?
- What is the expected recovery time?

The lung

Lobectomies of the lung also are called pulmonary lobectomies. Each part of the lung performs the same function: it exchanges oxygen for carbon dioxide in the blood. There are many different lobes of the lung, however, and some lobes exchange more oxygen than others. Lobes of the lung do not regenerate after they are removed. Therefore, removal of a large portion of the lung may cause a person to need oxygen or ventilator support for the rest of his or her life. However, removal of a small portion of the lung may result in very little change to the patient's quality of life. A test (a quantitative ventilation/perfusion scan, or quantitative V/Q scan) may be used before surgery to help determine how much of the lung can safely be removed.

The outcome of lung lobectomies also depends on the general health of the entire lung; emphysema and smoking would have a negative impact on the health of a patient's lung. The surgeon may perform the surgery with video assistance and special tools to decrease pain and speed patient recovery following surgery.

The liver

A lobectomy of the liver is also called a hepatic lobectomy. The liver plays a major role in digestion, in the transformation of food into energy, and in filtering and storing blood. It processes nutrients and drugs, produces bile, controls the level of glucose (sugar) in the blood, detoxifies blood, and regulates blood clotting. Unlike the brain and the lung, the liver may regrow, or regenerate, after part of the liver has been removed. In addition, since every part of the liver performs the same functions, the liver is the organ whose function is least likely to be severely affected by lobectomy, in the long term, because it regenerates. However, as the liver is central to the body's functions, removal of too much of the liver at once may result in coma or death.

Precautions

Brain lobectomies should not be performed unless the patient has been unable to control seizures through medication. Additionally, the seizures must be caused by a single, relatively small, localized part of the brain that can be resected without severe damage. Lung lobectomies should only be performed on patients with early stage non-small cell **carcinoma** of the lung, or as part of a combination of therapies at later stages. Since even a "complete removal" of the tumor does not result in an overwhelming survival rate after five years, other therapies also may be considered. Small cell cancer of the lung does not respond to surgical intervention. Patients with liver disease that is too extensive may need a liver transplant rather than a liver lobectomy. Patients with blood clotting problems, either due to chemotherapeutic agents or for other reasons, should have these problems addressed before surgery.

Preparation

Before surgery, patients should not take aspirin or ibuprofen for one week. Patients also should consult their physician about any blood-thinning medications such as coumadin or **warfarin**. The night before surgery, patients will usually be asked not to eat or drink after a certain time.

Aftercare

Each surgery offers different aftercare challenges. Patients may need to be hospitalized for some time after the operation. Patients with portions of their brain removed may require rehabilitation of a physical, mental, or emotional nature depending on the portion of the brain that has been removed. Patients who have had portions of their lungs removed probably will require a tube in their chest to drain fluid, and may require a machine to help them breathe. They also may require oxygen, either on a temporary or permanent basis. Patients who have had hepatic lobectomies also may have drainage tubes, and may also have initial dietary restrictions. Physicians should be consulted for the specifics of aftercare in each individual situation.

Risks

Specific risks vary from surgery to surgery and should be discussed with a physician. In general, any surgery requiring a general anesthetic may, uncommonly, result in death. Improperly performed brain surgery may result in permanent brain damage. Depending on the surgeon and the size of the tissue removed, patients may be at risk for some types of brain damage. As previously mentioned, patients having part of a lung removed may have difficulty breathing and may require the use of oxygen. Patients also may experience **infection** (**pneumonia**), or blood clots. Liver resection (surgery) may result in the following complications: coma, slow return of normal bowel function, and biliary leakage.

Normal results

Most patients who undergo temporal lobectomy experience few or no seizures after surgery (some estimates range from about 70% to about 90% success rate). Unfortunately, lung lobectomy is not as successful. 50% of cancer patients with completely removable stage I non-small cell cancer of the lung survive five years after the procedure. If the cancer has progressed beyond this stage, or if the cancer is not completely removable, the chances for survival drop significantly. The results of liver resection vary. The possible outcomes of each surgical type should be discussed with the patient's physician. Generally, the less severe the cancer, and the less tissue that needs to be removed, the better the outcome.

Abnormal results

Abnormal results vary from operation to operation and should be discussed thoroughly with the patient's physician before surgery. Patients who undergo temporal lobectomy may, rarely, die as a result of the operation (a complication in less than 1% of patients). Patients also may have problems with their vision, or problems with speech. Abnormal results from the removal of part of the lung could include pneumonia or blood clots (which may result in stroke, heart attack, or other problems) after the surgery. Also, a small percentage of patients undergoing lung lobectomy die during or soon after the surgery. The percentage of patients who suffer death varies from about 3–6% depending on the amount of lung tissue removed. Finally, abnormal outcomes from liver resection can include coma, death, and problems with liver function.

Resources

PERIODICALS

Namori, Hiroaki, et al. "Thoracoscopic Lobotomy for Lung Cancer with a Largely Fused Fissure." *Chest* 9, no. 10 (February 2003): 19–23.

Tatum, W. O., and S. R. Benbadis. "The Neurosurgical Treatment of Epilepsy." *Archives of Family Medicine* 9, no. 10 (November-December 2000): 1142–1147.

OTHER

*Harrison's Principles of Internal Medicine online, Chapter 90: Neoplasms of the lung.*http://www.harrisonsonline.com/.

Koike, Atsushi, M.A., Hiroyuki Shimizu, M.D., Ichiro Suzuki, M.D., Buichi Ishijima, M.D., and Morihiro Sugishita, Dr. H.S., Dr. M.S. "Preserved musical abilities following right temporal lobectomy." *Journal of Neurosurgery*. December 1996. [cited July 24, 2005]. http://www.c3.hu/~mavideg/jns/1-4-prev1.html.

"Lung Surgery." *Healthsquare.com*.http://www.healthsquare.com/htm.

Michael Zuck, Ph.D.
Teresa G. Odle

Lomustine

Definition

Lomustine is one of the anticancer (antineoplastic) drugs in a class called alkylating agents. It is available under the brand name CeeNU. Another commonly used name is CCNU.

Purpose

Lomustine is primarily used to treat **brain tumors** and **Hodgkin's disease**, which is a type of **cancer** that affects the lymph nodes and spleen.

Description

Lomustine chemically interferes with the synthesis of genetic material (DNA and RNA) of cancer cells, which prevents these cells from being able to reproduce and continue the growth of the cancer.

Recommended dosage

Lomustine is taken orally (in pill form). The dosage is typically 100–130 mg per square meter of body surface area once every 6 weeks. Lomustine should be taken on an empty stomach just prior to bedtime to prevent possible **nausea** and/or **vomiting**. Patients should avoid alcohol one hour before and shortly after taking lomustine.

KEY TERMS

Antineoplastic—A drug that prevents the growth of a neoplasm by interfering with the maturation or proliferation of the cells of the neoplasm.

Neoplasm—New abnormal growth of tissue.

Hodgkins disease—A disease characterized by enlargement of the lymph nodes and spleen.

Precautions

Lomustine can cause an allergic reaction in some people. Patients with a prior allergic reaction to lomustine should not take this drug.

Lomustine can cause harm to the fetus if a woman is taking this drug during pregnancy. Women of childbearing potential should use appropriate contraceptive measures to prevent pregnancy while on lomustine. There have been reports of infertility in men taking this drug due to testicular damage.

It is not known if lomustine is excreted in breast milk. Because of the potential of severe adverse effect, it is recommended that breastfeeding women should discuss with their physician the risk versus benefit of breastfeeding while taking lomustine.

Side effects

Common side effects of lomustine include nausea and/or vomiting, as well as an increased susceptibility to **infection** due to decreased production in the cells that fight infections. Patients should avoid crowds or exposure to any individuals who may have infections. Also, an increased risk of bleeding can occur due to decreased production of the platelets that are involved with the blood clotting process.

Less common side effects that may also occur include loss of appetite (**anorexia**), **diarrhea**, temporary hair loss (**alopecia**), and skin rash.

A doctor should be consulted immediately if the patient experiences any of the following effects:

- black, tarry or bloody stools
- blood in the urine
- confusion
- persistent cough
- fever and chills
- sore throat
- red spots on the skin

- shortness of breath
- unusual bleeding or bruising

Interactions

Lomustine should not be taken in combination with any prescription drug, over-the-counter drug, or herbal remedy without prior consultation with a physician.

Paul A. Johnson, Ed.M.

Loperamide *see* **Antidiarrheal agents**

Lorazepam

Definition

Lorazepam is a mild tranquilizer in the benzodiazepine class of drugs. It is used to treat anxiety, **nausea and vomiting**, insomnia, and seizures.

Purpose

Lorazepam is used:

- to treat anxiety
- to control muscle spasms that sometimes accompany severe pain
- to treat insomnia
- prior to the administration of chemotherapy to decrease the incidence of nausea and vomiting
- in combination with other drugs to help control nausea and vomiting associated with cancer treatment
- prior to surgery or other procedures to relieve anxiety, induce drowsiness and sedation, and reduce memories of the procedure
- in its injectable form, to control seizures

Description

Benzodiazepines depress the central nervous system primarily by enhancing the function of gamma-aminobutyric acid (GABA), a neurotransmitter that inhibits the transmission of nerve impulses in the brain and spinal cord. Lorazepam differs from other benzodiazepines, such as **diazepam** (Valium) and chlordiazepoxide (Librium), in that it is shorter-acting and does not accumulate in the body with repeated doses.

Lorazepam is available as 0.5-milligram (mg), 1-mg, and 2-mg tablets and in an intramuscular or intravenous injectable form. It is available as a generic drug.

U.S. brand names

- Ativan
- Lorzepam Intensol

Canadian brand names

- Ativan
- Apo-Lorazepam
- Novo-Lorazepam
- Nu-Loraz
- PMS-Lorazepam
- Riva-Lorazepam

International brand names

- Ativan
- Lorans
- Lorazepam
- Lorivan
- Sinestron
- Tavor
- Temesta

Recommended dosage

The lorazepam dosage is adjusted to the smallest dose that relieves symptoms. The usual recommended dosages are:

- 1–6 mg every 8–12 hours to relieve anxiety, with a maximum total daily dosage of 10 mg in two to three divided doses
- 0.05 mg per kilogram (kg) body weight every four to eight hours in infants and children for anxiety and sedation
- 2–4 mg at bedtime as a sleep aid
- 0.5–2 mg per day in divided doses for elderly or debilitated patients
- 0.5–1 mg every six to eight hours to control nausea and vomiting related to cancer or other medical treatments
- 2 mg 30 minutes prior to receiving chemotherapy and an additional 2 mg every four hours as needed to prevent stomach upset
- 0.05 mg per kg, up to 2 mg per intravenous dose, in children aged 2–15 prior to chemotherapy
- 2.5–5 mg prior to surgery

- 4 mg intravenously for seizures; increased to 8 mg in unresponsive patients

A missed dose should be taken as soon as possible, but two doses should not be taken at the same time. Lorazepam can be taken with or without food.

Precautions

Patients should not drive, operate machinery or appliances, or perform hazardous activities that require mental alertness until they have a sense of how lorazepam affects them. Lorazepam injection may impair performance and driving ability for 24–48 hours.

Lorazepam, like other drugs of this type, can cause physical and psychological dependence. Patients should not increase the dosage or frequency of this drug on their own, nor should they stop taking this medication suddenly. Instead, when stopping the drug, the dosage should gradually be decreased and then discontinued. Stopping lorazepam abruptly can cause agitation, irritability, insomnia, convulsions, and other withdrawal symptoms.

Pediatric

Lorazepam is not usually given to children under age 12. Children between the ages of 12 and 18 can be given oral lorazepam, although it is only approved as an antianxiety medication by the U.S. Food and Drug Administration (FDA) for those 18 and older. Intravenous lorazepam may be administered to children prior to **chemotherapy**.

Geriatric

Lorazepam injection may impair driving ability and performance for a longer period in older patients. The elderly dosage is normally lower, with a maximum initial dose of 2 mg.

Pregnant or breastfeeding

Pregnant women and those trying to become pregnant should not take lorazepam. This drug has been associated with fetal malformations when taken during the first three months of pregnancy. It can cause respiratory **depression** if administered near the time of delivery. Women should not breastfeed while taking lorazepam, since it passes into breast milk.

Other conditions and allergies

Lorazepam should not be used by patients with:

- narrow-angle glaucoma
- pre-existing depression of the central nervous system
- severe uncontrolled pain
- severe low blood pressure
- allergies to benzodiazepines

Lorazepam should be used with caution in patients with:

- kidney or liver disease
- myasthenia gravis
- lung disease
- alcohol intoxication
- a history of drug or alcohol abuse

Side effects

Drowsiness and sleepiness are common and expected effects of lorazepam. Possible side effects include dizziness, unsteadiness, clumsiness, or weakness. Patients may have difficulty walking and be prone to falls for up to eight hours after receiving a lorazepam injection, so they should request assistance.

Less common side effects of lorazepam include:

- decreased sex drive
- nausea
- headache
- insomnia
- rash
- vomiting
- dry mouth
- constipation
- yellowing eyes
- vision changes
- hallucinations
- redness and pain at the injection site
- high or low blood pressure and partial blockage of the airways following injection

Serious side effects that require a physician's attention include:

- depression
- confusion
- agitation
- nightmares
- impaired coordination
- personality changes
- changes in urinary patterns
- chest pain
- heart palpitations

Symptoms of lorazepam overdose include:

- confusion
- coma

QUESTIONS TO ASK YOUR PHARMACIST

- Will lorazepam interact with my other medications?
- Can I drink alcohol while taking lorazepam?
- What if I forget a dose?
- Can I take lorazepam on an as-needed basis?
- Can I take more than the prescribed dose?
- Can I stop taking lorazepam abruptly?

- slowed reflexes
- difficulty breathing

Geriatric

Patients over age 50 may experience greater and longer sedation after administration of lorazepam. These side effects may subside with continued use or dosage reduction.

Interactions

Alcohol and other central nervous system depressants can increase the drowsiness associated with lorazepam. Central nervous system depressants include some pain and over-the-counter (OTC) medications, as well as the herbs kava, St. John's wort, gotu kola, and valerian. Patients should check with their doctor before beginning any new medication, herb, or supplement. Alcohol should be avoided when taking lorazepam, since the drug diminishes alcohol tolerance.

Lorazepam injection may impair driving ability and performance for a longer period in those taking other central nervous system depressants, including some pain medications. Patients should refrain from alcohol for 24–48 hours after a lorazepam injection. When injected, lorazepam may also interact with **scopolamine**, causing drowsiness, odd behavior, and hallucinations.

Resources

BOOKS

Hales, Robert E., et al. *What Your Patients Need To Know About Psychiatric Medications*. Washington, DC: American Psychiatric Publishing, 2007.

Toufexis, Donna, and Sayamwong E. Hammac. *Anti-Anxiety Drugs*. New York: Chelsea House Publishers, 2006.

PERIODICALS

Giersch, Anne, et al. "Impairment of Contrast Sensitivity in Long-Term Lorazepam Users." *Psychopharmacology* 186, no. 4 (July 2006): 594–600.

Hung, Yi-Yung, and Tiao-Lai Huang. "Lorazepam and Diazepam Rapidly Relieve Catatonic Features in Major Depression." *Clinical Neuropharmacology* 29, no. 3 (May–June 2006): 144–147.

Izaute, M., and E. Bacon. "Effects of the Amnesic Drug Lorazepam on Complete and Partial Information Retrieval and Monitoring Accuracy." *Psychopharmacology* 188, no. 4 (November 2006): 472–481.

Kamboj, Sunjeev K., and H. Valerie Curran. "Neutral and Emotional Episodic Memory: Global Impairment After Lorazepam or Scopolamine." *Psychopharmacology* 188, no. 4 (November 2006): 482–488.

Pomara, Nunzio, et al. ldquo;Dose-Dependent Retrograde Facilitation of Verbal Memory in Healthy Elderly After Acute Oral Lorazepam Administration." *Psychopharmacology* 185, no.4 (May 2006): 487–494.

Yacoub, Adee, and Andrew Francis. "Neuroleptic Malignant Syndrome Induced by Atypical Neuroleptics and Responsive to Lorazepam." *Neuropsychiatric Disease and Treatment* 2, no. 2 (2006): 235–240.

OTHER

American Society of Health-System Pharmacists. "Lorazepam." *MedlinePlus*. http://www.nlm.nih.gov/medlineplus/druginfo/meds/a682053.html.

"Lorazepam." *University of Maryland Medical Center*. http://www.umm.edu/altmed/drugs/lorazepam-077600.htm

U.S. Food and Drug Administration. "Drug Details: Lorazepam." *Drugs@FDA*. http://www.accessdata.fda.gov/scripts/cder/drugsatfda/index.cfm?fuseaction=Search.DrugDetails.

ORGANIZATIONS

American Academy of Child & Adolescent Psychiatry, 3615 Wisconsin Avenue, NW , Washington, DC, 20016-3007, (202) 966-7300, (202) 966-2891, http://www.aacap.org.

National Institute of Mental Health, 6001 Executive Boulevard, Room 8184, MSC 9663, Bethesda, MD, 20892-9663, (301) 443-4513, (866) 615-6464 , (301) 443-4279, nimhinfo@nih.gov, http://www.nimh.nih.gov.

U.S. Food and Drug Administration, 10903 New Hampshire Ave., Silver Spring, MD, 20993-0002, (888) INFO-FDA, http://www.fda.gov.

Debra Wood, RN
Teresa G. Odle
Ajna Hamidovic, PharmD
Ruth A. Wienclaw, PhD
Margaret Alic, PhD

Loss of Appetite *see* **Anorexia**

Low molecular weight heparins

Definition

Low molecular weight heparins (LMWHs) belong to a class of medications known as blood thinners. They are used to stop blood clots from forming and growing.

Purpose

LMWHs are used to prevent and treat blood clots in persons undergoing certain types of surgery, recent heart attack, severe chest pain caused by disease of heart vessels usually from fat deposits (unstable angina), and people who have blood clots in their veins (also known as deep vein thrombosis or DVT) or lungs (also known as pulmonary embolism or PE). As of 2001, there are three drugs that belong to the class of LMWHs: enoxaparin, dalteparin, and tinzaparin. All three have the same mechanism of action, but differ in their doses, structures, and Food and Drug Administration (FDA) indicated uses.

Many **cancer** patients can become prone to hypercoagulation, or overactive thickening and clotting of the blood. This makes the patient more likely to experience deep vein thrombosis, possibly leading to death.

Description

LMWHs only became available in the mid-1990s, with enoxaparin (Lovenox) being the first and most studied drug in its class. Dalteparin (Fragmin) was the second LMWH to become available and tinzaparin (Innohep) is the latest addition to this class. These medicines work by inhibiting certain clotting factors in the blood (Factor Xa and thrombin) and preventing blood clots from forming and getting bigger.

LMWHs are closely related to **heparin**, which is one of the oldest blood thinners available. These drugs have an advantage over heparin in that they have longer duration in the body, more predictable effects after a given dose, require less blood tests to check for their effectiveness and side effects, and do not have to be given in the hospital setting only. LMWHs have been found to be safe and effective in blood clot prevention after general surgery, orthopedic surgery, neurosurgery, multiple trauma, hip fracture, certain types of stroke, unstable angina, heart attack and treatment DVT and PE. These drugs are usually given with **warfarin** (Coumadin) for treatment of blood clots and with aspirin for prevention of complications after heart attack or angina attack. Besides their use for blood clot prevention and treatment, there have been some research studies in animals and humans to suggest that they may prevent cancer by decreasing the blood supply needed for the tumor to grow. The effects of LMWHs on patients with cancer and blood clots are being investigated. In 2004, clinical trails suggested that LMWHs might interfere with tumor growth and cancer spread, but further study was needed.

KEY TERMS

Deep vein thrombosis—Also known as DVT, a condition in which a blood clot (thrombus) formed in one part of the circulation, becomes detached and lodges at another point (usually in one of the veins of the legs or arms). People may feel pain, redness, and swelling at the site where the blood clot lodges in. This condition is treated with blood thinning drugs such as LMWHs, heparin, or warfarin.

Pulmonary embolism—Also known as PE, a condition in which a blood clot usually formed in of the leg veins becomes detached and lodges in the lung artery or one of its branches. Patients may be coughing up blood and experience trouble breathing. This condition is treated with blood thinning drugs such as LMWHs, heparin, or warfarin.

Recommended dosage

Administration

These medicines are given by injection beneath the skin (subcutaneous injection) and should not be injected directly into the vein or muscle. Injections can be given around the navel, upper thigh or buttock. The injection site should be changed daily. Massaging of the site before injection with an ice cube can decrease excessive bruising.

Doses and indications differ between three medicines. These drugs can not be used interchangeably for one another.

Adults

PREVENTION OF BLOOD CLOTS AFTER ORTHOPEDIC SURGERY. The usual dose of tinzaparin is 50 units per kg daily starting two hours before surgery and continuing for 7–10 days. Doses of 75 units per kg per day have also been studied.

PREVENTION OF BLOOD CLOTS AFTER HIP OR KNEE REPLACEMENT SURGERY. Doses vary between different agents. The usual enoxaparin dose is 30 mg every 12 hours starting 12–24 hours after surgery in patients undergoing hip or knee surgery. Alternatively, 40 mg once a day with the first dose given approximately 12 hours before surgery can be used in patients undergoing hip replacement surgery. The average duration of the initial phase of treatment is 7–10 days (up to 14 days). After the initial phase, 40 mg once a day for three weeks is recommended.

For people undergoing hip replacement surgery, 5,000 units of dalteparin are given 10–14 hours before surgery, then 5,000 units 4–8 hours after surgery, followed by 5,000 units daily. The therapy is usually continued for five to ten days (up to 14 days). A physician should be consulted for alternative dosing regimens.

PREVENTION OF DVT IN PATIENTS AT HIGH RISK FOR BLOOD CLOTS AFTER ABDOMINAL SURGERY.. Enoxaparin is usually given at a dose of 40 mg once daily with the first dose given two hours before surgery for seven to ten days, up to 12 days.

In patients who are at moderate to high risk of blood clots, the usual dose of dalteparin is 2,500 units daily generally given for five to ten days. The first dose should be given one to two hours before surgery. In patients who are at high to very high risk of blood clots (those with cancer or history of DVT or PE) 5,000 units are given on the evening before surgery, followed by 5,000 units/day for five to ten days. A physician should be consulted for alternative dosing schedules.

Tinzaparin is usually dosed at 3,500 units daily starting two hours before surgery and continuing for seven to ten days.

TREATMENT OF DVT WITH OR WITHOUT PE. Enoxaparin doses of 1 mg per kg twice a day are given when people are treated at home. People who are treated in the hospital can be given 1 mg per kg twice a day or 1.5 mg per kg at the same time once a day. Warfarin is usually given to finish treatment and the two drugs overlap for about 72 hours until good response to warfarin is confirmed by blood tests.

Tinzaparin is usually dosed at 175 units per kg daily for six days or until good response to warfarin is confirmed by blood tests.

UNSTABLE ANGINA OR HEART ATTACK. In patients who are also getting aspirin the usual dose of enoxaparin is 1 mg per kg every 12 hours for a minimum of two days (usually two to eight days).

The usual dose of dalteparin in people who are also getting aspirin is 120 units per kg (up to a maximum 10,000 units) every 12 hours. Treatment should continue until the patient is stable for five to eight days.

Children

TREATMENT OF DVT WITH OR WITHOUT PE. Children younger than two months of age should receive enoxaparin 1.5 mg per kg every 12 hours. Children older than two months of age should receive enoxaparin 1 mg per kg every 12 hours. A physician will do a blood test four to six hours after the dose to check for effectiveness.

PREVENTION OF BLOOD CLOTS. The usual dose of enoxaparin is 0.75 mg per kg every 12 hours for children younger than two months and 0.5 mg per kg every 12 hours for children older than two months of age. A physician will do a blood test four to six hours after the dose to check for effectiveness.

Precautions

The use of LMWHs should be avoided in persons undergoing any procedure involving spinal puncture or anesthesia. Using these medicines before these procedures has caused severe bruising and bleeding into the spine and can lead to paralysis.

The use of these medicines should be avoided in patients with allergies to LMWHs, heparin, or pork products, allergies to sulfites or benzyl alcohol, people with active major bleeding, and people with a history of heparin-induced low blood platelet count (also known as heparin-induced **thrombocytopenia** or HIT).

LMWHs should be used with caution in the following persons:

- people with bleeding disorders
- people with a history of recent stomach ulcers
- people who recently had brain, spine, or eye surgery
- people on other blood thinners (such as warfarin, aspirin, ibuprofen, naproxen) because of increased risk of bleeding
- people with kidney or liver disease (the dose of LMWHs may need to be decreased)
- breast-feeding mothers (it is not known if these medicines cross into breast milk)
- women who are pregnant, unless benefits to the mother outweigh the risks to the baby

A doctor should be contacted immediately if any of these symptoms develop:

- tingling, weakness, numbness or pain
- blood in the urine or stool
- itching, swelling, skin rash, trouble breathing
- unusual bleeding or bruising

A physician may perform blood tests during therapy with LMWHs to prevent side effects. Blood tests to check for effectiveness of these medicines are usually not needed, except in children, people with kidney disease, and overweight persons.

Side effects

The most common side effects of LMWHs include irritation and pain at the injection site, easy bruising and bleeding, **fever**, increase in liver enzyme tests usually without symptoms, and allergic reactions. Severe painful erection sometimes requiring surgery has been reported with tinzaparin in some patients. LMWHs can lower platelet counts, which may necessitate discontinuation.

Interactions

LMWHs should be used with caution in people on other oral blood thinners (aspirin, non-steroidal anti-inflammatory drugs, warfarin, and ticlopidine) because of increased risk of bleeding. If using both drugs together is necessary, the patients must be closely monitored.

Resources

PERIODICALS

"Low-molecular Weight Heparins May Interfere With Tumor Growth and Metastasis." *Drug Week* (July 2, 2004): 269.

Olga Bessmertny, Pharm.D.
Teresa G. Odle

Lumbar puncture

Definition

Lumbar puncture (LP) is the technique of using a needle to withdraw cerebrospinal fluid (CSF) from the spinal canal. CSF is the clear, watery liquid that protects the central nervous system from injury and cushions it from the surrounding bone structure. It contains a variety of substances, particularly glucose (sugar), protein, and white blood cells from the immune system.

Purpose

Lumbar puncture (spinal tap) is used to diagnose some malignancies, such as certain types of brain **cancer** and leukemia, as well as other medical conditions that affect the central nervous system. It is sometimes used to assess patients with certain psychiatric symptoms and conditions.

It is also used for injecting **chemotherapy** directly into the CSF. This type of treatment is called intrathecal therapy. Other medical conditions diagnosed with lumbar puncture include:

- viral and bacterial meningitis
- syphilis, a sexually transmitted disease
- bleeding (hemorrhaging) around the brain and spinal cord
- multiple sclerosis, a disease that affects the myelin coating of the nerve fibers of the brain and spinal cord
- Guillain-Barré syndrome, an inflammation of the nerves

Precautions

In some circumstances, a lumbar puncture to withdraw a small amount of CSF for analysis may lead to serious complications. Lumbar puncture should be performed only with extreme caution, and only if the benefits are thought to outweigh the risks, in certain conditions. For example, in people who have blood clotting (coagulation) or bleeding disorders or who are on anticoagulant treatment, lumbar puncture can cause bleeding that can compress the spinal cord. The term for this condition is spinal subdural hematoma, and it is a rare complication. However, it is of concern to some cancer patients whose low platelet counts (**thrombocytopenia**) make them more susceptible to bleeding. In some cases, these patients are given a platelet transfusion prior to lumbar puncture, but this procedure is still under investigation. A 1984–88 study, supported in part by the National Cancer Institute, researched the risk of lumbar puncture on children with acute lymphoblastic leukemia (ALL). No serious lumbar puncture complications were observed in this study of over 5,000 children.

Lumbar puncture has been shown to be less precise than some other methods in monitoring intracranial fluid pressure. A transducer provides more accurate information about changes in the flow of blood and cerebrospinal fluid within the brain.

A traumatic lumbar puncture (TLP) occurs when a blood vessel is inadvertently ruptured during the procedure. If this happens as part of a diagnostic

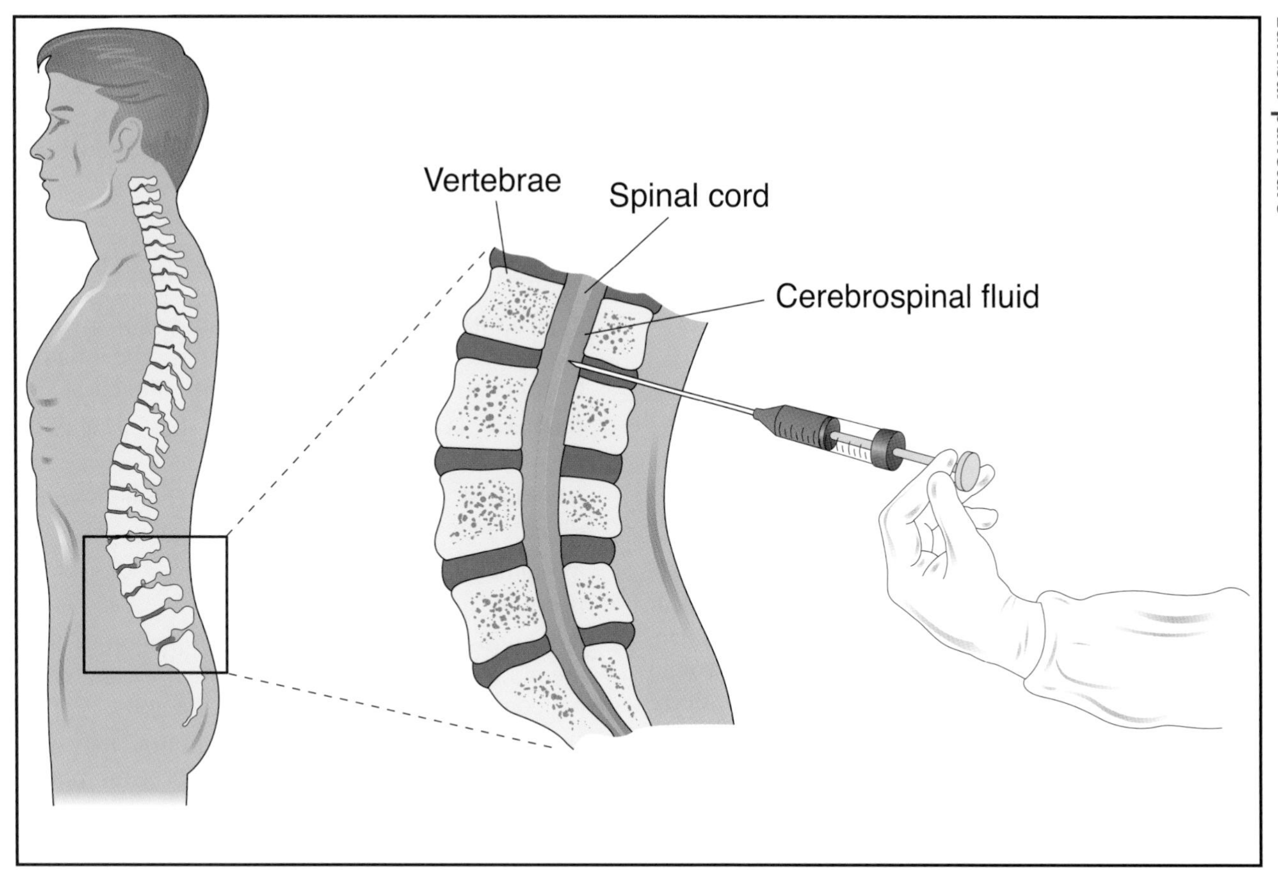

During a lumbar puncture, or spinal tap, the physician inserts a hollow thin needle in the space between two vertebrae of the lower back and slowly advances it toward the spine. The cerebrospinal fluid pressure is then measured and some fluid is withdrawn for laboratory analysis. *(Illustration by Electronic Illustrators Group. Cengage Learning, Gale.)*

leukemia workup, there is the potential of contaminating the CSF specimen that has been removed with leukemia cells, causing a false positive test result.

If there is a large brain tumor or other mass, removal of CSF can cause pressure shifts within the brain (herniation), causing compression of the brain stem and other vital structures, and leading to irreversible brain damage or death. These problems are easily avoided by checking blood coagulation through a blood test and by doing a **computed tomography** scan (CT) or **magnetic resonance imaging** (MRI) scan before attempting the lumbar puncture. In addition, a lumbar puncture procedure should never be performed at the site of a localized skin **infection** on the lower back because the infection may be introduced into the CSF and may spread to the brain or spinal cord.

Description

In a lumbar puncture, the area of the spinal column used to obtain the CSF sample is in the lumbar spine, or lower section of the back. In rare instances, such as a spinal fluid blockage in the middle of the back, a doctor may perform a spinal tap in the neck. The lower lumbar spine (usually between the vertebrae known as L4–5) is preferable because the spinal cord stops near L2, and a needle introduced below this level will miss the spinal cord and encounter only nerve roots, which are easily pushed aside.

A lumbar puncture takes about 15–30 minutes. Patients can undergo the test in a doctor's office, laboratory, or outpatient hospital setting. Sometimes it requires an inpatient hospital stay. If the patient has severe osteoarthritis of the spine, is extremely uncooperative, or obese, it may be necessary to introduce the spinal needle using x-ray guidance.

In order to get an accurate sample of cerebrospinal fluid, it is critical that a patient is in the proper position. The spine must be curved to allow as much space as possible between the lower vertebrae, or bones of the back, for the doctor to insert a lumbar puncture needle between the vertebrae and withdraw a

QUESTIONS TO ASK THE DOCTOR

- What is the purpose of my lumbar puncture?
- What aftercare will be needed?
- Will lumbar puncture be used for chemotherapy, and if so, how often will I receive treatments?
- What are the risks for diagnostic procedures or treatments through lumbar puncture?
- What do the test results mean?
- What techniques are suggested to relax children before and after a lumbar puncture?

small amount of fluid. The most common position is for the patient to lie on his or her side with the back at the edge of the exam table, head and chin bent down, knees drawn up to the chest, and arms clasped around the knees. (Small infants and people who are obese may need to curve their spines in a sitting position.) People should talk to their doctors if they have any questions about their position because it is important to be comfortable and to remain still during the entire procedure. In fact, the doctor will explain the procedure to the patient (or guardian) so that the patient can agree in writing to have it done (informed consent). If the patient is anxious or uncooperative, a short-acting sedative may be given.

During a lumbar puncture, the doctor drapes the back with a sterile covering that has an opening over the puncture site and cleans the skin surface with an antiseptic solution. Patients receive a local anesthetic to minimize any pain in the lower back.

The doctor inserts a thin hollow needle in the space between two vertebrae of the lower back and slowly advances it through ligamentous tissues toward the spine. A steady flow of clear cerebrospinal fluid, normally the color of water, will begin to fill the needle as soon as it enters the spinal canal. The doctor measures the cerebrospinal fluid pressure with a special instrument called a manometer and withdraws several vials of fluid for laboratory analysis. The amount of fluid collected depends on the type and number of tests needed to diagnose a particular medical disorder.

In some cases, the doctor must remove and reposition the needle. This occurs when there is not an even flow of fluid, the needle hits bone or a blood vessel, or the patient reports sharp, unusual pain.

KEY TERMS

Acute lymphoblastic leukemia (ALL)—A type of leukemia, also called acute lymphocytic leukemia, primarily in children, affecting lymphocytes.

Encephalitis—An inflammation or infection of the brain and spinal cord caused by a virus or as a complication of another infection.

Guillain-Barré syndrome—An inflammation involving nerves that affects the extremities. The inflammation may spread to the face, arms, and chest.

Immune system—Protects the body against infection.

Intrathecal therapy—Injecting chemotherapy directly into the CSF using lumbar puncture.

Manometer—A device used to measure fluid pressure.

Meningitis—An infection or inflammation of the membranes or tissues that cover the brain and spinal cord, and caused by bacteria or a virus.

Multiple sclerosis—A disease that destroys the covering (myelin sheath) of nerve fibers of the brain and spinal cord.

Spinal canal—The cavity or hollow space within the spine that contains cerebrospinal fluid.

Thrombocytopenia—Reduced platelet levels.

Vertebrae—The bones of the spinal column. There are 33 along the spine, with five (called L1–L5) making up the lower lumbar region.

Preparation

Patients can go about their normal activities before a lumbar puncture. Experts recommend that patients relax before the procedure to release any muscle tension, since the lumbar puncture needle must pass through muscle tissue before it reaches the spinal canal. A patient's level of relaxation before and during the procedure plays a critical role in the test's success. Relaxation may be difficult for those patients who face frequent lumbar punctures, such as children with leukemia. In these cases, it is especially important for the child to receive psychological support before and after each procedure. It may be helpful to praise a child who remained still and quiet during the procedure, and to remind the child of his or her good behavior before the next lumbar puncture.

Aftercare

After the procedure, the doctor covers the site of the puncture with a sterile bandage. Patients must avoid sitting or standing and remain lying down for as long as six hours after the lumbar puncture. They should also drink plenty of fluids to help prevent lumbar puncture headache, which is discussed in the next section.

Risks

The most common side effect of lumbar puncture is a headache. This problem occurs in 10–20% of adult patients and in up to 40% of children. It is caused by decreased CSF pressure related to a small leak of CSF through the puncture site. These headaches usually are a dull pain, although some people report a throbbing sensation. A stiff neck and **nausea** may accompany the headache. A lumbar puncture headache typically begins within a few hours to two days after the procedure and usually persists a few days, although it can last several weeks or months.

In some cases, the headache can be prevented by lying flat for an hour after the lumbar puncture, and taking in more fluids for 24 hours after the procedure. Since an upright position worsens the pain, lying flat also helps control the pain, along with prescription or non–prescription pain relief medication, preferably one containing caffeine. In rare cases, the puncture site leak is "patched" using the patient's own blood. People may also experience back pain. Headaches and backaches appear to be more common in adolescents than in younger children, and more common in girls than in boys.

Patients who receive **anticancer drugs** through lumbar puncture sometimes have **nausea and vomiting**. Intrathecal **methotrexate** can cause mouth sores. Some of these symptoms may be relieved by anti-nausea drugs prescribed by the physician.

In a very few cases, lumbar puncture in infants can lead to such complications as paraplegia. These complications are associated with the smaller size of the infant's central nervous system and increased difficulty in avoiding certain parts of the spinal cord when performing an LP.

People should talk to their doctors about complications from a lumbar puncture. In most cases, this procedure is safe and effective. Some patients experience pain, difficulty urinating, infection, or leakage of cerebrospinal fluid from the puncture site after the procedure.

Normal results

Normal CSF is clear and colorless. It may be straw or yellow–colored if there is excess protein, which may occur with cancer or inflammation. It may be cloudy in infections; blood–tinged if there was recent bleeding; or yellow to brown (xanthochromic) if caused by an older instance of bleeding.

A series of laboratory tests analyze the CSF for a variety of substances to rule out cancer or other medical disorders of the central nervous system. The following are normal values for commonly tested substances:

- CSF pressure: 50–180 mm H_2O
- Glucose: 40–85 mg/dL
- Protein: 15–50 mg/dL
- Leukocytes (white blood cells) total less than 5 per mL
- Lymphocytes (specific type of white blood cell): 60–70%
- Monocytes (a kind of white blood cell): 30–50%
- Neutrophils (another kind of white blood cell): none

Normally, there are no red blood cells in the CSF unless the needle passes though a blood vessel on route to the CSF. If this is the case, there should be more red blood cells in the first tube collected than in the last.

Abnormal results

A lumbar puncture is sometimes used as part of a diagnostic cancer workup. Abnormal test result values in the pressure or any of the substances found in the cerebrospinal fluid may suggest a number of medical problems including a tumor or spinal cord obstruction; hemorrhaging or bleeding in the central nervous system; infection from bacterial, viral, or fungal microorganisms; or an inflammation of the nerves. If there is a tumor in the meninges (membranes around the brain and spinal cord), the CSF may have higher protein levels, lower glucose levels, and a mild increase in lymphocytes (pleocytosis). It is important for patients to review the results of a cerebrospinal fluid analysis with their doctor and to discuss any treatment plans.

See also Acute lymphocytic leukemia; Brain and central nervous system tumors.

Resources

BOOKS

Braunwald, Eugene, et al., editors. *Harrison's Principles of Internal Medicine*. 15th ed. New York: McGraw-Hill, 2001.

PERIODICALS

Czosnyka, M., and J. D. Pickard. "Monitoring and Interpretation of Intracranial Pressure." *Journal of Neurology, Neurosurgery, and Psychiatry* 75 (June 2004): 813–821.

Ebinger, F., C. Kosel, J. Pietz, and D. Rating. "Headache and Backache after Lumbar Puncture in Children and Adolescents: A Prospective Study." *Pediatrics* 113 (June 2004): 1588–1592.

Gajjar, Amar, et al. "Traumatic Lumbar Puncture at Diagnosis Adversely Affects Outcome in Childhood Acute Lymphoblastic Leukemia." *Blood* 15 (November 2000): 3381–84.

Howard, Scott C., et al. "Safety of Lumbar Puncture for Children With Acute Lymphoblastic Leukemia and Thrombocytopenia." *Journal of the American Medical Association (JAMA)* 284 (November 2000): 2222-24.

Tubbs, R. S., M. D. Smyth, J. C. Wellons, III, and W. J. Oakes. "Intramedullary Hemorrhage in a Neonate after Lumbar Puncture Resulting in Paraplegia: A Case Report." *Pediatrics* 113 (May 2004): 1403–1405.

Zun, L. S., R. Hernandez, R. Thompson, and L. Downey. "Comparison of EPs' and Psychiatrists' Laboratory Assessment of Psychiatric Patients." *American Journal of Emergency Medicine* 22 (May 2004): 175–180.

ORGANIZATIONS

American Academy of Neurology. 1080 Montreal Ave., St. Paul, MN 55116–2325. (800) 879-1960. http://www.aan.com.

Martha Floberg Robbins
Rebecca J. Frey, Ph.D.

Lumpectomy

Definition

A lumpectomy is a type of surgery for **breast cancer**. It is considered "breast-conserving" surgery because in a lumpectomy, only the malignant tumor and a surrounding margin of normal breast tissue are removed. Lymph nodes in the armpit (axilla) also may be removed. This procedure is called **lymph node dissection**.

Purpose

Lumpectomy is a surgical treatment for newly diagnosed breast **cancer**. It is estimated that at least 50% of women with breast cancer are good candidates for this procedure. The location, size, and type of tumor are of primary importance when considering breast cancer surgery options. The size of the breast is another factor the surgeon considers when recommending surgery. The patient's psychological outlook, as well as her lifestyle and preferences, should also be taken into account when treatment decisions are made.

The extent and severity of a cancer is evaluated or "staged" according to a fairly complex system. Staging considers the size of the tumor and whether the cancer has spread to other areas, such as the chest wall, the lymph nodes, and/or to distant parts of the body. Women with early stage breast cancers are usually better candidates for lumpectomy. In most cases, a course of **radiation therapy** after surgery is part of the treatment. **Chemotherapy** or **antiestrogens** also may be prescribed.

Many studies have compared the survival rates of women who have had removal of a breast (**mastectomy**) with those who have undergone lumpectomy and radiation therapy. The data demonstrate that for women with comparable stages of breast cancer, survival rates are similar between the two groups, but the risk of the cancer recurring in the breast is slightly higher with lumpectomy. A 2003 study confirmed that younger women who have lumpectomies have a higher risk of tumor recurrence than those who have mastectomies.

In some instances, women with later stage breast cancer may be able to have lumpectomy. Chemotherapy may be administered before surgery to decrease tumor size and the chance of spread in selected cases.

Precautions

A number of factors may prevent or prohibit a breast cancer patient from having a lumpectomy. The tumor itself may be too large or located in an area where it would be difficult to remove with good cosmetic results. Sometimes several areas of cancer are found in one breast, so the tumor cannot be removed as a single lump. A cancer that has already attached itself to nearby structures, such as the skin or the chest wall, needs more extensive surgery.

Certain medical or physical circumstances also may eliminate lumpectomy as a treatment option. Sometimes lumpectomy may be attempted, but the surgeon is unable to remove the tumor with a sufficient amount of normal tissue surrounding it. This may be termed "persistently positive margins," or "lack of clear margins," referring to the margin of unaffected tissue around the tumor. Lumpectomy is not used for women who have had a previous lumpectomy and have a recurrence of the breast cancer.

The need for radiation therapy after lumpectomy makes this surgery medically unacceptable for some

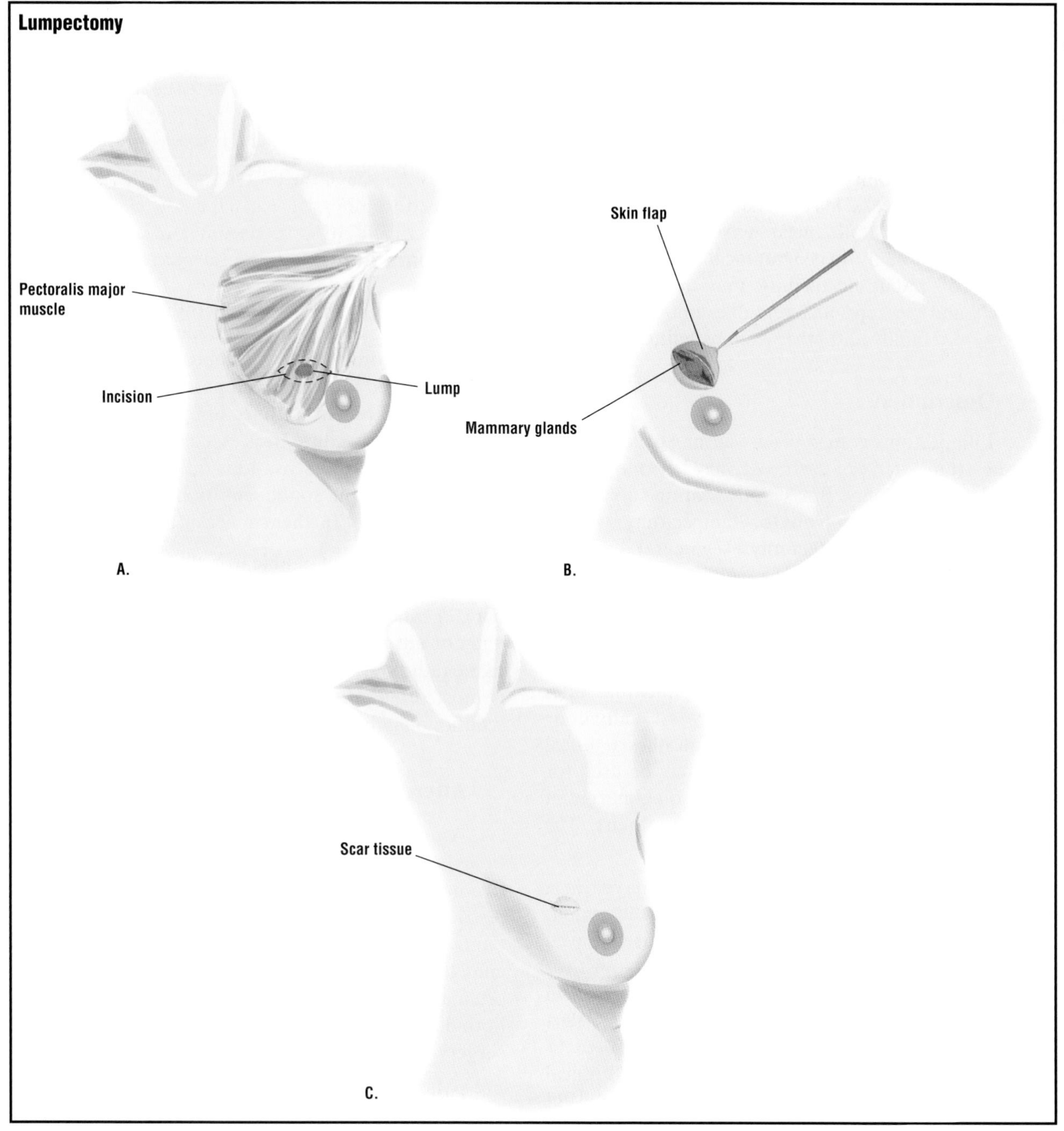

During a lumpectomy, a small incision is made around the area of the lump (A). The skin is pulled back, and the tumor removed (B). The incision is closed (C). *(Illustration by GGS Information Services. Cengage Learning, Gale.)*

women. For instance, radiation therapy cannot be administered to pregnant women because it may injure the fetus. If, however, delivery would be completed prior to the need for radiation, pregnant women may undergo lumpectomy. Women with collagen vascular disease, such as lupus erythematosus or scleroderma, would experience scarring and damage to their connective tissue if exposed to radiation treatments. A woman who has already had therapeutic radiation to the chest area for other reasons cannot have additional exposure for breast cancer therapy.

Some women may choose not to have a lumpectomy for other reasons. They may strongly fear a recurrence of breast cancer, and may consider a lumpectomy too risky. Others feel uncomfortable with a breast that has had a cancer, and they experience more peace of mind with the entire breast removed.

The need for radiation therapy may also be a barrier due to non-medical concerns. Some women simply fear this type of treatment and choose more extensive surgery so that radiation will not be required. The commitment of time, usually five days a week for six weeks, may not be acceptable for others. This may be due to financial, personal, or job-related constraints. Finally, in geographically isolated areas, a course of radiation therapy may require lengthy travel, and perhaps unacceptable amounts of time away from family and other responsibilities.

Description

Lumpectomy is an imprecise term. Any amount of tissue, from 1–50% of the breast, may be removed and called a lumpectomy. Breast conservation surgery is a frequently used synonym for lumpectomy. Partial mastectomy, **quadrantectomy**, segmental excision, wide excision, and tylectomy are other, less commonly used names for this procedure.

A lumpectomy is frequently done in a hospital setting (especially if lymph nodes are to be removed at the same time), but specialized outpatient facilities are sometimes preferred. The surgery is usually done while the patient is under general anesthesia. Local anesthetic with additional sedation may be used for some patients. The tumor and surrounding margin of tissue is removed and sent to the pathologist. The surgical site is closed.

If axillary lymph nodes were not removed in a prior **biopsy**, a second incision is made in the armpit. The fat pad that contains lymph nodes is removed from this area and is also sent to the pathologist for analysis. This portion of the procedure is called an axillary lymph node dissection; it is critical for determining the stage of the cancer. Typically, 10 to 15 nodes are removed, but the number may vary. Surgical drains may be left in place in either location to prevent fluid accumulation. The surgery may last from one to three hours.

The patient may stay in the hospital one or two days, or return home the same day. This generally depends on the extent of the surgery and the medical condition of the patient, as well as physician and patient preferences. A woman usually goes home with a small bandage. The inner part of the surgical site usually has dissolvable stitches. The skin may be sutured or stitched; or the skin edges may be held together with steristrips, which are special thin, clear pieces of tape.

KEY TERMS

Lymph node—A small mass of tissue in the form of a knot or protuberance. They are the primary source of lymph fluid, which serves in the body's defense by removing toxic fluids and bacteria.

Preparation

Routine preoperative preparations, such as having nothing to eat or drink the night before surgery, are typically ordered for a lumpectomy. Information about expected outcomes and potential complications is also part of preparation for lumpectomy, as it is for any surgical procedure. It is especially important that women know about sensations they might experience after the operation, so the sensations are not misinterpreted as signs of further cancer or poor healing.

If the tumor is not able to be felt (not palpable), a pre-operative localization procedure is needed. A fine wire, or other device, is placed at the tumor site, using x ray or ultrasound for guidance. This is usually done in the radiology department of a hospital. The woman is most often sitting up and awake, although some sedation may be administered.

Aftercare

After a lumpectomy, patients are usually cautioned against lifting anything that weighs more than five pounds for several days. Other activities may be restricted (especially if the axillary lymph nodes were removed) according to individual needs. Pain is often enough to limit inappropriate motion. Women are often instructed to wear a well-fitting support bra both day and night for approximately one week after surgery.

Pain is usually well controlled with prescribed medication. If it is not, the patient should contact the surgeon, as severe pain may be a sign of a complication, which needs medical attention. A return visit to the surgeon is normally scheduled approximately ten days to two weeks after the operation. Studies have shown that women improve their survival rates after lumpectomy if they stop smoking.

Radiation therapy is usually started as soon as feasible after lumpectomy. Other additional treatments, such as chemotherapy or hormone therapy, may also be prescribed. The timing of these is specific to each individual patient.

Risks

The risks are similar to those associated with any surgical procedure. Risks include bleeding, **infection**, asymmetry, anesthesia reaction, or unexpected scarring. A lumpectomy also may cause loss of sensation in the breast. The size and shape of the breast will be affected by the operation. Fluid can accumulate in the area where tissue was removed, requiring drainage.

If lymph node dissection is performed, there are several potential complications. A woman may experience decreased feeling in the back of her armpit. She may also experience other sensations, including numbness, tingling, or increased skin sensitivity. An inflammation of the arm vein, called phlebitis, can occur. There may be injury to the nerves controlling arm motion.

Approximately 2–10% of patients develop lymphedema (swelling of the arm) after axillary lymph node dissection. This swelling of the arm can range from mild to very severe. It can be treated with elastic bandages and specialized physical therapy, but it is a chronic condition, requiring continuing care. Lymphedema can arise at any time, even years after surgery.

A new technique often eliminates the need for removing many axillary lymph nodes. **Sentinel lymph node mapping** and biopsy is based on the idea that the condition of the first lymph node in the network, which drains the affected area, can predict whether the cancer may have spread to the rest of the nodes. It is thought that if this first, or sentinel, node is cancer-free, there is no need to look further. Many patients with early-stage breast cancers may be spared the risks and complications of axillary lymph node dissection as the use of this approach continues to increase.

Normal results

When lumpectomy is performed, it is anticipated that it will be the definitive surgical treatment for breast cancer. Other forms of therapy, especially radiation, are often prescribed as part of the total treatment plan. A 2003 study reported that radiation of the entire breast produces better results than radiation of part of the breast. The expected outcome after lumpectomy and radiation is no recurrence of the breast cancer, however, women who have had lumpectomies, particularly those who were young at the time of treatment, should continue to see their physicians for regular breast cancer check-ups, since the cancer can recur.

Abnormal results

An unforeseen outcome of lumpectomy may be recurrence of the breast cancer, either locally or distally (in a part of the body far from the original site). Recurrence may be discovered soon after lumpectomy or years after the procedure. For this reason, it is important for patients to be regularly and closely monitored by their physicians. A 2003 report showed that **magnetic resonance imaging** (MRI) is accurate in detecting any cancer left in the breast after lumpectomy. Women should continue to have regular mammograms. While the scar tissue from lumpectomy and radiation therapy can make mammograms less comfortable, a special cushion was approved by the U.S. Food and Drug Administration in 2003 that reduces discomfort in women who have had breast conserving surgery.

Resources

BOOKS

Love, Susan M., with Karen Lindsey. *Dr. Susan Love's Breast Book*. 3rd ed. Cambridge: Perseus Publishing, 2000.

Robinson, Rebecca Y., and Jeanne A. Petrek. *A Step-by-Step Guide to Dealing With Your Breast Cancer*. New York: Carol Publishing Group, 1999.

PERIODICALS

Ford, Steve. "Lumpectomy Associated With Higher Long-term Risk of Recurrence than Mastectomy." *Practice Nurse* November 28, 2003: 50.

Jancin, Bruce. "Cushion Lessens Mammogram Pain After Lumpectomy (Pain Decreased 54%)." *OB GYN News* February 15, 2003: 9 - 11.

"MR Accurate in Detecting Residual Disease Following Lumpectomy." *Women's Health Weekly* May 29, 2003: 14.

Norton, Patrice G.W. "More Data Support Breast Conservation Over Mastectomy (For Phase I or II Cancer)." *Family Practice News* January 15, 2003: 31.

"Smoking Decreases Survival of Patients Treated with Lumpectomy and Radiation." *Cancer Weekly* November 11, 2003: 36.

"Study: Whole-breast Irradiation After Lumpectomy Has Clear Long-term Benefits." *Cancer Weekly* November 11, 2003: 39.

Ellen S. Weber, M.S.N.
Teresa G. Odle

Lung biopsy

Definition

Lung **biopsy** is a procedure for obtaining a small sample of lung tissue for examination. The tissue is usually examined under a microscope, and may be sent to a microbiological laboratory for culture. Microscopic examination is performed by a pathologist.

Purpose

A lung biopsy is usually performed to determine the cause of abnormalities, such as nodules that appear on chest **x rays**. It can confirm a diagnosis of **cancer**, especially if malignant cells are detected in the patient's sputum or bronchial washing. In addition to evaluating lung tumors and their associated symptoms, lung biopsies may be used to diagnose lung infections, especially tuberculosis and Pneumocystis **pneumonia**, drug reactions, and chronic diseases of the lungs such as sarcoidosis and pulmonary fibrosis.

A lung biopsy can be used for treatment as well as diagnosis. **Bronchoscopy**, a type of lung biopsy performed with a long, flexible slender instrument called a bronchoscope, can be used to clear a patient's air passages of secretions and to remove airway blockages.

Demographics

Lung cancer is the leading cause of cancer-related deaths in the United States. About 213,380 patients were newly diagnosed with lung cancer in 2007 (about 114,760 in men and 98,620 in women). It is expected to claim nearly 160,390 lives in 2007 (89,510 in men and 70,880 in women). Lung cancer kills more people than cancers of the breast, prostate, colon, and pancreas combined. Cigarette smoking accounts for nearly 90% of cases of lung cancer in the United States.

Description

Overview

The right and left lungs are separated by the mediastinum, which contains the heart, trachea, lymph nodes, and esophagus. Lung biopsies sometimes involve **mediastinoscopy**.

Types of lung biopsies

Lung biopsies are performed using a variety of techniques, depending on where the abnormal tissue is located in the lung, the health and age of the patient, and the presence of lung disease. A bronchoscopy is ordered if a lesion identified on the x ray seems to be located on the wall (periphery) of the chest. If the suspicious area lies close to the chest wall, a needle biopsy can be done. If both methods fail to diagnose the problem, an open lung biopsy may be performed. When there is a question about whether the lung cancer or suspicious mass has spread to the lymph nodes in the mediastinum, a mediastinoscopy is performed.

BRONCHOSCOPIC BIOPSY. During the bronchoscopy, a thin, lighted tube (bronchoscope) is passed from the nose or mouth, down the windpipe (trachea) to the air passages (bronchi) leading to the lungs. Through the bronchoscope, the physician views the airways, and is able to clear mucus from blocked airways, and collect cells or tissue samples for laboratory analysis.

NEEDLE BIOPSY. The patient is mildly sedated, but awake during the needle biopsy procedure. He or she sits in a chair with arms folded in front on a table. An x-ray technician uses a computerized axial tomography (CAT) scanner or a fluoroscope to identify the precise location of the suspicious areas. Markers are placed on the overlying skin to identify the biopsy site. The skin is thoroughly cleansed with an antiseptic solution, and a local anesthetic is injected to numb the area. The patient will feel a brief stinging sensation when the anesthetic is injected.

The physician makes a small incision, about half an inch (1.25 cm) in length. The patient is asked to take a deep breath and hold it while the physician inserts the biopsy needle through the incision into the lung tissue to be biopsied. The patient may feel pressure, and a brief sharp pain when the needle touches the lung tissue. Most patients do not experience severe pain. The patient should refrain from coughing during the procedure. The needle is withdrawn when enough tissue has been obtained. Pressure is applied at the biopsy site and a sterile bandage is placed over the incision. A chest x ray is performed immediately after the procedure to check for potential complications. The entire procedure takes 30–60 minutes.

OPEN BIOPSY. Open biopsies are performed in a hospital operating room under general anesthesia. Once the anesthesia has taken effect, the surgeon makes an incision over the lung area, a procedure called a **thoracotomy**. Some lung tissue is removed and the incision is closed with sutures. Chest tubes are placed with one end inside the lung and the other end protruding through the closed incision. Chest tubes are used to drain fluid and blood, and re-expand the lungs. They are usually removed the day after the procedure. The entire procedure normally takes about an hour. A chest x ray is performed immediately after the procedure to check for potential complications.

VIDEO-ASSISTED THORACOSCOPIC SURGERY. A minimally-invasive technique, video-assisted thoracoscopic surgery (VATS) can be used to biopsy lung and mediastinal lesions. VATS may be performed on selected patients in place of open lung biopsy. While the patient is under general anesthetia, the surgeon makes several small incisions in the his or her chest wall. A thorascope, a thin, hollow, lighted tube with a tiny video camera mounted on it, is inserted through one of the small incisions. The other incisions allow the surgeon to insert special instruments to retrieve tissue for biopsy.

MEDIASTINOSCOPY. This procedure is performed under general anesthesia. A 2–3 inch (5–8 cm) incision is made at the base of the neck. A thin, hollow, lighted tube, called a mediastinoscope, is inserted through the incision into the space between the right and the left lungs. The surgeon removes any lymph nodes or tissues that look abnormal. The mediastinoscope is then removed, and the incision is sutured and bandaged. A mediastinoscopy takes about an hour.

Diagnosis/Preparation

Diagnosis

Before scheduling a lung biopsy, the physician performs a careful evaluation of the patient's medical history and symptoms, and performs a physical examination. Chest x rays and sputum **cytology** (examination of cells obtained from a deep-cough mucus sample) are other diagnostic tests that may be performed. An electrocardiogram (EKG) and laboratory tests may be performed before the procedure to check for blood clotting problems, **anemia**, and blood type, should a transfusion become necessary.

Preparation

During a preoperative appointment, usually scheduled within one to two weeks before the procedure, the patient receives information about what to expect during the procedure and the recovery period. During this appointment or just before the procedure, the patient usually meets with the physician (or physicians) performing the procedure (the pulmonologist, interventional radiologist, or thoracic surgeon).

A chest x ray or CAT scan of the chest is used to identify the area to be biopsied.

About an hour before the biopsy procedure, the patient receives a sedative. Medication may also be given to dry up airway secretions. General anesthesia is not used for this procedure.

For at least 12 hours before the open biopsy, VATS, or mediastinoscopy procedures, the patient should not eat or drink anything. Prior to these procedures, an intravenous line is placed in a vein in the patient's arm to deliver medications or fluids as necessary. A hollow tube, called an endotracheal tube, is passed through the patient's mouth into the airway leading to the lungs. Its purpose is to deliver the general anesthetic. The chest area is cleansed with an antiseptic solution. In the mediastinoscopy procedure, the neck is also cleansed to prepare for the incision.

Smoking cessation

Patients who will undergo surgical diagnostic and treatment procedures should be encouraged to stop smoking and stop using tobacco products. The patient needs to make the commitment to be a nonsmoker after the procedure. Patients able to stop smoking several weeks before surgical procedures have fewer postoperative complications. **Smoking cessation** programs are available in many communities. The patient should ask a health care provider for more information if he or she needs help with smoking cessation.

Informed consent

Informed consent is an educational process between health care providers and patients. Before any procedure is performed, the patient is asked to sign a consent form. Prior to signing the form, the patient should understand the nature and purpose of the diagnostic procedure or treatment, its risks and benefits, and alternatives, including the option of not proceeding with the test or treatment. During the discussions, the health care providers are available to answer the patient's questions about the consent form or procedure.

Aftercare

Needle biopsy

Following a needle biopsy, the patient is allowed to rest comfortably. He or she may be required to lie flat for two hours following the procedure to prevent the risk of bleeding. The nurse checks the patient's status at two-hour intervals. If there are no complications after four hours, the patient can go home once he or she has received instructions about resuming normal activities. The patient should rest at home for a day or two before returning to regular activities, and should avoid strenuous activities for one week after the biopsy.

Open biopsy, VATS, or mediastinoscopy

After an open biopsy, VATS, or mediastinoscopy, the patient is taken to the recovery room for observation. The patient receives oxygen via a face mask or nasal cannula. If no complications develop, the patient is taken to a hospital room. Temperature, blood oxygen level, pulse, blood pressure, and respiration are monitored. Chest tubes remain in place after surgery to prevent the lungs from collapsing, and to remove blood and fluids. The tubes are usually removed the day after the procedure.

The patient may experience some grogginess for a few hours after the procedure. He or she may have a sore throat from the endotracheal tube. The patient may also have some pain or discomfort at the incision site, which can be relieved by pain medication. It is common for patients to require some pain medication for up to two weeks following the procedure.

After receiving instructions about resuming normal activities and caring for the incision, the patient usually goes home the day after surgery. The patient should not drive while taking narcotic pain medication.

Patients may experience **fatigue** and muscle aches for a day or two because of the general anesthesia. The patient can gradually increase activities, as tolerated. Walking is recommended. Sutures are usually removed after one to two weeks.

The physician should be notified immediately if the patient experiences extreme pain, light-headedness, or difficulty breathing after the procedure. Sputum may be slightly bloody for a day or two after the procedure. Heavy or persistent bleeding requires evaluation by the physician.

Risks

Lung biopsies should not be performed on patients who have a bleeding disorder or abnormal blood clotting because of low platelet counts, or prolonged prothrombin time (PT) or partial thromboplastin time (PTT). Platelets are small blood cells that play a role in the blood clotting process. PT and PTT measure how well blood is clotting. If clotting times are prolonged, it may be unsafe to perform a biopsy because of the risk of bleeding. If the platelet count is lower than 50,000/cubic mm, the patient may be given a platelet transfusion as a temporary relief measure, and a biopsy can then be performed.

In addition, lung biopsies should not be performed if other tests indicate the patient has enlarged alveoli associated with emphysema, pulmonary hypertension, or enlargement of the right ventricle of the heart (cor pulmonale).

The normal risks of any surgical procedure include bleeding, **infection**, or pneumonia. The risk of these complications is higher in patients undergoing open biopsy procedures, as is the risk of pneumothorax (lung collapse). In rare cases, the lung collapses because of air that leaks in through the hole made by the biopsy needle. A chest x ray is done immediately after the biopsy to detect the development of this potential complication. If a pneumothorax occurs, a chest tube is inserted into the pleural cavity to re-expand the lung. Signs of pneumothorax include shortness of breath, rapid heart rate, or blueness of the skin (a late sign). If the patient has any of these symptoms after being discharged from the hospital, it is important to call the health care provider or emergency services immediately.

Bronchoscopic biopsy

Bronchoscopy is generally safe, and complications are rare. If they do occur, complications may include spasms of the bronchial tubes that can impair breathing, irregular heart rhythms, or infections such as pneumonia.

Needle biopsy

Needle biopsy is associated with fewer risks than open biopsy because it does not involve general anesthesia. Some **hemoptysis** (coughing up blood) occurs in 5% of needle biopsies. Prolonged bleeding or infection may also occur, although these are very rare complications.

Open biopsy

Possible complications of an open biopsy include infection or pneumothorax. If the patient has very severe breathing problems before the biopsy, breathing may be further impaired following the operation. Patients with normal lung function prior to the biopsy have a very small risk of respiratory problems resulting from or following the procedure.

Mediastinoscopy

Complications due to mediastinoscopy are rare. Possible complications include pneumothorax or bleeding caused by damage to the blood vessels near the heart. Mediastinitis, infection of the mediastinum, may develop. Injury to the esophagus or larynx may occur. If the nerves leading to the larynx are injured, the patient may be left with a permanently hoarse voice. All of these complications are rare.

Normal results

Normal results indicate no evidence of infection in the lungs, no detection of lumps or nodules, and cells that are free from cancerous abnormalities.

WHO PERFORMS THIS PROCEDURE AND WHERE IS IT PERFORMED?

Fiberoptic bronchoscopy is performed by pulmonologists, physician specialists in pulmonary medicine. CAT guided needle biopsy is done by interventional radiologists, physician specialists in radiological procedures. Thoracic surgeons perform open biopsies and VATS. Specially trained nurses, x-ray, and laboratory technicians assist during the procedures and provide pre- and postoperative education and supportive care.

The procedures are performed in an operating or procedure room in a hospital.

Abnormal results of needle biopsy, VATS, and open biopsy may be associated with diseases other than cancer. Nodules in the lungs may be due to active infections such as tuberculosis, or may be scars from a previous infection. In 33% of biopsies using a mediastinoscope, the biopsied lymph nodes prove to be cancerous. Abnormal results should always be considered in the context of the patient's medical history, physical examination, and other tests such as sputum examination, and chest x rays before a final diagnosis is made.

Morbidity and mortality rates

The risk of death from needle biopsy is rare. The risk of death from open biopsy is one in 3,000 cases. In mediastinoscopy, death occurs in fewer than one in 3,000 cases.

Alternatives

The type of alternative diagnostic procedures available depend upon each patient's diagnosis.

Some people may be eligible to participate in **clinical trials**, research programs conducted with patients to evaluate a new medical treatment, drug, or device. The purpose of clinical trials is to find new and improved methods of treating different diseases and special conditions. For more information on current clinical trials, visit the National Institutes of Health's ClinicalTrials.gov at http://www.clinicaltrials.gov or call (888) FIND-NLM [(888) 346-3656] or (301) 594- 5983.

The National Cancer Institute (NCI) has conducted a clinical trial to evaluate a technology—low-dose helical computed tomography—for its effectiveness in screening for lung cancer. One study concluded that this test is more sensitive in detecting specific conditions related to lung cancer than other screening tests.

QUESTIONS TO ASK THE DOCTOR

- Why is this procedure being performed?
- Are there any alternative options to having this procedure?
- What type of lung biopsy procedure is recommended?
- Is minimally invasive surgery an option?
- Will the patient be awake during the procedure?
- Who will be performing the procedure? How many years of experience does this physician have? How many other lung biopsies has the physician performed?
- Can medications be taken the day of the procedure?
- Can the patient have food or drink before the procedure? If not, how long before the procedure should these activities be stopped?
- How long is the hospitalization?
- After discharge, how long will it take to recover from the procedure?
- How is pain or discomfort relieved after the procedure?
- What types of symptoms should be reported to the physician?
- When can normal activities be resumed?
- When cam driving be resumed?
- When can the patient return to work?
- When will the results of the procedure be given to the patient?
- How often are follow-up physician visits needed after the procedure?

Resources

BOOKS

Abeloff, MD et al. *Clinical Oncology*. 3rd ed. Philadelphia: Elsevier, 2004.

Mason, RJ et al. *Murray & Nadel's Textbook of Respiratory Medicine*. 4th ed. Philadelphia: Saunders, 2007.

ORGANIZATIONS

American Association for Respiratory Care (AARC). 11030 Ables Lane, Dallas, TX 75229. E-mail: info@aarc.org. http://www.aarc.org.

American Cancer Society. 1599 Clifton Road, N.E., Atlanta, GA 30329. (800) 227-2345 or (404) 320-3333. http://www.cancer.org.

American College of Chest Physicians. 3300 Dundee Road, Northbrook, IL 60062-2348. (847) 498-1400. http://www.chestnet.org.

American Lung Association and American Thoracic Society. 1740 Broadway, New York, NY 10019-4374. (800) 586-4872 or (212) 315-8700. http://www.lungusa.org and http://www.thoracic.org.

Cancer Research Institute. 681 Fifth Avenue, New York, NY 10022. (800) 992-2623. http://www.cancerresearch.org.

Lung Line National Jewish Medical and Research Center. 14090 Jackson Street, Denver, CO 80206. (800) 222-5864. E-mail: lungline@njc.org. http://www.nationaljewish.org.

National Cancer Institute (National Institutes of Health). 9000 Rockville Pike, Bethesda, MD 20892. (800) 422-6237. http://www.nci.nih.gov.

National Heart, Lung and Blood Institute. Information Center. P.O. Box 30105, Bethesda, MD 20824-0105. (301) 251-2222. http://www.nhlbi.nih.gov.

OTHER

Dailylung.com. http://www.dailylung.com.

Chest Medicine On-Line. http://www.priory.com/chest.htm.

National Lung Health Education Program. http://www.nlhep.com.

Pulmonary Forum. http://www.pulmonarychannel.com.

Pulmonarypaper.org. P.O. Box 877, Ormond Beach, FL 32175. (800) 950- 3698. http://www.pulmonarypaper.org.

Barbara Wexler
Angela M. Costello
Rosalyn Carson-DeWitt, MD

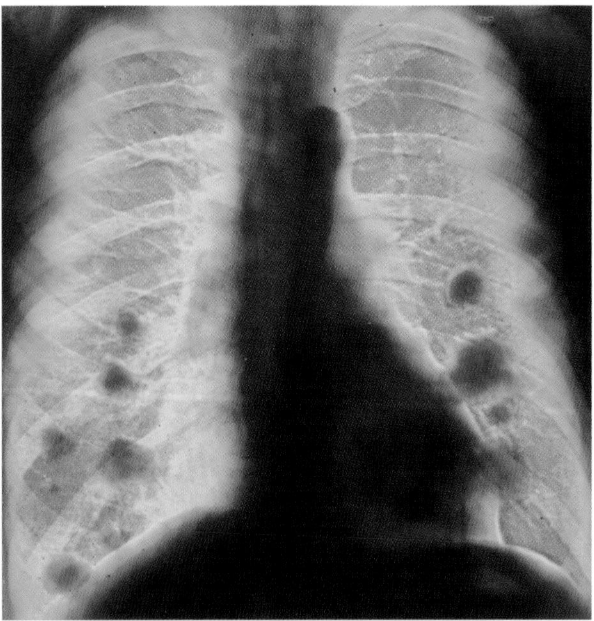

False-color chest x ray showing evidence of cancerous masses (orange shadows) in both lungs. *(Copyright CNRI, Science Source/Photo Researchers, Inc. Reproduced by permission.)*

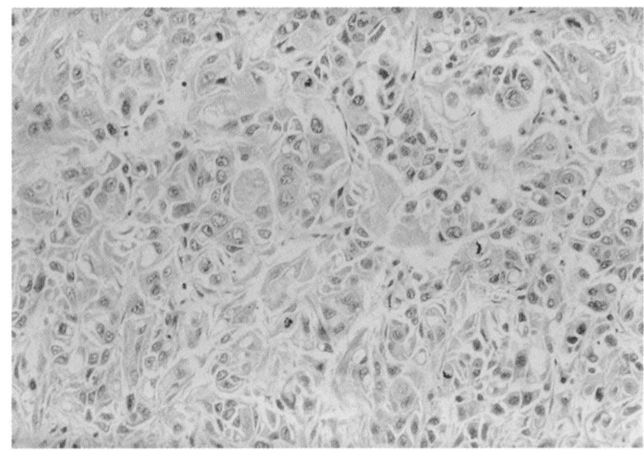

Large-cell anaplastic carcinoma of the lung. *(Copyright Biophoto Associates, Science Source/Photo Researchers, Inc. Reproduced by permission.)*

Lung cancer, non-small cell

Definition

Non-small cell lung **cancer** (NSCLC) is a disease in which the cells of the lung tissues grow uncontrollably and form tumors.

Demographics

Worldwide, lung cancer is the most common cancer in males, and the fifth most common cancer in women. The worldwide mortality rate for patients with lung cancer is 86%. In the United States, lung cancer is the leading cause of death from cancer among both men and women. The World Health Organization estimates that the worldwide mortality from lung cancer will increase to three million by the year 2025. Of those three million deaths, almost two and a half million will result from non-small cell lung cancer.

The American Cancer Society (ACS) estimates that 219,440 Americans will develop lung cancer in 2009, 116,090 men and 103,350 women. Of these patients, 159,000 will die of the disease.

The incidence of lung cancer is beginning to fall in developed countries. This may be a result of antismoking campaigns. In developing countries, however, rates continue to rise, which may be a consequence of both industrialization and the increasing use of tobacco products.

Description

There are two kinds of lung cancers, primary and secondary. Primary lung cancer starts in the lung itself, and is divided into **small cell lung cancer** and non-small cell lung cancer. Small cell lung cancers are shaped like an oat and called oat-cell cancers; they are aggressive, spread rapidly, and represent 20% of lung cancers. Non-small cell lung cancer represents almost 80% of all primary lung cancers. Secondary lung cancer is cancer that starts somewhere else in the body (for example, the breast or colon) and spreads to the lungs.

The lungs

The lungs are located along with the heart in the chest cavity. The lungs are not simply hollow balloons but have a very organized structure consisting of hollow tubes, blood vessels and elastic tissue. The hollow tubes, called bronchi, are highly branched, becoming smaller and more numerous at each branching. They end in tiny, blind sacs made of elastic tissue called alveoli. These sacs are where the oxygen a person breathes in is taken up into the blood, and where carbon dioxide moves out of the blood to be breathed out.

Normal healthy lungs are continually secreting mucus that not only keeps the lungs moist, but also protects the lungs by trapping foreign particles like dust and dirt in breathed air. The inside of the lungs is covered with small hairlike structures called cilia. The cilia move in such a way that mucus is swept up out of the lungs and into the throat.

Lung cancer

Most lung cancers start in the cells that line the bronchi, and can take years to develop. As they grow larger they prevent the lungs from functioning normally. The tumor can reduce the capacity of the lungs, or block the movement of air through the bronchi in the lungs. As a result, less oxygen gets into the blood and patients feel short of breath. Tumors may also block the normal movement of mucus up into the throat. As a result, mucus builds up in the lungs and **infection** may develop behind the tumor. Once lung cancer has developed it frequently spreads to other parts of the body.

The speed at which non-small cell tumors grow depends on the type of cells that make up the tumor. The following three types account for the vast majority of non-small cell tumors:

- Adenocarcinomas are the most common and often cause no symptoms. Frequently they are not found until they are advanced.
- Squamous cell carcinomas usually produce symptoms because they are centrally located and block the lungs.
- Undifferentiated large cell and giant cell carcinomas tend to grow rapidly, and spread quickly to other parts of the body.

Causes and symptoms

Causes

Tobacco smoking accounts for 87% of all lung cancers. Giving up tobacco can prevent most lung cancers. Smoking marijuana **cigarettes** is considered another risk factor for cancer of the lung. Second hand smoke also contributes to the development of lung cancer among nonsmokers.

Certain hazardous materials that people may be exposed to in their jobs have been shown to cause lung cancer. These include asbestos, coal products, and radioactive substances. Air pollution may also be a contributing factor. Exposure to radon, a colorless, odorless gas that sometimes accumulates in the basement of homes, may cause lung cancer in a tiny minority of patients. In addition, patients whose lungs are scarred from other lung conditions may have an increased risk of developing lung cancer.

Symptoms

Lung cancers tend to spread very early, and only 15% are detected in their early stages. The chances of early detection, however, can be improved by seeking medical care at once if any of the following symptoms appear:

- a cough that does not go away
- chest pain
- shortness of breath
- recurrent lung infections, such as bronchitis or pneumonia
- bloody or brown-colored spit or phlegm (sputum)
- persistent hoarseness
- significant weight loss that is not due to dieting or vigorous exercise; fatigue and loss of appetite
- unexplained fever

Although these symptoms may be caused by diseases other than lung cancer, it is important to consult a doctor to rule out the possibility of lung cancer.

If lung cancer has spread to other organs, the patient may have other symptoms such as headaches, bone fractures, pain, bleeding, or blood clots.

Diagnosis

Physical examination and diagnostic tests

The doctor will first take a detailed medical history and assess risk factors. During a complete physical examination the doctor will examine the patient's throat to rule out other possible causes of hoarseness or coughing, and will listen to the patient's breathing and chest sounds.

If the doctor has reason to suspect lung cancer, particularly if the patient has a history of heavy smoking or occupational exposure to irritating substances, a chest x ray may be ordered to see if there are any masses in the lungs. Special imaging techniques, such as **computed tomography** (CT) scans or **magnetic resonance imaging** (MRI), may provide more precise information about the size, shape, and location of any tumors.

Sputum analysis

Sputum analysis is a noninvasive test that involves microscopic examination of cells that are coughed up from the lungs. This test can diagnose at least 30% of lung cancers, even if tumors are not visible on chest **x rays**. In addition, the test can detect cancer in its very early stages, before it spreads to other regions. The sputum test does not provide any information about the location of the tumor.

Lung biopsy

Lung biopsy is the most definitive diagnostic tool for cancer. It can be performed in three different ways. **Bronchoscopy** involves the insertion of a slender, lighted tube, called a bronchoscope, down the patient's throat and into the lungs. This test allows the doctor to see the tubes inside the lungs, and to obtain samples of lung tissue. If a needle **biopsy** is to be performed, the location of the tumor is first identified using a computerized tomography (CT) scan or magnetic resonance imaging (MRI). The doctor then inserts a needle through the chest wall and collects a sample of tissue from the tumor. In the third procedure, known as surgical biopsy, the chest wall is opened up and a part of the tumor, or all of it, is removed. A doctor who specializes in the study of diseased tissue (a pathologist) examines the tumor to identify the cancer's type and stage.

Treatment

Staging

Treatment for non-small cell lung cancer depends primarily on the stage of the cancer. Staging is a process that tells the doctor if the cancer has spread and the extent of its spread. The most commonly used treatments are surgery, **radiation therapy**, and **chemotherapy**.

Non-small cell lung cancer has six stages:

- Occult carcinoma. Cancer cells have been found in the sputum, but no tumor has yet been found.
- Stage 0. A small group of cancerous cells have been found in one location.
- Stage I. The cancer is only in the lung and has not spread anywhere else.
- Stage II. The cancer has spread to nearby lymph nodes.
- Stage III. The cancer has spread to more distant lymph nodes, and/or other parts of the chest like the diaphragm.
- Stage IV. The cancer has spread to other parts of the body.

Surgery

Surgery is the standard treatment for the earlier stages of non-small cell lung cancer. The surgeon will decide on the type of surgery, depending on how much of the lung is affected. There are three different types of surgical procedures:

- Wedge resection is the removal of a small part of the lung.
- Lobectomy is the removal of one lobe of the lung. (The right lung has three lobes and the left lung has two lobes.)
- Pneumonectomy is the removal of an entire lung.

Lung surgery is a major procedure and patients can expect to experience pain, weakness in the chest, and shortness of breath. Air and fluid collect in the chest after surgery. As a result, patients will need help to turn over, cough, and breath deeply. Patients should be encouraged to perform these activities because they help get rid of the air and fluid and speed up recovery. It can take patients several months before they regain their energy and strength.

Radiotherapy

Patients whose cancer has progressed too far for surgery (Stages III and IV) may receive radiotherapy. Radiotherapy involves the use of high-energy rays to kill cancer cells. It is used either by itself or in combination with surgery or chemotherapy. The amount of radiation used depends on the size and the location of the tumor.

Radiation therapy may produce such side effects as tiredness, skin rashes, upset stomach, and **diarrhea**. Dry or sore throats, difficulty in swallowing, and loss of hair in the treated area are all minor side effects of radiation. These may disappear either during the course of the treatment or after the treatment is over.

Chemotherapy

Chemotherapy is also given to patients whose cancer has progressed too far for surgery. Chemotherapy is medication that is usually given intravenously to kill cancer cells. These drugs enter the bloodstream and travel to all parts of the body, killing cancer cells that have spread to different organs. Chemotherapy is used as the primary treatment for cancers that have spread beyond the lung and cannot be removed by surgery. It can also be used in addition to surgery or radiation therapy.

Chemotherapy for NSCLC has made significant advances since the early 1980s in improving the patient's quality of life as well as length of survival. Newer cytotoxic (cell-killing) agents developed in the 1990s, such as the taxanes, are typically combined with either **cisplatin** or **carboplatin** as first-line therapy for non-small cell lung cancer.

Newer drugs for lung cancer include gefinitib (Iressa) and **pemetrexed** (Alimta). The FDA approved gefinitib in May 2003 as a treatment for patients with NSCLC who have not responded to platinum-based or taxane chemotherapy. It is taken by mouth and works by inhibiting an enzyme involved in the growth of tumor cells. Pemetrexed, which is given by injection, was approved by the FDA in February 2004 for the treatment of **mesothelioma**, a type of lung cancer caused by exposure to asbestos fibers. However, the drug appears to be effective in treating other types of lung cancer as well.

Chemotherapy is also used as palliative treatment for non-small cell lung cancer. Palliative refers to any type of therapy that is given to relieve the symptoms of a disease but not to cure it.

Clinical trials

Patients diagnosed with non-small cell lung cancer should discuss participating in **clinical trials** with their doctor. There are many clinical trials currently underway that are investigating all different stages of the disease. These trials are studying various new treatment options including:

- Chemotherapy with new drugs, and combinations of drugs
- Courses of chemotherapy prior to surgery
- Radiotherapy after surgery
- Chemotherapy and radiotherapy in combination

Information on open clinical trials is available on the Internet from the National Cancer Institute at http://cancertrials.nci.nih.gov.

Alternative and complementary therapies

Because non-small cell lung cancer has a poor prognosis with conventional medical treatment, many patients are willing to try complementary and alternative therapies. These therapies are used to try to reduce stress, ease side effects and symptoms, or control disease. Two treatments sometimes used are shark cartilage and **mistletoe**. Although shark cartilage is thought to interfere with the tumor's blood supply, clinical trials have so far been inconclusive. Mistletoe is a poisonous plant that has been shown to kill cancer cells in the laboratory. Again, however, clinical trials with cancer patients have been inconclusive.

Patients who decide to try complementary and alternative therapies should tell their doctors. Some of these therapies may interfere with conventional treatment.

Coping with cancer treatment

The side effects associated with treatment of non-small cell lung cancer can be severe. Patients should ask their doctors about medications to treat **nausea and vomiting**, and other side effects. It is particularly important to eat a nutritious diet and to drink plenty of fluids. In addition, most patients report feeling very tired and should get plenty of rest.

Patients should consider joining local support groups with people who are coping with the same experiences. Many people with cancer find they can share thoughts and feelings with group members that they do not feel comfortable sharing with friends or family. Support groups are also a good source of information about coping with cancer.

Prognosis

The prognosis for non-small cell lung cancer is better if the disease is found early, and removed surgically. For patients whose disease is caught in Stage I, the survival rate five years after surgery ranges from 60–80%. Up to 55% of Stage II patients are alive after

QUESTIONS TO ASK YOUR DOCTOR

- What kinds of diagnostic studies will be required to ascertain the type and spread of this tumor?
- Could there be a genetic component to this tumor? Should other family member be tested?
- What types of treatments are available?
- What types of side effects from treatments can I expect? What are your recommendations to help me deal with those side effects?
- Am I eligible for any clinical trials? Would these be helpful to consider?
- Are there any lifestyle changes that I should make?
- What type of diet should I follow? Are there foods I should avoid?
- Should I avoid any medications?
- How often should I be checked after treatment has ended?
- Is there a support group that I can join to hear about other people's experiences with this disorder?

five years, but only about 30% of Stage III patients make it to five years. Unfortunately, 85% of patients already have at least Stage III cancer by the time they are diagnosed. Many of these patients have disease that is too advanced for surgery. Despite treatment with radiotherapy and chemotherapy, the five-year survival for patients with inoperable disease is extremely low.

Prevention

The best way to prevent lung cancer is not to start smoking or to quit smoking. Secondhand smoke from other people's tobacco should also be avoided. Appropriate precautions should be taken when working with cancer-causing substances (carcinogens). Testing houses for the presence of radon gas, and removing asbestos from buildings have also been suggested as preventive strategies.

Resources

BOOKS

Abeloff, MD et al. *Clinical Oncology*. 3rd ed. Philadelphia: Elsevier, 2004.

Goldman L, Ausiello D., eds. *Cecil Textbook of Internal Medicine*. 23rd ed. Philadelphia: Saunders, 2008.

Mason, RJ et al. *Murray & Nadel's Textbook of Respiratory Medicine*. 4th ed. Philadelphia: Saunders, 2007.

PERIODICALS

Cohen, M. H., G. A. Williams, R. Sridhara, et al. "United States Food and Drug Administration Drug Approval Summary: Gefitinib (ZD1839; Iressa) Tablets." *Clinical Cancer Research* 10 (February 15, 2004): 1212–1218.

Fossella, F. V. "Pemetrexed for Treatment of Advanced Non-Small Cell Lung Cancer." *Seminars in Oncology* 31 (February 2004): 100–105.

Frampton, J. E., and S. E. Easthope. "Gefitinib: A Review of Its Use in the Management of Advanced Non-Small-Cell Lung Cancer." *Drugs* 64 (2004): 2475–2492.

Ramalingam, S., and C. P. Belani. "State-of-the-Art Chemotherapy for Advanced Non-Small Cell Lung Cancer." *Seminars in Oncology* 31 (February 2004): 68–74.

Rigas, J. R. "Taxane-Platinum Combinations in Advanced Non-Small Cell Lung Cancer: A Review." *Oncologist* 9, Supplement 2 (2004): 16–23.

OTHER

American Cancer Society (ACS). *Cancer Facts & Figures 2004*. http://www.cancer.org/downloads/STT/CAFF_finalPWSecured.pdf.

FDA News, February 5, 2004. "FDA Approves First Drug for Rare Type of Cancer." http://www.fda.gov/bbs/topics/NEWS/2004/NEW01018.html.

ORGANIZATIONS

Alliance for Lung Cancer Advocacy, Support and Education. PO Box 849 Vancouver, WA 98666. (800) 298-2436. http://www.alcase.org.

American Lung Association. 1740 Broadway New York, NY 10019. (212) 315-8700. http://www.lungusa.org.

National Cancer Institute (National Institutes of Health). 9000 Rockville Pike, Bethesda, MD 20892. (800) 422-6237. http://www.nci.nih.gov.

National Center for Complementary and Alternative Medicine (National Institutes of Health). PO Box 8218, Silver Spring, MD 20907-8218. (888) 644-6226. http://nccam.nih.gov.

Lata Cherath, PhD
Alison McTavish, M.Sc.
Rebecca J. Frey, PhD

Lung cancer, small cell

Definition

Small cell lung **cancer** is a disease in which the cells of the lung tissues grow uncontrollably and form tumors.

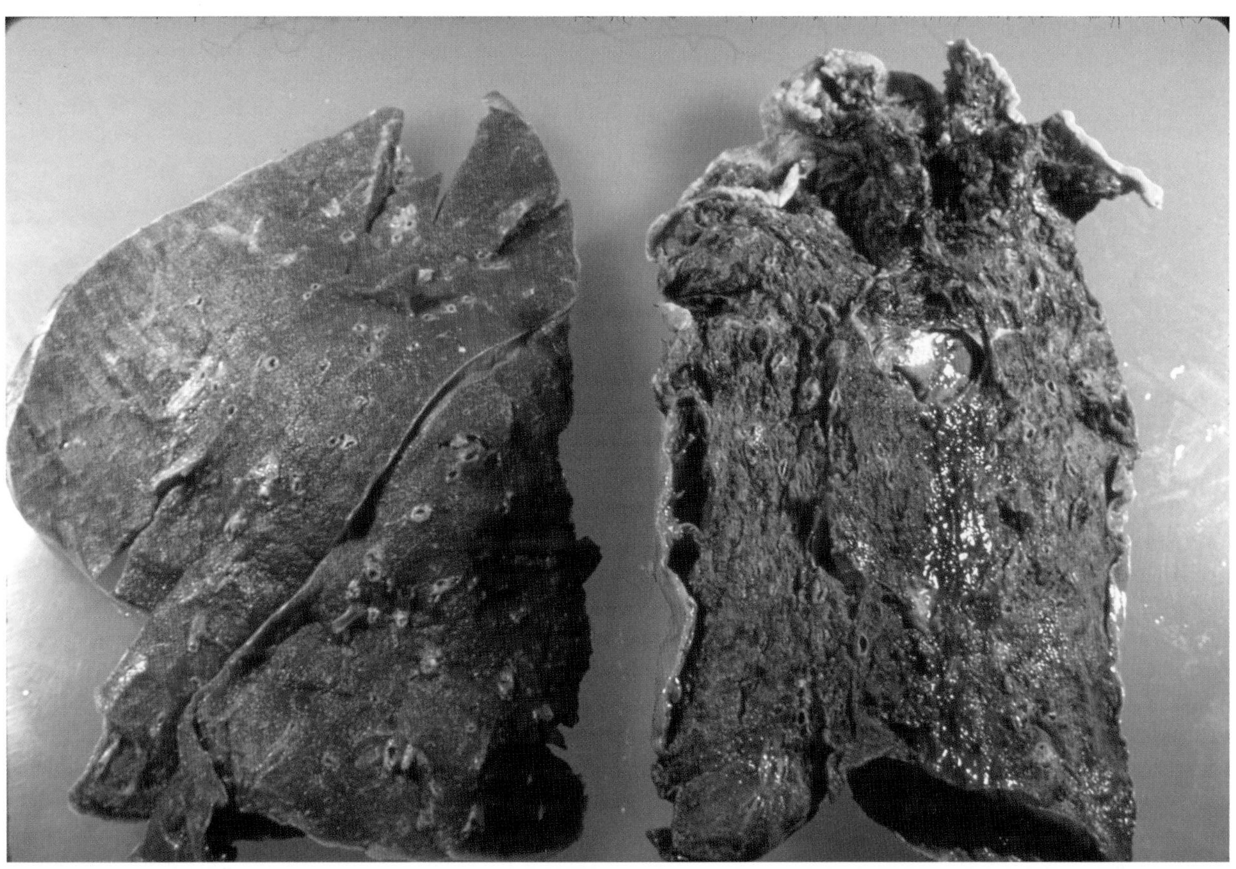

A normal lung (left) and the lung of a cigarette smoker (right). *(© by A. Glauberman/Science Source/Photo Researchers, Inc. Reproduced by permission.)*

Demographics

Lung cancer is a growing global epidemic. Worldwide, lung cancer is the second most common cancer among both men and women and is the leading cause of cancer death in both sexes. The worldwide mortality rate for patients with lung cancer is 86%. Of the 160,000 deaths from lung cancer that occur annually in the United States, about 40,000 are caused by small cell lung cancer. Although there are differences in mortality rates between ethnic groups, this is mainly due to differences in smoking habits.

Description

Lung cancer is divided into two main types: small cell and non-small cell. Small cell lung cancer is the least common of the two, accounting for only about 10–15% of all lung cancers. In the past, the disease was called oat cell cancer because, when viewed under a microscope, the cancer cells resemble oats. This type of lung cancer grows quickly and is more likely to spread to other organs in the body.

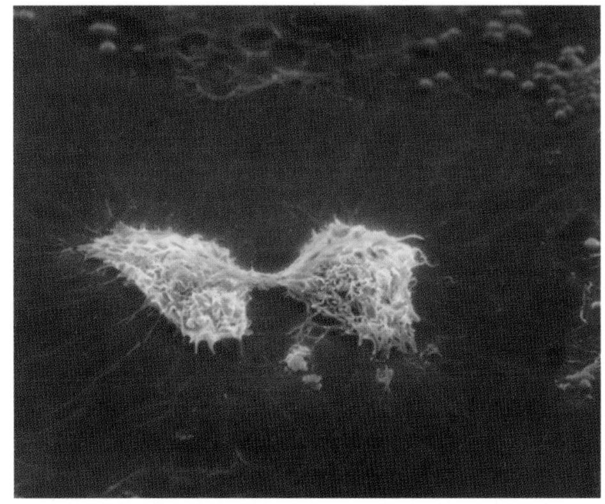

Lung cancer cells dividing. *(Custom Medical Stock Photo. Reproduced by permission.)*

The lungs are located along with the heart in the chest cavity. The lungs are not simply hollow balloons, but have a very organized structure consisting of hollow tubes, blood vessels, and elastic tissue. The hollow tubes, called bronchi, are multi-branched, becoming smaller and more numerous at each branching. They end in tiny, blind sacs made of elastic tissue called alveoli. These sacs are where the oxygen a person breathes in is taken up into the blood, and where carbon dioxide moves out of the blood to be breathed out.

Normal, healthy lungs are continually secreting mucus that not only keeps the lungs moist, but also protects the lungs by trapping foreign particles like dust and dirt in breathed air. The inside of the lungs is covered with small, hair-like structures called cilia. The cilia move in such a way that mucus is swept up out of the lungs and into the throat.

Small cell lung tumors usually start to develop in the central bronchi. They grow quickly and prevent the lungs from functioning at their full capacity. Tumors may block the movement of air through the bronchi in the lungs. As a result, less oxygen gets into the blood and patients feel short of breath. Tumors may also block the normal movement of mucus into the throat. As a result, mucus builds up in the lungs and **infection** may develop behind the tumor.

Causes and symptoms

Causes

Tobacco smoking accounts for nearly 90% of all lung cancers. The risk of developing lung cancer is increased for smokers who start at a young age, and for those who have smoked for a long time. The risk also increases as more **cigarettes** are smoked, and when cigarettes with higher tar content are smoked. Smoking marijuana cigarettes is also a risk factor for lung cancer. These cigarettes have a higher tar content than tobacco cigarettes.

Certain hazardous materials that people may be exposed to in their jobs have been shown to cause lung cancer. These include asbestos, coal products, and radioactive substances. Air pollution may also be a contributing factor. Exposure to radon, a colorless, odorless gas that sometimes accumulates in the basement of homes, may cause lung cancer in some patients. In addition, patients whose lungs are scarred from other lung conditions may have an increased risk of developing lung cancer.

Although the exact cause of lung cancer is not known, people with a family history of lung cancer appear to have a slightly higher risk of contracting the disease.

Symptoms

Small cell lung cancer is an aggressive disease that spreads quickly. Symptoms depend on the tumor's location within the lung, and on whether the cancer has spread to other parts of the body. More than 80% of small cell lung cancer patients have symptoms for only three months or less, and few cases are detected early. The following symptoms are the most commonly reported by small cell lung cancer patients at the time of their diagnosis:

- a persistent cough
- chest pain
- shortness of breath and wheezing
- persistent hoarseness
- fatigue and loss of appetite

Although some patients may experience bloody spit or phlegm, this symptom is more commonly seen in patients with other types of lung cancer.

Small cell tumors often press against a large blood vessel near the lungs called the superior vena cava (SVC), causing a condition known as SCV syndrome. This condition may cause patients to retain water, cough, and have shortness of breath. Because small cell lung cancer often spreads quickly to the bones and central nervous system, patients may also have **bone pain**, headaches, and seizures.

Small cell lung cancer can cause several hormonal disorders. About 40% of patients begin to secrete an anti-diuretic hormone at the wrong time. This hormone causes the body to retain water, which may result in the patient experiencing confusion, seizures, or coma. Less common are the development of **Cushing's syndrome** and the Eaton-Lambert syndrome. Symptoms of Cushing's syndrome include obesity, severe **fatigue**, high blood pressure, backache, high blood sugar, easy bruising, and bluish-red stretch marks on the skin. Eaton-Lambert syndrome is a neuromuscular disorder that causes muscle weakness, fatigue, and a tingling sensation on the skin. All of these hormonal disorders usually diminish after the lung tumor is successfully treated.

Diagnosis

If lung cancer is suspected, the doctor will take a detailed medical history that checks both symptoms and risk factors. During a complete physical examination, the doctor will examine the patient's throat to rule out other possible causes of hoarseness or coughing, and listen to the patient's breathing and the sounds made when the patient's chest and upper back are tapped. A chest x ray may be ordered to check for masses in the lungs. Special imaging techniques, such as **computed tomography** (CT) scans or **magnetic resonance imaging** (MRI), may provide more precise information about the size, shape, and location of any tumors.

Sputum analysis involves microscopic examination of the cells that are either coughed up from the lungs, or are collected through a special instrument called a bronchoscope. The sputum test does not, however, provide any information about the location of the tumor and must be followed by other tests.

Lung biopsy is the most definitive diagnostic tool for cancer. It can be performed in several different ways. The doctor can perform a **bronchoscopy**, which involves the insertion of a slender, lighted tube, called a bronchoscope, down the patient's throat and into the lungs. In addition to viewing the passageways of the lungs, the doctor can use the bronchoscope to obtain samples of the lung tissue. In another procedure known as a needle **biopsy**, the location of the tumor is first identified using a CT scan or MRI. The doctor then inserts a needle through the chest wall and collects a sample of tissue from the tumor. In the third procedure, known as surgical biopsy, the chest wall is opened up and a part of the tumor, or all of it, is removed for examination.

Treatment

Staging

Staging procedures are important in lung cancer because they tell doctors whether patients have disease only in their lungs, or whether the cancer has spread to other parts of the body. To establish the cancer stage, doctors have to perform various tests. These may include **bone marrow aspiration and biopsy**, CT scans of the chest and abdomen, MRI scans of the brain, and radionuclide bone scans. All of these tests determine the extent to which the cancer has spread. Once the stage is determined, doctors can decide on a course of treatment, and can have a better idea of the patient's prognosis.

Unlike other types of lung cancer, the staging of small cell lung cancer is relatively simple. This is because approximately 70% of patients already have metastatic disease when they are diagnosed, and small differences in the amount of tumor found in the lungs do not change the prognosis. Small cell lung cancer is usually divided into three stages:

- Limited stage: The cancer is found only in one lung and in lymph nodes close to the lung.
- Extensive stage: The cancer has spread beyond the lungs to other parts of the body.
- Recurrent stage: The cancer has returned following treatment.

Without treatment, small cell lung cancer has the most aggressive clinical course of any type of pulmonary tumor, with median survival from diagnosis of only 2–4 months. Compared with other cell types of lung cancer, small cell lung cancer has a greater tendency to be widely disseminated by the time of diagnosis, but is much more responsive to **chemotherapy** and irradiation.

Treatment of small cell lung cancer depends on whether the patient has limited, extensive, or recurrent disease. Treatment usually involves radiotherapy and chemotherapy. Surgery is rarely used for this type of lung cancer because the tumor is usually too advanced.

Patients with limited-stage disease are usually treated with chemotherapy. Combinations of two or more drugs have a better effect than treatment with a single drug. Up to 90% of patients with this stage of disease will respond to chemotherapy. The chemotherapy most commonly prescribed is a combination of the drugs **etoposide** (Vepesid) and **cisplatin** (Platinol). Combining chemotherapy with chest radiotherapy and/or occasionally surgery has also prolonged survival for limited-stage patients.

In addition to chest radiotherapy, some patients are also treated with **radiation therapy** to the brain, even if no cancer is found there. This treatment, called prophylactic cranial irradiation (PCI), is given to prevent tumors from forming in the brain. The combination of etoposide and cisplatin chemotherapy with chest radiation therapy and PCI has increased the two-year survival of limited-stage small cell lung cancer patients to almost 50%.

Combinations of different chemotherapy agents are also used for treating extensive-stage small cell lung cancer. However, compared with limited-stage patients, the percentage of extensive-stage patients who respond to therapy is lower. Commonly used drug combinations include **cyclophosphamide** (Cytoxan), **doxorubicin** (Adriamycin), and **vincristine** (Oncovin), or etoposide and cisplatin. The addition of radiation therapy to chemotherapy does not improve survival in these patients. However, radiation therapy is used for the palliative (pain relief) treatment of symptoms of metastatic lung cancer, particularly brain and bone tumors.

Patients who have recurrent small cell lung cancer often become resistant to chemotherapy. These patients are treated with palliative radiotherapy. Their doctor may also recommend that they take part in a clinical trial of a new therapy. Patients whose relapse occurs more than six months after their initial treatment, however, may still respond to traditional chemotherapy.

Coping with cancer treatment

The side effects associated with treatment of small cell lung cancer can be severe. Patients should ask their doctor about medications to treat **nausea and vomiting** and other side effects. It is particularly important to eat a nutritious diet and to drink plenty of fluids. In addition, most patients report feeling very tired and should get plenty of rest.

Clinical trials

Most of the improvements in the survival of patients with small cell lung cancer are the result of **clinical trials**. Ongoing trials are investigating new chemotherapy and radiotherapy regimens. In addition, entirely new types of therapy, such as gene therapy and biological therapy, are now being tested. Patients with a lung cancer diagnosis should ask their doctor about participating in a clinical trial.

Information on open clinical trials is available on the Internet from the National Cancer Institute at http://cancertrials.nci.nih.gov.

Alternative treatment

Many cancer patients have tried using shark cartilage to treat their disease. Shark cartilage is thought to interfere with the tumor's blood supply. A clinical trial using this treatment in lung cancer patients is ongoing. Information on this and other alternative treatments is available on the Internet from the National Center for Complementary and Alternative Medicine.

Patients who decide to try complementary and alternative therapies should tell their doctor. Some of these therapies may interfere with conventional treatment.

Prognosis

Small cell lung cancer is a very aggressive disease. Without treatment, limited-stage patients will survive for three to six months, while extensive-stage patients will survive six to 12 weeks. However, small cell lung cancer is much more responsive to chemotherapy and radiation therapy than other types of lung cancer. Among patients treated with chemotherapy, 70–90% have a major response to treatment.

Survival in patients responding to therapy is four to five times longer than in patients without treatment. In addition, two years after the start of therapy, about 10% of patients remain free of disease. In general, women tend to have a better prognosis than men. Patients whose disease has spread to the central nervous system or liver have a much worse prognosis. Although the overall survival at five years is 5–10%, survival is higher in patients with limited stage disease. About 70% of patients who are disease free after two years do not relapse. After five to 10 disease-free years, relapses are rare.

QUESTIONS TO ASK YOUR DOCTOR

- What kinds of diagnostic studies will be required to ascertain the type and spread of this tumor?
- Could there be a genetic component to this tumor? Should other family member be tested?
- What types of treatments are available?
- What types of side effects from treatments can I expect? What are your recommendations to help me deal with those side effects?
- Am I eligible for any clinical trials? Would these be helpful to consider?
- Are there any lifestyle changes that I should make?
- What type of diet should I follow? Are there foods I should avoid?
- Should I avoid any medications?
- How often should I be checked after treatment has ended?
- Is there a support group that I can join to hear about other people's experiences with this disorder?

Prevention

The best way to prevent lung cancer is either not start smoking, or quit smoking. Secondhand smoke from other people's tobacco should also be avoided. Appropriate precautions should be taken when working with substances that can cause cancer (carcinogens). Testing houses for the presence of radon gas, and removing asbestos from buildings have also been suggested as preventive strategies.

Resources

BOOKS

Abeloff, MD et al. *Clinical Oncology*. 3rd ed. Philadelphia: Elsevier, 2004.

Goldman L, Ausiello D., eds.*Cecil Textbook of Internal Medicine*. 23rd ed. Philadelphia: Saunders, 2008.

Mason, RJ et al. *Murray & Nadel's Textbook of Respiratory Medicine*. 4th ed. Philadelphia: Saunders, 2007.

ORGANIZATIONS

Alliance for Lung Cancer Advocacy, Support, and Education. P.O. Box 849, Vancouver, WA 98666. (800) 298-2436. http://www.alcase.org.

American Lung Association.1740 Broadway New York, NY 10019. (212) 315-8700. http://www.lungusa.org.

National Cancer Institute (National Institutes of Health). 9000 Rockville Pike, Bethesda, MD 20892. (800) 422-6237. http://www.nci.nih.gov.

National Center for Complementary and Alternative Medicine (National Institutes of Health). P.O. Box 8218, Silver Spring, MD 20907-8218. (888) 644-6226. http://nccam.nih.gov.

Lata Cherath, PhD
Alison McTavish, MSc

Lung metastasis *see* **Metastasis**

Lung surgery *see* **Lobectomy; Pneumonectomy; Thoracotomy**

Lymph node biopsy

Definition

A lymph node **biopsy** is a procedure in which all or part of a lymph node is removed and examined to determine if there is **cancer** within the node.

Purpose

The lymph system is the body's primary defense against **infection**. It consists of the spleen, tonsils, thymus, lymph nodes, lymph vessels, and the clear, slightly yellow fluid called lymph. These components produce and transport white blood cells called lymphocytes and macrophages that rid the body of infection. The lymph system is also involved in the production of antibodies. Antibodies are proteins that fight bacteria, viruses, and other foreign materials that enter the body.

The lymph vessels are similar to veins, only instead of carrying blood as veins do, they circulate lymph to most tissues in the body. Lymph nodes are about 600 small, bean-shaped collections of tissue found along the lymph vessel. They produce cells and proteins that fight infection, and clean and filter lymph. Lymph nodes are sometimes called lymph glands, although they are not true glands. When someone talks about having swollen glands, they are actually referring to lymph nodes.

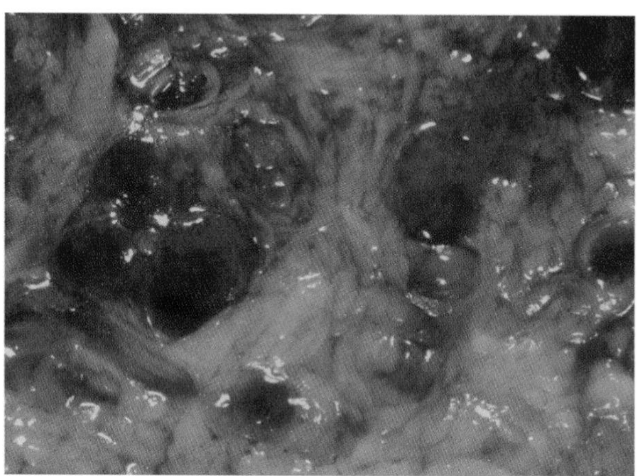

Close-up view of normal lymph nodes and fatty tissue. *(Custom Medical Stock Photo. Reproduced by permission.)*

Normal lymph glands are no larger than 0.5 in (1.3 cm) in diameter and are difficult to feel. However, lymph nodes can enlarge to greater than 2.5 in (6 cm) and can become sore. Most often the swelling is caused by an infection, but it can also be caused by cancer.

Cancers can metastasize (spread) through the lymph system from the site of the original tumor to distant parts of the body where secondary tumors are formed. The purpose of a lymph node biopsy is to determine the cause of the swelling and/or to see if cancer has begun to spread through the lymph system. This information is important in staging the cancer and devising a treatment plan.

Precautions

Women who are pregnant should inform their doctor before a lymph node biopsy, although pregnancy will not affect the results.

Description

There are three kinds of lymph node biopsy. **Sentinel lymph node mapping** and biopsy is a promising new technique that is discussed in its own entry. Fine needle aspiration (FNA) biopsy, often just called needle biopsy, is done when the lymph node of interest is near the surface of the body. A hematologist (a doctor who specializes in blood diseases) usually performs the test. In FNA biopsy, a needle is inserted through the

QUESTIONS TO ASK THE DOCTOR

- What kind of biopsy are you going to do?
- What will this tell me about my cancer?
- If you are doing an open biopsy, will you be removing any other structures at the same time?
- If you are, how will that affect my recovery from the operation?

skin and into the lymph node, and a sample of tissue is drawn out of the node. This material is preserved and sent to the laboratory for examination.

Advantages of a needle biopsy are that the test is minimally invasive. Only a local anesthetic is used, the procedure generally takes less than half an hour, and there is little pain afterwards. The disadvantage is that cancer may not be detected in the small sample of cells removed by the needle.

Open lymph node biopsy is a surgical procedure. It is done by a surgeon under general anesthesia on lymph nodes in the interior of the body and under local anesthesia on surface lymph nodes where FNA biopsy is considered inadequate. Once there is adequate anesthesia, the surgeon makes a small cut and removes either the entire lymph node or a slice of tissue that is then sent to the laboratory for examination. Results in both kinds of biopsies take one to three days.

Open biopsy can be advantageous in that it is easier to detect and identify the type of cancer in a large piece of tissue. Also, lymph nodes deep in the body can be sampled. Disadvantages include a longer recovery time, soreness at the biopsy site for several days, and the use of deeper anesthesia, increasing the risks to the patient. The procedure is done in a hospital or outpatient surgery center and takes about an hour, with additional time to recover from general anesthesia.

Preparation

No particular preparation is necessary for a needle biopsy. For an open biopsy, patients need standard pre-operative blood tests and other tests to evaluate general health. The doctor should be informed about any medications (prescription, non-prescription, or herbal) the patient is taking, as well as past bleeding problems or allergies to medication or anesthesia.

KEY TERMS

Lymph nodes—Small, bean-shaped organs located throughout the lymphatic system. The lymph nodes store special cells that can trap cancer cells or bacteria that are traveling through the body in lymph. Also called lymph glands.

Lymphocytes—Small white blood cells that bear the major responsibility for carrying out the activities of the immune system; they number about 1 trillion.

Malignant—Cancerous. Cells tend to reproduce without normal controls on growth and form tumors or invade other tissues.

Spleen—An organ located at the left side of the stomach that acts as a reservoir for blood cells and produces lymphocytes and other products involved in fighting infection.

Thymus—An organ near the base of the neck that produces cells that fight infection. It is at its largest at puberty, then declines in size and function during adult life.

Tonsils—Small masses of tissue at the back of the throat.

Aftercare

Little aftercare is needed in a needle biopsy other than a bandage to keep the biopsy site clean. Patients who have general anesthesia for an open biopsy often feel drowsy and tired for several days following the procedure, and should not plan to drive home after biopsy. The incision site must be kept clean and dry, and a follow-up visit to check on healing is usually necessary.

Risks

There are few risks associated with lymph node biopsy. The main risks are excessive bleeding (usually only in people with blood disorders) and allergic reaction to general anesthesia (rare). Occasionally the biopsy site becomes infected.

Normal results

Normal lymph nodes are small and flat. When examined under the microscope, they show no signs of cancer or infection.

Abnormal results

Abnormal lymph nodes are usually enlarged and contain cancerous (malignant) cells and/or show signs of infection.

See also Lymph node dissection; Radical neck dissection.

Resources

OTHER

ThriveOnline. [cited June 12, 2001]. http://thriveonline.oxygen.com/medical/library/article/003933.html.

ORGANIZATIONS

American Cancer Society. National Headquarters, 1599 Clifton Road NE, Atlanta, GA 30329. 800(ACS)-2345). http://www.cancer.org.

Cancer Information Service. National Cancer Institute, Building 31, Room 10A19, 9000 Rockville Pike, Bethesda, MD 20892. (800)4-CANCER. http://www.nci.nih.gov/cancerinfo.

Tish Davidson, A.M.

Lymph node dissection

Definition

Lymph node dissection (lymphadenectomy) is the surgical removal of lymph nodes in order to assess the spread of **cancer**.

Purpose

The lymph system is the body's primary defense against **infection**. It consists of the spleen, tonsils, thymus, lymph nodes, lymph vessels, and the clear, slightly yellow fluid called lymph. These components produce and transport cells and proteins that help rid the body of infection.

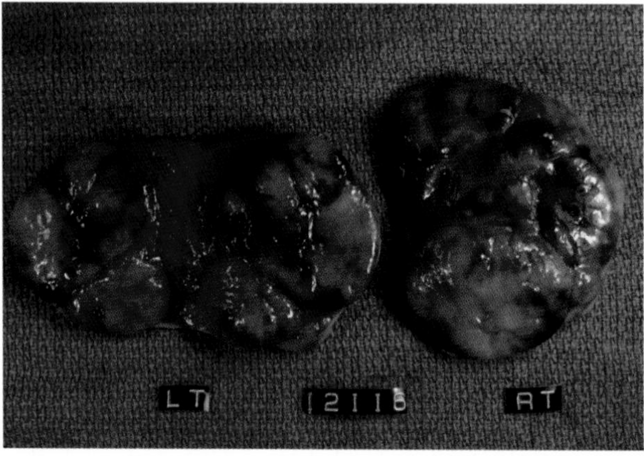

Diseased lymph nodes. *(Custom Medical Stock Photo. Reproduced by permission.)*

The lymph vessels are similar to veins, only instead of carrying blood as veins do, they circulate lymph to tissues in the body. There are about 600 small, bean-shaped collections of tissue found along the lymph vessels. These are called lymph nodes. They produce cells and proteins that fight infection. They also clean and filter foreign cells, such as bacteria or cancer cells, out of the lymph.

Cancer cells can break off from the original tumor and metastasize (spread) through the lymph system to distant parts of the body, where secondary tumors are formed. The purpose of a lymph node dissection is to remove the lymph nodes that have trapped cancer cells so that the extent of spread can be determined. Lymph node dissection is done for many different types of cancers, including cancers of the head and neck, breast, prostate, testes, bladder, colon, and lung.

About 200 lymph nodes are in the head and neck and another 30 to 50 are in the armpit. More are located in the groin area. Lymph nodes are sometimes called lymph glands, although they are not true glands. When someone talks about having swollen glands, they are referring to swollen lymph nodes.

Normally lymph nodes are no larger than 0.5 in (1.3 cm) in diameter and are difficult to feel. However, when lymph nodes trap bacteria or cancer cells, they can increase in size to greater than 2.5 in (6 cm). Most often, hot and painful swollen nodes are caused by trapped bacteria. Swollen lymph nodes caused by cancer are usually painless.

Precautions

This operation usually will not be performed if the cancer has already metastasized to another site. In this case, removing the lymph nodes will not effectively contain the cancer. As with any surgery, women who are pregnant should inform their doctors before a lymph node dissection.

Description

Lymph node dissection is usually done by a surgeon in a hospital setting, under general anesthesia. An incision is made and tissue is pulled back to reveal the lymph nodes. The surgeon is guided in what to remove by the location of the original cancer. Sample lymph nodes may be sent to the laboratory for examination. If the excised nodes do contain malignant cells, this would indicate that the cancer has spread beyond the original site, and recommendations can then be made regarding further therapy.

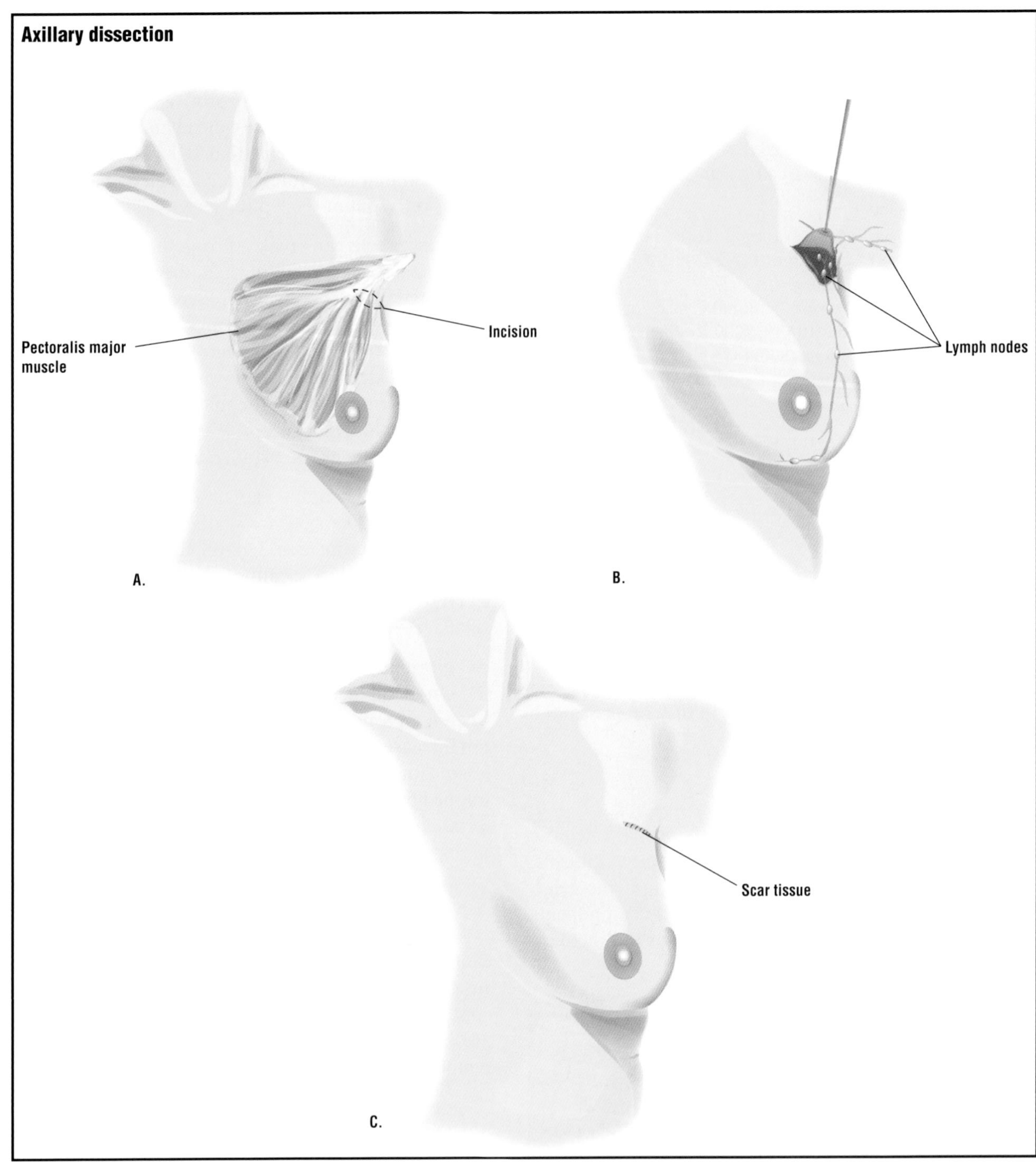

(Illustration by Argosy Publishing. Cengage Learning, Gale.)

Preparation

Tests may be done before the operation to determine the location of the cancer and which nodes should be removed. These tests may include lymph node biopsies, CT (**computed tomography**) scans, and MRI scans. In addition, standard pre-operative blood and liver function tests are performed. The patient will meet with an anesthesiologist before the operation, and should notify the anesthesiologist about all drug allergies and all medication (prescription, non-prescription, or herbal) that he or she is taking.

QUESTIONS TO ASK THE DOCTOR

- How will you determine which lymph nodes should be removed?
- How should I prepare for this procedure?
- Are there precautions I can take to help prevent lymphedema?
- How will lymph node dissection affect my daily life?
- Will you be removing anything else besides lymph nodes during this operation?
- About how long will I have to stay in the hospital?
- Will having my lymph nodes removed increase my chances of getting infections?

KEY TERMS

Computed tomography (CT or CAT) scan—Using x rays taken from many angles and computer modeling, CT scans help determine the size and location of tumors and provide information on whether they can be surgically removed.

Magnetic resonance imaging (MRI)—MRI uses magnets and radio waves to create detailed cross-sectional pictures of the interior of the body.

Malignant—Cancerous. Cells tend to reproduce without normal controls on growth and form tumors or invade other tissues.

Metastasize—Spread of cells from the original site of the cancer to other parts of the body where secondary tumors are formed.

Aftercare

How long a person stays in the hospital after lymph node dissection depends on how many lymph nodes were removed, their location, and whether surgery to remove the primary tumor or other structures was performed at the same time. Drains are inserted under the skin to remove the fluid that accumulates after the lymph nodes have been removed, and patients are usually able to return home with the drains still in place. Some patients are able to leave the same day or the day following the procedure.

An accumulation of lymph fluid that causes swelling, a condition known as lymphedema, is the most feared side effect of lymph node dissection. If swelling occurs, patients should consult their doctors immediately. Swelling may indicate that a new tumor is blocking a lymph vessel, or that a side effect of lymph node dissection is present. Treatment for lymphedema in people with cancer is different than treatment of lymphedema that arises from other causes. In cancer patients, it is essential to alleviate swelling without spreading cancer cells to other parts of the body, therefore an oncologist (cancer specialist) should be consulted before beginning any treatment.

Risks

People who have lymph nodes removed are at increased risk of developing lymphedema, which can occur in any part of the body where lymph accumulates in abnormal quantities. When the amount of fluid exceeds the capacity of the lymph system to move it through the body, it leaks into the tissues and causes them to swell. Removing lymph nodes and lymph vessels through lymph node dissection increases the likelihood that the capacity of the lymph transport system will be exceeded.

Lymphedema can occur days or weeks after lymph node dissection. **Radiation therapy** also increases the chance of developing lymphedema, so those people who have radiation therapy following lymph node dissection are at greatest risk of experiencing this side effect. Lymphedema slows healing, causes skin and tissue damage, and when left untreated can result in the development of hard or fibrous tissue. People with lymphedema are also at risk for repeated infection, because pools of lymph in the tissues provide a perfect spot for bacteria to grow. In severe cases, untreated lymphedema can develop into a rare form of cancer called lymphangiosarcoma.

Other risks associated with lymph node dissection are the same as for all major surgery: potential bleeding, infection, and allergic reaction to anesthesia.

Normal results

Normal lymph nodes are small and flat and show no cancerous cells under the microscope.

Abnormal results

Abnormal lymph nodes are enlarged and show malignant cells when examined under the microscope.

See also Lymph node biopsy; Radical neck dissection.

Resources

ORGANIZATIONS

American Cancer Society, National Headquarters. 1599 Clifton Rd. NE, Atlanta, GA 30329. 800(ACS)-2345. http://www.cancer.org.

Cancer Information Service. National Cancer Institute. Building 31, Room 10A19, 9000 Rockville Pike, Bethesda, MD 20892. (800) 4-CANCER. http://www.nci.nih.gov/cancerinfo/index.html.

National Lymphedema Network. Latham Square, 1611 Telegraph Ave., Suite 1111, Oakland, CA 94612-2138. (800) 541-3259. http://www.lymphnet.org.

Tish Davidson, A.M.

Lymphangiogram, lymph node angiogram

see **Lymphangiography**

Lymphangiography

Definition

Lymphangiography is a type of diagnostic testing technique in which **x rays** (called lymph node angiograms) and the injection of a contrast medium (a substance that provides a contrast between the tissue or organ being filmed and the medium) are used to visualize lymphatic circulation and the lymph nodes.

Purpose

The lymphatic system consists of tissues, organs, and vessels that aid in circulating body fluids and defending the body from damage by foreign substances such as viruses, bacteria, or fungi. However, certain cancers may also spread through the lymphatic system. Thus, lymphangiography is sometimes used to:

- diagnose the presence or spread of tumors, lymphatic cancer (lymphoma), and other cancers
- distinguish primary lymphedema (when swelling in the lymphatic system arises from missing or impaired lymphatic vessels) from secondary lymphedema (swelling caused by damaged lymph vessels or lymph nodes that have been removed)
- localize tumors for surgical removal
- assess the effectiveness of chemotherapy and radiation therapy in treating problems associated with metastatic (spreading) cancer

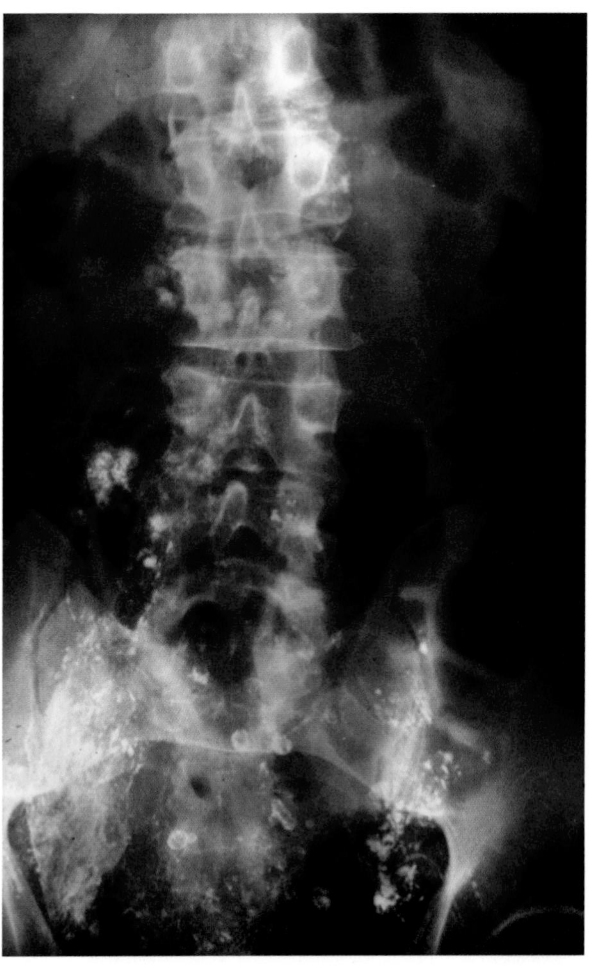

False-color lymphangiogram of the abdomen of a person suffering from lymphoma. *(Copyright Mehau Kulyk, Science Source/Photo Researchers, Inc. Reproduced by permission.)*

Although the results of lymphangiography are considered reliable, additional tests, studies, and clinical observations are necessary to determine a precise diagnosis. By itself, lymphangiography misses **cancer** in about 20% of cases. One of the major drawbacks of lymphangiography is its failure to fill certain lymphatic channels and groups of lymph nodes—a failure that may be due to **infection**, injury, or tumor spread. When this filling failure occurs, certain segments of the lymphatic system in the abdomen and pelvis cannot be visualized; thus, metastatic disease can be neither confirmed nor ruled out.

Since the late 1990s, conventional lymphangiography (using an iodine oil-based contrast agent) has been used almost exclusively for the staging of urologic pelvic and testicular malignancies. The test may demonstrate metastases within lymph nodes of normal size that are missed on **computed tomography** (CT)

QUESTIONS TO ASK THE DOCTOR

- What is the purpose of the test?
- How long will the test take?
- Will I be sedated or get anesthesia before the test?
- Is there anything special I need to do before the test?
- Can I drive myself home after testing?
- When will I get the results?

KEY TERMS

Contrast medium—A substance that provides a contrast between the tissue or organ being filmed and the medium.

Lymph node—A rounded, encapsulated body consisting of an accumulation of lymphatic tissue; found in lymphatic vessels.

Lymphoma—A type of lymphatic cancer.

Metastases—Cancer cells that have spread from the primary site of malignancy to another location in the body.

imaging. Technical innovations in nuclear diagnostics and computer imaging largely replaced lymphangiography with simpler, safer, and more reliable techniques of visualizing the lymphatic system (such as lymphangioscintigraphy, or isotope lymphography).

Precautions

Because of the possibility of an adverse reaction to the contrast medium, lymphangiography is usually not administered to patients with lung problems, heart disease, or severe kidney or liver disease.

Individuals with allergies to shellfish, iodine, or dye used in other diagnostic tests may receive steroids or antihistamines before the test to decrease the risk of allergic reactions.

Description

Lymphangiography testing may be done on an inpatient or outpatient basis. A sedative may be given to help the patient relax. After the skin of each foot is cleaned with an antiseptic, a blue indicator dye (which does not show up on x rays) is injected between the first, second, and third toes of each foot. The dye spreads into the lymphatic system in about 15 to 30 minutes. The thin, bluish lines that appear on the top of each foot delineate the lymphatic vessels. Next, a local anesthetic is injected, and a small incision is made into one of the larger blue lines in each foot. A needle or catheter (a thin flexible tube) is inserted into a vessel in each foot, and an oil-based contrast medium (such as Ethiodol) is injected at a slow, steady rate. A feeling of pressure may occur as the contrast medium is injected, but the patient must lie still to avoid dislodging the needle.

A fluoroscope (a device consisting of a fluorescent screen on which the shadows of objects that come between the screen and an attached x-ray apparatus can be viewed) is used to monitor the progress of the contrast medium as it spreads slowly (taking about 60 to 90 minutes) through the lymphatic system, traveling up the legs, into the groin, and along the back of the abdominal cavity. After the contrast agent is injected, the catheter is removed and the incisions are stitched and bandaged. Then x rays are taken of the legs, pelvis, abdomen, and chest areas. The following day, an additional set of x rays is obtained.

After the test, the patient's skin, feces, and urine may have a bluish tint for two to three days (until the marker dye disappears), and there may be some discomfort behind the knees and in the groin area. Test results are reported to the doctor or patient from a few hours to a few days after the procedure.

Preparation

There is usually no special preparation needed before lymphangiography—such as restrictions in diet, activity, or medication intake. However, some facilities may require a clear liquid diet for a specified period of time before the test. In addition, for comfort reasons, patients may be asked to empty their bladders before testing. A patient undergoing lymphangiography (or a close family member) must sign a consent form before the test is administered.

Aftercare

After testing, the patient's blood pressure, pulse, breathing status, and temperature are monitored at regular intervals until they are stable. Any lung complications are noted, such as hoarseness or shortness of breath, chest pain, low blood pressure, low-grade **fever**, and blueness of lips and nailbeds due to clotting of the dye.

Bedrest for at least 24 hours following the test is recommended, with feet elevated to help reduce swelling at the incision sites. The incision sites may be sore for several days, and ice packs may be applied to these sites to further reduce swelling. The patient should also inspect the incision sites for infection. Sterile dressings should remain in place for two days, and the incision sites should be kept dry until after the sutures are removed (7 to 10 days after the test).

Risks

There is a risk of infection or bleeding caused by introducing the needle or tube through the skin or an allergic reaction—usually not serious— to the contrast medium. There is also a slight risk of oil embolism (obstruction of a blood vessel) due to the oil-based contrast medium. The contrast medium eventually seeps from the lymphatic channels into the general circulation, where it may travel to, and lodge in, the lungs.

There is some radiation exposure involved in the procedure. Although pregnant women and children are particularly sensitive to these risks, physicians may order the procedure when the benefits appear to outweigh the risks.

Normal results

Normal test results indicate no anatomical or functional abnormalities.

Abnormal results

Abnormal results may indicate:

- filariasis (a tropical disease caused by worms living in the lymphatic system)
- Hodgkin's or non-Hodgkin's lymphoma (cancers of the lymphatic system)
- inflammation
- metastatic cancer
- primary lymphedema
- retroperitoneal tumors (tumors lying outside of the peritoneum—the membrane lining the abdominal cavity)
- trauma

Resources

BOOKS

Fischbach, Frances Talaska. *A Manual of Laboratory and Diagnostic Tests.* 6th ed. Philadelphia: Lippincott Williams and Wilkins, 2000.

PERIODICALS

Bellin, Marie-France, Catherine Beigelman, and Sophie Precetti-Morel. "Iron Oxide-Enhanced MR Lymphography: Initial Experience." *European Journal of Radiology* June 2000: 257–264.

Winterer, Jan Thorsten, Ulrich Blum, Stephan Boos, Stavros Konstantinides, and Mathia Langer. "Cerebral and Renal Embolization After Lymphangiography in a Patient with Non-Hogkin's Lymphoma: Case Report." *Radiology* February 1999: 381–385.

ORGANIZATIONS

American College of Radiology. http://www.acr.org.

Lymphoma Research Foundation of America. http://www.lymphomafocus.org.

Genevieve Slomski, Ph.D.

Lymphocyte immune globulin

Definition

Lymphocyte **immune globulin** is a drug used to suppress the immune system. Lymphocyte immune globulin is also known by the generic name anti-thymocyte globulin (ATG) and the brand names Atgam and Thymoglobulin. Atgam first received FDA approval in 1981 and Thymoglobulin in 1999. As of 2009, no generic preparations are available.

Purpose

Lymphocyte immune globulin is used to treat aplastic **anemia** and to prevent rejections during **bone marrow transplantation**. This drug has also been used experimentally to treat advanced **non-Hodgkin's lymphomas** and cutaneous T-cell lymphomas.

Description

This drug suppresses the immune system by slowing down T cells, cells critical in immunity. Without them, the immune system is essentially paralyzed. Lymphocyte immune globulin contains antibodies that attach to T cells and prevent them from working properly. This drug also decreases the number of T cells in the blood.

Lymphocyte immune globulin is made by vaccinating an animal with immature human T cells, then collecting the antibodies made against them. Atgam is made in horses and Thymoglobulin in rabbits.

Atgam is labeled for use only in kidney transplantation and aplastic anemia, and Thymoglobulin is

KEY TERMS

Adult respiratory distress syndrome (ARDS)—A lung disease characterized by widespread lung abnormalities, fluid in the lungs, shortness of breath, and low oxygen levels in the blood.

Antibodies—Proteins made by the immune system that attach to targeted molecules and cells.

Aplastic anemia—Failure of the bone marrow to make enough blood cells.

Blood cells—Cells found in the blood, including red blood cells that carry oxygen, white blood cells that fight infections, and platelets that help the blood to clot.

Bone marrow—A group of cells and molecules found in the centers of some bones. It makes all of the cells found in the blood, including the cells involved in immunity.

Graft-vs-host disease (GVHD)—A disease that develops when immune cells in transplanted bone marrow attack the body.

Immune system—The cells and organs that defend the body against infections.

Pulmonary edema—A disease characterized by excessive fluid in the lungs and difficulty breathing.

Sepsis—An infection that has spread into the blood.

Serum sickness—A type of allergic reaction against blood proteins. Serum sickness develops when the immune system makes antibodies against proteins that are not normally found in the body.

Skin test—A test used to diagnose allergies.

T lymphocyte or T cell—A type of white blood cell. Helper T cells aid other cells of the immune system, while cytotoxic T cells destroy abnormal body cells, including those that have been infected by a virus.

Thrombocytopenia—Too few platelets in the blood.

specifically approved only for kidney transplantation. The effectiveness of either drug for treating aplastic anemia in **cancer** patients, however, is unknown.

Lymphocyte immune globulin is often used off-label to treat graft-versus-host disease (GVHD) after bone marrow transplantation. The drug has been beneficial for GVHD patients in some studies, but its effectiveness has not been conclusively demonstrated. In some **clinical trials**, it is also being used to prepare the patient's body for bone marrow transplantation. This drug produces short partial remissions of some lymphomas in published experiments.

Recommended dosage

The usual dose of Atgam in adults is 10–30 mg/kg (1 kilogram is 2.2 pounds). Doses of 5–25 mg/kg have been given to a few children. Thymoglobulin, which is about 10 times stronger, has a recommended dose of 1–1.5 mg/kg in adults. Typically these drugs are given daily or every other day for several days or weeks. They are injected into the blood over several hours, under close supervision in the hospital or clinic.

Precautions

Patients should not take Atgam if they are allergic to horse proteins or Thymoglobulin if they are allergic to rabbit proteins. Patients should tell their doctors about any current or previous blood cell problems and about all their prescription and over-the-counter drugs.

Lymphocyte immune globulin can make infections more serious. Patients should check with their doctors if they have any symptoms of an **infection**, such as chills, **fever**, or sore throat. They should also avoid people with contagious diseases and anyone recently vaccinated with an oral polio vaccine. The drug decreases the effectiveness of vaccinations given just before or during treatment. Some types of **vaccines** are not safe to receive while taking this drug.

Lymphocyte immune globulin does not interact with any specific foods. However, patients should check with their doctor for specific recommendations for eating and drinking before the treatment.

Patients should be careful in planning their activities, as this drug can cause dizziness.

Side effects

Thymoglobulin and Atgam have very similar side effects. However, Thymoglobulin is approximately twice as likely to decrease the number of white blood cells and three times as likely to result in malaise. Dizziness is much more common with Atgam. Other numerous side effects caused by both drugs include:

- Chills or fever in most patients
- Risk of developing an infection, which has been seen in up to 30% of patients, and sepsis in approximately 10%
- Risk of bleeding, due to thrombocytopenia (seen in 30–45% of patients)

- Rarely, anemia or the destruction of white blood cells other than T cells
- Pain, swelling, and redness where the drug is injected (minimized by injecting the drug into the faster-moving blood in a large vein)
- Allergic reactions (Serious allergic reactions can cause difficulty breathing, swelling of the tongue, a drop in blood pressure, or pain in the chest, sides, or back. Severe allergic reactions are potentially life-threatening, but rare; milder allergic reactions can result in itching, hives, or rash. Skin tests are often done to predict the likelihood of an allergic reaction, but are not foolproof.)
- Serum sickness, an immune reaction against the drug (Can result in fever, chills, muscle and joint aches, rash, blurred vision, swollen lymph nodes, or kidney problems; serum sickness is common when lymphocyte immune globulin is used alone for aplastic anemia, but fairly rare when it is combined with other drugs that suppress immunity.)
- Headaches, pain in the abdomen, diarrhea, nausea or vomiting, fluid retention, weakness, rapid heartbeats, or an abnormal increase in blood potassium (these side effects develop in more than a fifth of all patients during treatment)
- Uncommon side effects such as kidney damage, high blood pressure, heart failure, lethargy, abnormal sensations such as prickling in the skin, seizures, pulmonary edema, and adult respiratory distress syndrome
- Risk of developing lymphoma or leukemia, if the immune system is greatly suppressed for a long time

Side effects in pregnant or nursing women

The effects of this drug on an unborn child are unknown. Doctors are not sure if this drug reaches breast milk.

Methods of preventing or reducing side effects

Drugs such as antihistamines, acetaminophen, and **corticosteroids** can prevent or decrease some side effects, including fevers, chills, and allergic reactions. **Antibiotics** may help to prevent infections.

Interactions

Combining this drug with other medications that suppress the immune system (including **chemotherapy**) can severely suppress immunity. Drugs that slow blood clotting, such as aspirin, can increase the risk of bleeding. Any drug that reduces the symptoms of an infection, including aspirin and acetaminophen, can increase the risk that a serious infection will go undetected.

See also Myelosuppression; Immune response; Infection and sepsis; Neuropathy.

Anna Rovid Spickler, D.V.M., Ph.D.

Lymphoma

Definition

Lymphoma is the name of a diverse group of cancers of the lymphatic system, a connecting network of glands, organs and vessels whose principle cell is the lymphocyte.

Description

When lymphoma occurs, cells in the lymphatic system grow abnormally. They divide too rapidly and grow without any order or control. Too much tissue is formed and tumors begin to grow. Because there is lymph tissue in many parts of the body, the **cancer** cells may involve the liver, spleen, or bone marrow.

Two general types of lymphoma are commonly recognized: **Hodgkin's disease** or Hodgkin's lymphoma (HD), and **Non-Hodgkin's lymphoma** (NHL). The two are distinguished by cell type. These differ significantly in respect of their natural histories and their response to therapy. Hodgkin's disease tends to be primarily of nodal origin. Non-Hodgkin's lymphomas, unlike HD, can spread beyond the lymphatic system.

See also AIDS-related cancers.

Kate Kretschmann

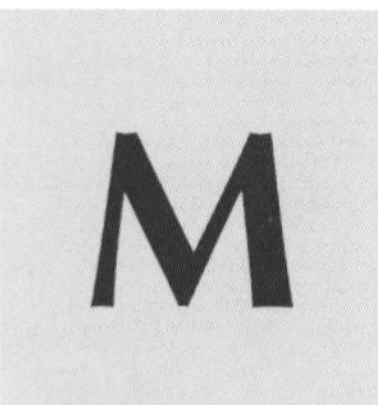

Magnetic resonance imaging

Definition

Magnetic resonance imaging (MRI) is one of the newest, and perhaps most versatile, medical imaging technology available. Doctors can get highly refined images of the body's interior without surgery using MRI. By using strong magnets and pulses of radio waves to manipulate the natural magnetic properties in the body, this technique makes better images of organs and soft tissues than those of other brain scanning technologies. MRI is particularly useful for imaging the brain and spine, as well as the soft tissues of joints and the interior structure of bones, as well as the liver. The entire body is visible with MRI, and the technique poses few known health risks.

Purpose

MRI was developed in the 1980s. Its technology has been developed for use in magnetic resonance **angiography** (MRA), magnetic resonance spectroscopy (MRS), and, more recently, magnetic resonance cholangiopancreatography (MRCP). MRA was developed to study blood flow, whereas MRS can identify the chemical composition of diseased tissue and produce color images of brain function. MRCP is evolving into a potential non-invasive alternative for the diagnostic procedure **endoscopic retrograde cholangiopancreatography** (ERCP).

Advantages

DETAIL. MRI creates precise images of the body based on the varying proportions of magnetic elements in different tissues. Very minor fluctuations in chemical composition can be determined. MRI images have greater natural contrast than standard **x rays**, **computed tomography** scan (CT scan), or ultrasound, all of which depend on the differing physical properties of tissues. This sensitivity allows MRI to distinguish fine variations in tissues deep within the body. It is also particularly useful for spotting and distinguishing diseased tissues (tumors and other lesions) early in their development. Often, doctors prescribe an MRI scan to more fully investigate earlier findings of other imaging techniques.

SCOPE. The entire body can be scanned, from head to toe and from the skin to the deepest recesses of the brain. Moreover, MRI scans are not obstructed by bone, gas, or body waste, which can hinder other imaging techniques. (Although the scans can be degraded by motion such as breathing, heartbeat, and bowel activity.) The MRI process produces cross-sectional images of the body that are as sharp in the middle as on the edges, even of the brain through the skull. A close series of these two-dimensional images can provide a three-dimensional view of the targeted area. Along with images from the cross-sectional plane, the MRI can also provide images sagitally (from one side of the body to the other, from left to right for example), allowing for a better three-dimensional interpretation, which is sometimes very important for planning a surgical approach.

SAFETY. MRI does not depend on potentially harmful ionizing radiation, as do standard x ray and computer tomography scans. There are no known risks specific to the procedure, other than for people who might have metal objects in their bodies.

Despite its many advantages, MRI is not routinely used because it is a somewhat complex and costly procedure. MRI requires large, expensive, and complicated equipment; a highly trained operator; and a doctor specializing in radiology. Generally, MRI is prescribed only when serious symptoms or negative results from other tests indicate a need. Many times another test is appropriate for the type of diagnosis needed.

Uses

Doctors may prescribe an MRI scan of different areas of the body.

BRAIN AND HEAD. MRI technology was developed because of the need for brain imaging. It is one of the few imaging tools that can see through bone (the skull) and deliver high quality pictures of the brain's delicate soft tissue structures. MRI may be needed for patients with symptoms of a brain tumor, stroke, or **infection** (like meningitis). MRI may also be needed when cognitive or psychological symptoms suggest brain disease (like Alzheimer's or Huntington's diseases, or multiple sclerosis), or when developmental retardation suggests a birth defect. MRI can also provide pictures of the sinuses and other areas of the head beneath the face. In adult and pediatric patients, MRI may be better able to detect abnormalities than compared to computed tomography scanning.

SPINE. Spinal problems can create a host of seemingly unrelated symptoms. MRI is particularly useful for identifying and evaluating degenerated or herniated spinal discs. It can also be used to determine the condition of nerve tissue within the spinal cord.

JOINT. MRI scanning is most commonly used to diagnose and assess joint problems. MRI can provide clear images of the bone, cartilage, ligament, and tendon that comprise a joint. MRI can be used to diagnose joint injuries due to sports, advancing age, or arthritis. MRI can also be used to diagnose shoulder problems, such as a torn rotator cuff. MRI can also detect the presence of an otherwise hidden tumor or infection in a joint, and can be used to diagnose the nature of developmental joint abnormalities in children.

SKELETON. The properties of MRI that allow it to see through the skull also allow it to view the inside of bones. Accordingly, it can be used to detect bone **cancer**, inspect the marrow for leukemia and other diseases, assess bone loss (osteoporosis), and examine complex fractures.

HEART AND CIRCULATION. MRI technology can be used to evaluate the circulatory system. The heart and blood flow provides a good natural contrast medium that allows structures of the heart to be clearly distinguished.

THE REST OF THE BODY. Whereas computed tomography and ultrasound scans satisfy most chest, abdominal, and general body imaging needs, MRI may be needed in certain circumstances to provide better pictures or when repeated scanning is required. The progress of some therapies, like **liver cancer** therapy, needs to be monitored, and the effect of repeated x-ray exposure is a concern.

Precautions

MRI scans and metal

MRI scanning should not be used when there is the potential for an interaction between the strong MRI magnet and metal objects that might be imbedded in a patient's body. The force of magnetic attraction on certain types of metal objects (including surgical steel) could move them within the body and cause serious injury. Metal may be imbedded in a person's body for several reasons.

MEDICAL. People with implanted cardiac pacemakers, metal aneurysm clips, or who have broken bones repaired with metal pins, screws, rods, or plates must tell their radiologist prior to having an MRI scan. In some cases (like a metal rod in a reconstructed leg), the difficulty may be overcome.

INJURY. Patients must tell their doctors if they have bullet fragments or other metal pieces in their body from old wounds. The suspected presence of metal, whether from an old or recent wound, should be confirmed before scanning.

OCCUPATIONAL. People with significant work exposure to metal particles (e.g., working with a metal grinder) should discuss this with their doctors and radiologists. The patient may need prescan testing—usually a single, regular x ray of the eyes to see if any metal is present.

Chemical agents

Chemical agents designed to improve the picture or allow for the imaging of blood or other fluid flow during MRA may be injected. In rare cases, patients may be allergic to, or intolerant of, these agents, and these patients should not receive them. If these chemical agents are to be used, patients should discuss any concerns they have with their doctor and radiologist.

Side effects

The potential side effects of magnetic and electric fields on human health remain a source of debate. In particular, the possible effects on an unborn baby are not well known. Any woman who is, or may be, pregnant, should carefully discuss this issue with her doctor and radiologist before undergoing a scan.

As with all medical imaging techniques, obesity greatly interferes with the quality of MRI.

Description

In essence, MRI produces a map of hydrogen distribution in the body. Hydrogen is the simplest

KEY TERMS

Angiography—Any of the different methods for investigating the condition of blood vessels, usually via a combination of radiological imaging and injections of chemical tracing and contrast agents.

Gadolinium—A very rare metallic element useful for its sensitivity to electromagnetic resonance, among other things. Traces of it can be injected into the body to enhance the MRI pictures.

Hydrogen—The simplest, most common element known in the universe. It is composed of a single electron (negatively charged particle). It is the nuclear proton of hydrogen that makes MRI possible by reacting resonantly to radio waves while aligned in a magnetic field.

Ionizing radiation—Electromagnetic radiation that can damage living tissue by disrupting and destroying individual cells. All types of nuclear decay radiation (including x rays) are potentially ionizing. Radio waves do not damage organic tissues they pass through.

Magnetic field—the three-dimensional area surrounding a magnet, in which its force is active. During MRI, the patient's body is permeated by the force field of a superconducting magnet.

Radio waves—Electromagnetic energy of the frequency range corresponding to that used in radio communications, usually 10,000 cycles per second to 300 billion cycles per second. Radio waves are the same as visible light, x rays, and all other types of electromagnetic radiation, but are of a higher frequency.

element known, the most abundant in biological tissue, and one that can be magnetized. It will align itself within a strong magnetic field, like the needle of a compass. The earth's magnetic field is not strong enough to keep a person's hydrogen atoms pointing in the same direction, but the superconducting magnet of an MRI machine can. This comprises the magnetic part of MRI.

Once a patient's hydrogen atoms have been aligned in the magnet, pulses of very specific radio wave frequencies are used to knock them back out of alignment. The hydrogen atoms alternately absorb and emit radio wave energy, vibrating back and forth between their resting (magnetized) state and their agitated (radio pulse) state. This comprises the resonance part of MRI.

The MRI equipment records the duration, strength, and source location of the signals emitted by the atoms as they relax and translates the data into an image on a television monitor. The state of hydrogen in diseased tissue differs from healthy tissue of the same type, making MRI particularly good at identifying tumors and other lesions. In some cases, chemical agents such as gadolinium can be injected to improve the contrast between healthy and diseased tissue.

A single MRI exposure produces a two-dimensional image of a slice through the entire target area. A series of these image slices closely spaced (usually less than half an inch) makes a virtual three-dimensional view of the area.

Magnetic resonance spectroscopy (MRS) is different from MRI because MRS uses a continuous band of radio wave frequencies to excite hydrogen atoms in a variety of chemical compounds other than water. These compounds absorb and emit radio energy at characteristic frequencies, or spectra, which can be used to identify them. Generally, a color image is created by assigning a color to each distinctive spectral emission. This comprises the spectroscopy part of MRS. MRS is still experimental and is available only in a few research centers.

Doctors primarily use MRS to study the brain and disorders like epilepsy, Alzheimer's disease, **brain tumors**, and the effects of drugs on brain growth and metabolism. The technique is also useful in evaluating metabolic disorders of the muscles and nervous system.

Magnetic resonance angiography (MRA) is another variation on standard MRI. MRA, like other types of angiography, looks specifically at fluid flow within the blood (vascular) system, but does so without the injection of dyes or radioactive tracers. Standard MRI cannot make a good picture of flowing blood, but MRA uses specific radio pulse sequences to capture usable signals. The technique is generally used in combination with MRI to obtain images that show both vascular structure and flow within the brain and head in cases of stroke, or when a blood clot or aneurysm is suspected.

MRI technology is also being applied in the evaluation of the pancreatic and biliary ducts in a new study called magnetic resonance cholangiopancreatography (MRCP). MRCP produces images similar to that of endoscopic retrograde cholangiopancreatography (ERCP), but in a non-invasive manner. Because MRCP is new and still very expensive, it is not readily available in most hospitals and imaging centers.

Regardless of the exact type of MRI planned, or area of the body targeted, the procedure involved is basically the same. In a special MRI suite, the patient lies down on a narrow table and is made as comfortable as possible. Transmitters are positioned on the body and the table moves into a long tube that houses the magnet. The tube is as long as an average adult lying down, and is open at both ends. Once the area to be examined has been properly positioned, a radio pulse is applied. Then a two-dimensional image corresponding to one slice through the area is made. The table then moves a fraction of an inch and the next image is made. Each image exposure takes several seconds and the entire exam will last anywhere from 30 to 90 minutes. During this time, the patient must remain still as movement can distort the pictures produced.

Depending on the area to be imaged, the radio-wave transmitters will be positioned in different locations.

- For the head and neck, a helmet-like covering is worn on the head.
- For the spine, chest, and abdomen, the patient will be lying on the transmitters.
- For the knee, shoulder, or other joint, the transmitters will be applied directly to the joint.

Additional probes will monitor vital signs (like pulse, respiration, etc.) throughout the test.

The procedure is somewhat noisy and can feel confining to many patients. As the patient moves through the tube, the patient hears a thumping sound. Sometimes, music is supplied via earphones to drown out the noise. Some patients may become anxious or feel claustrophobic while in the small, enclosed tube. Patients may be reassured to know that throughout the study, they can communicate with medical personnel through an intercom-like system.

Recently, open MRIs have become available. Instead of a tube open only at the ends, an open MRI also has opening at the sides. Open MRIs are preferable for patients who have a fear of closed spaces and become anxious in traditional MRI machines. Open MRIs can also better accommodate obese patients, and allow parents to accompany their children during testing.

If the chest or abdomen is to be imaged, the patient will be asked to hold his to her breath as each exposure is made. Other instructions may be given to the patient as needed. In many cases, the entire examination will be performed by an MRI operator who is not a doctor. However, the supervising radiologist should be available to consult as necessary during the exam, and will view and interpret the results sometime later.

Preparation

In some cases (such as for MRI brain scanning or MRA), a chemical designed to increase image contrast may be given immediately before the exam. If a patient suffers from anxiety or claustrophobia, drugs may be given to help the patient relax.

The patient must remove all metal objects (watches, jewelry, eye glasses, hair clips, etc.). Any magnetized objects (like credit and bank machine cards, audio tapes, etc.) should be kept far away from the MRI equipment because they can be erased. The patient cannot bring any personal items such as a wallet or keys into the MRI machine. The patient may be asked to wear clothing without metal snaps, buckles, or zippers, unless a medical gown is worn during the procedure. The patient may be asked not to use hair spray, hair gel, or cosmetics that could interfere with the scan.

Aftercare

No aftercare is necessary, unless the patient received medication or had a reaction to a contrast agent. Normally, patients can immediately return to their daily activities. If the exam reveals a serious condition that requires more testing or treatment, appropriate information and counseling will be needed.

Risks

MRI poses no known health risks to the patient and produces no physical side effects. Again, the potential effects of MRI on an unborn baby are not well known. Any woman who is, or may be, pregnant, should carefully discuss this issue with her doctor and radiologist before undergoing a scan.

Normal results

A normal MRI, MRA, MRS, or MRCP result is one that shows the patient's physical condition to fall within normal ranges for the target area scanned.

Abnormal results

Generally, MRI is prescribed only when serious symptoms or negative results from other tests indicate a need. There often exists strong evidence of a condition that the scan is designed to detect and assess. Thus, the results will often be abnormal, confirming the earlier diagnosis. At that point, further testing and appropriate medical treatment is needed. For example, if the MRI indicates the presence of a brain tumor, an MRS may be prescribed to determine the type of tumor so that aggressive treatment can begin immediately without the need for a surgical biospy.

Resources

BOOKS

Faulkner, William H. *Tech's Guide to MRI: Basic Physics, Instrumentation and Quality Control*. Malden: Blackwell Science, 2001.

Fischbach, F. T. *A Manual of Laboratory and Diagnostic Tests*. 6th ed. Philadelphia: Lippincott, 1999.

Goldman, L., and Claude Bennett, editors. *Cecil Textbook of Medicine*. 21st ed. Philadelphia: W. B. Saunders, 2000: pp 977–970.

Roth, Carolyn K. *Tech's Guide to MRI: Imaging Procedures, Patient Care and Safety*. Malden: Blackwell Science, 2001.

PERIODICALS

Carr-Locke, D., et al. "Technology Status Evaluation: Magnetic Resonance Cholangiopancreatography." *Gastrointestinal Endoscopy* (June 1999): 858–61.

Kurt Richard Sternlof

Male breast cancer

Definition

Male **breast cancer** is a malignant tumor that forms in a man's breast.

Demographics

Breast **cancer** in men is rare, accounting for less than 1% of all breast cancers. Still, the American Cancer Society predicts that about 1,910 American men will be diagnosed with the disease and 440 men will die of it in 2009. Although studies show the number of breast cancer cases in women has decreased in the United States and Europe since the 1960s, the number of breast cancer cases in men have not decreased, but remained stable or slightly increased.

The rate of increase in cases begins and steadily rises at age 50 for men. However, the average age for male breast cancer is between 60 and 70 years old, with a median age of 67 years. Men often are diagnosed at a later stage than women.

KEY TERMS

Lymph node—One of a number of small, bean-shaped structures that run along the lymphatic system of vessels. The lymph nodes trap cancer cells, along with other cells and fluids.

Malignant—Causing worsening or death. Malignant tumors can invade other tissues and organs and spread to other areas of the body.

Description

Breast cancer is rare in men, but can be serious and fatal. Many people believe that only women can get breast cancer, but men have breast tissue that also can develop cancer. When men and women are born, they have a small amount of breast tissue with a few tubular passages called ducts located under the nipple and the area around the nipple (areola). By puberty, female sex hormones cause breast ducts to grow and milk glands to form at the ends of the ducts. But male hormones eventually prevent further breast tissue growth. Although male breast tissue still contains some ducts, it will have only a few —or no— lobules. Near the breasts of men and women are axillary lymph nodes. These are underarm small structures shaped like beans that collect cells from lymphatic vessels. Lymphatic vessels carry lymph, a clear fluid that contains fluid from tissues, cells from the immune system, and various waste products throughout the body. The axillary lymph nodes are important to breast cancer patients, as they play a role in the spread and staging of breast cancer.

Breast cancer is much more common in women, mostly because women have many more breast cells that can undergo cancerous changes and because women are exposed to the effects of female hormones.

Infiltrating ductal **carcinoma** is the most common type of breast cancer in men. It is a type of **adenocarcinoma**, or a type of cancer that occurs in glandular tissue. Infiltrating ductal carcinoma starts in a breast duct and spreads beyond the cells lining the ducts to other tissues in the breast. Once the cancer begins spreading into the breast, it can spread to other parts of the body. This distant spread is called **metastasis**. When breast cancer metastasizes to other areas of the body, it can cause serious, life-threatening consequences. For example, breast cancer might spread to the liver or lungs. About 80–90% of all male breast cancers are infiltrating ductal carcinomas.

Ductal carcinoma in situ (DCIS) is not common; it accounts for about 10% of all male breast cancers. It also is an adenocarcinoma. In situ cancers remain in the immediate area where they began, so DCIS remains confined to the breast ducts and does not spread to the fatty tissues of the breast. This means it is likely found early. DCIS also may be called intraductal carcinoma.

Other types of breast cancer are very rare in men. Adenocarcinomas that are lobular (forming in the milk glands or lobules) only occur in about 2% of male breast cancer cases because men normally do not have milk gland tissues. Inflammatory breast cancer, a serious form of breast cancer in which the breast looks red and swollen and feels warm, also occurs rarely. Paget's disease of the nipple, a type of breast cancer that grows from the ducts beneath the nipple onto the nipple's surface, only accounts for about 1% of female breast cancers. However, slightly more men have this form of breast cancer than women. Sometimes, Paget's disease is associated with another form of breast cancer.

Although not a form of cancer, but a benign condition, gynecomastia is important to mention. It is the most common of all male breast disorders and can be associated with male breast cancer in a rare condition called Klilnefelter's syndrome. Gynecomastia most often occurs in teenage boys when their hormones change during puberty. Older men also may experience the condition when their hormone balance changes as they age. Gynecomastia is an increase in the amount of breast tissue, or breast tissue enlargement. If a man has Klinefelter's syndrome, he can develop gynecomastia and increased risk of breast cancer.

Causes and symptoms

Scientists do not know what causes most cases of male breast cancer. However, excellent progress is being made in genetic research and in understanding how genes instruct cells to grow, divide, and die. For example, researchers have now mapped all of the genes in the human body. Genes are part of the body's DNA, which is the chemical that instructs the cells. When DNA or genes carry defects (mutations), they activate changes in the cells, such as rapid cell division, that lead to cancer. Some genes, called tumor suppression genes, cause cells to die. Scientists have identified some genetic mutations that are risk factors for breast cancer. In other cases, environmental, or outside, factors are thought to increase a man's risk for breast cancer.

Mutations of at least two versions of a tumor suppressor gene (BRCA1 and BRCA2) have been identified as causes of breast cancer in women. In men, the BRCA2 mutation is considered responsible for about 15% of breast cancers. Men can inherit genes from either parent. Studies have shown that BRCA1 also may increase a man's risk for breast cancer, but its role is less certain. These mutations have been shown to increase other cancers in men, including **prostate cancer**. Klinefelter's syndrome is a rare genetic cause of breast cancer in men. It results from inheriting an additional X chromosome.

Several other factors also may cause male breast cancer. Some conditions, such as the liver disease cirrhosis, can cause an imbalance in a man's hormones, producing high levels of the female hormone estrogen, which can lead to breast cancer. Exposure to some substances such as high amounts of radiation may contribute to male breast cancer. A 2004 report studied why a cluster of breast cancer cases occurred among a small group of men who worked in the basement office of a multi-story office building. The study linked their breast cancer to exposure to high magnetic fields from a nearby electrical switchgear room in their work space.

Many men do not realize they can develop breast cancer; they ignore the symptoms. The most common symptom is a mass, or lump in the chest area, particularly around the nipple. The lump will be firm, not tender or painful. Other signs that may warn of male breast cancer include:

- Skin dimpling or puckering
- Changes in the nipple, such as drawing inward (retraction)
- Nipple discharge of any kind
- Redness or scaling of the nipple or breast skin
- Abnormal swelling (or lump) of the breast, nipple, or chest muscle
- Prolonged rash or irritation of the nipple that may indicate Paget's disease

Diagnosis

Physicians follow the same steps for diagnosing breast cancer in men as in women, except that routine screening of breast cancer is not done in men. Once symptoms are noticed, however, physicians will proceed in the same way. The physician will conduct a thorough medical history and examination, including questions that may identify risk factors for breast cancer, such as male or female relatives with the disease. The medical history also helps gather details on possible symptoms for breast cancer.

The physician also performs a clinical breast examination. This helps locate and study a lump or suspicious area. The physician will feel (palpate) a mass to get an idea of its size, texture, likely location and relation to surrounding skin, muscles and tissues. At this point, the physician already will begin to look for signs that the cancer may have spread to other organs and to the lymph nodes. The physician will palpate lymph nodes and the liver, for instance, to see if they are enlarged.

The next step in diagnosis usually is a diagnostic mammogram. **Mammography** is an x ray of the breast. Mammograms are performed by radiologic technologists who take special training in the procedure. Mammograms are evaluated by radiologists, physicians who receive medical training specifically in interpreting **x rays**. If the initial mammogram shows suspicious findings, the radiologist may order magnification views to more closely look at the suspicious area. Mammograms can accurately show the tissue in the breast, even more so in men than women, because men do not have dense breasts or benign cysts in their breasts that interfere with the diagnosis.

The radiologist also might recommend an ultrasound to follow up on suspicious findings. Ultrasound often is used to image the breasts. Also known as sonography, the technique uses high-frequency sound waves to take pictures of organs and functions in the body. Sound wave echoes can be converted by computer to an image and displayed on a computer screen. Ultrasound does not use radiation. A technologist will perform the ultrasound; it will be evaluated by the radiologist.

Biopsies, which involve removing a sample of tissue, are the only definite way to tell if a mass is cancerous. At one time, surgical biopsies were the only option, requiring removal of all or a large portion of the lump in a more complicated procedure. Today, fine-needle aspiration **biopsy** and core biopsies can be performed. In fine-needle aspiration biopsy, a thin needle is inserted to withdraw fluid from the mass. The physician may use ultrasound or other imaging guidance to locate the mass if necessary. The fluid is tested in a laboratory under a special microscope to determine if it is cancerous.

A core biopsy is similar, but involves removing a small cylinder of tissue from the mass through a slightly larger needle. Core biopsy may require local anesthesia. These biopsy techniques usually can be performed in a physician office or outpatient facility. The cells in biopsy samples help physicians determine if the lump is cancerous and the type of breast cancer. A tissue sample also may be used for assigning a grade to the cancer and to test for certain proteins and receptors that aid in treatment and prognosis decisions.

If there is discharge from the nipple, the fluid also may be collected and analyzed in a laboratory to see if cancer cells are present in the fluid.

Diagnosis of breast cancer spread may require additional tests. For example, a **computed tomography** (CT) scan may be ordered to check organs such as the liver or kidney for possible metastasized cancer. A chest x ray can initially check for cancer spread to the lungs. Bone scans are nuclear medicine procedures that look for areas of diseased bone. **Magnetic resonance imaging** (MRI) has been increasingly used in recent years as a follow-up study to mammograms when findings are not clear. However, for metastatic breast cancer, they are more likely to be ordered to check for cancer in the brain and spinal cord. **Positron emission tomography** (PET) scans also have become more common in recent years.

Staging

After cancer has been definitively diagnosed, the next step is staging. Staging helps clarify details about the tumor, the adjacent and distant lymph nodes that may be affected, and the adjacent and distant organs that may be affected. This information helps determine what type of treatment is most appropriate.

The first step in staging may utilize a technique called **sentinel lymph node biopsy**. The sentinel node is the first one the cancer cells are likely to reach, so it is the first one checked for cancerous cells. Using a radioactive substance and blue dye injected into the area around the tumor, physicians can track the path of the cells and stage the cancer. The technique has been used for many years on women with breast cancer; research in 2004 showed it worked well for predicting lymph node status in men as well.

Cancer staging systems help physicians compare treatments and research and identify patients for **clinical trials**. Most of all, they help physicians determine treatment and prognosis for individual patients by describing how severe a patient's cancer is in relation to the primary tumor. The most common system used for cancer is the American Join Committee on Cancer (AJCC) TNM system, which bases staging largely on the spread of the cancer. T stands for tumor and describes the tumor's size and spread locally, or within the breast and to nearby organs. The letter N stands for lymph nodes and describes the cancer's possible spread to and within the lymph node system. In some descriptions below, the cancer may have been found by sentinel node biopsy as microscopic disease in nodes that are in the breasts (rather than the armpits). For simplification, these findings have been grouped with the axillary lymph nodes. M stands for metastasis to note if the cancer has spread to distant organs. Further letters and numbers may follow these three letters to describe number of lymph nodes involved, approximate tumor sizes, or other information. The following is a summary of breast cancer stages:

Stage 0: Tis, N0, M0: Ductal carcinoma in situ (DCIS). This is the earliest and least invasive form of breast cancer; the cancer cells are located within a duct and have not invaded surrounding fatty tissue.

Stage I: T1, N0, M0: The tumor is less than 1 in. in diameter (2 cm or less) and has not spread to lymph nodes or distant organs.

Stage IIA: T0, N1, M0/T2, NO, MO: No tumor is found or the tumor is smaller than 2 cm and cancer is found in one to three axillary lymph nodes (even if no tumor is found), or the tumor is between 2 and 5 cm in diameter but has not spread to the axillary lymph nodes. The cancer has not spread to distant organs.

Stage IIIB: T2, N1, M0/T3, NO, MO: The tumor is between 2 and 5 cm in diameter and has spread to one to three axillary lymph nodes or the tumor is larger than 5 cm, has not grown into the chest wall or spread to the lymph nodes or distant organs.

Stage IIIA: T0-2, N2, M0/T3, N1, MO: The tumor is smaller than 5 cm in diameter and has spread to four to nine axillary lymph nodes or the tumor is larger than 5 cm and has spread to one to nine axillary lymph nodes. The cancer has not spread to distant organs.

Stage IIIB: T4, N0-2, M0: The tumor has grown into the chest wall or the skin and may have spread to no lymph nodes or as many as nine lymph nodes. Cancer has not spread to distant sites.

Stage IIIC: T0-4, N3, MO: The tumor is any size, has spread to 10 or more axillary lymph nodes or to one or more lymph nodes under or above the collarbone (clavicle) on the same side as the breast tumor. The cancer has not spread to distant organs.

Inflammatory breast cancer: Classified as stage III, unless it has spread to distant organs or lymph nodes not near the breast (which would classify it as Stage IV).

Stage IV: T0-4, N0-3, M1: Regardless of the tumor's size, the cancer has spread to distant organs, such as the liver, bones, or lung, or to lymph nodes far from the breast.

Treatment

If the axillary lymph nodes were identified as containing cancer at the time of the sentinel **lymph node biopsy**, they will be removed in an **axillary dissection**. Sometimes, this is done at the time of the biopsy.

For Stage I, surgery often is the only treatment needed for men. Women often have lumpectomies, which remove as little surrounding breast tissue as possible, to preserve some of their breast shape. For men, this is less of a concern, and **mastectomy**, or surgical removal of the breast, is performed in 80% of all male breast cancers. Men with Stage I tumors larger than 1 cm may receive additional (adjuvant) **chemotherapy**.

Men with Stage II breast cancer also usually receive a mastectomy. If they have cancer in the lymph nodes, they probably will receive adjuvant therapy. Those with estrogen receptor-positive tumors may receive hormone therapy with **tamoxifen**. The treatment team may recommend adjuvant **radiation therapy** if the cancer has spread to nearby lymph nodes and/or to the skin.

Stage III breast cancer requires mastectomy followed by adjuvant therapy with tamoxifen when hormones are involved. Most patients with Stage III disease also will require chemotherapy and radiation therapy to the chest wall.

Men with Stage IV breast cancer will require systemic therapy, or chemotherapy and perhaps hormonal therapy that works throughout the body to fight the cancer in the breast, as well as the cancer cells that have spread. Patients also may receive immunotherapy to help patients fight **infection** following chemotherapy. Radiation and surgery also may be used to relieve symptoms of the primary cancer and areas where the cancer may have spread. The treatment team also may have to diagnose specific treatments for the metastatic cancers, depending on their sites.

If male breast cancer recurs in the breast or chest wall, it can be treated with surgical removal and followed by radiation therapy. An exception is recurrence in the same area, where additional radiation therapy can damage normal tissue. Recurrence of the cancer in distant sites is treated the same as metasteses found at the time of diagnosis.

Alternative and complementary therapies

Many alternative and complementary therapies can help cancer patients relax and deal with pain, though none to date have been shown to treat or prevent male breast cancer. For example, traditional

Chinese medicine offers therapies that stress the importance of balancing energy forces. Many studies also show that guided imagery, prayer, meditation, laughter, and a positive approach to cancer can help promote healing. Early studies have shown that soy and flaxseed may have some preventive properties for breast cancer. However, these trials have been conducted in women. When looking for these therapies, cancer support groups suggest asking for credible referrals and working with the medical treatment team to coordinate alternative and complementary care.

Coping with cancer treatment

It is difficult for some men to accept and cope with a breast cancer diagnosis, since it is a relatively rare and unexpected disease among men. It is important that men work closely with their treatment team to talk about the their concerns and to carefully follow all instructions for care. Support groups and family support are critical in coping with a breast cancer diagnosis.

Eating a nutritious diet, stopping use of tobacco, and limiting use of alcohol, can help in recovery from breast cancer. Beginning a regular exercise program when the treatment team recommends also helps.

Clinical trials

Research currently is underway to test various chemotherapy combinations for male breast cancer at different stages. A clinical trial also is underway to investigate a vaccine for treating patients with metastatic breast cancer. The National Institutes of Health list clinical trials by disease type, including those for which they are recruiting patients. Choosing to participate in a clinical trial is a decision that involves the patient, family, and treatment team.

Prognosis

Prognosis for male breast cancer varies, depending on stage. Generally, prognosis is poorer for men than for women, because men tend to show up for diagnosis when their breast cancer has reached a later stage. The average five-year survival rate for Stage I cancers is 96%. For Stage II, it is 84%. Stage III cancers carry an average five-year survival rate of 52%, and by Stage IV, the rate drops to 24%.

Prevention

Some forms of male breast cancer cannot be prevented. But detecting the cancer at an early stage can prevent serious complications, such as spread to distant organs. Men who have a history of breast cancer in their family should pay particular attention to the symptoms of breast cancer and seek immediate medical evaluation. Physicians may be able to test the blood of men with family history for presence of the BRCA2 gene so they may more carefully watch for early signs of breast cancer. Avoiding exposure to radiation also may help present some male breast cancers.

QUESTIONS TO ASK YOUR DOCTOR

- What kinds of diagnostic studies will be required to ascertain the type and spread of this tumor?
- How far has my cancer advanced; what stage is it in?
- Could there be a genetic component to this tumor? Should other family member be tested?
- What types of treatments are available?
- What types of side effects from treatments can I expect? What are your recommendations to help me deal with those side effects?
- Am I eligible for any clinical trials? Would these be helpful to consider?
- Are there any lifestyle changes that I should make?
- How often should I be checked after treatment has ended?
- Is there a support group that I can join to hear about other people's experiences with this disorder?

Resources

BOOKS

Abeloff, MD et al. *Clinical Oncology*. 3rd ed. Philadelphia: Elsevier, 2004.

Khatri, VP and JA Asensio. *Operative Surgery Manual*. 1st ed. Philadelphia: Saunders, 2003.

Townsend, CM et al. *Sabiston Textbook of Surgery*. 17th ed. Philadelphia: Saunders, 2004.

PERIODICALS

"Cluster of Male Breast Cancer Linked to Electromagnetic Field Exposure." *Cancer Weekly* (Sept. 21, 2004):98.

"Largest Study of its Kind Finds Male Breast Cancer on the Rise." *Cancer Weekly* (June 15, 2004):32.

"SLN Biopsy Predicts Axillary Lymph Node Status in Male Breast Cancer Patients." *Clinical Oncology Week* (Aug. 2, 2004):15.

Stoppani, Jim. "Male Breast Cancer." *Muscle & Fitness* (December 2004):194.

OTHER

"Breast Cancer News. New Findings About Male Breast Cancer." Web page. Susan G. Komen Cancer Foundation, 2003.

"Facts For Life. Alternative and Complementary Therapy." Brochure/Web page. Susan G. Komen Cancer Foundation, 2004.

"Facts For Life. Breast Cancer in Men." Brochure/Web page. Susan G. Komen Cancer Foundation, 2004.

"How Is Breast Cancer in Men Diagnosed?" Web page. American Cancer Society, 2004.

"How Is Breast Cancer in Men Staged?" Web page. American Cancer Society, 2004.

"Male Breast Cancer (PDQ): Treatment, Patient Version." Web page. National Cancer Institute, 2003.

ORGANIZATIONS

American Cancer Society. 800-ACS-2345. http://www.cancer.org.

The Susan G. Komen Breast Cancer Foundation. 5005 LBJ Freeway, Ste, 250, Dallas, TX 75244. 800-I'M AWARE. http://www.komen.org.

Y-ME National Breast Cancer Organization. 212 W. Van Buren, Ste. 1000, Chicago, IL. 60607-3098. 800-221-2121. http://www.y-me.org.

Teresa G. Odle

Malignant melanoma *see* **Melanoma**

Malignant fibrous histiocytoma

Definition

Malignant fibrous histiocytoma (MFH), although rare, is the most common abnormal growth of soft tissue (**sarcoma**) in adults.

Description

MFH occurs as a painless mass most commonly in the skin, arms, legs, kidneys, or the pancreas. More rarely MFH may occur in the bones, heart, breasts, or inside the skull.

When MFHs spread (metastasize) to other organs, the most common site is the lung, but **metastasis** to local lymph nodes and to bone have also been reported.

MFHs tend to be slow growing and slow to metastasize.

Local recurrence of MFH after surgery to remove the initial tumor is common because MFHs grow along the fat layers that separate different layers of soft tissue. Often, an MFH is not completely removed because it has crossed, undetected, from one fat layer to another neighboring layer.

KEY TERMS

Liver function tests (LFTs)—Blood tests that measure the blood serum levels of several enzymes produced by the liver.

Sarcoma—A form of cancer that arises from within the supportive tissues, such as bone, cartilage, fat, or muscle.

Demographics

MFHs are diagnosed in six of every one million people each year. MFHs can occur in people of any age, but they are extremely rare in children.

MFHs occur in a slightly higher frequency in Caucasians than in people of African descent or Asians. No relationship of MFHs appear to exist to any geographic region. Males are affected in slightly higher numbers than are females.

MFHs of the skin are seen almost exclusively in sun-exposed areas of the skin in elderly patients.

People affected with certain genetic diseases, such as neurofibromatosis, have a higher incidence of MFHs than unaffected people.

MFHs of the bone are seen almost exclusively in people who have a pre-existing skeletal disorder such as Paget disease or fibrous dysplasia of bone.

Causes and symptoms

The cause, or causes, of MFHs are not known. An elevated risk for the development of MFHs has been linked to the chemical phenoxyacetic acid found in herbicides; to clorphenols found in wood preservatives; and to exposure to asbestos. People who have been exposed to high doses of radiation are also more prone to develop MFHs than the remainder of the population. Research is ongoing to determine if there is a genetic cause of MFHs.

The only direct symptom of MFHs is the presence of an abnormal mass, but some patients may also experience:

- abnormally high levels of a certain type of white blood cells (eosinophils) in the blood
- low blood sugar (hypoglycemia)
- fever
- abnormal liver function tests

QUESTIONS TO ASK THE DOCTOR

- Which type of MFH do I have?
- What is the size of my tumor?
- Will I require chemotherapy or radiation treatments to shrink my tumor prior to its removal?
- What is the likelihood of my type of MFH coming back?
- How often should I seek follow-up examinations?

Diagnosis

Prior to removal, MFHs are extremely difficult to distinguish from the other forms of **soft tissue sarcoma**. The definitive diagnosis of MFH usually occurs after a tumor has been surgically removed. This diagnosis is accomplished by conducting microscopic examinations on the tumor.

Treatment team

Treatment for MFHs is mostly surgical or observational. Surgeries to remove MFHs are generally performed by orthopedic surgeons. MFHs rarely require any chemotherapies or radiation therapies, however, when these treatments are called for they are directed by a medical oncologist and administered by health care personnel who specialize in these fields.

Clinical staging, treatments, and prognosis

MFHs are divided into three grades based on the appearance of the tissue within the tumor. Low grade tumors may closely resemble the surrounding normal tissue. Intermediate and high grade tumors may have little resemblance to normal tissue.

Additionally, MFHs are divided into two clinical stages based on size. Stage one MFHs are those tumors that are under 5 cm (2 in) in diameter. Stage two MFHs are those tumors larger than 5 cm (2 in) in diameter.

A treatment plan is determined after the grade and stage of the tumor has been established. High and intermediate grade tumors generally, regardless of the stage, are surgically removed. Low grade, stage one, tumors may be observed for development to a higher grade or stage rather than removed if it is determined that the risks of anesthetic and surgery outweigh the risk of the tumor to the individual patient.

Stage one MFHs are generally removed by wide local excision. This technique involves the surgical removal of the tumor and an area of healthy surrounding tissue that is approximately the same size as the tumor itself.

Stage two MFHs require wide surgical excision with the removal of wider margins of healthy tissue than those margins removed in the excision of smaller tumors. In some instances, stage two MFHs may require **amputation**.

Post-operative treatment of MFH patients may include **chemotherapy** or **radiation therapy**, especially in cases of MFH of the bones and in cases of metastasis to the lungs.

In cases of large MFHs, the patient may undergo radiation treatments prior to surgery in an attempt to shrink the size of the tumor prior to excision.

Overall survival from MFH is approximately 75% five-year disease-free survival. The prognosis is generally poorer if:

- the disease has metastasized to the lungs or bones
- complete tumor removal is not accomplished, or is not possible
- the patient is of an advanced age
- the tumor is large
- the location of the tumor is somewhere other than the arms or legs
- the tumor is located deep in the body, rather than superficially

Alternative and complementary therapies

There are no effective alternative treatments for MFHs other than surgical removal with or without chemotherapy or radiation treatments.

Coping with cancer treatment

Most patients who undergo wide local excision to remove their tumors can resume their normal activities within a few days of the operation.

The loss of a limb may produce feelings of grief that are similar to that felt upon the death of a spouse or close family member. Patients who must undergo amputation to remove their **cancer** may require extended psychological care to help them to deal with this grief and to help them develop a new, healthy, **body image**. These patients may also require extended physical therapy to learn to operate without the missing limb or to learn to use a prosthetic device.

Clinical trials

There were 40 **clinical trials** underway, in early 2001, aimed at the treatment of MFHs and other soft tissue sarcomas. More information on these trials, including contact information, may be found by conducting a clinical trial search at the website of the National Cancer Institute, CancerNet: http://cancernet.nci.nih.gov/trialsrch.shtml.

Prevention

Because the causes of MFHs are not known, there is no known prevention.

Special concerns

Repeat surgery may be necessary for MFHs because these tumors sometimes redevelop. Careful monitoring by the medical team will be required.

Resources

ORGANIZATIONS

Center for Orthopedic Oncology and Musculoskeletal Research, Washington Cancer Institute. 110 Irving St. NW, Washington, DC 20010. (202) 877-3970. [cited July 5, 2005]. <http:// www.sarcoma.org.

Sarcoma Alliance. 775 East Blithedale #334, Mill Valley, CA 94941. (415) 381-7236. [cited July 23, 2005]. http:// www.sarcomafoundation.com.

Paul A. Johnson, Ed.M.

MALT lymphoma

Definition

MALT lymphomas are solid tumors that originate from cancerous growth of immune cells that are recruited to secretory tissue such as the gastrointestinal tract, salivary glands, lungs, and the thyroid gland.

Demographics

MALT lymphomas occur at a frequency of about 1.5 per 100,000 people per year in the United States and account for about 10% of all non-Hodgkin's lymphomas. The frequency varies among different populations. For example, in parts of Italy the frequency of MALT lymphomas is as high as 13 per 100,000 people per year. This can in part be attributed to different rates of **infection** with H. pylori. However, other hereditary, dietary, or environmental factors are almost certainly involved.

Description

The digestive tract is generally not associated with lymphoid tissue, with the exception of small collections of lymphocytes such as Peyer's patches. A specific kind of white blood cell, B-lymphocytes, can accumulate in response to infections of the digestive tract and other secretory tissues, or as a result of autoimmune conditions such as Sjgren's syndrome. When the growth of these lymphocytes is maintained through continued infection or autoimmune disease, a malignant cell can arise and replace the normal lymphocytes. These lymphomas, derived from mucosa-associated lymphoid tissue (MALT), most commonly arise in the stomach. Their growth seems to be dependent upon continuous stimulation of the immune system by an infectious agent, such as H. pylori, or some other entity, termed an antigen, that the body recognizes as foreign. This antigen-driven growth permits these tumors to be treated by eliminating the stimulus that generated the original, normal **immune response**. In the stomach they are associated, in greater than 90% of all cases, with the bacteria called Helicobacter pylori (H. pylori). This bacteria is also associated with peptic stomach irritation, ulcers, and gastric **cancer**. MALT lymphomas are generally indolent, that is, they grow slowly and cause little in the way of symptoms. Those MALT lymphomas that arise in the stomach in response to H. pylori infections are generally successfully treated with **antibiotics**, which eliminate the bacteria.

Causes and symptoms

The majority of MALT lymphomas appear to be the result of infectious agents, most commonly H. pylori in the stomach. It is not known if infectious agents also cause MALT lymphomas outside of the stomach. In some cases, such as in the thyroid, MALT lymphomas seem to arise in patients who have autoimmune diseases, which make their immune systems treat their own tissue as foreign or antigenic. It is believed that there must be additional factors, in addition to infection or autoimmunity, that influence the development of MALT lymphomas. For example, in the United States, where infections with H. pylori are quite common, less than one in 30,000 people who have H. pylori in their stomachs develop MALT lymphomas. In addition, individuals who develop MALT lymphomas are more likely to develop other forms of cancer. This would suggest that there might be genetic factors predisposing individuals to develop MALT lymphomas or other tumors in response to environmental or infectious agents.

In general, patients have stomach pain, ulcers, or other localized symptoms, but rarely do they suffer from systemic complaints such as **fatigue** or **fever**.

Diagnosis

The indolent nature of most MALT lymphomas means that the majority of patients are diagnosed at early stages with relatively nonspecific symptoms. In the case of gastric MALT lymphomas, the physician will then have a gastroenterologist perform an endoscopy to examine the interior of the stomach. MALT lymphomas are then recognized as areas of inflammation or ulceration within the stomach. It is unusual for masses recognizable as tumors to be seen upon examination. Definitive diagnosis of MALT **lymphoma** requires a **biopsy**, in which a bit of tissue is removed from the stomach or other involved site. Examination of this tissue by a pathologist is the first step in distinguishing among the possible diagnoses of inflammation, indolent lymphoma, or a more aggressive form of cancer, such as gastric cancer or a rapidly growing **non-Hodgkin's lymphoma**. The pathologist evaluates the type of lymphoid cells that are present in the biopsy to establish the nature of the lesion. In addition, it is essential that the pathologist determine whether or not the lymphoma has grown beyond the borders of the mucosa, which lines the stomach or other gland.

Treatment

The best staging system to employ for MALT lymphomas is still the subject of discussion. However, it is standard practice that patients presenting with MALT lymphomas should be evaluated in a similar manner to individuals with nodal lymphomas, the more common type of lymphoma that originates at sites within the lymphoid system. These procedures include a complete history and physical, blood tests, chest **x rays**, and **bone marrow biopsy**. This evaluation will permit the oncologist to determine if the disease is localized or if it has spread to other sites within the body.

In general, the prognosis for patients with MALT lymphomas is good, with overall five-year survival rates that are greater than 80%. The features that are most closely related to the outlook for newly diagnosed individual patients are: whether the **primary site** is in the stomach or is extra-gastric; if the disease has spread beyond the initial location; and whether the histologic evaluation of the initial tumor biopsies is consistent with a low-grade, slowly growing lesion, as compared to a high-grade lesion that is more rapidly growing. In general, the histologic grade is the most important feature, with high-grade lesions requiring the most aggressive treatment.

Treatment of MALT lymphomas differs from that of most lymphomas. In the most common type of MALT lymphomas—low-grade lesions originating in the stomach—treatment with antibiotics to eliminate H. pylori leads to complete remissions in the majority of patients. The effectiveness of this treatment is indistinguishable from surgery, **chemotherapy**, **radiation therapy**, or a combination of surgery with drugs or irradiation. Approximately one-third of patients in this group have evidence of disseminated disease, where lymphoma cells are detected at sites in addition to the gastric mucosa. The response of these patients to antibiotic treatment is not significantly different from that for individuals with localized disease. For both groups a complete remission is achieved in about 75% of patients, who remain, on average, free of disease for about 5 years.

Clinical trials are underway and mostly concentrate upon optimizing treatment of gastric MALT lymphomas that involve H. pylori. The aspects of treatment being addressed are the most effective antibiotics and the use of antacids to modulate irritation in the stomach. These protocols have been designed to follow the natural history of gastric lymphomas and to establish the biological features that predict treatment response to antibiotics and duration of remission.

Prognosis

Patients with MALT lymphomas arising outside of the digestive tract also have good prognoses. Effective treatment for these lymphomas has been achieved with local radiation, chemotherapy, and/or interferon. Surgery followed by chemotherapy or radiation is also effective with nongastrointestinal MALT lymphomas. Overall these patients have five-year survival rates greater than 90%.

While the outlook for patients with MALT lymphomas is good, difficulties in diagnosis and staging have left the optimal treatment a matter of continued study. This is an especially open question for those patients who fail to respond to antibiotic therapy, or whose disease recurs. It may be the case that in these patients, the MALT lymphoma may have already progressed to a point where high-grade lesions, not observed in the original biopsies, were resistant to the initial treatment. The best treatment for these patients remains to be established. IN general, these patients are treated with chemotherapy in a similar manner to patients with other types of lymphoma.

QUESTIONS TO ASK YOUR DOCTOR

- What kinds of diagnostic studies will be required to ascertain the type and spread of this tumor?
- Could there be a genetic component to this tumor? Should other family member be tested?
- What types of treatments are available?
- What types of side effects from treatments can I expect? What are your recommendations to help me deal with those side effects?
- Am I eligible for any clinical trials? Would these be helpful to consider?
- Are there any lifestyle changes that I should make?
- What type of diet should I follow? Are there foods I should avoid?
- Should I avoid any medications?
- How often should I be checked after treatment has ended?
- Is there a support group that I can join to hear about other people's experiences with this disorder?

Given the success of antibiotics, and the good prognosis for gastric MALT lymphomas in general, no sufficient body of evidence exists to determine the best chemotherapy for patients who fail to achieve a complete and lasting remission upon initial treatment. At present, a chemotherapeutic regime designated CHOP includes the anti-cancer drugs **cyclophosphamide**, **doxorubicin**, **vincristine**, and prednisone. Similar drug combinations are being used for patients whose MALT lymphomas do not respond to antibiotic treatment.

Prevention

There are currently no commonly accepted means to prevent MALT lymphomas. While the H. pylori infections are associated with this and other gastric disease, the eradication of H pylori in asymptomatic individuals is not currently recommended for prevention of MALT lymphomas or gastric cancer.

Resources

BOOKS

Abeloff, MD et al. *Clinical Oncology*. 3rd ed. Philadelphia: Elsevier, 2004.

Feldman, M, et al. *Sleisenger & Fordtran's Gastrointestinal and Liver Disease*. 8th ed. St. Louis: Mosby, 2005.

Goldman L, Ausiello D., eds. *Cecil Textbook of Internal Medicine*. 23rd ed. Philadelphia: Saunders, 2008.

ORGANIZATIONS

American Cancer Society. 800-ACS-2345. http://www.cancer.org.

Warren Maltzman, Ph.D.

Mammography

Definition

Mammography is the study of the breast using x ray. The actual test is called a mammogram. There are two types of mammograms. A screening mammogram is ordered for women who have no problems

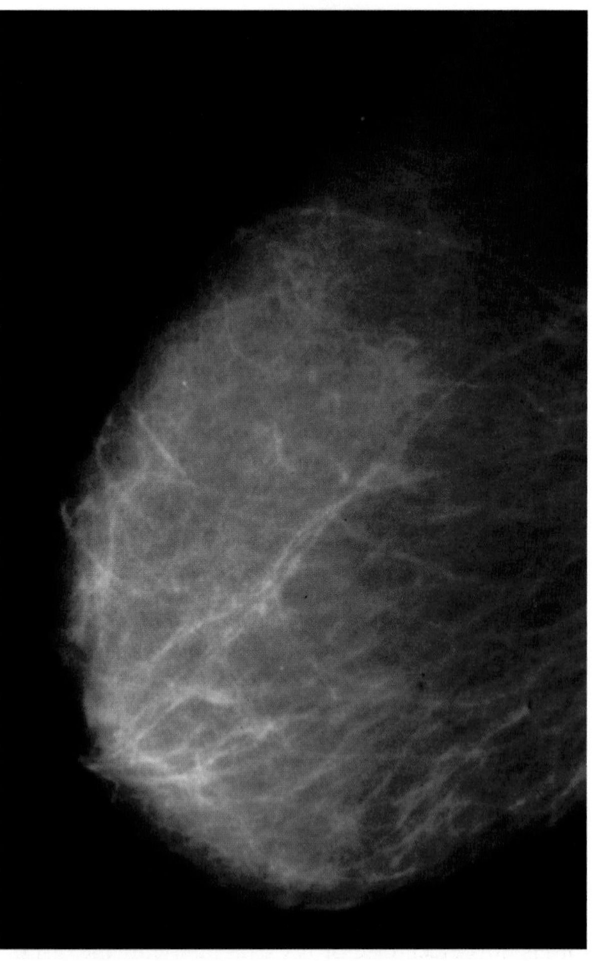

Color-enhanced mammogram of the left breast of a 73-year-old woman showing normal tissue. *(Copyright SIU, Science Source/Photo Researchers, Inc. Reproduced by permission.)*

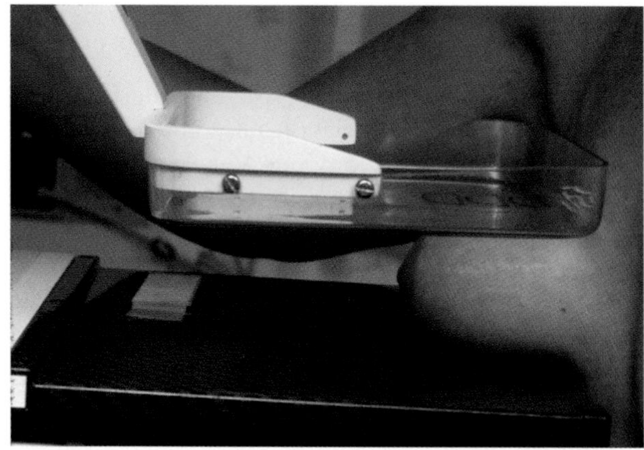

Mammogram. Breast compressed with compression paddle. *(Copyright SIU, Science Source/Photo Researchers, Inc. Reproduced by permission.)*

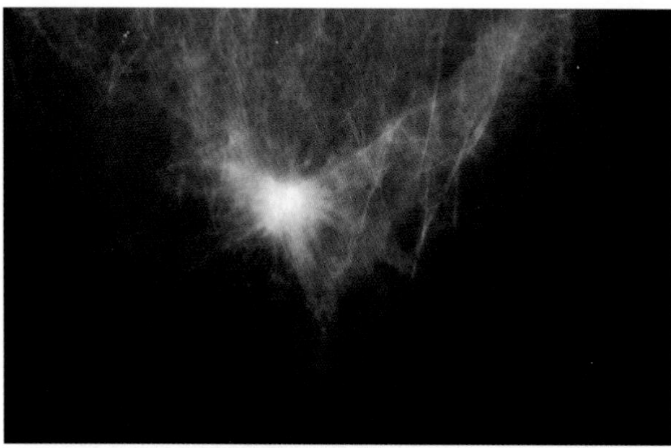

A mammogram of the right breast of a 72-year-old woman reveals carcinoma. *(Custom Medical Stock Photo. Reproduced by permission.)*

with their breasts. It consists of two x-ray views of each breast. A diagnostic mammogram is for evaluation of new abnormalities or of patients with a past abnormality requiring follow-up (i.e. a woman with **breast cancer** treated with **lumpectomy**). Additional **x rays** from other angles or special views of certain areas are taken.

Purpose

The purpose of screening mammography is breast **cancer** detection. A **screening test**, by definition, is used for patients without any signs or symptoms in order to detect disease as early as possible. Many studies have shown that having regular mammograms increases a woman's chances of finding breast cancer in an early stage, when it is more likely to be curable. It has been estimated that a mammogram may find a cancer as much as two years before it can be felt. The American Cancer Society, American College of Radiology, American College of Surgeons and American Medical Association recommend annual mammograms for every woman beginning at age 40.

QUESTIONS TO ASK THE DOCTOR

- What do the results mean?
- If there is something abnormal, shouldn't we immediately find out what it is?
- What future care will I need?

Screening mammograms are not usually recommended for women under age 40 who have no special risk factors and a normal physical breast examination. Below age 40, breasts tend to be "radiographically dense," which means it is difficult to see many details. In 2003, a new technique that introduces radiographic contrast into digital mammograms was proving useful at improving visibility of breast cancer in younger women. Screening mammograms can detect cancers in their earliest stages and greatly reduce mortality, particularly among women age 40 to 69. In fact, a study in 2003 found that women age 40 and older who had annual screening mammograms had better breast cancer prognoses because their cancers were diagnosed at earlier stages than women who had mammograms less often.

Some women are at increased risk for developing breast cancer, such as those with multiple relatives who have the disease. The 2003 American Cancer Society guidelines stated that women at increased risk might benefit from earlier screening mammograms and more frequent intervals for screening. However, the society suggested that evidence was not strong enough at that time to support making specific recommendations concerning screening examinations.

Diagnostic mammography is used to evaluate an existing problem, such as a lump, discharge from the nipple, or unusual tenderness in one area. The cause of the problem may be definitively diagnosed from this study, but further investigation using other methods often is necessary. This test is also used to evaluate findings from screening mammography tests.

Description

A mammogram may be offered in a variety of settings. Hospitals, outpatient clinics, physician's

KEY TERMS

Breast biopsy—A procedure in which suspicious tissue is removed and examined by a pathologist for cancer or other disease. The breast tissue may be obtained by open surgery or through a needle.

Radiographically dense—Difficult to see details of breast tissue on x ray.

offices, or other facilities may have mammography equipment. In the United States, since October 1, 1994, only places certified by the U.S. Food and Drug Administration (FDA) are legally permitted to perform, interpret, or develop mammograms.

In addition to the usual paperwork, a woman will be asked to fill out a form seeking information relevant to her risk of breast cancer and special mammography needs. The woman is asked about personal and family history of cancer, details about menstruation, child bearing, birth control, breast implants, other breast surgery, age, and hormone replacement therapy. Information about Breast Self Examination (BSE) and other breast health issues are usually available at no charge.

At some centers, a technologist may perform a physical examination of the breasts before the mammogram. Whether or not this is done, it is essential for the patient to tell the technologist about any lumps, nipple discharge, breast pain, or other concerns.

Clothing from the waist up is removed and a hospital gown or similar covering is put on. The woman stands facing the mammography machine. The technologist exposes one breast and places it on a plastic or metal film holder about the size of a placemat. The breast is compressed as flat as possible between the film holder and a rectangle of plastic (called a paddle), which presses down onto the breast from above. The compression should only last a few seconds, just enough to take the x ray. Good compression can be uncomfortable, but it is necessary to ensure the clearest view of all breast tissues.

Next, the woman is positioned with her side toward the mammography unit. The film holder is tilted so the outside of the breast rests against it, and a corner touches the armpit. The paddle again holds the breast firmly as the x ray is taken. This procedure is repeated for the other breast. A total of four x rays, two of each breast, are taken for a screening mammogram. Additional x rays, using special paddles, different breast positions, or other techniques are usually taken for a diagnostic mammogram.

The mammogram may be seen and interpreted by a radiologist right away, or it may not be reviewed until later. If there are any questionable areas or an abnormality, extra x rays may be recommended. These may be taken during the same appointment. More commonly, especially for screening mammograms, the woman is called back on another day for these additional films.

A screening mammogram usually takes approximately 15 to 30 minutes. A woman having a diagnostic mammogram can expect to spend up to an hour at the mammography facility.

The cost of mammography varies widely. Many mammography facilities accept "self referral." This means women can schedule themselves without a physician's referral. However, some insurance policies do require a doctor's prescription to ensure payment. Medicare will pay for annual screening mammograms for all women with Medicare who are age 40 or older and a baseline mammogram for those age 35 to 39.

A digital mammogram is performed in the same way as a traditional exam, but in addition to the image being recorded on film, it is viewed on a computer monitor and stored as a digital file.

Preparation

The compression or squeezing of the breast for a mammogram is a concern for some women, but necessary to render a quality image. Even with concerns about pain, a 2003 study said that three-fourths of women reported the pain associated with a mammogram as four on a 10-point scale. Mammograms should be scheduled when a woman's breasts are least likely to be tender. One week after the menstrual period is usually best. The MQSA regulates equipment compression for consistency and performance.

Women should not put deodorant, powder, or lotion on their upper body on the day the mammogram is performed. Particles from these products can get on the breast or film holder and may look like abnormalities on the mammogram film.

Aftercare

No special aftercare is required.

Risks

The risk of radiation exposure from a mammogram is considered virtually nonexistent. Experts are unanimous that any negligible risk is far outweighed by the potential benefits of mammography.

Some breast cancers do not show up on mammograms, or "hide" in dense breast tissue. A normal (or negative) study is not a guarantee that a woman is cancer-free. Mammograms find about 85–90% of breast cancers.

"False positive" readings are also possible, and 5–10% of mammogram results indicate the need for additional testing, most of which confirms that no cancer is present.

Normal results

A mammography report describes details about the x ray appearance of the breasts. It also rates the mammogram according to standardized categories, as part of the Breast Imaging Reporting and Data System (BIRADS) created by the American College of Radiology (ACR). A normal mammogram may be rated as BIRADS 1 or negative, which means no abnormalities were seen. A normal mammogram may also be rated as BIRADS 2 or benign findings. This means that one or more abnormalities were found but are clearly benign (not cancerous), or variations of normal. Some kinds of calcification, lymph nodes, or implants in the breast might generate a BIRADS 2 rating. A BIRADS 0 rating indicates that the mammogram is incomplete and requires further assessment.

Abnormal results

Many mammograms are considered borderline or indeterminate in their findings. BIRADS 3 means an abnormality is present and probably (but not definitely) benign. A follow-up mammogram within a short interval of six months is suggested. This helps to ensure that the abnormality is not changing, or is "stable." This stability in the abnormality indicates that a cancer is probably not present. If the abnormality were a cancer, it would have grown in the interval between mammograms. Some women are uncomfortable or anxious about waiting and may want to consult with their doctor about a having a **biopsy**. BIRADS 4 means suspicious for cancer. A biopsy is usually recommended in this case. BIRADS 5 means an abnormality is highly suggestive of cancer. The suspicious area should be biopsied.

Often, screening mammograms are followed up with additional imaging. The reasons are numerous; they may mot mean the radiologist suspects a cancerous lesion, only that he or she cannot make a clear diagnosis from the screening mammogram views. The most common imaging methods are additional views on the mammogram, sometimes called magnification views, and ultrasound. In recent years, some patients have received **magnetic resonance imaging** (MRI) of the breast. A new technique called dual-energy contrast enhanced digital subtraction mammography is reported to find cancers that may be missed by conventional mammography. It may be ordered in the future as a follow-up study.

Resources

BOOKS

"Contrast Mammography Reveals Hard-to-find Cancers." *Cancer Weekly* (October 14, 2003): 34.

Henderson, Craig. *Mammography & Beyond. Developing Technologies for the Early Detection of Breast Cancer: A Non-technical Summary*. Washington, DC: National Academy Press, 2001.

Love, Susan M., with Karen Lindsey. *Dr. Susan Love's Breast Book*. 3rd ed. Boulder, CO: Perseus Book Group, 2000.

PERIODICALS

Smith, Robert A., et al. "American Cancer Society Guidelines for Breast Cancer Screening: Update 2003." *Cancer* (May-June 2003): 141-170.

ORGANIZATIONS

American Cancer Society. 1599 Clifton Rd., Atlanta, GA 30329. (800) ACS-2345. http://www.cancer.org.

Federal Drug Administration. 5600 Fishers lane, Rockville, MD 20857. (800) 532-4440. http://www.fda.gov.

National Cancer Institute. Office of Cancer Communications. Bldg. 31, Room 10A31, Bethesda, MD 20892. NCI/Cancer Information Service: (800) 4-CANCER. http://cancernet.nci.nih.gov.

Ellen S. Weber, M.S.N.
Teresa G. Odle

Mantle cell lymphoma

Definition

Mantle cell **lymphoma** (MCL) is a rare type of **non-Hodgkin's lymphoma** (NHL) characterized under the microscope by expansion of the mantle zone area of the lymph node with a homogeneous (structurally similar) population of malignant small lymphoid cells. These cancerous cells have slightly irregular nuclei and very little cytoplasm, and are mixed with newly made normal lymphocytes (white blood cells) that travel from the bone marrow to the lymph nodes and spleen. Unlike normal lymphocytes, they do not mature properly and become cancerous instead.

KEY TERMS

Anemia—A condition caused by a reduction in the amount of red blood cells produced by the bone marrow. Its symptoms are general weakness and lack of energy, dizziness, shortness of breath, headaches, and irritability.

Antibody—A protein (immunoglobulin) produced by plasma cells (mature B cells) to fight infections in the body. They are released into the circulatory system in response to specific antigens and thus target those antigens that induced their production.

Antigen—An antigen is any substance which elicits an antibody response. As such, they are substances that stimulate a specific immune response of the body and are capable of reacting with the products of that response. Antigens may be foreign chemical substances or proteins located on the surface of viruses, bacteria, toxins, tumors and other infectious agents.

B-Cell lymphocyte—A type of lymphocyte (white blood cell). B cells react to the presence of antigens by dividing and maturing into plasma cells.

B-cell lymphomas—Non-Hodgkin's lymphomas that arise from B cells.

Blood cell—Cellular component of blood. There are three general types: white blood cells, red blood cells, and platelets, all which are produced in the bone marrow.

Cytoplasm—The organized complex of organic and inorganic substances external to the nuclear membrane of a cell.

DNA—Deoxyribonucleic acid are nucleic acids that are the part of the cell nucleus that contains and controls all genetic information.

Edema—Swelling of a body part caused by an abnormal buildup of fluids.

Gene—The specific site on a chromosome, consisting of protein and DNA responsible for the transmittal and determination of hereditary characteristics.

Gene therapy—The use of genes to treat cancer and other diseases.

Immune system—The system within the body, consisting of many organs and cells, that recognizes and fights foreign cells and disease.

Lymph—A milky white liquid responsible for carrying the lymphocytes in the lymphatic vessels.

Lymphatic system—Tissues and organs such as the bone marrow, spleen, thymus and lymph nodes that produce and store cells to fight infection and disease. Also includes the lymphatic vessels that carry lymph.

Lymphocyte—A type of white blood cell that defends the body against infection and disease. Lymphocytes are found in the bloodstream, the lymphatic system, and lymphoid organs. The two main types of lymphocytes are the B cells (produced in the bone marrow) and the T cells (produced in the thymus).

Lymphoma—Cancers that starts in the lymphatic system. Lymphomas are classified into two categories: Hodgkin's Disease and the non-Hodgkin's lymphomas.

Monoclonal antibody—An antibody raised against a specific antigen. Monoclonal antibodies are being used to target chemotherapy or radioactive substances directly to cancer cells.

Non-Hodgkin's lymphomas—Lymphomas characterized by different types of cancerous lymphatic cells, excluding those characterized by Hodgkin's disease.

Remission—A complete or partial disappearance of the signs and symptoms of cancer, usually in response to treatment.

Stem cell—Primitive cell found in the bone marrow and in the blood stream. Stem cells become different types of mature blood cells, thus enabling them to rejuvenate the circulatory and immune systems.

Stem cell transplant—Treatment procedure by which young blood stem cells are collected from the patient (autologous) or another matched donor (allogeneic). High-dose chemotherapy and/or radiation is given, and the stem cells are reinserted into the patient to rebuild his or her immune system.

Demographics

Each year, mantle cell lymphoma cases are only about 6% of all NHL diagnoses. Mantle cell lymphoma is rare in persons under the age of 50. The average age of a Mantle cell lymphoma patient is 65. Most patients are men; out of 1,000 persons diagnosed with MCL, approximately 33% will be women. This **cancer** has the shortest average survival of all lymphoma types.

Description

The body's immune system produces two types of lymphocytes or white blood cells: the B cells which are made in the bone marrow and the T cells which are made in the thymus. Both types of cells are found in the lymph, the clear liquid that bathes tissues and circulates in the lymphatic system. Lymphomas are cancers that occur in this lymphatic system and B-Cell lymphomas—also called non-Hodgkin's lymphomas—include follicular lymphomas, small non-cleaved cell lymphomas (Burkitt's lymphomas), marginal zone lymphomas (MALT lymphomas), small lymphocytic lymphomas, large cell lymphomas and also mantle cell lymphomas.

Mantle cell lymphoma accounts for 5% to 10% of all lymphomas diagnosed and 5% of B-cell lymphomas. There are three subsets of MCL cells: the mantle zone type, the nodular type, and the blastic or blastoid (immature) type. These various types often occur together to some degree, and approximately 30% to 40% of diagnoses are of mixed mantle and nodular type. As MCL develops further, the non-cancerous mantle centers also become invaded by cancerous cells. In about 20% of these cases, the cells become larger, and of the blastic type.

Extensive debates are ongoing concerning the grade of this cancer. European classification used to classify it as a low-grade cancer because it is initially slow-growing, while American classification considered it intermediate based on patients' shorter average survival rate. The combined European-American classification (REAL), is still discussing the status of mantle cell lymphoma. This is due to the mixed nature of MCL cells. Blastic type-MCL seems to be considered as a high-grade cancer because it spreads at about the rate of other lymphomas belonging to that category. The studies currently attempting to describe the precise nature of these cells will be key to any general agreement that is finally reached.

Causes and symptoms

The cause of MCL appears to be breakage in chromosome 11. A small piece of chromosome 11 is then transferred to chromosome 14. About 85% of all MCL patients display this chromosomal abnormality.

As a result of this chromosomal abnormality (deemed a reciprocal translocation), B cell lymphoma cells produce abnormally large quantities of a protein that encourages rapid cell growth.

Many of its symptoms are shared by other lymphomas as well and patients generally complain of **fatigue**, **anemia**, low grade fevers, **night sweats**, **weight loss**, rashes, digestive disturbances, chronic sinus irritation, recurrent infections, sore throat, shortness of breath, muscle and bone aches and edema.

More specific symptoms include spleen enlargement (in about 60–80% of cases), particularly with nodular-type MCL. Swollen lymph nodes are an early-stage symptom, even though the general health of the patient is good. Mild anemia is also common. Some patients also report lower back pain, and burning pain in the legs and testicles. As MCL becomes more advanced, the lymph nodes increase in volume, and the general symptoms become more pronounced.

In the end stage of MCL, neurologic symptoms appear, indicating that the MCL has spread to the central nervous system.

Diagnosis

MCL is very similar to several other lymphoma types and special care must be taken with the diagnosis. It should not be made from blood or bone marrow specimens alone. It is believed that immunologic tests are required to make the correct diagnosis. Immunophenotyping is one such test, it is used to determine what kind of surface molecules are present on cells, and thus, the exact type of lymphoma from a tissue sample. The Lymphoma Research Foundation of America recommends that several opinions be sought from recognized mantle cell experts to confirm the accuracy of the diagnosis.

At the time of diagnosis, mantle cell lymphoma has usually spread into other tissues such as the lymph nodes, spleen, bone marrow (up to 90% of cases), or to Waldeyer's ring (the ring of adenoid, palatine and lingual tonsils at the back of the mouth) or to the gastrointestinal tract. MCL can also spread to the colon, in which case it is diagnosed as multiple lymphomatous polyposis.

Treatment

There is no formal staging system for mantle cell lymphoma and no standard treatment has yet been adopted for MCL patients. Patients have been treated with surgery, radiation, single drug or combination **chemotherapy** and stem cell transplants. CHOP is one of the most common chemotherapy regimens for treating MCL. It derives its name from the combination of drugs used: **Cyclophosphamide** (cytoxan, neosar), adriamycin (**doxorubicin** or Hydroxydoxorubicin), **vincristine** (Oncovin), and Prednisone.

Alternative and complementary therapies

Because MCL is a cancer of the lymphatic system, **immunologic therapies** are often used, or combined with the more conventional radiation and chemotherapy treatments. Immunological therapies take advantage of the body's immune system. The immune system is a network of specialized cells and organs that defends the body against foreign invaders (antigens) by producing special "defense" proteins, an example of which are the antibodies. These substances recognize and attach to the antigens, usually found on the surface of cells and destroy them. There are reports of immunological therapies being used for MCL using interferon, one such natural substance produced by the body in response to a virus. Numerous studies show that **interferons** can stimulate the immune system to fight the growth of cancer, but there has not yet been enough evidence produced to see it emerge as a strong candidate for MCL treatment.

Other immunological therapies based on **monoclonal antibodies** (MABs or MOABs) have recently emerged, such as Rituxan (**rituximab**). MABs work on cancer cells in the same way natural antibodies work, by identifying and binding to the target cells, alerting other cells in the immune system to the presence of the cancer cells. MABs are very specific for a particular antigen, meaning that one designed for a B-cell lymphoma will not work on T-cell lymphomas. MABs used alone may enhance a patient's **immune response** to the cancer but they are thought to be more efficient when combined to another form of therapy, such as a chemotherapeutic drug. This way, the cancer is attacked on two fronts: chemical attack from the chemotherapy and immune response attack stimulated by the MAB.

Clinical trials

Clinical trials addressing the needs of MCL patients are very recent because the mantle cell lymphoma subtype has only recently been defined. There are now several trials being carried out in the United States specifically for mantle cell. Some other trials designed for patients with lymphomas may also accept mantle cell patients. Ongoing trials in this area are cheifly concerned with investigating monoclonal antibodies. Information regarding clinical trials can be obtained through the Clinical Trials web site listed at the end of this entry.

The following clinical protocols are specifically designed for MCL patients:

- The MD Anderson Protocol (high-dose chemotherapy with or without stem cell transplant)
- Rituxan, by itself or with CHOP
- Bexxar
- Oncolym
- Flavopiridol
- Phenylacetate

QUESTIONS TO ASK YOUR DOCTOR

- What kinds of diagnostic studies will be required to ascertain the type and spread of this tumor?
- Could there be a genetic component to this tumor? Should other family member be tested?
- What types of treatments are available?
- What types of side effects from treatments can I expect? What are your recommendations to help me deal with those side effects?
- Am I eligible for any clinical trials? Would these be helpful to consider?
- Are there any lifestyle changes that I should make?
- What type of diet should I follow? Are there foods I should avoid?
- Should I avoid any medications?
- How often should I be checked after treatment has ended?
- Is there a support group that I can join to hear about other people's experiences with this disorder?

Prognosis

There is no cure for mantle cell lymphoma. As with other slow-growing lymphomas, spontaneous remissions have been reported. Unfortunately, the median survival rate is only three to four years. All mantle cell lymphoma experts agree that the long-term prognosis of MCL patients receiving conventional treatment is poor, and that there is an urgent need for new, improved therapies.

Prevention

Because the cause of MCL is unknown, no prevention measures can be recommended.

Coping with cancer treatment

It is important to have a caregiver system when receiving medical treatment for MCL, and it is just as important to have a network of support for coping with the non-medical aspects of the cancer. Friends, relatives, coworkers and health professionals all can provide help, as well as the national cancer associations, some specifically addressing the needs of lymphoma patients. Please refer to the Resources section at the end of this entry for contact information.

Because MCL is a cancer that usually involves chemotherapy and **radiation therapy**, it can be severely damaging to organ function and long-term resistance. In addition to the immediate side effects of these treatments, other effects appear after treatment is completed, one of which, called Post-Cancer Fatigue (PCF), is often seen with lymphoma patients. This is fatigue that persists after treatment and can sometimes be extreme. The medical team will be able to offer the best advice to deal with PCF.

See also Acute lymphocytic leukemia; Central nervous system lymphomas.

Resources

BOOKS

Abeloff, MD et al. *Clinical Oncology*. 3rd ed. Philadelphia: Elsevier, 2004.

Hoffman R. et al. *Hematology: Basic Principles and Practice*. 4th ed. Philadelphia: Elsevier, 2005.

OTHER

Lymphoma Information Network Website. 7 June 2001. [cited July 5, 2009]. http://www.lymphomainfo.net/nhl/types/mantle.html.

National Institutes of Health Clinical Trials. [cited July 5, 2009]. http://www.clinicaltrials.gov.

ORGANIZATIONS

American Cancer Society. 800-ACS-2345. http://www.cancer.org.

Monique Laberge, Ph.D.

Mastectomy

Definition

Mastectomy is the surgical removal of the breast for the treatment or prevention of **breast cancer**.

Purpose

Mastectomy is performed as a surgical treatment for breast **cancer**. The severity of a breast cancer is evaluated according to a complex system called staging. This takes into account the size of the tumor and whether it has spread to the lymph nodes, adjacent tissues, and/or distant parts of the body. A mastectomy usually is the recommended surgery for more advanced breast cancers. Women with earlier stage breast cancers, who might also have breast-conserving surgery (**lumpectomy**), may choose to have a mastectomy. In the United States, approximately 50,000 women a year undergo mastectomy.

The size, location, and type of tumor are important considerations when choosing the best surgery to treat breast cancer. The size of the breast is also an important factor. A woman's psychological concerns and lifestyle choices should also be considered when making a decision.

There are many factors that make a mastectomy the treatment of choice for a patient. Large tumors are difficult to remove with good cosmetic results. This is especially true if the woman has small breasts. Sometimes multiple areas of cancer are found in one breast, making removal of the whole breast necessary. The surgeon is sometimes unable to remove the tumor with a sufficient amount, or margin, of normal tissue surrounding it. In this situation, the entire breast needs to be removed. Recurrence of breast cancer after a lumpectomy is another indication for mastectomy.

Radiation therapy is almost always recommended following a lumpectomy. If a woman is unable to have radiation, a mastectomy is the treatment of choice. Pregnant women cannot have radiation therapy for fear of harming the fetus. A woman with certain collagen vascular diseases, such as systemic lupus erythematosus or scleroderma, would experience unacceptable scarring and damage to her connective tissue from radiation exposure. Any woman who has had therapeutic radiation to the chest area for other reasons cannot tolerate additional exposure for breast cancer therapy.

The need for radiation therapy after breast-conserving surgery may make mastectomy more appealing for nonmedical reasons. Some women fear radiation and choose the more extensive surgery so radiation treatment will not be required. The commitment of time, usually five days a week for six weeks, may not be acceptable for other women. This may be due to financial, personal, or job-related factors. In geographically isolated areas, a course of radiation therapy may require lengthy travel and perhaps unacceptable amounts of time away from family or other responsibilities.

Some women choose mastectomy because they strongly fear recurrence of the breast cancer, and lumpectomy seems too risky. Keeping a breast that has contained cancer may feel uncomfortable for some

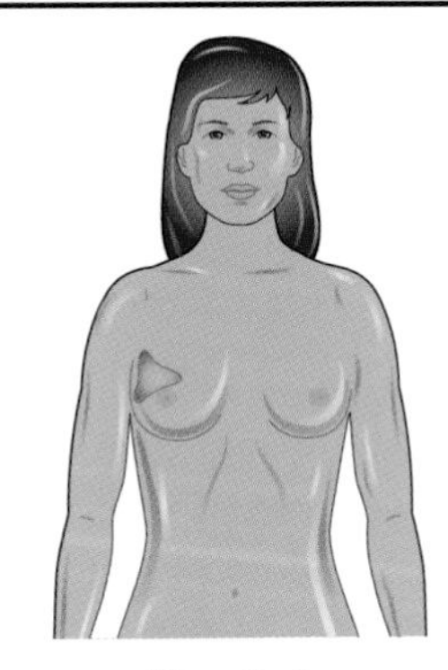

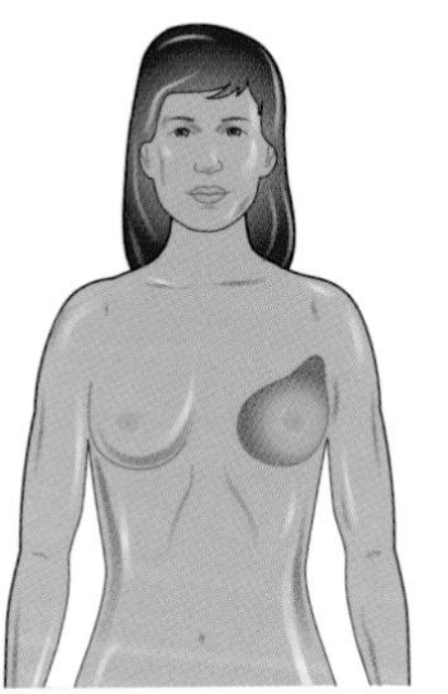

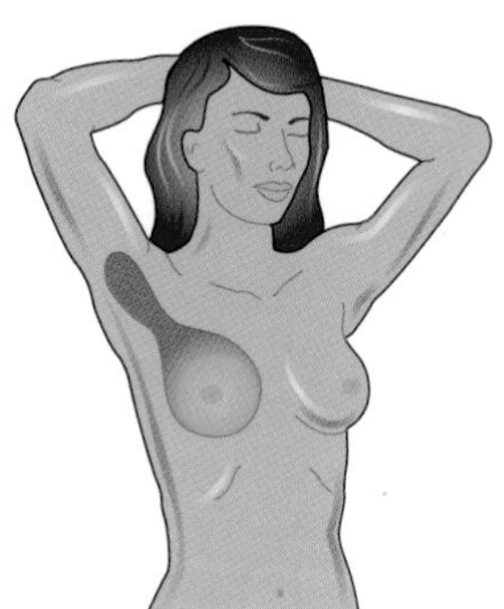

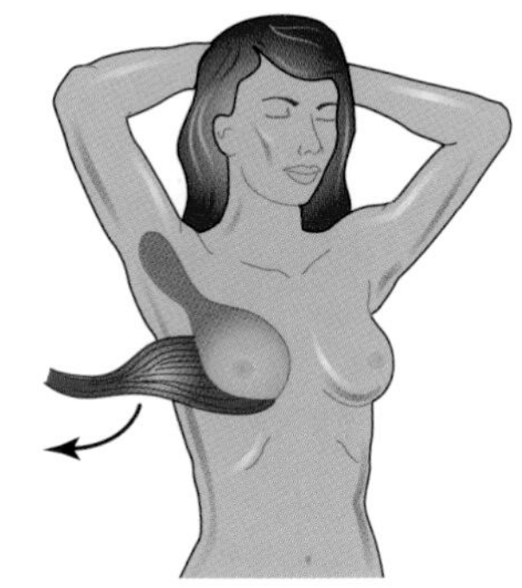

There are four types of mastectomies: partial mastectomy, or lumpectomy, in which the tumor and surrounding tissue is removed; simple mastectomy, where the entire breast and some axillary lymph nodes are removed; modified radical mastectomy, in which the entire breast and axillary lymph nodes are removed; and the radical mastectomy, where the entire breast, axillary lymph nodes, and chest muscles are removed. *(Illustration by Electronic Illustrators Group. Cengage Learning, Gale.)*

patients. They prefer mastectomy, so the entire breast will be removed.

The issue of prophylactic or preventive mastectomy, or removal of the breast to prevent future breast cancer, is controversial. Women with a strong family history of breast cancer and/or who test positive for a known cancer-causing gene may choose to have both breasts removed. Patients who have had certain types of breast cancers that are more likely to recur may elect to have the unaffected breast removed. Although there is some evidence that this procedure can decrease the chances of developing breast cancer, it is not a guarantee. It is not possible to be certain that all breast tissue has been removed. There have been cases where breast cancers have occurred after both breasts have been removed.

Studies have shown that women who choose preventive mastectomy generally are satisfied with their choice, but also believe they lacked enough information before deciding, particularly about the surgery, **genetic testing**, and **breast reconstruction**. A study released in 2003 concerning women who underwent radical mastectomy of one breast and chose surgical removal of the other breast as a preventive measure found that 83% were highly satisfied with their decision.

Precautions

The decision to have mastectomy or lumpectomy should be carefully considered. It is important that the woman be fully informed of all the potential risks and benefits of each surgical treatment before making a choice.

Description

There are several types of mastectomies. The radical mastectomy, also called the Halsted mastectomy, is rarely performed today. It was developed in the late 1800s, when it was thought that more extensive surgery was most likely to cure cancer. A radical mastectomy involves removal of the breast, all surrounding lymph nodes up to the collarbone, and the underlying chest muscle. Women were often left disfigured and disabled, with a large defect in the chest wall requiring skin grafting, and significantly decreased arm sensation and motion. Unfortunately, and inaccurately, it is still the operation many women picture when the word mastectomy is mentioned.

Surgery that removes breast tissue, nipple, an ellipse of skin, and some axillary or underarm lymph nodes, but leaves the chest muscle intact, is usually called a **modified radical mastectomy**. This is the most common type of mastectomy performed today. The surgery leaves a woman with a more normal chest shape than the older radical mastectomy procedure, and a scar that is not visible in most clothing. It also allows for immediate or delayed breast reconstruction.

In a **simple mastectomy**, only the breast tissue, nipple, and a small piece of overlying skin are removed. If a few of the axillary lymph nodes closest to the breast are also taken out, the surgery may be called an extended simple mastectomy.

QUESTIONS TO ASK THE DOCTOR

- What are my options for degree of treatment? Is it advisable to consider lumpectomy instead of a mastectomy procedure?
- What are the cosmetic implications of this surgery? What are my options for reconstruction?
- How soon after the procedure will I be able to return to normal activities?
- Is there a support group in the area where I could talk with other women who have undergone this procedure?

KEY TERMS

Axillary—Located in or near the armpit.

Lymphedema—Swelling caused by an accumulation of fluid from faulty lymph drainage.

Mastectomy, modified radical— Total mastectomy with axillary lymph node dissection, but with preservation of the pectoral muscles.

Mastectomy, radical—Removal of the breast, pectoral muscles, axillary lymph nodes, and associated skin and subcutaneous tissue.

Mastectomy, simple—Removal of only the breast tissue, nipple and a small portion of the overlying skin.

There are other variations on the term mastectomy. A skin-sparing mastectomy uses special techniques that preserve the patient's breast skin for use in reconstruction, although the nipple is still removed. Total mastectomy is a confusing expression, as it may be used to refer to a modified radical mastectomy or a simple mastectomy. In 2003, surgeons reported on a new technique that spared the nipple in many women with early stage breast cancer.

Many women choose to have breast reconstruction performed in conjunction with the mastectomy. The reconstruction can be done using a woman's own abdominal tissue, or using saline-filled artificial expanders, which leave the breast relatively flat but partially reconstructed. Additionally, there are psychological benefits to coming out of the surgery with the first step to a reconstructed breast. Immediate reconstruction will add time and cost to the mastectomy procedure, but the patient can avoid the physical impact of a later surgery.

A mastectomy is typically performed in a hospital setting, but specialized outpatient facilities sometimes are used. The surgery is done under general anesthesia. The type and location of the incision may vary according to plans for reconstruction or other factors, such as old scars. As much breast tissue as possible is removed. Approximately 10 to 20 axillary lymph nodes are usually removed. All tissue is sent to the pathology laboratory for analysis. If no immediate reconstruction is planned, surgical drains are left in place to prevent fluid accumulation. The skin is sutured and bandages are applied.

The surgery may take from two to five hours. Patients usually stay at least one night in the hospital, although outpatient mastectomy is increasingly performed for about 10% of all patients. Insurance usually covers the cost of mastectomy. If immediate reconstruction is performed, the length of stay, recovery period, insurance reimbursement, and fees will vary. In 1998, the Women's Health and Cancer Rights Act required insurance plans to cover the cost of breast reconstruction in conjunction with a mastectomy procedure.

Preparation

Routine preoperative preparations, such as not eating or drinking the night before surgery, typically are ordered for a mastectomy. On rare occasions, the patient also may be asked to donate blood in case a blood transfusion is required during surgery. The patient should advise the surgeon of any medications she is taking. Information regarding expected outcomes and potential complications also should be part of preparation for a mastectomy, as for any surgical procedure. It is especially important that women know about sensations they might experience after surgery, so they are not misinterpreted as a sign of poor wound healing or recurrent cancer.

Aftercare

In the past, women often stayed in the hospital at least several days. Now many patients go home the same day or within a day or two after their mastectomies. Visits from home care nurses can sometimes be arranged, but patients need to learn how to care for themselves before discharge from the hospital. Patients may need to learn to change bandages and/or care for the incision. The surgical drains must be attended to properly; this includes emptying the drain, measuring fluid output, moving clots through the drain, and identifying problems that need attention from the doctor or nurse. If the drain becomes blocked, fluid or blood may collect at the surgical site. Left untreated, this accumulation may cause **infection** and/or delayed wound healing.

After a mastectomy, activities such as driving may be restricted according to individual needs. Pain is usually well controlled with prescribed medication. Severe pain may be a sign of complications, and should be reported to the physician. A return visit to the surgeon is usually scheduled seven to 10 days after the procedure.

Exercises to maintain shoulder and arm mobility may be prescribed as early as 24 hours after surgery. These are very important in restoring strength and promoting good circulation. However, intense exercise should be avoided for a time after surgery in order to prevent injury. The specific exercises suggested by the physician will change as healing progresses. Physical therapy is an integral part of care after a mastectomy, aiding in the overall recovery process.

Emotional care is another important aspect of recovery from a mastectomy. A mastectomy patient may feel a range of emotions including **depression**, negative self-image, grief, fear and anxiety about possible recurrence of the cancer, anger, or guilt. Patients are advised to seek counseling and/or support groups and to express their emotions to others, whether family, friends, or therapists. Assistance in dealing with the psychological effects of the breast cancer diagnosis, as well as the surgery, can be invaluable for women.

Measures to prevent injury or infection to the affected arm should be taken, especially if axillary lymph nodes were removed. There are a number of specific instructions directed toward avoiding pressure or constriction of the arm. Extra care must be exercised to avoid injury, to treat it properly if it occurs, and to seek medical attention promptly when appropriate.

Additional treatment for breast cancer may be necessary after a mastectomy. Depending on the type of tumor, lymph node status, and other factors, **chemotherapy**, radiation therapy, and/or hormone therapy may be prescribed.

Risks

Risks that are common to any surgical procedure include bleeding, infection, anesthesia reaction, or unexpected scarring. After mastectomy and axillary **lymph node dissection**, a number of complications are possible. A woman may experience decreased feeling in the back of her armpit or other sensations including numbness, tingling, or increased skin sensitivity. Some women report phantom breast symptoms, experiencing **itching**, aching, or other sensations in the breast that has been removed. There may be scarring around where the lymph nodes were removed, resulting in decreased arm mobility and requiring more intense physical therapy.

Approximately 10–20% of patients develop lymphedema after axillary lymph node removal. This swelling of the arm, caused by faulty lymph drainage, can range from mild to very severe. It can be treated with elevation, elastic bandages, and specialized physical therapy. Lymphedema is a chronic condition that requires continuing treatment. This complication can arise at any time, even years after surgery. A new technique called **sentinel lymph node mapping** and **biopsy** can eliminate the need for removing many lymph nodes.

Normal results

A mastectomy is performed as the definitive surgical treatment for breast cancer. The goal of the procedure is that the breast cancer is completely removed and does not recur.

Abnormal results

An abnormal result of a mastectomy is the incomplete removal of the breast cancer or a recurrence of the cancer. Other abnormal results include long-lasting (chronic) pain or impairment that does not improve after several months of physical therapy.

Resources

BOOKS

Robinson, Rebecca Y., and Jeanne A. Petrek. *A Step-by-Step Guide to Dealing With Your Breast Cancer.* New York: Carol Publishing Group, 1999.

PERIODICALS

"American Women Still Having Too Many Mastectomies." *Women's Health Weekly* February 6, 2003: 10.

Frost, Marlene, et al. "Long-term Satisfaction and Psychological and Social Function Following Bilateral Prophylactic Mastectomy." *Journal of the American Medical Association* July 20, 2000: 319-24.

"Majority Satisfied with Prophylactic Mastectomy Decision." *AORN Journal* November 2003: 773.

"Studies Compare Mastectomy, Lumpectomy Survival Rates." *Clinican Reviews* January 2003: 24.

OTHER

ibreast.org. 15 Apr. 2001. [cited June 12, 2009]. http://www.breastcancer.org.

Living Beyond Breast Cancer. 15 Apr. 2001. [cited June 12, 2009]. http://www.lbbc.org.

ORGANIZATIONS

American Cancer Society. 1599 Clifton Rd., NE, Atlanta, GA 30329-4251. (800) 227-2345. http://www.cancer.org.

National Lymphedema Network. 2211 Post St., Suite 404, San Francisco, CA 94115-3427. (800) 541-3259 or (415) 921-1306. http://www.wenet.net/~lymphnet/.

Y-ME National Organization for Breast Cancer Information and Support. 18220 Harwood Ave., Homewood, IL 60430. 24-hour hotlines: (800) 221-2141 or (708) 799-8228.

Ellen S. Weber, M.S.N.
Teresa G. Odle

Matrix metalloproteinase inhibitors

Definition

Matrix metalloproteinases are a class of enzymes that can break down proteins, such as collagen and gelatin. Since these enzymes require zinc or calcium atoms to function, they are referred to as metalloproteinases. Matrix metalloproteinases function in tumor cell invasion and **metastasis**, wound healing, and angiogenesis (supplying the tumor with blood). They are normally found in the spaces between cells (extracellular) in tissues and are involved in degrading extracellular matrix proteins like collagens and gelatins. The extracellular matrix compartments are the primary barriers to tumor growth and spread. Matrix metalloproteinase inhibitors are selective inhibitors of matrix metalloproteinases. These agents inhibit tumor metastasis and angiogenesis.

Description

Matrix metalloproteinases have been linked to cancers such as breast, ovarian, colorectal, and lung. Synthetic matrix metalloproteinase inhibitors are being explored for use in **cancer prevention** and treatment because of their demonstrated antimetastatic and antiangiogenic properties. Matrix metalloproteinase inhibitors include compounds such as: Marimastat (BB-2516), COL-3, BAY 12-9566, and KB-R7785. Marimastat (BB-2516) was the first orally bioavailable matrix metalloproteinase inhibitor to enter **clinical trials** in the field of oncology. Developing nontoxic, orally active, MMP inhibitors is important because these compounds will likely need chronic administration in combination with other therapies.

Crystal Heather Kaczkowski, MSc.

Mechlorethamine

Definition

Mechlorethamine is a **chemotherapy** medicine used to treat **cancer** by destroying cancerous cells. Mechlorethamine is marketed as the brand name Mustargen. It is also commonly known as nitrogen mustard.

Purpose

Mechlorethamine is approved by the Food and Drug Administration (FDA) to treat **Hodgkin's disease** and non-Hodgkins' lymphomas. It is also approved for certain types of leukemia, malignant lymphomas, and lung cancer. Mechlorethamine has been used to relieve symptoms caused by a build up of cancerous fluid in the lungs, abdomen, and around the heart.

Description

Mechlorethamine is one of the first chemotherapy drugs discovered to have an effect on cancer cells. **Clinical trials** with this agent began in the 1940s. Mechlorethamine is a member of the group of chemotherapy drugs known as alkylating agents. Alkylating agents interfere with the genetic material (DNA) inside the cancer cells, more specifically through cross-linking DNA strands, and prevent them from further dividing and growing more cancer cells. Mechlorethamine is commonly combined with other chemotherapy agents to treat cancer.

Recommended dosage

A mechlorethamine dose can be determined using a mathematical calculation that measures a person's body surface area (BSA). This number is dependent upon a patient's height and weight. The larger the person, the greater the body surface area. BSA is measured in the units known as square meter (m^2). The body surface area is calculated and then multiplied by the drug dosage in milligrams per square meter (mg/m^2). This calculates the actual dose a patient is to receive.

KEY TERMS

Anemia—A red blood cell count that is lower than normal.

Antidote—A drug given to reverse the negative effects of another drug.

Chemotherapy—Specific drugs used to treat cancer.

Deoxynucleic acid (DNA)—Genetic material inside of cells that carries the information to make proteins that are necessary to run the cells and keep the body functioning smoothly.

Food and Drug Administration (FDA)—The government agency that oversees public safety in relation to drugs and medical devices, and gives the approval to pharmaceutical companies for commercial marketing of their products.

Intravenous—To enter the body through a vein.

Metastatic—Cancer that has spread to one or more parts of the body.

Neutropenia—A white blood cell count that is lower than normal.

Mechlorethamine is a yellowish liquid that is injected directly into a vein over a period of one to five minutes. It can also be applied onto the skin as an ointment for certain conditions.

Mechlorethamine is combined with other chemotherapeutic drugs **vincristine** (oncovin), **procarbazine**, and prednisone for treatment of Hodgkin's disease. The dose of mechlorethamine used in this regimen is 6 mg per square meter on day 1 and day 8 of a treatment cycle. This regimen is referred to as MOPP, and was one the initial regimens that caused a breakthrough in the treatment of Hodgkin's disease.

Mechlorethamine can also be infused into certain compartments in the body where cancerous fluid has accumulated. The dose for this treatment is based on a patient's weight in kilograms (1 kilogram is 2.2 pounds). Mechlorethamine is given at a dose of 0.2 to 0.4 mg per kilogram of body weight, infused directly into the area where the fluid is building up.

Precautions

Patients should notify their doctors if they have had any previous allergic reactions to chemotherapy treatment or if they have received **radiation therapy**.

Blood counts should be monitored regularly while on mechlorethamine therapy. During a certain time period after receiving mechlorethamine, there may be an increased risk of getting infections. Caution should be taken to avoid unnecessary exposure to crowds and people with infections.

Patients who may be pregnant or are trying to become pregnant should tell their doctors before receiving mechlorethamine. Chemotherapy can cause men and women to become sterile, or unable to have children.

Patients should check with their doctors before receiving live virus **vaccines** while on chemotherapy.

Patients should increase their intake of fluids while on this medication.

Side effects

One of the most common side effects from receiving mechlorethamine is **nausea and vomiting**. The **nausea** and **vomiting** can begin within one hour from receiving the drug. Patients will be given **antiemetics** before and after receiving mechlorethamine to help prevent or decrease this side effect.

A common side effect from taking mechlorethamine is low blood cell counts (**myelosuppression**). When the white blood cell count is lower than normal (**neutropenia**), patients are at an increased risk of developing **fever** and infections. The platelet blood count can also be decreased. Platelets are blood cells in the body that cause clots to form to stop bleeding. When the platelet count is low, patients are at an increased risk for bruising and bleeding. Low red blood cell counts (**anemia**), make people feel tired, dizzy, and lacking in energy.

Less common side effects from mechlorethamine include **diarrhea**, loss of appetite (**anorexia**), mouth sores, liver problems, metallic taste in the mouth, fever, ringing in the ears or hearing loss, and inflammation at the injection site. Allergic reactions have been reported, some of them severe anaphylactic reactions.

Damage to nerves and nervous system tissues is uncommon with mechlorethamine therapy. However, some reports do exist of nerve damage that has resulted in numbness and tingling in the hands and feet.

Mechlorethamine can cause skin reactions. When applied on top of the skin, the area can become red, swollen, brown colored, itchy, and have a burning sensation.

Hair loss (**alopecia**), irritation, and change of color of the vein where the drug was injected can occur. If the drug is not given directly into the vein, or is accidentally injected into surrounding areas of tissue, an antidote must be administered to that area as soon as possible. The area will become painful, gray-colored, and the tissue will begin to die. This is considered a severe reaction, and medical personnel must be notified immediately.

Interactions

Radiation therapy along with mechlorethamine administration can cause severe damage to the bone marrow.

Nancy J. Beaulieu, R.Ph., B.C.O.P.

Meclizine

Definition

Meclizine is an antihistamine commonly used to control **nausea**, **vomiting** and dizziness. It is known by the over-the-counter name Bonine. In the United States, the prescription brand name is Antivert.

Purpose

Meclizine may be given to help control **nausea and vomiting** that often occurs with **cancer** treatment, other medical conditions, or motion sickness. It is also used as part of palliative care for patients with terminal cancer.

More recently, meclizine has been reported to be effective in the treatment of panic disorder.

Description

Meclizine acts as a central nervous system depressant. It is believed its therapeutic actions occur due to the drug's drying effects and its ability to depress conduction of nerve messages in the inner ear. Meclizine begins working about one hour after ingestion. It continues being effective for eight to 24 hours.

Recommended dosage

The dosage to control nausea and vomiting associated with cancer treatment is 25–50 mg, every eight to 12 hours. When used to manage dizziness, patients generally take 25–100 mg daily in divided doses. Patients should not double up on this medication if a dose is missed.

KEY TERMS

Antihistamine—Agent that blocks or counteracts the action of histamine, which is released during an allergic reaction.

Palliative—Referring to treatments that are intended to relieve pain and other symptoms of disease but not to cure.

Precautions

Patients with glaucoma, an enlarged prostate, bladder or bowel obstructions, or asthma or other breathing difficulties should discuss with the doctor the risks and benefits associated with this drug before taking it. Those who have experienced an allergic reaction to meclizine should not take it. The FDA recommends that youngsters under age 12 should not take this drug, except under the direction of a physician. Pregnant women and those trying to become pregnant should not take this medication. Animal reproductive studies have shown some deformities at elevated doses. Women who are breastfeeding should discuss this medication with their doctors prior to taking it.

Side effects

Meclizine may cause drowsiness and **fatigue**. Drowsiness is the most common adverse reaction. Alcohol and other central nervous system depressants, such as pain medication and tranquilizers, may increase this effect. Patients should refrain from drinking alcoholic beverages, and avoid driving or operating machinery or appliances when taking this drug. Less frequently, the drug also may produce the opposite effect. Excitability, nervousness, restlessness, mood enhancement and difficulty sleeping may develop. Rarely, it may cause a patient to see or hear things that are not present (hallucinations). Despite being used to treat nausea and vomiting, it may produce this effect. It may also cause constipation, **diarrhea**, an upset stomach or a poor appetite (**anorexia**). Other side effects include frequent or difficult urination, incomplete emptying of the bladder, low blood pressure, a rapid heart rate or palpitations. It may cause vision changes, a dry nose and throat, ringing in the ears, and a rash or hives. Some of the side effects may be more pronounced in older adults.

Side effects may decrease as the body adjusts to the medication. Ice chips or sugarless hard candy or gum may help relieve the dry mouth. If the feeling of a dry mouth persists for more than two weeks, the doctor should be notified.

Interactions

Central nervous system depressants, including alcohol, may increase drowsiness associated with meclizine. Pain medications, other antihistamines, seizure medications, sleeping pills and muscle relaxants can depress the central nervous system. Taking this drug with some medications used to treat **depression** may increase the risk of side effects. Patients should inform the doctor of all medications being taken. Patients should not start or stop any drugs without the approval of the doctor. The herbal supplement henbane may increase some of meclizine's side effects, including dry mouth and difficulty urinating.

Resources

BOOKS

Beers, Mark H., MD, and Robert Berkow, MD, editors. "Care of the Dying Patient." In *The Merck Manual of Diagnosis and Therapy*. Whitehouse Station, NJ: Merck Research Laboratories, 2007.

Beers, Mark H., MD, and Robert Berkow, MD, editors. "Motion Sickness." Section 20, Chapter 282 In *The Merck Manual of Diagnosis and Therapy*. Whitehouse Station, NJ: Merck Research Laboratories, 2004.

PERIODICALS

Kuykendall, J. R., and R. S. Rhodes. "Auditory Hallucinations Elicited by Combined Meclizine and Metaxalone Use at Bedtime." *Annals of Pharmacotherapy* 38 (November 2004): 1968–1969.

Sansone, R. A., and C. D. Sears. "The Successful Use of Meclizine in Panic Disorder." *Journal of Clinical Psychiatry* 65 (September 2004): 1285–1286.

OTHER

Food and Drug Administration. "Taming Tummy Turmoil." FDA Publication No. 96-3219. http://www.fda.gov/fdac/reprints/tummy.html.

ORGANIZATIONS

United States Food and Drug Administration (FDA). 5600 Fishers Lane, Rockville, MD 20857-0001. (888) INFO-FDA. www.fda.gov.

Debra Wood, R.N.
Rebecca J. Frey, Ph.D.

Mediastinal tumors

Definition

A mediastinal tumor is a growth in the central chest cavity (mediastinum), which separates the lungs and contains the heart, aorta, esophagus, thymus, and trachea. Mediastinal tumors are also known as neoplasms of the mediastinum.

Mediastinal tumors

Cancer type	Occurs in
Thymomas	Anterior mediastinum, almost always form where heart and major vessels meet
Teratomas	Anterior mediastinum, along the center of the body between the skull and kidneys
Lymphomas	Anterior and middle mediastinum
Thyroid tumors	Thyroid (anterior mediastinum)
Mesenchymal tumors (soft tissue tumors)	Middle mediastinum
Carcinomas	Middle mediastinum
Neurogenic tumors (developing in nerve cells)	Posterior mediastinum
Malignant schwannomas	Posterior mediastinum
Neuroblastomas	Posterior mediastinum

(Table by GGS Creative Resources. Cengage Learning, Gale.)

Description

Growths that originate in the mediastinum are called primary mediastinal tumors. Most of them are composed of reproductive (germ) cells or develop in thymic, neurogenic (nerve), lymphatic, or mesenchymal (soft) tissue.

Secondary (metastatic) mediastinal tumors originate in the lung, stomach, esophagus, and trachea, and spread through the lymphatic system to the chest cavity.

Although still relatively rare, malignant mediastinal tumors are becoming more common. Usually diagnosed in patients between 30 and 50 years old, they can develop at any age and arise from any tissue that exists in or passes through the chest cavity.

The mediastinum is traditionally divided into superior, anterior, middle, and posterior compartments, and is also described as having anterosuperior, middle, and posterior divisions. Boundaries of these divisions are not fixed, and they frequently overlap.

The anterosuperior compartment contains a vein and the thymus gland, superior vena cava, aortic arch, and thyroid gland. More than half (54%) of mediastinal tumors in adults and 43% of those in children occur in the anterosuperior compartment.

The middle mediastinum contains the pericardium, heart, nerves of the diaphragm (phrenic nerves), trachea, main bronchial stem, and lung hila. Twenty percent of adult mediastinal tumors and 18% of those in children occur in this division.

The posterior mediastinum contains the sympathetic chain, vagus nerve (which controls the heart, larynx, and gastrointestinal tract), thoracic duct (which drains lymph from the abdomen, legs, and left side of the head and chest), descending thoracic aorta, and the esophagus. Slightly more than one fourth (26%) of adult mediastinal tumors and 40% of those in children occur in the posterior mediastinum.

Each of these compartments also contains lymph nodes and fatty tissue.

Types of cancers

Anterior mediastinal tumors

The most common anterior mediastinal tumors are thymomas, teratomas, lymphomas, and thyroid tissue that has become enlarged or displaced (ectopic).

THYMOMAS. The cause of most adult mediastinal tumors and 15% of those in children, thymomas almost always form at the spot where the heart and great vessels meet. These tumors usually develop between the ages of 40 and 60.

About half of the people who have thymomas do not have any symptoms. Between 35 and 50% experience symptoms of **myasthenia gravis**, such as

- weakness of the eye muscles
- drooping of one or both eyelids (ptosis)
- fatigue

Early treatment of these slow-growing tumors is very effective. Most are benign, but thymomas can metastasize and should always be considered cancerous.

TERATOMAS. Most common in young adults, teratomas are made up of embryonic (germ) cells that did not develop normally and do not belong in the part of the body where the tumor is located. Found along the center of the body between the skull and kidneys, teratomas account for:

- 10–15% of primary mediastinal tumors
- 70% of germ cell tumors in children
- 60% of germ cell tumors in adults

Teratomas may be solid or contain cysts. Malignant teratomas usually develop between the ages of 30 and 40, and almost all (90%) of them occur in men.

At least 90% of patients with these tumors experience:

- chest pain
- cough
- fever
- shortness of breath

These symptoms may not appear until the tumor has grown very large.

LYMPHOMAS. These tumors account for 10–20% of anterior mediastinal tumors. Although lymphomas are the second most common mediastinal tumor in children, they are usually diagnosed between the ages of 30 and 40. Nonsclerosing **Hodgkin's disease** causes most adult mediastinal lymphomas.

Some patients with lymphomas do not have symptoms. Others cough or experience chest pain.

THYROID TUMORS. Most mediastinal thyroid tumors grow out of goiters and occur in women between the ages of 50 and 60. About 75% of these tumors extend to the windpipe (trachea). The rest extend behind it.

Mediastinal thyroid tumors are encapsulated and do not metastasize.

Middle mediastinal tumors

Tumors of the middle mediastinum include lymphomas, mesenchymal tumors, and carcinomas.

MESENCHYMAL TUMORS. Also called soft tissue tumors, mesenchymal tumors originate in connective tissue within the chest cavity. These tumors account for about 6% of primary mediastinal tumors. More than half (55%) of them are malignant.

The most common mesenchymal tumors are lipomas, liposarcomas, fibromas, and fibrosarcomas.

Posterior mediastinal tumors

Tumors of the posterior mediastinum include: neurogenic tumors, mesenchymal tumors, and endocrine tumors.

NEUROGENIC TUMORS. Representing 19–39% of mediastinal tumors, neurogenic tumors can develop at any age. They are most common in young adults.

Adult neurogenic tumors are usually benign. In children, they tend to be malignant and tend to metastasize before symptoms appear.

MALIGNANT SCHWANNOMAS. Also known as malignant sheath tumors, malignant sarcomas, and neurosarcomas, these tumors develop from the tube (sheath) enclosing the peripheral nerves that transmit impulses from the central nervous system (CNS) to muscles and organs.

Usually large and painful, these rare, aggressive tumors may invade the lungs, bones, and aorta.

NEUROBLASTOMAS. The most common malignant tumors of early childhood, neuroblastomas generally occur before the age of two. These tumors usually develop in the adrenal glands, neck, abdomen, or pelvis.

Neuroblastomas often spread to other organs. Most patients have symptoms that relate to the part of the body the tumor has invaded. Likelihood of survival is greatest in patients who are less than a year old and whose tumor has not spread.

Symptoms

About 40% of people who have mediastinal tumors do not have any symptoms. When symptoms exist, they usually result from pressure on an organ that the tumor has invaded, and indicate that the tumor is malignant.

The symptoms most commonly associated with mediastinal tumors are:

- chest pain
- cough
- shortness of breath

A person who has a mediastinal tumor may be hoarse, cough up blood (**hemoptysis**), or have:

- fatigue
- difficulty swallowing (dysphagia)
- night sweats
- systemic lupus erythematosus
- inflamed muscles (polymyositis)
- ulcerative colitis
- rheumatoid arthritis
- thyroid problems (thyroiditis, thyrotoxicosis,)
- fever
- glandular disorders (panhypopituitarism, adenopathy)
- high blood pressure
- low blood sugar (hypoglycemia)
- breast development in males (gynecomastia)
- wheezing
- vocal cord paralysis
- heart problems (superior vena cava syndrome, pericardial tamponade, arrhythmias)
- neurologic abnormalities
- weight loss

and other immune, autoimmune, and endocrine system disorders.

Blood disorders associated with these tumors include abnormally high levels of calcium (**hypercalcemia**), abnormally low numbers of:

- circulating blood cells (cytopenia)
- normal red blood cells (pernicious anemia)
- antibodies (hypogammaglobulinemia)

and an inability to produce red blood cells (red-cell aplasia).

Diagnosis

Imaging studies

Routine **x rays** often detect mediastinal tumors. Doctors use **computed tomography** (CT) scans of the chest to determine tumor size and location, extent of disease, the tumor's relationship to nearby organs and tissues, and whether the tumor contains cysts or areas of calcification.

Magnetic resonance imaging (MRI) is more effective at clarifying the relationship between a tumor and nearby blood vessels, but is far more costly and time-consuming than CT scanning.

Other tests

Injecting radioactive substances into the patient's blood (radioimmunoassay) enables doctors to measure levels of hormones and other substances a tumor secretes and identify specific tumor types, evaluate the effectiveness of therapy, and monitor possible tumor recurrence.

Invasive procedures

Imaging studies play the most important role in initial diagnosis of mediastinal tumors, but before doctors can determine the most effective treatment for any tumor, they must know what kind of cells it contains.

Although invasive diagnostic procedures have been largely replaced by less invasive techniques (such as CT-guided percutaneous needle **biopsy**), some patients still require surgery.

MEDIASTINOSCOPY. Performed under general anesthesia, this relatively simple procedure enables doctors to accurately diagnose 80–90% of mediastinal tumors, and 95–100% of anterior mediastinal tumors.

Mediastinoscopy is especially useful in providing the large tissue specimens needed to diagnose lymphomas.

MEDIASTINOTOMY. Doctors perform mediastinotomy by using a lighted tube to:

- examine the center of the chest and nearby lymph nodes
- remove tissue for biopsy
- determine whether cancer has spread from the spot where it originated. Similar to mediastinoscopy, this procedure begins with a small incision next to the breastbone, rather than in the patient's neck.

Mediastinotomy also enables doctors to examine the lymph nodes closest to the heart and lungs. **Cancer** that originates in the left upper lobe of the lung often spreads to these nodes.

THORACOTOMY. Although some surgeons still perform this procedure to diagnose mediastinal tumors, **thoracoscopy** may be used instead in certain situations. In a **thoracotomy**, the physician gains access to the chest cavity by cutting through the chest wall. Thoracotomy allows for study, examination, treatment, or removal of any organs in the chest cavity. Tumors and metastatic growths can be removed, and a biopsy can be taken, through the incision. Thoracotomy also gives access to the heart, esophagus, diaphragm, and the portion of the aorta that passes through the chest cavity.

THORACOSCOPY. This 100% accurate, minimally invasive procedure is performed under general anesthesia. Enabling the surgeon to view the entire mediastinum, thoracoscopy may be used when a mediastinal tumor touches the mediastinal pleura. However, this procedure has limited applications.

Thoracoscopy cannot be performed on a patient who has thick scar tissue.

Treatment

Doctors use surgery, radiation, and single-agent or combination **chemotherapy** to treat mediastinal tumors.

Thymomas

A patient whose **thymoma** is surgically removed (resected) has the best chance of survival. To lessen the likelihood of new tumors developing (reseeding), surgeons do not recommend biopsy, and try to remove the tumor without puncturing the capsule that encloses it.

RADIATION. Thymomas respond well to radiation, which is used:

- to treat all stages of disease
- before or after surgical resection
- to treat recurrent disease.

The course of treatment lasts three to six weeks. The most common complications of **radiation therapy** are formation of scar tissue in the lungs (pulmonary fibrosis), inflammation of the pericardium (pericarditis), and inflammation of the spinal cord (myelitis).

CHEMOTHERAPY. The use of chemotherapy to treat invasive thymomas is becoming more common. One or more drugs may be administered before or after surgery. Synthetic hormones (**corticosteroids**) can reverse the progression of tumors that do not respond to chemotherapy.

Teratomas

Teratomas are removed surgically. Chemotherapy and radiation are not used to treat these tumors. The prospect for long-term cure is excellent, and these tumors rarely recur.

Lymphomas

These tumors do not require surgery, except to make the diagnosis. Doctors treat them with chemotherapy and radiation.

Thyroid tumors

Doctors generally treat thyroid tumors with surgical resection, chemotherapy, and/or radiation.

Fibrosarcomas

Fibrosarcomas cannot usually be resected and do not respond well to chemotherapy.

Malignant schwannomas

Multiagent chemotherapy is used to treat these aggressive tumors, which tend to recur following surgery. The 5-year survival rate is 75%.

Neuroblastomas

Because these tumors sometimes regress spontaneously, doctors may postpone treatment if the patient has no symptoms or the tumor is not growing.

In other cases, doctors remove these tumors even before symptoms appear. Risks associated with removing these tumors from the spinal canal include:

- injury to the spinal cord or anterior spinal artery
- uncontrolled bleeding in the spinal canal
- decreased blood supply (ischemia) to tissues and organs.

See also CT-guided biopsy; Fibrosarcoma; Neuroblastoma; Thyroid cancer.

Resources

OTHER

Mullen, Brian F., et al. "Anterior mediastinal masses." *Virtual Hospital.* [cited July 23, 2009]. http://www.vh.org/Providers/Textbooks/Lung Tumors/PathologicTypes/Text/AnteriorMediastinal Masses.html.

Maureen Haggerty

Mediastinoscopy

Definition

Mediastinoscopy is a surgical procedure that allows physicians to view areas of the mediastinum, the cavity behind the breastbone that lies between the lungs. The organs in the mediastinum include the heart and its vessels, the lymph nodes, trachea, esophagus, and thymus.

Mediastinoscopy is most commonly used to detect or stage **cancer**. It is also ordered to detect **infection**, and to confirm diagnosis of certain conditions and diseases of the respiratory organs. The procedure involves insertion of an endotracheal (within the trachea) tube, followed by a small incision in the chest. A mediastinoscope is inserted through the incision. The purpose of this equipment is to allow the physician to directly see the organs inside the mediastinum, and to collect tissue samples for laboratory study.

Purpose

Mediastinoscopy is often the diagnostic method of choice for detecting **lymphoma**, including **Hodgkin's disease**. The diagnosis of sarcoidosis (a chronic lung disease) and the staging of lung cancer can also be accomplished through mediastinoscopy. Lung cancer staging involves the placement of the cancer's progression into stages, or levels. These stages help a physician study cancer and provide consistent definition levels of cancer and corresponding treatments. The lymph nodes in the mediastinum are likely to show if lung cancer has spread beyond the lungs. Mediastinoscopy allows a physician to observe and extract a sample from the nodes for further study. Involvement of these lymph nodes indicates diagnosis and stages of lung cancer.

Mediastinoscopy may also be ordered to verify a diagnosis that was not clearly confirmed by other methods, such as certain radiographic and laboratory studies. Mediastinoscopy may also aid in certain surgical biopsies of nodes or cancerous tissue in the mediastinum. In fact, the surgeon may immediately perform a surgical procedure if a malignant tumor is

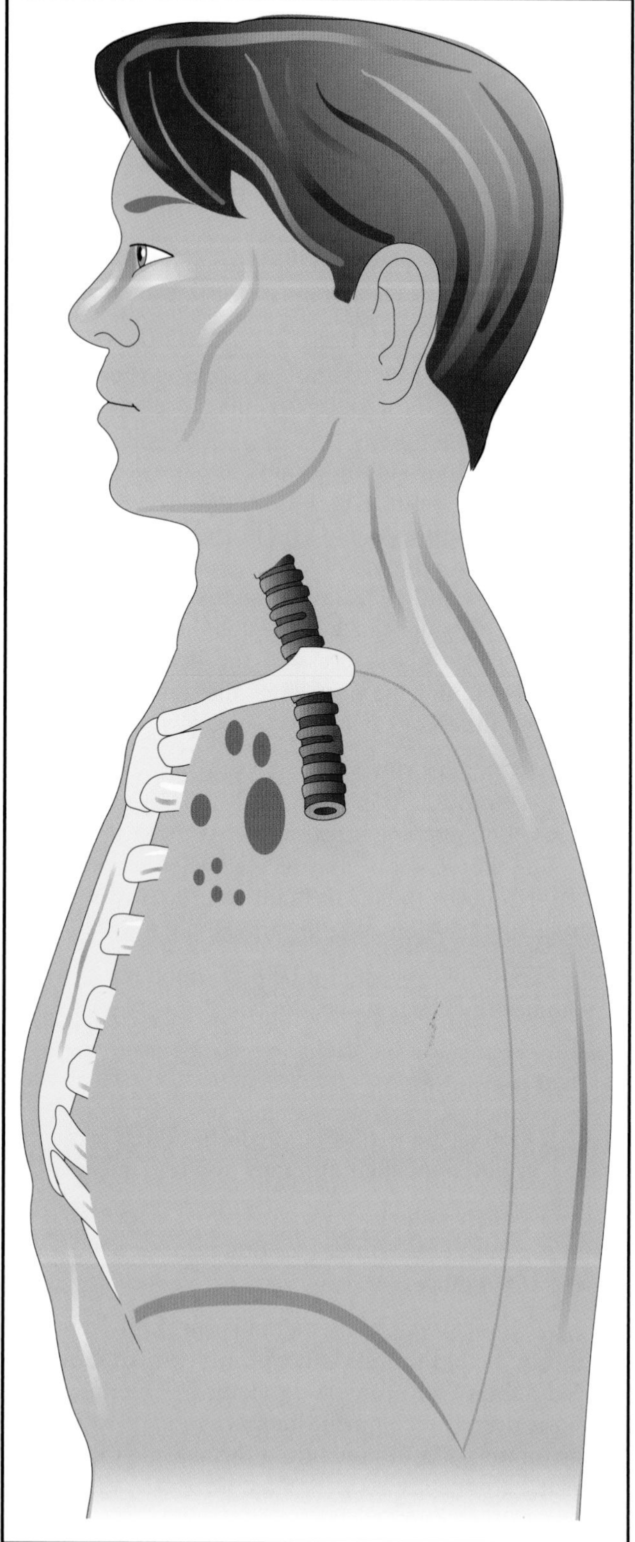

A mediastinoscopy is a surgical procedure most commonly used to detect or stage cancer in the lungs and the surrounding areas. *(Illustration by Electronic Illustrators Group. Cengage Learning, Gale.)*

QUESTIONS TO ASK THE DOCTOR

- Why do I need this test?
- Is the test dangerous?
- How do I prepare for the test?
- How long will the test take?
- Will I get general or local anesthesia?
- How soon will I get my test results?

confirmed while the patient is undergoing mediastinoscopy, thus combining the diagnostic exam and surgical procedure into one operation when possible.

Advancements in **computed tomography** (CT) and **magnetic resonance imaging** (MRI) techniques, as well as the new developments in **ultrasonography**, have led to a decline in the use of mediastinoscopy. In addition, better results of fine-needle aspiration (drawing out fluid by suction) and core-needle **biopsy** (using a needle to obtain a small tissue sample) investigations, along with new techniques in **thoracoscopy** (examination of the thoracic cavity with a lighted instrument called a thoracoscope) offer additional options in examining mediastinal masses. Mediastinoscopy may be required, however, when these other methods cannot be used or when the results they provide are inconclusive.

Precautions

Because mediastinoscopy is a surgical procedure, it should only be performed when the benefits of the exam's findings outweigh the risks of surgery and anesthesia. Patients who previously had mediastinoscopy should not receive it again if there is scarring present from the first exam.

Several other medical conditions, such as impaired cerebral circulation, obstruction or distortion of the upper airway, or thoracic aortic aneurysm (abnormal dilation of the thoracic aorta) may also preclude mediastinoscopy. Anatomic structures that can be compressed by the mediastinoscope may complicate these pre-existing medical conditions.

Description

Mediastinoscopy is usually performed in a hospital under general anesthesia. An endotracheal tube is inserted first, after local anesthesia is applied to the throat. Once the patient is under general anesthesia, a small incision is made usually just below the neck or at the notch at the top of the breastbone. The surgeon may clear a path and feel the patient's lymph nodes first to evaluate any abnormalities within the nodes. Next, the physician will insert the mediastinoscope through the incision. The scope is a narrow, hollow tube with an attached light that allows the surgeon to see inside the area. The surgeon can insert tools through the hollow tube to help perform biopsies. A sample of tissue from the lymph nodes or a mass can be extracted and sent for study under a microscope or on to a laboratory for further testing.

KEY TERMS

Endotracheal—Placed within the trachea, also known as the windpipe.

Hodgkin's disease—A malignancy of lymphoid tissue found in the lymph nodes, spleen, liver, and bone marrow.

Lymph nodes—Small round structures located throughout the body; contain cells that fight infections.

Pleural space—Space between the layers of the pleura (membrane lining the lungs and thorax).

Sarcoidosis—A chronic disease characterized by nodules in the lungs, skin, lymph nodes and bones; however, any tissue or organ in the body may be affected.

Thymus—An unpaired organ in the mediastinal cavity that is important in the body's immune response.

In some cases, analysis of the tissue sample which shows malignancy will suggest the need for immediate surgery while the patient is already prepared and under anesthesia. In other cases, the surgeon will complete the visual study and tissue extraction and stitch the small incision closed. The patient will remain in the surgery recovery area until it is determined that the effects of anesthesia have lessened and it is safe for the patient to leave the area. The entire procedure should take about an hour, not counting preparation and recovery time. Studies have shown that mediastinoscopy is a safe, thorough, and cost-effective diagnostic tool with less risk than some other procedures.

Preparation

Patients are asked to sign a consent form after having reviewed the risks of mediastinoscopy and known risks or reactions to anesthesia. The physician will normally instruct the patient to fast from midnight before the test until after the procedure is completed. A physician may also prescribe a sedative the night before the exam and before the procedure. Often a local anesthetic will be applied to the throat to prevent discomfort during placement of the endotracheal tube.

Aftercare

Following mediastinoscopy, patients will be carefully monitored to watch for changes in vital signs or indications of complications of the procedure or the anesthesia. A patient may have a sore throat from the endotracheal tube, temporary chest pain, and soreness or tenderness at the site of incision.

Risks

Complications from the actual mediastinoscopy procedure are relatively rare—the overall complication rate in various studies has been 1.3–3.0%. However, the following complications, in decreasing order of frequency, have been reported:

- hemorrhage
- pneumothorax (air in the pleural space)
- recurrent laryngeal nerve injury, causing hoarseness
- infection
- tumor implantation in the wound
- phrenic nerve injury (injury to a thoracic nerve)
- esophageal injury
- chylothorax (chyle—a milky lymphatic fluid—in the pleural space)
- air embolism (air bubble)
- transient hemiparesis (paralysis on one side of the body)

The usual risks associated with general anesthesia also apply to this procedure.

Normal results

In the majority of procedures performed to diagnose cancer, a normal result involves evidence of small, smooth, normal-appearing lymph nodes and no abnormal tissue, growths, or signs of infection. In the case of lung cancer staging, results are related to the severity and progression of the cancer.

Abnormal results

Abnormal findings may indicate lung cancer, tuberculosis, the spread of disease from one body part to another, sarcoidosis (a disease that causes nodules, usually affecting the lungs), lymphoma (abnormalities in the lymph tissues), and Hodgkin's disease.

Resources

BOOKS

Fischbach, Frances Talaska. *A Manual of Laboratory and Diagnostic Tests.* 6th ed. Philadelphia: Lippincott Williams and Wilkins, 2000.

PERIODICALS

Deslauriers, Jean, and Jocelyn Gregoire. "Clinical and Surgical Staging of Non-Small Cell Lung Cancer." *Chest,* Supplement (April 2000): 96S–103S.

Tahara R. W., et al. "Is There a Role for Routine Mediastinoscopy in Patients With Peripheral T1 Lung Cancers?" *American Journal of Surgery* (December 2000): 488–491.

ORGANIZATIONS

Alliance for Lung Cancer Advocacy, Support, and Education. P.O. Box 849, Vancouver, WA 98666. 800–298–2436. http://www.alcase.org.

American Cancer Society. 1599 Clifton Rd. NE, Atlanta, GA 30329. 800–ACS–2345 http://www.cancer.org.

American Lung Association. 1740 Broadway, New York, NY 10019–4374. 800–LUNG–USA (800–586–4872). http://www.lungusa.org.

Teresa G. Odle

Medroxyprogesterone acetate

Definition

Medroxyprogesterone acetate (MPA) is used during **cancer** therapy to stop new cell growth in some cancers. It is also used outside of cancer treatment as a contraceptive. MPA is known by many different brand names in the United States including Amen, Depo-Provera, Provera, Prodasone, and Progeston.

Purpose

MPA is used to treat some advanced, hormone-responsive cancers of the breast, kidney, and lining of the uterus.

Description

MPA is a synthetic derivative of the female hormone progesterone. In healthy women, progesterone plays a major role in preparing the uterus for pregnancy. MPA has been approved by the Food and Drug Administration (FDA), and its use in cancer treatment is usually covered by insurance. Outside the area of cancer treatment, it is used to prevent pregnancy.

Exactly why MPA stops tumor growth is unclear. Many cancerous tumors are sensitive to hormones. It appears that MPA, in some way, changes the hormonal climate of the tumor so that cells stop responding to other hormones and proteins that would normally stimulate their growth. This drug cannot tell the difference between normal cells and cancer cells, so some normal cells are also killed during treatment. But since

KEY TERMS

Endometrial cancer—Cancer of the uterus.

Food and Drug Administration (FDA)—The government agency that oversees public safety in relation to drugs and medical devices, and gives the approval to pharmaceutical companies for commercial marketing of their products.

cancer cells generally grow more rapidly than normal cells, more cancer cells are killed. MPA is considered very effective and relatively non-toxic.

MPA is usually given to women whose **breast cancer** has returned or whose cancer does not respond to **tamoxifen** or **toremifene**. Both drugs are **antiestrogens**, or agents that antagonize the actions of estrogen. For these women, it is an alternative to the new aromatase inhibiting drugs (anastrozole, letrozole, or aromasin). Aromatase is one of the enzymes involved in steroid biosynthesis. In **endometrial cancer** (cancer of the uterus), MPA is sometimes used when cancer has spread (metastasized) beyond the uterus or is inoperable.

Recommended dosage

MPA comes as tablets or as a liquid that is given as an intramuscular injection. For breast cancer, it is usually given as a tablet once a day at the same time each day. Occasionally, MPA is given in divided doses that are spaced evenly throughout the day. For kidney and uterine cancer, MPA is usually given as a shot once a week at first, then later once a month.

By 2001, **clinical trials** were underway testing the use of MPA in women with both breast and endometrial cancer. The selection of clinical trials underway changes frequently. Current information on clinical trials and where they are being held is available by entering the search term "medroxyprogesterone acetate" at the following web sites:

- National Cancer Institute: http://cancertrials.nci.nih.gov or (800) 4-CANCER
- National Institutes of Health Clinical Trials: http://clinicaltrials.gov
- Center Watch: A Clinical Trials Listing: http://www.centerwatch.com

Precautions

People taking MPA daily should take it at the same time each day. The time of day is unimportant, but the regular spacing of the dose is important.

Women taking MPA should not get pregnant. It is believed that MPA causes birth defects in babies born to mothers who are taking this drug during the first four months of pregnancy.

Side effects

The number and severity of side effects vary widely among people. Not only is it dependent on each person's own unique body chemistry, side effects vary with the type of cancer, the health of the patient, and the other drugs being given. There is no way to predict who will experience side effects of MPA.

among the more common side effects are:

- increased appetite and weight gain
- nausea
- swelling and fluid retention in the hands, legs, and breast
- breakthrough vaginal bleeding
- muscle cramps
- fatigue
- emotional or mood changes
- headaches

A less common, but serious, side effect is the development of blood clots that can lead to heart attack or stroke. People who have a history of clotting problems are not good candidates for using MPA.

Interactions

Aminoglutethimide (Cytadren: an inhibitor of steroid biosynthesis), when given with MPA, decreases the effectiveness of MPA.

Tish Davidson, A.M.

Medulloblastoma

Definition

Medulloblastoma is a solid, cancerous tumor originating in the cerebellum of the brain. It is also known as a primitive neuroendocrine tumor.

Description

Medulloblastoma is the most common cancerous brain tumor of childhood. It accounts for 20% to 25% of all childhood tumors. Medulloblastomas can occur soon after birth and into puberty, but most tumors occur either before age ten or sometime in the late

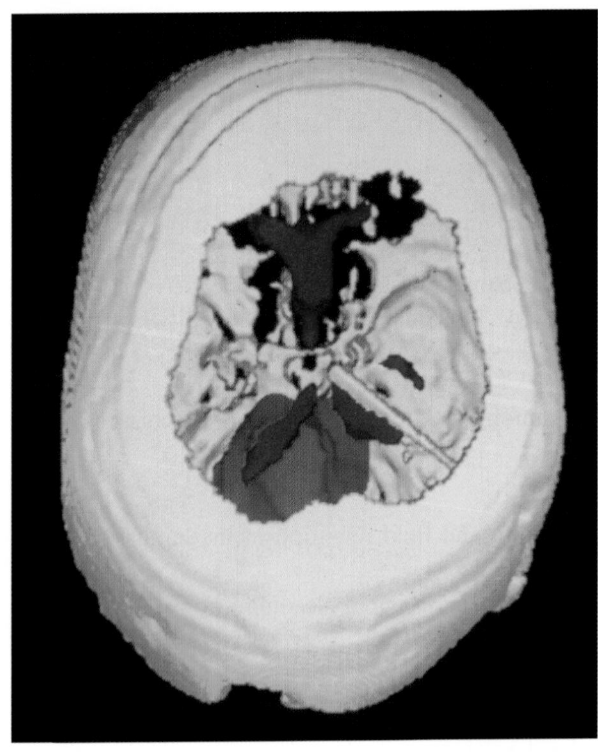

Colorized three-dimensional computed tomography brain scan showing a medulloblastoma tumor (red). *(Copyright CNRI/Science Photo Library, Science Source/Photo Researchers, Inc. Reproduced by permission.)*

teens or early twenties. If these tumors are left untreated, they can spread to other areas of the brain and to the spine.

Medulloblastomas occur in the area of the brain known as the cerebellum. The cerebellum, located in the back of the brain above the neck, is the area of the brain responsible for controlling and integrating movement. A person could move his or her muscles without the aid of the cerebellum, but those movements would be clumsy and disorganized. Medulloblastoma tumors in the cerebellum can cause loss of functioning of the cerebellum, leading to this uncoordinated movement, called cerebellar ataxia.

If medulloblastomas are not detected early, they may spread **cancer** throughout the brain or spinal cord. If the cancer spreads to the spinal cord, a child may begin experiencing severe back pain, difficulty walking, and the inability to control bladder and bowel functions.

Demographics

As stated earlier, medulloblastoma is a childhood cancer, occurring mainly in the first ten years of life. About half of all medulloblastomas occur in children aged five or younger. Boys tend to develop the tumors more than girls at a rate of approximately two to one. There are no current studies comparing the incidence of medulloblastoma between different racial and ethnic groups.

KEY TERMS

Ataxia—The inability to perform voluntary, coordinated muscular movements.

Cerebellum—The portion of the brain lying superior to the spinal cord, involved in coordinating voluntary muscular movements.

Chemotherapy—The application of certain medicinal chemicals to treat specific diseases, including cancer.

Radiation therapy—The use of high-energy ionizing radiation in the treatment of cancerous tumors.

Causes and symptoms

Besides being male, there are no other known risk factors for medulloblastoma. This type of tumor can occur in association with two rare types of genetically linked family cancer syndromes. Gorlin's syndrome and Turcot's syndrome. Gorlin's syndrome is caused by a defect in a gene known as PTC located on chromosome 9. This defect can cause medulloblastoma as well as cancers of the skin and ovary. Turcot's syndrome is caused by a defective gene known as APC, and can present with cancer of the intestinal tract as well as medulloblastoma. It should again be stated that both of these syndromes are quite rare and only account for a fraction of medulloblastoma cases seen and reported.

Medulloblastoma can present in many ways. In infants, symptoms of the tumor can include an unusual increase in head size, **vomiting**, irritability, and lethargy. Since all infants generally have these symptoms at one time or another, it can be difficult for a parent or even a health care worker to recognize the initial presentation of medulloblastoma in babies and toddlers.

In older children and teenagers, medulloblastoma can present the same as in infants or much differently. Non-specific symptoms such as **nausea and vomiting**, headache, and vague visual disturbances can be the first sign of a tumor in the cerebellum. Other, more striking signs can be double vision, sudden difficulty writing, and problems walking and moving that worsen over time.

Diagnosis

The diagnosis of medulloblastoma is made with both clinical observation and **imaging studies**. If a parent has noticed some of the signs and symptoms listed above, then a visit to a pediatrician is certainly warranted. During the office visit, various specialized neurological tests will be done to see if there is any sign of a problem in the cerebellum or surrounding brain structures.

If there are indications of a tumor, then imaging studies can be done to see if a tumor can be detected. The two types of imaging studies done to detect medulloblastoma are **magnetic resonance imaging** (MRI) and **computed tomography** (CT) scan. The MRI uses a high-strength magnetic field to visualize the brain, and is very useful for detecting medulloblastomas. The CT scan uses x-ray images reconstructed by computer. Like the MRI, a CT scan is also useful for detecting **brain tumors** as well as tumors that may have spread to the spine.

Treatment team

The treatment of medulloblastoma is optimally carried out in a medical center that has experience in treating this often difficult-to-treat cancer. Treatment and treatment planning is usually carried out by a multidisciplinary team of cancer specialists, including a pediatric oncologist (a doctor specializing in the treatment of **childhood cancers**), a pediatric neurosurgeon (a doctor specializing in childhood brain surgery), as well as a pediatric neurologist and radiation oncologist (a doctor specializing in the use of radiation to treat cancer).

Clinical staging, treatment, and prognosis

The staging of childhood brain tumors has become important to the selection of treatment plans, as well as giving information to make a more accurate prognosis. For medulloblastoma, there are four stages defined, as follows:

- T1: the tumor is less than 3 cm in diameter.
- T2: the tumor is greater than 3 cm in diameter and has invaded one other brain structure in addition to the cerebellum.
- T3: the tumor has invaded two other brain structures besides the cerebellum.
- T4: the tumor has spread down into the midbrain or upper spinal cord.

The treatment options for medulloblastoma have changed significantly over the past few decades. The first treatment option for medulloblastoma was surgery, and this is still the most common treatment. Surgeons try to remove the entire tumor, although this is sometimes not possible. After the surgery is completed, further treatment will depend upon whether or not the child has been placed in an "average risk" or "high risk" group. An average-risk child is defined as three years or older, with the tumor initially confined to the cerebellum with little to no tumor left after surgery. A high-risk child is defined as a child under three years of age, with the tumor initially spread into other areas of the brain besides the cerebellum, and with some of the tumor remaining in the brain after surgery.

Children in the average-risk group will often have **radiation therapy** applied to the area in their brain where the medulloblastoma tumor was, especially if the surgeon was not able to remove all of the tumor. Using radiation on children younger than three years may result in the child having growth retardation along with learning disabilities.

Because of the possible side effect of radiation, especially in children younger than three years of age, the use of certain medications called **chemotherapy** is being used more frequently for medulloblastoma. Researchers have found that medulloblastoma tumors are highly sensitive to chemotherapy, giving hope that chemotherapy can be used instead of radiation, especially for children at average risk. For children at high risk, the current recommendation is to use both radiation and chemotherapy, since this combination has been shown to improve overall survival rates for high-risk children.

In 1930, the anticipated survival rate for a child with medulloblastoma after surgery was less than 2%. Today, with the use of better surgical techniques, radiation, and chemotherapy, the prognosis for children in the average risk group has increased to a 60% survival rate over a five-year period. Children in the high-risk group do not fare as well, having a 30–35% survival rate over a five-year period.

Alternative and complementary therapies

Alternative and complementary therapies are those that fall outside the scope of traditional, first-line therapies such as surgery, chemotherapy and radiation. Complementary therapies are meant to supplement those traditional therapies with the objective of relieving symptoms. Alternative therapies are nontraditional, unproven attempts to cure the disease.

Common complementary therapies used in many types of cancer include aromatherapy, massage, meditation, music therapy, prayer, and certain forms of exercise. These therapies have the objective of reducing anxiety and increasing a patient's feeling of well-being.

Numerous alternative therapies exist in cancer treatment. Plant extracts, **vitamins**, protein therapies, and natural substances such as **mistletoe** and shark cartilage have all been touted as cancer-fighting remedies. However, some alternative therapies, such as Laetrile, can produce dangerous side effects and have shown no anticancer activity in **clinical trials**. Patients interested in alternative therapies should consult their doctors to ensure that the products are safe, especially for children, and do not interfere with regular cancer treatment.

Coping with cancer treatment

During treatment, a child's health will be followed by the team of physicians involved. Those physicians will be able to monitor the child for any side effects from the treatments, especially if the child is receiving chemotherapy. The most frequent side effects of chemotherapy can include **nausea** and vomiting, **diarrhea**, **fatigue**, and hair loss (**alopecia**). With medications, physicians can often treat some of the side effects, especially nausea, vomiting, and diarrhea.

Cancer treatment can be especially frightening for a young child. Family support is critical, and parents should consult their physician about any organizations in the area that can help their child cope with the effects of medulloblastoma and its treatment.

Clinical trials

There are many clinical trials being done to help better the treatment options for medulloblastoma. Some of the most promising ones are studies in which peripheral stem cell transplantation is used. This is a technique in which certain cells in the body known as stem cells are used to replace other, depleted cells, such as the immune cells and blood cells that are destroyed when chemotherapy is used. It is hoped that with stem cell use, physicians will be able to use higher doses of chemotherapy in order to destroy the medulloblastoma cancer.

Prevention

There are currently no known ways to prevent medulloblastoma. Those who have the very rare genetic disorders which predisposes them to medulloblastoma, Gorlin's and Turcot's syndrome, should be especially aware of any signs or symptoms of medulloblastomas. Children of parents with these genetic disorders should have routine screening done by a pediatrician for any signs of a brain tumor.

See also Bone marrow transplantation; Childhood cancers.

Resources

BOOKS

Abeloff, Martin, James O. Armitage, Allen S. Lichter, and John E. Niederhuber. *Clinical Oncology*. New York: Churchill Livingstone, 2000.

OTHER

National Cancer Institute CancerTrials. [cited July 23, 2009]. http://cancertrials.nci.nih.gov.

ORGANIZATIONS

American Brain Tumor Association. Suite 146, 2720 River Rd., Des Plaines, IL 60018. (800) 886-2282. http://www.abta.org.

National Cancer Institute, National Institutes of Health. Building 31, Room 10A31, 31 Center Dr., MSC 2580, Bethesda, MD 20892-2580. (800) 4-CANCER. http://www.nci.nih.gov.

St. Jude Children's Research Hospital. 332 N. Lauderdale St., Memphis, TN 38105. (901) 495-3300. http://www.stjude.org.

Edward R. Rosick, D.O., M.P.H.

Megestrol acetate

Definition

Megestrol acetate is used to treat unexplained **weight loss** during **cancer** therapy and to stop new cell growth in some cancers. Megestrol acetate is also known by the brand name Megace.

Purpose

Megestrol acetate is used to treat some advanced hormone-responsive cancers of the breast, kidney, and uterus. It is also used in larger doses to help reverse weight loss for which there is no other treatable cause.

Description

Megestrol acetate is a synthetic derivative of the female hormone progesterone. In healthy women, progesterone plays a major role in preparing the uterus for pregnancy. It has been approved by the Food and Drug Administration (FDA), and its use is usually covered by insurance.

Exactly why megestrol acetate stops tumor growth is unclear. Many tumors are sensitive to hormones. It appears that megestrol acetate, in some way, changes the hormonal climate of the tumor so that cells stop responding to other hormones and proteins that would normally stimulate their growth. This drug

KEY TERMS

Food and Drug Administration (FDA)—The government agency that oversees public safety in relation to drugs and medical devices, and gives the approval to pharmaceutical companies for commercial marketing of their products in the United States.

Hormone—A chemical released by a gland that travels through the circulatory system and affects only the tissues at a distance from its release point that have receptors for the chemical.

Progesterone—A female hormone that prepares the uterus for pregnancy.

cannot tell the difference between normal cells and cancer cells, so some normal cells are also killed during treatment. But since cancer cells grow more rapidly than normal cells, more cancer cells are killed.

Megestrol acetate has another independent use in cancer treatment. In high doses, it is used to counteract weight loss that does not occur for any other treatable reason. Megestrol acetate appears to bring about weight gain through increased fat storage.

Recommended dosage

Megestrol acetate comes in both liquid and tablet form. To treat weigh loss, the standard dosage is a single dose given in the morning with breakfast. Many clinical studies are underway to examine the best use of megestrol acetate in severe weight loss. Most of these studies are for people who are losing weight because they suffer with AIDS. However, the selection of **clinical trials** underway changes frequently. Current information on what clinical trials are available and where they are being held can be found by entering the search term "megestrol acetate" at the following websites:

- National Cancer Institute: http://cancertrials.nci.nih.gov or (800) 4-CANCER
- National Institutes of Health Clinical Trials: http://clinicaltrials.gov
- Center Watch: A Clinical Trials Listing: http://www.centerwatch.com

To reduce tumor growth, the dose of megestrol acetate is individualized, and depends on the type of cancer, the patient's body weight and general health, what other drugs are being given, and the way the cancer responds to hormones. A standard dose of Megace to treat **breast cancer** is 160 mg/day divided into four doses. A standard dose for **endometrial cancer** (cancer of the uterus) is 40–320 mg/day in divided doses. Treatment normally continues for about two months.

Precautions

Women taking megestrol acetate should not get pregnant. Megestrol acetate is believed to cause birth defects in babies born to mothers who are taking the drug. A patient assistance program is available through Bristol Meyer Squibb, the manufacturer of this drug at (800) 332-2056.

Side effects

Megestrol acetate has several rare but serious side effects. Some people have been reported to develop **Cushing's syndrome**. This is a hormonal imbalance in which people (usually women) develop fatty deposits in the face and neck, lose bone mass (osteoporosis), stop menstruating, develop diabetes, high blood pressure, and other signs of fluid and salt (electrolyte) imbalances.

Other common side effects of megestrol acetate include:

- worsening of diabetic symptoms
- pain in the chest or abdomen
- infection
- sarcoma (tumors of the skin or connective tissue)
- irregular heartbeat
- fluid retention
- breakthrough vaginal bleeding
- blood clots in legs or lungs
- nausea or constipation
- dry mouth or increased salivation
- abnormal white blood cell count
- confusion or abnormal thinking
- emotional and psychological changes
- rash, itching, abnormal sweating, or skin disorders
- cough, sore throat, lung disorders
- hair loss (alopecia)
- uncontrolled urination or urinary tract infection
- male impotence

Interactions

No specific interactions with other pharmaceuticals have been reported in people using megestrol acetate. However, many drugs interact with nonprescription (over-the-counter) drugs and herbal remedies as well as prescription drugs. Patients should always tell their health care providers about all remedies they are taking. Patients should also mention if they are on a special diet such as low salt or high protein.

Tish Davidson, A.M.

Melanoma

Definition

Melanoma is a type of **skin cancer**. The **cancer** cells form in melanocytes, the pigmented cells that give skin its color. In malignant melanoma, melanocytes become cancerous and may spread throughout the body and invade other organs and tissues. Initially melanoma begins on the surface of the skin. If left untreated, melanoma can cause illness that may be fatal; however, if caught early, melanoma may be treatable with surgery, **chemotherapy**, **radiation therapy**, and immunotherapy.

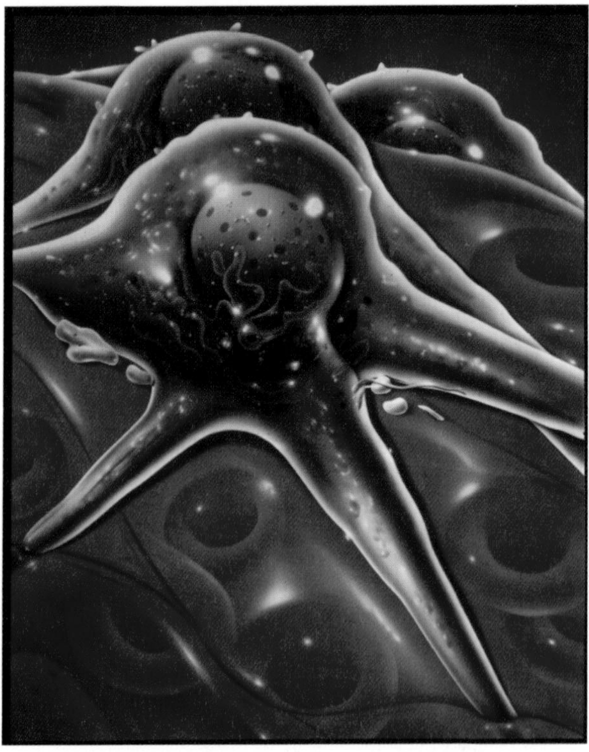

Melanoma. *(Photo Researchers, Inc. Reproduced by permission.)*

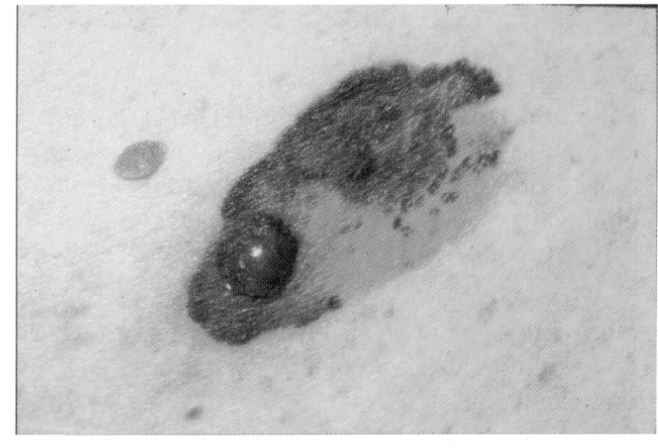

A close-up image of a malignant melanoma on a patient's back. *(Custom Medical Stock Photo. Reproduced by permission.)*

Demographics

Melanoma accounts for only 4 percent of skin cancers in the United States; however, it is responsible for 75 percent of deaths from skin cancer. About 8,500 Americans die each year from melanoma, 5,500 men and 3,000 women. Although melanoma is more common in women than men up to age 40, in adults over 40 it is more common in men. The average age of Americans at the time of diagnosis of melanoma is 53 years; however, it is the most common cancer in women between the ages of 25 and 29, and is second only to **breast cancer** in women between the ages of 30 and 34. In the United States, melanoma affects Caucasians twenty times more often than African Americans, and six times more often than Hispanics.

In the United States, one in 85 people are expected to develop melanoma during their lifetime. According to National Cancer Institute (NCI) estimates, 68,720 cases of melanoma were expected to be newly diagnosed in the United States in 2009. Melanoma was considered a rare form of cancer until the 1970s, but its rate among Caucasians in the United States has tripled since 1985. It is presently the sixth most common cancer in the United States. The current lifetime risk for developing invasive melanoma is 1 case for every 60 Americans, a 2,000% increase since 1930. This risk rises to 1 case for every 32 Americans if early-stage melanoma (Stage 0 below) is included. For Canada, doctors estimate that there are 10 to 13 cases of melanoma per 100,000 people. An estimated 4,300 new cases were diagnosed in Canadians in 2005, with 800 reported deaths.

The highest rates of melanoma in the world, however, are not found in the United States or Canada but in Australia, New Zealand, and Israel. There are approximately 57 cases of melanoma per 100,000 people per year in Australia each year and 40 cases per 100,000 people each year in Israel. The World Health Organization (WHO) reports that 160,000 cases of malignant melanoma are diagnosed worldwide each year, with 48,000 deaths.

One of the more unusual findings in the United States in recent years is the rapid increase of deaths from melanoma in older males. Although the death rate among younger men (44 years or younger) has dropped since the late 1990s, most likely as a result of public health education campaigns about the dangers of sun exposure, it has risen 66 percent in men between the ages of 45 and 64, and 157 percent in men over 65.

Description

The epidermis, the outermost and upper layer of the skin, contains melanocytes, the skin cells that make melanin, the pigment that gives skin its hue. Melanin is responsible for the color of a person's skin, hair, and eyes. There are between 1,000 and 2,000 melanocytes in each square millimeter of human skin. The difference in skin color between fair-skinned and darker-skinned people does not depend on the number of melanocytes in the skin but on their level of activity. When skin is exposed to the sun, the melanocytes become more active, produce more melanin, and cause the skin to darken—that is, they cause a suntan. When a cancerous tumor develops in tissue containing melanocytes, a person has melanoma.

Most cases of melanoma occur in the skin (cutaneous melanoma), but sometimes melanoma can also occur in the iris, the colored part of the eye—a condition known as ocular melanoma.

Cutaneous melanoma

Sometimes melanoma arises out of normal skin, but it can also develop in a mole (also called a nevus). Moles are benign growths or collections of melanocytes on the skin. According to the American Academy of Dermatology, individuals usually have about 30 moles on their skin.

The number and type of moles individuals have may increase the risk of developing melanoma. People with more than 50 moles or with moles that are unusual and irregular looking (doctors call these dysplastic or atypical moles) are at increased risk of developing melanoma.

There are four major types of cutaneous (skin-based) melanoma:

- Superficial spreading melanoma accounts for 70% of all cases of melanoma and typically occurs in younger people. This type of melanoma takes a long time to penetrate the top layer of skin, and the first sign of it is a flat or slightly raised skin lesion. The lesion may be discolored with irregular borders and may develop out of a previously benign mole. It is most likely to occur on the trunk in men, the legs in women, and the upper back in men and women.
- Lentigo maligna melanoma is another form of melanoma that is most often found in older adults. It begins as a flat or slightly raised tan, brown, or dark brown skin discoloration that remains close to the skin's surface. Once the malignancy spreads, it is referred to as lentigo maligna melanoma.
- Acral lentiginous melanoma is the most common type of melanoma in African Americans and Asians and is least common among Caucasians. The black or brown discoloration of acral letiginous melanoma first spreads on the surface of the skin, often under the nails or on the soles of the feet or palms of the hands.
- Nodular melanoma, which accounts for 10 to 15% of all melanoma cases, is the most aggressive form of melanoma, and by the time it is diagnosed, it may have spread to other areas of the body. This type of melanoma starts as a bump that is usually black. Most frequently nodular melanoma is found on the trunk, legs, and arms, and most often affects older people.

Superficial spreading melanoma, lentigo maligna melanoma, and acral lentiginous melanoma begin as in situ malignancies, which means they affect only the top layers of skin. Eventually, these forms of melanomas may become invasive and spread to other areas of the body. Nodular melanoma is often invasive by the time it is diagnosed, however.

Ocular melanoma

Ocular melanoma, or melanoma of the eye, is a cancer that develops in the parts of the eye that contain melanocytes—the iris and other nearby structures that belong to the middle pigmented layer of the eye. It affects about 6 persons per million per year in the United States and is most likely to develop in people with blue eyes and fair skin. Ocular melanoma is more common in Denmark and other Scandinavian countries than in the United States. It is slightly more common in men than in women. The average age of a person diagnosed with this type of melanoma is 55.

Ocular melanomas can grow slowly for years without producing any symptoms, although they eventually cause blurred vision, gradual loss of sight, and sometimes pain in the eye. This type of melanoma often spreads from the eye to the liver, lungs, or even the central nervous system before it is diagnosed. Most patients die from the spread of the cancer to these vital organs rather than from the effects of the cancer on the eye itself. About half of all patients diagnosed with ocular melanoma die within 10 years after diagnosis and treatment. The standard forms of treatment for this type of cancer are radiation therapy and surgical removal of the affected eye.

Risk factors

Malignant melanoma occurs in people of all ages and ethnicities. However, certain factors put people at greater risk for developing this disease, including the following:

- having fair skin
- having red or blond hair
- having blue or green eyes
- being older than 20 years; the rate rises sharply after age 50 and is highest among people in their 80s
- having excessive sun exposure, exposure to artificial ultraviolet light (such as in tanning beds), or a history of severe sunburns
- living in areas that get high levels of ultraviolet radiation, such as mountainous regions or countries closer to the equator.
- having a previous personal history of melanoma or another type of skin cancer.
- scars or burns on the skin. Fragile skin is more easily damaged by sun.
- exposure to certain chemicals in the environment, including arsenic and some types of weed killers.
- having a job that requires working outdoors during daylight hours.
- having a close relative with melanoma.
- having a high number of moles (50 or more).
- having moles that are unusual or irregular-looking.

Because the development of melanoma is usually related to sun exposure, people with less melanin and lighter skin, hair, and eyes are at greater risk. The disease is 10 times more common in whites than in African Americans.

Having certain procedures or health conditions that weaken the immune system may also predispose a person to developing melanoma. Compared to people in the general population, those who have undergone organ transplants have a threefold risk of melanoma. Having human immunodeficiency virus (HIV) or acquired immunodeficiency syndrome (AIDS), other forms of cancer, or autoimmune diseases that require immunosuppressive treatments can also increase a person's risk of developing malignant melanoma.

Causes and symptoms

Causes

ULTRAVIOLET RADIATION. The development of melanomas from normal skin is not completely understood as of 2009. Some researchers think there may be several different pathways to melanoma, depending on whether they occur on skin that is exposed to the sun only occasionally (such as the chest or back area in women) or on skin that is frequently exposed to the sun (head, face, neck, and hands). In general, melanoma is caused by the interaction of ultraviolet (UV) radiation from the sun and the melanin in melanocytes. UV radiation can damage the DNA in skin cells both directly and indirectly. Researchers have found that 92 percent of melanomas are caused by indirect damage to DNA and 8 percent by direct damage.

When the DNA in a skin cell is damaged by UV radiation, the cell can undergo a series of mutations that lead to abnormal multiplication of new cells. In some cases the changed DNA makes the cell more vulnerable to the damaging effects of UV radiation. About 40 percent of melanomas begin in moles, with the remaining 60 percent starting in normal skin.

Melanomas grow in two stages or phases. The first is a phase of outward or radial growth. The second phase, which is much more dangerous, is a phase of vertical growth into deeper layers of tissue. It is during this second phase of growth that melanomas become harder to treat and able to spread to other parts of the body.

ENVIRONMENTAL CHANGES. Melanoma was a rare form of cancer until the twentieth century. The earliest known surgical removal of a melanoma was performed in 1787 by a British surgeon, but the disease was little studied until the 1840s and 1850s, when two other British doctors described the stages of melanoma and found that it runs in some families. The connection between melanoma and sun exposure was not made until 1956, when an Australian doctor named Henry Lancaster found that high intensity of sunlight is a risk factor for melanoma. In the 1970s, scientists began to notice that the ozone layer—a layer of oxygen molecules consisting of three atoms of oxygen in the upper atmosphere—was becoming thinner. The ozone layer helps to block a high-energy type of ultraviolet radiation known as UVB from reaching the surface of the earth, so doctors began to wonder whether a thinner ozone layer could contribute to an increase in the rate of melanoma and other skin cancers.

As of 2009, however, doctors do not think that the rise in cases of melanoma since the 1980s is due primarily to changes in the ozone layer. One reason is that depletion of the ozone layer is most severe over Antarctica, which is not a heavily populated continent. Another is that recent advances in genetics indicate that heredity plays a larger role in melanoma than was thought to be the case in the 1980s. Still another reason for skepticism about the role of the ozone layer in melanoma is that recent studies indicate that a lower-energy form of ultraviolet radiation called UVA triggers the development of melanoma rather than the UVB blocked by the ozone layer. If this finding is accurate, then changes in the ozone layer are not related to melanoma. It is also likely that the increase in the number of reported cases of melanoma since the 1990s is due partly to better diagnostic instruments and earlier diagnosis.

Research into the rise in cases of melanoma is ongoing in the United States. According to a report published by the Department of Health and Human Services, the U.S. Climate Change Science Program for 2009 will include studies on the effect of UVA and UVB radiation on the skin, research into the effectiveness of various sunscreen products, and the role of genes in triggering the development of melanoma and other skin cancers.

GENETIC FACTORS. The development of melanoma is also thought to have a strong genetic link, since many people who develop melanoma also have family members with the disease. Researchers have identified mutations in genes on chromosomes 1, 9, and 12 as linked to familial melanoma, including a gene called BRAF that may play a role in the development of melanoma. A mutated form of BRAF, found in two-thirds of melanoma samples analyzed in one study, is thought to switch on the malignant cells, allowing them to grow and divide. Another gene mutation called p53 has also been associated with melanoma cases among families.

Symptoms

The first sign of melanoma is a mole, sore, lump, or growth found on the skin. Melanomas can occur anywhere on the body, but they are most often found on the backs of men and the legs of women. Generally, melanomas are black or brown, but may be red, skin-colored, or white. Some may develop pinkish or bluish patches mixed in with darker areas.

Changes in a mole's appearance over time may also indicate malignant melanoma. Sometimes, a growth or mole may bleed, ooze, or itch, which indicates malignancy. Having satellite moles, new moles that grow near an existing mole, may also point to this form of skin cancer.

Early-stage melanomas may itch or shed small flakes of skin, while more advanced melanomas may bleed or ooze fluid as well as itch. Advanced melanomas may also become hard or lumpy in texture. Melanomas do not, however, usually cause pain.

People with moles, lumps, or growths that fit these criteria should be checked by a doctor.

Diagnosis

Examination

For anyone who finds an abnormal mark or mole on the skin, the first step should be to contact their healthcare providers for a skin examination. About 80 percent of all skin cancers are first noticed by the patient. The doctor or nurse will carefully examine all moles, birthmarks, and pigmented areas over the person's entire body, including the back, legs, hands, feet, and scalp.

Doctors often use the "ABCDEs" when making a diagnosis of melanoma. They include:

- Asymmetry: Melanomas are usually asymmetrical, with one half different than the other.
- Border irregularity: The edges of a melanoma may be ragged or blurred.
- Color: A malignant melanoma often has several colors or shades, whereas benign moles are typically one color.
- Diameter: Cancerous moles are usually larger than a pencil eraser (about 6 millimeters).
- Evolving: An area of skin that has recently undergone changes.

A family doctor can often spot suspicious-looking changes in a patient's skin, but will usually refer the patient to a dermatologist for a definite diagnosis. Dermatologists are doctors with specialized training in diagnosing and treating skin disorders.

To diagnose cutaneous melanoma, a dermatologist will first use a dermatoscope, which is a special palm-sized instrument with a magnifying lens and built-in light. The use of dermatoscopes has increased the accuracy of diagnosing malignant melanoma by 20 percent, because the doctor can make digital images of suspicious moles or skin areas and save them for comparison with images from later checkups.

Tests

There are no blood tests as of 2009 that can be used to diagnose melanoma. The diagnosis is usually made by a combination of **imaging studies** and tissue analysis. Chest **x rays**, **computed tomography** (CT or CAT) scans, **magnetic resonance imaging** (MRI) scans, and **positron emission tomography** (PET) scans are tests that doctors use to determine the spread of melanoma throughout the patient's organs and tissues.

Procedures

BIOPSIES. If the dermatoscope images suggest that the patient may have melanoma, the next step is to take a sample of the abnormal mole or area of skin to be sent to a laboratory for analysis under a microscope. This procedure is called a **biopsy**. In the case of melanoma, the doctor will remove the entire mole rather than just a portion of it, so as to obtain an accurate measurement of its depth. Biopsies are done under topical or local anesthesia.

To evaluate whether the melanoma may have spread beyond the skin, the doctor may perform a **sentinel lymph node biopsy**. A sentinel lymph node is the lymph node closest to the melanoma, the one to which it is most likely to spread.

STAGING. Malignant melanoma is curable if caught early. When a melanoma is not removed in its early stages, however, cancer cells will start to grow downward from the skin surface and invade healthy tissue. The disease can then spread to other parts of the body, where it is difficult to control. Measuring a cancer's size, thickness, and likelihood of spreading is called staging. Melanomas are graded in five stages from 0 to 4. The chief factor in determining a patient's chances of recovery is the thickness of the melanoma. This is measured in millimeters and is called Breslow's depth, after the doctor who first connected it to the patient's chances of survival in 1970.

The five stages of melanoma and a person's chances of five-year survival at each stage are as follows:

- Stage 0: The cancerous cells are found only in the outer layer of skin and have not invaded deeper tissues. Survival rate is 99.9%.
- Stage 1: The melanoma is no more than 1/25 of an inch thick (1 millimeter) and has not spread to nearby lymph nodes. Five-year survival rate is 85–95%.
- Stage 2: The tumor is between 1 and 2 millimeters thick but has not spread to nearby lymph nodes. Survival rate is 40–85%.
- Stage 3: The melanoma has spread to nearby lymph nodes or to skin just outside the original tumor. Survival rate after five years is 25–60%.
- Stage 4: The melanoma cells have spread to other organs, to lymph nodes, or to skin areas far away from the original tumor. The five-year survival rate is 7–10%, with an average life expectancy of 6 to 9 months.

Young children are an exception to the survival rates for adults. For some reason that is not yet known as of 2009, survival in children is more closely related to age than to the thickness of the cancer, with younger children being less likely to survive than older children or teenagers.

Treatment

Traditional

SURGERY. The only definite cure for malignant melanoma is surgical removal of the cancerous mole or patch of skin before the melanoma reaches a Breslow depth of 1 millimeter. The surgeon will remove a margin of normal skin surrounding the melanoma as well as the tumor itself to make sure that no cancerous cells are left behind. A procedure known as microscopically controlled excision can be used to examine each layer of skin as it is removed to ensure that the proper amount is taken. Depending on the amount of skin removed, the cut is either closed with stitches or covered with a skin graft. When surgical excision is performed on visible areas, such as the face, cosmetic surgery may also be performed to minimize the scar. Other techniques for removing skin tumors include burning, freezing with dry ice (cryosurgery), or laser surgery. For skin cancer that is localized and has not spread to other areas of the body, excision may be the only treatment needed.

NONSURGICAL APPROACHES. Although chemotherapy is the normal course of therapy for most other types of advanced cancer, it is not usually effective and not usually used for advanced skin cancer. For advanced melanoma that has moved beyond the original tumor site, the local lymph nodes may be surgically removed. Immunotherapy in the form of interferon or interleukin is being used more often with success for advanced melanoma. There is growing evidence that radiation therapy may be useful for advanced melanoma. Other treatments under investigation for melanoma include gene therapy and vaccination. Recent studies have shown that the use of a vaccine prepared from a person's own cancer cells may be useful in treating advanced melanoma. For people previously diagnosed with skin cancers, the chances of getting additional skin cancers are high. Therefore, regular monthly self-examination, as well as frequent examinations by a dermatologist, are essential.

Alternative

There are no established alternative treatments for skin cancer. Preventive measures that can be helpful include minimizing exposure to the sun and sunburn, eating a diet high in **antioxidants** and supplementation with antioxidant nutrients.

Patients diagnosed with melanoma may benefit from some complementary therapies such as prayer, meditation, humor therapy, art therapy, pet therapy, and aromatherapy. While these approaches should not be used as replacements for conventional treatments, they can help to lift the patient's spirits following surgery.

"Look Good . . . Feel Better" is a free public service program approved by the American Cancer Society; it helps patients with any kind of cancer cope with changes in their looks related to cancer treatment. It began in 1987 when a doctor asked the president of the Personal Care Products Council to help a patient who was so depressed by her appearance during chemotherapy that she refused to leave her hospital room. The president sent a makeup artist to visit the patient, who was so delighted with her makeover that she began to respond better to her cancer treatment. Look Good . . . Feel Better has expanded to include programs for teens, men, and Spanish-speaking patients; groups are available in all 50 states, the District of Columbia, and Puerto Rico. The main website is http://www.lookgoodfeelbetter.org/.

Prognosis

Whether the melanoma has spread to the body's organs and the thickness of the lesion at the time of diagnosis have significant impact on the prognosis. The thicker the melanoma and the greater the spread, the worse the prognosis. Patients diagnosed and treated before their melanoma spreads to the lymph nodes have a 5-year survival rate of 91% however, those whose melanoma has spread to the lungs or liver have a 5-year survival rate of only 7–10%, with an average life expectancy of 6–9 months.

Other factors may also influence survival rates. For example, although melanoma among African Americans is rare, it is more lethal. Melanomas also tend to be thinner in females, so women have more favorable survival rates. In addition, older adults generally have shorter periods of survival after melanoma diagnosis.

QUESTIONS TO ASK YOUR DOCTOR

- How does my sun/ultraviolet light exposure history affect my risk of melanoma?
- How often do I need skin examinations for melanoma?
- Do I have any moles or lesions that I should watch carefully?
- How far has my melanoma spread beneath the skin?
- What is my prognosis, based on the stage of melanoma I have?
- Are there risks and side effects associated with cancer treatment?
- How should I care for my skin after melanoma treatment?
- What steps should I take to avoid sun exposure now that I have been treated for melanoma?

Prevention

Skin protection

People cannot change their skin type, but they can lower their risk of melanoma by taking the following precautions against sun exposure:

- Avoiding the use of tanning booths and sun lamps.
- Staying out of the sun between 10 A.M. and 4 P.M.
- Using a sunscreen with a sun protection factor (SPF) of 15 or higher every day. People with very fair skin should use a product with an SPF of 30 or higher.
- Applying sunscreen over the entire body 30 minutes before going outside, and reapplying the product every 2 hours.
- Using a lip balm that contains sunscreen.
- Wearing clothing that covers as much of the body as possible, including a broad-brimmed hat and sunglasses to protect the eyes.
- Keeping infants under 6 months out of the sun altogether, and using sunscreen on infants older than 6 months.

Because slightly more than half of melanomas do not start in moles, doctors do not think that removing normal moles in teenagers or young adults is a useful way to prevent melanoma.

Melanoma **vaccines** are undergoing **clinical trials** as biological therapies for patients with Stage 2 or Stage 3 melanoma, but the results will take several years to evaluate. As of 2009, none of these vaccines is being tested as a possible way to prevent melanoma.

Self-examination

Another important form of preventive care is regular self-examination of one's skin. The American Academy of Dermatology (AAD) outlines the steps:

- A person should first become familiar with his or her birthmarks, moles, freckles, and other skin blemishes in order to spot new growths or suspicious changes.
- Use a well-lit private room with a full-length mirror; take along a handheld mirror in order to see the back, buttocks, and other parts of the body that require a second mirror.
- It is important to check all parts of the body, not just those exposed to sunlight. Begin with the upper body, front and back; then the arms. Women should look underneath their breasts.
- Sitting in front of the mirror, examine the legs, genitals, soles of the feet, and the skin between the toes.
- Examine the back of the neck and scalp using the handheld mirror. Part the hair at intervals to check the entire scalp.

Nutrition/Dietetic concerns

Some research suggests that eating a diet rich in antioxidants, **folic acid**, fats, and proteins and whole, unprocessed foods may aid in the prevention of skin cancer such as melanoma. Specific plant flavonoids have also been studied for their skin-protective properties, including apigenin (found in vegetables, fruits, tea, and wine), curcumin (found in the spice turmeric), resveratrol (found in grape skins, red wine, and peanuts), and quercetin (found in apples and onions).

Health care team roles

A physician makes an initial diagnosis. A dermatologist and pathologist may confirm the diagnosis. A surgeon removes most lesions. A plastic and reconstructive surgeon may repair or minimize surgical scars. Nurses and nurse practitioners will participate in prevention education with patients.

Resources

BOOKS

Agarwala, Sanjiv S., and Vernon K. Sondak, eds. *Melanoma: Translational Research and Emerging Therapies.* New York: Informa Healthcare, 2008.

Buckmaster, Marjorie L. *Skin Cancer.* New York: Marshall Cavendish Benchmark, 2008.

Eldridge, Lynne, and David Borgeson. *Avoiding Cancer One Day at a Time: Practical Advice for Preventing Cancer.* Edina, MN: Beaver's Pond Press, 2006.

Kaufman, Howard L. *The Melanoma Book: A Complete Guide to Prevention and Treatment.* New York: Gotham Books, 2005.

Nouri, Keyvan. *Skin Cancer.* Columbus, OH: McGraw-Hill, 2007.

Poole, Catherine M. *Melanoma: Prevention, Detection, and Treatment*, 2nd ed. New Haven, CT: Yale University Press, 2005.

PERIODICALS

Crotty, Kerry. "Dermoscopy and Malignant Melanoma."*Australian Doctor* (June 22, 2007): 33.

Doben, A. R., and D. C. Macgillivray. "Current Concepts in Cutaneous Melanoma: Malignant Melanoma." *Surgical Clinics of North America* 89 (June 2009): 713–725.

Eggermont, A. M., and D. Schadendorf. "Melanoma and Immunotherapy." *Hematology/Oncology Clinics of North America* 23 (June 2009): 547–564.

Heinan, M. L. "Melanoma: Early Detection Saves Lives." *Journal of the American Academy of Physician Assistants* 22 (May 2009): 18, 21.

Ollila, D. W., et al. "Metastatic Melanoma Cells in the Sentinel Node Cannot Be Ignored." *Journal of the American College of Surgeons* 208 (May 2009): 924–929.

Smylie, M., et al. "Management of Malignant Melanoma: Best Practices." *Journal of Cutaneous Medicine and Surgery* 13 (March-April 2009): 55–73.

Wachter, Kerri. "UVA Mutations Tied to Malignant Melanoma."*Skin & Allergy News* (February 2007): 46.

Wargo, J. A., and K. Tanabe. "Surgical Management of Melanoma." *Hematology/Oncology Clinics of North America* 23 (June 2009): 565–581.

OTHER

American Academy of Dermatology (AAD). *Malignant Melanoma.* http://www.aad.org/public/publications/pamphlets/sun_malignant.html.

Centers for Disease Control and Prevention (CDC). *Skin Cancer: Questions and Answers.* http://www.cdc.gov/cancer/skin/chooseyourcover/qanda.htm.

National Cancer Institute (NCI). *What You Need to Know about Melanoma.* http://www.cancer.gov/cancertopics/wyntk/melanoma/allpages.

National Human Genome Research Institute (NHGRI). *Learning about Skin Cancer.* http://www.genome.gov/10000184.

National Library of Medicine (NLM). *Skin Cancer.* [online tutorial] http://www.nlm.nih.gov/medlineplus/tutorials/skincancerandmelanoma/htm/index.htm.

ORGANIZATIONS

American Academy of Dermatology, P.O. Box 4014, Schaumburg, IL, 60168-4014, 847-330-0230, 866-503-SKIN (503-7546), 847-240-1859, http://www.aad.org.

American Cancer Society, 250 Williams Street NW, Atlanta, GA, 30303, 800-ACS-2345 (227-2345), http://www.cancer.org.

National Cancer Institute, 6116 Executive Blvd., Room 3036A, Bethesda, MD, 20892-8322, 800-422-6237, cancergovstaff@mail.nih.gov, http://www.cancer.gov.

Skin Cancer Foundation, 149 Madison Ave., Suite 901, New York, NY, 10016, 212-725-5176, 212-725-5751, info@skincancer.org, http://www.skincancer.org.

Amy Sutton
Rebecca J. Frey, PhD

Melphalan

Definition

Melphalan is an anticancer (antineoplastic) agent. It also acts as a suppressor of the immune system. It is available under the brand name Alkeran.

Purpose

Melphalan is primarily used to treat **ovarian cancer** and **multiple myeloma**, which is a type of **cancer** of the bone marrow. It is also used to treat cancers that have metastasized to the liver.

Although not specifically labeled for use in the treatment of these cancers, melphalan is also used in some patients with:

- breast cancer
- cancers of the blood and lymph system
- endometrial cancer
- malignant melanoma
- Waldenström's macroglobulinemia

More recently, melphalan has been used to prevent rejection of transplanted stem cells in the treatment of metastatic **breast cancer** and renal cell **carcinoma**.

Description

Melphalan is a nitrogen mustard derivative and belongs to the group of alkylating anticancer agents. It chemically interferes with the synthesis of genetic material (DNA and RNA) of cancer cells, which prevents these cells from being able to reproduce and continue the growth of the cancer.

KEY TERMS

Antineoplastic—A drug that prevents the growth of a neoplasm by interfering with the maturation or proliferation of the cells of the neoplasm.

Neoplasm—New abnormal growth of tissue.

Recommended dosage

Melphalan may be taken either orally in pill form or as an injection in liquid form. The dosage prescribed may vary widely depending on the patient, the cancer being treated, and whether or not other medications are also being taken.

A typical dosage for multiple **myeloma** is 6 mg per day for two to three weeks. After this initial dose, the drug is halted for up to 4 weeks, then resumed at a dose of 2 mg per day, depending on blood counts of the drug in the patient's blood test.

A typical dosage for ovarian cancer is 0.2 mg per kilogram (2.2 pounds) of body weight once per day for five days.

Precautions

Melphalan should be taken with food to minimize stomach upset. Melphalan should always be taken with plenty of fluids.

Melphalan can cause an allergic reaction in some people. Patients with a prior allergic reaction to melphalan should not take the drug.

Melphalan can cause serious birth defects if either the man or the woman is taking this drug at the time of conception, or if the woman is taking this drug during pregnancy. Also, male sterility is a possible side effect of melphalan. This sterility may either be temporary or permanent.

Because melphalan is easily passed from mother to child through breast milk, breastfeeding is not recommended while melphalan is being taken.

Melphalan suppresses the immune system and interferes with the normal functioning of certain organs and tissues. For these reasons, it is important that the prescribing physician is aware of any of the following pre-existing medical conditions:

- a current case of, or recent exposure to, chicken pox
- herpes zoster (shingles)
- a current case, or history of, gout or kidney stones
- all current infections
- kidney disease

Because melphalan is such a potent immunosuppressant, patients taking this drug must exercise extreme caution to avoid contracting any new infections. They should do their best to:

- avoid any person with any type of infection
- avoid any person who has received a polio vaccine in the last two months
- avoid bleeding injuries, including those caused by brushing or flossing the teeth
- avoid contact of the hands with the eyes or nasal passages unless the hands have just been washed and have not touched anything else since this washing
- avoid contact sports or any other activity that could cause a bruising or bleeding injury

Side effects

There are no common side effects of melphalan. Side effects that may occur, however, include:

- increased susceptibility to infection
- nausea and vomiting
- diarrhea
- mouth sores
- skin rash, itching, or hives
- swelling in the feet or lower legs

A doctor should be consulted immediately if the patient experiences black, tarry, or bloody stools, blood in the urine, persistent cough, **fever** and chills, pain in the lower back or sides, painful or difficult urination, or unusual bleeding or bruising.

Interactions

Melphalan should not be taken in combination with any prescription drug, over-the-counter drug, or herbal remedy without prior consultation with a physician. It is particularly important that the prescribing physician be aware of the use of any of the following drugs:

- amphotericin B
- antithyroid agents
- azathioprine
- chloramphenicol
- colchicine
- flucytosine
- ganciclovir
- interferons
- plicamycin
- probenecid
- sulfinpyrazone
- zidovudine
- any radiation therapy or chemotherapy medicines

Resources

PERIODICALS

Alexander, H. R. Jr., S. K. Libutti, J. F. Pingpank, et al. "Hyperthermic Isolated Hepatic Perfusion using Melphalan for Patients with Ocular Melanoma Metastatic to Liver." *Clinical Cancer Research* 9 (December 15, 2003): 6343–6349.

Das-Gupta, E. P., G. M. Sidra, E. M. Bessell, et al. "High-Dose Melphalan Followed by Radical Radiotherapy for the Treatment of Massive Plasmacytoma of the Chest Wall." *Bone Marrow Transplantation* 32 (October 2003): 759–761.

Rothbarth, J., M. E. Pijl, A. L. Vahrmeijer, et al. "Isolated Hepatic Perfusion with High-Dose Melphalan for the Treatment of Colorectal Metastasis Confined to the Liver." *British Journal of Surgery* 90 (November 2003): 1391–1397.

Ueno, N. T., Y. C. Cheng, G. Rondon, et al. "Rapid Induction of Complete Donor Chimerism by the Use of a Reduced-Intensity Conditioning Regimen Composed of Fludarabine and Melphalan in Allogeneic Stem Cell Transplantation for Metastatic Solid Tumors." *Blood* 102 (November 15, 2003): 3829–3836.

ORGANIZATIONS

United States Food and Drug Administration (FDA). 5600 Fishers Lane, Rockville, MD 20857-0001. (888) INFO-FDA (463-6332). http://www.fda.gov.

Paul A. Johnson, Ed.M.
Rebecca J. Frey, Ph.D.

Memory change

Description

Many people with **cancer** experience memory changes—such as mild forgetfulness, an inability to concentrate on more than one task, or more severe memory loss—after undergoing **chemotherapy** or radiation treatments. In other cases, as in a person with a brain tumor, the cancer itself may cause memory changes. Surgical interventions, particularly for brain cancer, may also lead to memory loss.

Causes

Studies show that patients experience trouble with memory and language skills after chemotherapy. Scientists are searching for the exact cause, but they believe the chemotherapy agents may be associated with this side effect. The drugs are designed to attack cancer cells, but often kill healthy cells in the process. Researchers are studying whether chemotherapy agents may be damaging healthy brain cells. Others believe the cancer itself may be responsible for the memory changes.

Similarly, **radiation therapy** also may cause people with cancer to lose some mental abilities, including memory. Physicians use radiation waves to penetrate cancer cells and stop them from growing. During the process, the rays may damage some healthy tissue. The severity of damage depends on the dose and duration of the radiation treatments. In some cases, cells killed by radiation can form a tumor-like mass in the brain, which can lead to memory loss. Children who undergo radiation treatments for a brain tumor may have developmental delays later in life.

Other side effects of cancer, such as **fatigue**, pain, and **depression**, may lead to memory impairment as a person struggles to cope with cancer. Living with constant pain, for example, takes a great deal of energy and can cause a person to become more distracted than usual. Sometimes, especially in elderly patients, it can be difficult to tell if the memory changes are caused by an existing dementia or the cancer treatment.

Treatments

Depending on the type and intensity of cancer treatment, memory difficulties may fade over time. Some people, however, will experience a permanent loss. Families can help by offering useful strategies, such as making lists of daily tasks, using a calendar or daily organizer, reducing stress, and encouraging the person to ask for help if disoriented.

Patients scheduled for radiation therapy should discuss their concerns about memory loss with their physician before the treatment begins. The radiologists may be able to control the dosage to minimize damage to healthy cells. For instance, many hospitals use a gamma knife for brain cancer treatment. The device allows radiation therapists to simultaneously attack a tumor with high-energy rays from several different angles. The gamma knife sends a concentrated dose to the tumor without damaging surrounding brain tissue.

Occupational therapists can assist people who find that cancer-related memory changes are interfering with their ability to work or perform normal activities. Many people learn helpful coping strategies from other cancer survivors by joining a support group. Since more damage occurs in younger patients, children who go through radiation therapy for **brain tumors** may need extra tutoring, or special education programs when they go to school.

Alternative and complementary therapies

Often, when physicians prescribe medication to ease a person's pain or depression, the patient's memory may improve as well. Researchers also are studying the ability of the herb *gingko biloba* to increase mental sharpness. Although it has not yet been proven to be completely effective, some people with memory loss find it helpful. Since gingko can cause circulatory problems, it is important to check with a doctor before taking it.

Resources

PERIODICALS

Meyers, C. A. "Neurocognitive dysfunction in cancer patients." *Oncology* 14, no. 1 (January 2000): 81–82,85.

OTHER

American Cancer Society. "Chemotherapy's Effect on the Brain." *ACS News Today*. [cited July 13, 2009]. http://www2.cancer.org/zine/index.cfm?fn = 002_03241999_0.

American Cancer Society. "Complementary and Alternative Methods: Dietary and Herbal Remedies:Popular Herbs." [cited July 13, 2009]. http://www.cancer.org/alt_therapy/popherbs.html.

Liu, Li, M.D. "OncoLink FAQ: Long-Term Complications of Whole Brain Radiation." *OncoLink: University of Pennsylvania Cancer Center*. [cited July 13, 2009]. http://oncolink.upenn.edu/specialty/rad_onc/faq/faq_brainxrt.html.

Melissa Knopper, M.S.

Memory loss *see* **Memory change**

Meningioma

Definition

A meningioma is a benign tumor of the central nervous system that develops from cells of the meninges, the membranes that cover and protect the brain and spinal cord.

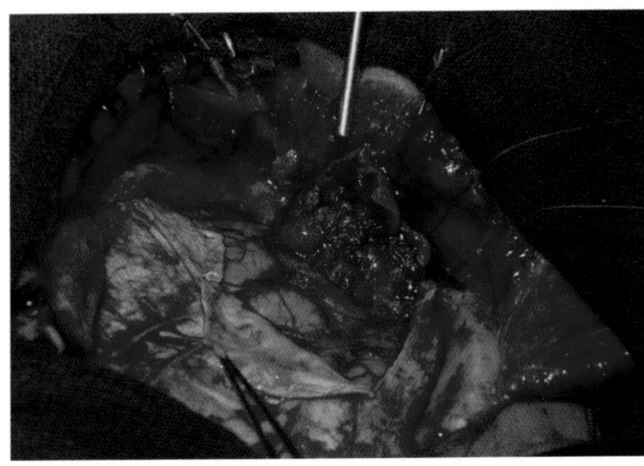

Brain surgery to remove an invasive meningioma. *(Custom Medical Stock Photo. Reproduced by permission.)*

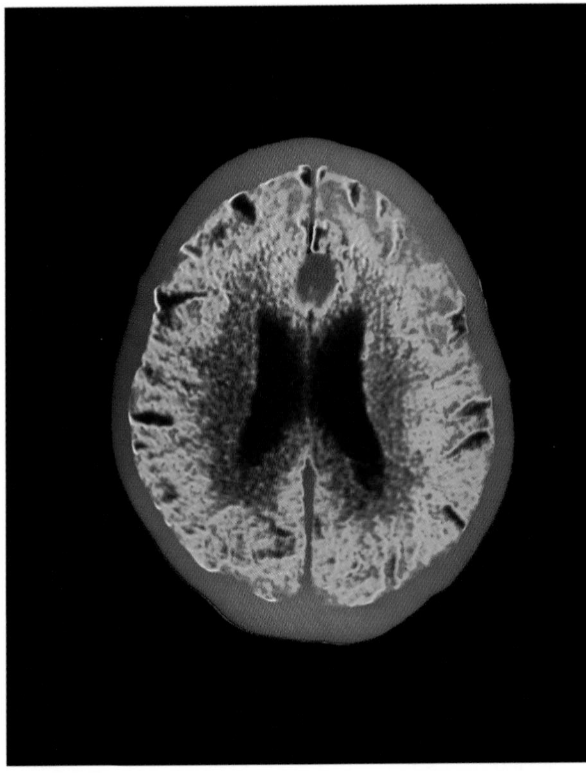

Colored computed tomography (CT) scan of the brain showing a meningioma. At upper center is the tumor (red). The cerebrum is colored yellow and light purple. *(Copyright Department of Clinical Radiology, Salisbury District Hospital, Science Source/Photo Researchers, Inc. Reproduced by permission.)*

KEY TERMS

Benign tumor—A growth that is non-cancerous.

Computed tomography (CT) scan—A method of imaging the inside of the body using x rays.

Magnetic resonance imaging (MRI)—A method of imaging the inside of the body using radio waves and a magnetic field.

Meninges—Membranes that cover and protect both the brain and spinal cord.

Neurofibromatosis—A rare, genetic disease that causes tumors to grow in the nervous system.

Radiotherapy—The use of radiation to treat a medical condition.

Description

The meninges

The delicate tissues of the brain and spinal cord are protected by a layer of bone and an inner covering called the meninges. The meninges are composed of three layers:

- dura mater
- arachnoid
- pia mater

The tough, thick dura mater forms the outer layer of the meninges and is attached to the bone of the skull and spinal cord. The arachnoid and pia mater layers are thinner and more delicate than the dura mater. The innermost pia mater layer is attached directly to the brain and spinal cord. Meningiomas arise from the middle arachnoid layer, and most remain attached to the dura mater by a dural tail.

Types of meningiomas

Meningiomas account for 15–20% of all **brain tumors**, and 25% of all spinal cord tumors. The World Health Organization (WHO) classifies meningiomas into 11 different categories according to their cell type. However, because there are so many different cell types and so much overlap between types, meningiomas are most often placed into three general categories, including benign, atypical, and malignant.

Benign meningiomas are by far the most common, accounting for more than 90% of all meningiomas. These tumors grow slowly and produce symptoms only if they become large enough to compress nearby brain tissue. In some patients, meningiomas can grow very large with almost no symptoms. This happens

QUESTIONS TO ASK THE DOCTOR

- Will I need to have surgery?
- Can I expect a full recovery after surgery?
- Will I need radiotherapy?
- How often will I need to return for an MRI or CT scan?
- How soon can I return to work after surgery?

because the tumor has grown very slowly and has gradually compressed the brain over time. Meningiomas can also cause fluid to build up in the brain, and can sometimes block veins. They may also grow into nearby bone, causing the bone to become thicker.

Up to 7% of meningiomas are classified as atypical. These tumors grow more quickly than benign meningiomas and are more likely to be symptomatic. Malignant meningiomas are fast-growing aggressive tumors and are the most rare, accounting for only about 2% of all meningiomas. It is extremely unusual for meningiomas to metastasize to other organs. When they do, the lungs are the most common site.

Only about one tenth of meningiomas are found in the spine. These slow-growing tumors cause symptoms when they begin to compress the spinal cord. Spinal meningiomas usually grow in the spinal canal between the neck and the abdomen, and are almost always benign.

Demographics

Only one person in every 50,000 is diagnosed with a symptomatic meningioma annually. Most of these patients are women. Women develop brain meningiomas almost twice as often as men and spinal meningiomas four to five times more often than men. The disease usually strikes middle-aged and elderly patients. Men are most affected between the ages of 50 and 60 years, while women are most affected between the ages of 60 and 70 years. Atypical and malignant meningiomas are more common in men. Meningiomas do not occur very often in children.

Causes and symptoms

Causes

Although no single factor has been found that causes meningiomas, several risk factors are known. Some patients have developed a meningioma after being exposed to radiation. These patients tend to be younger than typical meningioma patients, and their tumors often grow more quickly. According to one study, the average age of patients with radiation-induced meningiomas is 38 years.

There is also a genetic component to meningioma. Patients who suffer from neurofibromatosis, a rare genetic disease, often develop multiple meningiomas.

Since meningioma cells recognize the female sex hormone progesterone, some researchers believe that female sex hormones may play a role in the development of meningiomas. This possible link is still being investigated.

A group of researchers at the National Cancer Institute reported in 2004 that people in certain occupations have a higher than normal risk of developing meningiomas. These higher-risk occupations include auto body painting, industrial production supervision, teaching, business management, interior decorating and design, and career military service. Further research is needed to determine whether there is a common causal factor linking these different fields of work.

Symptoms

Up to 75% of meningiomas produce no symptoms because they grow slowly and remain small. Often, tumors are discovered only when patients are being investigated for an unrelated illness. When symptoms do appear, it results that the tumor has grown large enough to compress part of the brain or spinal cord.

Patients experience different symptoms depending on the location of the tumor. Most brain meningiomas are located either just below the top of the skull, or between the two hemispheres of the brain. If the tumor is located in these areas, symptoms include:

- headaches
- seizures
- dizziness
- problems with memory
- behavior changes
- protrusion of one or both eyeballs (exophthalmos)

More rarely, tumors are near sensory areas of the brain such as the optic nerve or close to the ears. Patients with these tumors experience vision or hearing losses.

Spinal meningiomas are usually found in the spinal column between the neck and the abdomen. The most common symptoms are:

- pain
- weakness and stiffness of the arms and legs
- episodes of partial paralysis

Diagnosis

Meningiomas are diagnosed using a painless non-invasive technique called **magnetic resonance imaging** (MRI). MRI works by exposing the patient to harmless radio waves and a magnetic field, which produce clear images of the brain and the spine that show the size and location of tumors. No special preparation is required for the test.

Diagnosis can also be made by computed tomography (CT) scan. The CT scan uses low-dose **x rays** to generate a picture of the inside of the body. Sometimes a dye is injected into the patient's vein to improve the visibility of tissues. If the meningioma has grown into nearby bone, a CT scan will show the extent of bone invasion better than MRI. Women who are pregnant, or who think they might be pregnant, should tell their doctors before having a CT scan.

Treatment team

The treatment team for a patient with a symptomatic meningioma may include a radiologist, a neurologist (specialist of the nervous system), and a neurosurgeon.

If surgery is necessary, a neurosurgeon will perform the procedure with the help of a surgical team. The team includes two or three nurses, and an anesthesiologist.

A small number of patients receive radiotherapy for their meningioma either because the tumor is too difficult to remove surgically, or because the surgeon had to leave some tumor behind. These patients will be referred to a radiation oncologist (specialist in giving radiation to cancer patients).

Clinical staging, treatments, and prognosis

Staging

Meningiomas are classified into three different grades depending upon the likelihood of recurrence and aggressive growth:

- Grade I: Low risk of recurrence and slow growth
- Grade II: Greater likelihood of recurrence and/or aggressive growth
- Grade III: High recurrence rates and aggressive growth.

The vast majority of meningiomas are grade I. Atypical tumors are grade II, and malignant tumors are grade III.

Medical therapies

Medical treatment for meningiomas is necessary when tumors cause symptoms. Fortunately, only about a quarter of meningiomas become symptomatic. Most patients are cured by surgery.

The objective of surgery is to remove not only the entire meningioma, but also the tail that attaches the tumor to the meninges. If the tumor has grown into bone, the bone is removed, too. If the tumor is in a difficult location in the brain, the surgeon may leave some tumor behind in order to preserve brain tissue.

The prognosis following brain meningioma treatment is very good. For the few patients who are not cured, prognosis depends on how completely the tumor is removed. If some tumor is left behind, recurrence is more likely, particularly for patients with grade II or grade III meningiomas. Ten years after surgery, 7–20% of patients with benign grade I tumors have a recurrence. For patients with malignant grade III tumors, up to 78% have a recurrence. A second surgery is sometimes necessary for patients with recurrent tumors.

Spinal meningioma is the most successfully treated meningioma, and the most successfully treated of all spinal tumors. Most of these tumors are removed completely, and they rarely recur. Even patients with quite severe symptoms fully recover after surgery.

For the few patients who are inoperable (usually because of tumor location), **radiation therapy** can stop the growth of tumors. Recently, stereotactic radiosurgery has been successfully used. This procedure uses images of the patient's skull to construct a frame that allows precise aiming of radiation, thus minimizing harm to nearby healthy tissue. Another option is fractionated radiotherapy, which also delivers precise doses of radiation to very small areas of tissue.

Not every patient with a meningioma receives surgery or radiation. Asymptomatic patients with small or slow-growing tumors can receive periodic MRI tests to check tumor growth. Treatment may also not be necessary for patients with mild or minimal symptoms.

Alternative and complementary therapies

Unlike many other cancers, conventional medical treatment of meningioma has very high success rates. As a result, alternative therapies are not commonly used for these tumors.

Coping with cancer treatment

When first diagnosed with a meningioma, many patients experience anxiety, resulting in nervousness, sleepless nights, and even **nausea**. However, patients can often relieve many of their fears by learning more about the disease and its course of treatment. Nevertheless, about 21% of patients with meningiomas develop psychiatric disorders, most commonly **depression** or an anxiety disorder.

The majority of meningioma patients are treated with surgery alone. Surgery will involve a hospital stay of at least a week. Before going home, patients are usually given medications to help prevent pain and swelling. Once home, patients can expect to feel some headache pain, and will become tired easily. If headaches and weakness become worse, a doctor should be contacted. Patients should make sure they get plenty of rest and eat a balanced, nutritious diet. Most patients can begin to resume their normal activities in about six to eight weeks.

Clinical trials

Chemotherapy is seldom given to meningioma patients because surgery (and/or radiotherapy) is usually successful. For patients with tumors that do not respond to these treatments, however, chemotherapy is available within a clinical trial.

Clinical trials have investigated several drugs to treat patients whose meningioma recurs following failure of both surgery and radiotherapy. **Hydroxyurea**, a drug used to treat some other cancers, has been shown to slow the growth of meningioma cells. Studies of hydroxyurea continue. Some trials have explored the link between meningioma and female sex hormones. **Tamoxifen**, an anti-estrogen drug used to fight **breast cancer**, has produced disappointing results. Trials using RU-486, an anti-progesterone agent, are underway. Information on these and other open clinical trials is available on the Internet from the National Cancer Institute at http://www.nci.nih.gov.

Prevention

The most avoidable risk factor for the development of meningioma is exposure to radiation. Children exposed to small amounts of radiation in the 1950s to treat tinea captis, a fungal **infection** of the scalp, developed meningiomas at an unusually high rate. There is also a clear relationship between radiation dose and meningioma: the higher the radiation dose, the greater the probability of developing a meningioma.

Special concerns

The very elderly

In very elderly people, the symptoms of a meningioma can be very similar to normal aging. These patients typically experience difficulty with learning and remembering things as a result of the tumor. Headaches, a classic symptom of a meningioma, are not usually reported. Treatment of very elderly patients may be difficult if the patient is too frail for surgery.

Children

On the rare occasions that meningiomas are diagnosed in children, they tend to be large, fast growing, and located in unusual positions. Treatment for children is the same as for adults: complete tumor removal with surgery and/or radiotherapy.

Neurofibromatosis

Neurofibromatosis (NF) is actually two different genetic diseases: NF Type 1 and NF Type 2. NF Type 2 is the more rare of the two diseases, affecting only one in 40,000 individuals. These patients often develop multiple brain meningiomas. Although there is no cure for NF, meningioma tumors can be removed with surgery.

Resources

BOOKS

Beers, Mark H., MD, and Robert Berkow, MD, editors. "Exophthalmos." In *The Merck Manual of Diagnosis and Therapy*. Whitehouse Station, NJ: Merck Research Laboratories, 2007.

Beers, Mark H., MD, and Robert Berkow, MD, editors. "Intracranial Neoplasms (Brain Tumors)." Section 14, Chapter 177 In *The Merck Manual of Diagnosis and Therapy*. Whitehouse Station, NJ: Merck Research Laboratories, 2004.

Greenberg, Harry S., et al., editors. *Brain Tumors*. New York: Oxford University Press, 1999.

Kleihues, Paul, and Webster K. Cavenee, editors. *World Health Organization Classification of Tumours: Tumours of the Nervous System*. Lyon: IARC Press, 2000.

PERIODICALS

Al-Mefty, O., C. Topsakal, S. Pravdenkova, et al. "Radiation-Induced Meningiomas: Clinical, Pathological, Cytokinetic, and Cytogenetic Characteristics." *Journal of Neurosurgery* 100 (June 2004): 1002–1013.

DeAngelis, Lisa M. "Brain Tumors." *New England Journal of Medicine* 344, no. 2 (January 11, 2001): 114–23.

Drummond, K. J., J. J. Zhu, and P. M. Black. "Meningiomas: Updating Basic Science, Management, and Outcome." *Neurologist* 10 (May 2004): 113–130.

Gupta, R. K., and R. Kumar. "Benign Brain Tumours and Psychiatric Morbidity: A 5-Years Retrospective Data Analysis." *Australian and New Zealand Journal of Psychiatry* 38 (May 2004): 316–319.

Rajaraman, P., A. J. De Roos, P. A. Stewart, et al. "Occupation and Risk of Meningioma and Acoustic Neuroma in the United States." *American Journal of Industrial Medicine* 45 (May 2004): 395–407.

Yamasaki, Fumiyuki, et al. "Recurrence of Meningiomas." *Cancer* 89, no. 5 (September 1, 2000): 1102–1110.

ORGANIZATIONS

American Brain Tumor Association. 2720 River Road, Des Plaines, IL 60018. (800) 886-2282. http://abta.org.

The Brain Tumor Society. 124 Watertown Street, Suite 3-H, Watertown, MA 02472. (800) 770-8287. http://www.tbts.org.

The Johns Hopkins Meningioma Society. Johns Hopkins University. Harvey 811, 600 North Wolfe Street, Baltimore, MD 21205-8811. (410) 614-2886. http://www.meningioma.org.

National Brain Tumor Foundation. 414 Thirteenth Street, Suite 700, Oakland, CA 94612-2603. (800) 934-2873. http://www.braintumor.org.

National Cancer Institute (National Institutes of Health). 9000 Rockville Pike, Bethesda, MD 20892. (800) 422-6237. http://www.nci.nih.gov.

Alison McTavish, M.Sc.
Rebecca J. Frey, Ph.D.

MENS, MEN syndrome *see* **Multiple endocrine neoplasia syndromes**

Meperidine

Definition

Meperidine, available as hydrochloride salt, is a narcotic analgesic, a classification term used to describe medications capable of producing a reversible **depression** of the central nervous system for pain control. Because of its potential for physical and psychological dependence, meperidine is a carefully controlled substance. It is commonly referred to by one of its brand names, Demerol.

Purpose

There are several possible indications for the administration of meperidine. It is commonly used for the relief of moderate to severe pain, particularly in obstetrics. Meperidine is also widely used preoperatively, and as an adjunct to anesthesia during surgery. Meperidine is not recommended for long-term management of chronic pain, such as pain caused by **cancer**, because of its potential for psychological and physical dependence.

KEY TERMS

Agonist—A drug that binds to cell receptors and stimulates activities normally stimulated by naturally occurring substances.

Endorphin—Short for endogenous morphine, it is a naturally occurring substance that binds to opioid receptors in the brain.

Narcotic analgesic—A classification of medications that relieves pain by temporarily depressing the central nervous system.

Opioid—A drug that possesses some properties characteristic of opiate narcotics but not derived from opium.

Patient controlled analgesic (PCA)—A device resembling an intravenous pump that allows patients to self-medicate within pre-established dosage parameters for pain control.

Description

Meperidine is a synthetic compound that acts as an agonist—meaning it attaches to opioid receptors in the central nervous system and stimulates physiologic activity normally stimulated by naturally occurring substances such as endorphins (short for endogenous morphine). Meperidine acts much like morphine, although constipation, suppression of the cough reflex, and smooth muscle spasm are all reduced with meperidine.

Meperidine is available in a banana-flavored syrup, in a tablet, and in a liquid form for injection. Oral meperidine tends to be less effective than the injectable form. When taking the syrup, patients should dilute it with approximately one half glass of water to reduce temporary anesthesia to the mouth and tongue.

Recommended dosage

The recommended dosage of meperidine depends on the purpose for which it is prescribed, as well as the population in whom it is administered. For example, elderly patients, or patients with underlying medical problems that increase side effects or decrease drug metabolism, should generally be given reduced dosages. Meperidine can be taken orally, in tablet or syrup form, intravenously (directly into a vein), or by injection into the muscle (intramuscularly) or connective tissue (subcutaneously).

Generally, repeated doses administered to manage pain should be given by injection intramuscularly. The subcutaneous route is acceptable for occasional administration. When given intravenously, meperidine should be diluted and administered very slowly. When taken in conjunction with phenothiazine or other tranquilizers, the dose should be decreased by as much as a half. Specific dosages are as follows.

FOR RELIEF OF MODERATE TO SEVERE PAIN. The recommended dosage for adults for pain relief is 50–150 mg every three to four hours by oral or intramuscular route. When given intravenously through a patient-controlled analgesia (PCA) device, an initial dose of 10 mg should be administered. The PCA should be programmed to administer between 1–5 mg every 6–10 minutes. If meperidine is given continuously through an intravenous line, the dose should be adjusted based on patient response to a range of 15–35 mg an hour. Children should be given 1–1.8 mg per kg (2.2 pounds) intramuscularly or subcutaneously.

FOR PREOPERATIVE MEDICATION. Adults may be given 50–100 mg of meperidine intramuscularly, or subcutaneously 30–90 minutes prior to surgery. Children's dosages should be reduced to 1–2 mg per kg through the same routes.

For obstetric pain control. The recommended dosage for control of regular (not sporadic) pain in this setting is 50–100 mg every 1–3 hours intramuscularly or subcutaneously.

Precautions

Other patients who should avoid meperidine use include those with previous hypersensitivity to narcotics, or those with underlying respiratory problems. Meperidine, even in recommended therapeutic doses, can decrease the respiratory drive. Conditions such as asthma or chronic obstructive pulmonary disease may increase the likelihood of respiratory difficulty. Meperidine can also impair judgment, and should not be used in individuals engaging in activities that require alertness, such as driving.

Because its effects on a fetus are unknown, meperidine is not recommended in pre-labor stage pregnant women. Even in labor, when it may be indicated for pain control, meperidine may cause respiratory depression of the mother and her baby, particularly premature babies. Meperidine is excreted in breast milk, and, if needed, should be administered several hours before breastfeeding to minimize ingestion by the infant.

Side effects

The most common adverse effects of meperidine are lightheadedness, dizziness, sedation, **nausea** and/or **vomiting**, and sweating. Less common, but more severe, side effects include respiratory depression and abnormally low blood pressure.

Interactions

Individuals who are taking, or who have recently taken, drugs called monoamine oxidase (MAO) inhibitors (a class of antidepressants), should not be given meperidine. Reactions have been reported in this population that are characterized by a variety of signs and symptoms including respiratory distress, coma, abnormally low or abnormally high blood pressure, hyperexcitability, and even death. If administration of a narcotic is required, it should be given in small, gradually increasing test doses under careful supervision.

Adverse effects such as respiratory depression and decreased blood pressure are more common when meperidine is administered in conjunction with other narcotic analgesics, anesthetics, phenothiazines, sedatives, or any other type of drug that suppresses the central nervous system. Alcohol should also be avoided.

Tamara Brown, R.N.

Mercaptopurine

Definition

Mercaptopurine is a medicine used to prevent the formation and spread of **cancer** cells. Mercaptopurine is also called 6-mercaptopurine or 6-MP, and is available under the brand name Purinethol.

Purpose

Mercaptopurine is used as part of the consolidation and maintenance treatment for **acute lymphocytic leukemia** (ALL) and acute myelocytic leukemia (AML).

Description

Mercaptopurine is an analog of purine, a component of DNA/RNA, and belongs to antimetabolites that prevent the biosynthesis, or utilization, of normal cellular metabolites. It has been used for several decades in combination with other **chemotherapy** drugs

KEY TERMS

Consolidation therapy—A stage in treatment of acute lymphocytic leukemia (ALL) that follows induction of remission. The purpose of this stage is to eliminate remaining cancer cells that cannot be detected by usual methods.

Inflammatory bowel disease (IBD)—This disease can be divided into two types: Crohn's disease and ulcerative colitis. Patients with Crohn's disease can have inflammation of the full thickness of the walls of the entire gastrointestinal tract. In patients with ulcerative colitis, the inflammation is limited to the surface of the walls of the large intestine and rectum.

Leukemia—A type of cancer caused by a progressive increase in abnormal blood-forming cells of the bone marrow.

Maintenance therapy—The last stage in treatment of ALL. The purpose of this stage is to provide long-term exposure to lower doses of drugs and to give the immune system time to kill the leukemia cells.

for the treatment of different types of acute adult and childhood leukemias (ALL and AML). It has also been shown to be effective for the treatment of inflammatory bowel disease (IBD) (which includes Crohn's disease and ulcerative colitis), certain types of arthritis, and polycythemia vera (above normal increase in red cells in the blood). Mercaptopurine helps to decrease the dose of steroids in patients with IBD, and to reduce their dependence on steroids to control symptoms of their disease. The medicine is taken up by red cells in the blood and works by decreasing the formation of certain genetic material (DNA and RNA) in patients with cancer and by altering the activity of the immune system in patients with IBD.

Recommended dosage

Doses vary between different chemotherapy protocols. The usual dose is 2.5 mg per kg (2.2 pounds) per day in adults and children (50 mg daily in an average 5-year old child or 100–200 mg daily in adults). The total daily dose is calculated to the nearest multiple of 25 mg and is given all at one time. Another way of dosing 6-MP is based on body surface area (BSA), and is usually 75 mg per square meter in children and 80–100 mg per square meter in adults.

Doses of 1.5–2.5 mg per kg per day is recommended for leukemia patients. For those patients with inflammatory bowel disease, doses of 1.5 mg per kg per day have been used in research studies.

Administration

This medicine is usually taken by mouth and should be given at the same time every day, preferably on an empty stomach (one hour before meals or two hours after meals). Children with leukemia should be taking this medicine at bedtime for maximum effectiveness. All patients should drink plenty of fluids (at least eight glasses of water per day) while taking this medication, unless otherwise directed by a physician.

Precautions

The use of 6-MP in pregnant women should be avoided whenever possible, especially during the first three months of pregnancy, as 6-MP can cause birth defects and spontaneous abortions.

As 6-MP can lower the body's ability to fight infections, patients are advised to avoid contact with people who have a cold, flu, or other infections.

Mercaptopurine should be used with caution in the following populations:

- people who had an allergic reaction to 6-MP in the past
- people at risk for pancreatitis (inflammation of the pancreas)
- breastfeeding mothers (it is not known if 6-MP crosses in to breast milk)
- people with liver or kidney disease
- people with gout (6-MP can exacerbate the symptoms of gout)
- people taking allopurinol for gout
- people with suppressed bone marrow (tissue filling the empty spaces inside the bone)

Patients are encouraged to stop taking 6-MP, and contact a physician immediately, if any of the following symptoms develop:

- fever, chills, or sore throat
- yellowing of the skin or eyes
- blood in the urine or stools
- black stools
- unusual bleeding or bruising
- stomach pain with nausea, vomiting, or loss of appetite

Patients taking 6-MP must see a physician before starting medication therapy, and also occasionally during therapy, to have blood tests for the monitoring of a complete blood count and kidney and liver functions.

Side effects

This is a very potent medicine that can cause serious side effects. These side effects include skin rash, **nausea**, **vomiting**, **diarrhea**, mouth sores, yellowing of the eyes or skin, clay-colored stools, dark urine, decreased ability to fight infections, pinpoint red dots on the skin, and darkening of the skin. **Nausea and vomiting**, diarrhea, and stomach pain are less common in children than in adults.

Interactions

Mercaptopurine can decrease the effectiveness of blood thinners such as **warfarin** (Coumadin).

The drug can exacerbate the symptoms of gout. The anti-gout medication, **allopurinol**, can increase blood levels of 6-MP and increase the risk of its side effects. The dose of 6-MP needs to be decreased, or its use should be avoided, in patients taking allopurinol, which interferes with the degradation of 6-MP.

Risk of liver disease may be increased in patients taking both **doxorubicin** (a cancer chemotherapy drug) and 6-MP. Other medicines that decrease the function of the liver can cause increased toxicity with 6-MP. Patients should inform their doctor or pharmacist about all the prescription drugs and over-the-counter medications that they are taking.

Olga Bessmertny, Pharm.D.

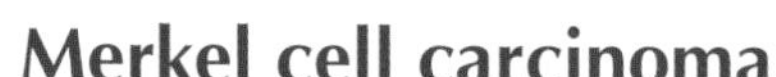

Merkel cell carcinoma

Definition

Merkel cell **carcinoma** (MCC) is a rare form of **cancer** that develops on, or just beneath, the skin and in hair follicles. It is also known as neuroendocrine cancer of the skin or trabecular cancer.

Description

Merkel cells are cells that lie in the middle layers of the skin. They are named for their discoverer, a German professor of anatomy named Friedrich Sigmund Merkel (1845–1919). These cells are organized around hair follicles and are believed to act as some type of touch receptors. MCC begins in these cells.

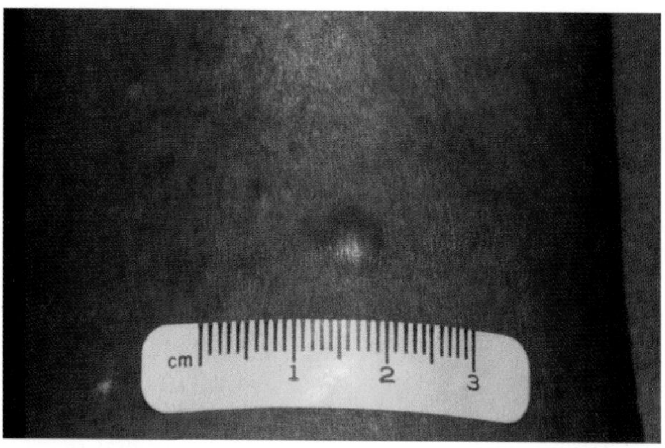

A Merkel cell tumor on a patient's leg. *(Custom Medical Stock Photo. Reproduced by permission.)*

MCC usually appears as firm shiny skin lumps, or tumors. These tumors are painless and can range in size from less than a quarter of an inch (0.6 cm) to over two inches (5.1 cm) in diameter. They may be red, pink, or blue. Tumors first appear on the head and neck in about 48% of cases, and less frequently on other sun-exposed parts of the body.

MCC is very aggressive, it spreads very rapidly, and it often invades other tissues and organs (metastasizes). The most common sites of **metastasis** of MCC are the lymph nodes, liver, bones, lungs, and brain. Metastasis to the lymph nodes generally occurs within seven to eight months after the first skin tumors appear. Nearly half of all people affected with MCC will develop systemic metastases within 24 months, and 67–74% of these people will die within five years.

Local recurrence of MCC after the removal of the primary tumor occurs in approximately one-third of all patients and is usually apparent within four months.

Several other names have been used to describe MCC, among these are: anaplastic carcinoma of the skin, apudoma, endocrine carcinoma of the skin, neuroendocrine carcinoma of the skin (NEC), primary small-cell carcinoma of the skin, primary undifferentiated carcinoma of the skin, and trabecular cell carcinoma. The two most commonly used names are MCC and NEC.

Demographics

MCC is seen almost exclusively (94% of known cases)in Caucasians. It affects males more often than females. Seventy-six percent of cases reported in the United States have been diagnosed in people older than 65, but MCC has also been seen in a child as young as seven and a woman as old as 97.

KEY TERMS

Merkel cells—Specialized cells of the skin that are located at the base of some hairs. These cells are believed to function as touch receptors. They are named for a nineteenth-century German professor of anatomy.

Metastasis—The migration of a cancer from its primary location to another, distant location in the body.

Neoplasm—Any new and abnormal growth of a tissue.

In 2003, the National Cancer Institute (NCI) compiled records of 1034 patients in the United States diagnosed with MCC. The number of new cases of MCC is expected to rise as the average life span continues to increase, exposure to the sun remains high, and MCC is recognized more often by medical practitioners.

Causes and symptoms

The cause of MCC has not been positively identified. It is believed to be caused by the skin damage associated with exposure to ultraviolet light from the sun.

Some researchers believe that Merkel cell carcinoma may also be associated with immunodeficiency syndromes, as six of the 1043 patients recorded in the United States developed MCC after being diagnosed with **chronic lymphocytic leukemia**.

The only symptom of primary MCC is the appearance of the characteristic tumors in the skin. Lymph node metastases show enlarged, firm, lymph nodes in the region of the primary tumor. Other systemic metastases show as masses in the affected organs. The location of the primary tumor is not related to the location of these systemic metastases.

Diagnosis

The diagnosis of MCC is performed by examining and testing a **biopsy** of the tumor. MCC is difficult to differentiate from several other forms of abnormal tissue growth (neoplasms). This diagnosis cannot be made just by examining the tumor cells under a microscope. It is done by performing a variety of chemical tests on these cells. Testing must be performed to make sure this is not metastatic oat-cell (lung) cancer.

QUESTIONS TO ASK THE DOCTOR

- What stage is my cancer in?
- How long will my radiation therapy treatments last after the tumor is removed?
- What are the possible side effects of the particular radiation or chemotherapy treatments that I will receive?
- How often should I continue to be checked for possible recurrence of MCC?

Treatment team

MCC is generally first identified by a microbiologist who examines a biopsy sample. Most MCC tumor removals are performed by dermatologists. Post-operative radiation treatments are generally ordered by the dermatologist and performed by a radiation therapist under the direction of a radiologist and/or a radiation physicist.

Because of the rapid and possibly invasive nature of MCC, patients are generally referred to a physician specializing in cancer (oncologist) to ensure that the disease has not spread to other parts of the body. **Chemotherapy** for MCC is considered investigational.

Clinical staging, treatments, and prognosis

MCC is classified into three clinical stages. Stage I MCC is defined as a disease that is localized to the skin. Stage II MCC is characterized by a spreading of the disease to the lymph nodes that are near the primary skin tumor or tumors. Stage III MCC is characterized by systemic metastases.

Treatment of stage I MCC involves wide local excision and follow-up **radiation therapy**. Wide local excision is a procedure in which the tumor and a small area of the surrounding healthy tissue are surgically removed. Since MCC is so aggressive, all patients are considered to be at high risk for recurrence and metastasis. For this reason, all patients will undergo radiation therapy of the lymph nodes near the site of the primary tumor that was removed. A technique called lymphoscintigraphy is used to determine the precise location of the lymph nodes that are most likely to be affected.

Treatment of stage II MCC is the same as for stage I MCC with the additional removal of the affected lymph nodes.

Treatment of stage III MCC is generally chemotherapy. But, because the number of known cases of MCC is relatively small, there is no generally prescribed chemotherapy regimen. It has been treated with **etoposide**, **cisplatin**, and **fluorouracil** with varying degrees of success.

The prognosis for patients affected with MCC is generally poor. Half will have a recurrence within two years and one-third will develop systemic involvement (stage III). The average time span from diagnosis of stage III MCC to death is eight months. The two-year survival rate for people affected with MCC is approximately 50%. Factors that improve the patient's length of survival include location of the tumor on the limbs rather than the face; localization of the disease; and female sex.

Alternative and complementary therapies

Naturopathic remedies believed by some to be beneficial in the prevention of skin cancers include regular cleansing by fasting, enema, or herbal supplements. Many naturopaths also recommend a daily scrubbing of the skin with a sauna brush prior to bathing to increase circulation. **Vitamins** A, C, and E, as well as zinc, are believed by some to be essential supplements to a high fiber diet in the prevention of skin damage. However, these remedies have not been proven effective in treating Merkel cell tumors. Traditional medical treatments which have succeeded include surgery, radiation therapy, chemotherapy, and rare success with stem cell transplant.

Coping with cancer treatment

The radiation therapy necessary for follow-up treatment after MCC tumor removal can become stressful for some patients. Additionally, most of these cancers occur in the head and neck region, and their removal can be very disfiguring. It is important that all patients receive adequate counseling and other psychological support prior to and during such treatments.

Clinical trials

In late 2009, there were 24 active trails for Merkel cell carcinoma.

Prevention

Because MCC is believed, at least in some cases, to be caused by long-term exposure to ultraviolet light, it may possibly prevented by avoiding sun exposure when possible and by wearing a PABA containing sunscreen daily.

Special concerns

MCC is very aggressive and can metastasize quickly. For these reasons, medical treatment needs to be sought quickly when MCC is suspected. Recurrence of MCC, either on the skin or in the lymph nodes or other bodily organs, is quite common. Therefore, it is extremely important that all MCC patients, even if they believe that they have no symptoms, have follow-up examinations monthly for at least two years after they have finished their initial radiation treatments.

Resources

PERIODICALS

Agelli, M., and L. X. Clegg. "Epidemiology of Primary Merkel Cell Carcinoma in the United States." *Journal of the American Academy of Dermatology* 49 (November 2003): 832–841.

Khan Durani, B., and W. Hartschuh. "Merkel Cell Carcinoma. Clinical and Histological Differential Diagnosis, Diagnostic Approach and Therapy." [in German] *Hautarzt* 54 (December 2003): 1171–1176.

Mortier, L., X. Mirabel, C. Fournier, et al. "Radiotherapy Alone for Primary Merkel Cell Carcinoma." *Archives of Dermatology* 139 (December 2003): 1587–1590.

Poulsen, M., and D. Rischin. "Merkel Cell Carcinoma—Current Therapeutic Options." *Expert Opinion in Pharmacotherapy* 4 (December 2003): 2187–2192.

Vlad, R., and T. J. Woodlock. "Merkel Cell Carcinoma After Chronic Lymphocytic Leukemia: Case Report and Literature Review." *American Journal of Clinical Oncology* 26 (December 2003): 531–534.

OTHER

CancerNet: Merkel Cell Cancer. [cited June 27, 2009]. http://www.cancer.med.upenn.edu/pdq/600611.html.

Skincancerinfo.com. [cited June 27, 2009].http://www.skincancerinfo.com.

ORGANIZATIONS

American Academy of Dermatology (AAD). P. O. Box 4014, Schaumburg, IL 60168-4014. (847) 330-0230. Fax: (847) 330-0050. http://www.aad.org.

American Cancer Society. (800) ACS-2345. http://www.cancer.org.

The Skin Cancer Foundation. 245 Fifth Ave., Suite #1403, New York, NY 10016. (800) SKIN-490. http://www.skincancer.org.

Paul A. Johnson, Ed.M.
Rebecca J. Frey, Ph.D.

Mesna

Definition

Mesna is a medicine that helps protect the inside lining of the bladder from damage due to certain **chemotherapy** drugs. Mesna may also be referred to as 2-mercaptoethane sulfonate, sodium salt, or Mesnex (its brand name).

Purpose

Mesna is a medicine that is approved by the Food and Drug Administration (FDA) for use in combination with the chemotherapy drug **ifosfamide** to protect the bladder lining from irritation due to the chemotherapy. It has also been shown useful in protecting the bladder lining when used in combination with large doses of the chemotherapy drug **cyclophosphamide**. Irritation to the bladder lining can cause bleeding and this is referred to as hemorrhagic cystitis. Mesna is not administered to treat **cancer**.

KEY TERMS

Acrolein—A breakdown product of the chemotherapy drugs ifosfamide and cyclophosphamide that concentrates in the bladder and irritates the bladder lining and causes bleeding.

Bladder—Organ in the body that collects urine from the kidneys.

Chemotherapy—Specific drugs used to treat cancer.

Food and Drug Administration—A government agency that oversees public safety in relation to drugs and medical devices. The FDA gives the approval to pharmaceutical companies for commercial marketing of their products.

Hemorrhagic cystitis—Irritation of the bladder lining that causes bleeding.

Nontoxic—Does not cause harm.

Description

Mesna is a clear, colorless solution with a foul odor. It is usually administered intravenously through a vein to prevent bleeding of the inside lining of the bladder. Sometimes it can be given to a patient to mix in a beverage and drink. When ifosfamide and cyclophosphamide are given, they break down in the body and form a poisonous substance called acrolein. Acrolein concentrates in the bladder and causes irritation that can lead to severe bleeding from the bladder into the urine. When mesna is administered it also concentrates in the bladder and combines with the toxic acrolein to form a nontoxic substance that is removed from the body by urinating.

Recommended dosage

Mesna is usually administered through a vein over at least five minutes. This same drug can also be mixed with a beverage and taken by mouth (flavored drinks like grape juice, cola, and chocolate milk are good choices to hide the taste of the mesna).

The mesna dose depends on the amount of chemotherapy drugs, ifosfamide or cyclophosphamide, that a patient receives. The mesna dose can vary with the time frame the chemotherapy drugs are being administered. The standard mesna dose is equal to 20% of the total ifosfamide dose given at three separate time intervals through a vein infused over at least five minutes. The first dose is right before the ifosfamide, often referred to as hour 0. The second dose is four hours after the start of the infusion and the third dose is eight hours after the start of the infusion. Mesna is given in this way each day the ifosfamide is administered.

Mesna can be given at a dose of 100% (the same dose as the ifosfamide) of the ifosfamide. This mesna would be mixed directly with the ifosfamide in the same intravenous infusion bag. This type of dosing may or may not have the patient receive a small dose of mesna right before or after the ifosfamide infusion.

Precautions

Mesna can cause allergic reactions that range from a mild rash to severe life-threatening, full-body allergic reactions. Patients with a known previous allergic reaction to mesna or thiol-like medicines should tell their doctor before receiving mesna.

Mesna that contains the preservative benzyl alcohol must not be used in premature babies or infants and must be used with caution in older children.

Mesna should prevent most bleeding from the bladder, however patients may be asked to check their urine for traces of blood with a chemical strip that is dipped into the urine sample.

Side effects

Side effects due only to the mesna are uncommon and difficult to determine since the drug is not given alone. However in clinical studies mesna has been known to cause **nausea and vomiting**, **diarrhea**, abdominal pain, and a bad taste in the mouth. Other reported side effects include; headache, **fatigue**, pain in arms and legs, drop in blood pressure, and allergic reactions.

All side effects a patient experiences should be reported to his or her doctor.

Interactions

Mesna can cause a false positive test of the urine for ketone bodies. This may be most important in diabetic patients who routinely check their urine for ketones.

Nancy J. Beaulieu, RPh.,BCOP

Mesothelioma

Definition

Mesothelioma is a rare form of **cancer**. In mesothelioma, malignant cells are found in the sac lining of the chest (the pleura) or the abdomen (the peritoneum). The majority of people with mesothelioma have a history of jobs that exposed them to asbestos, an insulation material.

Description

In the chest and abdominal cavities, as well as in the cavity around the heart (pericardial sac), there is a layer of specialized cells called mesothelial cells. These cells also surround the outer surface of most internal organs. These cells form tissue called mesothelium.

The mesothelium performs a protective function for the internal organs by producing a lubricating fluid that permits the organs to move around. For example, this fluid makes it easier for the lungs to move inside the chest while a person breathes. The mesothelium of the abdomen is known as the peritoneum, and the mesothelium of the chest is called the pleura. The pericardium refers to the mesothelium of the pericardial cavity.

There are three primary types of malignant mesotheliomas:

- Epithelioid. About 50–70% of mesotheliomas are of this type and have the best outlook for survival.

KEY TERMS

Asbestos—A group of naturally occurring fibrous minerals, found in soil and rocks around the world. These minerals are composed of magnesium, silicon, and other elements. Asbestos has been used as an insulating material since ancient times. Exposure to asbestos dust is the primary risk factor for developing mesothelioma.

- Sarcomatoid. Approximately 7–20% of cases are of this type.
- Mixed/biphasic. From 20–35% of mesothelioma cases fall into this category.

Approximately three-fourths of all mesotheliomas begin in the chest cavity and are known as pleural mesotheliomas. Peritoneal mesotheliomas begin in the abdomen, and make up around 10% to 20% of all cases. Mesotheliomas arising in the cavity around the heart are quite rare.

Demographics

Mesothelioma is a fairly rare form of cancer. According to the American Cancer Society, there are an estimated 2,000 to 3,000 new cases per year of the disease in the United States, but this figure seems to be rising. This rising figure is related to the widespread use of asbestos from the 1940s to the end of the 1970s. European researchers studying the disease expect deaths from mesothelioma to peak around the year 2020 and then drop off, because asbestos use has been cut back greatly since the early 1980s.

The average age of a person with mesothelioma is 50 to 70 years old. It affects men three to five times more often than women and is less common in African-Americans than in Caucasian Americans.

Causes and symptoms

The primary risk factor for developing mesothelioma is asbestos exposure. In the past, asbestos was used as a very effective type of insulation. The use of this material, however, has been declining since the link between asbestos and mesothelioma has become known. It is thought that when the fibers of asbestos are inhaled, some of them reach the ends of the small airways and penetrate into the pleural lining. There the fibers may directly harm mesothelial cells and eventually cause mesothelioma. If the fibers are swallowed, they can reach the abdominal cavity, where

QUESTIONS TO ASK THE DOCTOR

- What type of mesothelioma do I have?
- Has my cancer spread beyond the primary site?
- What stage is my cancer in? What treatment options are there?
- What is my prognosis?
- Are there experimental therapies I may benefit from? Where are they being performed?

they can contribute to the formation of peritoneal mesothelioma.

Exposure to certain types of radiation as well as to a chemical related to asbestos known as zeolite has also been related to incidences of mesothelioma.

The early symptoms of mesothelioma are often ignored, because they may be caused by a variety of ailments. These symptoms include:

- pain in the lower back or at the side of the chest
- shortness of breath
- difficulty swallowing
- cough
- fever
- fatigue
- abdominal pain, weight loss, and nausea and vomiting (symptoms of peritoneal mesothelioma)

Diagnosis

A doctor should be seen if a person experiences shortness of breath, chest pain, or pain or swelling in the abdomen. If these symptoms are present, the doctor may order an x ray of the abdomen or chest. The doctor will do a complete physical examination and take a thorough medical history. Then, one or more of the following methods may be used to ascertain whether mesothelioma is present.

- Imaging tests. These tests may include x rays, computed tomography (CT scans), or magnetic resonance imaging (MRI) to allow the doctor to visualize the area in question. These studies will help determine the location, size, and extent of the cancer.
- Pleural biopsy. Diagnosing mesothelioma requires an adequate biopsy specimen. However, because mesothelioma usually arises from the lower part of the diaphragmatic and/or parietal pleura, obtaining enough tissue may be difficult. A simple, or closed, pleural biopsy involves the insertion of a needle into the chest cavity to obtain tissue from the pleural membrane for analysis. This technique is minimally invasive and normally requires only local anesthesia. This technique, however, may not provide adequate material for the necessary stains of the tissue to make a diagnosis of mesothelioma. Moreover, since the biopsy is not done under direct vision, the sample may not be exactly in the area of the tumor. If the diagnosis cannot be made with this relatively noninvasive technique, an adequate tissue sample usually can be obtained via an open pleural biopsy. In this approach, a surgeon makes an incision on the patient's side and goes into the pleural space. This method allows maximum exploration of the pleural membranes as well. However, the technique requires general anesthesia.
- Thoracoscopy. A thoracoscopy, which is a relatively new technique, allows the doctor to look directly into the chest (pleural) cavity at the tumor and during the same operation to also take a tissue sample for laboratory analysis. The thoracoscopy is performed by making a small incision into the chest and using a tiny video camera to inspect the region. The doctor can then use forceps to obtain a tissue biopsy. A laparoscopy, a similar operation, is used to obtain a biopsy of a peritoneal tumor.
- Bronchoscopy. A bronchoscopy, which examines the airways, or a mediastinoscopy, which looks at the lymph nodes in the chest, allows the doctor to look at the area using a lighted tube. Samples may be taken with a needle and sent to the lab to find out if cancer cells are present. However, bronchoscopy and mediastinoscopy are not that effective for diagnosing mesothelioma, as the disease is seldom found within the airways or the lymph nodes.
- Surgery. This lets the doctor obtain a larger tumor sample or, on occasion, the entire tumor.

Diagnosing mesothelioma is often difficult, even with tissue biopsies. Microscopically, mesothelioma is often difficult to distinguish from several other forms of cancer. For this reason, certain laboratory tests are performed to help correctly diagnose mesothelioma. Some of these tests involve using antibodies to distinguish lung cancer from mesothelioma. Sometimes the tissue samples must be viewed under an electron microscope in order to get the correct diagnosis.

Treatment team

A person with symptoms of mesothelioma will most likely seek help from a primary physician initially. During the diagnostic phase, various technicians will perform the **imaging studies**. A specially trained physician—a thoracic surgeon or, rarely, a pulmonologist—performs other diagnostic tests like **pleural biopsy** and **thoracoscopy**. A pathologist will view the tissue samples and make the tissue diagnosis. Following diagnosis, the patient will be offered some form of treatment, which may entail surgery, **radiation therapy**, **chemotherapy**, or a combination of these. The patient may receive care from a thoracic surgeon, an anesthesiologist, medical and radiation oncologists, and specially trained nurses who administer chemotherapy.

Clinical staging, treatments, and prognosis

The treatment and outlook for those with mesothelioma depends a great deal on the stage of their cancer. Because the most frequently occurring type of mesothelioma is pleural, and it is also the one most studied, it is the only type for which a staging system exists. The following stages are based on a system known as the Butchart system, which divides mesothelioma into four stages:

- Stage I: Mesothelioma is found within the right or the left pleura and may also involve the lung, the pericardium, or the diaphragm on the same side.
- Stage II: In this stage, mesothelioma has spread to the chest wall or involves the esophagus, the heart, or the pleura on both sides. The lymph nodes in the chest may be involved as well.
- Stage III: Mesothelioma has gone through the diaphragm and into the lining of the abdominal cavity. Additional lymph nodes besides those in the chest may be involved.
- Stage IV: There is evidence that mesothelioma has spread through the bloodstream to distant organs or tissues.

Another system of staging mesothelioma is based on a TNM system (T = tumor, N = spread to lymph nodes, and M = metastasis). There are minor differences between this and the Butchart system. It is more detailed and precise, but the original Butchart system is still the one most often used to describe pleural mesotheliomas.

There are treatments available for all patients with malignant mesothelioma. The three kinds of treatment used are surgery, radiation therapy, and chemotherapy.

Surgery is a common treatment for mesothelioma. It is not an option unless the cancer is limited to one place and unless the person can withstand the surgery. During surgery, the physician may remove a portion of the lining of the chest (pleurectomy) or abdomen (peritonectomy) and some of the tissue surrounding it. Depending on the extent the disease has spread, a lung may also require removal (extrapleural **pneumonectomy**). Occasionally, a portion of the diaphragm is taken out as well. If treatment is not possible, other less invasive measures can be used to relieve the patient's symptoms. For example, a needle placed into the chest cavity (**thoracentesis**) can remove excess fluid in the chest. If recurrence of fluid causes symptoms, a nonsurgical or surgical method can be used to scar the lining of lung cavity and cause it to adhere to the lung. The procedure obliterates the pleural space and thus prevents the fluid from reaccumulating. (This procedure is called sclerosis or sclerotherapy.) These methods are called palliative, for they are not meant to cure the cancer but to improve symptoms.

Radiation therapy uses high-energy **x rays** to kill cancer cells and cause tumor shrinkage. It is rarely used as the primary treatment for pleural mesothelioma in those patients for whom surgery is not an option. It may also be used as an adjunct to surgery or as a method of alleviating various symptoms like trouble with swallowing, pain, and shortness of breath.

Chemotherapy involves the use of drugs to kill cancer cells. The most commonly used drugs are **doxorubicin**, **cisplatin**, and **methotrexate**. The medicines are delivered into a vein or taken by mouth. In the treatment of mesothelioma, they may also be injected directly into the chest or abdominal cavity. Chemotherapy may be given as the main treatment or may be an addition to surgery, depending on the type and stage of the cancer.

A new treatment being studied for early stages of mesothelioma confined to the chest is called intraoperative **photodynamic therapy**. This treatment uses special drugs that make cancer cells more sensitive to killing by a laser light. The drugs are given several days before surgery. During surgery, the special light is used to shine on the pleura.

By the time symptoms show up and mesothelioma is diagnosed, the disease is often advanced. The average survival period after diagnosis is about one year. If the cancer is found before it has spread and it is treated aggressively, about half of the patients will live two years, and approximately 20% will survive five years.

Alternative and complementary therapies

There are no proven effective alternative therapies for mesothelioma. Because the prognosis is often poor, many patients may be interested in trying other avenues of treatment. Patients should first consult with their physicians prior to trying any of these methods. There are many well-studied complementary treatments that may increase a patient's comfort and sense of well-being. These may include meditation to aid in relaxation, massage to decrease pain, and guided imagery to help prevent **nausea**.

Coping with cancer treatment

Coping with cancer treatment can be difficult and exhausting. It can be very helpful for the patient receiving therapy for mesothelioma to find a group of family and friends who can aid with household responsibilities, provide transportation, and give psychological support. The patient should not feel a need to rush back to normal activities after treatment is completed.

Clinical trials

A great deal of research is being performed in the area of mesothelioma. Much of the research is focused on finding out how asbestos changes the mesothelial cells to cause these cancers. In addition, new combinations of treatments are being tested, along with gene therapy. A variety of **clinical trials** are testing new chemotherapy drugs and immunotherapy. Some of these treatments use hormonelike substances called interleukins and **interferons** that activate the immune system.

Prevention

The best method of preventing mesothelioma is to avoid or limit exposure to asbestos. People who might experience asbestos exposure at work include miners, insulation manufacturers, construction workers, ship builders, and factory workers.

Special concerns

Mesothelioma is a serious disease with a poor long-term prognosis. Patients with this cancer should communicate their wishes regarding treatment to their family and physicians.

Resources

PERIODICALS

Apgar, Barbara. "Diagnosis of Malignant Pleural Mesothelioma." *American Family Physician* January 15, 2000: 536.

ORGANIZATIONS

American Cancer Society. (800) ACS-2345. http://www.cancer.org.

National Cancer Institute. Building 31, Room 10A31, 31 Center Drive, MSC 2580, Bethesda, MD 20892-2580. (800) 4-CANCER. http://www.nci.nih.gov.

Deanna Swartout-Corbeil, R.N.

Metastasis

Definition

The ability to invade and metastasize are the defining characteristics of a **cancer**. Invasion refers to the ability of cancer cells to penetrate through the membranes that separate them from healthy tissues and

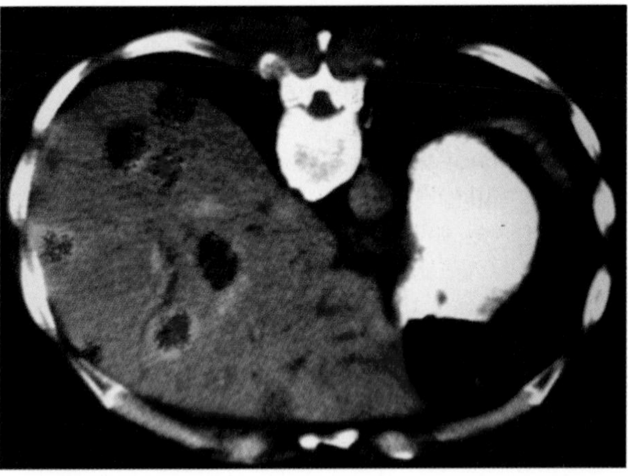

Computed tomography (CT) scan of abdomen revealing liver metastases from colon adenocarcinoma. *(Copyright Scott Camazine & Sue Trainor, Science Source/Photo Researchers, Inc. Reproduced by permission.)*

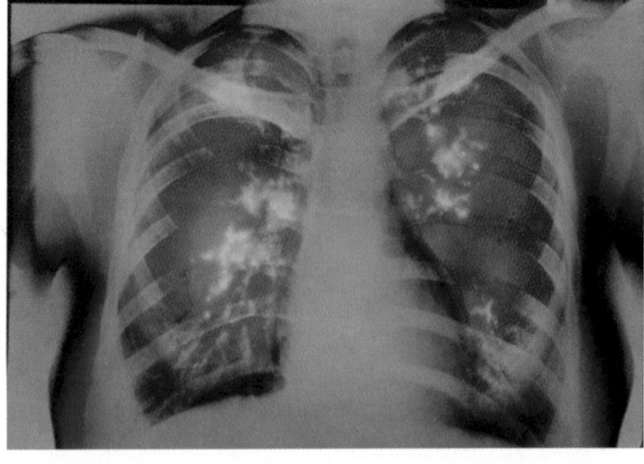

Color-enhanced x ray shows areas of cancer spread. *(Copyright AFIP, Science Source/Photo Researchers, Inc. Reproduced by permission.)*

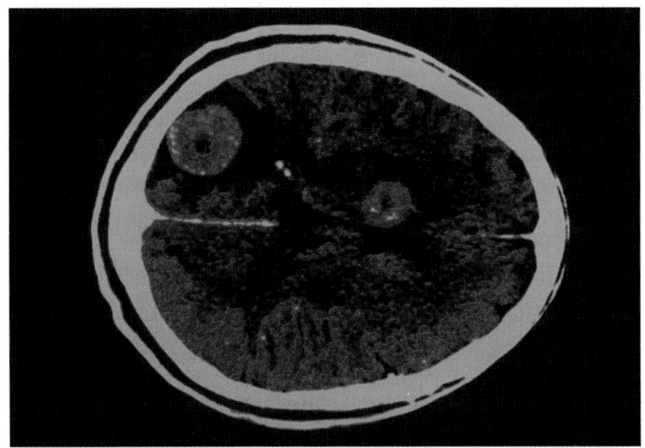

Computed tomography (CT) scan of 47-year-old female's brain showing adenocarcinoma of lung metastatic to brain. *(Copyright Scott/Brian Carmazine, Science Source/Photo Researchers, Inc. Reproduced by permission.)*

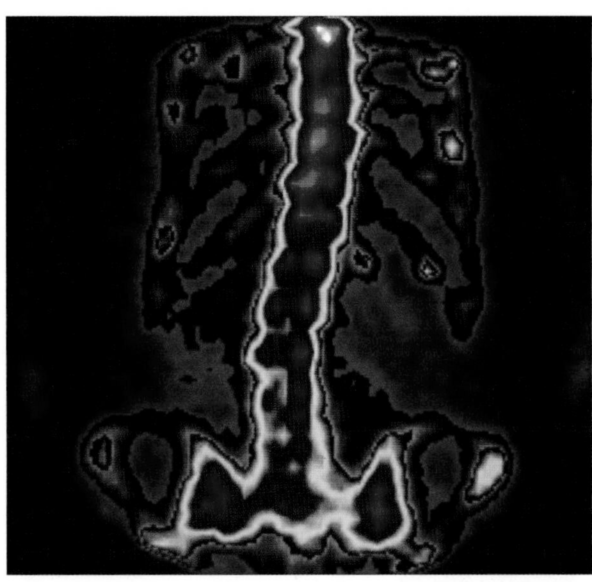

False-color scintigram (bone scan) of the human spine and ribs, revealing secondary cancers (metastases) in the vertebrae (backbones), arising from a primary cancer of the prostate gland. *(Copyright CNRI, Science Source/ Photo Researchers, Inc. Reproduced by permission.)*

blood vessels. Metastasis can refer either to the spread of cancer cells to other parts of the body, or to the condition produced by this spread. The English word metastasis (plural, metastases) comes from a Greek word that means "a change." The tumors produced by metastasis sometimes are called secondary tumors. metastasis is responsible for 90% of the deaths caused by cancer.

Description

Metastasis is a complex multi-step process that begins with changes in the genetic material of a cell (**carcinogenesis**) followed by the uncontrolled multiplication of altered cells. It continues with the development of a new blood supply for the tumor (angiogenesis), invasion of the circulatory system, dispersal of small clumps of tumor cells to other organs or parts of the body, and the growth of secondary tumors in those sites.

Carcinogenesis and genetic mutations

The first step in cancer development is a change or mutation of the DNA in the chromosomes of a cell. Mutations can be triggered by a number of different factors, including:

- Environmental carcinogens. Ultraviolet radiation from the sun is known to cause skin cancer. Chemical carcinogens include tobacco smoke, asbestos, and benzene. Ionizing radiation from x-ray therapy or atomic fallout, or industrial exposure to uranium or thorium are also associated with an increased risk of cancer.
- Viruses. Infection by a virus containing an oncogene is known to cause cancer in experimental animals. In humans, such viruses as human immunodeficiency virus (HIV), human papillomavirus (HPV), hepatitis B or C viruses, and Epstein-Barr virus (EBV) have been linked to Kaposi's sarcoma, anal cancer, certain types of lymphoma, primary liver cancer, and cancers of the genitals.
- Chronic irritation and inflammation. Chronic irritation of the skin, or chronic inflammation of the bladder or bile ducts caused by certain intestinal parasites, have been linked to cancers of the skin, bladder, or pancreas.
- Chromosomal rearrangement or damage. Oncogenes are genes found in the chromosomes of tumor cells. Activation of oncogenes is associated with the conversion of normal cells into cancer cells. Oncogenes sometimes are activated by chromosomal rearrangements. The so-called Philadelphia chromosome, an abnormality that involves a transposition of genetic material between the long arms of human chromosomes 9 and 22, is found in about 80% of patients with chronic myelocytic leukemia.
- Loss of tumor suppressor genes. Another type of genetic alteration that can lead to cancer is the inactivation of anti-oncogenes, or tumor suppressor genes. Under normal circumstances, tumor suppressor genes act like a brake on cell growth and division. If these genes are altered or lost, oncogenes can stimulate cells to multiply uncontrollably without

KEY TERMS

Angiogenesis—The process of forming new blood vessels that supply a tumor with nutrients and help to carry tumor emboli into the larger vessels of the circulatory system.

Apoptosis—The programmed self-destruction of a cell, which takes place when the cell detects some damage to its DNA. Apoptosis is sometimes called "cell suicide."

Basement membrane—A specialized layer of extracellular matrix that separates epithelial tissue from underlying connective tissue. Cancer cells must break through the basement membrane in order to migrate to other parts of the body and form metastases.

Embolus (plural, emboli)—A clump of tumor cells that breaks off from a primary tumor to travel through the circulatory system and lodge in a capillary in another part of the body. The process of forming emboli is called embolization.

Epithelium—The layer of tissue that covers body surfaces and lines the internal surfaces of body cavities, blood vessels, and hollow organs. Most cancer cells arise within epithelial tissue.

Extracellular matrix—A collection of connective tissue proteins and fibers that supports and nourishes body tissues. The extracellular matrix forms a physical barrier to the movement of tumor cells.

Extravasation—The process of reverse invasion in which tumor cells that have invaded the blood vessels and traveled to other organs force their way back out of the blood vessels and into the tissues surrounding their new site.

Micrometastasis (plural, micrometastases)—A term sometimes used to describe malignant tumor cells circulating in the blood or other metastases too small to be detected by a standard clinical examination.

Multicentric—A type of cancer that appears at several different sites in the patient's body simultaneously.

Oncogene—Any gene that is a factor in triggering the development of cancer. Oncogenes are mutated forms of proto-oncogenes, which are genes that promote the normal process of cell growth and division.

Replication—The process in which a cell duplicates or copies itself.

Tumor markers—Substances that occur in the blood, urine, or tissues of patients with certain types of cancer. Tumor markers may be produced either by the tumor itself or by the body in response to the tumor.

Tumor necrosis factor (TNF)—A protein that destroys cells showing abnormally rapid growth. TNF is used in immunotherapy to shrink tumors rapidly.

Tumor suppressor gene—A gene that encodes proteins that inhibit cell division and replication. Tumor suppressor genes are damaged or inactive in many types of cancer cells.

Vascular endothelial growth factor (VEGF)—A substance released by tumor cells that attracts vascular (blood vessel) cells to the tumor. The vascular cells then form new blood vessels within the tumor.

Vascularization—Another name for angiogenesis.

any opposition. In colorectal cancer, deletion of the DCC gene, which is a tumor suppressor gene located on the long arm of human chromosome 18, lowers the patient's chances of five-year survival by 30%.

Other mutations in a cell's DNA occur for reasons that are not yet fully understood.

Steps in the development of metastases

Cell alteration and replication

Most cancer cells originate within the epithelium, which is a layer of tissue that covers body surfaces and lines the inner surfaces of body cavities and blood vessels. Cancer cells in epithelial tissue are known to be genetically unstable and to have a high mutation rate. Most cancers, in fact, are the end result of multiple genetic alterations both in oncogenes and tumor suppressor genes. The activation of oncogenes is accompanied by the loss or deactivation of tumor suppressor genes, which means that one of the body's normal lines of defense against uncontrolled cell proliferation is disabled just when it is most needed.

Following these alterations in its genetic material, the cell replicates, or copies itself at a faster rate. In some instances, a mutation prevents the cell's apoptosis, or programmed self-destruction. Apoptosis, which is also sometimes called "cell suicide," normally occurs when a cell recognizes some damage to its DNA and

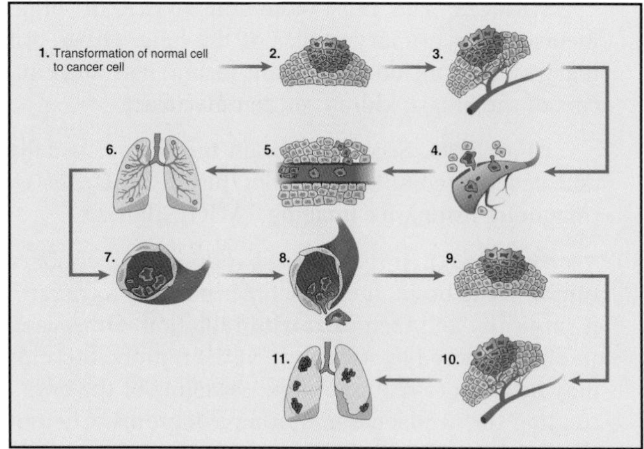

(1) A cell is transformed. (2) Cancerous cell proliferates and cells pile up to form a malignant tumor. (3) Angiogenesis: the tumor acquires a blood supply, which also allows (4) the cancer cells access into the circulatory system. (5) Cancer cells travel through the blood stream. (6) The cells stop in a capillary bed, and (7) adhere to the layer of cells that line the blood vessel. (8) The cells invade the essential, functional tissue of the organ surrounding the blood vessel. (9) In this new organ, cancer cells pile up to form secondary tumors, which (10) induce angiogenesis. (11) Metastases (secondary tumors) are now evident. *(Illustration by Argosy Publishing. Cengage Learning, Gale.)*

dies. The protein produced by the p53 gene ordinarily encourages apoptosis in cells with defective DNA, but these cells are more likely to survive and replicate if the p53 gene has been altered or deactivated.

Breaking through the basement membrane

Once a cancer develops, the first stage in the development of metastasis is the tumor's penetration of the basement membrane, which separates epithelial tissue from underlying connective tissue. The basement membrane is a specialized layer of extracellular matrix, which is a mass of connective tissue fibers and proteins that support and nourish the body's connective tissues. Under normal circumstances, the extracellular matrix is a barrier that keeps cells from moving away from their sites of origin. Cancer cells, however, secrete several different types of enzymes that digest the proteins in the basement membrane. When the membrane has been sufficiently weakened, the tumor can push through it.

Angiogenesis

Angiogenesis is the process in which a tumor creates its own blood supply by releasing growth factors—particularly a substance called vascular endothelial growth factor, or VEGF—that attract vascular cells that begin to migrate toward the tumor. The vascular cells eventually form new blood vessels within the tumor. Angiogenesis is sometimes called vascularization, which means blood vessel formation. Angiogenesis is a significant step in the development of metastasis for two reasons: the formation of blood vessels in the tumor supplies the tumor with nutrients that speed up its growth; these vessels also provide pathways for cancer cells to travel from the primary tumor to other organs. A similar process of vessel formation involves the lymph system.

Angiogenesis may occur at about the same time that the tumor breaks through the basement membrane, but it can also take place at an earlier point in the tumor's growth.

Invasion and embolization

After the tumor's new blood vessels have formed, individual cancer cells break off from the tumor and travel through these new vessels into the body's main circulatory system. These cells are sometimes called micrometastases. Even a small tumor can shed as many as a million cancer cells each day into the blood and lymph vessels. Most of these cells die soon after entering the blood stream or lymph vessels. Sometimes, however, the cancer cells may travel as small clumps of cells called emboli. A protein called fibrin, which ordinarily is formed when blood clots, surrounds each embolus. The fibrin appears to protect the embolus of cancer cells as it moves through the circulatory system, and may increase its chances for survival when it arrives in the capillaries (small blood vessels) that supply another organ or area of the body.

Extravasation and formation of secondary tumors

Extravasation refers to the cancer cell's breaking out through the wall of the capillary where it has been stopped and invading the tissue around the capillary. In order to extravasate, the tumor cell must attach itself to the wall of the capillary. Once it has attached itself, it can work its way through the tissue lining the blood vessel, the vessel wall itself, and the basement membrane covering the blood vessel. The tumor cell can then begin to replicate itself and start the process of angiogenesis, thus forming a metastasis or secondary tumor in its new location. The secondary tumor can eventually release its own cancer cells into the circulation and produce further metastases.

Most tumor cells do not survive in the blood stream long enough to extravasate and form metastases. The longer the cells are in the circulation, the more likely they are to die. The chances of a given tumor cell's surviving the journey and forming a metastasis in its new site have been variously estimated as one in 10,000 or as less than one in one million. Researchers have asked whether the tumor cells that do produce metastases are random survivors or whether they have special capacities for survival and reproduction. Recent studies indicate that cells from the same tumor vary in their metastatic potential; those that eventually form metastases have a higher degree of malignancy.

Diagnosis and monitoring of metastases

Some primary cancers, such as lung and ovarian cancers, begin to shed tumor cells that form metastases elsewhere in the body before the primary cancer is large enough to be detected by standard diagnostic techniques. Marker molecules that are given off by micrometastases circulating in the bloodstream can now be detected.

Tumor markers are substances produced either by tumors themselves or by the body in response to a tumor. The blood levels of tumor markers can be used to evaluate the recurrence or spread of cancer and the patient's response to treatment. Some commonly used tumor markers include: prostate-specific antigen (PSA) for **prostate cancer**; prostatic acid phosphatase (PAP) for prostate cancer that has metastasized, **testicular cancer** and leukemia; and CA 125 (Cancer antigen 125) for recurrence of **ovarian cancer**. It also detects cancers of the uterus, liver, pancreas, colon, cervix, lung, and digestive tract, as well as several others.

DNA analysis can be used to distinguish metastatic tumors from multicentric tumors. A multicentric cancer is one that appears simultaneously in several different parts of the body, as distinct from cancers with primary and secondary (metastatic) tumors. Mutations in the p53 tumor suppressor gene have been used as "genetic fingerprints" to identify differences between multicentric and metastatic tumors.

Specific types of metastases

Brain

SYMPTOMS. Metastatic tumors to the brain usually come to the doctor's attention in the same way as primary tumors—they cause increased pressure inside the head, disturbances of brain functions, or both. Common symptoms of brain metastases include headaches, seizures, loss of sensation or balance, or personality changes.

SOURCES. The most common source of brain metastases is primary cancer of the lung. Other primary sources include malignant melanomas and cancers of the breast, kidney, or digestive tract.

DIAGNOSIS. Secondary **brain tumors** are usually detected on (computed tomography) (CT) scans or (**magnetic resonance imaging**) (MRI) studies.

TREATMENT. If the patient has only one secondary tumor in the brain, it is sometimes possible to remove it surgically and then treat with radiation. Otherwise, radiation is used by itself to treat the tumors. Steroids may be given to reduce or lower swelling of the brain, treating the headaches and other symptoms. **Chemotherapy** has only a limited role in treating brain metastases, because most chemotherapy drugs cannot cross the blood-brain barrier. However, **intrathecal chemotherapy** (chemotherapy drugs injected directly into the spinal fluid) can have a role in treating brain metastases. Patients with multiple metastases in the brain or widespread cancer elsewhere in the body have a poor prognosis. Treatments that are still under evaluation include laser-assisted surgery and **biological response modifiers**.

Bone

SYMPTOMS. Primary bone cancers are less common than bone metastases. Bone metastases, in fact, are a common cause of pain in many patients with late-stage cancer. Metastases in the spine can compress the spinal cord and damage the nervous system. Bone metastases also make bones more prone to fracture.

SOURCES. Breast, lung, and prostate cancer are responsible for about 80% of bone metastases; over half of patients with these three types of primary cancer will develop bone metastases. Patients with lung cancer that has metastasized to bone live on average less than six months, but breast and prostate cancer patients may have lengthy periods of survival with bone metastases.

Bone metastases usually are caused by tumor cells carried through the bloodstream, and are typically multiple. About 70% of bone metastases occur in the ribs, spine, sacrum (lowest portion of spine, attached to pelvis), or head; most of the remainder occur in the long bones of the body.

DIAGNOSIS. Bone metastases usually are detected by bone scans, CT scans, or MRIs, and confirmed by a **biopsy**. In 2003, reports showed that **positron emission tomography** (PET) scans were effective in detecting certain types of bone mestasteses from lung and **breast cancer** and from **lymphoma**.

TREATMENT. Bone metastases are treated with hormonal or systemic chemotherapy and/or **radiation therapy**. Metastases in the spine may require surgical removal of part of the vertebrae (laminectomy) followed by radiation treatment to prevent compression of the spinal cord. Surgery also may be performed if there is a risk of fracture.

As of May 2005, two new drugs were approved show promise as treatments for bone metastases. One is a generic drug called clodronate, which is taken by mouth, and the other is a medication called Atrasentan. Atrasentan was tested on patients in advanced stages of bone metastases who were no longer responding to other forms of treatment.

Lung

SOURCES. Metastatic tumors in the lungs may result either from primary cancer of the lung or from malignancies elsewhere in the body that spread to the lungs through the circulatory system or by direct extension. The incidence of metastatic cancer to the lung is six in 100,000 people. Almost any type of cancer can metastasize to the lung, but the most common tumors that spread to the lung are breast cancer, sarcomas, **non-Hodgkin's lymphoma**, **neuroblastoma**, and **Wilms' tumor**. Between 20% and 54% of patients dying of cancer are found to have metastases in the lungs.

DIAGNOSIS. Diagnosis is usually the appearance of a group of masses on a chest x ray. Evaluation of lung metastases is first directed at diagnosing/locating the primary tumor.

TREATMENT. Secondary lung cancers are treated primarily by appropriate systemic therapy for the primary tumor. Surgery for secondary lung tumors may be beneficial if there are four or less metastases. Surgical removal of tumors metastatic to the lung is usually performed only if: the primary tumor is treatable, all metastases can be removed, chemotherapy or other nonsurgical approaches cannot be used, and if there are no metastases elsewhere in the patient's body. If the primary cancer is a malignant **melanoma** and there is only one secondary tumor, surgery may be an option. (Surgery is usually not performed if the primary cancer is a malignant melanoma and there is more than one secondary tumor.) The five-year survival rate for surgical treatment of secondary tumors to the lung is 20–35%.

Liver

The most common form of **liver cancer** is metastatic; in fact, metastases in the liver are often the first noticeable evidence of a primary cancer located elsewhere in the body. In the liver, finding multiple metastases is more common than finding a single tumor. The liver's important role within the circulatory system makes it a common stopping point for tumor emboli carried in the blood from other organs.

SOURCES. The most common sites of primary tumors that metastasize to the liver are the lungs, breasts, colon, pancreas, and stomach.

DIAGNOSIS. The diagnosis of metastatic liver cancer is usually difficult unless the patient's primary tumor is in advanced stages of disease. Ultrasound, CT scans, and liver function tests are used to screen patients with a known cancer for metastases in the liver, but the results are not fully reliable. A definitive diagnosis depends on biopsy of liver tissue.

TREATMENT. Metastatic cancer to the liver is considered incurable. Systemic chemotherapy may temporarily shrink tumors in the liver and extend the patient's life span but does not cure the cancer. Radiation treatment may relieve pain but is not otherwise helpful. Some doctors may recommend surgical removal of liver metastases, particularly if the primary tumor is in the colon and there is a solitary metastasis, but others do not favor this approach. The five-year survival rate for surgical removal of liver metastases is 20%-30%.

Metastatic cancers of unknown primary origin

Between 0.5% and 7% of all cancers are carcinomas of unknown primary origin, or CUPs. The patient's history and physical examination should be analyzed for signs of breast, prostate, pelvic, rectal, and **gastrointestinal cancers**. The pattern of spread of a CUP may indicate whether the primary tumor is above or below the diaphragm; lung metastases are twice as common with primary tumors found to be above the diaphragm, while liver metastases are more common if the **primary site** is below the diaphragm.

Metastases of unknown primary origin are usually treated by chemotherapy—either cisplatin/carboplatin, **doxorubicin** or paclitaxel. In most cases, the patient's prognosis is poor; the average length of survival is three to four months, with fewer than 10% of patients surviving five years. Male sex and involvement of the liver are negative factors in the prognosis.

Treatment

Surgery

Surgery as a method of cancer treatment has limitations in the therapy of metastatic cancer. It is sometimes used to remove large secondary tumors that are causing pain or interfering with body functions. It also may offer a survival advantage over other therapies, as with limited metastases to the lung or liver.

Chemotherapy

Chemotherapy is frequently used to treat micrometastases that have entered the patient's bloodstream or lymphatic system. Systemic chemotherapy is the only type of treatment that can act at multiple sites simultaneously. Because of some chemotherapy drugs' side effects and risks (for example, **nausea and vomiting**, some drugs are implicated in causing some cancers), the likelihood of tumor responsiveness needs to be balanced with the patient's quality of life when selecting chemotherapy.

Radiation

Radiation therapy can be effective in the treatment of metastatic disease, especially for metastases to the brain and bones. It is limited, however, because it treats only a limited area. One complication that is possible with radiation therapy is that it has been associated with an increased rate of secondary cancers in patients who have been previously treated for malignancies. The risk is particularly high in patients who were treated with a combination of radiation and chemotherapy.

Immunotherapy

Immunotherapy, or immunologic therapy, is a modality, or method, of cancer treatment that is still in its experimental stages. It mobilizes the patient's own immune system to fight cancer cells. Immunotherapy is being evaluated in the treatment of metastatic melanoma, renal cell **carcinoma**, breast tumors, and other tumors. Some of the substances that are being tested in **clinical trials** are produced by the human body, while others are made in laboratories. The major categories of substances used in immunotherapy include:

- Interferons. Interferons are proteins produced by virus-infected cells that limit further reproduction of the virus and stimulate resistance to the infection.
- Interleukins. Interleukins are small proteins that promote the growth and activation of the body's white cells. Interleukin-2, known as IL-2 or aldesleukin, is approved for the treatment of metastatic melanoma and renal cell carcinoma.
- Tumor necrosis factor (TNF). TNF is a protein that was discovered in 1975. It destroys cells that show unusually rapid growth and stimulates the production of interleukins.
- Monoclonal antibodies. Monoclonal antibodies are antibodies produced in laboratory-grown cell clones in order to achieve greater abundance and uniformity than are found in antibodies produced in the body.
- Vaccines. Cancer vaccines are intended to stimulate the body's killer T cells (a specialized type of white blood cell) to attack tumor cells. Some vaccines being tested are made from relatively rare white blood cells called dendritic cells; others are made from genetically altered tumor cells.

Newer therapies for metastatic cancer

Recent advances in understanding the process of metastasis have led to some new approaches to treatment.

GENE THERAPY. Some researchers are investigating ways to replace a mutated p53 tumor suppressor gene, or to inhibit an activated *ras* oncogene. Another approach involves the use of **angiogenesis inhibitors** to suppress metastatic tumors. An antibody to VEGF, called anti-VEGF, is presently being used in clinical trials for patients with late-stage colon, breast, and lung cancers. A second angiogenesis inhibitor that is being tested is endostatin.

Other researchers are studying substances that trigger apoptosis in defective cells or prevent the uncontrolled multiplication of tumor cells.

ISOLATED PERFUSION. Isolated perfusion is the treatment of metastatic melanoma and **sarcoma** to the extremities by isolating the vasculature (blood vessels) of the affected extremity, and then delivering high doses of chemotherapeutic drugs directly to the area of metastatic disease. The limb is then flushed before re-establishing circulation. With this technique, it becomes possible to deliver doses of drugs regionally that would otherwise be very toxic or lethal if delivered systemically.

HYPERTHERMIA. Hyperthermia is the use of therapeutic heat to treat cancers on and inside the body. The goal of hyperthermia is to shrink and destroy cancer without harming noncancerous cells. The treatment can be delivered directly to the tumor, to an area of the body, or to the whole body. Research has established that the effectiveness of some forms of radiation therapy and chemotherapy are enhanced when combined with hyperthermia. In 2001, the American Cancer Society acknowledged that hyperthermia could the cells of some cancers more responsive to treatment, but still considered the treatment experimental, especially in whole-body form. The National Institutes of Health are sponsoring ongoing clinical trials studying hyperthermia. Patients with extensive metastasis may not be good candidates for hyperthermia.

Alternative and complementary therapies

The National Center for Complementary and Alternative Medicine (NCCAM) is sponsoring new as well as ongoing trials of alternative treatments for metastatic cancer. One ongoing trial involves **PC-SPES**, a combination of eight Chinese herbs that is used to treat prostate cancer. Other trials are evaluating the use of herbal remedies to treat the side effects of chemotherapy. The National Cancer Institute (NCI) makes information about ongoing clinical trials available. Patients can contact the NCI or the NCCAM at the numbers and web sites listed below.

See also Cancer biology; Cancer genetics; Carcinogenesis; Hepatic arterial infusion.

Resources

BOOKS

Aminoff, Michael J., MD, FRCP. "Nervous System." Chapter 24 In *Current Medical Diagnosis & Treatment 2001*, edited by L. M. Tierney, Jr., MD, et al., 40th ed. New York: Lange Medical Books/McGraw-Hill, 2001.

Beers, Mark H., MD, and Robert Berkow, MD, editors. "Hematology and Oncology." Section 11 In *The Merck Manual of Diagnosis and Therapy*. Whitehouse Station, NJ: Merck Research Laboratories, 2007.

Chesnutt, Mark S., MD, and Thomas J. Prendergast, MD. "Lung." Chapter 9 in *Current Medical Diagnosis & Treatment 2001*, edited by L. M. Tierney, Jr., MD, et al., 40th ed. New York: Lange Medical Books/McGraw-Hill, 2001.

Rugo, Hope S., MD. "Cancer." Chapter 4 In *Current Medical Diagnosis & Treatment 2001*, edited by L. M. Tierney, Jr., MD, et al., 40th ed. New York: Lange Medical Books/McGraw-Hill, 2001.

Shaffrey, Mark E., MD, and Edward R. Laws, MD. "Brain Tumors." In *Conn's Current Therapy 2001*, edited by Robert E. Rakel, MD. and Edward T. Bope, MD. Philadelphia: W. B. Saunders Company, 2001.

PERIODICALS

Fidler, Isaiah J. "Melanoma Metastasis." *Cancer Control Journal* 2, no. 5 (2000).

"PET Effective in Detecting of Osseous Metastasis from Several Malignancies." *Cancer Weekly* December 30, 2003: 141.

OTHER

National Center for Environmental Research, U.S. Environmental Protection Agency. Web site: http://www.es.epa.gov/ncerqa.

ORGANIZATIONS

American Cancer Society (ACS). 1599 Clifton Road, NE, Atlanta, GA 30329. (404) 320-3333 or (800) ACS-2345. Fax: (404) 329-7530. http://www.cancer.org.

National Cancer Institute, Office of Cancer Communications. 31 Center Drive, MSC 2580, Bethesda, MD 20892-2580. (800) 4-CANCER (1-800-422-6237). TTY: (800) 332-8615. http://www.nci.nih.gov.

NIH National Center for Complementary and Alternative Medicine (NCCAM) Clearinghouse. P. O. Box 8218, Silver Spring, MD 20907-8218. TTY/TDY: (888) 644-6226. Fax: (301) 495-4957. http://www.nccam.nih.gov.

Office of Cancer Complementary & Alternative Medicine of the National Cancer Institute (OCCAM). Email: ncioccam1-r@mail.nih.gov. http://www.occam.nci.nih.gov.

Rebecca J. Frey, Ph.D.
Teresa G. Odle

Methadone *see* **Opioids**

Methotrexate

Definition

Methotrexate is a **folic acid** derivative that interferes with folic acid metabolism (folate antagonist). It is a cytotoxic agent (a chemical that is directly toxic to cells) with multiple characteristics and may be described as an antimetabolite, antineoplastic, and immunosuppressant. In the United States, methotrexate is also recognized by the trade names Folex and Mexate, or the generic name amethopterin.

Purpose

Methotrexate is administered to **cancer** patients diagnosed with various malignancies. These conditions may include **breast cancer**, lung cancer, non-metastatic bone cancer, cancers associated with the head and neck, **acute lymphocytic leukemia**, meningeal leukemia, advanced non-Hodgkin's lymphomas, and uterine tumors. Certain other cancers may be treated with methotrexate as prescribed by the oncologist.

Description

Methotrexate was granted FDA approval in 1986. Methotrexate is a highly effective chemical compound that targets a specific enzyme required by cells for normal function. When this enzyme activity is blocked by methotrexate, certain processes within the cell are

KEY TERMS

Antimetabolite—Anti-cancer drugs which prevent cells from growing and dividing by blocking the chemical reactions required in the cell to produce DNA.

Antineoplastic—Agents that inhibit or prevent the development of cancers by stopping the maturation and proliferation of malignant cells.

BCD—The combined chemotherapy treatment of bleomycin, cyclophosphamide, and dactinomycin.

Cytotoxic—Chemicals that are toxic to cells, and prevent their reproduction or growth.

Hodgkin's lymphoma—A human malignant disorder of lymph tissue that appears to originate in a particular lymph node and later spreads to the spleen, liver, and bone marrow.

Immunosupressant—Any chemotherapeutic agent which also has the effect of suppressing the immune system.

Leucovorin—The antidote for high dose treatments of methotrexate.

Lymphocytic leukemia—An acute form of childhood leukemia characterized by the development of abnormal cells in the bone marrow and lymph cells found in blood-forming tissues.

Metastatic—Refers to the spread of a cancer from its place of origin to another site in the body.

Oncologist—A physician who specializes in the diagnosis and treatment of patients with cancer.

shut down and cell death results. The growth of some normal cells may be affected by methotrexate. However, because this is a process associated with actively dividing cells, the accelerated rate at which cancer cells grow and divide make them more susceptible to the effects of methotrexate. Methotrexate may be given as a single agent, often followed by **leucovorin** rescue. Methotrexate may also be administered in a combination regimen with steroids to produce and maintain rapid remission of certain cancers or as part of an adjuvant therapy regimen with **doxorubicin**, **cisplatin**, or the BCD combination of **bleomycin**, **cyclophosphamide**, and **dactinomycin**.

Recommended dosage

Methotrexate is available is both injectable and tablet form. The injectable form may be given intravenously (IV), intramuscularly (IM), or intrathecal (directly into the spinal fluid). The dose amount varies over a wide range for patients receiving methotrexate. The final dose and treatment cycle will be determined by the oncologist based on what the medication is being used for, what cancer type is being treated, whether methotrexate is being used as a single agent or in concert with other **anticancer drugs**, and the method by which the medication is being administered. It is extremely important to take methotrexate in the correct timetable prescribed by the oncologist. If a dose is missed, the patient should not take the missed dose at a later time, or double the next prescribed dose. Rather, the patient should maintain the schedule prescribed and notify the oncologist about the missed dose.

Precautions

To maximize treatment effects, patients receiving methotrexate should observe certain guidelines. Including any modifications given by the oncologist, these guidelines should include regular visits with the oncologist and laboratory testing for white blood cell count, kidney, liver, and bone marrow function. Avoid any immunizations not approved or prescribed by the oncologist. Avoid contact with individuals taking or that have recently taken oral polio vaccine, or individuals that have an active **infection**. When necessary wear a protective facemask. Avoid prolonged or direct exposure to sunlight, as some patients experience an increased sensitivity. Ask for specific instructions on oral hygiene procedures to reduce the risk of gum abrasion, and avoid touching the eye and nasal areas unless hands have been properly washed immediately prior to contact. To reduce bleeding and bruising complications, patients should exercise extreme caution when handling sharp instruments and decline participation in contact sports. Prior to treatment, the patient's medical history should be thoroughly reviewed to avoid complications that might arise from previous conditions such as gout, kidney stones or kidney disease, liver disease, chickenpox, shingles, intestinal blockage, colitis, immunosupression, stomach ulcers, mouth sores, or a history of allergic reactions to various drugs. The oncologist should also be made aware if the patient is pregnant or if there is the possibility the patient might be pregnant, or if the patient is a breast-feeding mother. Only prescribed medications or over the counter (OTC) drugs approved by the oncologist should be taken by a patient receiving methotrexate.

Side effects

The beneficial effects of methotrexate are usually accompanied by less desirable side effects. Side effects correlate in severity with dose amount and length of treatment. It is important to encourage the patient to discuss any presenting side effects. Some side effects do not require medical attention, but still cause the patient concern. Side effects that fall into this category may include loss of hair (**alopecia**) and appetite (**anorexia**), **nausea** or **vomiting**, skin rash with **itching**, pale skin tone, and the appearance of boils or acne. These side effects tend to diminish as the body adjusts to the therapy, or if they become bothersome, the oncologist may prescribe interventions. Side effects that should be reported immediately to the oncologist include mouth sores; back, lower side, joint or stomach pain; **fever** or chills; headaches; bloody or dark urine; drowsiness; dizziness; black tarry stools; bloody stools or vomit; **diarrhea**; redness or pinpoint red spots on the skin; swelling of the feet or lower legs; the development of a cough or hoarseness; and shortness of breath.

Interactions

Anti-inflammatory medications should be avoided while the patient is receiving methotrexate. These drugs elevate the effects of methotrexate to potentially harmful levels. **Vaccines** should be avoided due to the immunosuppression action of methotrexate, and alcohol should be avoided to reduce the risk of liver complications.

Jane Taylor-Jones, Research Associate, M.S.

Methylphenidate

Definition

Methylphenidate is a mild central nervous system stimulant. It is the most commonly prescribed medication for treating children with attention-deficit/hyperactivity disorder (ADHD) and is also used to treat narcolepsy and certain other conditions.

Purpose

The primary use of methylphenidate, first developed in 1956, is in the treatment of ADHD in children and adults. ADHD is the most common childhood neurobehavioral disorder. Every year more than 2.5 million children are medicated for ADHD. Methylphenidate increases the release of the neurotransmitters norepinephrine and dopamine. Although the drug can cause restlessness in normal individuals, it generally calms children with ADHD, improving their ability to focus and helping to control motor restlessness, inattention, and impulsivity. Hyperactive children who take methylphenidate have improved self-control, make fewer errors in their schoolwork, and get along better with their peers. Children with ADHD often take methylphenidate only during the school year.

Methylphenidate is also used to prevent daytime sleep episodes in patients with severe narcolepsy. On occasion it is used to decrease sedation and lethargy from opioid pain medications and to help relieve **depression** in terminally ill patients. It is sometimes used to increase appetite and energy levels in **cancer** patients.

Description

Methylphenidate comes in a variety of strengths and forms:

- 5-, 10-, and 20-milligram (mg) tablets
- chewable tablets
- immediate-release tablets
- intermediate-acting (extended-release) 20-mg tablets
- long-acting (extended-release) capsules and tablets
- solutions
- skin patches for children aged 6–12

U.S. brand names

- Ritalin, Ritalin LA, Ritalin-SR
- Metadate CD, Metadate ER
- Methylin, Methylin ER
- Concerta (long-acting tablets)
- Daytrana (patch) p

Canadian brand names

- Ritalin, Ritalin SR
- PMS-Methylphenidate
- Riphenidate
- Concerta

International brand names

- Ritalin
- Ritalina
- Rubifen
- Concerta

Recommended dosage

Methylphenidate dosages depend on the form of the drug, body weight, and individual responses. For treating ADHD, regular tablet and solution forms are usually introduced with two low daily doses—preferably 35–45 minutes before breakfast and lunch—of 0.3 mg/kilogram (kg) of body weight or 2.5–5 mg per dose. The dosage is increased at weekly intervals by 0.1 mg/kg/dose or 5–10 mg/day, to a maximum of 2 mg/kg/day or 90 mg/day. The usual therapeutic dose is 0.5–1 mg/kg/day or 20–30 mg per day.

The recommended dosage for treating narcolepsy in adults is 5–20 mg two to three times a day, 30–45 minutes before meals.

The usual adult dose to counteract opiate side effects is 2.5–15 mg once or twice per day.

Methylphenidate should be taken exactly as directed. The last dose of the day should be short-acting and taken before 6 P.M. because it can interfere with sleep. Tablets should be swallowed whole: crushing or breaking them changes the absorption time. A missed dose should be taken as soon as possible, but two tablets should not be taken at the same time.

Precautions

It is relatively easy to become physically and/or psychologically dependent on methylphenidate, particularly if it is taken at higher dosages or for longer than necessary. Signs of physical dependency include:

- having to increase the dosage to achieve the same effect
- mental depression
- unusual behavior
- fatigue or weakness

Methylphenidate should be tapered off gradually before discontinuing. Halting the drug abruptly can cause withdrawal symptoms including:

- headache
- irritability
- nausea
- abnormal chewing and tongue movements
- anxiety
- agitation
- sleep disturbance
- depression
- paranoia
- suicidal thoughts

Patients should not drive or operate machinery or appliances until they understand how methylphenidate affects them, since it makes some people lightheaded or dizzy.

Methylphenidate may cause changes in the composition of the blood and in liver function. Patients should receive regular blood tests and blood pressure and pulse checks while taking this drug.

Pediatric

Methylphenidate has undergone more testing than any other drug prescribed for children. Although it is generally considered safe and effective for the treatment of ADHD, the increasing frequency with which it is prescribed for younger and younger children has caused a great deal of controversy. Some medical professionals believe that methylphenidate is over-prescribed. They call for better diagnostic procedures conducted by trained personnel, rather than relying on subjective observations by parents and teachers for diagnosing ADHD. Children should have a drug-free period ("drug holiday") for at least several weeks every year. Methylphenidate should not be prescribed for children under age six.

Methylphenidate can cause sudden death in children, teenagers, and adults, especially those with heart defects or other serious heart problems. The American Heart Association recommends that children be monitored for heart problems before administration of methylphenidate.

Pregnant or breastfeeding

Methylphenidate is in pregnancy category C, meaning that there have been no adequate studies in pregnant women. It is not usually prescribed for women in their childbearing years, unless the physician determines that the benefits outweigh the risks. It is not known whether methylphenidate passes into breast milk; however breastfeeding is not recommended while taking this drug.

Other conditions and allergies

Methylphenidate can cause sudden death, heart attack, or stroke, especially in those with heart defects or other serious heart problems. It should be used with caution in patients with high blood pressure or a history of seizures. Methylphenidate is contraindicated for patients with:

- severe anxiety, tension, or agitation
- severe depression
- mental or emotional instability

- certain other mental-health conditions
- a history of alcohol or drug abuse
- epilepsy
- Tourette's syndrome
- tic disorders
- glaucoma

Side effects

The most common side effects of methylphenidate are nervousness, sleep disturbances, rapid heartbeat, and increased blood pressure. Reducing the dose, changing the time of day the drug is taken, or having regular drug-free periods may reduce some side effects.

Other side effects of methylphenidate may include:

- agitation
- dizziness
- irritability
- vision changes
- drowsiness
- nausea
- vomiting
- loss of appetite
- stomach pain
- diarrhea
- heartburn
- dry mouth
- headache
- muscle tightness
- restlessness
- numbness, burning, or tingling in the hands or feet
- decreased sexual desire
- painful menstruation

Less common side effects of methylphenidate include:

- chest pain
- heart palpitations
- joint pain
- skin rash
- uncontrolled speech or movements
- blood in the urine or stool
- muscle cramps
- red dots on the skin
- bruising

At higher dosages or with long-term use, side effects of methylphenidate may include **weight loss** or mental changes such as confusion, false beliefs, mood changes, hallucinations, or dissociative symptoms.

QUESTIONS TO ASK YOUR PHARMACIST

- How should I give this medication to my child?
- What if my child misses a dose?
- What side effects are to be expected?
- Can I take my child off this drug whenever I want?
- Should my child have drug-free periods?

Symptoms of methylphenidate overdose include:

- inappropriate happiness
- sweating
- flushing
- headache
- fever
- fast, pounding, or irregular heartbeat
- widening of pupils
- dry mouth or nose
- vomiting
- agitation
- muscle twitching
- uncontrollable shaking of a part of the body
- confusion
- hallucinations
- loss of consciousness

Pediatric

The most serious pediatric side effect of methylphenidate is growth suppression. It may slow a child's rate of growth or weight gain. Other common side effects in children include insomnia, appetite loss, and stomach pains.

Interactions

Methylphenidate may have adverse interactions with many drugs including:

- amphetamines
- appetite suppressants
- caffeine
- cocaine
- asthma medications
- cold, sinus and hay fever medications
- nabilone
- pemoline

- monoamine oxidase inhibitors (MAOIs) and other antidepressants
- pimozide
- anticoagulants (blood thinners)
- anti-seizure drugs
- high blood pressure medications

Methylphenidate should not be taken within two weeks of having taken an MAOI.

Resources

BOOKS

Diller, Lawrence H. *The Last Normal Child: Essays on the Intersection of Kids, Culture, and Psychiatric Drugs.* Westport, CT: Praeger, 2006.

Iversen, Leslie L. *Speed, Ecstasy, Ritalin: The Science of Amphetamines.* New York: Oxford University Press, 2006.

Tone, Andrea, and Elizabeth Siegel Watkins. *Medicating Modern America: Prescription Drugs in History.* New York: New York University Press, 2007.

PERIODICALS

Ahuja, Anjana. "Ritalin? Does It Work?" *The Times* (London) (November 16, 2007): 6.

Godfrey, J. "The Prevalence and Correlates of Adult ADHD in the United States: Results from the National Comorbidity Survey Replication." *American Journal of Psychiatry* 163 (2006): 716–723.

Kessler, R. C., et al. "Safety of Therapeutic Methylphenidate in Adults: A Systematic Review of the Evidence." *Journal of Psychopharmacology* 23, no. 2 (March 2009): 194.

Rubin, Rita. "Sudden Death in Kids, ADHD Drugs Linked." *Miami Times* 86, no. 43 (June 24–30, 2009): 11B.

OTHER

American Society of Health-System Pharmacists. "Methylphenidate." *MedlinePlus.* http://www.nlm.nih.gov/medlineplus/druginfo/meds/a682188.html

"NIDA InfoFacts: Stimulant ADHD Medications—Methylphenidate and Amphetamines." *National Institute on Drug Abuse.* http://www.drugabuse.gov/infofacts/ADHD.html

"NIDA Study Shows That Methylphenidate (Ritalin) Causes Neuronal Changes in Brain Reward Areas." *National Institute on Drug Abuse.* http://www.drugabuse.gov/newsroom/09/NR2-02.html

Vetter, Victoria L., et al. "Cardiovascular Monitoring of Children and Adolescents With Heart Disease Receiving Medications for Attention Deficit/Hyperactivity Disorder: A Scientific Statement From the American Heart Association Council on Cardiovascular Disease in the Young, Congenital Cardiac Defects Committee, and the Council on Cardiovascular Nursing." *Circulation.* http://circ.ahajournals.org/cgi/content/full/117/18/2407

ORGANIZATIONS

American Academy of Pediatrics, 141 Northwest Point Blvd., Elk Grove Village, IL, 60007-1098, (874) 434-4000, (874) 434-8000, kidsdocs@aap.org, http://www.aap.org.

American Heart Association, 7272 Greenville Avenue, Dallas, TX, 75231, (800) 242-8721, http://www.americanheart.org.

National Institute on Drug Abuse (NIDA), 6001 Executive Boulevard, Room 5213, Bethesda, MD, 20892-9561, (301) 443-1124, information@nida.nih.gov, http://www.drugabuse.gov/NIDAHome.html.

U.S. Food and Drug Administration, 10903 New Hampshire Ave., Silver Spring, MD, 20993-0002, (888) INFO-FDA, http://www.fda.gov.

Debra Wood, RN
L. Fleming Fallon, Jr, MD, DrPH.
Margaret Alic, PhD

Methylprednisolone *see* **Corticosteroids**

Metoclopramide

Definition

Metoclopramide (Reglan, Octamide, Maxeran) is a drug used to prevent the **nausea and vomiting** caused by **cancer chemotherapy**, diabetic **neuropathy**, gastroesophageal reflux, and similar conditions. It has also been approved by the Food and Drug Administration (FDA) to treat the small bowel prior to intubation. Metoclopramide is one of the drugs most frequently used in palliative care for cancer patients.

Purpose

Nausea and **vomiting** are among the most common side effects of cancer chemotherapy. They are also among the most unpleasant and upsetting side effects for patients. If left untreated, persistent nausea and vomiting can lead to dehydration, dental decay, digestive abnormalities, and nutritional deficiencies. In addition, persistent vomiting may force some patients to stop taking their chemotherapy and risk a recurrence of their cancer. It is therefore very important that these symptoms be adequately treated.

The nausea and vomiting that occurs with chemotherapy is often divided into three types: anticipatory, acute, and delayed. Anticipatory nausea and vomiting usually occurs before or during chemotherapy. These symptoms are thought to be caused by anxiety, and often occur in patients who have been previously

KEY TERMS

Antiemetic—A drug that prevents nausea and vomiting.

Dyskinesia—A condition that causes a person to make abnormal, involuntary movements.

Palliative care—Care given to relieve pain and other symptoms of a disease but not to cure the disease.

treated with very toxic chemotherapy. Acute nausea and vomiting occurs within a few minutes to several hours after drug administration and usually stops within 24 hours. Delayed nausea and vomiting occurs several hours after chemotherapy, and can last several days.

Description

For the majority of patients, nausea and vomiting can be successfully treated with antiemetic medication. Metoclopramide is one of the most widely used and effective **antiemetics** for treating the delayed nausea and vomiting caused by chemotherapy. It has been used since the 1980s, and works in two ways. It affects a part of the brain known to trigger vomiting, and also affects the speed of intestinal motion. As a result, the stomach empties into the intestines more quickly, and the contents of the intestines move more quickly in the correct direction.

Metoclopramide is most often used in patients taking **cisplatin** (Platinol) chemotherapy. Cisplatin is used to treat a wide range of cancers including **bladder cancer**, **ovarian cancer** and **non-small cell lung cancer**. Compared with other cancer chemotherapy, cisplatin is often considered to cause the most severe nausea and vomiting. For 60–70% of patients taking cisplatin, however, metoclopramide provides adequate control of nausea and vomiting.

Recommended dosage

Although metoclopramide can be taken either orally or intravenously, cancer patients on chemotherapy usually receive the drug intravenously. Metoclopramide is usually given 30 minutes before chemotherapy, and then two more times after chemotherapy at two hour intervals.

The recommended dose varies from patient to patient, and depends on both the severity of nausea and vomiting, and on the toxicity of the drug. A higher dose will be given to patients with severe symptoms. Higher doses will also be given to patients receiving drugs such as cisplatin that are known to cause severe nausea and vomiting. Some patients receiving cisplatin may be given a combination of three different drugs to help combat their nausea: metoclopramide, **dexamethasone** (Dexone), and **lorazepam** (Ativan). The three work on different areas of the body and produce a greater effect together than they do when given separately.

Precautions

Metoclopramide can cause sleepiness and lack of concentration. Patients should avoid tasks that require mental alertness such as driving or operating machinery. Patients should also be aware that metoclopramide may enhance their response to alcohol and drugs that depress the central nervous system. Because metoclopramide can cause **depression**, patients with a history of serious clinical depression should take this drug only if absolutely necessary.

Metoclopramide can make the symptoms of Parkinson's disease worse, and patients with a history of seizures should not take metoclopramide, because the frequency and severity of the seizures may increase. The drug should also not be used in patients with intestinal problems such as bleeding, tears, or blockages. The safety of metoclopramide for pregnant women or children is unknown. The drug is found in the breast milk of lactating mothers.

Side effects

The most frequent side effects of metoclopramide are restlessness, drowsiness, and **fatigue**. These occur in about 10% of patients. Less common side effects include insomnia, headache, and dizziness. These occur in only 5% of patients. Feelings of anxiety or agitation may also occur, especially after a rapid intravenous injection of the drug. Some women may experience menstrual irregularities.

Metaclopramide therapy can cause some patients to make abnormal involuntary movements, a condition known as dyskinesia. These reactions are most common in young adults of 18–30 years of age, and often disappear about a day after the patient stops taking the drug. Among geriatric patients, particularly women, dyskinesia sometimes develops when patients stop taking metoclopramide after long term treatment.

Interactions

Patients who are also taking cabergoline (Dostinex), a drug used to treat hormonal problems and Parkinson's disease, should not take metoclopramide.

Because metoclopramide affects the functioning of the intestines, it can interfere with the absorption of certain drugs. The effect of digoxin (Lanoxin), for example, may be reduced, whereas the effects of other drugs like aspirin, **cyclosporine** (Neoral, Sandimmune, SangCya) and tetracycline (Minocin, Vibramycin) may be enhanced.

Resources

BOOKS

Karch, A. M. *Lippincott's Nursing Drug Guide*. Springhouse, PA: Lippincott Williams & Wilkins, 2003.

PERIODICALS

Duby, J. J., R. K. Campbell, S. M. Setter, et al. "Diabetic Neuropathy: An Intensive Review." *American Journal of Health-System Pharmacy* 61 (January 15, 2004): 160–173.

Nauck, F., C. Ostgathe, E. Klaschik, et al. "Drugs in Palliative Care: Results from a Representative Survey in Germany." *Palliative Medicine* 18 (March 2004): 100–107.

Steely, R. L., D. R. Collins Jr., B. E. Cohen, and K. Bass. "Postoperative Nausea and Vomiting in the Plastic Surgery Patient." *Aesthetic Plastic Surgery* 28 (January-February 2004): 29–32.

ORGANIZATIONS

American Society of Health-System Pharmacists (ASHP). 7272 Wisconsin Avenue, Bethesda, MD 20814. (301) 657-3000. http://www.ashp.org.

United States Food and Drug Administration (FDA). 5600 Fishers Lane, Rockville, MD 20857-0001. (888) INFO-FDA. http://www.fda.gov.

Alison McTavish, M.Sc.
Rebecca J. Frey, Ph.D.

Metronidazole *see* **Antibiotics**

Mistletoe

Description

Mistletoe is a parasitic evergreen plant that lives on trees such as oak, elm, fir, and apple. The parasitic plant has yellowish flowers, small yellowish green leaves, and waxy white berries. There are many species of this plant in the Viscacea and Loranthacea plant families. European mistletoe (*Viscum album*) and American mistletoe (*Phoradendron leucarpum*) are used as medical remedies. In addition to Europe and North America, mistletoe is also found in Australia and Korea.

Mistletoe berries are poisonous to cats and other small animals. There is, however, some debate about how toxic the berries are to humans, and there is controversy about whether it is safe to use mistletoe as a remedy. Mistletoe is also known as mystyldene, all-heal, bird lime, golden bough, and devil's fuge.

General use

Mistletoe is known popularly as the plant sprig that people kiss beneath during the Christmas season. That custom dates back to pagan times when, according to legend, the plant was thought to inspire passion and increase fertility.

Over the centuries, mistletoe has acquired a reputation as an all-purpose herbal remedy. In the seventeenth century, French herbalists prescribed mistletoe for nervous disorders, epilepsy, and the spasms known as the St. Vitus dance.

Mistletoe has also been used in folk medicine as a digestive aid, heart tonic, and sedative. It was used to treat arthritis, hysteria and other mental disturbances, **amenorrhea**, wounds, asthma, bed wetting, **infection**, and to stimulate glands.

For centuries, mistletoe also served as a folk medicine treatment for **cancer**, and as of early 2005, the plant is sometimes used in Europe to treat tumors. Iscador, an extract of the European mistletoe plant, is said to stimulate the immune system and kill cancer cells. It reportedly reduces the size of tumors and improves the quality of life. Iscador is one brand name of the mistletoe extract in Europe, and other brand names include Helixor and Eurixor.

Although in alternative medicine mistletoe is viewed as a multipurpose remedy, there is disagreement among medical experts about the safety and effectiveness of this herb. The number of possible interactions with other medications described below indicates that mistletoe should be used with caution.

Preparations

In alternative medicine, the leaves, twigs, and sometimes the berries of mistletoe are used. In Europe, mistletoe remedies range from tea made from mistletoe leaves to injections of Iscador. However, the berries may be poisonous and the herb may cause liver damage.

Since 2005 mistletoe has not been tested by the United States Food and Drug Administration (FDA), many experts urge caution until more research is completed.

Home remedies

Mistletoe tea may be an alternative treatment for conditions that include high blood pressure, asthma, epilepsy, nervousness, **diarrhea**, and amenorrhea. The tea is prepared by adding 1 tsp (5 g) of finely cut mistletoe to 1 cup (250 ml) of cold water. The solution is steeped at room temperature for 12 hours and then strained.

Mistletoe wine is prepared by mixing 8 tsp (40 g) of the herb into 34 oz (1 L) of wine. After three days, the wine can be consumed. Three to four glasses of medicinal wine may be consumed each day.

Mistletoe must be stored away from light and kept above a drying agent.

Cancer treatment

Iscador, the European extract, may be injected before surgery for cancers of the cervix, ovary, breast, stomach, colon, and lung. Cancer treatments can take several months to several years. The treatment is given by subcutaneous injection, preferably near the tumor. Iscador may be injected into the tumor, especially tumors of the liver, cervix, or esophagus.

The dosage of Iscador varies according to the patient's age, sex, physical condition, and type of cancer. The treatment usually is given in the morning three to seven days per week. As treatment continues, the dosage may be increased or adjusted.

Advocates of Iscador believe it can stimulate the immune system, kill cancer cells, inhibit the formation of tumors, and extend the survival time of cancer patients. They maintain that mistletoe can help prevent cancer and be complementary to standard medical cancer treatments. They also think that mistletoe could possibly repair the DNA that is decreased by **chemotherapy** and radiation.

AIDS treatment

Mistletoe extract has been used to combat AIDS, but its efficacy has not been medically confirmed as of 2005.

Precautions

Opinions are sharply divided on how safe and effective the herb is as a home remedy and in the treatment of conditions such as cancer and AIDS. There is controversy about which parts of the plants are poisonous. Although the berries are classified as poisonous in the United States, some sources say that eating berries is only dangerous for babies, and only if handfuls are consumed. Pregnant or breast-feeding women, however, should not use the plant.

According to a report from the Hepatitis Foundation International, mistletoe is toxic to the liver. However, the *PDR for Herbal Medicines* advises that there are no health hazards when mistletoe is taken properly and in designated therapeutic dosages.

People considering mistletoe should consult with their doctors or practitioners. Until there is definitive proof otherwise, there is a risk that the herbal remedies will conflict with conventional treatment.

Side effects

Mistletoe may be toxic to the liver. For people diagnosed with hepatitis, use of an herb such as mistletoe may cause additional liver damage. However, advocates of mistletoe maintain it is safe, at least under certain circumstances.

Commercial mistletoe extracts may produce fewer side effects. The body temperature may rise and there may be flu-like symptoms. The patient may experience **nausea**, abdominal pain, and (if given the extract injection) inflammation around the injection sight. Allergy symptoms may result.

Interactions

Mistletoe should not be used by people who take monoamine oxidase (MAO) inhibitor antidepressants such as Nardil. Potential reactions include a dangerous rise in blood pressure and a lowering of blood potassium levels (hypokalemia). In addition, mistletoe may interfere with the action of antidiabetic medications, to increase the activity of diuretics, and to increase the risk of a toxic reaction to aspirin or NSAIDs. Cancer patients considering mistletoe treatment should first consult with their doctors or practitioners.

Resources

PERIODICALS

Kroz, M., F. Schad, B. Matthes, et al. "Blood and Tissue Eosinophilia, Mistletoe Lectin Antibodies, and Quality of Life in a Breast Cancer Patient Undergoing Intratumoral and Subcutaneous Mistletoe Injection." [in German] *Forschende Komplementarmedizin und Klassische Naturheilkunde* 9 (June 2002): 160–67.

Maier, G., and H. H. Fiebig. "Absence of Tumor Growth Stimulation in a Panel of Sixteen Human Tumor Cell Lines by Mistletoe Extracts in Vitro." *Anticancer Drugs* 13 (April 2002): 373–79.

Mengs, U., D. Gothel, and E. Leng-Peschlow. "Mistletoe Extracts Standardized to Mistletoe Lectins in Oncology: Review on Current Status of Preclinical Research." *Anticancer Research* 22 (May-June 2002): 1399–1407.

Tabiasco, J., et al. "Mistletoe Viscotoxins Increase Natural Killer Cell-Mediated Cytotoxicity." *European Journal of Biochemistry* 269 (May 2002): 2591–2600.

ORGANIZATIONS

American Botanical Council. PO Box 201660, Austin, TX 78720. (512)331-8868. http://www.herbalgram.org.

Herb Research Foundation. 1007 Pearl St., Suite 200, Boulder, CO 80302. (303)449-2265. http://www.herbs.org.

National Cancer Institute (NCI). NCI Public Inquiries Office, Suite 3036-A, 6116 Executive Boulevard, MSC8322, Bethesda, MD, 20892.(800)422-6237. http://www.nci.nih.gov/cancerinfo/pdq/cam/mistletoe.

Liz Swain
Rebecca J. Frey, Ph.D.

Mithramycin *see* **Plicamycin**

Mitoguazone

Definition

Mitoguazone is an investigational (experimental) medicine used to stop growth of **cancer** and formation of new cancer cells.

Purpose

Mitoguazone may be effective in patients with acute leukemia, **chronic myelocytic leukemia**, **lymphoma**, **multiple myeloma**, **head and neck cancers**, **esophageal cancer**, and other types of malignancies.

Description

Mitoguazone, also known as MGBG, was discovered in 1898. The exact mechanism of MGBG action is not fully understood and a variety of mechanisms appear to be involved. Most likely, MGBG's antitumor activity comes from inhibition of spermine, a protein necessary for cell reproduction. This drug underwent numerous **clinical trials** in the early 1960s; however, the trials were discontinued due to severe toxicities noticed when MGBG was given on a daily basis. In these early research trials, MGBG was shown to have both anticancer and antiviral activity. Later, researchers discovered that MGBG has a long duration of action in the body and can be given less frequently. In 1976 MGBG enjoyed a rebirth when Southwest Oncology Group started using once weekly administration schedule of this agent in patients with lymphoma (Hodgkin's and non-Hodgkin's type), esophageal cancer, **prostate cancer** and other tumor types.

In addition to being effective as a single agent, MGBG was used in combination **chemotherapy** regimens containing **ifosfamide**, **methotrexate** and **etoposide** (also known as MIME regimen). The best results with MGBG have been obtained against **Hodgkin's** and **non-Hodgkin's lymphoma** using MIME regimen.

Mitoguazone appears particularly effective in patients who are malnourished and would be ideally suited for patients with AIDS-associated lymphomas. Another potential advantage of mitoguazone in patients with AIDS is its high penetration into the brain, since the brain is one area frequently involved by lymphoma in this patient population.

KEY TERMS

AIDS—Also known as acquired immunodeficiency syndrome, caused by the progression of HIV, and is the leading cause of death from HIV. AIDS is characterized by opportunistic diseases, including fungal infections, pneumocystis carinii pneumonia, non-Hodgkin's lymphoma, and other malignant or infectious illnesses.

Non-Hodgkin's lymphoma—Lymphomas are some of the most treatable cancers with cure rates around 50% in 1990s. Non-Hodgkin's lymphoma mainly affects people over 50 years of age and has been more difficult to treat than the Hodgkin's type. There has been an increase in non-Hodgkin's lymphoma cases in the last two decades in patients with HIV.

Recommended dosage

Adults

AIDS-ASSOCIATED NON-HODKIN'S LYMPHOMA. Doses vary between different chemotherapy protocols. One of the schedules used was 600 mg per square meter of body surface area given intravenously on days 1, 8, and then every two weeks.

Children

There is no data available on dosing and use of mitoguazone in children.

Precautions

To maximize treatment effects, patients receiving mitoguazone should observe certain guidelines. In addition to any modifications given by the oncologist, these guidelines should include regular visits with the oncologist and laboratory testing for white blood cell count, liver, and bone marrow function. Avoid any immunizations not approved or prescribed by the oncologist. When necessary wear a protective facemask. Use good oral hygiene to reduce incidence of mouth sores and avoid touching the eye and nasal areas unless hands have been properly washed immediately prior to contact. To reduce bleeding and bruising complications, patients should exercise extreme caution when handling sharp instruments and decline participation in contact sports. Prior to treatment, the patient's medical history should be thoroughly reviewed to avoid complications that might arise from previous conditions such as liver disease, chickenpox, shingles, peripheral **neuropathy** (tingling and weakness in hands or feet), suppressed immune system, stomach ulcers, mouth sores, or a history of allergic reactions to various drugs.

Contact a doctor immediately if any of these symptoms develop:

- signs of infection (fever, chills, sore throat)
- pain, numbness, and tingling in fingers or toes
- severe muscle weakness
- nausea, vomiting, and yellowing of the skin or eyes
- unresolved mouth sores
- mental status changes (euphoria, drowsiness, anxiety, emotional instability)
- unusual bleeding or bruising
- skin rash or itching

Side effects

The dose-limiting toxicity of MGBG is muscle weakness. The most common side effect of MGBG is flushing primarily on the face during infusion. Other toxicities associated with MGBG are usually mild, consisting of somnolence, tingling in the face or extremities, ringing in the ears, euphoria, mouth ulcers, **nausea**, **vomiting**, and **fatigue**. This drug also lacks significant **myelosuppression**, which makes it an ideal agent to consider for combination regimens.

Interactions

The drug and food interactions with MGBG have not been studied in research trials. There is a theoretical drug interaction between MGBG and pentamidine (a drug used to prevent and treat pneumocystis carinii **pneumonia** in AIDS patients). Pentamidine inhibits the same enzyme in the body as MGBG, which can enhance effects of MGBG. This interaction can either increase effectiveness of MGBG against cancer or put patients at higher risk of its side effects.

Olga Bessmertny, Pharm.D.

Mitomycin-C

Definition

Mitomycin-C is also known as mitomycin and MMC. It is an antineoplastic, or medicine that kills **cancer** cells. It is sold under the trade name Mutamycin.

Purpose

Mitomycin-C may be used to fight a number of different cancers, including cancer of the stomach, colon, rectum, pancreas, breast, lung, uterus, cervix, bladder, head, neck, eye, and esophagus.

It is impossible to provide a detailed description of how mitomycin-C may be combined with other medications in the treatment of each of these cancers, but some examples can be presented. In the treatment of **non-small cell lung cancer** (NSCLC), one therapeutic regimen that may be used is known as MT, which consists of mitomycin-C, **vindesine**, and **cisplatin**.

Mitomycin-C is sometimes used in patients with colorectal cancer metastatic to the liver. However, the side effects of mitomycin-C, especially those involving the bone marrow and **fatigue**, are so great that other medications may be tried first. In treating **breast cancer** metastatic to the liver, mitomycin is regarded as salvage therapy.

For advanced **stomach cancer**, the FAM regimen may be used, which consists of **fluorouracil**, **doxorubicin** (adriamycin), and mitomycin-C. Mitomycin-C may also be used for colorectal cancer metastatic to the liver in combination with other medicines.

More recently, mitomycin has been found effective in treating malignant **melanoma** of the eye.

In addition to cancer treatment, mitomycin is sometimes used as a topical application in eye surgery to prevent visual haze after operations on the cornea (the transparent exterior coat that covers the front of the eye where light enters). It is also used topically by some doctors to keep incisions in the ear drum open in children with recurrent ear infections without the need to place ventilation tubes in the incisions. This use of mitomycin is considered experiental.

Description

Mitomycin-C is an antitumor antibiotic. Mechanistically however, it belongs to DNA covalent binding (alkylating) agents. Mitomycin-C, upon bioactivation, kills cancer cells by disrupting the activity of DNA

KEY TERMS

Antineoplastic—A medicine given to kill cancer cells.

Salvage therapy—A term that refers to measures taken at a late point in the treatment process after other therapies have failed.

Topical—Referring to a medication or other preparation applied directly to the skin or other external body tissues..

within the cells. DNA is an acid that contains genetic material.

Recommended dosage

Twenty milligrams per square meter should be given intravenously every six to eight weeks when this medication is used alone. Alternately, five to ten milligrams per square meter may be given every six weeks when the drug is used in combination with other drugs. Mitomycin-C, **leucovorin**, and fluorouracil may be used to treat metastatic **rectal cancer**; this regimen includes an injection of 10 milligrams per square meter of mitomycin-C. When mitomycin-C is combined with vindesine and cisplatin in the treatment of non-small cell lung cancer, eight milligrams per square inch are administered intravenously on days one and twenty-nine of a six-week cycle.

Precautions

Because of the side effects associated with mitomycin-C, some physicians perform blood tests and order chest **x rays** (of the lungs) for patients receiving this therapy. The likelihood that lung problems will appear in patients receiving mitomycin-C increases if oxygen therapy and/or x-ray therapy are administered.

Patients receiving less than 60 mg of mitomycin-C are at reduced risk of developing a complex medical condition called cancer-associated hemolytic uremia syndrome (HUS). HUS is characterized by **anemia**, other blood defects, and kidney problems. Doctors should carefully observe patients receiving mitomycin-C, as cancer-related HUS is best treated early. However, HUS is not likely to develop until four or more months after the patient received the final dose of mitomycin-C. To achieve early diagnosis of HUS, the doctor may carefully monitor kidney function and blood levels. In addition, transfusions may be avoided as may be certain other procedures involving the blood, as these may increase the risk HUS will develop.

Side effects

The ability of the bone marrow to produce blood cells may be affected. This side effect can be serious. If it occurs, the doctor may decide to reduce the dose of medicine administered. However, mitomycin-C may cause delayed, rather than immediate, bone marrow suppression. Once such suppression does occur it may last for as many as eight weeks.

Major lung problems may occur. Such lung deficits may start as no more than cough, fatigue, and breathing problems. Doctors may conduct lung function tests and obtain x rays to observe whether lung problems are developing. If these lung problems do occur, **corticosteroids** may provide effective therapy. Stopping mitomycin-C therapy may also be recommended.

Mitomycin-C may also cause cancer-associated HUS.

In addition, there may be **nausea and vomiting**, loss of appetite (**anorexia**), stomach problems, fatigue, **fever**, hair loss (**alopecia**), and lung problems. If bleeding does occur, there may be damage to the surrounding skin.

Resources

BOOKS

Wilson, Billie A., Margaret T. Shannon, and Carolyn L. Stang. *Nurses Drug Guide 2000*. Stamford, CT: Appleton & Lange, 2000.

PERIODICALS

Brownstein, S. "Malignant Melanoma of the Conjunctiva." *Cancer Control* 11 (September-October 2004): 310–316.

d'Eredita, R. "Contact Diode Laser Myringotomy and Mitomycin C in Children." *Otolaryngology and Head and Neck Surgery* 130 (June 2004): 742–746.

Hashemi, H., S. M. Taheri, A. Fotouhi, and A. Kheiltash. "Evaluation of the Prophylactic Use of Mitomycin-C to Inhibit Haze Formation after Photorefractive Keratectomy in High Myopia: A Prospective Clinical Study." *BMC Ophthalmology* 4 (September 14, 2004): 12.

Loibl, S., G. von Minckwitz, K. Schwedler, et al. "Mitomycin C, 5-Fluorouracil and Folinic acid (Mi-Fu-Fo) as Salvage Chemotherapy in Breast Cancer Patients with Liver Metastases and Impaired Hepatic Function: A Phase II Study." *Anti-Cancer Drugs* 15 (August 2004): 719–724.

Rao, S., D. Cunningham, T. Price, et al. "Phase II Study of Capecitabine and Mitomycin C as First-Line Treatment in Patients with Advanced Colorectal Cancer." *British Journal of Cancer* 91 (August 31, 2004): 839–843.

Solomon, R., E. D. Donnenfeld, J. Thimons, et al. "Hyperopic Photorefractive Keratectomy with Adjunctive Topical Mitomycin C for Refractive Error after Penetrating Keratoplasty for Keratoconus." *Eye and Contact Lens* 30 (July 2004): 156–158.

ORGANIZATIONS

American Society of Health-System Pharmacists (ASHP). 7272 Wisconsin Avenue, Bethesda, MD 20814. (301) 657-3000. http://www.ashp.org.

United States Food and Drug Administration (FDA). 5600 Fishers Lane, Rockville, MD 20857-0001. (888) INFO-FDA. http://www.fda.gov.

Bob Kirsch
Rebecca J. Frey, Ph.D.

Mitotane

Definition

Mitotane (also known by the brand name Lysodren) is a medicine that has been proven to be effective in the treatment of **adrenocortical carcinoma**.

Purpose

Mitotane destroys cells of the adrenocortex. The adrenocortex, also called the adrenal cortex, is a section of adrenal gland that sits on top of the kidneys. Mitotane is usually used for patients whose **cancer** cannot be treated surgically and for patients whose cancer has metastasized.

Description

As a chemical, mitotane resembles the insecticides DDD and DDT, although mitotane does not harm people as these do. Scientists do not understand why, but the drug causes damage to the adrenocortex in such a way as to be helpful for some patients with adrenocortical tumors. In addition, mitotane restricts the ability of the gland to produce chemicals.

Recommended dosage

The dose of mitotane given to patients varies, although between four and eight grams (0.12–0.25 oz) per day is a typical dose. Patients vary in how much mitotane they tolerate, some patients tolerating two grams (0.1 oz) per day while others tolerate sixteen grams (0.5 oz) per day. The doses are given orally. At the beginning of the therapy, the patient may receive 500 milligrams of mitotane twice a day. At any one time a third or a quarter of an entire day's dose is taken. If the patient has difficulty tolerating a certain dose, the doctors may adjust this and use a somewhat smaller dose. Mitotane should be given for at least three months. If the medicine is effective, it may be continued indefinitely. However, most patients respond to the x-ray treatment of the pituitary gland and so do not need mitotane treatment to continue indefinitely.

Many doctors use mitotane in conjunction with **radiation therapy** directed to the pituitary gland, but other approaches to this medicine may also be taken.

KEY TERMS

Adrenocortex—The outer part of adrenal gland that sits on top of the kidneys.

Anorexia—A condition of uncontrolled lack or loss of desire for food.

Precautions

Many patients on mitotane should receive adrenocorticosteroids.

Side effects

Four out of five patients receiving mitotane experience **anorexia** and **nausea**. About one-third of patients experience lethargy and sleepiness. Roughly one in five develop skin problems with the medicine. However, patients who experience these side effects do not have to stop taking the medication, although the doctor may lower the dose the person is receiving.

Interactions

Mitotane should not be given with spironolactone (a diuretic/water pill).

Bob Kirsch

Mitoxantrone

Definition

Mitoxantrone, also known by its trade name Novantrone, is an anticancer agent effective against certain kinds of leukemias. It is also used in Multiple Sclerosis (MS), and was approved by the Federal Drug Administration in 1987.

Purpose

Mitoxantrone is used with other drugs to treat acute non-lymphocytic leukemia (ANLL), a category

KEY TERMS

Body surface area (BSA)—A measurement, based on a patient's height and weight, that helps determine appropriate chemotherapy dosages.

Mucositis—A severe, painful inflammation of the mucous membranes.

Myelosuppression—A condition in which bone marrow activity is diminished, resulting in decreased platelet, red blood cell, and white blood cell counts.

Remission—The time period during which symptoms of a disease are absent.

that includes myelogenous, promyelocytic, monocytic and erythroid acute leukemia. In adults, ANLL accounts for up to 85% of all adult leukemia cases. Mitoxantrone may also be used in the treatment of **acute lymphocytic leukemia**, **chronic myelocytic leukemia**, **ovarian cancer**, advanced or recurrent **breast cancer**, **prostate cancer**, and MS.

Description

Mitoxantrone is classified as an anthracycline antitumor antibiotic, and closely resembles another drug in this category, **daunorubicin**. Although its precise mechanism is not clear, mitoxantrone is cell cycle non-specific, meaning that it is toxic to cells that are dividing, as well as those that are not.

Recommended dosage

Mitoxantrone is given intravenously over a thirty-minute time period. **Chemotherapy** dosages are based on a person's body surface area (BSA), which is calculated in square meters using height and weight measurements. Drug dosages are ordered in milligrams per square meter (mg/m^2).

In patients with **cancer**, the recommended dosage for induction therapy is 12mg/ mg/m^2 administered on the first three days of treatment. After that time, another chemotherapy drug is usually infused. This course of treatment is often adequate to induce remission, but may be repeated if it does not. In the second induction course, the dosage remains the same, but mitoxantrone is given for two days, rather than three, followed by other chemotherapy agents. Dosages may be altered, depending on the level of bone marrow toxicity the patient develops.

For patients with solid tumors, such as advanced hormone-refractory prostate cancer, a single dose of 12mg/ mg/m^2 is administered, and repeated every three to four weeks. Recent studies show that mitoxantrone used with glucocorticoids has resulted in improved pain control and quality of life in men with prostate cancer.

Precautions

Mitoxantrone's use in children has not been studied sufficiently to determine whether its use is safe and effective. It should not be used in individuals who have experienced a previous reaction to it.

Mitoxantrone is excreted by the liver and kidneys. It may alter the appearance of urine, causing it to be a blue-green color for approximately 24 hours. The sclera, or whites of the eyes, may temporarily be blue-tinged. Patients should not be alarmed by this change, but should alert their doctors if it is prolonged or is accompanied by other symptoms.

Mitoxantrone should not be administered to pregnant women, as damage to the fetus may occur. Throughout treatment, women should use methods to prevent pregnancy. It is excreted in breast-milk, so breast-feeding should be avoided during treatment.

Side effects

Mitoxantrone can cause severe and sometimes rapid **myelosuppression** leading to decreased white blood cell, red blood cell, and platelet counts. Blood counts should be monitored frequently throughout treatment. The white blood cells tend to nadir, or drop to their lowest point, within ten to fourteen days after mitoxantrone is administered. Patients should also be examined for symptoms of low white blood cell count, which typically resemble those of an **infection**: sore throat, burning with urination, increased temperature, or swelling. Patients should also be carefully monitored for indications that platelet count is low. Symptoms may include unexplained bruises, bleeding or increased bleeding with menstruation, and headache.

Mitoxantrone can damage the heart, possibly causing changes that lead to congestive heart failure (CHF). Patients especially at risk are those previously treated with anthracyclines or radiation to the chest area, or those with an already existing heart condition. Symptoms to watch for include swelling of the hands and ankles, difficulty breathing, or heart palpitations.

Mitoxantrone can cause a severe, painful inflammation of the mucous membranes called **mucositis**.

The condition may develop within a week of treatment. A patient may experience a burning sensation in his or her throat, as well as mouth pain. Mucositis typically resolves in a few weeks on its own, but there are measures one can take to hasten the process and provide comfort during healing. Hydration is very important to keep the mouth moist. Good oral hygiene is important—the teeth should be brushed with a very soft toothbrush, and flossed gently with unwaxed dental floss. (If bleeding occurs, using a toothbrush may not be safe. Patients should talk to their health care providers should this occur.) Your doctor or nurse may recommend a special mouthwash that helps relieve pain.

Patients undergoing treatment with mitoxantrone may be at risk for **tumor lysis syndrome**, a potentially life-threatening condition that develops when large numbers of cells rupture and release their contents into the blood stream. Preventative measures should be implemented to prevent adverse effects.

Interactions

Because mitoxantrone can alter normal blood counts, medications that contain aspirin should be avoided. Aspirin acts as a blood-thinner, and can predispose a person to bleeding. Patients should discuss all medications, whether they are prescribed or over-the-counter drugs, with their doctor to ensure there are no potential interactions. **Cytarabine**, another drug used to treat cancer, may increase the toxicity of mitixantrone if the drugs are used together.

Tamara Brown, R.N.

MMPI's *see* **Matrix metalloproteinase inhibitors**

Modified radical mastectomy

Definition

A surgical procedure that removes the breast, surrounding tissue, and nearby lymph nodes that are affected by **cancer**.

Purpose

The purpose for modified radical **mastectomy** is the removal of **breast cancer** (abnormal cells in the breast that grow rapidly and replace normal healthy tissue). Modified radical mastectomy is the most widely used surgical procedure to treat operable breast cancer. This procedure leaves a chest muscle called the pectoralis major intact. Leaving this muscle in place will provide a soft tissue covering over the chest wall and a normal-appearing junction of the shoulder with the anterior (front) chest wall. This sparing of the pectoralis major muscle will avoid a disfiguring hollow defect below the clavicle. Additionally, the purpose of modified radical mastectomy is to allow for the option of **breast reconstruction**, a procedure that is possible, if desired, due to intact muscles around the shoulder of the affected side. The modified radical mastectomy procedure involves removal of large multiple tumor growths located underneath the nipple and cancer cells on the breast margins.

Demographics

The highest rates of breast cancer occur in Western countries (more than 100 cases per 100,000 women) and the lowest among Asian countries (10–15 cases per 100,000 women). Men can also have breast cancer, but the incidence is much less when compared to women. There is a strong genetic correlation since breast cancer is more prevalent in females who had a close relative (mother, sister, maternal aunt, or maternal grandmother) with previous breast cancer. Increased susceptibility for development of breast cancer can occur in females who never breastfed a baby, had a child after age 30, started menstrual periods very early, or experienced menopause very late.

The American Cancer Society estimated that in 2009, 192,370 new cases of breast cancer would be diagnosed in the United States and 40,170 women would die as a result of the disease. Approximately one in eight women will develop breast cancer at some point in her life. The risk of developing breast cancer increases with age: women aged 30 to 40 have a one in 252 chance of developing breast cancer; women aged 40 to 50 have a one in 68 chance; women aged 50 to 60 have a one in 35 chance; and women aged 60 to 70 have a one in 27 chance—and these statistics do not even account for genetic and environmental factors.

Description

The surgeon's goal during this procedure is to minimize any chance of local/regional recurrence; avoid any loss of function; and maximize options for breast reconstruction. Incisions are made to avoid visibility in a low neckline dress or bathing suit. An

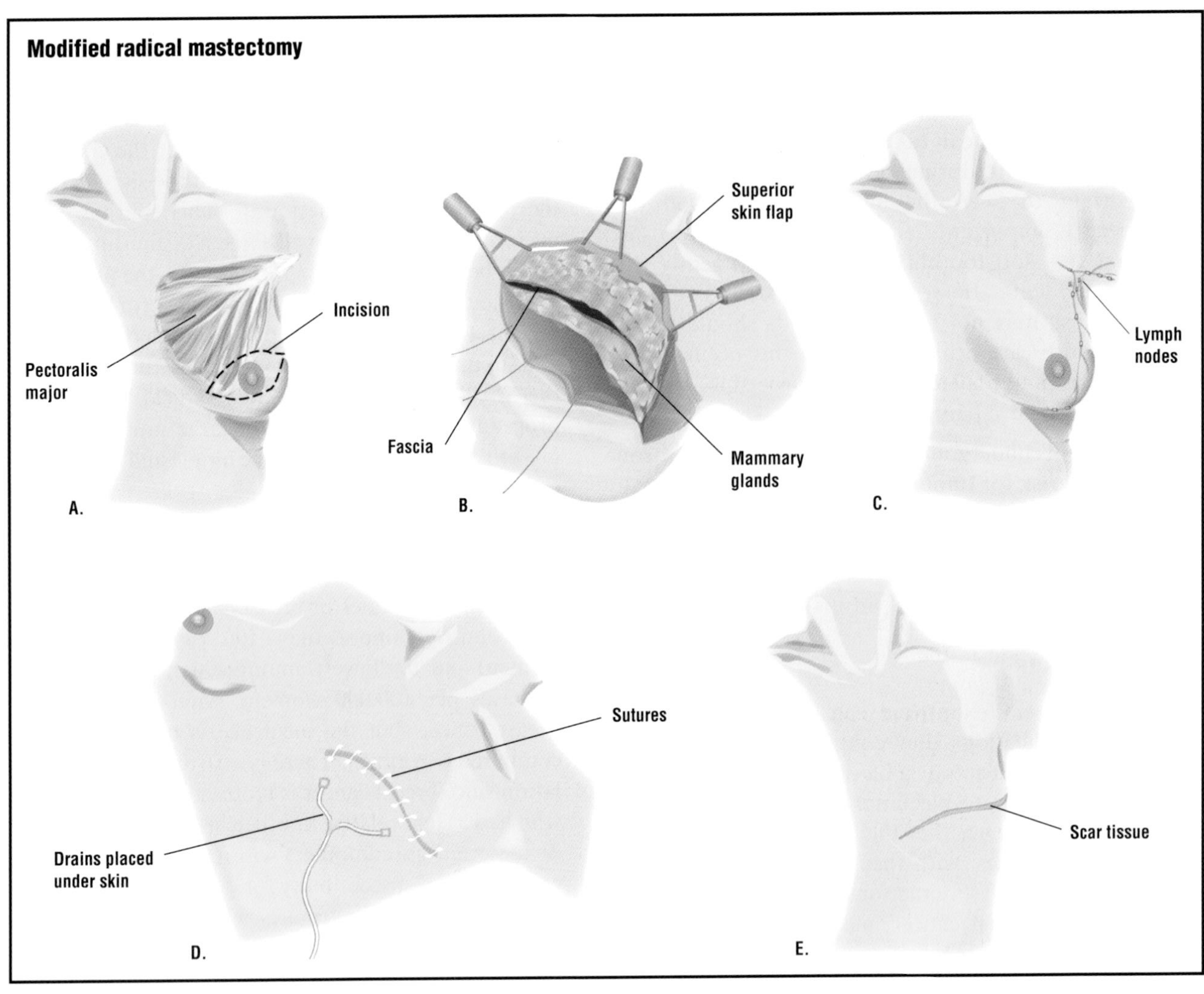

In a modified radical mastectomy, the skin on the breast is cut open (A). The skin is pulled back, and the tumor, lymph nodes, and breast tissue is removed (B and C). The incision is closed (D). *(Illustration by GGS Information Services. Cengage Learning, Gale.)*

incision in the shape of an ellipse is made. The surgeon removes the minimum amount of skin and tissue so that remaining healthy tissue can be used for possible reconstruction. Skin flaps are made carefully and as thinly as possible to maximize removal of diseased breast tissues. The skin over a neighboring muscle (pectoralis major fascia) is removed, after which the surgeon focuses in the armpit (axilla, axillary) region. In this region, the surgeon carefully identifies vital anatomical structures such as blood vessels (veins, arteries) and nerves. Accidental injury to specific nerves like the medial pectoral neurovascular bundle will result in destruction of the muscles that this surgery attempts to preserve, such as the pectoralis major muscle. In the armpit region, the surgeon carefully protects the vital structures while removing cancerous tissues. After axillary surgery, breast reconstruction can be performed, if desired by the patient.

Diagnosis and preparation

Modified radical mastectomy is a surgical procedure to treat breast cancer. In order for this procedure to be an operable option, a definitive diagnosis of breast cancer must be established. The first clinical sign for approximately 80% of women with breast cancer is a mass (lump) located in the breast. A lump can be discovered by monthly self-examination or by a health professional who can find 10–25% of breast cancers that are missed by yearly mammograms (a low radiation x ray of the breasts). A **biopsy** can be performed to examine the cells from a lump that is suspicious for cancer. The diagnosis of the extent of cancer and spread to regional lymph nodes determines the treatment course (i.e., whether surgery, **chemotherapy**, or **radiation therapy**, either singly or in combinations). Staging the cancer can estimate the amount of tumor, which is important not only for diagnosis but for prognosis (statistical outcome of the disease process). Patients with a type of breast cancer called ductal **carcinoma** in situ (DCIS), which is a stage 0 cancer, have the best outcome (nearly all these patients are cured of breast cancer). Persons who have cancerous spread to other distant places within the body (metastases) have stage IV cancer and the worst prognosis (potential for survival). Persons affected with stage IV breast cancer have essentially no chance for cure.

Persons affected with breast cancer must undergo the staging of the cancer to determine the extent of cancerous growth and possible spread (**metastasis**) to distant organs. Patients with stage 0 disease have non-invasive cancer with a very good outcome. Stages I and II are early breast cancer, without lymph node involvement (stage I) and with node positive results (stage II). Persons with stage III disease have locally advanced disease and about a 50% chance for five-year survival. Stage IV disease is the most severe since the breast cancer cells have spread through lymph nodes to distant areas and/or other organs in the body. It is very unlikely that persons with stage IV metastatic breast cancer survive 10 years after diagnosis.

It is also imperative to assess the degree of cancerous spread to lymph nodes within the armpit region. Of primary importance to stage determination and regional lymph node involvement is identification and analysis of the sentinel lymph node. The sentinel lymph node is the first lymph node to which any cancer would spread. The procedure for sentinel node biopsy involves injecting a radioactively labeled tracer (technetium 99) or a blue dye (isosulphan blue) into the tumor site. The tracer or dye will spread through the lymphatic system to the sentinel node, which should be surgically removed and examined for the presence of cancer cells. If the sentinel node and one or two other neighboring lymph nodes are negative, it is very likely that the remaining lymph nodes will not contain cancerous cells, and further surgery may not be necessary.

Once a breast lump (mass) has been identified by **mammography** or physical examination, the patient should undergo further evaluation to histologically (studying the cells) identify or rule out the presence of cancer cells. A procedure called fine-needle aspiration allows the clinician to extract cells directly from the lump for further evaluation. If a diagnosis cannot be established by fine-needle biopsy, the surgeon should perform an open biopsy (surgical removal of the suspicious mass). Preparation for surgery is imperative. The patient should plan for both direct care and recovery time after modified radical mastectomy. Preparation immediately prior to surgery should include no food or drink after midnight before the procedure. Post-surgical preparation should include caregivers to help with daily tasks for several days.

Aftercare

After breast cancer surgery, women should undergo frequent testing to ensure early detection of cancer recurrence. It is recommended that annual mammograms, physical examination, or additional tests (biopsy) be performed annually. Aftercare can also include psychotherapy since mastectomy is emotionally traumatic. Affected women may be worried or have concerns about appearance, the relationship with their sexual partner, and possible physical limitations. Community-centered support groups usually made up of former breast cancer surgery patients can be a source of emotional support after surgery. Patients may stay in the hospital for one to two days. For about five to seven days after surgery, there will be one or two drains left inside to remove any extra fluid from the area after surgery. Usually, the surgeon will prescribe medication to prevent pain. Movement restriction should be specifically discussed with the surgeon.

Risks

There are several risks associated with modified radical mastectomy. The procedure is performed under general anesthesia, which itself carries risk. Women may have short-term pain and tenderness. The most frequent risk of breast cancer surgery (with extensive lymph node removal) is edema, or swelling of the arm, which is usually mild, but the presence of fluid can increase the risk of **infection**. Leaving some lymph nodes intact instead of removing all of them may help lessen the likelihood of swelling. Nerves in the area may be damaged. There may be numbness in the arm or difficulty moving shoulder muscles. There is also the risk of developing a lump scar (keloid) after surgery. Another risk is that surgery did not remove all the cancer cells and that further treatment may be necessary (with chemotherapy and/or radiotherapy). By far, the worst risk is recurrence of cancer. However, immediate signs of risk following surgery include **fever**, redness in the incision area, unusual drainage from the incision, and increasing pain. If any of these signs develop, it is imperative to call the surgeon immediately.

WHO PERFORMS THE PROCEDURE AND WHERE IS IT PERFORMED?

The procedure is typically performed by a surgeon who has received five years of general surgery training and additional training in the specialty of surgical oncology. A surgeon who specializes in the area has expertise in removing cancerous tissues or areas. The procedure is performed in a hospital and requires that the hospital have a surgical care unit. In the surgical care unit, the patient will be treated by a team of professionals that includes, but is not limited to, physicians, nurses, physician assistants, and medical assistants.

QUESTIONS TO ASK THE DOCTOR

- What is the prognosis for the stage (0, I, II, III, IV) of my type of cancer?
- Will my movement be restricted after surgery?
- What care will I need on a daily basis following surgery?
- When should we set up a follow-up consultation/examination?
- Will I require other treatment (chemotherapy and/or radiation therapy) following surgery?
- What kind of mental-health treatment should I pursue (psychotherapy, community-centered support groups, etc.) following surgery?
- What options do I have for breast reconstruction? When would that treatment begin?

Normal results

If no complications develop, the surgical area should completely heal within three to four weeks. After mastectomy, some women may undergo breast reconstruction (which can be done during mastectomy). Recent studies have indicated that women who desire cosmetic **reconstructive surgery** have a higher quality of life and better sense of well-being than those who do not utilize this option.

Morbidity and mortality rates

The outcome of breast cancer is very dependent of the stage at the time of diagnosis. For stage 0 disease, the five-year survival is almost 100%. For stage I (early/lymph node negative), the five-year survival is alsom almost 100%. For stage II (early/lymph node positive), the five-year survival decreases to 81-92%. For stage III disease (locally advanced), the five-year survival is 54-67%. For women with stage IV (metastatic) breast cancer, the five-year survival is about 20%.

Approximately 17% of patients develop lymphedema after axillary **lymph node dissection**, while only 3% of patients develop lymphedema after sentinel node biopsy. Five percent of women are unhappy with the cosmetic effects of the surgery.

Alternatives

There are no real alternatives to mastectomy. Surgical requirement is clear since mastectomy is recommended for tumors with dimensions over 2 in (5 cm). Additional treatment (adjuvant) is typically recommended with chemotherapy and/or radiation therapy to destroy any remaining cancer during surgery. Modified radical mastectomy is one of the standard treatment recommendations for stage III breast cancer.

Resources

BOOKS

Abeloff, MD et al. *Clinical Oncology*. 3rd ed. Philadelphia: Elsevier, 2004.

Khatri, VP and JA Asensio. *Operative Surgery Manual*. 1st ed. Philadelphia: Saunders, 2003.

Townsend, CM et al. *Sabiston Textbook of Surgery*. 17th ed. Philadelphia: Saunders, 2004.

ORGANIZATIONS

American Cancer Society. (800) ACS-2345. http://www.cancer.org.

Cancer support groups. http://www.cancernews.com.

Y-ME National Breast Cancer Organization. http://www.y-me.org.

Laith Farid Gulli, MD
Nicole Mallory, MS, PA-C

Mohs' surgery

Definition

Mohs' surgery, also called Mohs' micrographic surgery, is a precise surgical technique that is used to remove all parts of cancerous skin tumors while preserving as much healthy tissue as possible. It is named for Frederic Edward Mohs, an American surgeon (1910–).

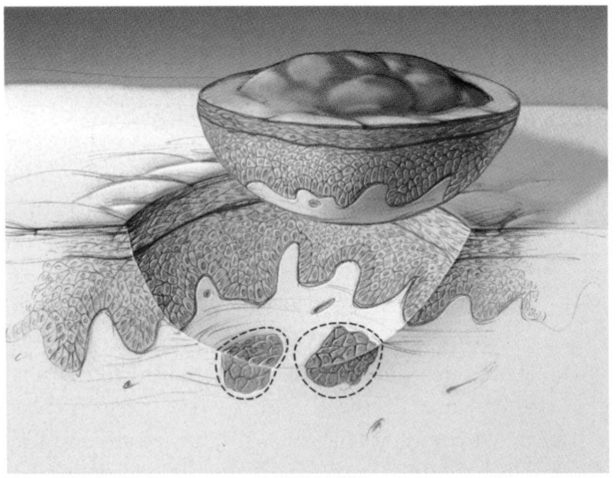

Mohs' surgery is used to remove skin cancer tumors of many types, including melanoma. Here, the main portion of the tumor is excised (debulked) using a spoon-shaped tool (curette). Further layers of tissue will be removed as necessary. *(Custom Medical Stock Photo. Reproduced by permission.)*

QUESTIONS TO ASK THE DOCTOR

- How long have you been performing Mohs' surgery?
- Will you use the fresh-tissue or fixed-tissue technique?
- Will I have to alter the use of my current medications for this procedure?
- What will you do if you don't find the border of the cancerous lesion?
- How will the wound be repaired?
- Will I need a plastic surgeon to repair the wound?
- What is the cure rate for this type of cancer when treated by Mohs' surgery?
- What is the chance that the tumor will recur?
- How often will I have follow-up appointments?

Purpose

Mohs' surgery is used to treat such skin cancers as **basal cell carcinoma**, **squamous cell carcinoma of the skin**, **melanoma**, Bowen's disease, extramammary Paget's disease, **leiomyosarcoma**, **laryngeal cancer**, **malignant fibrous histiocytoma**, microcystic adnexal **carcinoma**, mucoepidermoid carcinoma, and **Merkel cell carcinoma**.

Malignant skin tumors may appear as strange-looking asymmetrical shapes. The tumor may have long finger-like projections that extend across the skin (laterally) or down into the skin. Because these extensions may be composed of only a few cells, they cannot be seen or felt. Standard surgical removal (excision) may miss these cancerous cells leading to recurrence of the tumor. To assure removal of all cancerous tissue, a large piece of skin needs to be removed. This causes a cosmetically unacceptable result, especially if the **cancer** is located on the face. Mohs' surgery enables the surgeon to precisely excise the entire tumor without removing excessive amounts of the surrounding healthy tissue.

Precautions

To reduce the risk of bleeding, the use of non-steroidal anti-inflammatory medications, alcohol, vitamin E, and fish oil tablets should be avoided prior to the procedure. Patients who use the anti-coagulants aspirin, coumadin, or **heparin**, should consult with the prescribing physician before changing their use of these drugs.

Description

There are two types of Mohs' surgery: fresh-tissue technique and fixed-tissue technique. Seventy-two percent of surgeons who perform Mohs' surgery use only the fresh-tissue technique. The remaining surgeons use both techniques; however, the fixed-tissue technique is used in fewer than 5% of the patients. The main difference between the two techniques has to do with the preparation steps.

Fresh-tissue technique

Fresh-tissue Mohs' surgery is performed under local anesthesia for tumors of the skin. The area to be excised is cleaned with a disinfectant solution and a sterile drape is placed over the site. The surgeon may outline the tumor using a surgical marking pen or a dye. A local anesthetic (lidocaine plus epinephrine) is injected into the area. Once the local anesthetic has taken effect, the main portion of the tumor is excised (debulked) using a spoon-shaped tool (curette). To define the area to be excised and allow for accurate mapping of the tumor, the surgeon makes identifying marks around the wound. These marks may be made with stitches, staples, fine cuts with a scalpel, or temporary tattoos. One layer of tissue is carefully excised

KEY TERMS

Debulking—The removal of the major portion of a tumor by surgery so that the remainder of the tumor can be treated more effectively, usually by chemotherapy or radiation therapy.

Fixative—A chemical that preserves tissue without destroying or altering the structure of the cells.

Fixed—A term used to describe chemically preserved tissue. Fixed tissue is dead so it does not bleed or sense pain.

Mohs' excision—Referring to the excision of one layer of tissue during Mohs' surgery. Also called stage.

(first Mohs' excision), cut into smaller sections, and taken to the laboratory for analysis.

If cancerous cells are found in any of the tissue sections, a second layer of tissue is removed (second Mohs' excision). Because only the section(s) that have cancerous cells are removed, healthy tissue can be spared. The entire procedure, including surgical repair of the wound, is performed in one day. Surgical repair may be performed by the Mohs' surgeon, a plastic surgeon, or other specialist. In certain cases, wounds may be allowed to heal naturally.

Fixed-tissue technique

With fixed-tissue Mohs' surgery, the tumor is debulked as described above. Trichloracetic acid is applied to the wound (to control bleeding) followed by a preservative (fixative) called zinc chloride. The wound is dressed and the tissue is allowed to fix for 6 to 24 hours, depending on the depth of the tissue involved. This fixation period is painful. The first Mohs' excision is performed as above; however, anesthesia is not required because the tissue is dead. If cancerous cells are found, fixative is applied to the affected area for an additional 6 to 24 hours. Excisions are performed in this sequential process until all cancerous tissue is removed. Surgical repair of the wound may be performed once all fixed tissue has sloughed off, usually a few days after the last excision.

Preparation

Under certain conditions, such as the location of the skin tumor or health status of the patient, **antibiotics** may be taken prior to the procedure (prophylactic antibiotic treatment). Patients are encouraged to eat prior to surgery and bring along snacks in case of a lengthy procedure.

Aftercare

Patients should expect to receive specific wound care instructions from their physicians or surgeons, but generally, wounds that have been repaired with absorbable stitches or skin grafts are kept covered with a bandage for one week. Wounds that were repaired using nonabsorbable stitches are covered with a bandage, which should be replaced daily until the stitches are removed one to two weeks later. Patients with nonabsorbable stitches may shower. Signs of **infection** (e.g., redness, pain, drainage) should be reported to the physician immediately.

Risks

Using the fresh-tissue technique on a large tumor requires large amounts of local anesthetic, which can be toxic. Complications of Mohs' surgery include infection, bleeding, scarring, and nerve damage.

Normal results

Mohs' surgery provides high cure rates for malignant skin tumors. For instance, the five-year cure rate for basal cell carcinoma treated by Mohs' surgery is greater than 99%. The frequency of recurrence is much lower with Mohs' surgery (less than 1%) than with conventional surgical excision.

Abnormal results

Tumors spread in unpredictable patterns. Sometimes a seemingly small tumor is found to be quite large and widespread, resulting in a much larger excision than was anticipated. Technical errors, such as those involving processing and interpretation of the tissue sections, may lead to local recurrence of cancer.

Resources

BOOKS

Beers, Mark H., MD, and Robert Berkow, MD, editors. "Dermatologic Disorders: Malignant Tumors." In *The Merck Manual of Diagnosis and Therapy*. Whitehouse Station, NJ: Merck Research Laboratories, 2007.

Gross, Kenneth, Howard Steinman, and Ronald Rapini, editors. *Mohs Surgery: Fundamentals and Techniques*. St. Louis: Mosby, 1999.

PERIODICALS

Abbate, M., N. C. Zeitouni, M. Seyler, et al. "Clinical Course, Risk Factors, and Treatment of Microcystic

Adnexal Carcinoma: A Short Series Report." *Dermatologic Surgery* 29 (October 2003): 1035–1038.
Anthony, Margaret. "Surgical Treatment of Nonmelanoma Skin Cancer." *AORN Journal* March 2000: 552–64.
Lewis, R., and P. G. Lang, Jr. "Delayed Full-Thickness Skin Grafts Revisited." *Dermatologic Surgery* 29 (November 2003): 1113–1117.
Nouri, K., J. T. Trent, B. Lowell, et al. "Mucoepidermoid Carcinoma (Adenosquamous Carcinoma) Treated with Mohs Micrographic Surgery." *International Journal of Dermatology* 42 (December 2003): 957–959.
Silapunt, S., S. R. Peterson, J. Alcalay, and L. H. Goldberg. "Mohs Tissue Mapping and Processing: A Survey Study." *Dermatologic Surgery* 29 (November 2003): 1109–1112.

Belinda Rowland, Ph.D.
Rebecca J. Frey, Ph.D.

Monoclonal gammopathy of undetermined significance *see* **Multiple myeloma**

Monoclonal antibodies

Definition

Monoclonal antibodies are proteins produced in the laboratory from a single clone of a B cell, the type of cells of the immune system that make antibodies.

Description

Antibodies, also known as immunoglobulins (Igs), are proteins that help identify foreign substances to the immune system, such as a bacteria or a virus. Antibodies work by binding to the foreign substance to mark it as foreign. The substance that the antibody binds to is called an antigen. All monoclonal antibodies of a particular type bind to the same antigen, which distinguishes them from polyclonal antibodies.

The structure of most antibodies can be divided into two parts: the section that binds the antigen and a section that identifies the type of antibody. This second region is called a constant region, because it is essentially the same within the same type of antibody. The most common type of antibody is IgG (immunoglobulin gamma), which is found in the blood and body fluids. For **cancer** treatments, monoclonal antibodies are often humanized. This involves using human sequences for the constant regions and using mouse or other animal-derived sequence for the binding region. Humanization reduces the immune reaction of the patient to the antibody itself.

When used as a treatment for cancer, there are three general strategies with monoclonal antibodies. One uses the ability of the antibodies to bind to the cancer cells having the tumor antigens on their surface. The immune system will see the cancer cells marked with bound antibodies as foreign and destroy them. A second strategy is to use the antibodies to block the binding of cytokines or other proteins that are needed by the cancerous cells to maintain their uncontrolled growth. Monoclonal antibodies designed to work like this bind to the receptors for the cytokine that are on the tumor cell surface. As doctors don't completely understand how monoclonal antibodies work as drugs, both strategies may help rid the body of the tumor cells.

A final strategy involves special antibodies that are linked (conjugated) to a substance that is deadly to the cancer cells. Both radioactive isotopes, like yttrium 90, and toxins produced by bacteria, like pseudomonas exotoxin, have been successfully conjugated to antibodies. The antibodies are then used to specifically destroy the tumor cells with the radioactivity or toxic substance. The use of monoclonal antibodies is a useful approach to cancer therapy and as scientists learn more about the function of the immune system and cancer, new antibodies and new strategies promise to become more and more effective.

Michelle Johnson, M.S., J.D.

Morphine *see* **Opioids**
MRI *see* **Magnetic resonance imaging**

Mucositis

Description

Mucositis involves the inflammation of the lining of the mouth and digestive tract, and frequently occurs in **cancer** patients after **chemotherapy** and **radiation therapy**. The cheek, gums, soft plate, oropharynx, top and sides of tongue, and floor of the mouth may be affected, as well as the esophagus and rectal areas. Along with redness and swelling, patients typically experience a strong, burning pain.

Although there are factors that increase the likelihood and severity of mucositis, there is no reliable manner to predict who will be affected. Not only is mucositis more common in elderly patients, the degree of breakdown is often more debilitating. The severity of mucositis tends to be increased if a patient exercises poor oral hygiene or has a compromised nutritional status. A preexisting **infection** or irritation to the mucous membrane may also result in a more severe case of mucositis.

Causes

The precise mechanism by which cancer treatment induces mucositis is not clear, but it is believed to damage the rapidly dividing epithelial cells in the mucous membranes. This damage leads to inflammation and swelling, and then actual breakdown of the mucosa, the lining of the mouth and digestive tract. Another theory is that the body's natural defenses are weakened. For example, the immunoglobulin IgA is normally found in saliva. In patients who developed mucositis after undergoing cancer treatment with **methotrexate**, IgA levels in saliva were decreased.

The types of drug used to treat cancer and the schedule by which they are given influence the risk of developing mucositis. **Doxorubicin** and methotrexate, for example, frequently cause mucositis. The chemotherapy agent **fluorouracil** does not usually severely affect the mucous membranes when administered in small doses over continuous intravenous (IV) infusion. When the schedule is adjusted so that a higher dose is given over a shorter period of time (typically over five days), fluorouracil can cause very severe, painful, dose-limiting cases of mucositis. Patients undergoing treatment with high-dose chemotherapy and bone marrow rescue usually develop mucositis.

In addition, mucositis also tends to develop in radiation therapy administered to the oral cavity, or in dosages that exceed 180 cGy per day over a five-day period. Combination therapy, either multiple chemotherapy agents or chemotherapy and radiation therapy to the oral cavity, can increase the incidence of mucositis.

Treatments

Because there is no real cure for mucositis, treatment is aimed at prevention and management of symptoms. Mucositis typically resolves a few weeks after treatment as the cells regenerate, and treatment cessation is only occasionally required. In some cases, drug therapy will be altered so that a less toxic agent is given.

Patients at risk for mucositis should be meticulous about their oral hygiene, brushing frequently with a soft toothbrush and flossing carefully with unwaxed dental floss. If bleeding of the gums develops, patients should replace their toothbrushes with soft toothettes or gauze. Dentures should also be cleaned regularly. Patients should be well-hydrated, drinking fluids frequently and rinsing the mouth several times a day. Mouthwashes that contain alcohol or hydrogen peroxide should be avoided as they may dry out the mouth and increase pain. Lips should also be kept moist. Physical irritation to the mouth should be avoided. If time permits, dental problems, such as cavities or ill-fitting dentures, should be resolved with a dentist prior to beginning cancer treatment. Patients are generally more comfortable eating mild, medium-temperature foods. Spicy, acidic, very hot or very cold foods can irritate the mucosa. Tobacco and alcohol should also be avoided.

Hospital personnel and the patients themselves should inspect the mouth frequently to look for signs and symptoms of mucositis. Evidence of mucositis (inflammation, white or yellow shiny mucous membranes developing into red, raw, painful membranes) may be present as early as four days after chemotherapy administration.

Sodium bicarbonate mouth rinses are sometimes used to decrease the amount of oral flora and promote comfort, though there is no scientific evidence that this is beneficial. Typically, patients will rinse every few hours with a solution containing 1/2 teaspoon (tsp) salt and 1/2 tsp baking soda in one cup of water.

Pain relief is often required in patients with mucositis. In some cases, rinsing with a mixture of maalox, xylocaine, and diphenhydramine hydrochloride relieves pain. However, because of xylocaine's numbing effects, taste sensation may be altered. Worse, it may reduce the body's natural gag reflex, possibly causing problems with swallowing. Coating agents such as kaopectate and aluminum hydroxide gel may also help relieve symptoms. Rinsing with benzydamine has also shown promise, not only in managing pain, but also in preventing the development of mucositis. More severe pain may require liquid tylenol with codeine, or even intravenous opioid drugs. Patients with severe pain may not be able to eat, and may also require nutritional supplements through an I.V. (intravenous line).

Alternative and complementary therapies

A treatment called **cryotherapy** has shown promise in patients being treated with fluorouracil administered in the aforementioned five-day, high-dose schedule. Patients continuously swish ice chips in their mouth during the thirty-minute infusion of the drug, causing the blood vessels to constrict, thereby reducing the drug's ability to affect the oral mucosa.

Chamomile and **allopurinol** mouthwashes have been tried in the past to manage mucositis, but studies have found them to be ineffective. Biologic response modifiers are being evaluated to determine their possible role in managing mucositis. Recent studies using topical antimicrobial lozenges have shown promise as well, but more research is needed.

Resources

BOOKS

Abeloff, M., et al., editors. "Oral Complications." In *Clinical Oncology*. 2nd ed. New York, NY: Churchill Livingstone Publishers, 2004.

PERIODICALS

Balducci, L., and M. Corcoran. *Hematology/Oncology Clinics of North America* February 2000: 193–203.

Epstein, J., and A. Chow. *Infectious Disease Clinics of North America* December 1999: 901–18.

Tamara Brown, R.N.

Multiple endocrine neoplasia syndromes

Definition

The multiple endocrine neoplasia (MEN) syndromes are three related disorders in which two or more of the hormone-secreting (endocrine) glands of the body develop tumors. Commonly affected glands are the thyroid, parathyroids, pituitary, adrenals, and pancreas. Two common cancers are medullary **thyroid cancer** and gastrinomas. MEN is sometimes called familial multiple endocrine neoplasia (FMEN) and previously has been known as familial endocrine adenomatosis.

Description

The three forms of MEN are MEN1 (Wermer's syndrome), MEN2A (Sipple syndrome), and MEN2B (previously known as MEN3). Each form leads to excessive growth of normal cells (hyperplasia) and overactivity of a number of endocrine glands. Excessive growth can result in the formation of tumors (neoplasia) that are either benign (noncancerous) or malignant (cancerous). Overactive endocrine glands increase the secretion of hormones into the bloodstream. Hormones are important chemicals that control and instruct the functions of different organs. Their levels in the body are carefully balanced to maintain normal functioning of many vital processes, including metabolism, growth, timing of reproduction, and the composition of blood and other body fluids.

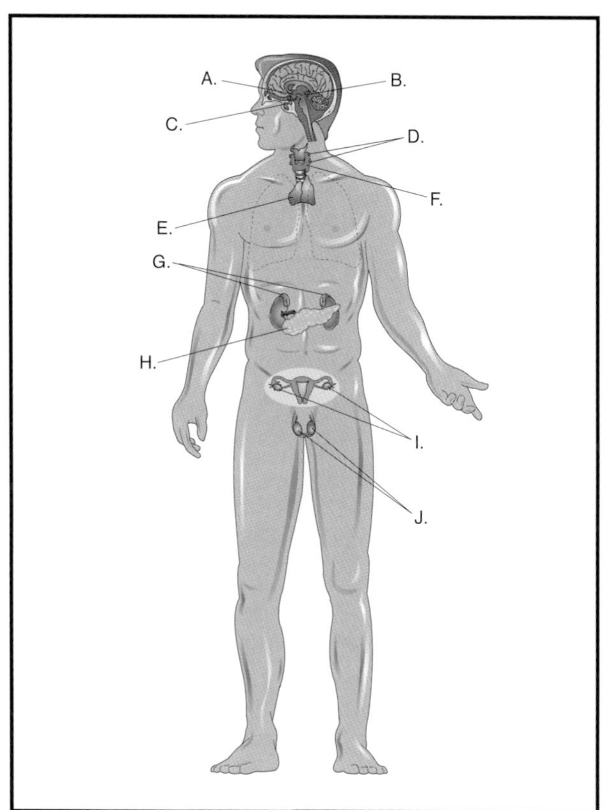

The human endocrine system: A. Hypothalamus. B. Pineal. C. Pituitary. D. Parathyroid. E. Thymus. F. Thyroid. G. Adrenals. H. Pancreas. I. Ovaries (female). J. Testes (male). *(Illustration by Electronic Illustrators Group. Cengage Learning, Gale.)*

All three forms are genetic disorders. They result when an abnormal form of a gene is inherited from one parent. The gene causing MEN1, named the MEN1 gene, was isolated in 1997. Both types of MEN2 are caused by mutations of the RET (REarranged during Transfection) gene. MEN1 and MEN2 are both autosomal dominant genetic conditions, meaning that an individual needs only one defective copy of the MEN1 gene or the RET gene to develop the associated disorder. In all forms, the children of an affected individual have a 50% chance of inheriting the defective gene.

The three forms of MEN are further distinguished by the endocrine glands affected. MEN1 is characterized by conditions of the parathyroid glands, pancreas, and pituitary gland. Patients with MEN2 commonly experience a form of thyroid **cancer** and **adrenal tumors**.

MEN1

Enlarged and overactive parathyroid glands, a condition called hyperparathyroidism, is present in 90–97% of MEN1 gene carriers and is usually the

KEY TERMS

Endocrine—A term used to describe the glands that produce hormones in the body.

Exocrine—A term used to describe organs that secrete substances outward through a duct.

Hyperplasia—An overgrowth of normal cells within an organ or tissue.

Medullary thyroid cancer (MTC)—A slow-growing tumor of which about 20% are associated with MEN2.

Neoplasm—An abnormal formation of tissue; for example, a tumor.

Oncogene—A gene with a mutation that causes cell growth and division, leading to the formation of cancerous tumors.

Pheochromocytoma—A tumor of the medullary of the adrenal gland.

RET (REarranged during Transfection) gene—Located on chromosome 10q11.2, mutations in this gene are associated with two very different disorders, the multiple endocrine neoplasia (MEN) syndromes and Hirschsprung disease.

Tumor suppressor gene—A type of gene that instructs cells on the appropriate time to die. A mutation can turn off the gene, resulting in cell growth and tumor formation.

QUESTIONS TO ASK THE DOCTOR

- Are the tumors associated with this condition cancerous?
- Can one endocrine tumor spread to other endocrine glands?
- What are the long-lasting effects of this disorder?
- What are the long-lasting effects of treatment?
- After treatment, what are the chances that a condition will recur?
- Are there alternative treatments to surgery?
- Will I need to take hormone supplements, if so, for how long?
- Will this disorder affect my ability to have children?
- What is the current status of predictive gene testing?
- Who in my family should be tested for this disorder?

first condition to develop. The four parathyroid glands are located in the neck region, with a pair of the glands on either side of the thyroid. They produce parathyroid hormone, which regulates calcium and phosphorus levels. Hyperparathyroidism leads to elevated levels of the hormone, resulting in high blood calcium levels (**hypercalcemia**), which can cause kidney stones and weakened bones. All four parathyroid glands tend to develop tumors, but most tumors are benign and **parathyroid cancer** is rare. Hyperparathyroidism may be present during the teenage years, but most individuals are affected by age 40.

Pancreatic tumors occur in 40–75% of individuals with the MEN1 gene. The pancreas, which sits behind the stomach, has two parts, an endocrine part and an exocrine part. Tumors in MEN1 occur only in the endocrine pancreas. Among the hormones secreted are ones that lower and raise blood sugar levels—insulin and glucagons—and the hormone gastrin, which is secreted into the stomach to aid in digestion. Thirty to 35% of pancreatic tumors are malignant, and they are the tumors most likely to cause cancer in MEN1 patients. Gastrin-producing tumors (gastrinomas) are the most common tumors that form, representing about 50% of the MEN1 pancreatic tumors. Other tumors that form are insulin-producing tumors (insulinomas), representing 25–30%, and glucagon-producing tumors (glucagonomas), representing 5–10%.

Gastrinomas can cause recurring upper gastrointestinal ulcers, a condition called **Zollinger-Ellison syndrome**. About half of MEN1 patients with a pancreatic condition develop this syndrome. Insulinomas raise the insulin level in the blood and can lead to hypoglycemia, or low blood sugar (glucose), resulting in glucose levels that are too low to fuel the body's activity. Glucagonomas can cause high blood sugar levels, or hyperglycemia.

Pituitary tumors are the third most common condition in MEN1, occurring in about 50% of MEN1 patients. Fewer than 5% of these tumors are malignant. The pituitary gland, located at the base of the brain, secretes many hormones that regulate the function of other endocrine glands. The most common tumors forming in MEN1 patients are prolactin-producing tumors (prolactinomas) and growth hormone–secreting tumors, which lead to a condition known as acromegaly.

Association of multiple endocrine neoplasias with other conditions

Form	Associated diseases/conditions
MEN 1 (Wermer's syndrome)	Parathyroid hyperplasia Pancreatic islet cell carcinomas, Pituitary hyperplasia Thymus, adrenal, carcinoid tumors (less common)
MEN 2A (Sipple syndrome)	Medullary thyroid carcinoma, Pheochromocytoma Parathyroid hyperplasia
MEN 2B	Medullary thyroid carcinoma, Pheochromocytoma Parathyroid hyperplasia Swollen lips Tumors of mucous membranes (eyes, mouth, tongue, nasal cavities) Enlarged colon Skeletal problems such as spinal curving
Familial medullary thyroid carcinoma	Medullary thyroid carcinoma

(Table by GGS Creative Resources. Cengage Learning, Gale.)

MEN2

Patients with MEN2A and MEN2B experience two main symptoms, medullary thyroid cancer (MTC) and a medullary adrenal tumor known as **pheochromocytoma**. Additional symptoms distinguish the two forms of MEN2. Twenty percent of MEN2A patients develop parathyroid tumors, which have not been reported for MEN2B. As in MEN1, parathyroid tumors in MEN2A affect all four glands and are usually benign. MEN2B is further characterized by the occurrence of benign tumors of the tongue, nasal cavities, and other facial surfaces (mucosal neuromas) and by a condition known as marfanoid habitus. Marfanoid habitus features a characteristic appearance resulting from severe wasting of the proximal muscles. A distinct facial appearance—an elongated face with a thick forehead, wide-eyed look, and broad nose—is often noted at birth. Gastrointestinal, skeletal, and pigmentation abnormalities may also occur. Mucosal neuromas occur in all MEN2B patients, and marfanoid habitus occurs in 65%. About 5% of MEN2 cases are MEN2B.

Ninety-five percent of MEN2A patients and 90% of MEN2B patients develop medullary thyroid **carcinoma** (MTC). Medullary thyroid carcinoma forms from the C-cells of the thyroid. C-cells make the hormone **calcitonin**, which is involved in regulating the calcium levels in the blood and calcium absorption by the bones. The thyroid, which is located in the front of the neck between the Adam's apple and the collarbone, also secretes hormones that are essential for the regulation of body temperature, heart rate, and metabolism.

Medullary thyroid carcinoma causes high blood levels of calcitonin. In MEN2B, MTC develops earlier and is more aggressive than in MEN2A. It has been described in MEN2B patients younger than one year, whereas in MEN2A patients it is likely to occur between the ages of 20 and 40.

Pheochromocytoma is found in 50% of MEN2A patients and 45% of MEN2B patients. A tumor of the medulla portion of the adrenal gland, it is usually a slow-growing and benign adrenal tumor. The two flat adrenal glands, one situated above each kidney, secrete the hormones epinephrine and norepinephrine to increase heart rate and blood pressure, along with other effects. Excessive secretion of these adrenal hormones can cause life-threatening hypertension and cardiac arrhythmia. Tumors form on both adrenal glands in 50% of MEN2 patients diagnosed with a pheochromocytoma. Tumor malignancy is very rare.

Demographics

MEN syndromes are rare. MEN1 occurs in about three to twenty persons out of 100,000, and MEN2 occurs in about three out of 100,000 people. Both MEN1 and MEN2 show no geographic, racial, or ethnic trend, and men and women have an equal chance of acquiring the MEN syndromes.

Ninety-eight percent of MEN1 gene carriers will develop varying combinations of tumors by age 30, but cancer has not been reported in patients younger than 18. Seventy percent of MEN2A gene carriers will have symptoms by age 70, with most diagnoses occurring between the ages of 30 and 50. MEN2B can occur before one year of age, but most symptoms appear anytime between the ages of 20 and 70.

Causes and symptoms

MEN1

MEN1 is caused by mutations of the MEN1 gene. The MEN1 gene encodes for a previously unknown protein named menin. The role of menin in tumor formation in endocrine glands is not known. But the MEN1 gene is thought to be one of a group of genes known as a tumor suppressor gene. A patient who inherits one defective copy of a tumor suppressor gene from either parent has a strong predisposition to the disease because of the high probability of incurring a second mutation in at least one dividing cell. That cell no longer possesses even one normal copy of the gene. When both copies are defective, tumor suppression fails and tumors develop.

A number of different mutations have been discovered in the MEN1 gene, but people having the same mutation do not always develop the same endocrine conditions. Members within a single family can show different sets of conditions. The symptoms of MEN1 depend on the endocrine condition present:

- Hyperparathyroidism: weakness, fatigue, constipation, kidney stones, loss of appetite (anorexia), and bone and joint pain.
- Gastrinoma: peptic ulcers of the stomach and small intestine, diarrhea, and weight loss.
- Insulinoma: hypoglycemia characterized by weakness, shakiness, fast heartbeat, and difficulty concentrating.
- Glucagonoma: hyperglycemia characterized by inflammation of the tongue or stomach, anemia, weight loss, diarrhea, and blood clots.
- Prolactinoma: secretion of milk in women who are not nursing, headaches, sweating, fatigue, weight gain, fertility problems in men and women, and visual problems.
- Acromegaly: enlarged hands and feet, enlarged face, thickened oily skin, fatigue, sweating, bone and joint pain, weight gain, and high blood sugar.

MEN2

Both types of MEN2 are caused by mutations of the RET gene. The RET gene is a cancer-causing gene, or an oncogene. A number of different mutations lead to MEN2A, but only one specific genetic alteration leads to MEN2B.

Unlike for MEN1, the likelihood of developing different conditions in MEN2A is associated with specific mutations of the RET gene. Family history can indicate which conditions current family members are likely to develop. The symptoms of MEN2 are those that accompany hyperparathyroidism, MTC, and pheochromocytoma:

- Medullary thyroid cancer: enlargement of thyroid or neck swelling; lumps or nodules in the neck, pain in the neck region going to the ears, persistent cough unrelated to a cold, cough with bleeding, diarrhea or constipation, hoarseness, and difficulty swallowing or breathing.
- Pheochromocytoma: headaches, sweating, chest pains, feelings of anxiety.

The conditions of MEN2B patients show a variety of additional symptoms, including the occurrence of mucosal neuromas and marfanoid habitus, which is characterized by an elongated face, a thick forehead, and poor muscle development.

Diagnosis

The occurrence of one endocrine condition does not immediately lead to a suspicion of MEN syndromes. Diagnoses is based on the occurrence of one or more endocrine conditions and a family history of MEN1 or MEN2.

Since 1994, **genetic testing** using DNA technology has been available for both MEN1 and MEN2. The identification of the MEN1 gene in 1997 has made genetic screening for this gene more accurate.

A blood sample is usually analyzed for DNA testing, although other tissue can be used. The sample is sent to a laboratory that specializes in DNA diagnosis. There a geneticist will perform several tests on the DNA collected from the cells in blood sample. The exact tests performed will depend on whether MEN1 or MEN2 is suspected. Because different regions of the RET gene are associated with different endocrine conditions in MEN2A, several regions of the gene are examined. A positive result means the defective gene is present, and a negative result means the defective gene is not present.

The test results for the RET gene mutations are more reliable than for the MEN1 gene because detection techniques for identifying MEN1 are still being developed. A clinical diagnosis of MEN2 is confirmed with genetic testing 90–95% of the time. Even when a genetic test is negative, family medical records will be carefully reviewed to confirm the presence of MEN2, and periodic screening of related conditions will likely continue until age 30 or 40. The time required to obtain the test results for MEN2 is about 2–4 weeks, but MEN1 results will likely take longer because there are fewer diagnostic labs set up for MEN1 analysis.

Those considered at risk for MEN1 or MEN2 based on genetic tests or family history are offered preventative surgery, regular screening for associated endocrine conditions, or a combination of these treatment options. Conditions are screened following the accepted procedure for each condition. Diagnosis is based on clinical features and on testing for elevated hormone levels.

MEN1

Hyperparathyroidism is diagnosed when high levels of calcium and intact parathyroid hormone are measured in a blood sample. Normal values of calcium for adults is 4.4–5.3 mg/dl (milligrams per deciliter), and normal values of parathyroid hormone are 10–55 pg/ml (picograms per milliliter). Prior to the parathyroid test, no food should be eaten for at least six hours. An x ray of bones may be taken and then examined by a radiologist for signs of low bone density. An x ray of the abdominal region can reveal kidney stones. Patients should be screened yearly.

Diagnosis of a gastrinoma follows established procedures and includes measuring the levels of gastrin in the blood and the level of stomach gastic acid production. Hypoglycemia associated with insulinomas is diagnosed by measuring blood glucose levels. This test may be administered while a patient is experiencing symptoms related to low insulin levels or during a supervised period of fasting. Depending on the type of test given, no food should be eaten from 6–12 hours prior to the test. Normal glucose levels range between 64–128 mg/dl. Blood glucagon levels above the normal range of 50–100 pg/ml can indicate hyperglycemia, which is associated with glucagonomas. Large pancreatic tumors are identified using **computed tomography** (CT scans) or radionuclide imaging, but **ultrasonography** conducted during surgery is the best method for detecting small tumors. There is no accepted system for staging the pancreatic tumors associated with MEN1.

Prolactinomas, the pituitary tumors most often associated with MEN1, are diagnosed when prolactin levels are greater than 20 ng/l (nanograms per liter). A tumor is identified using **magnetic resonance imaging** (MRI). Tumors secreting excess growth hormone are diagnosed when hormone levels are above the upper normal range of 3 ng/l and from observable changes in physical appearance.

MEN2

Medullary thyroid carcinoma is diagnosed by measuring calcitonin levels in blood and urine samples and from a **biopsy** of any thyroid nodules. Levels of calcitonin above 50 pg/ml can indicate the presence of MTC. Patients showing normal calcitonin levels may require a different test, in which calcitonin is measured at regular intervals after an injection of pentagastrin, a synthetic hormone.

Fine needle aspiration is the biopsy procedure used to diagnose MTC and other forms of thyroid cancer. A sample of cells is removed from a nodule, and the cells are then examined under a microscope by a pathologist to determine if cancer cells are present. MTC has four stages, based on the size of the tumor and where the cancer has spread. Tumor staging follows the system established for other forms of thyroid cancer.

A high level of epinephrine relative to norepinephrine indicates a pheochromocytoma on one or both adrenal glands. A CT scan, an MRI, or radionuclide imaging will be performed to locate the tumor.

Diagnosis of hyperparathyroidism in MEN2A patients is identical to its diagnosis for MEN1 patients, but with screening recommended every two to three years.

Treatment team

Conditions of MEN syndromes are first diagnosed by a pathologist who interprets blood and urine samples collected at a doctor's office or a clinic. Depending on the specific condition, a doctor specializing in conditions of the endocrine gland (an endocrinologist) may be consulted. When MEN syndromes are suspected, a genetic counselor will help prepare a patient for the genetic testing procedures and results. A geneticist will perform and interpret genetic tests. Since MEN syndromes often require surgery, the surgical team will likely consist of a surgeon experienced in operating on endocrine glands.

Clinical staging, treatments, and prognosis

No comprehensive treatment is available for genetic disorders such as MEN, but the symptoms of many conditions are treatable. Surgical removal of tumors is the recommended treatment for most conditions, and most MEN patients will require more than one endocrine gland surgery during a lifetime.

An important distinction between an endocrine condition in MEN patients and the same condition in patients not diagnosed with MEN is that endocrine tumors for MEN patients are likely to arise in many locations of a single gland or on multiple glands. Treatment options that work for patients with a single endocrine condition may not be effective in MEN patients. Surgery is often more extensive for MEN patients.

Genetic testing can exclude family members who do not have mutations of the RET or MEN1 gene. The advantage of testing is the early treatment and improved outcomes for those who carry the defective gene and relief from unnecessary anxiety and clinical testing for those not having the defective gene.

MEN1

A common approach to treating MEN1 is with regular screening. Surgical procedures may be delayed until a patient has developed clinical symptoms caused by excess hormone or an easily identifiable tumor.

There are two surgical options for MEN1 patients showing multiple symptoms of hyperparathyroidism or for patients having high blood calcium levels (hypercalcemia), even when no symptoms of the condition are present. All parathyroid tissue is identified and removed and parathyroid tissue is implanted in the forearm, or the surgeon removes three parathyroids and one half of the fourth. After surgery, blood calcium levels are regularly tested to ensure that the remaining parathyroid tissue has not enlarged and caused the condition to return. If hyperparathyroidism recurs, a portion of the remaining tissue is removed until calcium levels return to normal or all the remaining tissue is removed. For MEN1 patients, recurrence is likely within 15 years of the first surgery. Patients with no parathyroid tissue must take daily calcium and vitamin D supplements to prevent hypercalcemia.

There are two views on the best screening strategy for pancreatic tumors in MEN1 patients. One approach is yearly screening, particularly for gastrinomas. This strategy emphasizes the earliest possible detection and surgical removal of tumors. The other approach is screening every 2–3 years, with the reasoning that although tumors are detected at a later stage, they can be better managed with drugs and, if necessary, with surgery.

Surgical removal of insulinomas and glucagonomas, as well as of other less commonly occurring pancreatic tumors in MEN1 patients, is generally the recommended treatment because these tumors are difficult to treat with medication.

The best treatment option for gastrinomas is complex because in MEN1 patients there can be multiple gastrinomas of varying sizes on the pancreas and upper portion of the small intestine (duodenum), and they have a tendency to recur. Most doctors support the use of medication to control the condition and do not recommend surgical intervention. Common treatment of symptoms is the use of drugs that block acid production, called acid pump inhibitors. Others recommend surgery that includes removal of the duodenum and a section of the pancreas and cutting nerves to the section of the stomach involved in acid secretion. Surgery is supported as a way to reduce the risk for **metastasis**. In some cases, gastrin levels and gastric acid levels returned to normal, and MEN1 patients experienced no symptoms after the surgery. A treatment no longer recommended is removal of the entire stomach. Malignant gastrinomas cause death in 10% to 20% of MEN1 patients with this condition, and 30–50% will eventually spread to the liver.

Treatment of pituitary tumors in MEN1 patients rarely involves surgery. For prolactinomas, medications are effective in returning prolactin levels to normal and preventing tumor growth.

MEN2

Medullary thyroid carcinoma is the primary concern for those testing positive for the RET gene mutations. Since genetic testing became available for MEN2, two approaches have emerged to manage this cancer. Some recommend removing the entire thyroid gland (thyroidectomy) before any symptoms occur, although doctors disagree at what age to perform this surgery. This strategy emerged owing to a number of cases in which thyroids removed from identified MEN2 patients showing no clinical signs of MTC were found to be cancerous. Preventative thyroid surgery is offered to those with RET gene mutations beginning at age 5. Some recommend surgery after age 10, unless calcitonin tests are positive earlier. They contend that surgery before age 10 may increase the chance of damaging the larynx or the parathyroids.

The second approach is yearly blood calcitonin testing beginning in early childhood. A thyroidectomy is performed after the first abnormal calcitonin test. There is only a 10% chance of recurrence 15–20 years after surgery for those identified using this method. The advantage of this method is to delay surgery until it is necessary. The disadvantages are the cost and discomfort of yearly testing. Also, the first detection of elevated levels of calcitonin in the blood may occur after the cancer has already reached an advanced stage.

A thyroidectomy is the standard treatment for all stages of MTC. If MTC is diagnosed in an advanced stage, the spread of the cancer may have already occurred. Metastasis is very serious in MTC because **chemotherapy** and **radiation therapy** are not effective in controlling metastasis. Further tests are likely to include a CT scan and an MRI.

All MTC patients must take thyroid hormone medication for the rest of their lives in order to maintain normal body functions. Follow-up treatment to assure that the cancer has not recurred includes monitoring the levels of calcitonin in the blood. The survival rate 10 years after the initial diagnosis is 46%. If the cancer is detected using genetic screening before the patient shows signs of having the disease, surgical removal of the thyroid gland can cure MTC.

Pheochromocytoma may occur after the MTC diagnosis by as much as 20 years. Pheochromocytoma in MEN2 can be cured by surgical removal of the affected adrenal gland. If a pheochromocytoma occurs on only one gland, there is some debate on whether to remove both adrenal glands or only the affected gland. Fifty percent of MEN2 patients who underwent removal of one adrenal gland developed a pheochromocytoma in the other gland within 10 years. Because malignancy is rare, most doctors recommend removing the affected glands first and then monitoring hormone levels to see if a second tumor occurs. If both glands are removed, hormone replacement therapy is required.

Alternative and complementary therapies

There are no alternative treatments specifically targeted for people with MEN syndromes, although cow and shark cartilage treatments are being investigated as a way to decrease tumor growth in some cancers. These treatments are administered orally, by injection, or as an enema, but studies of the effectiveness of this treatment for humans are inconclusive.

Coping with cancer treatment

The surgery that most MEN syndromes patients will face can cause anxiety and fear. Patients should discuss their concerns about an operation with their personal physician, the surgeon, nurses, and other medical personnel. Getting specific answers to questions can provide a clear idea of what to expect immediately after the surgery as well as any long-term changes in quality of life.

Clinical trials

Clinical studies of MEN syndromes focus on understanding the genes involved in the inheritance of MEN1 and MEN2 and on the unique treatment needs for the endocrine gland conditions occurring in MEN patients. One ongoing study investigates new imaging techniques for locating pheochromocytomas, particularly in MEN2 patients. Contact information:

National Institute of Child Health and Human Development (NICHD), 9000 Rockville Pike, Bethseda, MD 20892. (800) 411-1222

A second clinical trial is a genetic-analysis study of known and suspected individuals with MEN1. Participants are offered genetic counseling with an option for involvement in research designed to improve genetic counseling services. Contact information:

National Institute of Diabetes and Digestive and Kidney Diseases (NIDDK), 9000 Rockville Pike, Bethseda, MD 20892. (800) 411-1222

Prevention

There is no preventive measure to block the occurrence of the genetic mutations that cause MEN syndromes. Medullary thyroid carcinoma, one of the most serious conditions of MEN2, can be prevented by thyroidectomy.

Special concerns

It is important to seek professional genetic counseling before proceeding with genetic testing, particularly for children. Adults may have to make treatment decisions for children.

Genetic tests are often expensive. Whether or not **health insurance** will cover the costs of counseling and testing will depend on individual policies. Some insurance companies cover the costs only when a patient shows symptoms of a condition. Genetic tests raise issues of privacy. Most states in the United States have legislation that restricts the use of genetic test results by insurance companies and employers.

See also Cancer genetics; Familial cancer syndromes; Pancreatic cancer, endocrine; Thyroid cancer.

Resources

PERIODICALS

Hoff, A. O., G. J. Cote, and R. F. Gagel. "Multiple Endocrine Neoplasias." *Annual Review of Physiology* 62 (2000): 377–411.

Noll, Walter W. "Utility of RET Mutation Analysis in Multiple Endocrine Neoplasia Type 2." *Archives of Pathology and Laboratory Medicine* 123 (1999): 1047–9.

OTHER

Labs Performing MEN Testing. http://endocrine.mdacc.tmc.edu.

ORGANIZATIONS

Canadian MEN Society. P.O. Box 100, Meola, SK, Canada SOM 1XO. (306) 892-2080.

The Genetic Alliance (formerly the Alliance of Genetic Support Groups). 4301 Connecticut Ave. NW, Suite 404, Washington, DC 20008-2304. (202) 966-5557, (800) 336-GENE.

G. Victor Leipzig
Monica McGee, M.S.

Multiple myeloma

Definition

Multiple **myeloma** is a **cancer** in which antibody-producing plasma cells grow in an uncontrolled and invasive (malignant) manner.

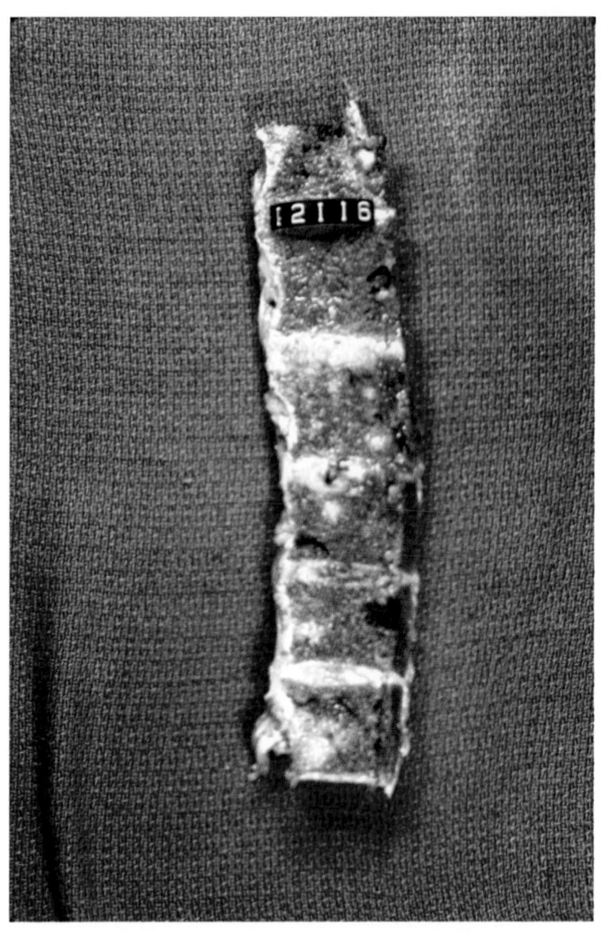

Portion of spine from patient with multiple myeloma. In this disease, malignant plasma cells spread through the bone marrow and hard outer portions of the body's large bones. As malignant plasma cells increase in the bone marrow, replacing normal marrow, they exert pressure on the bone. Bones become soft and may fracture; spinal bones may collapse. *(Custom Medical Stock Photo. Reproduced by permission.)*

Description

Multiple myeloma, also known as plasma cell myeloma, is the second-most common cancer of the blood. It is the most common type of plasma cell neoplasm. Multiple myeloma accounts for approximately 1% of all cancers and 2% of all deaths from cancer. Multiple myeloma is a disease in which malignant plasma cells spread through the bone marrow and hard outer portions of the large bones of the body. These myeloma cells may form tumors called plasmacytomas. Eventually, multiple soft spots or holes, called osteolytic lesions, form in the bones.

Bone marrow is the spongy tissue within the bones. The breastbone, spine, ribs, skull, pelvic bones, and the long bone of the thigh all are particularly rich in marrow. Bone marrow is a very active tissue that is responsible for producing the cells that circulate in the blood. These include the red blood cells that carry oxygen, the white blood cells that develop into immune system cells, and platelets, which cause blood to clot.

Plasma cells and immunoglobulins

Plasma cells develop from B lymphocytes or B cells, a type of white blood cell. B cells, like all blood cells, develop from unspecialized stem cells in the bone marrow. Each B cell carries a specific antibody that recognizes a specific foreign substance called an antigen. Antibodies are large proteins called immunoglobulins (Igs), which recognize and destroy foreign substances and organisms such as bacteria. When a B cell encounters its antigen, it begins to divide rapidly to form mature plasma cells. These plasma cells are all identical (monoclonal). They produce large amounts of identical antibody that are specific for the antigen.

Malignant plasma cells

Multiple myeloma begins when the genetic material (DNA) is damaged during the development of a stem cell into a B cell in the bone marrow. This causes the cell to develop into an abnormal or malignant plasmablast, a developmentally early form of plasma cell. Plasmablasts produce adhesive molecules that allow them to bond to the inside of the bone marrow. A growth factor, called interleukin-6, promotes uncontrolled growth of these myeloma cells in the bone marrow and prevents their natural death. Whereas normal bone marrow contains less than 5% plasma cells, bone marrow of an individual with multiple myeloma contains over 10% plasma cells.

In most cases of multiple myeloma, the malignant plasma cells all make an identical Ig. Igs are made up of four protein chains that are bonded together. Two of the chains are light and two are heavy. There are five classes of heavy chains, corresponding to five types of Igs with different immune system functions. The Igs from myeloma cells are nonfunctional and are called paraproteins. All of the paraproteins from any one individual are monoclonal (identical) because the myeloma cells are identical clones of a single plasma cell. Thus, the paraprotein is a monoclonal protein or M-protein. The M-proteins crowd out the functional Igs and other components of the immune system. They also cause functional antibodies, which are produced by normal plasma cells, to rapidly break down. Thus, multiple myeloma depresses the immune system.

In about 75% of multiple myeloma cases, the malignant plasma cells also produce monoclonal light

KEY TERMS

Amyloidosis—A complication of multiple myeloma in which amyloid protein accumulates in the kidneys and other organs, tissues, and blood vessels.

Anemia—Any condition in which the red blood cell count is below normal.

Antibody—Immunoglobulin produced by immune system cells that recognizes and binds to a specific foreign substance (antigen).

Antigen—Foreign substance that is recognized by a specific antibody.

B cell (B lymphocyte)—Type of white blood cell that produces antibodies.

Bence-Jones protein—Light chain of an immunoglobulin that is overproduced in multiple myeloma and is excreted in the urine.

Beta 2-microglobulin—Protein produced by B cells; high concentrations in the blood are indicative of multiple myeloma.

Cryoglobulinemia—Condition triggered by low temperatures in which protein in the blood forms particles, blocking blood vessels, leading to pain and numbness of the extremities.

Electrophoresis—Use of an electrical field to separate proteins in a mixture (such as blood or urine), on the basis of the size and electrical charge of the proteins.

Hemoglobin—Protein in red blood cells that carries oxygen.

Hypercalcemia—Abnormally high levels of calcium in the blood.

Hyperviscosity—Thick, viscous blood, caused by the accumulation of large proteins, such as immunoglobulins, in the serum.

Immunoglobulin (Ig)—Antibody; large protein produced by B cells that recognizes and binds to a specific antigen.

M-protein—Monoclonal or myeloma protein; paraprotein; abnormal antibody found in large amounts in the blood and urine of individuals with multiple myeloma.

Malignant—A characteristic of cancer cells that grow uncontrollably and invade other tissues.

Monoclonal—Identical cells or proteins; cells (clones) derived from a single, genetically distinct cell, or proteins produced by these cells.

Monoclonal gammopathy of undetermined significance (MGUS)—Common condition in which M-protein is present, but there are no tumors or other symptoms of disease.

Neoplasm—Tumor made up of cancer cells.

Osteoblast—Bone-forming cell.

Osteoclast—Cell that absorbs bone.

Osteolytic lesion—Soft spot or hole in bone caused by cancer cells.

Osteoporosis—Condition in which the bones become weak and porous, due to loss of calcium and destruction of cells.

Paraprotein—M-protein; abnormal immunoglobulin produced in multiple myeloma.

Plasma cell—Type of white blood cell that produces antibodies; derived from an antigen-specific B cell.

Platelet—Cell that is involved in blood clotting.

Stem cell—Undifferentiated cell that retains the ability to develop into any one of numerous cell types.

chains, or incomplete Igs. These are called Bence-Jones proteins and are secreted in the urine. Approximately 1% of multiple myelomas are called nonsecretors because they do not produce any abnormal Ig.

Osteolytic lesions

About 70% of individuals with multiple myeloma have soft spots or lesions in their bones. These lesions can vary from quite small to grapefruit-size. In part, these lesions occur because the malignant plasma cells rapidly outgrow the normal bone-forming cells. In addition, malignant myeloma cells produce factors that affect cells called osteoclasts. These are the cells that normally destroy old bone, so that new bone can be produced by cells called osteoblasts. The myeloma cell factors increase both the activation and the growth of osteoclasts. As the osteoclasts multiply and migrate, they destroy healthy bone and create lesions. Osteoporosis, or widespread bone weakness, may develop.

Demographics

There are more than 40,000 multiple myeloma patients in the United States. The American Cancer Society predicts an additional 14,400 new cases in

QUESTIONS TO ASK THE DOCTOR

- What stage of multiple myeloma do I have and what does it mean?
- What are my treatment options?
- What are the side effects of treatment?
- Are there clinical trials that may be appropriate for me?
- How long can I expect to survive?
- Is my cancer likely to recur?

2001. About 11,200 Americans will die of the disease in 2001. Multiple myeloma is one of the leading causes of cancer deaths among African-Americans.

In Western industrialized countries, approximately four people in 100,000 develop multiple myeloma. The incidence of multiple myeloma among African Americans is 9.5 per 100,000, about twice that of Caucasians. Asians have a much lower incidence of the disease. In China, for example, the incidence of multiple myeloma is only one in 100,000. The offspring and siblings of individuals with multiple myeloma are at a slightly increased risk for the disease.

At diagnosis, the average age of a multiple myeloma patient is 68 to 70. Although the average age at onset is decreasing, most multiple myelomas still occur in people over 40. This cancer is somewhat more prevalent in men than in women.

Causes and symptoms

Associations

The cause of multiple myeloma has not been determined. However, a number of possible associations have been identified:

- decreased immune system function; the immune systems of older individuals may be less efficient at detecting and destroying cancer cells
- genetic (hereditary) factors, suggested by the increased incidence in some ethnic groups and among family members
- occupational factors, suggested by the increased incidence among agricultural, petroleum, wood, and leather workers, and cosmetologists
- long-term exposure to herbicides, pesticides, petroleum products, heavy metals, plastics, and dusts such as asbestos
- radiation exposure, as among Japanese atomic bomb survivors, nuclear weapons workers, and medical personnel such as radiologists
- Kaposi's sarcoma-associated herpes virus (also called human herpes virus-8 or HHV-8), found in the blood and bone marrow cells of many multiple myeloma patients

Early symptoms

The accumulation of malignant plasma cells can result in tiny cracks or fractures in bones. Malignant plasma cells in the bone marrow can suppress the formation of red and white blood cells and platelets. About 80% of individuals with multiple myeloma are anemic due to low red blood cell formation. Low white blood cell formation results in increased susceptibility to **infection**, since new, functional antibodies are not produced. In addition, normal circulating antibodies are rapidly destroyed. Low platelet formation can result in poor blood clotting. It is rare, however, that insufficient white blood cell and platelet formations are presenting signs of multiple myeloma.

These factors cause the early symptoms of multiple myeloma:

- pain in the lower back or ribs
- fatigue and paleness due to anemia (low red blood cell count)
- frequent and recurring infections, including bacterial pneumonia, urinary-tract and kidney infections, and shingles (herpes zoster)
- bleeding

Bone destruction

Bone pain, particularly in the backbone, hips, and skull, is often the first symptom of multiple myeloma. As malignant plasma cells increase in the bone marrow, replacing normal marrow, they exert pressure on the bone. As overly active osteoclasts (large cells responsible for the breakdown of bone) remove bone tissue, the bone becomes soft. Fracture and **spinal cord compression** may occur.

Plasmacytomas (malignant tumors of plasma cells) may weaken bones, causing fractures. Fractured bones or weak or collapsed spinal bones, in turn, may place unusual pressure on nearby nerves, resulting in nerve pain, burning, or numbness and muscle weakness. Proteins produced by myeloma cells also may damage nerves.

Calcium from the destroyed bone enters the blood and urine, causing **hypercalcemia**, a medical condition in which abnormally high concentrations of calcium compounds exist in the bloodstream. High calcium affects nerve cell and kidney function. The symptoms of hypercalcemia include:

- weakness and fatigue
- depression
- mental confusion
- constipation
- increased thirst
- increased urination
- nausea and vomiting
- kidney pain
- kidney failureHypercalcemia affects about one-third of multiple myeloma patients.

Serum proteins

The accumulation of M-proteins in the serum (the liquid portion of the blood) may cause additional complications, such as hyperviscosity syndrome, or thickening of the blood (though rare in multiple myeloma patients). Symptoms of hyperviscosity include:

- fatigue
- headaches
- shortness of breath
- mental confusion
- chest pain
- kidney damage and failure
- vision problems
- Raynaud's disease

(Raynaud's phenomenon, can affect any part of the body, but particularly the fingers, toes, nose, and ears.)

Cryoglobulinemia occurs when the protein in the blood forms particles under cold conditions. These particles can block small blood vessels and cause pain and numbness in the toes, fingers, and other extremities during cold weather.

Amyloidosis is a rare complication of multiple myeloma. It usually occurs in individuals whose plasma cells produce only Ig light chains. These Bence-Jones proteins combine with other serum proteins to form amyloid protein. This starchy substance can invade tissues, organs, and blood vessels. In particular, amyloid proteins can accumulate in the kidneys, where they block the tiny tubules that are the kidney's filtering system. Indicators of amyloidosis include:

- carpal tunnel syndrome
- kidney failure
- liver failure
- heart failure

Diagnosis

Blood and urine tests

Often, the original diagnosis of multiple myeloma is made from routine blood tests that are performed for other reasons. Blood tests may indicate:

- anemia
- abnormal red blood cells
- high serum protein levels
- low levels of normal antibody
- high calcium levels
- high blood urea nitrogen (BUN) levels
- high creatinine levels

Urea and creatinine normally are excreted in the urine. High levels of urea and creatinine in the blood indicate that the kidneys are not functioning properly to eliminate these substances.

Protein electrophoresis is a laboratory technique that uses an electrical current to separate the different proteins in the blood and urine on the basis of size and charge. Since all of the multiple myeloma M-proteins in the blood and urine are identical, electrophoresis of blood and urine from a patient with multiple myeloma shows a large M-protein spike, corresponding to the high concentration of monoclonal Ig. Electrophoresis of the urine also can detect Bence-Jones proteins.

Bones

A **bone marrow aspiration** utilizes a very thin, long needle to remove a sample of marrow from the hip bone. Alternatively, a **bone marrow biopsy** with a larger needle removes solid marrow tissue. The marrow is examined under the microscope for plasma cells and tumors. If 10–30% of the cells are plasma cells, multiple myeloma is the usual diagnosis.

X rays are used to detect osteoporosis, osteolytic lesions, and fractures. **Computed tomography** (CAT or CT) scans can detect lesions in both bone and soft tissue. **Magnetic resonance imaging** (MRI) may give a more detailed image of a certain bone or a region of the body.

Treatment team

After the initial diagnosis, the treatment team for multiple myeloma may include a hematologist (a specialist in diseases of the blood) and an oncologist or cancer specialist. If radiation is used in treatment, a radiation oncologist may join the team. The treatment of multiple myeloma involves complex decisions, and obtaining second opinions from additional specialists may be important.

Clinical staging, treatments, and prognosis

Related disorders

Monoclonal gammopathy of undetermined significance (MGUS) is a common condition in which a monoclonal Ig is detectable. However, there are no tumors or other symptoms of multiple myeloma. MGUS occurs in about 1% of the general population and in about 3% of those over age 70. Over a period of years, about 16–20% of those with MGUS will develop multiple myeloma or a related cancer called malignant **lymphoma**.

Occasionally, only a single plasmacytoma develops, either in the bone marrow (isolated plasmacytoma of the bone) or other tissues or organs (extramedullary plasmacytoma). Some individuals with solitary plasmacytoma may develop multiple myeloma.

Clinical stages

The Durie-Salmon system is used to stage multiple myeloma. Stage I multiple myeloma requires all of the following (1 gram = approx. 0.02 pints, 1 deciliter = approx. 0.33 fluid ounces):

- hemoglobin (the oxygen-transporting molecule of red blood cells) above 10 grams/deciliter (g/dl)
- serum calcium below 12 mg/dl
- normal bone structure or only isolated plasmacytoma
- low M-protein, based on established guideline levels of Ig protein chains

Approximately 5% of multiple myeloma cases are not progressing at diagnosis, and may not progress for months or years. This is called smoldering myeloma. These patients have stage I blood chemistry but no symptoms.

Stage II multiple myeloma fits neither stage I nor stage III. Stage III multiple myeloma meets one or more the following criteria:

- hemoglobin below 8.5 g/dl
- serum calcium above 12 mg/dl
- advanced bone lesions
- high M-protein

Each stage is subclassified as A or B, based on serum creatinine indicators of normal or abnormal kidney function. Most patients have stage III multiple myeloma at diagnosis.

Prognostic indicators

Prognostic indicators for multiple myeloma may be used instead of, or in addition to, the staging system described above. Prognostic indicators are laboratory tests that help to define the stage of the disease at diagnosis, and its progression during treatment. These indicators are:

- plasmablastic multiple myeloma (presence of plasmablasts, the precursor malignant plasma cells)
- plasma cell labeling index (the percentage of plasma cells that are actively dividing)
- beta 2-microglobulin, a protein secreted by B cells that correlates with the myeloma cell mass (also indicates kidney damage)

Treatment

Since multiple myeloma often progresses slowly, and since the treatments can be toxic, the disease may not be treated until M-protein levels in the blood are quite high. In particular, MGUS and smoldering myeloma may be followed closely but not treated. Solitary plasmacytomas are treated with radiation and/or surgery and followed closely with examinations and laboratory tests.

CHEMOTHERAPY. **Chemotherapy**, or treatment with anti-cancer drugs, is used for multiple myeloma. MP, a combination of the drugs **melphalan** and prednisone, is the standard treatment. Usually, the drugs are taken by mouth every 3 to 4 weeks for 6 to 9 months or longer, until the M-protein levels in the blood stop decreasing. MP usually results in a 50% reduction in M-protein.

Dexamethasone, a corticosteroid, sometimes is used to treat the elderly or those in poor health. It can drop the M-protein levels by 40% in untreated individuals and by 20–40% in patients who have not responded to previous treatment. Other chemotherapy drugs, including **cyclophosphamide**, **carmustine**, **doxorubicin**, **vincristine**, and **chlorambucil**, may be used as well.

Multiple myeloma usually recurs within a year after the end of chemotherapy. Although the chemotherapy can be repeated after each recurrence, it is progressively less responsive to treatment.

Side effects of chemotherapy may include:

- anemia
- hair loss (alopecia)
- nausea and vomiting
- diarrhea
- mood swings
- swelling
- acne

These side effects disappear after treatment is discontinued.

OTHER DRUG TREATMENTS. **Bisphosphonates** are drugs that inhibit the activity of osteoclasts. These drugs can slow the progression of bone disease, reduce pain, and help prevent bone fractures. Different types of bisphosphonates inhibit osteoclasts in different ways. They also reduce the production of interleukin-6 by bone marrow cells. Laboratory studies suggest that bisphosphonates may kill or inhibit the growth of multiple myeloma cells. Pamidronate is the most common bisphosphonate for treating multiple myeloma.

The drug **thalidomide** appears to have several anti-myeloma activities. Thalidomide affects the immune system in various ways and it appears to inhibit myeloma cells, both directly and indirectly. It also inhibits the growth of new blood vessels that are needed by tumors. However, if thalidomide is taken during pregnancy, it can cause severe birth defects or death of the fetus.

The drug **allopurinol** may be used to reduce high blood levels of uric acid that result from kidney dysfunction. Diuretics can improve kidney function. Infections require prompt treatment with **antibiotics**.

BONE AND PERIPHERAL BLOOD STEM CELL TRANSPLANTATION. Bone marrow or peripheral blood stem cell transplantations (PBSCT) are used to replace the stem cells of the bone marrow following high-dosage chemotherapy. Chemotherapy destroys the bone marrow stem cells that are necessary to produce new blood cells. In an autologous transplant, the patient's bone marrow stem cells or peripheral blood stem cells (immature bone marrow cells found in the blood) are collected, treated with drugs to kill any myeloma cells, and frozen prior to chemotherapy. Growth factors are used to increase the number of peripheral stem cells prior to collection. A procedure called apheresis is used to collect the peripheral stem cells. Following high-dosage chemotherapy, the stem cells are reinjected into the individual. In an allogeneic transplant, the donor stem cells come from a genetically related individual such as a sibling.

OTHER TREATMENTS. Blood transfusions may be required to treat severe **anemia**.

Plasmapheresis, or plasma exchange transfusion, may be used to thin the blood to treat hyperviscosity syndrome. In this treatment, blood is removed and passed through a machine that separates the plasma, containing the M-protein, from the red and white blood cells and platelets. The blood cells are transfused back into the patient, along with a plasma substitute or donated plasma.

Multiple myeloma may be treated with high-energy x rays directed at a specific region of the body. **Radiation therapy** is used for treating bone pain.

Alternative and complementary therapies

Interferon alpha, an immune-defense protein that is produced by some white blood cells and bone marrow cells, can slow the growth of myeloma cells. It usually is given to patients following chemotherapy, to prolong their remission. However, interferon may have toxic effects in older individuals with multiple myeloma.

Once multiple myeloma is in remission, calcium and vitamin D supplements can improve bone density. It is important not to take these supplements when the myeloma is active. Individuals with multiple myeloma must drink large amounts of fluid to counter the effects of hyperviscous blood.

Prognosis

The prognosis for individuals with MGUS or solitary plasmacytoma is very good. Most do not develop multiple myeloma. However, approximately 15% of all patients with multiple myeloma die within three months of diagnosis. About 60% respond to treatment and live for an average of two and a half to three years following diagnosis. Approximately 23% of patients die of other illnesses associated with advanced age.

The prognosis for a given individual may be based on the prognostic indicators described above. The median survival for those without plasmablasts, and with a low plasma cell labeling index (PCLI) and low beta 2-microglobulin, is 5.5 years. The median survival for patients with plasmablastic multiple myeloma, or with a high PCLI (1% or greater) and high beta 2-microglobulin (4 or higher), is 1.9 and 2.4 years, respectively. Many multiple myeloma patients are missing part or all of chromosome 13. The deletion of this chromosome, along with high beta 2-microglobulin, leads to a poor prognosis.

With treatment, multiple myeloma may go into complete remission. This is defined as:

- M-protein absent from the blood and urine
- myeloma cells not detectable in the bone marrow
- no clinical symptoms
- negative laboratory tests

However, with very sensitive testing, a few myeloma cells are usually detectable and eventually lead to a recurrence of the disease, in the bone or elsewhere in the body.

Coping with cancer treatment

Techniques such as biofeedback, guided imagery, and meditation may be helpful for reducing stress and relieving pain. Pain medication is usually prescribed for multiple myeloma. Back or neck braces may help relieve bone pain. Exercise, if possible, is important for retaining calcium in the bones.

Clinical trials

There are hundreds of ongoing **clinical trials** for the treatment of multiple myeloma. These take place throughout the United States and are sponsored by both government and industry. Clinical trials of treatments for multiple myeloma include:

- thalidomide
- thalidomide-like drugs that affect the immune system in various ways
- skeletal targeted radiotherapy (STP), in which a radioactive element is attached to a drug that binds to bone
- new anti-cancer drugs
- new combinations of drugs
- new chemotherapies in combination with PBSCT
- combinations of PBSCT, interleukin-2, and interferon alpha
- treatments for disease resulting from PBSCT (graft-versus-host disease)
- bone marrow transplantations
- immunotherapies, including vaccines, to destroy remaining myeloma cells after high-dosage chemotherapy and PBSCT
- treatments for MGUS

Prevention

There are no clearly established risk factors for multiple myeloma and it is possible that a combination of factors interact to cause the disease. Thus, there is no method for preventing multiple myeloma.

Special concerns

Since there is a high probability that multiple myeloma will recur after treatment, patients are followed carefully. Blood tests, x rays, and other **imaging studies** may be used to check for a recurrence.

See also Bone marrow transplantation; Immunoelectrophoresis; Pheresis; Protein electrophoresis.

Resources

BOOKS

Holland, Jimmie C., and Sheldon Lewis. *The Human Side of Cancer: Living with Hope, Coping with Uncertainty.* New York: HarperCollins, 2000.

OTHER

"About Myeloma." *Multiple Myeloma Research Foundation.* [cited June 15, 2009]. http://www.multiplemyeloma.org/aboutmyeloma.html.

Complementary and Alternative Therapies for Leukemia, Lymphoma, Hodgkin's Disease and Myeloma. The Leukemia and Lymphoma Society. [cited June 15, 2009]. http://www.leukemia-lymphoma.org.

Facts and Statistics About Leukemia, Lymphoma, Hodgkin's Disease and Myeloma. The Leukemia and Lymphoma Society. [cited March 15, 2009]. http://www.leukemia-lymphoma.org.

"Multiple Myeloma and Other Plasma Cell Neoplasms." *CancerNet.* National Cancer Institute. [cited April 16, 2009]. http://cancernet.nci.nih.gov.

"Multiple Myeloma." *Cancer Resource Center.* American Cancer Society. [cited June 15, 2009]. http://www3.cancer.org/cancerinfo.

ORGANIZATIONS

International Myeloma Foundation. 12650 Riverside Dr., Suite 206, North Hollywood, CA 91607. (800) 452-CURE. (818) 487-7455. http://www.myeloma.org. Information and support for patients and families and the scientific and medical communities.

The Leukemia and Lymphoma Society. 600 Third Avenue, New York, NY 10016. (800) 955-4572. (914) 949-5213. http://www.leukemia-lymphoma.org. Information, support, and guidance for patients and health care professionals.

Multiple Myeloma Research Foundation. 11 Forest Street, New Canaan, CT 06840. (203) 972-1250. http://www.multiplemyeloma.org. Information and research funding.

Margaret Alic, Ph.D.

Muromonab-CD3

Definition

Muromonab-CD3 is a mouse-derived (murine) monoclonal antibody that specifically binds to the CD3 (T3) protein found on the surface of T cells. It is a protein known to be necessary for activation (immune responses) of T cells. Muromonab-CD3 is marketed in the United States under the Orthoklone OKT3 brand name.

KEY TERMS

Antibody—A protective protein made by the immune system in response to an antigen; also called an immunoglobulin.

Cytokine—A protein produced by cells of the immune system that help boost immune function.

hOKT3—A humanized version of the muromonab-CD3 antibody.

Humanization—Fusing the constant and variable framework region of one or more human immunoglobulins with the binding region of an animal immunoglobulin; done to reduce human reaction against the fusion antibody.

Interleukin-2—A cytokine responsible for the activation of B and T cells of the immune system that induces growth and maturation of those cells.

Monoclonal antibody—Genetically engineered antibodies specific for one antigen.

Purpose

Muromonab-CD3 is believed to have two effects when it binds to the CD3 protein on the surface of T cells. In the short term the T cells are activated and begin to excrete cytokines—small proteins that boost immune function. In the long term, function of the T cells is eliminated because access to the CD3 protein is blocked and binding by the antibody encourages removal of the cell from the bloodstream by the immune system.

When using muromonab-CD3 to treat **cancer**, doctors are seeking the short-term effect by boosting the activity of T cells against tumor antigens. In this setting muromonab-CD3 is not administered directly to the patient. Rather, it is used to stimulate white blood cells (lymphocytes) that have been removed from the patient, treated outside the body, then reinfused (infused back into the patient). In the test tube the binding of the antibody to the CD3 protein stimulates the T cells so they can begin the cell-mediated destruction of the tumor cells upon reentry into the patient's bloodstream. Often, the T cells used for this treatment are either preselected to be specific against the proteins found on the tumor surface (tumor antigens) or are genetically engineered before reinfusion to express the desired tumor-antigen specific receptors. This is often followed by stimulation of T-cell division using interleukin-2.

Clinical trials using this stimulated lymphocyte treatment are ongoing for **astrocytoma**, **oligodendroglioma**, nonmetastatic **kidney cancer**, metastatic **melanoma**, **Kaposi's sarcoma** (a twin study), and advanced epithelial **ovarian cancer**.

Description

In late 1986, Muromonab-CD3 was the first monoclonal antibody approved for use by the FDA as an immunosuppressive drug in kidney transplantation. The use of this drug in transplantation is based on the long-term effect of antibody binding, blocking cellular interaction with the CD3 protein known to be necessary to activate T cells involved in the rejection of transplanted tissue. As of mid-2001, it had not been approved for use as a cancer therapy. However, there were at least five active clinical trials to test its ability to activate lymphocytes outside the body in preparation for reinfusion.

A second use of the muromonab-CD3 antibody to treat cancer required the development of a humanized monoclonal antibody called hOKT3, using the same binding sites as muromonab-CD3. This treatment involves direct administration of the antibody to the patient. The humanized antibody retains the murine sequences at the antibody's two binding sites, but has human sequences in the other areas of the antibody molecule. This allows the monoclonal antibody to be directly administered to the patient without the immune reaction against the mouse antibodies seen when muromonab-CD3 is used. hOKT3 was used in a clinical trial of 24 patients against a wide variety of cancers. Although testing the antibody's function as a therapy was not the main goal of the study, three patients with cancers of the peritoneum cavity (lower abdomen) did see a clinical improvement.

Recommended dosage

To treat cancer, muromonab-CD3 is not administered directly to the patient. However, a similar humanized antibody, hOKT3, has been given to patients during a clinical trial. The most effective dosage in the trial was three doses of 800 micrograms every two weeks in a 10-minute infusion, but further study is necessary to confirm this finding.

Precautions

As the two uses of muromonab-CD3 are still in the clinical trial stage, the exact precautions for this drug (or the humanized version, hOKT3) are not yet known. However, for monoclonal antibody treatment in general, preexisting heart conditions and arrhythmias can make taking this drug more dangerous. Vaccination during the treatment session is also not recommended, given the T-cell depletion that occurs during treatment.

Side effects

During clinical trials the majority of side effects occurred during the first administration of activated T cells or humanized antibody. These side effects included flu-like symptoms, headache, dizziness, and shortness of breath. The humanized antibody also caused edema (collection of fluid) in all three patients who exhibited a clinical benefit from the treatment.

Interactions

Still in the early clinical trial stages in 2001, muromonab-CD3 had not been studied to determine interactions with other drugs.

Michelle Johnson, M.S., J.D.

Myasthenic syndrome of Lambert-Eaton *see* **Lambert-Eaton myasthenic syndrome**

Myasthenia gravis

Description

Myasthenia gravis (MG) is an autoimmune disease that causes muscle weakness. It affects the neuromuscular junction, interrupting the communication between nerve and muscle, and thereby causing weakness. People with MG may have difficulty moving their eyes, walking, speaking clearly, swallowing, and even breathing, depending on the severity and distribution of weakness. Increased weakness with exertion, and improvement with rest, is a characteristic feature of MG.

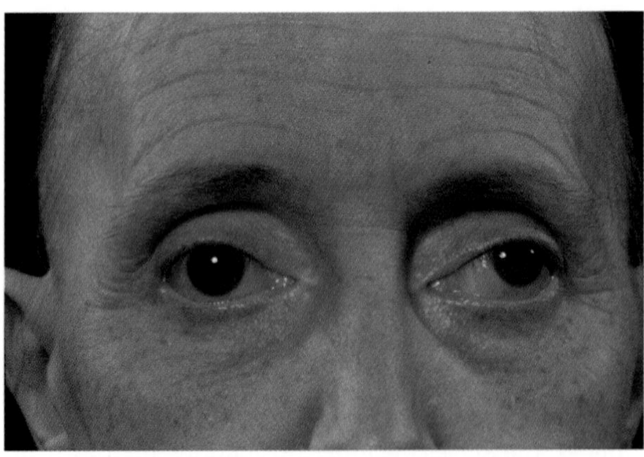

Face of a person afflicted with myasthenia gravis. Half of patients with thymoma (a cancer of the thymus) also have myasthenia gravis. *(Custom Medical Stock Photo. Reproduced by permission.)*

About 30,000 people in the United States are affected by MG. It can occur at any age, but is most common in women who are in their late teens and early twenties, and in men in their sixties and seventies.

MG has been associated with malignant **thymoma**, a disease in which **cancer** cells are found in the tissues of the thymus.

Causes

Myasthenia gravis is an autoimmune disease, meaning that it is caused by the body's own immune system. In MG, the immune system attacks a receptor on the surface of muscle cells. This prevents the muscle from receiving the nerve impulses that normally make it respond. MG affects "voluntary" muscles, which are those muscles under conscious control responsible for movement. It does not affect heart muscle or the "smooth" muscle found in the digestive system and other internal organs.

A muscle is stimulated to contract when the nerve cell controlling it releases acetylcholine molecules onto its surface. The acetylcholine lands on a muscle protein called the acetylcholine receptor. This leads to rapid chemical changes in the muscle which cause it to contract. Acetylcholine is then broken down by acetylcholinesterase enzyme, to prevent further stimulation.

In MG, immune cells create antibodies against the acetylcholine receptor. Antibodies are proteins normally involved in fighting **infection**. When these antibodies attach to the receptor, they prevent it from receiving acetylcholine, decreasing the ability of the muscle to respond to stimulation.

Why the immune system creates these self-reactive "autoantibodies" is unknown, although there are several hypotheses:

- During fetal development, the immune system generates many B cells that can make autoantibodies, but B cells that could harm the body's own tissues are screened out and destroyed before birth. It is possible that the stage is set for MG when some of these cells escape detection.
- Genes controlling other parts of the immune system, called MHC genes, appear to influence how susceptible a person is to developing autoimmune disease.
- Infection may trigger some cases of MG. When activated, the immune system may mistake portions of

the acetylcholine receptor for portions of an invading virus, though no candidate virus has yet been identified conclusively.

- About 10% of those with MG also have thymomas, or tumors of the thymus gland. The thymus is a principal organ of the immune system, and researchers speculate that thymic irregularities are involved in the progression of MG. A definite relationship exists between MG and thymoma: of patients with MG, 15% also have thymoma, and of patients with thymoma, 50% have MG.

Treatment

While there is no cure for myasthenia gravis, there are a number of treatments that effectively control symptoms in most people. Even though no rigorously tested treatment trials have been reported and no clear consensus exists on treatment strategies, MG is one of the most treatable immune disorders. Several factors require consideration before initiating treatment, such as the severity, distribution, and rapidity of the MG progression.

Edrophonium (Tensilon) is a drug used to block the action of acetylcholinesterase, prolonging the effect of acetylcholine and increasing strength. An injection of edrophonium rapidly leads to a marked improvement in most people with MG. An alternate drug, neostigmine, may also be used.

Pyridostigmine (Mestinon) is usually the first drug tried. Like edrophonium, pyridostigmine blocks acetylcholinesterase. It is longer-acting, taken by mouth, and well-tolerated. Loss of responsiveness and disease progression combine to eventually make pyridostigmine ineffective in tolerable doses in many patients.

Thymectomy, or removal of the thymus gland, has increasingly become a standard form of treatment for MG. Up to 85% of people with MG improve after thymectomy, with complete remission eventually seen in about 30%. The improvement may take months or even several years to fully develop. Thymectomy is not usually recommended for children with MG, since the thymus continues to play an important immune role throughout childhood.

Immune-suppressing drugs are used to treat MG if patient response to pyridostigmine and thymectomy is not adequate. These drugs include **corticosteroids** such as prednisone, and the non-steroids **azathioprine** (Imuran) and **cyclosporine** (Sandimmune).

Plasma exchange may also be performed to treat the condition or to strengthen very weak patients before thymectomy. In this procedure, blood plasma is removed and replaced with purified plasma free of autoantibodies. It can produce a temporary improvement in symptoms, but is too expensive for long-term treatment. Another blood treatment, intravenous immunoglobulin therapy, is also used. In this procedure, large quantities of purified immune proteins (immunoglobulins) are injected. For unknown reasons, this leads to symptomatic improvement in up to 85% of patients. It is also too expensive for long-term treatment. There are indications that IVIg is an effective immunoglobulin for some categories of MG patients.

People with weakness of the bulbar muscles may need to eat softer foods that are easier to chew and swallow. In more severe cases, it may be necessary to obtain nutrition through a feeding tube placed into the stomach (gastrostomy tube).

Alternative and complementary therapies

No alternative therapies have been shown to be effective for the treatment of MG. Reports claiming that herbal remedies or alternative treatments alleviate or cure MG have not been corroborated by properly controlled **clinical trials**, which are required to evaluate the benefit of such treatments.

Among complementary MG therapies, prescription of low dose atropine can help relieve the cramping and **diarrhea** often caused by the drug Mestinon. Propantheline bromide (ProBanthine) is a drug similar to atropine, and it may also be prescribed to treat gastrointestinal discomfort. Caution must be taken not to take too much atropine because it cancels the beneficial effects of the anticholinesterase drugs. Ephedrine is sometimes also used with anticholinesterase therapy to strengthen the muscle tissue of MG patients.

Resources

PERIODICALS

Bedlack, R. S., and D. B. Sanders. "How to handle myasthenic crisis. Essential steps in patient care." *Postgraduate Medicine* 107 (April 2000): 211–214.

Carrieri, P. B., E. Marano, A. Perretti, and G. Caruso. "The thymus and myasthenia gravis: immunological and neurophysiological aspects." *Annals of Medicine* 31, Supplement 2 (October 1999): 52–56.

Davitt, B. V., G. A. Fenton, and O. A. Cruz. "Childhood myasthenia." *Journal of Ophthalmic and Nursing Technology* 19 (March-April 2000): 74–81.

Richard Robinson
Monique Laberge, Ph.D.

Mycophenolate mofetil

Definition

Mycophenolate mofetil (brand name CellCept) is a drug that has been shown to inhibit tumor growth in rodents, and that may prove useful in treating tumors in humans.

Purpose

The Food and Drug Administration (FDA) approved the use of mycophenolate mofetil in August 2000 for use in patients undergoing liver transplants, and the drug is used primarily to ease the acceptance of a transplanted organ by a recipient. The drug makes acceptance of the transplanted organ more likely because it prevents the recipient from mounting an **immune response** to the organ, or treating it like a foreign invader. The drug also seems to have the ability to inhibit tumor growth, and may prove effective in treating certain kinds of **cancer**.

In laboratory studies, mycophenolate mofetil has inhibited tumor growth in cancers of the pancreas, colon, lung, and blood. The value of the drug for anticancer therapy is still being evaluated.

In addition to its use in treating cancer, mycophenolate mofetil has been used by dermatologists to treat pyoderma gangrenosum, a rare skin disorder of unknown origin characterized by ulcerated areas on the legs. Pyoderma gangrenosum is associated with systemic diseases in about half the patients diagnosed with it, and mycophenolate mofetil has been found to be effective in treating these patients either alone or in combination with prednisone.

Mycophenolate mofetil is reported to be effective in relieving pain in patients with cluster headache; however, this use of the drug is considered investigational.

Description

Mycophenolate mofetil suppresses, or prevents activity of, cells in the lymphatic system, both T cells and B cells. Under normal circumstances, T cells mount an immune response by reacting directly with foreign materials in the body and B cells release compounds that attack foreign materials. But during a transplant, T cells and B cells can cause a reaction that leads to the rejection of a donor organ.

KEY TERMS

B cell—A type of cell in the lymphatic system that contributes to immunity by releasing compounds that attack foreign bodies, such as bacteria and viruses.

Clearance—A measure of the rate at which a drug or other substance is removed from the blood.

Intravenous line—A tube that is inserted directly into a vein to carry medicine directly to the blood stream, bypassing the stomach and other digestive organs that might alter the medicine.

Kilogram—Metric measure that equals 2.2 pounds.

Lymphatic system—The system that collects and returns fluid in tissues to the blood vessels and produces defensive agents for fighting infection and invasion by foreign bodies.

Milligram—One-thousandth of a gram, and there are one thousand grams in a kilogram. A gram is the metric measure that equals about 0.035 ounces.

Mutant—Altered, not normal.

T cell—A cell in the lymphatic system that contributes to immunity by attacking foreign bodies, such as bacteria and viruses, directly.

Recommended dosage

The drug is given orally and by intravenous line. Dosages given for cancer therapy are experimental. To prevent immune response during organ transplants, the drug is dispensed in capsules of 250 mg, tablets of 500 mg, and by intravenous line in doses of 500 mg. Time intervals between dosages are determined according to the rate of the drug's breakdown in the patient's body.

Precautions

Mycophenolate mofetil is known to cause or may cause lymphomas and **skin cancer**. The benefit of taking the drug must be weighed against the increased risk of the cancers it causes.

It is critical for the patient's doctor to monitor blood levels carefully when using this drug, as patients vary widely in their rate of clearance of mycophenolate mofetil, particularly when it is given in combination with other immunosuppressants.

Side effects

In addition to increasing the risk of lymphomas and skin cancer, mycophenolate mofetil may cause a number of other unwanted reactions. They include dizziness, headache, trembling, as well as pain in the chest, swelling (edema), and high blood pressure (hypertension). Many digestive tract upsets from constipation to **diarrhea** to **vomiting** are also possible side effects. There is also a chance of hemorrhage, or uncontrolled bleeding in the digestive tract.

Interactions

Taking the drug is likely to make oral contraceptives ineffective and another form of birth control should be used. Stomach medications that contain magnesium and aluminum hydroxides, such as antacids, can block the uptake of mycophenolate mofetil across the gut. They should be avoided. As always, the physician in charge of the care plan should be told of every drug a patient is taking so that the potential for interactions can be avoided. The drug is considered superior to some others used as a suppressant of the immune response in transplants because it does not show as many drug interactions as other drugs do. But the short list of interactions might be in part related to its limited time on the market, and interactions that are yet unidentified.

Resources

BOOKS

Wilson, Billie A., Margaret T. Shannon, and Carolyn L. Stang. *Nurses Drug Guide 2000*. Stamford, CT: Appleton & Lange, 2000.

PERIODICALS

Fireman, M., A. F. DiMartini, S. C. Armstrong, and K. L. Cozza. "Immunosuppressants." *Psychosomatics* 45 (July-August 2004): 354–360.

Jackson, J. Mark, MD, and Jeffrey P. Callen, MD. "Pyoderma Gangrenosum." *eMedicine* August 4, 2003. http://www.emedicine.com/DERM/topic367.htm.

Lee, M. R., and A. J. Cooper. "Mycophenolate Mofetil in Pyoderma Gangrenosum." *Journal of Dermatological Treatment* 15 (September 2004): 303–307.

Rozen, T. D. "Complete But Transient Relief of Chronic Cluster Headache with Mycophenolate Mofetil." *Headache* 44 (September 2004): 818–820.

Shaw, L. M., A. Nawrocki, M. Korecka, et al. "Using Established Immunosuppressant Therapy Effectively: Lessons from the Measurement of Mycophenolic Acid Plasma Concentrations." *Therapeutic Drug Monitoring* 26 (August 2004): 347–351.

ORGANIZATIONS

American Society of Health-System Pharmacists (ASHP). 7272 Wisconsin Avenue, Bethesda, MD 20814. (301) 657-3000. http://www.ashp.org.

United States Food and Drug Administration (FDA). 5600 Fishers Lane, Rockville, MD 20857-0001. (888) INFO-FDA. www.fda.gov.

Diane M. Calabrese
Rebecca J. Frey, PhD

Mycosis fungoides

Definition

Mycosis fungoides is a **skin cancer** characterized by patches, plaques, and tumors where cancerous T lymphocytes have invaded the skin.

Description

Mycosis fungoides, the most common type of **cutaneous T-cell lymphoma**, originates from a type of white blood cell called a T lymphocyte or T cell. In mycosis fungoides, cancerous T cells accumulate in the skin. These cells and the skin irritation they create become visible as growths or changes in the skin's color or texture.

Mycosis fungoides usually develops and progresses slowly. It often begins as an unexplained rash that can wax and wane for years. Whether this stage represents early mycosis fungoides or a precancerous stage is controversial. The classic symptoms of mycosis fungoides are red, scaly skin patches that develop into raised plaques, then into large, mushroom-shaped tumors. The patches often originate on parts of the body that are covered by clothing and sometimes

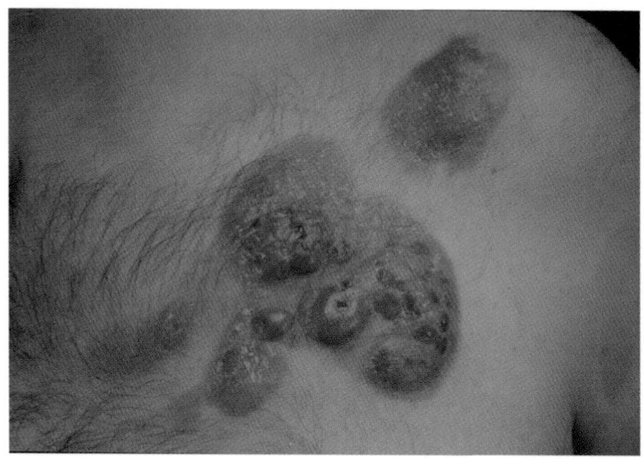

Red, scaly plaque on skin of patient with mycosis fungoides. *(Custom Medical Stock Photo. Reproduced by permission.)*

KEY TERMS

Acyclovir—A drug used to kill viruses.

Antibody—A protein made by the immune system. Antibodies attach to target molecules and can be useful as drugs.

Biopsy—A sample of an organ taken to look for abnormalities. Also, the technique used to take such samples.

Computed tomography (CT)—A special x-ray technique that produces a cross-sectional image of the body.

Cutaneous T-cell lymphoma—A type of skin cancer originating from T lymphocytes.

Electron beam—A type of radiation composed of electrons. Electrons are tiny, negatively charged particles found in atoms.

Hypericin—A chemical derived from plants that kills cells after being activated by visible light.

Interferon alpha—A chemical made naturally by the immune system and also manufactured as a drug.

Local anesthetic—A liquid used to numb a small area of the skin.

Lymph node—A small organ full of immune cells that are found in clusters throughout the body. Lymph nodes are where reactions to infections usually begin.

Myelosuppression—A decrease in blood cell production from the bone marrow. This can result in anemia, an increased risk of infections, or bleeding tendencies.

Oncologist—A doctor who specializes in the treatment of cancer.

Pancreatitis—Inflammation of the pancreas. This disease is potentially serious and life-threatening.

Pathologist—A doctor who specializes in examining cells and other parts of the body for abnormalities.

Precancerous—Abnormal and with a high probability of turning into cancer, but not yet a cancer.

Remission—A decrease in the symptoms of the cancer. In a complete remission, there is no longer any evidence of the cancer, although it may still be there.

Retinoids—Drugs related to vitamin A.

T lymphocyte or T cell—A type of white blood cell. Some T cells, known as helper T cells, aid other cells of the immune system. Other T cells, called cytotoxic T cells, fight viruses and cancer.

Ultraviolet light—Light waves that have a shorter wavelength than visble light, but longer wavelength than x rays. UVA light is closer to visible light than UVB.

White blood cells—The cells in the blood that fight infections. There are several types of white blood cells. Also called immune cells.

improve when they are exposed to sunlight. **Itching** can be intense.

As the **cancer** progresses, the cancer cells lose their affinity for the skin and spread to nearby lymph nodes and other internal organs. The normal T cells also start to disappear. Because T cells are very important in immunity, this leaves the patient susceptible to infections. Treatment at an earlier stage of the disease can often stop or slow this progression.

Sézary syndrome is a variant of mycosis fungoides. Sézary syndrome is characterized by red, thickened skin and large numbers of cancer cells in the blood.

Demographics

Mycosis fungoides is usually diagnosed after the age of 50, but has been seen as early as childhood. Mycosis fungoides develops twice as often in men as in women and is more common in people of African than of European origin.

Causes and symptoms

Environmental chemicals, virus infections, allergies, and genes have all been suggested as possible causes of this cancer.

The symptoms of mycosis fungoides include:

- Patches: patches are red or brown, sometimes scaly, flat areas. There may be one patch or many. Patches may itch and can resemble psoriasis, eczema, allergies, or other skin diseases. Some patients do not have a patch stage.
- Plaques: plaques are red or brown, sometimes scaly, raised areas. Itching is usually more intense than during the patch stage. The hair sometimes falls out in the affected skin. If the face is involved, the facial features can change.
- Tumors: tumors can originate from plaques, red skin, or normal skin. They are usually reddish brown or purple. The itching can diminish, but the

QUESTIONS TO ASK THE DOCTOR

- What stage is my cancer?
- If it is treated, is my cancer likely to progress?
- Which treatment(s) do you recommend?
- What are the side effects of these treatments?
- Can you recommend anything to help with those side effects?
- How should I prepare for the treatment?
- Are there any other treatments which might work as well?
- Do you expect me to go into remission and, if so, how long can I expect it to last?
- How often should I return for check-ups?

tumors may develop painful open sores or become infected. Some tumors can become very large. Patches, plaques, and tumors can co-exist.

- Erythrodermic form: in the erythrodermic form, the skin becomes red, thickened, and sometimes peels and flakes. The palms and soles thicken and may crack. Itching is usually intense. More than 90% of the time, the erythrodermic form is associated with Sézary syndrome.
- Other, more rare symptoms are also seen, including itching alone.

Diagnosis

A physical examination, history of the symptoms, blood tests, and skin **biopsy** are usually the key to diagnosing this cancer. The blood tests examine the health of the internal organs and look for cancer cells in the blood. The skin biopsy checks for the typical microscopic changes seen in this disease. This biopsy is a brief, simple procedure often done in the doctor's office. After numbing the skin with an injection of local anesthetic, the doctor snips out one or more tiny pieces of abnormal skin. The skin samples are sent to a trained pathologist for examination, and results may take up to a week to come back.

During its early stages, mycosis fungoides can be very difficult to diagnose. The symptoms resemble other skin diseases and numerous biopsies may be needed before the typical features are found. Special stains and DNA tests on the skin sample may find the cancer a little earlier.

To stage this cancer, the lymph nodes are checked for abnormal size or texture and, if necessary, biopsied. The doctor may also recommend x-ray studies of the chest, **computed tomography**, or biopsies of the internal organs to look for cancer cells.

Treatment team

Patients diagnosed with mycosis fungoides are often referred to an oncologist. A dermatologist may also become involved. Depending on the treatment chosen, the team may include other specialists, such as a radiation oncologist, specially trained nurses, a dietitian, or a social worker.

Clinical staging, treatments, and prognosis

Staging

In stage I, the lymph nodes look normal and cancer cells cannot be found in the internal organs. In stage IA, patches or plaques cover less than 10% of the skin. In stage IB, they are present on more than 10%.

In stage IIA, some of the lymph nodes look swollen or abnormal. Patches or plaques may cover any amount of skin. In stage IIB, the lymph nodes may or may not look abnormal, but there is at least one tumor on the skin. Neither the lymph nodes nor the internal organs contain detectable cancer cells in stage IIA or IIB.

In stage III, the skin looks thickened, red and sometimes scaly. The lymph nodes sometimes look abnormal, but no cancer cells can be detected in them or within internal organs.

In stage IVA and IVB, the skin may have patches, plaques, tumors, or widespread reddening. In stage IVA, cancer cells have been found in the lymph nodes but not in other internal organs. In stage IVB, cancer cells have been found in internal organs and sometimes the lymph nodes.

Treatment

Mycosis fungoides is rarely cured. Instead, most treatments are aimed at controlling the symptoms, improving the quality of life, and preventing the disease from progressing into later stages. This cancer responds well to a variety of therapies and frequently goes into remission, particularly if it is caught early. Even in stage IV, treatment can significantly improve the symptoms in the skin.

In stages III and IV, treatments directed against the cancer cells in the skin may be combined with **chemotherapy** or other therapies against metastatic cells. Experimental treatments are sometimes offered, especially in stage III or stage IV. If the cancer relapses, re-treatment may be possible or other therapies can be tried.

One treatment option for early cancers is ultraviolet B (UVB) light. UVB light can treat mycosis fungoides patches, but not plaques or tumors. About 70% of patients go into complete remission and 15% into partial remission. The side effects can include itching, sunburn, aging of the skin, and a risk of developing other skin cancers. The eyes must be protected from UVB light.

Psoralen and ultraviolet A (PUVA) photochemotherapy is an option for all stages, although earlier stages usually have a better response. In PUVA, the drug methoxypsoralen is taken before exposure to ultraviolet A (UVA) light. The drug sensitizes the cancer cells to the light. The complete remission rate with this treatment is 62–90%. The side effects may include itching, dry skin, sunburn, **nausea**, nail discoloration, and a risk of developing other skin cancers. The eyes must be protected to prevent damage to the retina and possibly cataracts.

Total skin electron-beam irradiation (TSEB) is also effective for all stages. TSEB is a type of radiation treatment that uses beams of electrons to irradiate the skin. The electrons stop at the skin and do not penetrate deeper tissues. Up to 80% of patients in stages II and III will respond. The side effects can include flaking of the skin, **alopecia** or hair loss (usually temporary), loss of sweat glands, skin irritation, blisters, dryness, temporary loss of the nails, and a risk of developing other skin cancers. These side effects limit the number of times this treatment can be given. TSEB is not available everywhere.

Other types of radiation—for instance, focused electron beam irradiation or **x rays** —can shrink or destroy some tumors or plaques.

Mechlorethamine (nitrogen mustard) is a drug that can be painted onto the skin to suppress the cancer. A thin layer is applied to the whole skin at bedtime, then washed off in the morning. The side effects can include dryness, skin irritation, darkening of the skin, allergies to the ingredients, and possibly a risk of other skin cancers. Half to 80% of mycosis fungoides patients in stage IA and 25–75% of patients in stage IB or IIA go into complete remission. In stage IIB, the complete remission rate is up to 50%. In stage III, it is 20–40% and, in stage IV, up to 35%. In stages III and IV, this treatment is used to decrease the skin symptoms and is often combined with other treatments.

Carmustine (BCNU) is an alternative drug. Its effectiveness is similar to mechlorethamine. In addition to side effects in the skin, this drug may cause **myelosuppression**.

Bexarotene is a drug used for cases that do not respond to other treatments. About 40% of patients have a complete or partial remission. The side effects may include dryness of the mucous membranes, aching joints or muscles, headaches, **fatigue**, and increased fragility of the skin. One of the most serious side effects is an increase in the fats in the blood, which can lead to pancreatitis.

Aldesleukin fusion toxin contains a poison that damages cells, attached to a molecule that directs that poison to T cells. About 10% of patients have complete remissions and 40% respond to some extent. The side effects can include chills, nausea, fluid retention, and allergic reactions to the drug.

Chemotherapy is sometimes combined with other therapies for stages III and IV. In stage IV, chemotherapy is directed against the metastatic cells in the lymph nodes or internal organs. Approximately 60% of mycosis fungoides patients in stage IV respond to single drugs, but the remission usually lasts less than six months. No cures have been reported, and it is not certain whether chemotherapy lengthens survival.

Corticosteroids are sometimes added to other treatments. These drugs decrease skin irritation and can destroy T cells. Fifty percent of patients have complete remissions on corticosteroids and 40% have partial remissions.

Supportive therapies can also help. Antihistamines or other drugs can decrease the itching. Mild moisturizing soaps and moisturizers can also combat the dryness and itching. If **infection** sets in, **antibiotics** may be necessary.

Prognosis

If mycosis fungoides is caught early, the prognosis is very good. If treatment begins during stage IA, most patients can expect to live as long as someone of the same age and gender who does not have this cancer. Median survival in stage IA is at least 20 years and most people die of diseases unrelated to the cancer. The overall 5-year survival in stage I is 80–90%. In stage II, five-year survival is 60–70%. As tumors develop and the cancer cells spread internally, the prognosis becomes worse. Five-year survival drops to 30% in stage IIB, 40–50% in stage III, and 25–35% in stage IV. Cancer cells can spread into almost any organ in the later stages of mycosis fungoides. Once this happens, many patients die of cancer complications, particularly skin infections that spread into the blood. Overall, half of mycosis fungoides patients live for at least 10 years after their cancer is diagnosed.

Alternative and complementary therapies

Complementary treatments can decrease stress, reduce the side effects of cancer treatment, and help patients feel more in control. For instance, some people find activities such as biofeedback, hypnosis, pet therapy, yoga, massage, pleasant distractions, meditation and prayer, mild physical exercise, or visualization helpful. Patients should check with their doctors before starting any complementary or alternative treatment. This is particularly important for alternative treatments that attempt to cure the cancer, boost the immune system, or reduce the side effects of conventional treatments. Some alternative treatments may interfere with the standard medical treatments or be dangerous when they are combined.

Coping with cancer treatment

Many of the treatments used for mycosis fungoides can dry and irritate the skin. Some ways to help are:

- Wear soft, loose clothing over the affected areas.
- Protect the skin from the sun.
- Don't scratch or rub the affected areas.
- Check with a doctor or nurse before using lotions, moisturizers, sunscreens, or cosmetics on the area.
- If allowed, use moisturizer and a moisturizing soap.

Clinical trials

Because mycosis fungoides is unlikely to be cured with the standard treatments, all patients with this disease are candidates for **clinical trials**. Patients should check with their medical insurers before enrolling in a clinical trial. Insurers may not pay for some treatments; however, this varies with the insurer and each individual case.

Some clinical trials are testing new drugs, including some retinoids, acyclovir, and hypericin.

In extracorporeal photochemotherapy, the white blood cells are exposed to a chemical called a psoralen, temporarily separated from the rest of the blood and treated with UVA light, then returned to the body. This treatment may stimulate the immune system to destroy the cancer cells.

Interferon alpha is a drug that is injected into plaques and tumors. About 55% of patients have some response and 17% go into complete remission. The side effects may include fevers, fatigue, loss of appetite (**anorexia**), decreases in the number of white blood cells, or irregular heartbeats.

Antibodies can block important molecules on the cancer cells or carry poisons or radioactive molecules to the cancer.

Some clinical trials are testing whether **bone marrow transplantation** can produce lasting remissions.

Prevention

The risk factors for mycosis fungoides are unknown and there is no known means of prevention.

Special concerns

Because mycosis fungoides is rarely cured, patients must usually return periodically for checkups or treatments to maintain the remission. Between visits, patients should also be alert for skin infections. These infections can spread into the blood and become serious if they are not controlled. Because mycosis fungoides can affect the appearance, patients may wish to discuss cosmetic concerns with a doctor, other professional, or support group. Mycosis fungoides increases the risk of developing other types of lymphocyte cancers.

See also Body image; Lymph node biopsy.

Resources

BOOKS

Habermann, Thomas M., and Mark R. Pittelkow. "Cutaneous T-Cell Lymphoma." In *Clinical Oncology*, edited by Martin D. Abeloff, James O. Armitage, Allen S. Lichter, and John E. Niederhuber, 2nd ed. Philadelphia: Churchhill Livingstone, 2004, pp.2720-40.

Wood, Gary S., and Seth R. Stevens. "Cutaneous T Cell Lymphomas." In *Conn's Current Therapy; Latest Approved Methods of Treatment for the Practicing Physician*, edited by Robert E. Rakel, et al., 52nd ed. Philadelphia: W. B. Saunders, 2000, pp.766-70.

PERIODICALS

Duvic, Madeleine, and Jennifer C. Cather. "Emerging New Therapies for Cutaneous T-Cell Lymphoma." *Dermatologic Clinics* 18, no. 1 (January 2000): 147-55.

Elmer, Kathleen B., and Rita M. George. "Cutaneous T- Cell Lymphoma Presenting as Benign Dermatoses." *American Family Physician* 59, no. 10 (15 May 1999): 2809-13.

Pujol, Ramon M., Fernando Gallardo, Enric Llistosella, Aurora Blanco, Lluis Bernado, Ramon Bordes, Josep F. Nomdedeu, and Octavio Servitje. "Invisible Mycosis Fungoides: A Diagnostic Challenge." *Journal of the American Academy of Dermatology* 42, no. 2 (February 2000): 324-8.

OTHER

"Mycosis Fungoides and the Sézary Syndrome Treatment—Health Professionals." *CancerNet*. National Cancer Institute. [cited June 7, 2009]. http://cancernet.nci.nih.gov/pdq.html.

"Radiation Therapy and You: A Guide to Self-Help During Cancer Treatment." *CancerNet*. National Cancer Institute. [cited June 7, 2009]. http://cancernet.nci.nih.gov./peb/radiation.

ORGANIZATIONS

The Cutaneous Lymphoma Network. Judi Van Horn, R.N., Editor. c/o Department of Dermatology, University of Cincinnati, P.O. Box 670523, Cincinnati, OH 45267-0523. (513) 558-6805. This organization produces a newsletter with articles on this cancer, information on support groups, and opportunities for contact with other mycosis fungoides patients.

The Mycosis Fungoides Foundation. P.O. Box 374, Birmingham, MI, 48102-0374. (248) 644-9014. http://MFFoundation.org.

Anna Rovid Spickler, D.V.M., Ph.D.

Myelodysplastic syndrome

Definition

Myelodysplastic syndrome (MDS) is a disease that is associated with decreased production of blood cells. Blood cells are produced in the bone marrow, and the blood cells of people with MDS do not mature normally. There are three major types of blood cells—red blood cells, white blood cells and platelets. Patients with MDS can have decreased production of one, two, or all three types of blood cells.

Description

Overview

Blood cells are used in the body for many different and important functions, such as carrying oxygen (red blood cells), fighting **infection** (white blood cells), and controlling bleeding (platelets). Blood cells are formed and stored in the bone marrow, which is the spongy tissue inside large bones. Stem cells, or immature blood cells, are stored in the bone marrow and have the ability to develop into all three types of mature blood cells. When the body needs a specific type of blood cell, the bone marrow uses its stockpile of stem cells to produce the kind of mature cells needed for that particular situation.

In patients who have MDS, blood cells fail to mature normally. In other words, the bone marrow is unable to develop a normal amount of mature blood cells, and is also not able to increase blood cell production when mature cells are needed. Sometimes, even the cells that are produced do not function normally. The marrow eventually becomes filled with the immature cells (blasts) and there is not room for the normal cells to grow and develop. MDS therefore causes a shortage of functional blood cells.

Subtypes of MDS

MDS is divided into five different subtypes that are classified according to the number and appearance of blast cells in the bone marrow. It is important for doctors to know the type of MDS a patient has, because each subtype affects patients differently and requires specific treatment. The International Prognostic Scoring System (IPSS) can help the doctor to determine the best treatment for an individual patient. The subtypes are as follows:

- Refractory anemia (RA). Bone marrow with less than 5% blast cells and abnormal red blood cell blasts.
- Refractory anemia with ring sideroblasts (RARS). Bone marrow with less than 5% blasts and characteristic abnormalities in red blood cells.
- Refractory anemia with excess blasts (RAEB). Bone marrow with 5–20% blast cells, and higher risk of changing into acute leukemia over time.
- Refractory anemia with excess blasts in transformation (RAEBT). Bone marrow with 21–30% blast cells. This form is most likely to change into acute leukemia.
- Chronic myelomonocytic leukemia (CMMoL). Marrow with 5–20% blasts and excess monocytes (a specific type of white blood cell).

Demographics

Approximately 15,000 new cases are diagnosed annually in the United States. The average age at diagnosis is 70. The most common types are RA and RARS. It is rare to have MDS before age 50. MDS is slightly more common in males than in females.

Causes and symptoms

Causes

There is no clear cause for the majority of MDS cases, which is referred to as primary or *de novo* myelodysplastic syndrome. In some cases, however, MDS results from earlier **cancer** treatments such as radiation and/or **chemotherapy**. This type of MDS is called secondary or treatment related MDS, is often seen three to seven years after the exposure, and usually occurs in younger people.

Other possible causative agents for MDS include exposure to radiation, cigarette smoke or toxic chemicals such as benzene. Children with pre-existing chromosomal abnormalities such as Down syndrome have a higher risk of developing MDS. MDS does not appear to run in families, nor can it be spread to other individuals.

Symptoms

MDS symptoms are related to the type of blood cells that the body is lacking. The earliest symptoms are usually due to **anemia**, which results from a shortage of mature red blood cells. Anemia causes patients to feel tired and out of breath because there is a lack of cells transporting oxygen throughout the body. MDS may also lead to a shortage of white blood cells resulting in an increased likelihood of infections. Another symptom of MDS is increased bleeding (e.g. blood in stool, nose bleeds, increased bruises or bleeding gums) which is due to low level of platelets. These symptoms can occur in any combination, depending on a given patient's specific subtype of MDS.

Diagnosis

Blood tests

People who have MDS usually visit their primary care doctor first, with symptoms of **fatigue**, and are then referred to a hematologist (a physician who specializes in diseases of the blood). The diagnosis of MDS requires a complete analysis of the patient's blood and bone marrow, which is done by the hematologist. A complete blood count (CBC) is done to determine the number of each blood cell type within the sample. Low numbers of red blood cells, white blood cells, and or platelets are signs that a patient has MDS. Numerous other medical problems such as bleeding, nutritional deficiencies, or adverse reaction to a medication can also cause low blood counts. The hematologist will investigate other causes for low blood counts before assigning a diagnosis of MDS. Blood cells in patients with MDS can also be abnormal when viewed under the microscope.

Bone marrow aspiration and biopsy

A **bone marrow biopsy** is required to confirm the diagnosis of MDS and determine the correct MDS subtype. This procedure involves a needle used to take a sample of marrow from inside the bone. The area of the skin where the needle is inserted is numbed and sometimes the patient is also sedated. Patients may experience some discomfort but the procedure is safe and is over fairly quickly. Marrow samples are usually taken from the back of the hip bone (iliac crest). A sample of the marrow, known as an aspirate, and a small piece of bone are both removed with the needle.

A hematologist or a pathologist (a specialist in diagnosing diseases through cell examination) will carefully examine the bone marrow sample through a microscope. Microscopic examination allows the doctor to determine the number and type of blast cells within the marrow in order to identify the MDS subtype. Cells from the bone marrow are also sent for cytogenetic testing, which analyzes the cells' chromosomes. Forty to seventy percent of MDS patients have abnormal bone marrow chromosomes as a result of the disease. The pattern of these abnormalities can be used to predict how a patient will respond to a particular treatment. Thus, the full set of information provided by a bone marrow **biopsy** and CBC will ultimately allow the doctor to recommend the most effective treatment plan.

Clinical staging, treatments, and prognosis

International Prognostic Scoring System (IPSS) for MDS

Once a diagnosis of MDS is established, the doctor will calculate the IPSS score for each individual patient. The bone marrow blast percentage, chromosomal abnormalities and number of different blood types that are reduced determine the score. A score of 0 to 3.5 is assigned to each patient. Patients with lower score have a better prognosis and usually should not undertake treatment upon initial diagnosis. Patients with a higher score have more aggressive disease and should consider more aggressive treatment.

Treatments

SUPPORTIVE CARE. Treatment for MDS is tailored to the patient's age, general health, specific MDS subtype, and IPSS score. Treatment varies for each patient, but most treatment strategies are designed to control the symptoms of MDS. This approach is called supportive care and aims to improve the patient's quality of life.

Supportive care for the MDS patients commonly includes red blood cell transfusions to relieve symptoms related to anemia. Red cell transfusions are relatively safe and the physician will review risks and benefits with this approach. Transfusions of any type only last a certain amount of time and therefore need to be repeated at certain intervals. Platelet transfusions can also be a way to control excessive bleeding. The doctor will decide with each individual patient when it is appropriate to give a transfusion. **Antibiotics** are used when needed to combat infections that can occur more frequently in patients with low white blood cell counts.

BONE MARROW TRANSPLANTATION. **Bone marrow transplantation** (BMT) is a type of treatment that attempts to provide MDS patients with a cure. This strategy requires the patients to be in fairly good health and are therefore more likely to be used in younger patients. Bone marrow transplantation (BMT) has been found to be a successful treatment for MDS patients under the age of 50 (and some over 50 in good health). Following BMT, many patients are able to achieve long-term, disease-free survival. Unfortunately, most MDS patients cannot receive a traditional bone marrow transplant because of older age or because they do not have a suitable donor. Bone marrow donors are usually siblings or are obtained from the national bone marrow registry. "Mini"-bone marrow transplants use less intense chemotherapy, and are currently being tested in older patients who would otherwise not be candidates for traditional bone marrow transplants.

CHEMOTHERAPY. Chemotherapy has been used to treat some MDS patients; however, the disease often recurs after a period of time. This type of therapy uses cell-killing drugs that may also damage healthy cells in the body. Most chemotherapy drugs are associated with some side effects. For these reasons, chemotherapy is generally not used until the MDS becomes more aggressive or the patient has a high IPSS score.

GROWTH FACTORS. Growth factors are natural proteins that the body normally uses to control blood production. These substances stimulate the patient's bone marrow to produce healthy blood cells. Growth factors that stimulate white cell production are G-CSF (also called neupogen or **filgrastim**) and GMCSF (Leukine, **sargramostim**). In order to increase red cell production another growth factor, **erythropoietin** (Procrit) is used. These growth factors are safe with few side effects and are available only in the injectable form. The physician will decide if this treatment is appropriate for an individual patient.

Prognosis

The prognosis for MDS patients depends on the subtype of their disease and the IPSS score. Patients with RA, RARS or low IPSS score rarely develop leukemia and may live with disease for some years. The higher-risk patients including those with RAEB, RAEBt, CMMoL or high IPSS scores progress more rapidly, and require intensive therapy to control the disease.

Managing MDS requires frequent doctor appointments to monitor disease progression and to evaluate the response to treatment. Fortunately for many patients, recent advances in therapy have significantly enhanced their ability to cope with MDS. Experimental drugs and a better understanding of the disease are likely to improve the overall prognosis in the future.

Alternative and complementary therapies

There are no alternative therapies that have been proven to successfully treat MDS. Some of the available alternative drugs can have adverse side effects and therefore a physician should be informed if they are being used.

Clinical trials

Many **clinical trials** are available for MDS patients. These trials are testing new drugs or procedures in this condition. These treatments have not yet been proven to have success in this condition, but the principal investigators are hopeful that patients will benefit. The physician can discuss appropriate clinical trials with interested patients. Trials can involve new chemotherapy drugs, low-dose bone marrow transplantation and novel non-chemotherapy drugs. It is important for a patient to thoroughly understand the risks (listed in the consent form) before signing up for such treatments.

Prevention

MDS is usually impossible to prevent. Being careful about daily activities and avoiding the use of aspirin-like products that thin the blood may prevent secondary complications of MDS such as bruising and bleeding. Practicing good hygiene and avoiding crowds or people with infections can sometimes prevent infections. A well-balanced diet is recommended to increase overall energy.

Special concerns

MDS is the subject of extensive research, and new treatments are under development. In addition to treatment by their local hematologist or oncologist, motivated patients can pursue experimental treatments at major medical centers.

Resources

BOOKS

Aguayo, Alvaro, Jorge Cortes, and Hagop Kantarjian. "Myelodysplastic Syndromes," In *Cancer Management: A Multidisciplinary Approach*, edited by Richard Pazdur, et al., 4th ed. PRR, Inc, 2000.

ORGANIZATIONS

Aplastic Anemia Foundation of America. P.O. Box 613, Annapolis, MD 21404. (800)747-2820. http://www.aplastic.org.

Leukemia Society of America. 600 Third Avenue, New York, NY 10016. (800)955-4LSA. http://www.leukemia.org.

Myelodysplastic Syndromes Foundation. 464 Main Street, P.O. Box 477, Crosswicks, NJ 08515. (800) MDS-0839. http://www.mds-foundation.org.

Andrea Ruskin, M.D.

Myelofibrosis

Definition

Myelofibrosis is a rare disease of the bone marrow in which collagen builds up fibrous scar tissue inside the marrow cavity. This is caused by the uncontrolled growth of a blood cell precursor, which results in the accumulation of scar tissue in bone marrow. Myelofibrosis goes by many names including idiopathic myelofibrosis, agnogenic myeloid metaplasia, chronic myelosclerosis, aleukemic megakaryocytic myelosis, and leukoerythroblastosis.

Description

Myelofibrosis can be associated with many other conditions including **breast cancer**, **prostate cancer**, **Hodgkin's disease**, non-Hodgkin's lymphomas, acute myelocytic leukemia, **acute lymphocytic leukemia**, **hairy cell leukemia**, **multiple myeloma**, **myeloproliferative diseases**, tuberculosis, Gaucher's disease, and Paget's disease of bone. Myelofibrosis typically becomes progressively worse and can cause death.

In myelofibrosis, abnormal cells (hematopoietic stem cells) grow out of control and begin to produce both immature blood cells and excess scar (fibrous) tissue. The fibrous tissue builds up (fibrosis) primarily in the bone marrow, the place where blood cells are produced. The fibrous tissue interferes with the production of normal blood cells. The outcome of this is that the blood made by the bone marrow is of poor quality. To compensate for this, blood cell production occurs in other parts of the body (extramedullary hematopoiesis), but most notably in the spleen and liver. This causes enlargement of the spleen (splenomegaly) and the liver (hepatomegaly). Extramedullary hematopoiesis is not effective and, combined with the reduced production of blood cells by the bone marrow, a condition called **anemia** results.

The abnormal stem cells can spread throughout the body, settle in other organs, and form tumors that produce more abnormal blood cells and fibrous tissue. These tumors are most commonly found in the adrenals, kidneys, lymph nodes, breast, lungs, skin, bowel, thymus, thyroid, prostate, and urinary tract.

KEY TERMS

Anemia—Low numbers of red blood cells in the blood.

Benzene—A colorless volatile flammable toxic liquid hydrocarbon used as a solvent and as a motor fuel.

Biopsy—Surgical removal of tissue for microscopic examination.

Fibrosis—Buildup of scar tissue.

Glucocorticoid therapy—Treatment using corticoids that are anti-inflammatory and immunosuppressive.

Leukemia—Cancer of white blood cells.

Portal hypertension—Extreme pressure on the blood vessels of the liver.

Stem cell—A cell that has the ability to become many different specialized cells.

Demographics

Most patients with myelofibrosis are over 50 years old; the average age at diagnosis is 65 years. However, myelofibrosis can occur at any age. Myelofibrosis occurs with equal frequency in women and men, but in children it affects girls twice as often as it does boys.

Causes and symptoms

Myelofibrosis is caused by an abnormality in a single stem cell, which causes it to grow out of control. Myelofibrosis tumors that have originated from a single cell are called monoclonal. The cause of the stem cell abnormality is unknown. Persons who were exposed to benzene or high doses of radiation have developed myelofibrosis. There may be an association between myelofibrosis and autoimmune diseases, such as systemic lupus erythematosus and scleroderma, in which the immune system treats certain molecules of the body as foreign invaders.

Symptoms usually appear slowly over a long period of time. About one quarter of all patients with myelofibrosis have no symptoms (asymptomatic). An enlarged spleen discovered at an annual medical examination may be the first clue. Symptoms of myelofibrosis include:

- fatigue
- weight loss
- paleness
- fever
- sweating
- weakness
- heart palpitations
- shortness of breath
- itching
- feeling full after eating a small amount of food
- stomach pain or discomfort
- pain in the left shoulder or upper left portion of the body
- unexpected bleeding
- bone pain, especially in the legs

Diagnosis

Because symptoms are similar to other diseases (mostly leukemias), myelofibrosis is not easy to diagnose. The doctor would use his or her hands to feel (palpate) for enlargement of the spleen and liver. Blood tests and urine tests would be performed. **Bone marrow aspiration and biopsy** can help make a diagnosis, but they often fail because of the fibrosis. X-ray imaging and **magnetic resonance imaging** (MRI) may be performed.

Treatment

Many asymptomatic patients, if stable, do not require treatment. There is no cure for myelofibrosis, although **bone marrow transplantation** is curative in some cases. Treatment is aimed at reducing symptoms and improving quality of life.

Medications

Male hormones (androgens) can be used to treat anemia but, in women, these drugs can cause the development of male characteristics (e.g., hair growth on the face and body). Glucocorticoid therapy is also an effective treatment of anemia and can improve myelofibrosis in children. Nutrients that stimulate blood formation (hematinics), such as iron, **folic acid**, and vitamin B_{12}, may reduce anemia. **Cancer-chemotherapy** (usually **hydroxyurea**) can decrease splenomegaly and hepatomegaly, reduce symptoms of myelofibrosis, lessen anemia, and sometimes reduce bone marrow fibrosis. The bone marrow of myelofibrosis patients is often not strong enough to withstand the harsh chemotherapy drugs, so this treatment is not always an option. Interferon-alpha has been shown to reduce spleen size, reduce **bone pain**, and, in some cases, increase the number of blood platelets (structures involved in blood clotting).

Other treatments

In certain cases, the enlarged spleen may be removed (**splenectomy**). Conditions that warrant splenectomy include spleen pain, the need for frequent blood transfusion, very low levels of platelets (**thrombocytopenia**), and extreme pressure in the blood vessels of the liver (portal hypertension).

Radiation therapy is used to treat splenomegaly, spleen pain, bone pain, tumors in certain places such as next to the spinal cord, and fluid accumulation inside the abdomen (**ascites**). Patients who are not strong enough to undergo splenectomy are often treated with radiation therapy.

Bone marrow transplantation may be used to treat some patients with myelofibrosis. This procedure may be performed on patients who are less than 50 years old, have a poor life expectancy, and have a brother or sister with blood-type similarities.

Patients with severe anemia may require blood transfusions.

Prognosis

Similar to leukemias, myelofibrosis is progressive and often requires therapy to control the disease. Myelofibrosis can progress to acute lymphocytic leukemia or **lymphoma**. Although a number of factors to predict the survival time have been proposed, advanced age or severe anemia are consistently associated with a poor prognosis. The average survival rate of patients diagnosed with myelofibrosis is five years. Death is usually caused by **infection**, bleeding, complications of splenectomy, heart failure, or progression to leukemia. Spontaneous remission is rare.

Prevention

Persons who have been exposed to radiation, benzene, or radioactive thorium dioxide (a chemical used during certain diagnostic radiological procedures) are at risk for myelofibrosis.

Resources

BOOKS

Lichtman, Marshall. "Idiopathic Myelofibrosis (Agnogenic Myeloid Metaplasia)." In *Williams Hematology*, edited by Ernest Beutler, et al. New York: McGraw Hill, 2001, pp.1125-36.

Mavroudis, Dimitrios, and John Barrett. "Myelofibrosis (Agnogenic Myeloid Metaplasia)." In *Bone Marrow Failure Syndromes*, edited by Neal Young. Philadelphia: W.B. Saunders Company, 2000, pp.122-34.

Peterson, Powers. "Myelofibrosis." In *Practical Diagnosis of Hematologic Disorders*, edited by Carl Kjeldsberg. Chicago: ASCP Press, 2000, pp.477-9.

Belinda Rowland, Ph.D.
J. Ricker Polsdorfer, M.D.

Myeloma

Definition

Cancer that arises in the bone marrow and involves plasma cells, a type of white blood cell that produces proteins called immunoglobulins.

Kate Kretschmann

Myeloproliferative diseases

Definition

The myeloproliferative diseases are four conditions—essential thrombocythemia, polycythemia vera, **chronic myelocytic leukemia**, and agnogenic myeloid metaplasia—characterized by overproduction of normal-looking blood cells.

Because chronic myelocytic leukemia has its own individual entry, it is not covered in depth in this entry.

Description

The prefix "myelo-" refers to marrow. Bone marrow, a reddish substance in the middle of some bones, produces blood cells. In the myeloproliferative diseases, the body makes too many blood cells. Blood contains red blood cells to carry oxygen, white blood cells to fight infections, and platelets to begin blood clotting. Myeloproliferative diseases develop when a myeloid progenitor cell—a cell that makes red blood cells, platelets, and certain types of white blood cells—becomes overactive. The abnormal progenitor cell continues to make normal blood cells, but it makes too many of them. This excess of blood cells results in varying symptoms, depending on the progenitor cell involved.

Other problems develop when some of the abnormal myeloid progenitor cells travel to the spleen, liver, or lymph nodes and begin making blood cells there. Most often, they migrate to the spleen. An enlarged spleen can crowd other organs in the abdomen and cause discomfort or digestive troubles. It is also susceptible to painful damage from blocked arteries. Massively swollen spleens can use large amounts of energy and cause muscle wasting and **weight loss**.

In the later stages of myeloproliferative diseases, the bone marrow can become scarred. This may leave no space for progenitor cells. As a result, blood cell production can drop to dangerously low levels. The abnormal progenitor cells may also mutate and develop into leukemia. These two serious complications are rare in some myeloproliferative diseases but very common in others.

Types of myeloproliferative disease

The four myeloproliferative diseases include essential thrombocythemia, polycythemia vera, chronic myelocytic leukemia, and agnogenic myeloid metaplasia.

In essential thrombocythemia (primary thrombocythemia), the myeloid progenitor cell makes too many platelets. Blood containing too many platelets may either clot too easily or too slowly. Blood that clots too easily can lead to a variety of health problems, including strokes or heart attacks. Blood that clots too slowly can cause symptoms such as easy bruising, frequent nosebleeds, bleeding from the gums, or life-threatening hemorrhages. Excessive numbers of platelets can also cause headaches or erythromelalgia, an unusual condition characterized by warmth, redness and pain in the hands or feet. Typically, patients with this disease have long periods without symptoms, interspersed with clotting or bleeding episodes. Some patients may have no symptoms at all. Rarely, this disease ends in scarring of the bone marrow or leukemia. Patients with bone marrow scarring have symptoms identical to agnogenic myeloid metaplasia.

KEY TERMS

Androgen—A drug related to the male sex hormones.

Autoimmune disease—A disease that develops when white blood cells attack normal cells or organs.

Biopsy—A sample of an organ taken to look for abnormalities. Also, the technique used to take such samples.

Bone marrow—A group of cells and molecules found in the centers of some bones. It makes all of the cells found in the blood.

Computed tomography (CT)—A special x-ray technique that produces a cross-sectional image of the organs inside the body.

Corticosteroids—A class of drugs, related to hormones naturally found in the body, that suppresses the immune system. One example is prednisone, sold under many brand names including Deltasone.

Erythromelalgia—A condition characterized by warmth, redness and pain in the hands and especially the feet.

Erythropoietin—A drug that stimulates the bone marrow to make more red blood cells. It is also known as epoetin alfa.

Extracorporeal photochemotherapy—A technique in which the white blood cells are exposed to a chemical called a psoralen, temporarily separated from the rest of the blood and treated with UVA light, then returned to the body.

Gout—A painful swelling of the joints that results from an accumulation of uric acid. This disease often affects the big toe.

Granulocyte—One of three types of white blood cells (neutrophils, eosinophils, and basophils) that contain visible granules.

Lymph node—A small organ full of white blood cells, found in clusters throughout the body. Lymph nodes are where reactions to infections usually begin.

Median—A type of average. The median is the number in the middle of a sequence of numbers.

Myeloid progenitor cell—A cell normally found in the bone marrow that makes red blood cells, platelets, and some white blood cells (granulocytes and monocytes).

Phlebotomy—The removal of blood.

Platelets—Tiny fragments of cells that begin the blood clotting process. They are found in the blood.

Red blood cells—The cells in the blood that carry oxygen.

Spleen—An organ in the abdomen near the stomach. The spleen makes white blood cells, stores red blood cells, and removes old blood cells from the circulation.

Transfusion—A transfer of blood or blood products from one person to another.

Ultrasound—A technique that uses sound waves to form an image of organs inside the body.

White blood cells—The cells in the blood that fight infections. There are several types of white blood cells. Also known as immune cells.

In polycythemia vera (primary polycythemia, Vaquez disease), the bone marrow makes too many red blood cells. Large numbers of red blood cells can make the blood too thick. Viscous blood flows sluggishly, pools in the veins, and delivers oxygen poorly. Patients may experience headaches, dizziness, **fatigue**, chest pains, or weakness and cramping in the calves while walking. The abnormal blood flow can also result in bleeding tendencies or blood clotting inside the veins. Many patients also have increased numbers of white blood cells or platelets, but most symptoms are caused by the sluggish blood flow. The spleen often enlarges. Polycythemia rarely leads to leukemia, but occasionally ends in bone marrow scarring.

In chronic myelocytic leukemia (chronic myelogenous leukemia), the myeloid progenitor cell makes a type of white blood cell called a granulocyte. With this condition, platelets can also increase. In the early stages of this disease, the white blood cells look outwardly normal. However, in 90–95% of patients, two chromosomes—number 9 and number 22— inside the progenitor cell have broken and exchanged parts. This chromosome rearrangement is known as the Philadelphia chromosome, and this genetic abnormality destabilizes these cells and inevitably they become cancerous.

Agnogenic myeloid metaplasia (idiopathic **myelofibrosis**, myelofibrosis with myeloid metaplasia) begins like other myeloproliferative diseases, with overproduction of blood cells. However, bone marrow scarring develops very quickly and causes most of the symptoms. Blood cell numbers drop, causing fatigue and weakness from **anemia**. Many of the cells found in

QUESTIONS TO ASK THE DOCTOR

- Does my condition require treatment?
- What treatment would you recommend I try?
- What risks and side effects should I expect?
- How will it affect my quality of life?
- Are there any alternative treatments that might work equally well?
- Are there any activities I should avoid? For how long?
- Are there any symptoms I should watch for? Who should I contact if I experience them? How urgent is it to let someone know immediately?

the blood are also immature or oddly shaped. Although myeloid progenitor cells in the spleen and liver can partly compensate, the enlargement of these organs creates additional problems. Occasionally, this disease also ends in leukemia.

Demographics

Essential **thrombocytopenia**, polycythemia vera, and agnogenic myeloid metaplasia are usually diagnosed late in life, at an average (median) age of 60.

Essential thrombocythemia may be slightly more common in women and agnogenic myeloid metaplasia and polycythemia vera slightly more common in men; however, estimates vary. At one time, polycythemia vera was thought to develop more often in Jews. More recent statistics do not confirm this.

Causes and symptoms

No consistent chromosomal abnormalities have been discovered in essential thrombocythemia, polycythemia vera, or agnogenic myeloid metaplasia. The causes of these diseases are unknown.

Myeloproliferative diseases share many features, such as enlargement of the spleen and abnormalities in blood clotting. Symptoms that can be seen in any of these diseases include:

- fatigue
- poor appetite (anorexia)
- weight loss
- night sweats
- fullness in the stomach after eating only a small amount
- abdominal pain or discomfort, especially in the upper left side
- nosebleeds, bleeding from the gums, easy bruising, or intestinal bleeding
- symptoms of blood clots including strokes, heart attacks, pain and swelling in the legs, or difficulty breathing
- disturbances in vision

Other symptoms of essential thrombocythemia can include:

- weakness
- dizziness
- headaches
- prickling or tingling in the skin
- erythromelalgia (warmth, redness, and pain in the extremities)

Other symptoms of polycythemia vera can include:

- headaches
- dizziness
- ringing in the ears
- pain in the chest (angina)
- weakness or cramping pains in the legs that disappear during rest
- redness of the face
- a blue tinge to the skin and other body surfaces (cyanosis)
- high blood pressure
- itching, especially after a warm bath or shower
- tingling or prickling of the skin
- erythromelalgia
- ulcers
- kidney stones
- gout

Other symptoms of agnogenic myeloid metaplasia can include:

- fever
- gout
- bone pain

Diagnosis

The diagnosis of a myeloproliferative disease relies mainly on a physical examination, examination of a blood sample, and sometimes a **bone marrow biopsy**. In the blood samples, the doctor will find excessive numbers of the cells characteristic of each disease. Chromosome studies on the blood can often distinguish chronic myelocytic leukemia from the other three diseases. Bone marrow samples reveal increased cell production and sometimes scarring. An enlarged spleen can often be detected during a physical examination, but occasionally ultrasound or **computed tomography** scans may be necessary.

Myeloproliferative diseases can resemble normal reactions to infections and other diseases. Various tests may be done to rule out such diseases.

Clinical staging, treatments, and prognosis

Staging

There is no staging system for essential thrombocythemia, polycythemia vera, or agnogenic myeloid metaplasia.

Treatments

ESSENTIAL THROMBOCYTHEMIA. Treatments for essential thrombocythemia lower the risk of bleeding or blood clots. One option is **hydroxyurea** (Hydrea), a drug that suppresses platelet production. Hydroxyurea has few side effects but can occasionally cause a rash, intestinal upsets, sores on the skin, or a **fever**. This drug may also slightly increase the risk of leukemia. **Anagrelide** (Agrylin), an alternative, is effective in more than 90% of patients. It does not promote leukemia but can cause dizziness, headaches, fluid retention, rapid heartbeats, **diarrhea**, and rare cases of heart failure. Hydroxyurea and anagrelide both increase the risk of miscarriages during the first trimester in pregnant women.

A patient under 60 who has never had a blood clot has a 3% chance of developing one in the future. Some doctors recommend treatment for these patients only during high-risk situations such as surgery. Low doses of aspirin are sometimes used to control symptoms such as erythromelalgia.

POLYCYTHEMIA VERA. Periodically removing small amounts of blood, called phlebotomy, is a safe and very effective way to treat polycythemia vera. In some studies, phlebotomy has increased the risk of blood clotting. However, this may not occur when the hematocrit (the percentage of red blood cells in the blood) is kept below 45% in men and 43% in women. Phlebotomy can result in symptoms of iron deficiency such as abnormal food cravings (particularly a craving for ice).

Patients who are unlikely to develop blood clots may not need any other treatments. Patients with a higher risk of clotting are sometimes given hydroxyurea. This drug has relatively few side effects, but it may increase the chance of developing leukemia. In some studies, 3–5% of patients taking hydroxyurea eventually developed leukemia, compared to 1.5–2% treated with phlebotomy alone. Alternatives to hydroxyurea include interferon alpha and anagrelide. These drugs do not increase the risk of leukemia, but they tend to have more side effects. Interferon alpha may be particularly difficult to tolerate. Its side effects include flu-like symptoms (fever, chills, postnasal drip and poor appetite), fatigue, weight loss, **depression**, insomnia, memory loss, and **nausea**.

Radioactive phosphorus is used mainly in elderly patients who do not expect to need many years of treatment. In 80–90% of patients, this treatment can suppress the disease symptoms for six months to several years. However, up to 17% of patients develop leukemia within 15 years.

Other symptoms of polycythemia vera are treated with a variety of drugs. **Itching** is sometimes suppressed by phlebotomy, but antihistamines are often needed as well. Other options include extracorporeal photochemotherapy, hydroxyurea, or interferon alpha. **Allopurinol** (Zyloprim) prevents kidney stones and gout. Aspirin can suppress the symptoms of erythromelalgia.

One of the most difficult complications to treat is enlargement of the spleen. In the early stages of the disease, this enlargement can often be controlled by phlebotomy. Later, interferon alpha, hydroxyurea, or surgical removal may be necessary. Surgery to remove a very large spleen is difficult and can be fatal in up to 10% of patients. Complications can include infections, bleeding, serious blood clotting, or increased numbers of white blood cells and platelets. Radiation treatments directed at the spleen may be another option, but they can suppress the bone marrow.

AGNOGENIC MYELOID METAPLASIA. Agnogenic myeloid metaplasia can be cured by a bone marrow transplant from a healthy donor. In patients eligible for this treatment, it is successful in about a third. **Bone marrow transplantation** may not be feasible for many patients, particularly those who are older or in poor health. This procedure can have serious or fatal complications including infections, organ damage, and bleeding. In addition, compatible donors are not available for all patients.

Other treatments for this disease are not curative and are mainly intended to improve the quality of life. Anemia is often treated with regular transfusions of red blood cells. Adverse effects can include heart failure or damage to the liver from excess iron. Drugs can sometimes make red blood cells last longer. **Corticosteroids** combined with an androgen (**fluoxymesterone**) are effective in about a third of all patients.

Danazol, another androgen, works in about 20%. These drugs may damage the liver and can produce masculine traits in women. Injections of **erythropoietin**, a hormone that stimulates red blood cell production, also work in a few patients.

About half of all patients with anemia improve after surgical removal of the spleen (**splenectomy**). This surgery can also help patients who have abdominal discomfort, weight loss, muscle wasting, or high blood pressure in the liver. However, it can be dangerous and sometimes fatal. Removal of the spleen may make the disease progress more quickly, but this is not certain.

A painfully enlarged spleen can also be treated with hydroxyurea, interferon alpha, or radiation treatments. Hydroxyurea has few side effects, but it may increase the risk of leukemia. Interferon alpha shrinks the spleen in 30–50% of patients, but has many side effects. Radiation treatments can decrease the symptoms for three to six months, but sometimes fatally suppress the blood-producing cells.

Prognosis

Patients with essential thrombocythemia can expect a near normal life-span. Average (median) survival is 12 to 15 years. The chance of developing either leukemia or serious scarring of the bone marrow is less than 5%.

Without treatment, patients with polycythemia vera usually die from bleeding or blood clotting within months. With treatment, average (median) survival is about 10 years in older patients and more than 15 years in younger patients. Many patients can reach their normal life expectancy if they do not develop bone marrow scarring or leukemia. The risk of bone marrow scarring after 10 years is approximately 15–20%. If polycythemia vera is treated with phlebotomy alone, the risk of developing leukemia is 2%.

Unless they receive a successful bone marrow transplant, most patients with agnogenic myeloid metaplasia become progressively worse. The anemia becomes more severe and the liver and spleen continue to swell. Average (median) survival in this disease is 3.5 to 5.5 years, but survival is often unpredictable and may be much longer or much shorter. Leukemia develops in about 5–20% of patients. In other patients, death occurs from heart failure, infections, bleeding or blood clots.

Alternative and complementary therapies

In traditional Chinese and Japanese medicine, herbal preparations are used to treat symptoms of chronic illnesses such as fatigue, loss of appetite, and **night sweats**, or to decrease red blood cell formation in polycythemia vera. Patients who are interested in non-traditional complementary remedies should discuss them with their doctors. Some may have dangerous side effects or be harmful when combined with traditional therapies.

Coping with cancer treatment

Acetaminophen and antidepressant drugs can help reduce some of the side effects of interferon alpha. Taking this drug at night may also make it easier to tolerate.

Clinical trials

The following therapies are being tested in **clinical trials**. Patients should check with their medical insurers before enrolling in a clinical trial. Insurers may not pay for some treatments but this varies with the insurer and each individual case.

Interferon alpha injections are being tested in essential thrombocythemia. This drug can lower platelet numbers and decrease the size of the spleen in about 80% of patients.

Several new drugs are in clinical trials. **Thalidomide** and SU5416 are being tested in patients with agnogenic myeloid metaplasia. R115777 and 12-O-tetradecanoylphorbol-13-acetate (TPA) are in clinical trials open to patients with various myeloproliferative diseases.

Another possible treatment for agnogenic myeloid metaplasia is to purify the normal progenitor cells and return them to the body after destroying the abnormal progenitor cells with **chemotherapy**.

Prevention

The following environmental factors have been linked to myeloproliferative diseases:

- working as an electrician or in a petroleum manufacturing plant
- prolonged use of dark hair dyes
- exposure to nuclear bomb blasts or thorium dioxide

Special concerns

Whether polycythemia vera, essential thrombocythemia, and agnogenic myeloid metaplasia progress to leukemia is influenced by the specific treatment strategies. Patients should be aware that some treatments, particularly radioactive phosphorus, can substantially increase the risk of developing **cancer**.

See also Acute myelocytic leukemia; Bone marrow aspiration and biopsy; Cytogenetic analysis; Cytology; Chromosome rearrangements; Hypercoagulation disorders; Myelosuppression; Radiation therapy; Ultrasonography.

Resources

BOOKS

Aster, Jon, and Vinay Kumar. "White Cells, Lymph Nodes, Spleen, and Thymus." In *Robbins Pathologic Basis of Disease*, edited by Ramzi S. Cotran, Vinay Kumar, and Tucker Collins, 6th ed. Philadelphia: W.B. Saunders, 1999, pp. 645-85.

Spivak, Jerry L. "Polycythemia vera." In *Conn's Current Therapy; Latest Approved Methods of Treatment for the Practicing Physician*, edited by Robert E. Rakel, et al., 53rd ed. Philadelphia: W. B. Saunders, 2001, pp.469-73.

Tefferi, Ayalew, and Murray N. Silverstein. "Myeloproliferative Diseases." In *Cecil Textbook of Medicine*, edited by Lee Goldman and J. Claude Bennett, 21st ed. Philadelphia: W.B. Saunders, 2000, pp. 935-41.

PERIODICALS

Saiki, I. "A Kampo Medicine, Juzen-taiho-to—Prevention of Malignant Progression and Metastasis of Tumor Cells and the Mechanism of Action." *Biological and Pharmaceutical Bulletin* 23, no. 6 (June 2000): 677-88.

OTHER

Besa, Emmanuel C., and Ulrich Woermann. "Polycythemia Vera." *eMedicine Journals*. eMedicine.com, Inc. [cited May 17, 2009]. http://emedicine.com/MED/topic1864.htm.

The MPD-Support-L Webpage. [cited May 23, 2009]. http://members.aol.com/mpdsupport.

"Myelofibrosis." *The Merck Manual of Diagnosis and Therapy*. 2009 Merck and Co., Inc. [cited May 17, 2009]. http://www.merck.com/pubs/mmanual/section11/chapter130/130c.htm.

"Myeloproliferative Disorders Treatment—Health Professionals." *CancerNet*. National Cancer Institute. [cited May 9, 2009]. http://cancernet.nci.nih.gov/pdq.html.

ORGANIZATIONS

MPD-Net Online Support Group from Myeloproliferative Diseases Research Center, Inc. 115 East 72nd Street, New York, NY 10021. http://inform.acor.org/mpd/index.htm.

The National Organization for Rare Disorders. P.O. Box 8923, New Fairfield, CT 06812-8923. (800) 999-6673. http://www.rarediseases.org.

Anna Rovid Spickler, D.V.M., Ph.D.

Myelosuppression

Definition

Myelosuppression is a decrease in the production of blood cells.

Description

Normal blood contains large numbers of cells, including red blood cells to carry oxygen and white blood cells to fight infections. The blood also contains platelets, tiny cell fragments that initiate blood clotting. These cells and fragments are made in the bone marrow, a reddish substance found in the centers of some bones. Healthy bone marrow makes large numbers of red blood cells, white blood cells, and platelets each day to replace those that wear out. In myelosuppression, the bone marrow makes too few of these cells.

A decrease in the number of red blood cells, called **anemia**, is very common in **cancer** patients. A drop in white blood cell numbers is often a problem during **chemotherapy**. One type of white blood cell, called a neutrophil, is usually affected most severely. A decrease in these cells is called **neutropenia**. Because neutrophils are responsible for defending the body against bacteria, neutropenia increases the chance of an **infection**. **Thrombocytopenia**, a drop in the number of platelets in the blood, is more rare; platelet numbers become low enough to cause problems in less than 10% of cancer patients.

Myelosuppression is a painless condition, but the decreases in important blood cells can result in **fatigue**, an increased risk of infections, or excessive bleeding. The consequences vary from mild to life-threatening, depending on how low the blood cell numbers fall.

Causes and symptoms

The most common cause of myelosuppression is cancer treatment. Many of the drugs used in chemotherapy temporarily suppress the bone marrow. Therapeutic **x rays** that reach the bone marrow are also destructive. Cancer cells can also cause myelosuppression. Some cancers invade the bone marrow and crowd out the cells normally found there. Others can suppress the bone marrow without invasion. Nutritional deficiencies, common in cancer patients, also slow blood cell production as do viruses and some non chemo drugs.

Myelosuppression usually starts seven to ten days after an injury to the bone marrow. However, the bone

KEY TERMS

Anemia—Too few red blood cells in the blood.

Blood cells—The red blood cells and white blood cells found in the blood.

Bone marrow—A group of cells and molecules found in the centers of some bones. It makes all of the cells found in the blood.

Erythropoietin—A growth factor that stimulates the bone marrow to make more red blood cells. It is also known as epoetin alfa.

Granulocyte colony-stimulating factor (G-CSF)—A growth factor that stimulates the bone marrow to make neutrophils and some other types of white blood cells. It is also known as filgrastim.

Granulocyte-macrophage colony-stimulating factor (GM-CSF)—A growth factor that stimulates the bone marrow to make neutrophils and some other types of white blood cells. It is also known as sargramostim or molgramostim.

Growth factor—A chemical that stimulates body cells to grow or make more cells. Growth factors are found naturally in the body, but can also be manufactured and used as drugs.

Interleukin 11 (IL-11)—A growth factor that stimulates the bone marrow to make platelets. It is also known as oprelvekin.

Neutropenia—Too few neutrophils in the blood.

Neutrophil—A type of white blood cell that destroys bacteria.

Packed red blood cells—Blood that has had the fluid portion (plasma) removed.

Platelets—Tiny fragments of cells that begin the blood clotting process. They are found in the blood.

Red blood cells—The cells in the blood that carry oxygen.

Thrombocytopenia—Too few platelets in the blood.

Transfusion—A transfer of blood or blood products from one person to another.

Transfusion reaction—An allergic reaction to some of the cells or proteins in another person's blood.

White blood cells—The cells in the blood that fight infections. There are several types of white blood cells.

marrow generally returns to normal within the next few weeks. Less often, cumulative damage can be caused. Occasionally, irreversible damage causes permanent myelosuppression. Very intensive chemotherapy or radiation can destroy all of the cells in the bone marrow.

The symptoms of myelosuppression depend on the type of blood cell that is depleted, and the severity of the depletion. Low red blood cells results in anemia, which can cause severe fatigue. Low white blood cells results in an increased risk of serious infection, which may manifest in **fever** and symptoms specific to the area of the infection. Low platelet count results in an increased risk of bruising and bleeding, including severe hemorrhage.

Treatments

Myelosuppression is not always treated, especially if it is mild.

If the myelosuppression is a result of chemotherapy or **radiation therapy**, the cancer treatments may be stopped, delayed, or reduced to give the bone marrow a chance to recover. This may mean that the full dose of the treatment is not received.

Careful monitoring of possible neutropenia in cancer patients is important. If a cancer patient has a fever and other signs of possible infection, the physician may treat the patient with injected **antibiotics**, possibly for several days.

Red blood cells or platelets can be replaced by transfusions, packed red blood cells, or platelets. These treatments can be very effective in the short term; however, the transfused cells are short-lived and the treatment may need to be repeated. There is a small chance of a transfusion reaction and a slight risk of infection by a virus carried in the blood. Transfusions of white blood cells are ineffective and rarely given.

Injections of growth factors may also be effective. Growth factors are chemicals, found naturally in the body, that stimulate the bone marrow to make blood cells. Each type of growth factor affects specific blood cells. Several are being manufactured as drugs. They include **erythropoietin**, granulocyte colony-stimulating factor (G-CSF, or **filgrastim**), granulocyte-macrophage colony-stimulating factor (GM-CSF, or **sargramostim**), and interleukin 11 (**oprelvekin**). Erythropoietin injections stimulate red blood cell production. They can decrease the need for a transfusion and improve the quality of life. This drug has few side effects if the kidneys are healthy, but it may not be effective if the body is already making enough natural erythropoietin. G-CSF and GM-CSF can speed the return of neutrophils. Their side effects include **bone pain**, fevers, rashes, muscle pains, and **nausea**. Interleukin 11 can increase platelet numbers. Its side effects may include fluid retention, a rapid heartbeat, red eyes, and difficulty breathing. Growth factors are expensive and several injections are usually needed.

Complete destruction of the bone marrow is incompatible with life. If the bone marrow is severely damaged, a bone marrow transplant may be necessary.

Supportive therapy can help to minimize the effects of myelosuppression. If nutrition is a contributing factor, iron or vitamin supplements may be beneficial. Antibiotics can aid in preventing infections. Some patients find that mild exercise and enjoyable distractions help with fatigue.

Prognosis

The prognosis of myelosuppression depends on the reason for it, its reversibility, and its severity. Certainly, severe myelosuppression can result in a level of anemia incompatible with life, serious, life-threatening infections, and massive bleeding. Frequently, however, the effects of myelosuppression can be ameliorated through treatments that address the underlying deficiency, as well as by stopping any medications or exposures that may be implicated in its etiology.

Prevention

Myelosuppression may not be totally preventable, for example in the case of an individual who must receive chemotherapy or radiation. However, some treatments may proactively prevent the meylosuppression from becoming severe.

QUESTIONS TO ASK YOUR DOCTOR

- What is causing the myelosuppression?
- Should other medications or treatment that may be worsening the myelosuppression be stopped or postponed?
- What types of treatments are available?
- What types of side effects from treatments can I expect? What are your recommendations to help me deal with those side effects?
- Am I eligible for any clinical trials? Would these be helpful to consider?

See also Anemia; Bone marrow transplantation; Transfusion therapy.

Resources

BOOKS

Abeloff, MD et al. *Clinical Oncology*. 3rd ed. Philadelphia: Elsevier, 2004.

Hoffman R. et al. *Hematology: Basic Principles and Practice*. 4th ed. Philadelphia: Elsevier, 2005.

PERIODICALS

Rolston, Kenneth V.I. "The Infectious Diseases Society of America 2002 Guidelines for the Use of Antimicrobial Agents in Patients With Cancer and Neutropenia: Salient Features and Comments." *Clinical Infectious Diseases* July 15, 2004: S44–S49.

Anna Rovid Spickler, D.V.M., Ph.D.

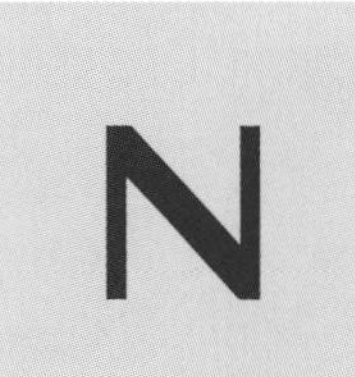

Nasal cancer

Definition

Nasal **cancer** is any cancer that occurs within the nose, either in the nasal vestibule (the immediate interior of the nose, just beyond the nostrils), or the nasal cavity (the deep interior of the nose). Many different types of cancer can occur within the nose, and the type of treatment and the chance of cure will vary according the type of cancer that occurs.

Description

Nasal cancers are very rare, making up less than 2% of all tumors of the respiratory tract in the United States. Less than 50 cases a year are diagnosed in the United States. Although squamous cell **carcinoma** is the most common type of cancer that occurs within the nose, many other types can also occur, including **adenocarcinoma**, **melanoma**, different kinds of sarcomas, inverted papilloma, **lymphoma**, and esthesioneuroblastoma.

Squamous cell carcinomas arise from skin tissue. They are the most common type and are often the result of either cigarette smoking or occupational exposure to dusts or chemical fumes. Adenocarcinomas are malignancies that resemble glandular tissue. Nasal adenocarcinomas are also often associated with occupational exposure to dusts or chemical fumes. T-cell lymphomas (Non-Hodgkins) in the nasal area are strongly associated with a virus (**Epstein-Barr virus**, EBV). Although nasal T-cell lymphomas are fairly common in some parts of the world, they are very rare in the United States.

Inverted papillomas are associated with another virus (**human papilloma virus**, HPV) and arise from benign but locally invasive nasal polyps. They are rare, comprising only about 0.5% of all nasal tumors. Although a definite association with HPV has been shown, a tumor may require interaction of the virus with chemicals or other factors, which appear to cause transformation of the inverted papilloma into squamous cell carcinoma in the nose. Esthesioneuroblastoma is a very rare nasal tumor, with less than 200 cases reported in the last 25 years. They are tumors that arise in the nerves in the nose, and have occurred most commonly in teenagers and senior citizens.

Demographics

Although the overall risk of nasal cancer is quite low (since this type of cancer is very rare), relative risks for some specific groups are fairly high. For example, nasal T-cell lymphomas are virus-associated and occur in high incidence in Asia and South America. Nasal squamous cell carcinomas occur much more frequently in cigarette smokers and individuals who have **occupational exposures** to dusts or chemical fumes, especially in Europe. Consumption of salted and pickled foods creates an increased relative risk of nasal cancer in Asia. Nasal cancers are also more frequent in some African populations that use mahogany wood in cooking fires.

In the United States, nasal cancers are rare. There are no significant racial differences in incidence. Males experience all types of nasal cancer in significantly greater numbers than women, probably due to more occupational exposure to agents that can cause these types of cancer. Most nasal cancers occur in people over 40, although the rare esthesioneuroblastoma has occurred in relatively high percentages in adolescents.

Causes and symptoms

All cancers are caused when a genetic mutation is made in a gene that is involved in the control of cell division. This mistake can arise naturally, can be inherited, or it can be caused by a virus, by sunlight or other radiation, or by some chemical that a person is exposed to, usually through eating, drinking or breathing. For nasal cancers, all of these factors have been shown to play a part.

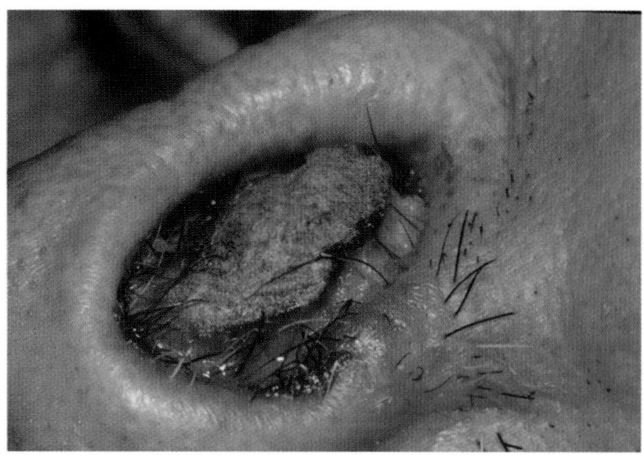

Cancerous tumor in nose. *(Custom Medical Stock Photo. Reproduced by permission.)*

The use of tobacco products has been strongly associated with the occurrence of nasal adenocarcinomas and squamous cell carcinomas. Chronic occupational exposures to leather, wool, or wood dust or chemical mixtures, particularly nickel, dioxane, nitrosamine, chromium used in dye manufacturing, mustard gas, rubbing alcohol, or formaldehyde, have a demonstrated association with nasal adenocarcinomas and squamous cell carcinomas as well. Some rare nasal T-cell lymphomas have been shown to be very strongly associated with a virus (Epstein-Barr Virus, EBV). Some nasal malignancies (about 5%) begin as inverted papillomas, a locally aggressive tumor which does not usually metastasize but which may turn malignant. These are also thought to be caused by a virus, although a different one: Human papilloma virus (HPV). Some nasal cancers have a strong hereditary component: people with genetic alterations that cause hereditary **retinoblastoma** have a much higher incidence of nasal cancers than average, which indicates that the genetic change that caused their original disease may also contribute to nasal cancer.

People with nasal cancer may think that they have a cold or chronic sinus infections. They may experience a feeling of stuffiness or blockage in the nose, persistent nasal drainage, or frequent nose bleeds. Other symptoms can occur if the tumor has invaded other tissues around the nose, particularly the orbit of the eye or the base of the skull. Other symptoms which may occur include:

- double vision
- bulging of the eye
- a lump on the face or around the eye
- loose teeth
- frequent headaches

KEY TERMS

Carcinoma—Any malignant tumor.

Endoscopy—A diagnostic procedure in which a miniature videocamera on the end of a flexible tube is inserted into internal body cavities so that the physician can view the internal structures.

Lymphoma—A type of cancer that arises in the lymph nodes.

Nasal polyp—A non-cancerous mass that grows out from the inner lining of the nasal cavity.

Sarcoma—A tumor that arises from bone or connective tissue.

Squamous cell carcinoma—A malignancy that arises from outer skin cells.

In advanced stages, patients with nasal cancers may suffer from **fatigue**, **weight loss**, lack of appetite (**anorexia**), and **fever**.

Diagnosis

When otherwise unexplainable symptoms lead a doctor to suspect that a patient may have nasal cancer, often he or she will arrange for endoscopic examination of the nasal cavity (and possibly the sinuses) in order to see if there is a tumor. Definite diagnosis requires a **biopsy**, in which a small piece of the tumor is cut out and examined to see what types of cells it contains. After a nasal cancer is diagnosed (depending on the type of cancer), many doctors will ask the patient to have an x ray, **computed tomography** scanning (CT scans), or **magnetic resonance imaging** (MRI). These techniques visualize the tumor and show the doctor how much the tumor has invaded surrounding tissues. Because treatment for nasal cancer, as well as **paranasal sinus cancer**, involves surgery in a small, complex space which requires the surgeon to set very precise surgical boundaries, and because most nasal cancers are advanced by the time a patient sees a doctor, it is very important that the doctor evaluate the tumor thoroughly before planning treatment. If the tumor appears to have invaded other tissues, often a doctor will schedule a surgical exploration of the tumor in order to better evaluate the cancer, with the goal of constructing the best possible treatment plan. Sometimes, in addition, surgical exploration is necessary to determine whether the position and invasion of the tumor into surrounding tissue makes surgical removal of the tumor impossible.

QUESTIONS TO ASK THE DOCTOR

- Can you explain what kind of cancer I have?
- Can you explain the grade and stage of my cancer? What are the chances that it will come back?
- How was this cancer diagnosed?
- What is my prognosis?
- How much will the surgery alter my facial appearance?
- What treatments are we going to pursue? What happens if these don't work?
- Do you have experience in treating this type of cancer?
- Is there anything I can do to optimize treatment? Are there any particular side effects I should expect?
- Are there complementary therapies that you would recommend? Any other things that would help me cope with the diagnosis or treatment?
- How often will I need further check-ups? Is there anything I can do to keep this cancer from coming back?

Treatment team

As the understanding of cancer grows and new treatment approaches are developed, the complexity of cancer treatment also increases. Today, a multidisciplinary approach to cancer treatment is considered necessary for effective patient care. People involved in the treatment of a nasal cancer will typically include the referring physician, an otolaryngologist, a medical oncologist, a pathologist, and a nurse. If **radiation therapy** is pursued, a radiation oncologist, radiation therapist, radiation nurse, radiation physicist, and a dosimetrist will also be involved. Treatment will also probably include a psychologist, nutritionist, social worker and chaplain. For nasal cancers, a reconstructive or plastic surgeon may be necessary for optimum cosmetic results after removal of a nasal tumor. If surgical removal of the eye is necessary, specialists in prosthetic eye replacement will be necessary as well.

Clinical staging, treatments, and prognosis

When a cancer develops, the original tumor can spread, usually through the blood or lymph system, to other parts of the body. Since the cancer spreads through the lymph system, often the lymph nodes in the area of the original tumor are the first other sites where cancerous cells can be found. Common other places that metastatic disease may appear are the lungs, the liver, and the bones.

One of the foremost goals of a doctor's assessment of a cancer patient is to determine how far the cancer has already spread and how likely it is to spread further, both of which are key factors in the likelihood that the patient will be cured. The assessment of the tumor's spread is termed staging, and the assessment of how aggressive the cancer cells are is termed grading.

Staging of nasal cancers is performed by visual inspection of tumors (maybe through endoscopy) or visualization of tumors by imaging techniques like **x rays**, MRIs, or CT scans. The doctor may also attempt to feel for tumors manually. This information will be used to create an official stage for the tumor that is a standardized expression of how much the tumor has already spread.

Because tumors of the nasal vestibule and cavity are rare, and because they are comprised of so many different types, no one staging system has been defined for use with these cancers. Cancers of the paranasal sinuses have a defined staging system based on the TNM system, and this system is often used for describing nasal cancers. The T in the TNM system represents the growth of the local tumor, N describes the spread of the tumor to the lymph nodes, and M describes the spread, or **metastasis**, of the cancer to distant body sites. The cancer is given various numbered ratings in each letter category, and these are used to create a standardized stage. Generally, tumors with no invasion of local tissues are described as Stage I, while tumors with minimal invasion of local tissues are identified as Stage II. Tumors that have extensive local invasion or that have spread to the lymph nodes but which have not metastasized are described as Stage III or early Stage IV (A and B). Stage IVC tumors are any tumors which have metastasized.

Most nasal cancers (up to 80%) have already spread to other body sites by the time the symptoms prompt a patient to see their doctor. This fact, combined with the fact that the area is anatomically complex and tightly constructed, makes it very important that the first attempt at treatment is well-planned, with input from a multidisciplinary team and thorough evaluation of the cancer before treatment is begun.

Since cancers of the nasal cavity and vestibule include many different types of cancers, treatment will vary depending on the type of cancer involved, where it is located, and the extent to which it has already spread. Because of this, and because of the complexity of the anatomy in the area and the multitude of other important structures that may be involved in later stages, treatment of nasal cancers is highly individualized, with no firm standard practice guidelines.

For most nasal cancers, treatment will involve surgical removal of the tumor followed by four to five weeks of radiation therapy. In advanced cancers, preoperative radiation therapy may also be employed. However, since radiation therapy has proven very effective for nasal cancers and because radiation has better cosmetic results than surgical removal of a tumor, for many nasal cancers (especially T-cell lymphomas and esthesioneuroblastomas), radiation will be the initial treatment option. If the doctor decides to remove as much of the tumor as possible surgically, radiation therapy (external) will usually be used for four to five weeks after surgery in order to destroy any remaining cancerous tissue. One exception is the case of inverted papillomas, for which surgical excision alone is usually employed. Surgery, because of the tight anatomical area in which a surgeon must work, may also involve more recent techniques like cryosurgery (freezing tissue) or laser surgery.

Tumors initially treated by either radiation or surgery alone may, if they come back, be treated by the untried option or by employing both. External radiation may be supplemented, especially in advanced nasal vestibule cancer, by internal radioactive implants. In addition, advanced stage or recurrent nasal cancer may be treated by **chemotherapy**, usually involving a combination of drugs. Drugs are used in combination in most chemotherapy because combinations of different drugs (with different side effects) deliver the highest cancer-destroying effect, while minimizing the chance for a serious adverse reaction to the therapy. The drug combinations used in nasal cancer vary on the type of cancer, and may include one or all of the drugs **cisplatin**, **fluorouracil**, **bleomycin**, or **methotrexate**. In addition, nasal cancers described as Stage III or IV will probably be treated with preventative radiation therapy of the neck area, in order to destroy cancerous cells which may have traveled to the lymph nodes.

Although nasal cancers are made up of many different types of cancer, all types of nasal cancers are considered aggressive. The majority of nasal cancers, because symptoms mimic upper respiratory illnesses and because symptoms often do not occur until the cancer has already filled up the nasal cavity and has invaded surrounding tissues, are already in advanced stages when a patient seeks medical help. For this reason, and because treatment is difficult because of the complexity of the anatomical area, fewer than half of nasal cancer patients survive. If the first treatment attempt is successful, and a patient is cancer-free at two years, however, chances improve greatly.

Nasal cancer is unusual in that, although many patients have metastasis to the lymph nodes or beyond (usually to the lungs), metastasis is not usually the reason for a patient's death. Most nasal cancer patients who succumb to the disease die from invasion of the tumor into vital areas of the brain.

Alternative and complementary therapies

Alternative and complementary therapies are treatments that are not traditional, first-line therapies like surgery, chemotherapy, and radiation. Complementary therapies are those that are meant to supplement traditional therapies and usually have the objective of relieving symptoms or helping cancer patients cope with the disease or traditional treatments. Alternative therapies are nontraditional treatments that are chosen instead of traditional treatments in an attempt to cure the disease. Alternative therapies have typically not been proven to be effective in the same way that traditional drugs are evaluated, in **clinical trials**.

Common complementary therapies that may be employed by patients with nasal cancer are art therapy, massage, meditation, visualization, music therapy, prayer, t'ai chi, and yoga or other forms of exercise, which reduce anxiety and can increase a patient's feeling of well-being.

Numerous alternative therapies exist in cancer treatment, but none has been proven in clinical trials to be effective. Laetril, a product of apricot seeds, is probably one of the most well known. Laetril contains a form of cyanide that may be released by tumor enzymes and may then act to kill cancerous cells. Laetril is not approved for use in the United States, although it is available in Mexico. The National Cancer Institute (NCI) sponsored two trials of Laetril in the late 1970s and early 1980s, but found Laetril to be ineffective and concluded that no further study of the substance was necessary. **Vitamins** and other nutritional elements like vitamins A, C, and E, and selenium are thought to act as **antioxidants**. Vitamin E, melatonin, aloe vera, and a compound called beta-1,3-glucan are reported to stimulate the immune system. Natural substances like garlic, ginger, and shark cartilage are also commonly held to shrink tumors, with less defined modes of action.

Antineoplastons are believed by some to be another alternative approach to a cancer cure. Antineoplastons are small proteins which may act as molecular messengers and which may be absent from the urine and blood of many cancer patients. Proponents believe that replacing these proteins may have beneficial effects. The NCI has been unable to draw definitive conclusions about the usefulness of antineoplastons as a therapy because no large-scale clinical trials of the therapy have been completed.

Coping with cancer treatment

Treatment of nasal cancers commonly includes surgery, radiation therapy and chemotherapy. Although the use of chemotherapy and radiation therapy in addition to surgery has improved the chance of survival for nasal cancer patients, both of these treatments unavoidably result in damage to some healthy tissues and other undesirable side effects.

Fatigue is a very common side effect of both radiation therapy and chemotherapy. Side effects of the actual treatments combine with the natural depletion of the body's resources as it fights off the disease and normal psychological consequences of the disease such as **depression** to make coping with fatigue a very significant aspect of dealing with cancer treatment. The best way to deal with these symptoms is to cut back on stressful activities and take plenty of time to allow the body to heal. It is also important to try to maintain a well-balanced, nutritious diet, and to exercise. Patients should avoid as much extra stress as possible and should limit visitors, if needed, to avoid being overtired. At the same time, it is also important for psychological health for the patient to pursue their interests as much as possible and to avoid becoming isolated.

The biggest problem for those undergoing radiation therapy is the development of dry, sore, "burned" skin in the area being treated. (Radiation does not hurt during treatment and does not make the person radioactive.) Skin in the treatment area will become red, get itchy and sore, and may blister and peel, becoming painful. Patients with fair skin or those who have undergone previous chemotherapy have a greater risk of more serious reactions. Dry, itchy or sore skin is temporary, but affected skin may be more sensitive to sun exposure for the rest of the patient's lifetime, so a good sunscreen and a hat should be used whenever affected skin is exposed to sunlight.

Other effects, specific to the nasal area, may also occur. Sometimes very thick mucus is produced that may be difficult to cough up. Some patients become hoarse and find it difficult to eat. It is important for patients to keep well-hydrated by drinking plenty of fluids and to eat as much protein as possible. If patients cannot eat enough to maintain a high-protein diet, liquid high-protein drinks should be consumed. Patients may be more susceptible to upper respiratory infections after treatment, so some physicians will prescribe preventative **antibiotics**. If eating is extremely painful, tylenol can be consumed in milk about 30 minutes before a meal for pain relief. Patients should be prepared for the fact that symptoms of radiation treatment can persist for up to a month after the last treatment.

Some of the more common side effects of chemotherapy include hair loss, and **nausea and vomiting**. Hair loss (**alopecia**) is a difficult part of dealing with cancer treatment for most patients, especially women. Hair may thin out gradually, or it may fall out in big clumps. To slow down the rate of hair loss, avoid any unnecessary sources of damage to the hair, like curling, blow-drying, or chemical treatments.

Different patients choose different ways of coping with the loss of their hair. Some patients may find they are more comfortable hiding hair loss with a wig; it is a good idea to cut off a lock of hair before hair loss begins in case a wig is later desired. Some patients may choose to remain bald, or may want to choose hats or scarves instead of wigs. In any case, it is important to remember that the loss of hair is a sign that the medication is doing its job, and that hair loss is temporary. Hair usually begins regrowth within a few months of the end of intensive chemotherapy, although it may come in a different color or texture than the original hair.

Nausea and **vomiting** are other fairly common side effects of many chemotherapy drugs. (Radiation to the brain or the GI tract can also cause nausea and vomiting.) After a few courses of chemotherapy drugs, some patients will become nauseated just from thinking about an upcoming treatment or from smelling certain odors. Drugs that combat nausea and vomiting can be prescribed, but are often not effective for anticipatory nausea. If nausea and vomiting are a problem, heavy, regular meals should be avoided in favor of small, frequent snacks made up of light but nourishing foods like soup. Avoiding food smells and other strong odors may help.

Desensitization, hypnosis, guided imagery, and relaxation techniques may be used if nausea and vomiting are severe. These techniques help to identify the triggers for the nausea and vomiting, decrease patient anxiety, and distract the patient from thinking about getting sick. Acupressure bands, commonly used for seasickness, and acupuncture, may also provide some relief for some patients.

Both radiation therapy and chemotherapy treatments require a substantial level of commitment from the patient in terms of time and emotional energy. Fear and anxiety are major factors in coping with cancer in general and these cancer treatments. The feelings are completely normal. Some patients find that concentrating on restful, pleasurable activities like hobbies, prayer, or meditation is helpful in decreasing negative emotions. It is also very important that patients have people to whom they can express their fears and other negative emotions. Support groups may help to provide an environment where fears can be freely expressed and understood.

Clinical trials

Clinical trials are studies in which new treatments for disease are evaluated in human patients. Current clinical trials for nasal cancer patients are concentrating on the addition of chemotherapy to the more common treatments of surgery and radiation therapy, either before or after those treatments, in order to improve cure rates or to lessen the side effects of radiation.

Nasal cancer patients are also being recruited for a clinical trial evaluating an alternative therapy known as antineoplaston therapy.

Prevention

Although mutations in genetic material happen frequently, most of these do not result in cancer. This is because a healthy body repairs most mistakes before a cancer develops and because, if a cancer does develop, the immune system of a healthy body will usually destroy it. In general, therefore, a healthy lifestyle that includes exercise, plenty of sleep, a diet rich in fruits and vegetables, regular health screenings and the avoidance of stress, excessive sun exposure, tobacco use, or excessive **alcohol consumption** will help to prevent most cancers.

Since nasal cancers, in particular, are often caused by chemical exposures, many of these cancers are preventable by avoiding excessive inhalation of wood dust or chemical mixtures and by avoiding use of all tobacco products. (Nasal cancers resulting from wood dust appear to require high-dose, long-term exposure, especially to hardwoods.)

One type of nasal cancer appears to be virus-associated and is more prevalent in people with a history of nasal polyps. People who are diagnosed with nasal polyps should discuss their removal with their physicians and have existing polyps checked regularly in order to detect a malignant polyp as quickly as possible.

Patients with nasal cancer can increase their chances of a cure by making sure that they see their doctors for all scheduled follow-up appointments. This is especially important for the first two years (when most recurrences of nasal cancer occur), but it is also important to maintain follow-up beyond that. Many nasal cancer patients experience a second tumor somewhere else in the upper respiratory tract.

Special concerns

One of the unique aspects of dealing with nasal cancer is the fact that surgical removal of a nasal tumor can result in substantial facial disfigurement. Patients who are dealing with this aspect of nasal cancer are forced to cope with the substantial emotional burden of disfigurement in addition to the other emotional ramifications of the disease.

People with facial disfigurement may be forced to cope with negative reactions from other people in public places, including staring, whispering, rude remarks or averted eyes, and other avoidance of interpersonal interaction.

In addition, the loss of the accustomed appearance will be experienced much like a bereavement. Patients will probably initially feel numb, then experience intense, overwhelming feelings of sadness, fear, and anger. The period characterized by intense, almost unbearable emotions is usually followed by a period of time when the patient feels completely empty, fatigued, and apathetic. Given time, most patients will come to an acceptance of their new reality and begin to enjoy old friends and activities again. It is important not to expect patients in such circumstances to immediately accept their situation or to suppress the natural emotions that accompany the change in their appearance. Patients can ease the process by trying to focus on one day at a time and by finding people who can help them work through the process by listening and accepting their emotions. It is very important that a patient dealing with these changes have friends or family members to whom they can express their feelings of grief and anger. A support group might also be helpful.

See also Cryotherapy; Tumor grading; Tumor staging.

Resources

BOOKS

Buckman, R. *What You Really Need to Know About Cancer*. Baltimore: Johns Hopkins University Press, 1999.

ORGANIZATIONS

American Cancer Society, 1599 Clifton Road, NE, Atlanta, GA 30329-4251. (800)586-4872 http://www.cancer.org.

National Cancer Institute, 9000 Rockville Pike, Bethesda, Maryland, 20892. (800)422-6237. <http:www.nci. nih.gov.

The Wellness Community, 10921 Reed Harman Highway, Cincinnati, Ohio, 45242 (888)793-9355. http://www. wellness-community.org.

Wendy Wippel, M.Sc.

Nasopharyngeal cancer

Definition

Nasopharyngeal **cancer** is an uncontrolled growth of cells that begins in the nasopharynx, the passageway at the back of the nose.

Description

The nasopharynx connects the nose (hence, naso) to the pharynx, the shared passageway for air and food at the back of the nose and mouth. Air moves through the pharynx on its way into and out of the trachea, the tube that carries air to the lungs. Food passes through the pharynx on its way to the esophagus, the muscular tube that carries food to the stomach.

Although it is possible for people to breathe through the mouth, breathing through the nose is better. The nose warms and moistens air, and the interior of the nose has hairs to filter particles from the air. Thus, any blockage, such as a tumor or cancer in the nasopharynx, interferes with normal breathing.

Not all tumors that grow in the nasopharynx are malignant. Many are benign, but the tumors still cause problems because they often grow into the vessels that supply blood to the nose. Malignant cancers in the nasopharynx grow from squamous, or flat, epithelial cells. Epithelial cells form body coverings, such as skin. Cancers that originate in epithelial cells are known as carcinomas.

Demographics

Nasopharyngeal cancer is rare in most parts of the world. The exception is in Southeast Asia, where there are as many as 40 new cases each year for every 100,000 people. In other parts of the world, there are as few as one new case per year for every 100,000 people. Men are at a greater risk than women. Although all age groups can be affected by this cancer, like many other cancers, people over the age of 40 tend to be more susceptible.

KEY TERMS

Biopsy—A diagnostic procedure in which a tissue sample is removed from the body for examination.

Computed tomography (CT)—A radiographic technique in which multiple x-ray images assembled by a computer to give a three-dimensional image of a structure.

Endoscope—Instrument designed to allow direct visual inspection of body cavities, a sort of microscope in a long access tube.

Magnetic resonance imaging (MRI)—Magnetic fields and radio frequency waves are used to image internal structures of the body.

Nasoscope—A type of endoscope designed specifically to be inserted through the nose and used for examination of the nasal cavity.

Causes and symptoms

Several factors put people at risk for nasopharyngeal cancer. One is an **infection** with a type of herpes virus called **Epstein-Barr virus** (EBV). Another factor is genetic make-up, or inherited DNA. Finally, anything that introduces radioactive elements into the diet or respiratory pathway increases the risk of developing this cancer.

In certain parts of China, the soil has a high concentration of uranium and thorium, which break down into radioactive elements such as radium and radon. The elements are taken up by trees, which are burned for wood and become airborne. They also dissolve in water, and fish and plants draw them up. The fish are eaten. Some of the plants are used for tea. The scenario seems to increase the risk of nasopharyngeal cancer, but the exact way in which it does is not known.

In all parts of the world, people who work in sawmills or with wood products have a higher likelihood of acquiring nasopharyngeal cancer. Sawdust or chemicals in the wood may contribute to its development.

Recently, E. Lopez-Lizarraga demonstrated that **human papilloma virus** (HPV) is often present in people who contract nasopharyngeal cancer. Neither this link nor the others cited show a precise cause and effect, however. Some of the links may mask true causes. For example, in the HPV study, subjects who had HPV infection also tended to have poor oral hygiene. And in the case of EBV, infection with the virus is so common that some researchers are now investigating whether there is a unique strain of the

QUESTIONS TO ASK THE DOCTOR

- In what stage is this cancer?
- What is the outlook for a patient with my profile?
- What are the side effects of the treatments that are recommended? Which treatment gives the best combination of survival and quality of life?
- Is there a clinical trial for which I am eligible?

EBV that puts individuals at greater risk for nasopharyngeal cancer.

Symptoms of nasopharyngeal cancer include:

- lump in the nose or neck
- headaches
- ear pain
- numbness on the side of the face
- difficulty breathing
- difficulty speaking

Diagnosis

A physician examines the nasopharynx in various ways, usually starting with an instrument such as a nasoscope. The nasoscope allows a look at the inside of the nasal cavity. Palpating, or touching, lymph nodes in the neck to check for enlarged ones is also part of the examination.

If suspicious growths are found, a **biopsy** is done to take a tissue sample. Different types of biopsy can be used. An incision may be made to obtain tissue, or a needle with a small diameter may be inserted into a suspicious mass to obtain cells, especially if there is a lump in the neck.

Computed tomography (CT) and **magnetic resonance imaging** (MRI) scans are also used. They help determine whether the cancer has spread from the walls of the nasopharynx. MRI offers a good way to examine the tonsils and the back of the tongue, which are soft tissues. CT is used as a way of studying the jaw, which is bone.

Treatment team

Generally, physicians with special training in the organs of the nose and throat take initial responsibility for the care of a patient with nasopharyngeal cancer. They are called otolaryngologists, or occasionally, otorhinolaryngologists. Otolaryngologists are usually labeled ENT (for ear, nose, and throat) specialists. An ENT specializing in cancer will probably lead the team, accompanied by radiation therapists and oncologists.

Clinical staging, treatments, and prognosis

Stage I describes a cancer that has not spread. It is not in the lymph nodes and is localized in the nasopharynx. Stage II describes a larger cancer, one that affects more than half the area of the nasopharynx, that is not in the lymph nodes. Stage III nasopharyngeal cancer has spread beyond the nasopharynx; it might affect the oropharynx, the cavity at the back of the mouth, or part of the throat. Or, it might have spread to the lymph nodes. Stage IV involves one or more of the following indications:

- spread of cancer to a site near the original site, such as the bones and nerves of the head
- more than one lymph node with cancer
- spread to other parts of the body, such as the larynx, the trachea, the bronchi, the esophagus, or more distant points, such as the lungs

The outlook for recovery from nasopharyngeal cancer is better the earlier the stage in which the cancer is diagnosed. For stage I and stage II, radiation or **chemotherapy** treatment of the affected area is sometimes all that is required to halt the cell growth. Decisions about which method to use depend on many factors, but the tolerance a patient has for radiation or chemotherapy and the size of the tumor are important.

Often, the most promising treatment option for a person with nasopharyngeal cancer is a clinical trial. The outlook for early stage diagnoses of nasopharyngeal cancer is good. The five-year survival rate is over 80% for small cancers, which are typically in Stage I. Cancers that are larger, but have not spread to the lymph nodes, usually have survival rate of 50% or more. Unfortunately, about half of all people diagnosed with nasopharyngeal cancer are not diagnosed until the cancer is advanced, which leads to a poorer prognosis.

Coping with cancer treatment

The patient should be an active member of the treatment team, listening to information and making decisions about which course of treatment to take. Premier cancer centers encourage such a role.

Appetite might be affected before, during, and after treatment. Before treatment, the presence of a tumor can interfere with chewing and swallowing food, and food might not seem as appealing as it once did. During treatment, particularly radiation treatment, the treated nasopharynx will be sore, and eating and breathing may be difficult.

Patients should also seek out a support network to help them cope with the psychological implications of cancer. In addition to family and friends, local support organizations can offer guidance, answer questions, and link newly diagnosed patients with others who have survived a similar experience.

Alternative and complementary therapies

Any technique, such as yoga, meditation, or biofeedback, that helps a patient cope with anxiety over the condition and discomfort from treatment is useful and should be explored as an option. Many herbal remedies are available to ease the symptoms of **nausea** that accompany treatment; the physician, however, should be notified of any remedies, herbal or otherwise, that are taken.

Clinical trials

There are a number of **clinical trials** currently in progress, especially with **biological response modifiers** (BMR), or substances that take advantage of the capabilities of the body's own immune system. **Aldesleukin** is one BMR that has been used to fight nasopharyngeal cancer, with inconclusive results. The Cancer Information Service at the National Institutes of Health offers information about clinical trials that are looking for volunteers. The service offers a toll-free number at (800) 422-6237.

Prevention

The link between HPV and nasopharyngeal cancer suggests that any precaution taken to avoid contracting sexually transmitted diseases, such as the use of condoms, affords protection. Radon gas levels should be checked in homes, and measures taken to reduce them if they are high. Individuals working with wood, especially those exposed to sawdust and chemicals, should wear protective respiratory covers, such as a breathing mask.

Special concerns

Additional cancers that begin in the nasopharynx can start in the lymph cells found there. Because of their origin, these cancers are called lymphomas.

See also Oral cancer; Oropharyngeal cancer.

Resources

PERIODICALS

Lopez-Lizarraga, E., et al. "Human Papilloma Virus in Tonsillar and Nasopharyngeal Carcinoma: Isolation of HPV Subtype 31."*Ear, Nose, and Throat Journal* 79 (December 2000): 942–4.

OTHER

Oral Cavity and Pharyngeal Cancer. Online text. American Cancer Society. [cited July 6, 2005]. http://www3.cancer.org.

ORGANIZATIONS

SPOHNC, Support for People with Oral and Head and Neck Cancer. P.O. Box 53, Locust Valley, NY 11560-0053. (800) 377-0928. http://www.spohnc.org.

Diane M. Calabrese

Nausea and vomiting

Description

Nausea and vomiting are recognized as two separate and distinct conditions. Nausea is the subjective, unpleasant feeling or urge to vomit, which may or may not result in vomiting. Vomiting is the forceful expelling of the contents of the stomach and intestines through the mouth. To some, nausea is a more distressing symptom than vomiting. Nausea and vomiting are major problems for patients being treated with **cancer**, with approximately 50% of patients experiencing nausea and vomiting as a result of cancer treatments even though **antiemetics** (anti-nausea and vomiting medications) were used. In addition, more than 50% of cancer patients experience nausea and vomiting as a result of progression of the disease, or as a result of exposure to other therapies used to treat the cancer.

Not all patients diagnosed with cancer will experience nausea and vomiting. However, nausea and vomiting remain two of the side effects associated with cancer and cancer treatment that patients and their families fear the most. The negative aspects of nausea and vomiting can influence all facets of a patient's life. If nausea and vomiting are not controlled in the patient with cancer, the result can be serious metabolic problems such as disturbances in fluid and electrolyte balance and nutritional status. Psychological problems associated with nausea and vomiting include anxiety and **depression**. Uncontrolled nausea and vomiting can also lead to the decision by the patient to stop potentially curative cancer therapy.

Causes

The most common causes of nausea and vomiting in cancer patients include treatment with **chemotherapy** and **radiation therapy**; tumor spread to the gastrointestinal tract, liver, and brain; constipation; **infection**; and use of some **opioids**, which are drugs used to treat cancer pain. The mechanisms that control nausea and vomiting are not fully understood, but both are controlled by the central nervous system. Nausea is thought to arise from stimulation of the autonomic nervous system. It is theorized that chemotherapy causes vomiting by stimulating areas in the gastrointestinal tract and the brain. The areas in the brain that are stimulated are the chemoreceptor trigger zone (CTZ) and the emetic or vomiting center (VC). When the VC is stimulated, muscular contractions of the abdomen, chest wall, and diaphragm occur, which result in the expulsion of stomach and intestinal contents.

Chemotherapy-induced nausea and vomiting

Not all chemotherapeutic agents cause nausea and vomiting. Chemotherapy drugs vary in their ability or potential to cause nausea and vomiting. This variation is known as the emetogenic potential of the drug, or the potential of the drug to cause emesis. Chemotherapy drugs are classified as having severe (greater than 90% of patients exposed to this drug will experience nausea and vomiting), high (60–90% of patients will experience nausea and vomiting), moderate (30–60% will experience nausea and vomiting), low (10–30% will experience nausea and vomiting), and very low (less than 10% experience nausea and vomiting) emetogenic potential.

The incidence and severity of chemotherapy-induced nausea and vomiting varies and is related to the following factors: the emetogenic potential of the drug, the drug dosage, the schedule of administration of the drug, and the route of the drug. For example, even a drug with a low emetogenic potential may cause nausea and vomiting if given at higher doses. Factors that are associated with increased nausea and vomiting after chemotherapy include female gender, age greater than six in children, age less than 50 in adults, history of motion sickness, and history of vomiting in pregnancy.

When nausea and vomiting result from chemotherapy administration, the nausea and vomiting can be classified as anticipatory, acute, or delayed. Anticipatory nausea and vomiting occur prior to the actual chemotherapy treatment and are a response primarily to an environmental stimulus, such as a specific odor, which is then associated with the chemotherapy treatment in the future. That is, the smell of the odor alone can be enough to induce or trigger nausea and vomiting in the sensitized patient. Acute nausea and vomiting occur within 24 hours of administration of the chemotherapeutic agent. Delayed nausea and vomiting occur after the acute phase and may last 48 or more hours after chemotherapy administration.

Radiation therapy induced nausea and vomiting

Although not all patients receiving radiation therapy will experience nausea and vomiting, patients receiving radiation therapy to the gastrointestinal tract and brain are most likely to experience those side effects. Radiation therapy to the brain is believed to stimulate the CTZ, the VC, or both. The higher the radiation therapy dose and the greater the body surface area irradiated, the higher the potential for nausea and vomiting. Also, the larger the amount of gastrointestinal tract tissue exposed to radiation the more likely nausea and vomiting will occur. Nausea and vomiting associated with radiation therapy usually occurs one-half hour to several hours after treatment and usually does not occur on the days when the patient is not undergoing treatment.

Treatments

Pharmacologic management

The most commonly used intervention to manage nausea and vomiting in cancer patients is the use of antiemetic drugs. Many of these drugs work by inhibiting stimulation of the CTZ and perhaps the VC. Most of the drugs used today to clinically treat nausea and vomiting are classified into one of the following groups: dopaminergic antagonists, neurokinin receptor antagonists, **corticosteroids**, cannabinoids, and serotonin receptor antagonists. Antiemetics can be utilized as single agents or several drugs can be prescribed together as combination therapy.

Examples of dopaminergic antagonists include phenothiazines such as prochlorperazine (Compazine), substituted benzamides such as metaclopramide (Reglan), and butyrophenones such as droperidol (Inapsine) and haloperidol (Haldol). Side effects of the dopaminergic antagonists include extrapyramidal reactions (e.g., tremors, slurred speech, anxiety, distress, paranoia) and sedation. In 2004, the FDA approved a drug called aprepitant (Emend) for use in cancer patients. It is used in combination with other antiemetics for relief of acute and delayed nausea and vomiting caused by high-dose chemotherapy, most often caused by the chemotherapy drug **cisplatin**. Side effects of aprepitant include **fatigue**, dizziness, stomach pain, nausea, hiccups, **diarrhea**, constipation, and loss of appetite.

Steroids may be used to treat mild to moderately emetogenic chemotherapy. However, long-term corticosteroid use is considered inappropriate due to the multiple adverse effects associated with long-term use. Cannabinoids (substances similar to, or derived from, marijuana) may be effective in selected patients but are usually not prescribed as first line therapy due to generally low rates of effectiveness. Controversy continues to exist related to the use of cannabinoids, which may not be accepted cultural or societal practice for some patients. Side effects of cannabinoids include physical and psychogenic effects such as acute withdrawal syndrome, dizziness, dry mouth, sedation, depression, anxiety, paranoia, and panic.

The newest class of antiemetics is the serotonin or 5-HT_3 antagonists. In 2001, three serotonin receptor antagonists were available in the United States: granisetron (Kytril), ondansetron (Zofran), and dolasetron (Anzemet). Serotonin receptor antagonists are better tolerated, are generally more effective, and result in fewer side effects than previously available antiemetics. A common adverse effect of the serotonin antagonists is asthenia, a state of unusual fatigue and weakness. Asthenia usually occurs two to three days after treatment with serotonin antagonists and may last one to four days. Serotonin receptor antagonists may not be offered or made available to all patients due to the relatively high cost of the drugs. Controversy exists related to the optimal role of serotonin receptor antagonists. Some clinicians argue there is the potential for overuse of the serotonin receptor antagonists when used to treat patients who are not receiving chemotherapeutic agents with moderate to severe emetogenic potential and when less expensive agents would be as effective.

Another class of drugs, the **benzodiazepines** including **lorazepam** (Ativan), midazolam (Versed), and alprazolam (Xanax), may be used in conjunction with antiemetics in the prevention and treatment of anxiety and expected chemotherapy-induced nausea and vomiting. These agents appear to be especially effective in highly emetogenic regimens administered to children. The benzodiazepines have only modest antiemetic properties. Therefore, they are usually used as adjuncts to antiemetic agents. Adverse effects of the benzodiazepines include sedation, confusion, hypotension (unusually low blood pressure), and visual disturbances.

Alternative and complementary therapies

The use of antiemetics is considered the cornerstone of therapy to treat chemotherapy-induced vomiting. Nonpharmacologic therapies may be used in conjunction with pharmacologic agents to enhance the effects of the drugs. Nonpharmacologic strategies include behavioral interventions such as guided imagery, hypnosis, systematic desensitization, and attentional distraction. Dietary interventions such as eating cold or room temperature foods and foods with minimal odors while avoiding spicy, salty, sweet, or high-fat foods may be beneficial to some patients while undergoing chemotherapy treatments. Another dietary recommendation is the use of ginger or ginger capsules to decrease episodes of nausea and vomiting. Acupressure, specifically stimulation of the Nei-Guan point (P6) of the dominant arm or stimulation of the Inner Gate and ST36 or Three Miles point (below the knee and lateral—outside area—to the tibia) has proven helpful to some patients. Music therapy interventions have also been effective as diversional interventions to reduce incidence and severity of chemotherapy-induced nausea and vomiting.

Resources

BOOKS

Wickham, R. "Nausea and Vomiting." In *Cancer Symptom Management*, edited by C. H. Yarbro, M. H. Frogge, and M. Goodman. Boston: Jones and Bartlett Publishers, 1999, pp. 228–253.

PERIODICALS

American Society of Health-System Pharmacists. "ASHP Therapeutic Guidelines on the Pharmacologic Management of Nausea and Vomiting in Adult and Pediatric Patients Receiving Chemotherapy or Radiation Therapy or Undergoing Surgery." *American Journal of Health System Pharmacy* 56 (1999): 729–764.

Boothby, Lisa A., and Paul L. Doering. "New Drug Update 2003: Part 1." *Drug Topics* February 23, 2004: 54.

OTHER

"Nausea and Vomiting." *WebMDHealth*. WebMD. [cited June 26, 2009]. http.//www.my.webmd.com/content/article/1680.50839.

"Symptom Management: Nausea/Vomiting." *Oncolink*. Oncolink. [cited June 26, 2009]. http://www.oncolink.upenn.edu/support/nausea.

Melinda Granger Oberleitner, R.N., D.N.S.
Teresa G. Odle

Navelbine *see* **Vinorelbine**

Nephrectomy

Definition

A nephrectomy is a surgical procedure for the removal of a kidney or section of a kidney.

Purpose

Nephrectomy, or kidney removal, is performed on patients with severe kidney damage from disease, injury, or congenital conditions. These include **cancer** of the kidney (renal cell **carcinoma**); polycystic kidney disease (a disease in which cysts, or sac-like structures, displace healthy kidney tissue); and serious kidney infections. It is also used to remove a healthy kidney from a donor for the purposes of kidney transplantation.

Demographics

The HCUP Nationwide Inpatient Sample from the Agency for Healthcare Research and Quality (AHRQ)

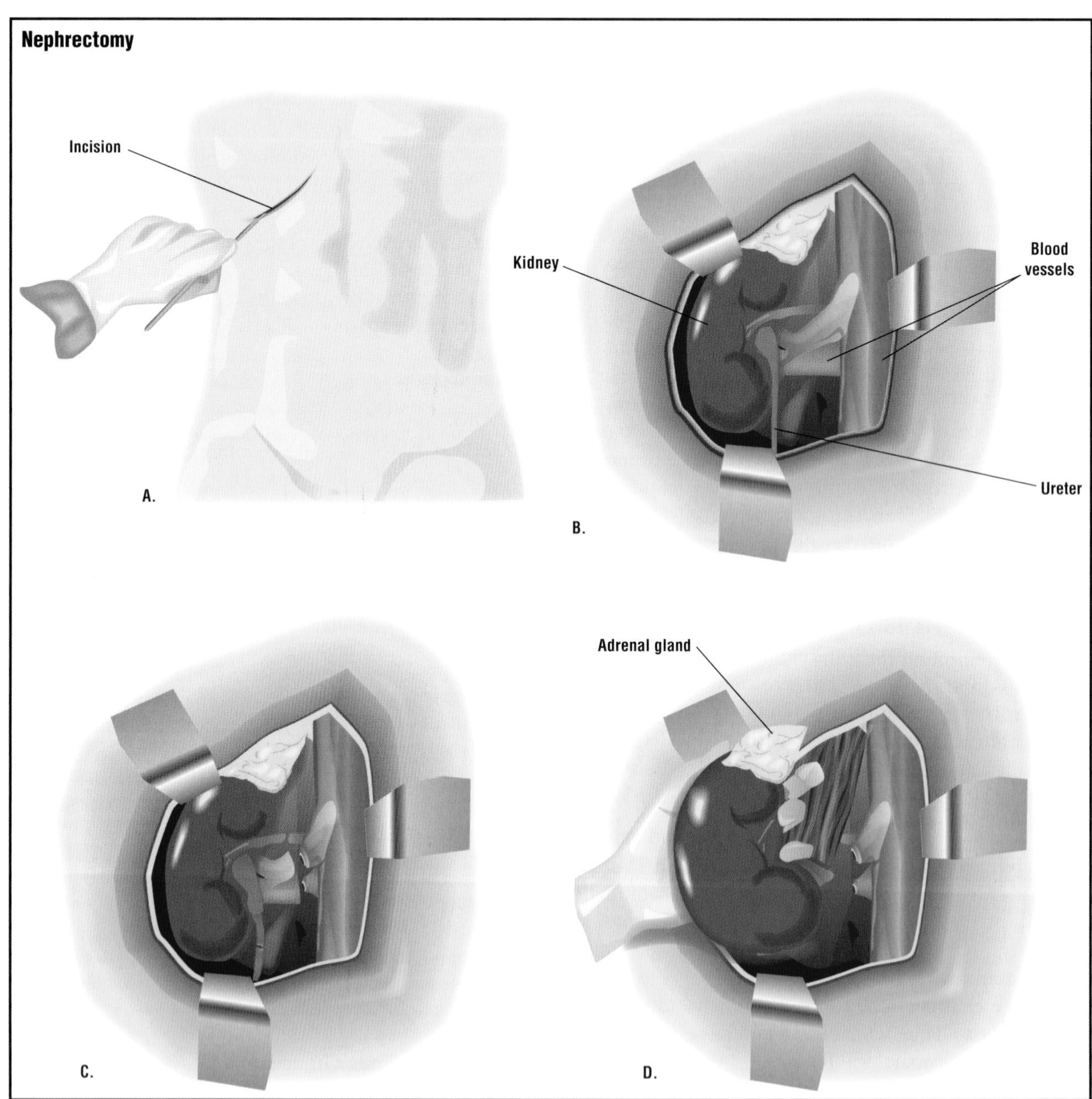

To remove a kidney in a nephrectomy procedure, an incision is made below the ribcage (A). The kidney is exposed (B) and connections to blood vessels and the ureter are severed (C). The kidney is removed in one piece (D). *(Illustration by GGS Information Services. Cengage Learning, Gale.)*

reports that 46,130 patients underwent partial or radical nephrectomy surgery for non-transplant-related indications in the United States in 2000. Patients with **kidney cancer** accounted for over half of those procedures. About 57,760 new cases of renal cell carcinoma were expected to be diagnosed in 2009, per the American Cancer Society.

According to the United Network for Organ Sharing (UNOS), 5,086 people underwent nephrectomy to become living kidney donors in 2007. Of these, 2,911 were male and 2,975 were female. Related donors were more common than non-related donors, with full siblings being the most common relationship between living donor and kidney recipients (28.5% of living donors).

Description

Nephrectomy may involve removing a small portion of the kidney or the entire organ and surrounding tissues. In partial nephrectomy, only the diseased or infected portion of the kidney is removed. Radical nephrectomy involves removing the entire kidney, a section of the tube leading to the bladder (ureter), the gland that sits atop the kidney (adrenal gland), and the fatty tissue surrounding the kidney. A simple nephrectomy performed for living donor transplant purposes requires removal of the kidney and a section of the attached ureter.

Open nephrectomy

In a traditional, open nephrectomy, the kidney donor is administered general anesthesia and a 6–10 in (15.2–25.4 cm) incision through several layers of muscle is made on the side or front of the abdomen. The blood vessels connecting the kidney to the donor are cut and clamped, and the ureter is also cut between the bladder and kidney and clamped. Depending on the type of nephrectomy procedure being performed, the ureter, adrenal gland, and/or surrounding tissue may also be cut. The kidney is removed and the vessels and ureter are then tied off and the incision is sutured (sewn up). The surgical procedure can take up to three hours, depending on the type of nephrectomy being performed.

Laparoscopic nephrectomy

Laparoscopic nephrectomy is a form of minimally invasive surgery that utilizes instruments on long, narrow rods to view, cut, and remove the kidney. The surgeon views the kidney and surrounding tissue with a flexible videoscope. The videoscope and surgical instruments are maneuvered through four small incisions in the abdomen, and carbon dioxide is pumped into the abdominal cavity to inflate it and improve visualization of the kidney. Once the kidney is isolated, it is secured in a bag and pulled through a fifth incision, approximately 3 in (7.6 cm) wide, in the front of the abdominal wall below the navel. Although this surgical technique takes slightly longer than a traditional nephrectomy, preliminary studies have shown that it promotes a faster recovery time, shorter hospital stays, and less post-operative pain.

A modified laparoscopic technique called hand-assisted laparoscopic nephrectomy may also be used to remove the kidney. In the hand-assisted surgery, a small incision of 3–5 in (7.6–12.7 cm) is made in the patient's abdomen. The incision allows the surgeon to place his hand in the abdominal cavity using a special surgical glove that also maintains a seal for the inflation of the abdominal cavity with carbon dioxide. This technique gives the surgeon the benefit of using his hands to feel the kidney and related structures. The kidney is then removed by hand through the incision instead of with a bag.

Diagnosis/Preparation

Prior to surgery, blood samples will be taken from the patient to type and crossmatch in case transfusion is required during surgery. A catheter will also be inserted into the patient's bladder. The surgical procedure will be described to the patient, along with the possible risks.

Aftercare

Nephrectomy patients may experience considerable discomfort in the area of the incision. Patients may also experience numbness, caused by severed nerves, near or on the incision. Pain relievers are administered following the surgical procedure and during the recovery period on an as-needed basis. Although deep breathing and coughing may be painful due to the proximity of the incision to the diaphragm, breathing exercises are encouraged to prevent **pneumonia**. Patients should not drive an automobile for a minimum of two weeks.

Risks

Possible complications of a nephrectomy procedure include **infection**, bleeding (hemorrhage), and post-operative pneumonia. There is also the risk of kidney failure in a patient with impaired function or disease in the remaining kidney.

Normal results

Normal results of a nephrectomy are dependent on the purpose of the procedure and the type of

WHO PERFORMS THE PROCEDURE AND WHERE IS IT PERFORMED?

If nephrectomy is required for the purpose of kidney donation, it will be performed by a transplant surgeon in one of over 200 UNOS-approved hospitals nationwide. For patients with renal cell carcinoma, nephrectomy surgery is typically performed in a hospital setting by a surgeon specializing in urologic oncology.

QUESTIONS TO ASK THE DOCTOR

- How many procedures of this type have you performed, and what are your success rates?
- Will my nephrectomy surgery be performed with a laparoscopic or an open technique?
- Will my nephrectomy be partial or radical, and what are the risks involved with my particular surgery?
- What will my recovery time be after the procedure?
- What are the chances that the transplant will be successful? (For those undergoing a nephrectomy to donate a kidney.)
- What are the odds of success, and will I require adjunctive treatment such as chemotherapy or immunotherapy? (For those undergoing a nephrectomy to treat kidney cancer.)

nephrectomy performed. Immediately following the procedure, it is normal for patients to experience pain near the incision site, particularly when coughing or breathing deeply. Renal function of the patient is monitored carefully after surgery. If the remaining kidney is healthy, it will increase its functioning over time to compensate for the loss of the removed kidney.

Length of hospitalization depends on the type of nephrectomy procedure. Patients who have undergone a laparoscopic radical nephrectomy may be discharged two to four days after surgery. Traditional open nephrectomy patients are typically hospitalized for about a week. Recovery time will also vary, on average from three to six weeks.

Morbidity and mortality rates

Survival rates for living kidney donors undergoing nephrectomy are excellent; mortality rates are only 0.03%—or three deaths for every 10,000 donors. Many of the risks involved are the same as for any surgical procedure: risk of infection, hemorrhage, blood clot, or allergic reaction to anesthesia.

For patients undergoing nephrectomy as a treatment for renal cell carcinoma, survival rates depend on several factors, including the stage of the cancer and the patient's overall health history. According to the American Cancer Society, the five-year survival rate for patients with stage I renal cell carcinoma is 96 percent, while the five-year survival rate for stage II kidney cancer is 82 percent. Stage III and IV cancers have metastasized, or spread, beyond the kidney and have a lower survival rate, 64 percent for stage III and about 23 percent for stage IV. **Chemotherapy**, radiation, and/or immunotherapy may also be required for these patients.

Alternatives

Because the kidney is responsible for filtering wastes and fluid from the bloodstream, kidney function is critical to life. Nephrectomy candidates diagnosed with serious kidney disease, cancer, or infection usually have few treatment choices aside from this procedure. However, if kidney function is lost in the remaining kidney, the patient will require chronic dialysis treatments or transplantation of a healthy kidney to sustain life.

Resources

BOOKS

Brenner, BM et al *Brenner & Rector's The Kidney*. 7th ed. Philadelphia: Saunders, 2004.

Wein, AJ et al. *Campbell-Walsh Urology*. 9th ed. Philadelphia: Saunders, 2007.

PERIODICALS

Johnson, Kate. "Laparoscopy is Big Hit With Living Donors." *Family Practice News* 31 (January 2001): 12.

ORGANIZATIONS

American Cancer Society. (800) 227-2345. http://www.cancer.org.

National Kidney Foundation. 30 East 33rd St., Suite 1100, New York, NY 10016. (800) 622-9010. http://www.kidney.org.

United Network for Organ Sharing (UNOS). 700 North 4th St., Richmond, VA 23219. (888) 894-6361. UNOS Transplant Connection: http://www.transplantliving.org.

OTHER

Living Donors Online. http://www.livingdonorsonline.org.

Paula Anne Ford-Martin

Nephrostomy

Definition

Nephrostomy is a procedure in which a catheter (plastic tube) is inserted through the skin and into the kidney to drain it of urine. Urine drains into a bag outside the body.

Purpose

The ureter is the tube that carries urine from the kidney to the bladder. When this tube is blocked, urine backs up into the kidney. Serious, irreversible kidney damage can occur because of this backflow of urine. **Infection** is also a common implication in this stagnant urine.

Nephrostomy is performed in several different circumstances:

- when the ureter is blocked by a kidney stone
- when the ureter is blocked by a tumor
- when there is a hole in the ureter or bladder and urine is leaking into the body
- as a diagnostic procedure to assess kidney anatomy
- as a diagnostic procedure to assess kidney function

Precautions

People preparing for a nephrostomy should review with their doctors all the medications they are taking. People taking anticoagulants (blood thinners such as Coumadin) may need to stop medication. People taking metformin (Glucophage) may need to stop taking the medication for several days before and after nephrostomy. Diabetics should discuss modifying their insulin doses because fasting is required before the procedure.

Description

Nephrostomy is done by an interventional radiologist or urologist with special training in the procedure. It can be done either as an inpatient or an outpatient procedure, depending on why it is needed. For most **cancer** patients, nephrostomy is an inpatient procedure that is covered by insurance.

First, the patient is given an anesthetic to numb the area where the catheter will be inserted. The doctor then inserts a needle into the kidney. There are several imaging technologies such as ultrasound and **computed tomography** that are used to help the doctor guide the needle into the correct place.

QUESTIONS TO ASK THE DOCTOR

- Why am I having a nephrostomy?
- How long do you think I will have to stay in the hospital?
- How long do you expect the catheter to stay in?
- How much help will I need in caring for the catheter?

Next, a fine guide wire follows the needle. The catheter, which is about the same diameter as IV tubing, follows the guide wire to its proper location. The catheter is then connected to a bag outside the body that collects the urine. The catheter and bag are secured so that the catheter will not pull out. The procedure usually takes one to two hours.

Preparation

Either the day before or on the day of the nephrostomy, blood samples will be taken. Other diagnostic tests done before the procedure vary depending on why the nephrostomy is being done, but the patient may have a computed tomography (CT) scan or ultrasound to help the doctor locate the blockage.

Patients should not eat for eight hours before a nephrostomy. On the day of the procedure, the patient will have an intravenous (IV) line placed in a vein in the arm. Through this the patient will receive **antibiotics** to prevent infection, medication for pain, and fluids. The IV line will remain in place after the procedure for at least several hours, and often longer.

Aftercare

Outpatients will be expected to stay about eight to 12 hours after the procedure to make sure the catheter is functioning properly. They should plan to have someone drive them home and stay with them at least the first 24 hours after the procedure. Inpatients may stay in the hospital several days. Generally people feel sore where the catheter is inserted for about a week to ten days.

Care of the catheter is important. The catheter will be located on the patient's back, so it may be necessary to have someone help with catheter care. The catheter should be kept dry and protected from water when taking showers. The skin around it should be kept clean, and the dressing over the area changed frequently. Special care is needed in handling the urine collection bag so that it does not dislodge the catheter.

Risks

Nephrostomy is an established and generally safe procedure. As with all operations, there is always a risk of allergic reaction to anesthesia, bleeding, and infection.

Normal results

In a successful nephrostomy, the catheter is inserted, and urine drains into the collection bag. How long the catheter stays in place depends on the reason for its insertion. In people with pelvic cancer or **bladder cancer** where the ureter is blocked by a tumor, the catheter will stay in place until the tumor is surgically removed. If the cancer is inoperable, the catheter may have to stay in place for the rest of the patient's life.

Abnormal results

Bruising at the catheter insertion site occurs in about half of people who have a nephrostomy. This is a minor complication. Major complications are infrequent, but include the tube becoming blocked or dislodged requiring tube replacement, bleeding and blood in the urine, and perforation of other organs.

Resources

ORGANIZATIONS

American Cancer Society. National Headquarters, 1599 Clifton Road NE, Atlanta, GA 30329. 800–ACS–2345. http://www.cancer.org.

Cancer Information Service. National Cancer Institute, Building 31, Room 10A19, 9000 Rockville Pike, Bethesda, MD 20892. –800–4–CANCER. http://www.nci.nih.gov/cancerinfo/index.html.

Tish Davidson, A.M.

Neuroblastoma

Definition

Neuroblastoma is a type of **cancer** that usually originates either in the tissues of the adrenal gland or in the ganglia of the abdomen or in the ganglia of the nervous system. (Ganglia are masses of nerve tissue or groups of nerve cells.) Tumors develop in the nerve tissue in the neck, chest, abdomen, or pelvis.

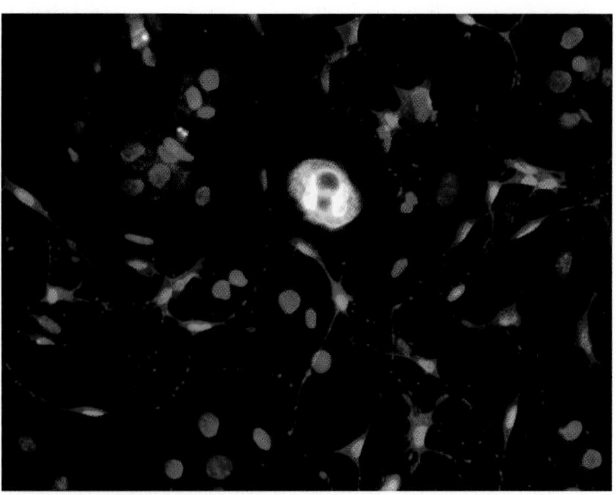

Immunofluorescent light micrograph of human neuroblastoma cancer cells. The normal epithelial cells appear green, the cytoplasm of neuroblastoma is red, and the nuclei are blue. *(Photograph by Nancy Kedersha. Science Source/Photo Researchers, Inc. Reproduced by permission.)*

Description

Neuroblastoma is one of the few cancer types known to secrete hormones. It occurs most often in children, and it is the third most common cancer that occurs in children. Approximately 7% of the **childhood cancers** diagnosed are neuroblastomas. Close to 50% of cases of neuroblastoma occur in children younger than two years old. The disease is sometimes present at birth, but is usually not noticed until later. By the time the disease is diagnosed, it has often spread to the lymph nodes, liver, lungs, bones, or bone marrow. Approximately one-third of neuroblastomas start in the adrenal glands.

Demographics

According to some reports, African-American children develop the disease at a slightly higher rate than Caucasian children (8.7 per million compared to 8.0 per million cases diagnosed).

Causes and symptoms

The causes of neuroblastoma are not precisely known. Current research holds that neuroblastomas develop when cells produced by the fetus (neuroblast cells) fail to mature into normal nerve or adrenal cells and keep growing and proliferating. The first symptom of a neuroblastoma is usually an unusual growth or lump, found in most cases in the abdomen of the child, causing discomfort or a sensation of fullness and pain. Other symptoms such as numbness and

KEY TERMS

Adjuvant chemotherapy—Treatment of the tumor with drugs after surgery to kill as many of the remaining cancer cells as possible.

Adrenal gland—Gland located above each kidney consisting of an outer wall (cortex) that produces steroid hormones and an inner section (medulla) that produces other important hormones, such as adrenaline and noradrenaline.

Alternative therapy—A therapy is generally called alternative when it is used instead of conventional cancer treatments.

Biopsy—A small sample of tissue removed from the site of the tumor to be examined under a microscope.

Complementary therapy—A therapy is called complementary when it is used in addition to conventional cancer treatments.

Conventional therapy—Treatments that are widely accepted and practiced by the mainstream medical community.

Disseminated—Spread to other tissues.

Hormone—A substance produced by specialized cells that affects the way the body carries out the biochemical and energy-producing processes required to maintain health (metabolism).

Localized—Confined to a small area.

Monoclonal antibody—A protein substance which is produced in the laboratory by a single population of cells. They are being tested as a possible form of cancer treatment.

Neoadjuvant chemotherapy—Treatment of the tumor with drugs before surgery to reduce the size of the tumor.

Neuroblast cells—Cells produced by the fetus which mature into nerve cells and adrenal medulla cells.

Resectable cancer—A tumor that can be surgically removed.

Salvage therapy—Treatment measures taken late in the course of a disease after other therapies have failed. It is also known as rescue therapy.

Staging system—A system based on how far the cancer has spread from its original site, developed to help the physician determine how best to treat the disease.

Unresectable cancer—A tumor that cannot be completely removed by surgery.

fatigue, arise because of pressure caused by the tumor. **Bone pain** also occurs if the cancer has spread to the bone. If it has spread to the area behind the eye, the cancer may cause protruding eyes and dark circles around the eyes; in a few cases, blindness may be the presenting symptom. Or paralysis may result from compression of the spinal cord. **Fever** is also reported in one case out of four. High blood pressure, persistent **diarrhea**, rapid heartbeat, reddening of the skin, and sweating occur occasionally. Some children may also have uncoordinated or jerky muscle movements, or uncontrollable eye movements, but these symptoms are rare. If the disease spreads to the skin, blue or purple patches are observed.

Diagnosis

A diagnosis of neuroblastoma usually requires blood and urine tests to investigate the nature and quantity of chemicals (neurotransmitters) released by the nerve cells. These are broken down by the body and released in urine. Additionally, scanning techniques are used to confirm the diagnosis of neuroblastoma. These techniques produce images or pictures of the inside of the body and they include **computed tomography** scan (CT scan) and **magnetic resonance imaging** (MRI). To confirm the diagnosis, the physician will surgically remove some of the tissue from the tumor or bone marrow (**biopsy**), and examine the cells under the microscope.

Treatment team

The treatment team usually consists of an oncologist specialized in the treatment of neuroblastoma, a surgeon to perform biopsies and possibly attempt surgical removal of the tumor, a **radiation therapy** team and, if indicated, a **bone marrow transplantation** team.

Clinical staging, treatments, and prognosis

Staging

Once neuroblastoma has been diagnosed, the physician will perform more tests to determine if the cancer has spread to other tissues in the body. This process, called staging, is important for the physician to determine how to treat the cancer and check liver and kidney function. The staging system for neuroblastoma is based on how far the disease has spread from its original site to other tissues in the body.

QUESTIONS TO ASK THE DOCTOR

- What treatment choices do we have?
- Has the neuroblastoma spread to other parts of the body?
- What is the stage of the cancer?
- Based on your experience in treating neuroblastoma, how long do you think my child will survive if there is no response to treatment or the cancer comes back?
- How long will it take to recover from treatment?
- Will my child develop any long-term risks or complications from the cancer or its treatment?
- Can you recommend a support group in my town for people who are coping with neuroblastoma?

Localized resectable (able to be cut out) neuroblastoma is confined to the site of origin, with no evidence that it has spread to other tissues, and the cancer can be surgically removed. Localized unresectable neuroblastoma is confined to the site of origin, but the cancer cannot be completely removed surgically. Regional neuroblastoma has extended beyond its original site, to regional lymph nodes, and/or surrounding organs or tissues, but has not spread to distant sites in the body. Disseminated neuroblastoma has spread to distant lymph nodes, bone, liver, skin, bone marrow, and/or other organs. Stage 4S (or IVS, or "special") neuroblastoma has spread only to liver, skin, and/or, to a very limited extent, bone marrow. Recurrent neuroblastoma means that the cancer has come back, or continued to spread after it has been treated. It may come back in the original site or in another part of the body.

Treatments

Treatments are available for children with all stages of neuroblastoma. More than one of these treatments may be used, depending on the stage of the disease. The four types of treatment used are:

- Surgery (removing the tumor in an operation)
- Radiation therapy (using high-energy x-rays to kill cancer cells)
- Chemotherapy (using drugs to kill cancer cells)
- Bone marrow transplantation (replacing the patient's bone marrow cells with those from a healthy person).

Surgery is used whenever possible, to remove as much of the cancer as possible, and can generally cure the disease if the cancer has not spread to other areas of the body. Before surgery, **chemotherapy** may be used to shrink the tumor so that it can be more easily removed during surgery; this is called neoadjuvant chemotherapy. Radiation therapy is often used after surgery; high-energy rays (radiation) are used to kill as many of the remaining cancer cells as possible. Chemotherapy (called **adjuvant chemotherapy**) may also be used after surgery to kill remaining cells. Bone marrow transplantation is used to replace bone marrow cells killed by radiation or chemotherapy. In some cases the patient's own bone marrow is removed prior to treatment and saved for transplantation later. Other times the bone marrow comes from a matched donor, such as a sibling.

One novel approach to treatment of neuroblastomas is therapy with desferoxamine (DFO), which is ordinarily used to treat iron poisoning. DFO has been shown to have antitumor activity in neuroblastomas and other cancers of the central nervous system. It is thought that the drug works by lowering the increased iron levels in the body associated with cancer.

As of 2004, there are significant differences in treatment protocols for neuroblastoma between the major North American study group (Children's Oncology Group) and its European counterpart, the Société Internationale d'Oncologie Pédiatrique (SIOP). These differences include biopsy techniques, the timing and extent of surgery, chemotherapy dosages, and the types of salvage therapy employed.

Prognosis

The chances of recovery from neuroblastoma depend on the stage of the cancer, the age of the child at diagnosis, the location of the tumor, and the state and nature of the tumor cells evaluated under the microscope. Infants have a higher rate of cure than do children over one year of age, even when the disease has spread. In general, the prognosis for a young child with neuroblastoma is good: the predicted five-year survival rate is approximately 85% for children who had the onset of the disease in infancy, and 35% for those whose disease developed later.

Alternative and complementary therapies

No alternative therapy has yet been reported to substitute for conventional neuroblastoma treatment. Complementary therapies—such as retinoic acid therapy—have been shown to be beneficial to patients when administered after a conventional course of chemotherapy or transplantation.

Coping with cancer treatment

Neuroblastoma is a childhood cancer and it must be recognized that children, adolescents and their families have very special needs. These are best met at cancer centers for children working in close contact with the treatment team and the primary care physician. These centers have experience in recognizing the unique needs of children having to cope with cancer and they are staffed by pediatric support professionals other than the oncology treatment team while being associated with a children's hospital.

Clinical trials

The National Cancer Institute supported over 157 neuroblastoma **clinical trials** to evaluate a variety of **anticancer drugs** either combined to other drugs or to other treatments. No fewer than 14 of these studies involve stem cell transplantation, alone or in combination with other forms of treatment. Other clinical trials are concerned with anticancer drugs that are still considered investigational.

Prevention

Neuroblastoma may be a genetic disease passed down from the parents. In 2004, a group of German researchers reported that a series of neuroblastomas demonstrated a consistent pattern of deletions and overrepresentations on chromosomes 3, 10, 17q, and 20. There is currently no known method for its prevention.

Special concerns

After completion of a course of treatment for neuroblastoma, physicians sometimes recommend that the child undergo an investigative operation. This procedure allows the treatment team to evaluate how effective treatment has been, and may offer an opportunity to remove more of the tumor if it is still present.

See also Bone marrow aspiration and biopsy.

Resources

BOOKS

Beers, Mark H., MD, and Robert Berkow, MD, editors. "Neuroblastoma." In *The Merck Manual of Diagnosis and Therapy*. Whitehouse Station, NJ: Merck Research Laboratories, 2007.

PERIODICALS

Alexander, F. "Neuroblastoma." *Urol. Clin. North. Am.* 27 (August 2000): 383–392.

Berthold, F., and B. Hero. "Neuroblastoma: current drug therapy recommendations as part of the total treatment approach." *Drugs* 59 (June 2000): 1261–1277.

Bockmuhl, U., X. You, M. Pacyna-Gengelbach, et al. "CGH Pattern of Esthesioneuroblastoma and Their Metastases." *Brain Pathology* 14 (April 2004): 158–163.

Dayani, P. N., M. C. Bishop, K. Plack, and P. M. Zeltzer. "Desferoxamine (DFO)—Mediated Iron Chelation: Rationale for a Novel Approach to Therapy for Brain Cancer." *Journal of Neurooncology* 67 (May 2004): 367–377.

Grosfeld, J. L."Risk-based management of solid tumors in children." *American Journal of Surgery* 180 (November 2000): 322–327.

Lau, J. J., J. D. Trobe, R. E. Ruiz, et al. "Metastatic Neuroblastoma Presenting with Binocular Blindness from Intracranial Compression of the Optic Nerves." *Journal of Neuroophthalmology* 24 (June 2004): 119–124.

Morgenstern, B. Z., A. P. Krivoshik, V. Rodriguez, and P. M. Anderson. "Wilms' Tumor and Neuroblastoma." *Acta Paediatrica Supplementum* 93 (May 2004): 78–84.

Pinkerton, C., R. Blanc, M. P. Vincent, C. Bergeron, B. Fervers, and T. Philip. "Induction chemotherapy in metastatic neuroblastoma—does dose influence response? A critical review of published data standards, options and recommendations (SOR) project of the National Federation of French Cancer Centres (FNCLCC)." *European Journal of Cancer* 36 (September 2000): 1808–1815.

ORGANIZATIONS

The American Cancer Society (1-800-ACS-2345) provides information on specific types of cancer and a variety of cancer-related subjects. Additionally, it distributes booklets which can help cope with cancer treatment. Examples are: After Diagnosis: A Guide for Patients and Families (Booklet, Code #9440); Caring for the Patient with Cancer at Home (Booklet, Code #4656); Understanding Chemotherapy: A Guide for Patients and Families (Booklet, Code #9458); Understanding Radiation Therapy: A Guide for Patients and Families (Booklet, Code #9459).

National Cancer Institute. Office of Cancer Communications, 31 Center Drive, MSC 2580, Bethesda, MD 20892-2580. 800-422-6237. <http://cancernet.nci.nih.gov/clinpdq/pif/Neuroblastoma_Patient.html.>.

National Institutes of Health & National Cancer Institute. *Young People With Cancer: A Handbook for Parents.* http://www.cancernet.nci.nih.gov/young_people/yngconts.html.

Lisa Christenson
Monique Laberge, Ph.D.
Rebecca J. Frey, Ph.D.

Neuroendocrine tumors

Definition

Neuroendocrine tumors are tumors that develop from the cells of the diffuse neuroendocrine system, such as the enterochromaffin (EC) cells. These tumors are characterized by the presence of cells that possess secretory granules and have the ability to secrete neurohormones.

Description

The endocrine system is a network of glands consisting of endocrine cells that produce hormones in the body. The neuroendocrine system cells are specialized endocrine cells of the nervous system and produce neurohormones. Neuroendocrine cells do not form a specific gland; instead, they are found distributed in a wide variety of body organs where they help regulate body function.

Neuroendocrine tumors therefore represent a large class of cancers that can occur wherever neuroendocrine cells are found throughout the body. They are sometimes called carcinoid tumors, but it would be more accurate to consider these tumors as a sub-category of the larger family of neuroendocrine tumors. Neuroendocrine tumors are most often found in the digestive system and the lung. Statistically, 38% occur in the appendix, 23% in the ileum, 13% in the rectum, and 11.5% in the bronchi. Neuroendocrine pancreatic tumors are rather rare cancers with an incidence of one to two cases per 100,000 people. They occur with the same frequency in men and women and the average age at diagnosis is 53 years. Neuroendocrine tumors are also known as apudomas, or tumors that contain apud cells. These cells release excessive amounts of a variety of neurohormones in the bloodstream with chemical composition that varies with location, as does their effect on the body. Neuroendocrine tumors therefore have symptoms that vary with location. Unlike other cancers that are located in a specific organ, the hormone-releasing action of these tumors causes other symptoms to appear in many other organs of the body as well. The majority of neuroendocrine tumors can give rise to metastases with time if they are left untreated.

The total incidence of neuroendocrine tumors is thought to be between five and nine million people in the United States. It is possible that these tumors are underreported because they grow slowly and do not always produce dramatic symptoms.

Types of cancers

Because they can occur wherever neuroendocrine cells are found, neuroendocrine tumors come in a wide variety of types and have been classified according to their site of origin, usually either as digestive system, pancreatic or lung neuroendocrine tumors.

Neuroendocrine tumors of the digestive system

The types of neuroendocrine tumors found in the digestive system are also indicative of their general location:

- Foregut neuroendocrine tumors. Foregut tumors arise in the stomach or duodenum (first part of the small intestine) and represent approximately 15–25% of neuroendocrine tumors.
- Midgut neuroendocrine tumors. Midgut tumors are the most common variety and they include small and large intestine tumors.
- Hindgut neuroendocrine tumors. Hindgut tumors occur less frequently and are found in parts of the colon and in the rectum.

Pancreatic neuroendocrine tumors

Most neuroendocrine pancreatic tumors produce multiple hormones but usually there is excessive production of only one hormone. This is why neuroendocrine pancreatic tumors are often classified according to the predominant hormone secreted or resulting symptoms observed. For example, insulinomas produce excessive amounts of insulin, and gastrinomas produce excessive amounts of the peptide gastrin. Glucagonomas are associated with skin lesions and irritation around the eyes, and somatostatinomas are associated with gallstones, slight diabetes and **diarrhea** or constipation.

Lung neuroendocrine tumors

There are four main types of neuroendocrine lung tumors:

- Small-cell lung cancer (SCLC). SCLC represents one of the most rapidly growing types of cancer.
- Large-cell neuroendocrine carcinoma. A rare form of cancer, similar to SCLC in prognosis and treatment, except that the cancer cells are unusually large.
- Typical carcinoid tumors. These types of neuroendocrine lung tumors grow slowly and do not often spread beyond the lungs.
- Atypical carcinoid tumors. Atypical lung carcinoids tumors grow faster than the typical tumors and are more likely to metastasize to other organs.

KEY TERMS

Apudoma—A tumor capable of Amine Precursor Uptake and Decarboxylation (APUD).

Bronchi—Air passages to the lungs.

Diffuse neuroendocrine system—Concept developed by Feyrter, a German pathologist, more than 60 years ago, to unify tumors that occur in various parts of the body and possess secretory activity as well as similar properties when examined under a microscope.

Epithelial cells—Cells that cover the surface of the body and line its cavities.

Gastrointestinal tract—The GI tract, also called the digestive tract, starts from the oral cavity (mouth) and proceeds to the esophagus, the stomach, the duodenum, the small intestine, the large intestine (colon), the rectum and the anus. It processes all the food we eat. Along its way, food is digested, nutrients are extracted and waste is eliminated from the body in the form of stool and urine.

Gland—An organ that produces and releases substances for use in the body, such as fluids or hormones.

Hormone—Chemical substances produced by endocrine glands and transported by the bloodstream to the organs which require them to regulate their function.

Ileum—The last portion of the small intestine.

Metastasis—The transfer of cancer from one location or organ to another one not directly related to it.

Nervous system—The network of nerve tissue of the body. It includes the brain, the spinal cord and the ganglia (group of nerve cells).

Neurohormone—A hormone produced by specialized neurons or neuroendocrine cells.

Neuron—Specialized cell of the nervous system, that transmits nervous system signals. It consists of a cell body linked to a long branch (axon) and to several short ones (dendrites).

Syndrome—A series of symptoms or medical events occurring together and pointing to a single disease as the cause.

Other classifications for neuroendocrine tumors

Additionally, neuroendocrine tumors are subclassified into "functionally active" and "functionally inactive" tumors. Functionally active neuroendocrine tumors display specific symptoms, such as the excessive release of specific neurohormones from the tumor cell, as described above for pancreatic neuroendocrine tumors.

A recent classification groups neuroendocrine tumors into two types, depending on the kind of cells they develop from:

- Group I (epithelial). This group includes neuroendocrine carcinomas, graded 1, 2, and 3. Grade 1 neuroendocrine carcinomas are also known as carcinoid tumors. Grade 2 include tumors such as atypical carcinoid tumors, medullary thyroid carcinomas, and some pancreatic endocrine tumors. Grade 3 includes small-cell as well as large-cell neuroendocrine carcinomas.
- Group II (neural). Group II neuroendocrine tumors include paragangliomas, neuroblastomas, primitive neuroectodermal tumors, medulloblastomas, retinoblastomas, pineoblastomas and peripheral neuroepitheliomas.

Diagnosis

The diagnosis of carcinoid syndrome is made by the measurement of 5-hydroxy indole acetic acid (5-HIAA) in the urine. 5-HIAA is a breakdown (waste) product of serotonin. If the syndrome is diagnosed, the presence of carcinoid tumor is a given. When the syndrome is not present, diagnosis may be delayed, due to the vague symptoms present. Diagnosis can sometimes take up to two years. It is made by performing a number of tests, and the specific test used depends on the tumor's suspected location. The tests that may be performed include gastrointestinal endoscopy, chest x ray, **computed tomography** scan (CT scan), **magnetic resonance imaging**, or ultrasound. A **biopsy** of the tumor is performed for diagnosis. A variety of hormones can be measured in the blood as well to indicate the presence of a carcinoid.

Treatment

The only effective treatment for carcinoid tumor, is surgical removal of the tumor. Although **chemotherapy** is sometimes used when **metastasis** has occurred, it is rarely effective. The treatment for carcinoid syndrome is typically meant to decrease the severity of symptoms. Patients should avoid stress as well as foods that bring on the syndrome. Some medications can be given for symptomatic relief; for example, tumors of the gastrointestinal tract may be treated with octreotide (Sandostatin) or lanreotide (Somatuline) to relieve such symptoms as diarrhea and flushing. These drugs are known as somatostatin analogs.

Liver transplantation is a treatment option for patients with neuroendocrine tumors that have metastasized only to the liver. As of 2004, this approach is reported to offer patients long disease-free periods and relief of symptoms.

Prognosis

The prognosis of carcinoid tumors is related to the specific growth patterns of that tumor, as well as its location. For example, a group of researchers at the University of Wisconsin reported in 2004 that patients with gastrointestinal tumors in the hindgut had longer periods of disease-free survival than those with foregut or midgut cancers. For localized disease the five-year survival rate can be 94%, whereas for patients where metastasis has occurred, the average five-year survival rate is 18%. It is not unusual for patients with carcinoid tumors to live 10 or 15 years after the initial diagnosis.

Prevention

Neuroendocrine tumors such as carcinoid tumors are rare, and no information consequently is yet available on cause or prevention.

See also Adenoma; Carcinoid tumors, gastrointestinal; Carcinoid tumors, lung; Cushing's syndrome; Endocrine system tumors; Lung cancer, small cell; Merkel cell carcinoma; Pancreatic cancer, endocrine; Parathyroid cancer; Pituitary tumors; Zollinger-Ellison syndrome.

Resources

BOOKS

Beers, Mark H., MD, and Robert Berkow, MD, editors. "Carcinoid Tumors." In *The Merck Manual of Diagnosis and Therapy*. Whitehouse Station, NJ: Merck Research Laboratories, 2007.

PERIODICALS

Ahlman, H., S. Friman, C. Cahli, et al. "Liver Transplantation for Treatment of Metastatic Neuroendocrine Tumors." *Annals of the New York Academy of Sciences* 1014 (April 2004): 265–269.

Chatal, J. F., M. F. Le Bodic, F. Kraeber-Bodere, C. Rousseau, and I. Resche. "Nuclear medicine applications for neuroendocrine tumors." *World Journal of Surgery* 24 (November 2000): 1285-1289.

Jensen, R. T. "Carcinoid and pancreatic endocrine tumors: recent advances in molecular pathogenesis,localization, and treatment." *Current Opinions in Oncology* 12 (July 2000): 368-377.

Oberg, K., L. Kvols, M. Caplin, et al. "Consensus Report on the Use of Somatostatin Analogs for the Management of Neuroendocrine Tumors of the Gastroenteropancreatic System." *Annals of Oncology* 15 (June 2004): 966–973.

Rougier, P., and E. Mitry. "Chemotherapy in the treatment of neuroendocrine malignant tumors." *Digestion* 62, Supplement 1 (2000): 73-78.

Singhal, Hemant, MD, and Alan A. Saber, MD. "Carcinoid Tumor, Intestinal." *eMedicine* April 13, 2004. http://www.emedicine.com/med/topic271.htm.

Van Gompel, J. J., R. S. Sippel, T. F. Warner, and H. Chen. "Gastrointestinal Carcinoid Tumors: Factors That Predict Outcome." *World Journal of Surgery* 28 (April 2004): 387–392.

Warner, R. R. P. "Exploring Carcinoid Tumors." *Coping with Cancer Magazine* January-February 2001: 49-50.

Warner, R. R. P., L. P. Angel, C. M. Divino, S. T. Brower, T. Damani. "Pancreatic Neuroendocrine Tumors: A Ten Year Experience." *Regulatory Peptides* 94 (October 2000): 51-56.

OTHER

The Carcinoid Cancer Online Support Group. To subscribe: http://www.LISTSERV@LISTSERV.ACOR.ORG.

European Neuroendocrine Tumor Network. http://www.tentelemed.com/eunet/home.html.

ORGANIZATIONS

The Carcinoid Cancer Foundation, Inc. 1751 York Avenue, New York, NY 10128. Phone:(888)722-3132 or (212)722-3132. Web site: http://www.carcinoid.org/.

Monique Laberge, Ph.D.
Rebecca J. Frey, Ph.D.

Neurofibromatosis *see*
Von Recklinghausen's neurofibromatosis

Neuropathy

Description

Neuropathy, also known as peripheral neuropathy, is an inflammation, injury, or degeneration of any nerve outside of the central nervous system. These nerves, known as the peripheral nerves, help the muscles to contract (motor nerves) and allow a range of sensations to be felt (sensory nerves). Peripheral nerves also help control some of the involuntary functions of the autonomic nerves, which regulate the sweat glands, blood pressure, and internal organs. Unfortunately, peripheral nerves are fragile and easily damaged. The symptoms of neuropathy depend upon the cause and on which nerve, or nerves, are involved.

In **cancer** patients, neuropathy may be a consequence of certain **chemotherapy** drugs, the cancers themselves, or other diseases and medications. If the sensory nerves are involved, the symptoms may include pain, numbness and tingling, burning, or a loss of feeling. If the motor nerves are affected, there may be weakness or paralysis of the muscles that control those nerves. These symptoms may begin gradually. Depending upon the specific nerves involved, symptoms can range from mild tingling or numbness in the fingers or toes to severe pain in the hands or feet. Patients may also describe these symptoms as burning, prickling, or pinching. Some patients report that the skin is so sensitive that the slightest touch is agonizing. They may also experience heaviness or weakness in the arms and legs. As neuropathy increases in severity, patients might have an unsteady gait and can have difficulty feeling the floor beneath them. Those with autonomic neuropathy might experience dizziness, constipation, difficulty urinating, impotence, vision changes, and hearing loss.

Causes

Neuropathy occurs in cancer patients for a number of reasons. The cancer itself may be infiltrating the nerves. Patients may have other diseases such as diabetes, nutritional imbalances, alcoholism, and kidney failure, which may also cause neuropathy. It is important for the physician to distinguish which factor is responsible, so the appropriate treatment can be initiated. The most common cause in cancer patients, however, is chemotherapy drugs. Neuropathy occurs in approximately 10–20% of cancer patients receiving chemotherapy. The most common chemotherapy drugs that cause neuropathy include:

- platinum compounds (e.g., cisplatin, carboplatin)
- taxanes (e.g., docetaxel and paclitaxel)
- vincristine

The following chemotherapy agents can also cause neuropathy, but the incidence is relatively small compared to the prior ones listed. These include:

- procarbazine
- cytosine Arabinoside (Ara C or cytarabine)
- metronidazole

Treatments

Not long ago, few options were available to prevent or stop the progress of peripheral neuropathy. Treatments are now available that can halt the development of chemotherapy-caused neuropathy or at least diminish its effects.

The only effective preventive therapy is the use of **amifostine** (Ethyol). Some of the side effects of this medication include temporary low blood pressure, and **nausea and vomiting**. Patients should have adequate fluid intake before and during the 15-minute intravenous administration of amifostine. Blood pressure readings should be taken every five minutes during the infusion. Chemotherapy is administered shortly after giving the amifostine so that the maximum amount of the drug is in the cells before the chemotherapy is started.

If neuropathy does develop, it may be necessary to discontinue the suspected chemotherapy drug causing it. Administration of amifostine may reverse the neuropathy or lessen its symptoms.

A variety of medications are available that can ease symptoms for those suffering from neuropathy. These medications include:

- Pain relievers. Pain medicines available over-the-counter, such as acetaminophen (Tylenol), and **nonsteroidal anti-inflammatory drugs** (NSAIDs) such as aspirin and ibuprofen (Advil, Motrin IB, Nuprin), can help to alleviate mild symptoms. For more severe symptoms, the physician may recommend a prescription NSAID.
- Tricyclic antidepressants. Certain antidepressant medications, including amitriptyline (Elavil), nortriptyline (Pamelor), desipramine (Norpramin) and imipramine (Tofranil), can help with mild to moderate symptoms.
- Antiseizure medications. Certain drugs intended to treat epilepsy, such as carbamazepine (Tegretol) and phenytoin (Dilantin), can be effective in treating jabbing, shooting pain.
- Other drugs. Mexiletine (Mexitil), a drug normally used to treat irregular heart rhythms, may help to relieve burning pain.

The physician or pharmacist should be consulted regarding potential side effects or interactions with other medications.

Alternative and complementary therapies

Several other drug-free techniques can be helpful in providing pain relief. These are frequently used in conjunction with medication. These include:

- Biofeedback. This therapy uses a special machine to teach the patient how to control certain responses that can reduce pain.
- Transcutaneous electronic nerve stimulation (TENS). The physician may prescribe this treatment that may prevent pain signals from reaching the

brain. It is generally more effective for acute pain than chronic pain.

- Acupuncture. This may be effective for chronic pain, including the pain of neuropathy.
- Hypnosis. The patient under hypnosis typically receives suggestions intended to decrease the perception of pain.
- Relaxation techniques. These techniques can help decrease the muscle tension that aggravates pain. They may include deep-breathing exercises, visualization, and meditation.

Resources

PERIODICALS

Ndubisi, Boniface U., et al. "A Phase II Open-Label Study to Evaluate the Use of Amifostine in Reversing Chemotherapy-Induced Peripheral Neuropathy in Cancer Patients—Preliminary Findings." *American Society of Clinical Oncology 1999 Annual Meeting* Abstract: 2326.

Pace, Brian, and Richard M. Glass. "Neuropathy." *JAMA, The Journal of the American Medical Association* 284 (November 1, 2000): 2276.

OTHER

Almadrones, Lois A. "Neurotoxicity: The Elephant on the Coffee Table." *Oncology Nursing Society Online Education* [cited June 28, 2009]. http://nt.ons.org/ONS/education/online/neurotoxicities/content/text_intro.htm.

Armstrong, Terri S. "Chemotherapy Induced Neurotoxicities." *Oncology Nursing Society Online Education.* [cited June 28, 2009]. http://nt.ons.org/ONS/education/online/neurotoxicities/content/text_topic1.htm.

"Nursing Management of Peripheral Neurotoxicity and Quality of Life Concerns." *Oncology Nursing Society Online Education.* [cited June 28, 2009]. http://nt.ons.org/ONS/education/online/neurotoxicities/content/text_topic4.htm.

"Peripheral Neuropathy." *MayoClinic.com* [cited June 28, 2009]. http:mayohealth.org/home?id = DS00131.

Thigpen, James T. "Medical Management of Peripheral Neurotoxicity and Prevention Strategies." *Oncology Nursing Society Online Education* [cited June 28, 2009]. http://nt.ons.org/ONS/education/online/neurotoxicities/content/text_topic3.htm.

Deanna Swartout-Corbeil, R.N.

Neurotoxicity

Definition

Neurotoxicity is the ability to damage or destroy neurons (nerve cells) in the brain and/or other parts of the nervous system. Radiation and a large number of naturally occurring and synthesized substances are neurotoxins. **Radiation therapy** and **chemotherapy** for treating **cancer**, as well as numerous diseases and disorders, are common causes of neurotoxicity. Neurotoxicity can lead to conditions called neuropathies. Peripheral neuropathies involve damage to the motor, sensory, or vasomotor nerves of the peripheral nervous system (the extremities). Cranial neuropathies involve damage to the brain. Polyneuropathies are noninflammatory degenerative nerve diseases that are usually caused by toxins such as lead.

Chemotherapy drugs associated with peripheral neuropathy

Name of drug
5-azacytidine
5-fluorouracil
Bortezomib (Velcade)
Cytarabine (in high doses)
Epothilones, such as ixabepilone (Ixempra)
Gemcitabine
Hexamethylmelamine
Ifosphamide
Lenalidomide (Revlimid)
Misonidazole
Plant alkaloids, such as vinblastine, vincristine, vinorelbine, and etoposide
Platinum drugs, such as cisplatin, carboplatin, and oxaliplatin
Suramin
Taxanes, including paclitaxel (Taxol) and docetaxel (Taxotere)
Teniposide (VM-26)
Thalidomide (Thalomid)

(Table by GGS Creative Resources. Cengage Learning, Gale.)

Demographics

There are no general demographics on neurotoxicity, since it involves exposure to any of a large number of substances that can harm the human nervous system. Although neurotoxicity is less common than neuropathies caused by genetic disorders, metabolic diseases, or inflammation, many cases of neurotoxicity are either sub-clinical or go undiagnosed. Medication-induced neurotoxicity accounts for only 2–4% of neuropathies. Toxic polyneuropathies (TxPN) are relatively infrequent in North America. The majority of them are caused by small-scale and often chance **occupational exposures** or by intentional or homicidal ingestion of neurotoxins.

Some statistics are available on the incidence of radiation-induced neurotoxicity in the United States:

- Brachial plexopathy (injury to the brachial plexus—the nerve bundles located on each side of the neck that give rise to the individual nerves controlling the

muscles of the shoulders, arms, and hands) has been estimated to occur in 1.8–4.9% of patients treated with radiation, most often for breast or lung cancer.
- Lumbosacral plexopathy (injury to the lumbosacral plexus—the network of nerves in the lower back region) occurs in 0.3–1.3% of patients receiving radiation therapy.
- The incidence of severe radiation-induced dementia from whole brain radiotherapy (WBRT) ranges from 11% in one-year survivors to 50% in those surviving for two years.

Description

Most neurotoxicity involves distal axonopathy—the degeneration or "dying back" of the axons of nerve cells, especially the longest peripheral nerves. However some neurotoxins cause demyelination of nerve cells or target specific types of nerve cells, such as Schwann cells, spinal ganglia, or autonomic neurons.

Neurotoxicity of the peripheral nervous system has some general features:

- The extent and severity of the neurotoxicity is related to the degree of exposure to the toxin.
- All individuals exposed to a given neurotoxin exhibit similar signs and symptoms.
- Neurotoxic illness usually occurs upon or shortly after exposure, with the common exceptions of organophosphates, which have a two–four-week latency period, and cisplatin, which sometimes has a two-month latency period.
- Improvement of symptoms usually begins as soon as exposure to the toxin ceases.

Occupational and/or environmental toxins may play a role in some progressive neurodegenerative disorders including:

- Parkinson's disease
- amyotrophic lateral sclerosis (Lou Gehrig's disease)
- multiple sclerosis
- dementia

Chemotherapy-induced (chemo-induced) peripheral **neuropathy** (CIPN) is a collection of neurotoxic symptoms caused by peripheral nerve damage from chemotherapy. Neurotoxicity is the dose-limiting factor for three common chemotherapy drugs—cisplatin, **vincristine**, and paclitaxel.

Radiation-induced neurotoxicity can involve both the central and peripheral nervous systems. Although peripheral nerves are relatively resistant to radiation-induced damage, the brachial and lumbosacral plexuses are susceptible. Radiation damage can be acute, sub-acute and transient, or progressive, permanent, and disabling. Radiation-induced damage may not become fully apparent until months or years after treatment.

Radiation-induced nerve damage depends on:

- the total radiation dose
- its duration
- the method of administration
- the volume of irradiated nerve tissue
- the amount of irradiated healthy tissue
- individual susceptibility

The most important determinant of radiation-induced neurotoxicity is the amount of healthy tissue that is irradiated:

- One-session radiosurgery targets little or no healthy tissue.
- Fractionated radiotherapy targets more healthy tissue, but the intervals between treatments may allow for more healing.
- Whole brain radiotherapy targets large areas of the brain and is more neurotoxic.
- Radiation-induced brachial plexopathy occurs when radiotherapy is directed at the chest, axillary (armpit) region, thorax, or neck.
- Radiation-induced lumbosacral plexopathy occurs when radiotherapy is directed at cancers in the abdominal and pelvic regions.

Risk factors

Radiation and/or chemotherapy for cancer treatment are major risk factors for neurotoxicity. Occupations involving toxic chemicals are also major risk factors.

Certain disorders can make individuals more or less susceptible to neurotoxins:

- Some patients are more vulnerable to neurotoxic drugs because of an underlying genetic or acquired neuropathy, such as neuropathies caused by cancer or HIV/AIDS.
- Some brain disorders in children may develop through interactions between genes and neurotoxic environmental triggers.
- Genetic impairments in metabolism sometimes either increase or decrease the neurotoxicity of certain drugs.
- Certain forms of genes that promote nerve cell survival can counter neurotoxicity.

Causes and symptoms

In as many as 25% of neuropathies the source of the neurotoxicity cannot be identified. Known sources of neurotoxicity include:

- heavy metals, such as lead and mercury
- certain foods and food additives
- pesticides
- industrial and household cleaning solvents
- chronic exposure to industrial chemicals such as ethylene oxide
- contaminated water
- cyanotoxins from blooms of cyanobacteria (blue-green algae) in drinking or recreational waters
- cosmetics
- venoms
- tetrodotoxin from pufferfish
- alcohol
- various recreational drugs and chemicals of abuse
- chronic or heavy use of kava (*Piper methysticum* G. Forst)
- a large number of pharmaceuticals
- radiation

Drugs are among the most common causes of neurotoxicity and a large number of drugs are associated with or suspected of being neurotoxic. Chemotherapy drugs associated with peripheral neuropathy include:

- 5-azacytidine
- 5-fluorouracil
- bortezomib (Velcade)
- cytarabine (in high doses)
- epothilones such as ixabepilone (Ixempra)
- gemcitabine
- hexamethylmelamine
- ifosphamide
- lenalidomide (Revlimid)
- misonidazole
- plant alkaloids such as vinblastine, vincristine, vinorelbine, and etoposide
- platinum drugs such as cisplatin, carboplatin, and oxaliplatin
- suramin
- taxanes including paclitaxel (Taxol) and docetaxel (Taxotere)
- teniposide (VM-26)
- thalidomide (Thalomid)

Antibiotics associated with peripheral neuropathy include:

- chloroquine
- chloramphenicol
- clioquinil
- dapsone
- ethambutol
- fluoroquinolones
- griseofulvin
- isoniazid (INH)
- mefloquine
- metronidazole
- nitrofurantoin
- nucleoside analogs
- podophyllin resin
- sulfonamides
- streptomycin

Cardiovascular drugs associated with peripheral neuropathy include:

- amiodarone
- enalapril
- hydralazine
- statins
- perhexiline
- propafenone

Drugs that act on the central nervous system and have been associated with peripheral neuropathy include:

- amitriptyline
- phenytoin
- chlorprothixene
- gangliosides
- gluthethimide
- lithium
- nitrous oxide
- phenelzine

Other drugs associated with peripheral neuropathy include:

- allopurinol
- almitrine
- botulinum toxin
- cimetidine
- clofibrate
- colchicine
- cyclosporin A
- dichloroacetate
- disulfiram

- etretinate
- gold salts
- immunosuppressants
- interferons alpha-2A and 2B
- penacillamine
- pyridoxine (if abused)
- sulphasalazine
- tacrolimus (FK506, ProGraf)
- zimeldine

Symptoms of neurotoxicity can appear immediately upon exposure to the toxin or they can develop later. The most common symptoms of neurotoxicity are pain, tingling, or numbness in the feet. Other symptoms may include:

- weakness, numbness in the limbs, possibly accompanied by restless leg syndrome
- difficulty walking
- sensory loss
- impaired reflexes
- vision loss
- headache
- memory loss
- cognitive or behavioral problems
- sexual dysfunction

Different neurotoxins have different effects on the nervous system:

- Exposure to lead or arsenic, the cardiac medications perhexiline and amiodarone, or the administration of tetanus toxoid or diphtheria toxin can cause demyelination of nerves.
- Both limited and long-term exposure to industrial chemicals, either in the workplace or the environment, can cause subtle pain and weakness; continued exposure can cause progressive neuropathy.
- Organophosphates, snake venom, or botulism can cause dysfunction in neuromuscular transmission.
- Trichloroethylene (TCE) and ethylene glycol can affect the nerves of the head and face.
- Reef fish and shellfish toxins can disrupt sodium channels in nerves.
- Cisplatin, antibiotics, and pyridoxine can cause sensory neuropathy.

CIPN can begin at any time during or after chemotherapy and sometimes worsens over the course of chemotherapy. It often affects both sides of the body in similar ways; for example, the toes of both feet may be affected. The neuropathy often starts in the feet and later appears in the hands, called a "stocking/glove distribution." CIPN can cause severe pain and affect daily movements, including walking or writing.

Symptoms of CIPN depend on which on which nerves are affected. Common symptoms include:

- pain
- numbness
- tingling or burning sensations
- weakness
- muscle shrinkage
- balance problems, tripping, or stumbling
- loss of reflexes
- increased sensitivity to temperature (usually cold) or pressure
- constipation
- difficulty urinating
- blood pressure changes
- difficulty swallowing

Severe problems from CIPN include:

- changes in heart rate
- breathing difficulties
- paralysis
- organ failure

Acute reactions to radiation normally occur during or immediately following therapy and are usually caused by swelling. Acute toxicity lessens with subsequent treatments. Symptoms of acute radiation neurotoxicity include:

- headache
- nausea
- vomiting
- drowsiness

Neurotoxicity from localized radiation therapy often involves specific neurologic deficits. Following radiation therapy to the neck or upper thorax, early-delayed neurotoxicity can result in a myelopathy characterized by an electric shock-like sensation radiating down the back and into the legs when the neck is flexed. This myelopathy resolves spontaneously. Radiation therapy for extraspinal tumors, such as Hodgkin **lymphoma**, can cause late-delayed symptoms such as progressive paralysis and sensory loss.

Symptoms of acute neurotoxicity from WBRT include hair loss (**alopecia**), **nausea**, **vomiting**, lethargy, middle-ear inflammation, and severe cerebral swelling. Some of these effects are transient, but others can last for months following radiation therapy. Late-delayed neurotoxicity reactions are usually permanent and may be progressive. They can vary from moderate to severe and can include:

- memory impairment
- confusion

- personality changes
- progressive dementia
- cerebral atrophy
- rarely, the development of new cancers

Diagnosis

Examination

Neurotoxicity is often diagnosed based solely on exposure to known neurotoxins. For patients who have undergone radiation therapy or chemotherapy, a diagnosis of neurotoxicity is usually obvious. In other cases diagnosis may be much more difficult. The physician will conduct a complete physical examination and a medical history focusing on drug use, medications, and occupational and environmental exposures. New medications begun in recent weeks or months are common causes of neurotoxicity. A neurological exam will be performed. Some neurotoxins are known to cause greater motor neuropathies than sensory neuropathies and others are known to affect sensory nerves more than motor nerves. When a potential source of the neurotoxicity can be identified, the dose, duration of exposure, and level of protection are estimated.

If the source of the neurotoxicity cannot be identified, the examination, as well as subsequent tests and procedures, may focus on identifying an underlying disease or condition. For example, peripheral neuropathy also can be caused by:

- cancer surgery
- tumors pressing on nerves
- infections that affect the nerves
- shingles
- diabetes
- low vitamin B levels
- some autoimmune disorders

Tests

Tests for neurotoxicity may include:

- facial nerve testing
- blink reflex testing
- blood and urine tests for the presence of known neurotoxins
- a variety of laboratory tests, depending on the suspected source of the neurotoxicity

Procedures

Diagnostic procedures may include:

- electromyography (EMG), which measures electrical activity associated with functioning skeletal muscle
- studies of nerve conduction, such as nerve conduction velocity (NVC) measurements
- nerve and/or muscle biopsies to obtain tissue for examination by a pathologist
- MRI or CT scans to visualize damage from neurotoxicity or rule out tumors

Treatment

Traditional

Treatment for neurotoxicity depends on the cause. The most important treatment is elimination or reduction of exposure to the neurotoxin. In cases of CIPN, treatment may be postponed, the doses of chemotherapy drugs lowered, or the drug that is causing the CIPN may be eliminated.

Drugs

Acute neurotoxicity from radiation therapy and pain from CIPN may be treated with:

- corticosteroids
- tricyclic antidepressants in smaller doses than are used to treat depression
- anticonvulsants
- numbing patches or topical creams, such as lidocaine patches or capsaicin cream, applied to the painful area
- opioids or narcotics for severe pain

Alternative

Alternative medicines for neurotoxicity include:

- alpha-lipoic acid
- evening primrose, which contains the omega-6 essential fatty acids linoleic acid and gamma-linoleic acid (GLA)
- vitamin E

Alternative treatments for neuropathic pain include:

- physical therapy
- acupuncture
- massage
- biofeedback
- relaxation therapy
- occupational therapy

Home remedies

Home remedies for neuropathy include:

- maintaining a balanced diet
- vitamin B supplements

QUESTIONS TO ASK YOUR DOCTOR

- How will you test for neurotoxicity?
- What is causing the neurotoxicity?
- Are there treatments that you can recommend?
- Are my symptoms likely to improve on their own?

- soaking in cool water
- applications of heat
- elevating or lowering limbs
- remaining seated as much as possible if the neuropathy is in the feet
- caring for the feet—checking often for open sores or using special shoes or inserts
- exercise
- avoiding anything that worsens the neuropathy, such as heat or cold or tight clothes or shoes
- avoiding alcohol, which can damage nerves and make the neuropathy worse
- controlling blood sugar, since high blood sugar can damage nerves

Prognosis

The prognosis for neurotoxicity varies tremendously depending on the neurotoxin, the degree and duration of exposure, and the severity of the damage to the nervous system. Depending on the circumstances, patients can fully recover following treatment, survive without full recovery, or die.

CIPN may be short-term and disappear after treatment stops, may take up to two years to completely resolve, or may develop into a chronic disorder requiring long-term treatment. Some cases may be both severe and permanent. The prognosis for CIPN depends on:

- the chemotherapy drug(s)
- the drug dose
- the total chemotherapy dose over time
- the patient's age
- a personal or family history of neuropathy
- the existence of other medical conditions that can cause neuropathy, such as diabetes or HIV infection

Prevention

Smaller chemotherapy doses over a longer period of time may help prevent CIPN:

- smaller doses two or three times per week, instead of a large dose once a week
- the same dose administered over six hours instead of over one hour
- the same dose as a continuous, very slow infusion over a few days

Possible preventions for CIPN that are being studied include:

- vitamin E, an antioxidant that may help protect against nerve damage caused by cisplatin and paclitaxel
- calcium and magnesium infusions before and after oxaliplatin
- the anticonvulsant drug carbamazepine, which may help treat as well as prevent CIPN
- various supplements, including amino acids and proteins, given before and after chemotherapy

Resources

BOOKS

Davidson, Philip William, Gary J. Myers, and Bernard Weiss, eds. *Neurotoxicity and Developmental Disabilities*. London: Elsevier, 2006.

DeAngelis, Lisa M., and Jerome B. Posner. *Neurological Complications of Cancer*, 2nd ed. New York: Oxford University Press, 2009.

Dobbs, Michael R. *Clinical Neurotoxicity*. Philadelphia: Saunders/Elsevier, 2009.

PERIODICALS

Visovsky C., et al. "Putting Evidence into Practice: Evidence-Based Interventions for Chemotherapy-Induced Peripheral Neuropathy." *Clinical Journal of Oncology Nursing* 11 (2007): 901-913.

Wickham, R. "Chemotherapy-Induced Peripheral Neuropathy: A Review and Implications for Oncology Nursing Practice." *Clinical Journal of Oncology Nursing* 11 (2007): 361-376.

OTHER

Kaplan, Robert J. "Radiation-Induced Brachial Plexopathy." *eMedicine*. http://emedicine.medscape.com/article/316497-overview.

"NINDS Neurotoxicity Information Page." *National Institute of Neurological Disorders and Stroke*. http://www.ninds.nih.gov/disorders/neurotoxicity/neurotoxicity.htm.

"Peripheral Neuropathy Caused by Chemotherapy." *American Cancer Society*. http://www.cancer.org/docroot/MBC/content/MBC_2_3x_Peripheral_Neuropathy_Caused_by_Chemotherapy.asp?sitearea = MBC

"Radiation Injury to the Brain." *International RadioSurgery Association*. http://www.irsa.org/radiation_injury.html

Rutchik, Jonathan S. "Toxic Neuropathy." *eMedicine.* http://emedicine.medscape.com/article/1175276-overview

Weimer, Louis H. "Medication-Induced Neuropathies." *The Neuropathy Association.* http://www.neuropathy.org/site/DocServer/Medication-Induced_Neuropathies.pdf?docID = 1604

ORGANIZATIONS

American Cancer Society, 1599 Clifton Road NE, Atlanta, GA, 30329-4251, (800) ACS-2345, http://www.cancer.org.

National Cancer Institute, NCI Public Inquiries Office, 6116 Executive Boulevard, Room 3036A, Bethesda, MD, 20006, (800) 4-CANCER, http://www.cancer.gov.

National Institute of Neurological Disorders and Stroke (NINDS), NIH Neurological Institute, PO Box 5801, Bethesda, MD, 20824, (301) 496-5751, (800) 352-9424, http://www.ninds.nih.gov/index.htm.

The Neuropathy Association, Inc., 60 East 42nd Street, Suite 942, New York, NY, 10165, (212) 692-0662, (212) 692-0668, info@neuropathy.org, http://www.neuropathy.org.

Margaret Alic, PhD

Neutropenia

Description

Neutropenia is an abnormally low level of neutrophils in the blood. Neutrophils are white blood cells (WBCs) produced in the bone marrow and comprise approximately 60% of the blood. These cells are critically important to an **immune response** and migrate from the blood to tissues during an **infection**. They ingest and destroy particles and germs. Germs are microorganisms such as bacteria, protozoa, viruses, and fungus that cause disease. Neutropenia is an especially serious disorder for **cancer** patients who may have reduced immune functions because it makes the body vulnerable to bacterial and fungal infections. White blood cells are especially sensitive to **chemotherapy**. The number of cells killed during **radiation therapy** depends upon the dose and frequency of radiation, and how much of the body is irradiated.

Neutrophils can be segmented (segs, polys, or PMNs) or banded (bands) which are newly developed, immature neutrophils. If there is an increase in new neutrophils (bands) this may indicate that an infection is present and the body is attempting a defense. Neutropenia is sometimes called agranulocytosis or granulocytopenia because neutrophils display characteristic multi-lobed structures and granules in stained blood smears.

QUESTIONS TO ASK THE DOCTOR

- What symptoms lead to this diagnosis?
- What can be expected with this condition and how long it last?
- What is the plan for treatment? Will it be covered by my insurance? Can it be done at home?
- What support and monitoring for home health care might be available? Would supervision be required? Would this be appropriate and what are the risks of complications? What are the costs?
- What are the side effects of treatment? Are there any drugs, foods, etc. that should not be taken during treatment? Should daily activities be modified?
- What complementary and alternative treatment methods have been shown to be helpful in addition to conventional medical treatments? Have any of these treatments been helpful to reduce symptoms and side effects from medication?
- Are complementary treatments easy to access and what is the cost of such treatments? Are these covered by my insurance as well?
- Where can a person get more information about this condition?
- What avenues for emotional and spiritual support might be available to help cope with this diagnosis?

The normal level of neutrophils in human blood varies slightly by age and race. Infants have lower counts than older children and adults. African Americans have lower counts than Caucasians or Asians. The average adult level is 1,500 cells/mm^3 of blood. Neutrophil counts (in cells/mm^3) are interpreted as follows:

- Greater than 1,000. Normal protection against infection.
- 500–1,000. Some increased risk of infection.
- 200–500. Great risk of severe infection.
- Lower than 200. Risk of overwhelming infection; requires hospital treatment with antibiotics.

Neutropenia has no specific symptoms except the severity of the patient's current infection. In severe neutropenia, the patient is likely to develop periodontal disease, oral and rectal ulcers, **fever**, and bacterial **pneumonia**. Fever recurring every 19–30 days suggests cyclical neutropenia.

Diagnosis is made on the basis of a white blood cell count and differential. The cause of neutropenia can be difficult to establish and depends on a combination of the patient's history, genetic evaluation, **bone marrow biopsy**, and repeated measurements of the WBC. However, in cancer patients it is usually an expected side effect of chemotherapy or radiation. The overall risk of infection is dependent upon the type of cancer an individual has as well as the treatment received. Patients at greater risk include those with hematologic malignancies, leukemia/lymphoma (cancers) and those who receive bone marrow transplants.

It is important to detect infections early. Some signs that indicate infection include:

- coughing and difficulty breathing, congestion
- an oral temperature greater than 105° with typical fever symptoms of chills and sweating
- problems in the mouth such as white patches, sore and swollen gums
- changes in urination or in stools
- drainage and pain from any cuts or tubes used in the cancer treatments such as catheters and feeding tubes
- an overall feeling of illness

Causes

Neutropenia may result from three processes:

Decreased WBC production

Lowered production of white blood cells is the most common cause of neutropenia. It can result from:

- Cancer, including certain types of leukemia.
- Radiation therapy.
- Medications that affect the bone marrow, including cancer drugs (chemotherapy), chloramphenicol (Chloromycetin), anticonvulsant medications, and antipsychotic drugs (Thorazine, Prolixin, and other phenothiazines). In hematopoietic stem cell transplantation (HSCT), high levels of total body irradiation (TBI) or chemotherapy are used to kill cancer cells, or these treatments may be combined. Two types of HSCT treatments are bone marrow transplantation (BMT) and peripheral blood stem cell transplantation (PBSCT). During the treatment process, the patient's normal bone marrow stem cells are killed along with the cancer cells. The stem cells are not able to mature into immune cells such as neutrophils, causing neutropenia. To reduce neutropenia, the normal stem cells from the patient may be removed prior to treatment and given back at a later time. Cells can also be supplied from another donor.
- Hereditary and congenital disorders that affect the bone marrow, including familial neutropenia, cyclic neutropenia, and infantile agranulocytosis.
- Exposure to pesticides.
- Vitamin B_{12} and folate (folic acid) deficiency.

Destruction of White Blood Cells

WBCs are used and die at a faster rate by:

- Acute bacterial infections in adults.
- Infections in newborns.
- Certain autoimmune disorders, including systemic lupus erythematosus (SLE).
- Penicillin, phenytoin (Dilantin), and sulfonamide medications (Benemid, Bactrim, Gantanol).

Sequestration and margination of WBCs

Sequestration and margination are processes in which neutrophils are removed from the general blood circulation and redistributed within the body. These processes can occur because of:

- Hemodialysis.
- Felty's syndrome, or malaria. The neutrophils accumulate in the spleen.
- Bacterial infections. The neutrophils remain in the infected tissues without returning to the bloodstream.

Special concerns

Often the infections that develop in a cancer patient are opportunistic infections. That is, the organisms responsible for the infection normally would not cause disease in a healthy person, but do so in a cancer patient because the immune system is weak. Several steps can be taken on a daily basis to reduce the risk of developing an infection.

Steps to Prevent Infection

- Care should be taken to keep the body clean. Hands should be washed after using the bathroom and before eating.
- Avoid stagnant or still water in the environment that might contain bacteria such as flower vases and birdbaths, or containers that may hold items such as dentures.
- Use antiseptic mouthwashes to cleanse the mouth. Use those that do not contain alcohol.

- Use deodorant. Antiperspirants will not allow the body to sweat, trapping bacteria within the body that may increase the risk of infection.
- Women with neutropenia should consider using sanitary napkins instead of tampons during their menstruation to help prevent possible infection such as toxic shock syndrome.
- Avoid others who are ill and large crowded areas where one might encounter illness.
- Avoid activities that may increase the chance of physical injury. Take care to protect the body by wearing gloves, shoes, and other items. Tend to all injuries as soon as possible.
- Neutropenic patients should consult their doctors before receiving any vaccinations.

Treatments

Treatment of neutropenia depends on the underlying cause.

Medications

Patients with fever and other signs of infection are treated with **antibiotics**. Some antibiotics used in the treatment of cancer patients include imipenem, meropenem, aminoglycoside, antipesudomonal penicillin, rifampin, and vancomycin. Combination therapy can be used that uses several types of antibiotics to stop the infection, but some of the drugs may be toxic or costly.

Patients receiving chemotherapy for cancer may be given drugs even in health to help restore the WBC to normal. A blood growth factor called **sargramostim** (Leukine, Prokine) stimulates WBC production. Another commonly used medication to reduce neutropenia in cancer patients is the cytokine G-CSF (granulocyte colony-stimulating factor, or **filgrastim** by Amgen-Roche). This substance is normally produced in the body at low levels. G-CSF helps the body produce more neutrophils to fight infection. This is especially useful in that many bacteria can not be killed by antibiotics due to antibiotic resistance.

Throughout the course of treatment it is important that the patient be monitored closely. This requires hospitalization for some patients, while others may be adequately treated at home.

Alternative and complementary therapies

A healthy lifestyle should be adopted that includes good nutrition, plenty of sleep, and appropriate levels of exercise. Avoid uncooked foods that may contain harmful bacteria. A nutritionist should be consulted to determine an appropriate, healthy diet.

Psychological stress can also weaken the immune system, making a person more susceptible to illness. It is important to find emotional support through family, friends, support groups, or through spiritual means.

See also Immunologic therapies; Infection and sepsis; Chronic myelocytic leukemia.

Resources

BOOKS

Janeway, Charles A., et al. *Immunobiology:The Immune System in Health and Disease*. London and New York: Current Biology Publications, Elsevier Science London/Garland Publishing, 1999.

PERIODICALS

Feld, Ronald. "Vancomycin as Part of Initial Empirical Antibiotic Therapy for Febrile Neutropenia in Patients with Cancer: Pros and Cons." *Clinical Infectious Diseases* 29 (1999): 503-7.

Rahiala, J., Perkkio, M., and Pekka Riikonen. "Prospective and Randomized Comparison of Early Versus Delayed Prophylactic Administration of Granulocyte Colony-Stimulating Factor (Filgrastim) in Children With Cancer." *Medical and Pediatric Oncology* 32 (1999): 326–30.

Rolston, Kenneth. "New Trends in Patient Management: Risk-based Therapy for Febrile Patients with Neutropenia." *Clinical Infectious Diseases* 29 (1999): 515–21

OTHER

American Cancer Society. http://www.cancer.org.

Mayo Clinic. http://www.mayoclinic.com.

National Neutropenia Network, Inc. http://www.neutropenia.org.

University of Pennsylvania Oncolink. http://www.oncolink.upenn.edu.

WebMd. http://www.webMD.com.

Rebecca Frey, Ph.D.
Jill Granger, M.S.

Night sweats

Description

Night sweats can be a side effect of **cancer** treatment or a symptom of certain cancers. Night sweats are part of a variety of symptoms referred to as vasomotor. Vasomotor symptoms stem from the body's thermoregulatory center, which is affected by circulating hormones.

Women may undergo **oophorectomy** (the surgical removal of one or both ovaries), either for **ovarian cancer** or when accompanied by hysterectomy for **endometrial cancer** or uterine **sarcoma**, as part of their cancer treatment. Pelvic radiation may also damage the ovaries. Removal or permanent damage to the ovaries results in immediate menopause. Many women with ovarian cancer have already gone through menopause, as a function of their age. However, when ovarian or reproductive tract cancer strikes a pre-menopausal woman, the immediate, versus gradual, loss of circulating hormones is dramatic, and is a concern in the immediate post-operative period. In an *American Cancer Society News Today* of January 29, 2001, the ACS reported on a study that found women undergoing systemic treatment for **breast cancer**, especially those on **tamoxifen**, reported a higher frequency and intensity of menopausal symptoms such as night sweats, hot flashes, and **fatigue**. Men may also experience vasomotor symptoms with metastatic **adenocarcinoma** of the prostate, or following removal of the prostate for **prostate cancer**.

Vasomotor symptoms such as night sweats add to the existing stress for individuals undergoing cancer treatment, as they can reduce the quality of sleep, make daily life very uncomfortable, and decrease the quality of life.

Night sweats can be a sign of **infection** in the immuno-compromised cancer patient, as well as being a symptom of undiagnosed cancer and early AIDS. Drenching night sweats may be a sign of Hodgkin's or non-Hodgkin's **lymphoma**, both in children as well as in adults. Night sweats may also be present with liver hemangioma tumors. Generalized symptoms such as night sweats, **fever**, chills, and sweating are sometimes referred to as B symptoms. Night sweats have also been associated with malignant **melanoma** and with metastatic compression of the optic nerve. Children who are ultimately diagnosed with a malignancy may present to a rheumatologist with a variety of symptoms, including night sweats. Night sweats in the absence of explained fever or perimenopause should be brought to the attention of one's health care provider for evaluation.

Causes

The ovary produces the hormone estrogen. When the ovary is removed, there is a dramatic termination of circulating estrogen, with symptoms such as night sweats, hot flashes, and vaginal dryness. Estrogen replacement therapy (ERT) can relieve these symptoms. However, the use of ERT is controversial with some cancers, because of the association with estrogen-receptor positive cancers. Women who are approaching menopause at the time of **chemotherapy** may lose ovarian function as a result of treatment, thus undergoing significant menopausal symptoms. The use of tamoxifen in postmenopausal women has been associated with an increase in vasomotor symptoms.

Hodgkin's and non-Hodgkin's lymphomas are cancers of the lymphatic system. Symptoms include night sweats, painless swelling in the lymph nodes, especially in the neck, underarm or groin, unexplained **weight loss**, recurrent fevers, and itchy skin. The night sweats in Hodgkin's disease appears to be related to an instability in the thermoregulatory center of the hypothalamus. Risk factors for Hodgkin's and non-Hodgkin's lymphomas include reduced immune function, transplant surgery, occupational exposure to herbicides and other toxic chemicals, Sjögren's syndrome, and **Epstein-Barr virus**.

Treatments

Some research has been conducted using estrogen-androgen replacement therapy. The concerns about ERT and estrogen-sensitive cancers remains the same. The androgen component assists in the healing process, as well as in a sense of well-being, sexual desire and arousal, and increased energy level. The use of androgens can result in hirsutism (growth of male-pattern hair), which may be dose-dependent.

Successful diagnosis of the cause of the night sweats can lead to proper treatment for the condition. Successful treatment of Hodgkin's or non-Hodgkin's lymphoma resolves the night sweats.

Alternative and complementary therapies

Acupuncture has been effective for both men and women. Individuals considering herbal remedies or supplements for reproductive-related night sweats associated with cancer treatment should seek the counsel of a knowledgeable practitioner. Substances that function through mimicking estrogenic properties could have an adverse effect in estrogen-sensitive tumors.

Resources

OTHER

Memorial Sloan-Kettering Cancer Center [cited July 18, 2009]. http://www.mskcc.org.

National Cancer Institute Cancer Trials [cited July 18, 2009]. <http://cancertrials.nci.nih.gov/system>.

Natural Health Village [cited July 18, 2009]. http://www.naturalhealthvillage.com.

ORGANIZATIONS

American Cancer Society. 800–ACS–2345. http://www.cancer.org.

National Cancer Institute. Building 31, Room 10A31, 31 Center Drive, MSC 2580, Bethesda, MD 20892–2580. 301–435–3848. http://www.nci.nih.gov.

National Center for Complementary and Alternative Medicine. NCCAM Clearinghouse, P.O. Box 8218, Silver Spring, MD 20907-8218. (888) 644-6226. <http://nccam.nih.gov>

Esther Csapo Rastegari, R.N., B.S.N., Ed.M.

Nilotinib

Definition

Nilotinib (Tasigna) is a second generation BCR-ABL inhibitor drug manufactured by Novartis Pharmaceuticals. It is used for the treatment of Philadelphia positive chronic myeloid leukemia (Ph+ CML).

Purpose

Nilotinib is used to treat chronic myeloid leukemia (CML), also called chronic myelogenous leukemia, in people who carry a specific genetic abnormality called the Philadelphia chromosome. CML is **cancer** that develops in myeloid cells in the bone marrow and results in the production of abnormal blood cells. These blood cells mature incorrectly or incompletely and live longer than normal so that they build up in the blood causing symptoms of CML.

CML accounts for 10–15% of all leukemias, and almost all CML is associated with a specific non-inherited genetic defect called the Philadelphia chromosome. When cells divide, their chromosomes double and also divide in order for each cell to have a complete set of genetic information. Sometimes during this doubling and division process material from one chromosome incorrectly gets attached to or exchanged with material from another chromosome. This process is called translocation. CML starts when part of chromosome 9 is exchanged with part of chromosome 22. The resulting abnormal chromosome 22 is known as the Philadelphia chromosome. People who have it are said to be Philadelphia chromosome positive or Ph+. Although it is not clear what factors cause this translocation, almost everyone with CML is Ph+.

As the result of the formation of the translocation between chromosomes 9 and 22, a new gene called bcr-abl is formed on the Philadelphia chromosome. This gene produces a tyrosine kinase protein called BCR-ABL. BCR-ABL causes myeloid cells to become cancer (malignant) cells. These malignant cells grow and reproduce abnormally. Nilotinib is a tyrosine kinase inhibitor. It interferes with the activities of the BCR-ABL protein and stops the production of cancerous myeloid cells while allowing the production of normal blood cells to continue.

Nilotinib is approved for use during the chronic (early) phase of CML and in the accelerated (second) stage of CML. As of October 2009, it is not approved for use in the blast (final) stage of the disease. It normally is used only after another tyrosine kinase inhibitor drug, **imatinib mesylate** (Gleevec), has been tried. Imatinib mesylate successfully treats CML in many people. Those people whose cancer does not respond to the drug or who cannot tolerate the side effects of imatinib mesylate may be treated with nilotinib. As of 2009, studies were underway to determine if nilotinib was useful in people who had not first received imatinib mesylate therapy.

Description

Nilotinib is sold in the United Sates and the European Union under the brand name of Tasigna. The drug was first approved by the United Sates Food and Drug Administration (FDA) on October 27. 2007 and by the European Union on November 17, 2007. The drug is also approved in the European Union to treat gastrointestinal stroma tumors, a type of digestive system cancer.

Nilotinib is a light yellow hard gel capsule with red printing. Each capsule has a strength of 200 mg. Capsules should be stored at controlled room temperature. Nilotinib continues to be tested in **clinical trials** in the United States for use against other cancers and in combination with other therapies. A list of clinical trials currently enrolling volunteers can be found at http://www.clinicaltrials.gov.

Recommended dosage

Nilotinib must be taken *exactly* as prescribed, and the dosage should not be changed or the drug discontinued except on order of a physician. The usual recommended dosage in patients with CML Ph+ is 400 mg taken twice daily 12 hour apart. Nilotinib capsules must be taken whole; they should never be crushed or divided. They may not be taken with food; nothing should be eaten for at least 2 hours before and one hour after the dose is taken. Grapefruit juice or dietary supplements containing extracts from grapefruit juice should not be used while taking this drug. Patients who forget to take a dose should not take a make-up dose. Instead they should skip the dose and then take the next dose at their regularly scheduled time.

There are special dosage recommendations and restrictions for use of nilotinib in some individuals including those with certain heart conditions, liver function abnormalities, suppression of normal production of blood cells in the bone marrow (**myelosuppression**), and those taking certain drugs. See Precautions and Drug Interacitons below for additional information.

The safety and effectiveness of this drug have not been established in children.

No information is available on overdosage.

Precautions

Nilotinib can cause serious and life-threatening side effects. Sudden deaths have occurred with the administration of nilotinib. The drug carries a black-box warning concerning administration of the drug. An electrocardiogram (ECG) and various blood tests must be done before the drug can safely be started.

The following black box warnings must be observed:

- Nilotinib can prolong a phase of the heart contraction cycle called the QT interval. This drug should not be used in patients with long QT interval. Heart monitoring (ECG) should be done before the drug is started, one week after starting the drug, when dosage is changed, and at regular intervals during treatment to check for long QT interval. Other drugs known to prolong the QT interval should be avoided. If long QT interval occurs, dosage must be substantially reduced or the drug must be discontinued.
- Nilotinib should not be given to individuals with low blood potassium levels (hypokalemia) and low blood magnesium levels (hypomagnesemia). Blood electrolyte levels should be checked regularly and levels corrected when possible.
- Nilotinib should be used with caution in patients with liver (hepatic) impairment.

The following precautions also should be observed:

- Severe decrease in the number of normal blood cells (myelosuppression) may occur. Decrease in the number of blood platelets (thrombocytopenia) may reduce the ability of the blood to clot and increase the risk of bleeding episodes. Decrease in the number of neutrophils (neutropenia) may decrease the ability of the body to fight infection. Decrease in the number of red blood cells (anemia) may reduce the ability of the blood to supply oxygen. Blood count should be monitored frequently; dosage may need to be reduced.
- Patients with a history of pancreatitis may have elevated serum lipase levels. Serum lipase should be monitored.
- Patients with impaired liver function may have a variety of abnormally elevated measures of liver function (e.g., bilirubin, alkaline phosphatase). Liver function should be monitored.
- Nilotinib can cause abnormal blood levels of phosphate, potassium, calcium, and sodium. Electrolytes should be monitored and corrected.
- Food increases the amount of nilotinib in the blood. All food should be avoided for 2 hours before and 1 hour after each dose.

QUESTIONS TO ASK YOUR DOCTOR OR PHARMACIST

- How long will I need to take this drug before you can tell if it helps for me?
- How often do I have to have blood work and other laboratory tests done to check the effect the drug is having?
- Is this drug safe to take with the other drugs that I am currently taking?
- What side effects should I watch for? When should I call the doctor about them?
- Are there any clinical trials of this drug combined with other therapies that might benefit me?

Pregnant or breastfeeding

Nilotinib is a pregnancy category D drug. Woman who are pregnant or who might become pregnant should not use nilotinib. It is not known whether the drug is excreted in breast milk. Women taking this drug should not breastfeed, as there is the potential for this drug to cause serious adverse effects on nursing infants.

Side effects

Nilotinib has many side effects, the most serious of which is sudden death. The two most common serious side effects reported during clinical trials were **thrombocytopenia** and **neutropenia** (see Precautions). Other common serious side effects included **pneumonia**, **fever**, elevated serum lipase levels, and intracranial hemorrhage (bleeding in the brain). Additional serious side effects included fluid retention around the heart (**pericardial effusion**) and lungs (**pleural effusion**), inflammation of the pancreas, and liver damage.

Common but less serious side effects reported in more than 10% of patients during clinical trials included rash, **nausea**, **vomiting**, constipation, **diarrhea**, and headache.

Interactions

Nilotinib is known to interact with many drugs and all food. If these drugs cannot be avoided, the dosage of nilotinib may need to be adjusted. All interactions are not known. Patients should provide their doctor and pharmacist with a complete list of all prescription and nonprescription drugs, herbs, and dietary supplements that they are taking.

When taken with nilotinib, these drugs are likely to increase the amount of nilotinib circulating in the blood.

- ketoconazole (Nizoral)
- itraconazole (Sporanox)
- ritonavir (Norvir)
- atazanavir sulfate (Reyataz)
- indinavir (Crixivan)
- nelfinavir (Viracept)
- saquinavir (Invirase)
- telithomycin (Ketek)
- erythromycin (E-mycin)
- clarithromycin (Biaxin)

When taken with nilotinib, these drugs are likely to decrease the amount of nilotinib circulating in the blood.

- dexamethasone (Decadron)
- phenytoin (Dilantin)
- carbamazepine (Tergretol)
- rifampin (Rimactane)
- phenobarbitol (Luminal)

Taking nilotinib with food increases the amount of drug in the blood.

Nilotinib contains a small amount of lactose as an inactive ingredient. Individuals who are lactose-intolerant should discuss this with their physician.

Resources

OTHER

"Detailed Guided Leukemia, Chronic Myeloid (CML)." American Cancer Society. 2009 [October 6, 2009]. http://www.cancer.org/docroot/CRI/CRI_2_3x.asp?rnav=cridg&dt=83.

"FDA Approval for Nilotinib." National Cancer Institute. October 20, 2007 [October 7, 2009]. http://www.cancer.gov/cancertopics/druginfo/fda-nilotinib.

"Leukemia, Adult Chronic." MedlinePlus. September 30, 2009 [October 7, 2009]. http://www.nlm.nih.gov/medlineplus/leukemiaadultchronic.html.

"Oncolink." Abramson cancer Center of the University of Pennsylvania. 2009 [October 7, 2009]. http://www.oncolink.upenn.edu.

ORGANIZATIONS

American Cancer Society, 1599 Clifton Rd., NE, Atlanta, GA, 30329, (404) 320-3333, (800) ACS-2345, http://www.cancer.org.

Leukemia & Lymphoma Society, 1311 Mamaroneck Avenue, Suite 310 , White Plains, NY, 10605, (800) 955-4572, http://www.leukemia-lymphoma.org.

National Cancer Institute Public Inquires Office., 6116 Executive Boulevard, Room 3036A, Bethesda, MD, 20892-8322, (800) 4-CANCER. TTY (800) 332-8615, http://www.cancer.gov.

Tish Davidson, A.M.

Nilutamide *see* **Antiandrogen**

Nitrogen mustard *see* **Mechlorethamine**

Non-Hodgkin's lymphoma

Definition

One of two general types of lymphomas (cancers that begin in lymphatic tissues and can invade other organs) differing from **Hodgkin's disease** (HD) by a lack of Hodgkin's-specific Reed-Sternberg cells.

Description

Non-Hodgkin's **lymphoma** (NHL) is a **cancer** of lymphocytes, a type of white blood cell that moves around the body as part of its role in the immune system. NHL is much less predictable than HD and is more likely to spread to areas beyond the lymph nodes.

NHL is comprised of approximately 10 subtypes and 20 different disease entities. Division is based on whether the lymphoma is low grade (progressing slowly) or high grade (progressing rapidly). NHL is also grouped according to cell type—B cells or T cells. Physicians can diagnose the type of lymphoma by performing a **biopsy**, in which a lymph node is removed and examined in the laboratory. Some of the Non-Hodgkin's lymphoma types include: **Burkitt's lymphoma**, diffuse large B-cell lymphoma, follicular center lymphoma, and **mantle cell lymphoma**.

Kate Kretschmann

Nonsteroidal anti-inflammatory drugs

Definition

Nonsteroidal anti-inflammatory drugs (NSAIDs) are a type of drug that reduce pain and inflammation.

Purpose

NSAIDs often are used to relieve mild to moderate pain for all types of **cancer**, as well as the pain of arthritis, menstrual cramps, sore muscles following exercise, and tension headaches. Most NSAIDs are available in over-the-counter formulations.

Ibuprofen and naproxen are two NSAIDs that are also used to bring down **fever** and treat the side effects of **radiation therapy**.

Description

This class of drugs eases discomfort by blocking the pathway of an enzyme that forms prostaglandins (hormones that cause pain and swelling). By doing so, the drugs lessen the pain in different parts of the body.

Some of the NSAIDs used in cancer treatment include: ibuprofen (Motrin, Advil, Rufen, Nuprin), naproxen (Naprosyn, Naprelan, Anaprox, Aleve), nabumetone (Relafen), ketorolac, sulindac and diclofenac (Cataflam, Voltaren). The class of drugs known as Cyclooxygenase-2 inhibitors that emerged in the late 1990s for dealing with arthritis pain, such as the brand names Celebrex and Vioxx, is also considered part of the group of NSAIDS.

If NSAIDs are not strong enough to keep a cancer patient comfortable, physicians often will combine them with such **opioids** (narcotics) as codeine. In later stages, doctors also may combine NSAIDs with stronger opioids like morphine, to treat very severe pain.

NSAIDs also may be used to prevent **colon cancer** and other types of cancer, although scientists are still studying this experimental approach (see entry on **chemoprevention**).

Recommended dosage

Patients typically take NSAIDs on an as-needed basis. Doses vary depending on the type of NSAID being used. For example, the most common type, ibuprofen, is available over the counter in 200mg caplets, which can be taken at regular intervals throughout the day. The maximum daily dose for ibuprofen is 1,200 mgs.

KEY TERMS

Cyclooxygenase-2 inhibitor—A type of drug, such as Celebrex, that reduces pain and inflammation. Also called a COX-2 inhibitor.

Enzyme—A type of protein that speeds up the chemical reactions in the body.

NSAIDs—A category of drugs that reduce pain, fever and swelling.

Opioids—A class of pain-killing drugs either derived directly from the opium poppy or from synthetic compounds resembling morphine. Opioids are also known as narcotics.

Prostaglandins—Hormones that cause pain and swelling in the body.

Precautions

Most doctors recommend taking NSAIDs with a full glass of water. Avoid taking these drugs on an empty stomach. Smoking **cigarettes** and drinking alcohol while taking NSAIDs may irritate the stomach.

People who take NSAIDs should notify their doctors before having surgery or dental work, since these drugs can prevent wounds from healing properly.

Women who are pregnant or breastfeeding should check with their doctors before taking NSAIDs, because they may be harmful to a developing fetus or a newborn.

Diabetics, people who take aspirin, blood thinners, blood pressure medications, or steroids also should check with their doctors before taking NSAIDs.

Side effects

Many NSAID users experience mild side effects, such as an upset stomach. In 4–7% of cases, more serious complications develop, such as stomach ulcers. Typically, elderly people experience the most serious complications.

Common side effects include stomach upset, constipation, dizziness and headaches.

More severe side effects include stomach ulcers and bleeding ulcers. If a person has black, tarry stools or starts **vomiting** blood, it may be caused by a bleeding ulcer.

Kidney dysfunction is another severe complication of long-term NSAID use. Signs of kidney problems include dark yellow, brown or bloody urine. NSAID use also may cause liver function problems over longer periods of time.

To guard against ulcers, physicians may ask patients to take NSAIDs with such anti-ulcer medications as omeprazole or misoprostol. Another option is to take the NSAID in a different, non-oral form. Often topical creams or suppositories are available. Finally, doctors may decide to switch to a different type of pain killer, such as a cyclooxygenase-2 (COX-2) inhibitor like Celebrex, which may be easier on the stomach. Some studies indicate that the use of COX-2 inhibitors may postpone the need to prescribe narcotic medications for severe pain.

Some patients who have had problems with side effects from NSAIDs may benefit from acupuncture as an adjunctive treatment in **pain management**. A recent study done in New York found that older patients with lower back pain related to cancer reported that their pain was relieved by acupuncture with fewer side effects than those caused by NSAIDs.

Interactions

NSAIDs can be taken with most other prescription and over-the-counter drugs without any harmful interactions. Certain drug combinations, however, should be avoided. For instance, when ibuprofen is combined with **methotrexate** (used for **chemotherapy** and arthritis treatment) or certain diabetic medicines and anti-depressants, it can amplify negative side effects. Patients should check with a pharmacist before taking NSAIDs with other drugs.

NSAIDs may also interact with certain herbal preparations sold as dietary supplements. Among the herbs known to interact with NSAIDs are bearberry (*Arctostaphylos uva-ursi*), feverfew (*Tanacetum parthenium*), evening primrose (*Oenothera biennis*), and gossypol, a pigment obtained from cottonseed oil and used as a male contraceptive. In most cases, the herb increases the tendency of NSAIDs to irritate the digestive tract. It is just as important for patients to inform their doctors of herbal remedies that they take on a regular basis as it is to give the doctors lists of their other prescription medications.

Resources

BOOKS

Beers, Mark H., MD, and Robert Berkow, MD, editors. "Drug Therapy in the Elderly." In *The Merck Manual of Diagnosis and Therapy*. Whitehouse Station, NJ: Merck Research Laboratories, 2007.

Pelletier, Dr. Kenneth R. *The Best Alternative Medicine, Part I: Western Herbal Medicine*. New York: Simon and Schuster, 2002.

Wilson, Billie Ann, RN, PhD, Carolyn L. Stang, PharmD, and Margaret T. Shannon, RN, PhD. *Nurses Drug Guide 2000*. Stamford, CT: Appleton and Lange, 1999.

PERIODICALS

Birbara, C. A., A. D. Puopolo, D. R. Munoz, et al. "Treatment of Chronic Low Back Pain with Etoricoxib, A New Cyclo-Oxygenase-2 Selective Inhibitor: Improvement in Pain and Disability—A Randomized, Placebo-Controlled, 3-Month Trial." *Journal of Pain* 4 (August 2003): 307–315.

Gordon, D. B. "Nonopioid and Adjuvant Analgesics in Chronic Pain Management: Strategies for Effective Use." *Nursing Clinics of North America* 38 (September 2003): 447–464.

Graf, C., and K. Puntillo. "Pain in the Older Adult in the Intensive Care Unit." *Critical Care Clinics* 19 (October 2003): 749–770.

Harris, R. E., R. T. Chlebowski, R. D. Jackson, et al. "Breast cancer and Nonsteroidal Anti-Inflammatory Drugs: Prospective Results from the Women's Health Initiative." *Cancer Research* 63 (September 15, 2003): 6096–6101.

Hatsiopoulou, O., R. I. Cohen, and E. V. Lang. "Postprocedure Pain Management of Interventional Radiology Patients." *Journal of Vascular and Interventional Radiology* 14 (November 2003): 1373–1385.

Meng, C. F., D. Wang, J. Ngeow, et al. "Acupuncture for Chronic Low Back Pain in Older Patients: A Randomized, Controlled Trial." *Rheumatology (Oxford)* 42 (December 2003): 1508–1517.

Perrone, M. R., M. C. Artesani, M. Viola, et al. "Tolerability of Rofecoxib in Patients with Adverse Reactions to Nonsteroidal Anti-Inflammatory Drugs: A Study of 216 Patients and Literature Review." *International Archives of Allergy and Immunology* 132 (September 2003): 82–86.

Raffa, R. B., R. Clark-Vetri, R. J. Tallarida, and A. I. Wertheimer. "Combination Strategies for Pain Management." *Expert Opinion in Pharmacotherapy* 4 (October 2003): 1697–1708.

Small, R. C., and A. Schuna. "Optimizing Outcomes in Rheumatoid Arthritis." *Journal of the American Pharmaceutical Association* 43, no. 5 Supplement 1 (September-October 2003): S16–S17.

Stephens, J., B. Laskin, C. Pashos, et al. "The Burden of Acute Postoperative Pain and the Potential Role of the COX-2-Specific Inhibitors." *Rheumatology (Oxford)* 42, Supplement 3 (November 2003): iii40–iii52.

ORGANIZATIONS

U. S. Food and Drug Administration (FDA). 5600 Fishers Lane, Rockville, MD 20857. (888) 463-6332. http://www.fda.gov.

Melissa Knopper, M.S.
Rebecca J. Frey, Ph.D.

NSAIDs *see* **Nonsteroidal anti-inflammatory drugs**

Nuclear medicine scans

Definition

A nuclear medicine scan is a test in which radioactive material is taken into the body and is used to create an image of a specific organ or bone.

Purpose

The purpose of a nuclear medicine scan is to locate areas of impaired function in the organ or bone being scanned. Nuclear medicine scans are widely used for diagnosis and monitoring of many different conditions. In the diagnosis and treatment of **cancer**, nuclear medicine scans are used to identify cancerous sites, for tumor localization and staging, and to judge response to therapy.

Precautions

Women who are pregnant or breast feeding should not undergo this test. A patient who is unable to remain still for an extended period of time may require sedation for a nuclear medicine scan.

Description

A nuclear medicine scan is an extremely sensitive test that can provide information about the structure and function of specific parts of the body. Types of nuclear scans include bone scans, heart scans, lung scans, kidney and bladder scans, thyroid scans, liver and spleen scans, and gallbladder scans. Brain scans are done to detect malignancy.

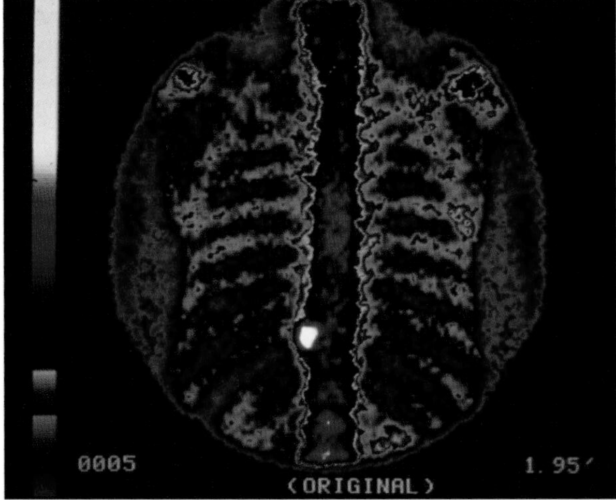

False-color bone scintigram (nuclear bone scan) of a person suffering from a secondary (metastatic) bone cancer (white area) affecting the dorsal spine. *(Copyright CNRI, Science Source/Photo Researchers, Inc. Reproduced by permission.)*

KEY TERMS

Tracer—A radioactive, or radiation-emitting, substance used in a nuclear medicine scan.

In a nuclear medicine scan, a small amount of radioactive material, or tracer, is injected or taken orally by the patient. After a period of time during which the radioactive material accumulates in one area of the body, a scan is taken by a special radiation detector, called a radionuclide scanner. This machine produces an image of the area for analysis by the medical team.

This test is performed in a radiology facility, either in a hospital department or an outpatient x-ray center. During the scan, the patient lies on his or her back on a table, but may be repositioned to the stomach or side during the study. The radionuclide scanner is positioned against the body part to be examined. Either the camera, the table, or both, may change position during the study. Depending on the type of scan, the procedure may take anywhere from 15 to 60 minutes. It is important for the patient not to move except when directed to do so by the technologist.

Preparation

The required preparation for nuclear medicine scans ranges from slight to none. The doctor may advise that certain prescription medications be discontinued before the test or that the patient not eat for three to four hours before the test. Depending on the type of test, a reference scan or specialized blood studies may be done before the scan is taken. Jewelry or metallic objects should be removed.

The patient should advise the doctor of any previously administered nuclear medicine scans, recent surgeries, sensitivities to drugs, allergies, prescription medications, and if there is a chance that she is pregnant.

Aftercare

No special care is required after the test. Fluids are encouraged after the scan to aid in the excretion of the radioactive material. It should be almost completely eliminated from the body within 24 hours.

Risks

The risks of nuclear medicine scans are very low. Most scans use the same or less amount of radiation as

QUESTIONS TO ASK THE DOCTOR

- How long will my scan take?
- How long will the tracer stay in my body?
- Will repeat scans be necessary?

a conventional x ray and the radioactive material is quickly passed through the body. Side effects or negative reactions to the test are very rare.

Normal results

A normal result is a scan that shows the expected distribution of the tracer and no unusual shape, size, or function of the scanned organ.

Abnormal results

Depending on the tracer and technique used, the scan can identify and image particular types of tumors or certain cancers. Too much tracer in the spleen and bones, compared to the liver, can indicate potential hypertension or cirrhosis. Liver diseases such as hepatitis may also cause an abnormal scan, but are rarely diagnosed from the information revealed by this study alone.

In a bone scan, a high concentration of tracer occurs in areas of increased bone activity. These regions appear brighter and may be referred to as "hot spots." They may indicate healing fractures, tumors, infections, or other processes that trigger new bone formation. Lower concentrations of tracer may be called "cold spots." Poor blood flow to an area of bone, or bone destruction from a tumor, may produce a cold spot.

See also Imaging studies; Magnetic resonance imaging.

Resources

OTHER

Virtual Hospital: Iowa Health Book: Diagnostic Radiology: Patient's Guide to Nuclear Medicine. [cited June 27, 2009]. http://www.vh.org/Patients/IHB/Rad/NucMed/PatGuideNucMed/PatGuideNucMed.html.

ORGANIZATIONS

Society of Nuclear Medicine. 1850 Samuel Morse Dr., Reston, Virginia 20190. (703) 708-9000. Fax (703) 708-9015. http://www.snm.org.

Ellen S. Weber, M.S.N.
Paul A. Johnson, Ed.M.

Nutritional support

Description

Achieving adequate nutritional support is difficult during **cancer** therapy or treatment. However, preservation of body composition and proper nutrition will help to maintain strength and may improve daily function and ability to cope with cancer therapies. Adequate nutrition may contribute to a patient feeling better and stronger and may help to fight off **infection**.

Malnutrition is a primary concern and is an important cause of illness in cancer patients due to difficulty consuming enough calories and nutrients. Protein-energy malnutrition (or protein-calorie malnutrition) is particularly problematic, which is the most common secondary illness in cancer patients. It occurs when a lack of protein and energy (calories) are consumed to sustain the body composition, instigating **weight loss**. When body stores are severely compromised, the body's functionality declines, which may lead to illness and perhaps death. Exhaustion, weakness, decreased resistance to infection, progress wasting, and difficulties tolerating cancer therapies may result from inadequate nutrition.

People with cancer commonly experience **anorexia**, which is characterized by a loss of appetite. Anorexia is the most predominate cause of malnutrition and deterioration in patients with cancer. Another common problem in cancer is weight loss and cachexia. Cachexia is a condition where the bodyweight wastes away, characterized by a constant loss of weight, muscle, and fat. It is known as a wasting syndrome and can occur in individuals who consume enough food, but due to disease complications, cannot absorb enough nutrients. Malnutrition, anorexia, and cachexia are serious in cancer patients and can lead to death.

Causes

There are many reasons for malnutrition in cancer patients, including the effect of the tumor, effect of treatment, or psychological issues such as **depression**. The growth of tumors in the digestive system may induce blockage, lead to **nausea and vomiting**, or cause poor digestion or absorption of nutrients.

Cancer therapies and their side effects may also lead to nutrition difficulties. For example, following surgery, malabsorption of protein and fat may occur. In addition, there may be an increased requirement for energy due to infection or **fever**.

QUESTIONS TO ASK THE DOCTOR

- What effect will the treatment or disease have on my body nutritionally (i.e., on the ability to eat, digest food, absorb nutrients, energy requirements)?
- How long will the negative side effects last?
- Is there a risk of malnutrition or weight loss with this type of cancer or treatment?
- What nutrients are most important to obtain during treatment?
- Are there any nutritional supplements that may be required?

Special concerns

Cancer patients should maintain an adequate intake of fluids, energy, and protein. The patient's nutrient requirements can be calculated by a dietitian or doctor because requirements vary considerably from patient to patient.

Enteral nutrition may be administered through a nose tube (or surgically placed tubes) for patients with eating difficulties due to upper gastrointestinal blockage such as difficulty swallowing, esophageal narrowing, tumor, stomach weakness, paralysis, or other conditions that preclude normal food intake. If the gastrointestinal tract is working and will not be affected by the cancer treatments, then enteral support is preferable. Parenteral nutrition (most often an infusion into a vein) can be used if the gut is not functioning properly or due to other reasons that prevent enteral feeding.

Treatments

Nutritional problems related to side effects should be addressed to ensure adequate nutrition and prevent weight loss. The following suggestions will provide some helpful hints on dealing with side effects such as loss of appetite, **nausea**, **vomiting**, **fatigue**, and **taste alteration**. To deal with appetite loss and weight loss:

- Eat more when feeling the hungriest.
- Eat foods that are enjoyed the most.
- Eat several small meals and snacks instead of three large meals.
- Have ready-to-eat snacks on hand such as cheese and crackers, granola bars, muffins, nuts and seeds, canned puddings, ice cream, yogurt, and hard boiled eggs.
- Eat high-calorie foods and high-protein foods.
- Begin with small portions during a meal to enjoy the satisfaction of finishing a meal. Have additional servings if still hungry.
- Eat in a pleasant atmosphere with family and friends if desired.
- Make sure to consume at least 8–10 glasses of water per day to maintain fluid balance.
- Consider commercial liquid meal replacements such as Ensure.
- Discuss with a physician the possibility of using appetite-increasing medications such Megace or Marinol.

Nausea is a common side effect of several cancer treatments including surgery, **chemotherapy**, biological therapy, and radiation. If nausea is problematic, the following methods may provide relief:

- Avoid fatty, fried, spicy, greasy, or hot foods with a strong odor.
- Eat small meals frequently but slowly.
- If nausea is particularly worse in the morning, consume dry toast or crackers before getting up.
- Try consuming such foods as clear liquids, toast, crackers, yogurt, sherbet, pretzels, oatmeal, skinned chicken (baked or broiled), angel food cake, and fruits and vegetables that are soft or bland.
- Drink beverages cool or chilled.
- Hot foods may add to nausea, so consume foods at room temperature or cooler.
- Drink or sip liquids (a straw may help) throughout the day, but not during meals. Try sucking on ice chips.
- Discuss with a physician the possibility of using antinausea medications (also called antiemetics) such Zofran or Kytril.

Vomiting may occur for several reasons due to the cancer itself, treatment, or emotional upset. If vomiting occurs, the following guidelines may help:

- Do not drink or eat until vomiting has subsided, then consume small amounts of clear liquids.
- When able to tolerate clear liquids, try to consume a full liquid diet (including dairy products unless they are difficult to digest). Begin with small quantities and gradually return to a regular diet if nausea and vomiting have dissipated.

If fatigue is preventing receiving adequate nutrition, the following strategies may help:

- Try using frozen, canned, or ready-to-use foods.
- Eat high-calorie foods.
- Have ready-to-eat snacks on hand such as cheese and crackers, granola bars, muffins, nuts and seeds,

canned puddings, ice cream, yogurt, and hard-boiled eggs.

- Consider using a service such as Meals on Wheels, a delivery or home care service.
- Invite friends or family over to assist with meal preparation.
- Consider commercial liquid meal replacements such as Ensure.

Taste changes can give foods a metallic or off flavor. Consider the following strategies to alleviate taste changes.

- If meats have a metallic taste, try other sources of protein such as dairy products, poultry, fish, seafood, peanut butter, eggs, seeds, nuts, tofu, and legumes.
- Use plastic utensils to decrease metallic flavor.
- Choose tart foods such as citrus juices, lemonade, cranberry juice, and pickles to help alleviate a metallic taste. If sore mouth and throat symptoms are also present, do not consume these foods.
- Consume a variety of foods.
- Try different seasonings, herbs, and sauces.
- Choose foods that look and smell good.
- Dilute drinks that are too strong or sweet with water.
- Rinse mouth often with baking soda and water.

Alternative and complementary therapies

There is no alternative or complementary nutritional therapy that has proven effective for **cancer prevention** or cancer treatment. However, the are several foods and nutraceuticals such as garlic, plant sterols, green and black tea polyphenols, and soybean products (soy isoflavones) that have shown promise in previous research for anticarcinogenic properties. Many of these products are actively being tested in **clinical trials** to elucidate anti-carcinogenic properties. As for prevention, past research has clearly demonstrated that intake of fruits and vegetables are correlated to a lower incidence rate for certain types of cancer. It is important to check with a dietitian or doctor before taking nutritional supplements or alternative therapies because they may interfere with cancer medications or treatments.

Resources

BOOKS

Quillin, Patrick, and Noreen Quillin. *Beating Cancer With Nutrition-Revised.* Sun Lakes, AZ: Bookworld Services, 2001.

PERIODICALS

Alberts, D.S., et al. "Lack of Effect of a High-Fiber Cereal Supplement on the Recurrence of Colorectal Adenomas." *New England Journal of Medicine* 2000: 1156–62.

Schatzkin, A., et al. "Lack of Effect of a Low-Fat, High-Fiber Diet on the Recurrence of Colorectal Adenomas." *New England Journal of Medicine* 2000: 1149–55.

Singletary, Keith. "Diet, Natural Products and Cancer Chemoprevention." *The Journal of Nutrition* 2000: 465S–466S.

ORGANIZATIONS

The National Cancer Institute (NCI). Public Inquiries Office, Building 31, Room 10A31, 31 Center Drive, MSC 2580, Betheseda, MD 20892-2580. (301)435-3848, 800-4-CANCER. http://cancer.gov/publications/. http://cancertrials.nci.nih.gov. http://cancernet.nci.nih.gov.

National Center for Complementary and Alternative Medicine (NCCAM). 31 Center Dr., Room #5B–58, Bethesda, MD 20892-2182. (800) NIH-NCAM. Fax (301) 495-4957. <http://nccam.nih.gov>.

Crystal Heather Kaczkowski, MSc.

Nystatin *see* **Antifungal therapy**

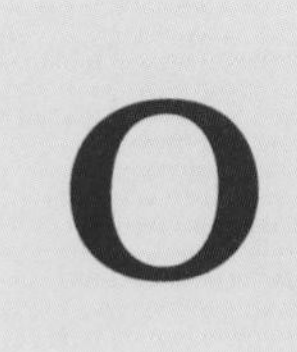

Occupational exposures and cancer

Definition

Occupational exposure to **cancer** occurs at the workplace. Some individuals develop cancer from exposure to certain substances at an indoor workplace such as a factory or a restaurant. Others may be exposed to carcinogenic substances while working primarily outdoors, such as construction or lawn maintenance workers.

Description

About 5% of cancer in men and 1% of cancer in women result from exposure to carcinogenic substances in their work environment. The most common cancers associated with occupational exposure are:

- lung and pleura
- bladder
- skin
- laryngeal
- nasal cavity
- leukemia
- throat
- lymphoma
- soft-tissue sarcomas
- liver

Causes

Tobacco smoking is considered the greatest risk factor for lung cancer. Individuals who do not smoke can still develop lung cancer. Employees in smoke-filled environments such as bars, restaurants, casinos, bingo halls, and bowling alleys are at greatest risk from second-hand smoke. Second-hand smoke is highly toxic. For instance, non-smokers who live with a smoker are at 30% greater risk of developing lung cancer than if they lived with a non-smoker. However, many states, and now other countries, have worked on laws to ban smoking in some work environments.

Asbestos is a known carcinogen. Individuals whose work exposes them to asbestos are seven times more likely to die from lung cancer. Asbestos workers who smoke are 50–90 times more likely to develop lung cancer than the average individual. Asbestos affects the lining of the lungs, causing malignant **mesothelioma**. Mesothelioma is considered incurable and fatal, and may not be detected until as long as 45 years after exposure. Asbestos still exists in schools, offices, factory buildings, and homes in the form of insulation. Workers who remove asbestos from buildings need to take special precautionary measures to avoid inhalation of asbestos fibers, and wear special clothing so that they do not bring home the dust on their clothes. Asbestos can affect railroad workers, ship builders, gas mask manufacturers, and workers in insulation factories. Because of the way in which asbestos in inhaled and processed in the body, it can also lead to cancers of the larynx, esophagus, pancreas, kidney, and colon.

Radon is another substance that can cause lung cancer. Houses or commercial properties that are built on soil containing radon may contain radon in gas form. Many inhaled chemicals put workers at risk. This includes uranium and talc miners and workers who are exposed to the chemicals arsenic, vinyl chloride, nickel chromates, coal products, mustard gas, and chloromethyl ethers. While these industries need to provide safety gear to protect workers from these substances, it is always best if the worker makes sure she or he is properly protected.

Workers who are exposed to diesel fumes, such as railroad crews and truck drivers, may have a 40% greater risk of lung cancer. Diesel fumes contain benzene, formaldehyde, and dioxins. Formaldehyde alone can cause respiratory cancers. It also is used as a sterilizing agent in dialysis units, disinfectant in operating

KEY TERMS

Carcinogen—A substance, method, or process that has been scientifically shown to be a causative factor in the development of a certain cancer.

Metastasize—The ability of a cancer to spread from its site of origin to other sites in the body. The more a cancer has metastasized, the worse is the individual's prognosis for cure.

Pleura—The pleura is a membrane that covers the lungs, and lines the chest cavity.

QUESTIONS TO ASK THE DOCTOR

- What type and stage is my cancer?
- What do you think is the cause of my cancer?
- Will I be able to work during my cancer treatment?
- Will I be able to go back to my same job after treatment is finished?
- If not, what kind of limitations will there be on my activity level?
- What kind of work will I be able to do when my treatment is over?
- Is anyone at home at risk for cancer or illness because of my work?

rooms, carpet and furniture glues, as well as for embalming.

Painters, printers, and chemists are also at increased risk for lung cancer because of their occupational exposure to certain chemicals. Employees exposed to fine silica particles also have an increased risk for lung cancer. Silica appears in sand, rock, and mineral ores, and is used in sandblasting, masonry work, tunnel construction, ceramics, laying railroad track, soap manufacturing, glass manufacturing, shipbuilding, and agriculture.

Bladder cancer from occupational exposure is most common in individuals working with radiation or dyes that involve the aromatic amine chemicals such as benzidine and beta naphthylamine. Factory workers involved in the production of these dyes, as well as those who use these dyes, such as hair colorists, and possibly even people who apply their own permanent hair dye at least once a month may be at increased risk for bladder cancer.

Chemicals used in the rubber, leather, textile, and paint industries can also be carcinogenic. The risk of bladder cancer rises with age, and smoking increases significantly the risk of developing bladder cancer. Individuals who have taken the herb *Aristocholia fangchi* as part of an herbal **weight loss** product may also be at higher risk for bladder cancer. Drinking at least 11 cups of fluid a day can decrease the risk of bladder cancer, as it increases urination and decreases the concentration and the amount of time that carcinogenic substances come into contact with the bladder lining.

There are several types of **skin cancer**, varying in aggressiveness. Basal and squamous cell cancers are considered very curable. **Melanoma** is the most serious type, and the most likely to metastasize. Exposure to ultraviolet rays, coal tar, pitch, creosote, arsenic, and radium can lead to skin cancer. Individuals whose work is primarily outdoors, such as employees of road and building construction, landscaping, outdoor painting, and beach and boating work are at greater risk. A 2004 study in Germany found a dose-dependent relationship with exposure. In other words, the more UV rays workers were exposed to, the higher their risk proportionately rose. Using sunscreen and protective clothing such as a long-sleeved shirt, long pants, and a wide-brimmed hat can decrease exposure.

Laryngeal cancer. Individuals whose work includes heavy exposure to wood dust, paint fumes, and asbestos, and workers exposed to certain chemicals in the metalworking, petroleum, plastic, and textile industries are at increased risk for laryngeal and hypopharyngeal cancers. Tobacco and heavy alcohol use can increase the risk for these cancers by as much as 100 times.

Farmers and others who have long-term exposure to herbicides and pesticides are at increased risk for leukemia. Children whose parent has **chronic lymphocytic leukemia** (CLL) have two to four times greater risk of getting CLL themselves. Long-term exposure to benzene places the employee at greater risk of developing acute leukemia. Herbicides and pesticides are both associated with the development of lymphomas, so workers involved in their production as well as their application are at increased risk. Children exposed to pesticides on a regular basis are significantly more likely to develop **non-Hodgkin's lymphoma** than children not exposed.

Farmers appear to have an increased incidence of **prostate cancer**. The reason is not yet clear. While some have suggested it may be due to a diet high in red meat and fatty foods, studies are investigating the link between prostate cancer and pesticides, fertilizers, chemical solvents, and farm equipment fumes. Salivary gland cancer may be linked to working with nickel alloy and silica dust, and exposure to radioactive substances.

Pancreatic cancer appears to be associated with significant exposure to pesticides, certain dyes, and chemicals found in gasoline. Occupational exposure to asbestos, cadmium, and organic solvents (especially trichloroethylene) seems to increase the risk of getting **kidney cancer**. Dioxin is a known carcinogen, and may be a causative factor in a variety of cancers. It is a byproduct in industrial processing that deals with chlorine and hydrocarbons, such as found in incinerators and paper and pulp factories.

Other chemicals linked with cancer are DDT and PCBs (polychlorinated biphenols). Health care professionals, both human and veterinary, may be exposed to carcinogenic substances in caring for their patients. Body fluid exposure can increase the risk of hepatitis B and hepatitis C, cause liver failure, and increase the risk of **liver cancer**. HIV can cause AIDS and increase the risk of a variety of malignant tumors. Chemicals in paint and paint solvents are also used in ceramic factories.

Electric and magnetic fields surround electric tools and machinery. Studies have been done to investigate whether these fields are harmful to humans. Research findings continue to be controversial, some showing an increased incidence of cancers, others not finding an association. However, federally funded research studies continue.

Special concerns

Cancers that originate in the workplace do not require different treatment than if the same cancer had developed from another source. However, workers who develop cancer through occupational exposure may not be able to return to the same job, perhaps not even the same company. This means that even if the individual has survived the cancer, and gone though all that treatment entails, they cannot pick up their life where they left it at the time of the cancer diagnosis. They may be disabled, and not be able to work at all, or they may have to retrain for work, either a different job within the same company, or a whole new job and environment.

If the person is older, he or she may be less employable after illness because of age. Depending on the type of cancer, it may be difficult to prove that the work environment was a causal factor in the development of the disease. This can make it harder to obtain work-related benefits. Consequently, financial concerns may be a great burden. Also, certain cancers may have developed from the inhalation of substances that were also brought home on the employee's clothing. Others in the family may have gotten ill as well. Fine dust particles can come home on workers' clothing, shoes, skin, hair, facial hair, tools or lunch boxes, and on the inside or outside of their cars.

Workers in any occupation need to be fully informed of the substances with which they come in contact. Federal regulations are in place to improve employee safety, but the regulations are ineffective if the employees do not utilize the protective clothing, masks, and other safety measures at their disposal. Individuals who learned their trade prior to the installation of many safety measures may find it difficult to *retrain* themselves with the new equipment. But not doing so may raise their risk of cancer.

While many cancers have an unknown source, cancers due to occupational exposures have known sources. This means that they are preventable, if proper safety equipment is used all of the time, and always used correctly.

Treatments

Treatments for cancers due to occupational exposure should be the same as for the same cancer developed from a different source. Treatment will depend on the type and stage of the cancer diagnosed, as well as the age and fertility needs of the patient. Access to treatment may vary, however, depending on the type of insurance the individual holds. Access to experimental treatments, or treatment that a **health insurance** deems experimental can vary.

Alternative and complementary therapies

Alternative therapy options for cancer due to occupational exposure should be the same as if the cancer developed from another source. Complementary treatments that improve the functioning of the body's immune system, or that decrease treatment side effects such as **nausea**, can be helpful. There may be different stresses in the life of the person with a work-related cancer. So therapies such as meditation, guided imagery, therapeutic touch, yoga, and t'ai chi can help deal with the stress of having cancer, going through treatment, and having to find alternative work options.

See also Environmental factors in cancer development.

Resources

BOOKS

Kimball, Chad T., editor. *Work Health and Safety Sourcebook. Health Reference Series*. Detroit: Omnigraphics, 2000.

Teeley, Peter, and Philip Bashe. *The Complete Cancer Survival Guide*. New York: Doubleday, 2000.

PERIODICALS

"Dose-dependent Risk of Skin Cancer With Occupational Exposure to UV Radiation." *Cancer Weekly* April 27, 2004: 184.

Michaud, D. S., et al. "Fluid Intake and the Risk of Bladder Cancer in Men." *The New England Journal of Medicine*. May 6, 1999: 1390–1397.

ORGANIZATIONS

American Cancer Society. (800) ACS-2345. http://www.cancer.org.

United States Department of Labor. Occupational Safety and Health Administration, 200 Constitution Ave., NW, Washington, D.C. 20210. http://www.osha.gov.

Esther Csapo Rastegari, R.N., B.S.N., Ed.M.
Teresa G. Odle

Octreotide *see* **Antidiarrheal agents**

Oligodendroglioma

Definition

Oligodendrogliomas are a rare form of **brain tumors**. The brain is made up of many supporting cells that are called glial cells. Any tumor of these glial cells is called a glioma. Oligodendrogliomas are tumors that arise from a type of glial cell called oligodendrocytes. These cells are the specialized cells of the brain that produce the fatty covering of nerve cells (myelin).

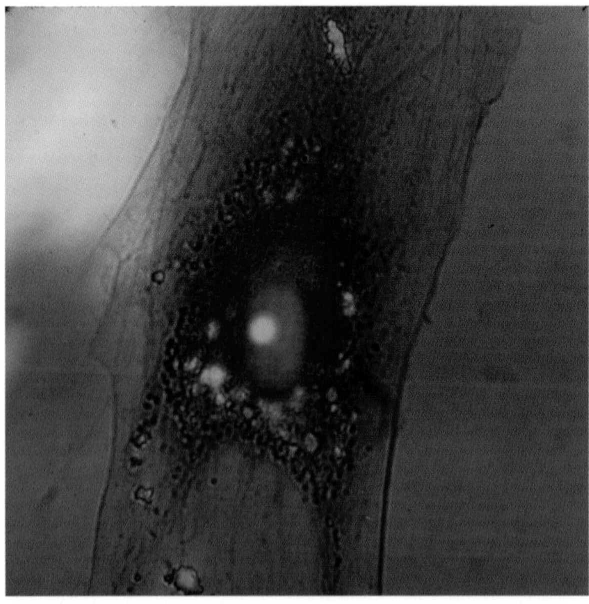

Malignant oligodendroglioma cells from the human brain. *(Copyright Cecil Fox, Science Source/Photo Researchers, Inc. Reproduced by permission.)*

KEY TERMS

Anaplastic oligodendroglioma—A form of oligodendroglioma that does not have a well-defined shape and grows very rapidly and aggressively.

Astrocytoma—A type of brain tumor that arises from the astrocytes, specialized brain cells that regulate the chemical environment of the brain and form the blood-brain barrier. These types of tumors are often mixed with oligodendrogliomas to form oligoastrocytomas.

Frontal lobes—The two lobes of the cerebrum of the brain that are responsible for cognitive thought processes (knowing, thinking, learning, and judging).

Glioma—Any tumor that arises from the supporting cells in the brain called glial cells.

Intracranial hypertension—A higher-than-normal pressure of the fluid in the skull.

Oligoastrocytoma—A type of brain tumor that is a mixture of oligodendroglioma and astrocytoma. This is also called a mixed glioma.

Spinal fluid shunt—A small tube that is surgically implanted to allow excess spinal fluid to drain directly into the abdominal cavity.

Temporal lobes—The two lobes of the cerebrum of the brain that are responsible for coordination, speech, hearing, memory, and awareness of time.

Well-differentiated tumor—A tumor that grows relatively slowly and in a well-defined shape.

Description

Oligodendrogliomas can grow in different parts of the brain, but they are most commonly found in the frontal or temporal lobes of the cerebrum. The frontal lobes are responsible for cognitive thought processes (knowing, thinking, learning, and judging). The temporal lobes are responsible for coordination, speech, hearing, memory, and awareness of time.

There are two types of oligodendroglioma: the well-differentiated tumor, which grows relatively slowly and in a defined shape; and the anaplastic oligodendroglioma, which grows much more rapidly and does not have a well-defined shape. Anaplastic

QUESTIONS TO ASK THE DOCTOR

- Which type of oligodendroglioma do I have?
- Is my tumor operable?
- What is the likelihood of my type of oligodendroglioma coming back?
- How often should I seek follow-up examinations?

oligodendrogliomas are much less common than well-differentiated oligodendrogliomas.

More common than either form of pure oligodendroglioma is the mixed glioma, or oligoastrocytoma. These mixed gliomas are a mixture of oligodendroglioma and **astrocytoma**. An astrocytoma is a tumor that arises from the astrocytes, specialized cells in the brain that regulate the chemical environment of the brain and help to form the blood–brain barrier.

Oligodendrogliomas and mixed gliomas account for approximately 4–5% of all primary brain tumors and 10% of all gliomas. A primary brain tumor is a tumor that begins in the brain, as opposed to a secondary (or metastatic) brain tumor, which originates in another organ and spreads (metastasizes) to the brain.

Demographics

Oligodendromas occur in approximately nine in every one million people. Oligodendrogliomas can occur in people of any age, but most occur in middle-aged adults.

Oligodendrogliomas occur with equal frequency in members of all races and ethnic groups. There does not appear to be any relation of oligodendrogliomas to any geographic region. For unknown reasons, men are affected by oligodendrogliomas in higher numbers than women.

Causes and symptoms

The cause, or causes, of oligodendrogliomas are not known; however, most people with these types of tumors have some type of genetic mutation on chromosome 1, chromosome 19, or on both chromosomes 1 and 19. Investigations are ongoing in an attempt to determine if these genetic factors, or other factors, cause oligodendrogliomas. Oligodendrogliomas are not contagious.

The symptoms of oligodenrogliomas are the result of increased pressure in the fluid within the skull (intracranial hypertension). These symptoms include:

- nausea
- vomiting
- irritability
- headache
- vision disturbances
- enlargement of the head
- seizures

Oligodendrogliomas may also be accompanied by a weakness or paralysis on the side of the body opposite to the side of the brain where the tumor is located. When the tumor is located in a frontal lobe, the patient may experience gradual changes in mood and personality. When it is located in a temporal lobe, the patient may experience difficulty with speech, hearing, coordination, and memory.

Diagnosis

The diagnosis of oligodendrogliomas begins in the doctor's office with a basic neurological examination. This examination involves:

- testing eye reflexes, eye movement, and pupil reactions
- testing hearing with a tuning fork or ticking watch
- reflex tests with a rubber hammer
- balance and coordination tests
- pin-prick and cotton ball tests for sense of touch
- sense of smell tests with various odors
- facial muscle tests (e.g., smiling, frowning, etc.)
- tongue movement and gag reflex tests
- head movement tests
- mental status tests (e.g., asking what year it is, who the President is, etc.)
- abstract thinking tests (e.g., asking for the meaning of a common saying, such as "every cloud has a silver lining.")
- memory tests (e.g., asking to have a list of objects repeated, asking for details of what a patient ate for dinner last night, etc.)

If the doctor suspects a brain tumor may be present, further diagnostic tests will be ordered. These tests are performed by a neurological specialist. Imaging tests that may be ordered include **computed tomography** (CT) and **magnetic resonance imaging** (MRI). Other tests may include a spinal tap, to examine the cerebrospinal fluid, and an electroencephalogram (EEG), which measures the electrical activity of the brain.

Treatment team

Treatment of any primary brain tumor, including oligodendrogliomas, is different from treating tumors in other parts of the body. Brain surgery requires much more precision than most other surgeries. Also, many medicinal drugs cannot cross the blood–brain barrier. Therefore, the therapies that are used to treat oligodendrogliomas, and the side effects of these therapies, are quite complex.

The most up-to-date treatment opportunities are available from experienced, multi-disciplinary medical professional teams made up of doctors, nurses, and technologists who specialize in **cancer** (oncology), neurology, medical imaging, drug or **radiation therapy**, and anesthesiology.

Clinical staging, treatments, and prognosis

Oligodendrogliomas and other primary brain tumors are diagnosed, or staged, in grades of severity from I to IV. Grade I tumors have cells that are not malignant and are nearly normal in appearance. Grade II tumors have cells that appear to be slightly abnormal. Grade III tumors have cells that are malignant and clearly abnormal. Grade IV, the most severe type of brain tumors, contain fast-spreading and abnormal cells. Well-defined oligodendrogliomas are generally stage I or stage II tumors. Anaplastic oligodenrogliomas are generally stage III or stage IV tumors.

The standard treatment for all grades of oligodendrogliomas is surgery to remove the tumor completely. This surgery is generally aided by an image guidance system that allows the surgeon to determine the most efficient route to location of the tumor. Approximately half of oligodendroglioma patients gain relief of the increased intracranial pressure after complete removal of their tumors. The other half require a spinal fluid shunt to allow drainage of the excess fluid.

In some instances of oligodendroglioma, the tumor is inoperable or cannot be completely removed. Patients with inoperable oligodendrogliomas are generally treated with radiation therapies. Oligodendrogliomas are among the only brain tumors that can be successfully treated with a type of **chemotherapy** called PCV (**Procarbazine**, CCNU or **lomustine**, and **Vincristine**). Chemotherapy is usually used only in cases of recurrent anaplastic oligodendrogliomas.

For patients with well-defined oligodendrogliomas, median survival exceeds 10 years. For patients with anaplastic dendrogliomas, median survival ranges from two to five years.

Alternative and complementary therapies

For oligodendrogliomas, there are no effective alternative treatments—treatments used instead of conventional treatments like surgery or chemotherapy.

Coping with cancer treatment

Most patients who undergo brain surgery to remove their tumors can resume their normal activities within a few days of the operation.

Clinical trials

There were 47 **clinical trials** underway by 2005, aimed at the treatment of oligodendrogliomas. More information on these trials, including contact information, may be found by conducting a clinical trial search at the web site of the National Cancer Institute, CancerNet http://cancernet.nci.nih.gov/trialsrch.shtml.

Prevention

Because the cause or causes of oligodenrogliomas are not known, there are no known preventions.

Special concerns

Repeat surgery may be necessary for oligodendrogliomas because these tumors sometimes redevelop. Careful monitoring by the medical team will be required. Also, if the tumor is located in the dominant hemisphere of the patient's brain, any treatment, especially surgery, requires special consideration and care not to disrupt the personality or other higher brain functions of the patient.

See also Brain and Central nervous system tumors.

Resources

OTHER

"Understanding Oligodendrogliomas: Information on Diagnosis, Treatment, Radiotherapy, Surgery and Chemotherapy." [cited June 27, 2005]. http://www.bacup.org.uk/info/oligodendroglioma.htm.

ORGANIZATIONS

American Brain Tumor Association. 2720 River Road, Suite 146, Des Plaines, IL 60018-4110. Telephone (800) 886-2282. http://www.abta.org/.

The Brain Tumor Society. 124 Watertown Street, Suite 3-H. Watertown, MA 02472. (617) 924-9997. Fax (617) 924-9998. http://www.tbts.org/.

National Brain Tumor Foundation. 785 Market Street, Suite 1600. San Francisco, CA 94103. Telephone 415-284-0208. http://www.braintumor.org/.

Paul A. Johnson, Ed.M.

Omega-3 fatty acids

Definition

Essential to human health, omega-3 fatty acids are a form of polyunsaturated fats that are not made by the body and must be obtained from a person's food.

Purpose

Eating foods rich in omega-3 fatty acids is part of a healthy diet and helps people maintain their health.

Description

In recent years, a great deal of attention has been placed on the value of eating a low fat diet. In some cases, people have taken this advice to the extreme by adopting a diet that is far too low in fat or, worse yet, a diet that has no fat at all. But the truth is that not all fat is bad. Although it is true that trans and saturated fats, which are found in high amounts in red meat, butter, whole milk, and some prepackaged foods, have been shown to raise a person's total cholesterol, polyunsaturated fats can actually play a part in keeping cholesterol low. Two especially good fats are the omega-3 fatty acids and the omega-6 fatty acids, which are polyunsaturated.

Two types of omega-3 fatty acids are eicosapentaenoic acid (EPA) and docosahexanoic acid (DHA), which are found mainly in oily cold-water fish, such as tuna, salmon, trout, herring, sardines, bass, swordfish, and mackerel. With the exception of seaweed, most plants do not contain EPA or DHA. However, alpha-linolenic acid (ALA), which is another kind of omega-3 fatty acid, is found in dark green leafy vegetables, flaxseed oil, fish oil, and canola oil, as well as nuts and beans, such as walnuts and soybeans. Enzymes in a person's body can convert ALA to EPA and DHA, which are the two kinds of omega-3 fatty acids easily utilized by the body.

Many experts agree that it is important to maintain a healthy balance between omega-3 fatty acids and omega-6 fatty acids. As Dr. Penny Kris-Etherton and her colleagues reported in their article published in the *American Journal of Nutrition* an over consumption of omega-6 fatty acids has resulted in an unhealthy dietary shift in the American diet. The authors point out that what used to be a 1:1 ratio between omega-3 and omega-6 fatty acids is now estimated to be a 10:1 ratio. This poses a problem, researchers say, because consuming some of the beneficial effects gained from omega-3 fatty acids are negated by an over consumption of omega-6 fatty acids. For example, omega-3 fatty acids have anti-inflammatory properties, whereas omega-6 fatty acids tend to promote inflammation. Cereals, whole grain bread, margarine, and vegetable oils, such as corn, peanut, and sunflower oil, are examples of omega-6 fatty acids. In addition, people consume a lot of omega-6 fatty acid simply by eating the meat of animals that were fed grain rich in omega-6. Some experts suggest that eating one to four times more omega-6 fatty acids than omega-3 fatty acids is a reasonable ratio. In other words, as dietitians often say, the key to a healthy diet is moderation and balance.

The health benefits of omega-3 fatty acids

There is strong evidence that omega-3 fatty acids protect a person against atherosclerosis and therefore against heart disease and stroke, as well as abnormal heart rhythms that cause sudden cardiac death, and possibly autoimmune disorders, such as lupus and rheumatoid arthritis. In fact, Drs. Dean Ornish and Mehmet Oz, renowned heart physicians, said in a 2002 article published in *O Magazine* that the benefits derived from consuming the proper daily dose of omega-3 fatty acids may help to reduce sudden cardiac death by as much as 50%. In fact, in an article published by *American Family Physician*, Dr. Maggie Covington, a clinical assistant professor at the University of Maryland, also emphasized the value of omega-3 fatty acids with regard to cardiovascular health and referred to one of the largest **clinical trials** to date, the GISSI-Prevenzione Trial, to illustrate her point. In the study, 11,324 patients with coronary heart disease were divided into four groups: one group received 300 mg of vitamin E, one group received 850 mg of omega-3 fatty acids, one group received the vitamin E and fatty acids, and one group served as the control group. After a little more than three years, "The group given omega-3 fatty acids only had a 45% reduction in sudden death and a 20% reduction in all-cause mortality," as stated by Dr. Covington.

According to the American Heart Association (AHA), the ways in which omega-3 fatty acids may reduce cardiovascular disease are still being studied. However, the AHA indicates that research as shown that omega-3 fatty acids:

- decrease the risk of arrthythmias, which can lead to sudden cardiac death
- decrease triglyceride levels
- decrease the growth rate of atherosclerotic plaque
- lower blood pressure slightly

In fact, numerous studies show that a diet rich in omega-3 fatty acids not only lowers bad cholesterol, known as LDL, but also lowers triglycerides, the fatty material that circulates in the blood. Interestingly, researchers have found that the cholesterol levels of Inuit Eskimos tend to be quite good, despite the fact that they have a high fat diet. The reason for this, research has found, is that their diet is high in fatty fish, which is loaded with omega-3 fatty acids. The same has often been said about the typical Mediterranean-style diet.

Said to reduce joint inflammation, omega-3 fatty acid supplements have been the focus of many studies attempting to validate its effectiveness in treating rheumatoid arthritis. According to a large body of research in the area, omega-3 fatty acid supplements are clearly effective in reducing the symptoms associated with rheumatoid arthritis, such as joint tenderness and stiffness. In some cases, a reduction in the amount of medication needed by rheumatoid arthritis patients has been noted.

More research needs to be done to substantiate the effectiveness of omega-3 fatty acids in treating eating disorders, attention deficit disorder, and **depression**. Some studies have indicated, for example, that children with behavioral problems and attention deficit disorder have lower than normal amounts of omega-3 fatty acids in their bodies. However, until there is more data in these very important areas of research, a conservative approach should be taken, specially when making changes to a child's diet. Parents should to talk to their child's pediatrician to ascertain if adding more omega-3 fatty acids to their child's diet is appropriate. In addition, parents should take special care to avoid feeding their children fish high in mercury. A food list containing items rich in omega-3 fatty acids can be obtained from a licensed dietitian.

A great deal of media attention has been focused on the high mercury levels found in some types of fish. People concerned about fish consumption and mercury levels can review public releases on the subject issued by the U. S. Food and Drug Administration (FDA) and the Environmental Protection Agency. Special precautions exist for children and pregnant or breastfeeding women. They are advised to avoid shark, mackerel, swordfish, and tilefish. However, both the U.S. Food and Drug Administration and the Environmental Protection Agency emphasis the importance of dietary fish. Fish, they caution, should not be eliminated from the diet. In fact, Robert Oh, M.D., stated in his 2005 article, which was published in *The Journal of the American Board of Family Practice* " With the potential health benefits of fish, women of childbearing age should be encouraged to eat one to two low-mercury fish meals per week."

Mercury levels and concerns about safety

Other concerns regarding fish safety have also been reported. In 2004, Hites and colleagues assessed organic contaminants n salmon in an article published in *Science*. Their conclusion that farmed salmon had higher concentrations of polychlorinated biphenyls than wild salmon prompted public concerns and a response from the American **Cancer** Society. Farmed fish in Europe was found to have higher levels of mercury than farmed salmon in North and South America; however, the American Cancer Society reminded the public that the "levels of toxins Hites and his colleagues found in the farmed salmon were still below what the U. S. Food and Drug Administration, which regulates food, considers hazardous." The American Cancer Society still continues to promote a healthy, varied diet, which includes fish as a food source.

Recommended dosage

The AHA recommends that people eat two servings of fish, such as tuna or salmon, at least twice a week. A person with coronary heart disease, according to the AHA, should consume 1 gram of omega-3 fatty acids daily through food intake, most preferably through the consumption of fatty fish. The AHA also states that "people with elevated triglycerides may need 2 to 4 grams of EPA and DHA per day provided as a supplement," which is available in liquid or capsule form. Ground or cracked flaxseed can easily be incorporated into a person's diet by sprinkling it over salads, soup, and cereal.

Sources differ, but here are some general examples:

- 3 ounces of pickled herring = 1.2 grams of omega-3 fatty acids
- 3 ounces of salmon = 1.3 grams of omega-3 fatty acids
- 3 ounces of halibut = 1.0 grams of omega-3 fatty acids
- 3 ounces of mackerel = 1.6 grams of omega-3 fatty acids
- 1 1/2 teaspoons of flaxseeds = 3 grams of omega-3 fatty acids

Precautions

In early 2004, the U.S. Food and Drug Administration, along with the the Environmental Protection Agency, issued a statement that women who are or may be pregnant, as well as breastfeeding mothers and children, should avoid eating some types of fish thought to contain high levels of mercury. Fish that typically contain high levels of mercury are shark, swordfish, and mackerel, whereas shrimp, canned light tuna, salmon, and catfish are generally thought to have low levels of mercury. Because many people engage in fishing as a hobby, women should be sure before they eat any fish caught by friends and family that the local stream or lake is considered low in mercury.

Conflicting information exists whether it is safe for patients with macular degeneration to take omega-3 fatty acids in supplement form. Until more data becomes available, it is better for people with macular degeneration to receive their omega-3 fatty acids from the food they eat.

Side effects

Fish oil supplements can cause **diarrhea** and gas. Also, the fish oil capsules tend to have a fishy aftertaste.

Interactions

Although there are no significant drug interactions associated with eating foods containing omega-3 fatty acids, patients who are being treated with blood-thinning medications shouldn't take omega-3 fatty acid supplements without seeking the advice of their physicians. Excessive bleeding could result. For the same reason, some patients who plan to take more than 3 grams of omega-3 fatty acids in supplement form should first seek the approval of their physicians.

Resources

PERIODICALS

Albert, C. M., Hennekens, C. H., O'Donnell, C. J., et al. "Fish consumption and risk of sudden cardiac death." *Journal of the American Medical Association* 279 (1998): 23–28.

Covington, M. B. "Omega-3 Fatty Acids." *American Family Physician* 70 (2004): 133–140.

Harris, W. S. "N-3 fatty acids and serum lipoproteins: human studies." *American Journal of Clinical Nutrition* 65 (1997): 1645–1654.

Hites, R. A., Foran, J. A., Carpenter, D. O., et al. W. S. "Global assessment of organic contaminants in farmed salmon." *Science* 303 (1997): 226–229.

Kris-Etherton, P. M., Harris, W. S., Appel, L. J., and American Heart Association Nutrition Committee. "Fish consumption, fish oil, omega-3 fatty acids, and cardiovascular disease." *Circulation* 106 (2003): 2747–2757.

Kris-Etherton, P. M., Taylor, D. S., Yu-Poth, S., et al. "Polyunsaturated fatty acids in the food chain in the United States. " *American Journal of Clinical Nutrition* 71 (2000): 1795–1885.

Oh, R. "Practical applications of fish oil (omega-3 fatty acids) in primary." *The Journal of the American Board of Family Practice* 18 (2005): 28–36.

Ornish, Dean and Oz, Mehmet. "Caution: Strong at Heart." *O: The Oprah Magazine* November 2002:163–168.

ORGANIZATION

American Cancer Society. "Is Salmon Safe?" *American Cancer Society*. 28 Jan 2004 American Cancer Society. [24 Feb 2009] http://www.cancer.org/.

American Heart Association. "American Heart Association Recommendation: Fish and Omega-3 Fatty Acids." *American Heart Association*, 2005. American Heart Association. [22 Feb 2009] http://www.americanheart.org/.

Health and Age. "Omega-3 Fatty Acids." *Health and Age* 2005 [22 Feb 2009]. http://www.healthandage.com/html/res/com/ConsSupplements/Omega3FattyAcidscs.html.

Kris-Etherton, P. M., Harris, W. S., Appel, L. J., and American Heart Association Nutrition Committee. "American Heart Association Statement: New Guidelines Focus on Fish, Fish Oil, Omega-3 Fatty Acids." *American Heart Association*. 18 November 2002. American Heart Association. [22 Feb 2009] http://www.americanheart.org/.

U.S. Food and Drug Administration. "What You Need to Know About Mercury in Fish and Shellfish." *U.S. Food and Drug Administration*. March 2004. U.S. Food and Drug Administration. [22 Feb 2009] http://www.cfsan.fda.gov/~dms/admehg3.html.

Lee Ann Paradise

Ommaya reservoir

Definition

The Ommaya reservoir is a plastic, dome–shaped device, with a catheter (thin tubing) attached to the underside used to deliver **chemotherapy** (**anticancer drugs**) to the central nervous system (CNS or brain and spinal cord).

Purpose

Chemotherapy may be administered to patients by various methods, depending on the type of **cancer** being treated. Some cancer types respond well to chemotherapy given by intravenous (IV) injection, and some cancer types may be treated with oral medication. In both cases, the chemotherapy reaches its target site systemically (carried by the blood). Cancers that affect the CNS pose a special challenge. Systemically delivered drugs seldom reach the CNS because of a network of blood vessels that surround the brain. This protective shield is called the blood–brain barrier. It acts as a filtering device for the brain by blocking the passage of foreign substances from the blood to the CNS. To avoid the obstacle created by the blood–brain barrier, alternative delivery treatments must be used. These treatments are collectively called **intrathecal chemotherapy** treatments. These treatments require injecting the chemotherapy directly into the cerebrospinal fluid (CSF). The CSF is the clear fluid surrounding the CNS. An oncologist (a physician specializing in cancer study and treatment) will determine the frequency of the treatment schedule and will decide if it is better for the patient to receive intrathecal chemotherapy injections directly into the spinal column or through an Ommaya reservoir implanted in the brain. The Ommaya reservoir may be used in several ways. Its primary function is to facilitate the uniform delivery of the intrathecal chemotherapy. By implanting the Ommaya reservoir, multiple rounds of chemotherapy may be given through a single access site, thereby increasing patient comfort and reducing the stress and pain associated with repeated spinal injections. The Ommaya reservoir also serves as a sampling site for removal of CSF. Samples are withdrawn an analyzed for the presence of abnormal cells. Some physicians utilize the reservoir to deliver pain medication, and more recently, trials have been conducted to test the efficacy of using the Ommaya reservoir to deliver gene therapy (treating a disease caused by a malfuncting gene, by introducing a normal gene back into the diseased individual) to cancer patients.

Precautions

High-dose chemotherapy drugs such as **methotrexate** may produce toxic effects if the reservoir or catheter becomes compromised. For infants and children being considered as candidates for an Ommaya reservoir implant, the age of the patient should be considered. Some studies have suggested that infants may be at a higher risk for post–treatment neurologic and endocrinologic problems, cognitive (learning) disabilities, and higher infant mortality when high–dose chemotherapy agents are administered via the Ommaya reservoir. These conditions are significantly reduced in adult patients. Any patient compromised by a pre–existing suppressed immune system should make the physician aware of this condition so the choice of chemotherapy and specific protocols for administering the drugs are employed.

Description

Placement of the Ommaya reservoir requires a minor surgical procedure with the patient placed under general anesthesia. The procedure is performed in the hospital by a neurosurgeon (a physician specially trained to perform surgery on the brain or spinal cord). The reservoir is placed under the scalp with the catheter positioned into the cavity of the brain where the CSF is formed. Once in place, chemotherapy treatments using the Ommaya reservoir may be conducted as outpatient visits either in the hospital, the home, or a satellite clinic staffed by specially trained healthcare professionals. To perform an Ommaya reservoir tap (CSF sampling and chemotherapy delivery) requires 15–20 minutes with little or no pain to the patient. Basic guidelines for the tap include:

- Remove hair from over the reservoir area.
- Gently pump the reservoir to allow the reservoir to fill with CSF.
- Clean the area with alcohol and iodine solution, maintaining a sterile field.
- The healthcare professional will insert a small needle into the reservoir and slowly withdraw a sample of CSF.
- The chemotherapy will be delivered by slowly injecting the prescribed medication into the reservoir.
- The needle is removed and the site covered with sterile gauze.
- Light pressure is applied, and the reservoir is gently pumped to enhance uniform distribution of the chemotherapy into the CSF.
- The site is covered with a Band–Aid.

Preparation

Placement of the Ommaya reservoir will require a minimal stay in the hospital. The surgeon will provide detailed pre–operative instructions for the patient prior to the hospital visit. Post–operative recovery

KEY TERMS

Blood–brain barrier—The blood vessel network surrounding the brain that blocks the passage of foreign substances into the brain.

Central nervous system (CNS)—The body system composed of the brain and spinal cord.

Cerebrospinal fluid (CSF)—The fluid surrounding the brain and spinal cord.

Chemotherapy—Anticancer drugs

Intrathecal chemotherapy—Chemotherapy that must be given directly into the CSF.

QUESTIONS TO ASK THE DOCTOR

- What makes me a good candidate for the Ommaya reservoir?
- What types of chemotherapy will I receive?
- How often will the treatments be scheduled, and will there be side effects after each one?
- How will I know if the Ommaya reservoir is working properly?
- Is this device and procedure covered by insurance?

will monitor vital signs and watch for possible side effects from the anesthesia. Before the patient is discharged, an initial round of chemotherapy administered via the Ommaya reservoir will be performed to assure the device is working properly. No special preparations are required for routine scheduled chemotherapy treatments.

Aftercare

Following an Ommaya tap, the patient may participate in all normal activities. Hair may be washed. There are no special requirements for care of the reservoir site; however, a physician should be notified if symptoms appear such as a spike in **fever**, headaches with or without **vomiting**, neck stiffness, tenderness, redness, or drainage at the access site of the reservoir.

Risks

The most common risks associated with the use of the Ommaya reservoir primarily deal with complications due to malposition or malfunction of the device. Either condition may result in blockage or leakage of the catheter, leading to improper drug delivery. Lesions may develop along the catheter, **infection** may develop, and chemotherapy may reach toxic levels. In cancer patients scheduled for surgical intervention, who have previously received chemotherapy via an Ommaya reservoir, there is some evidence of increased perioperative morbidity (a diseased condition existing at the time of surgery).

Normal results

Patients may expect successful delivery of the intrathecal chemotherapy during each treatment session with minimal discomfort. It should be noted, however, that the chemotherapy delivered by the Ommaya reservoir works on cells that are actively growing and dividing. This means both cancer cells and certain normal cell types may be affected and may result in side effects. Depressed blood cell counts may lower resistance to infection and increase susceptibility to bruising and bleeding. There may be an overall decrease in energy levels. Hair loss (**alopecia**) may occur, and cells of the digestive tract may be damaged resulting in bouts of **nausea**, vomiting, and mouth sores. For female patients, symptoms of menopause may develop, and in males, sperm production may stop.

Abnormal results

Severe complications associated with drug delivery could occur. Due to improper function of the reservoir, toxic levels of chemotherapy could induce behavioral abnormalities, confusion, dementia, irritability, convulsions, sensory impairment, damage to pulmonary and renal function, and patient death.

Resources

BOOKS

Meyer, Fredric B. *Atlas of Neurosurgery, Basic Approaches to Cranial and Vascular Procedures*. Philadelphia: Churchill Livingstone, 1999.

PERIODICALS

Hakim, A., et al. "Ommaya Catheter–Related Staphylococcus Epidermidis Cerebritis and Recurrent Bacteremia Documented by Molecular Typing." *European Journal of Clinical Microbiology and Infectious Disease* 19 (2000): 875–877.

Stone, J.A., et al. "Leukoencephalopathy Complicating an Ommaya Reservoir and Chemotherapy." *Neuroradiology* 41 (1999): 134–136.

OTHER

Adult Brain Tumor Treatment Information for Physicians. CancerLinksUSA com, Inc. [cited April 1, 2009]. http://cancerlinksusa.com.

What is a Brain Tumor? Johns Hopkins University. [cited April 1, 2009]. http://www.med.jhu.edu.

Jane Taylor-Jones, M.S., Research Associate

Oncologic emergencies

Definition

Oncologic or oncological emergencies are serious, life-threatening metabolic and structural complications of **cancer** and its treatments.

Demographics

As both the incidence of cancer and cancer survival rates increase, so does the frequency of oncologic emergencies. However demographic information is limited:

- Tumor lysis syndrome (TLS) is the most common metabolic oncologic emergency in children: 42% of children with intermediate- or high-grade non-Hodgkin lymphomas have laboratory evidence of TLS, although only 6% exhibit symptoms; 70% of children with acute leukemia who receive high-dose chemotherapy for advanced disease have laboratory evidence of TLS, although only 3% have symptoms.
- Hypercalcemia (excess blood calcium) of malignancy affects 20–30% of all cancer patients and 40–50% of those with breast cancer or multiple myeloma.
- Febrile (feverish) neutropenia (deficiency in neutrophils, a type of white blood cell) is one of the most common complications related to cancer treatment, especially chemotherapy, and is a contributing factor in 50% of deaths associated with leukemia, lymphomas, and solid tumors.
- Hyperleukocytosis—dangerously high levels of circulating white blood cells—is the most common hematologic overproduction syndrome requiring emergency treatment in pediatric cancer patients. It is present at diagnosis in 13–22% of patients with acute non-lymphocytic leukemia (ANLL), almost all children with chronic myelogenous leukemia, and 6–15% of children with acute lymphoid leukemia (ALL).
- As many as 10–15% of cancer patients have some degree of pericardial effusion—leakage of fluid from around the heart—and it is a frequent cause of death in patients with otherwise treatable cancers.
- Extravasation injuries—leakage of chemotherapy drugs from a vein into the surrounding tissues—occurs in 0.1–6.5% of chemotherapy infusions.
- Up to 50% of patients undergoing chemotherapy for colon cancer become severely dehydrated from vomiting, diarrhea, and inflammation of mucus membranes.

Description

Oncologic emergencies are a very diverse collection of conditions. Some develop over a period of months, whereas others develop very quickly and can cause paralysis and death in just a few hours. It is not unusual for cancer to be first diagnosed because of an oncologic emergency. Oncologic emergencies also can cause severe pain—an additional oncologic emergency.

Sometimes oncologic emergencies are categorized according to their origins or the affected organ(s); however most often they are classified as:

- metabolic
- hematologic
- structural or mechanical
- cancer-treatment-related or chemotherapy side effects
- infections

The most common metabolic oncologic emergencies include:

- tumor lysis syndrome, a potentially lethal complication of cancer treatment characterized by excess uric acid, potassium, and phosphate in the blood (hyperuricemia, hyperkalemia, and hyperphosphatemia, respectively), with renal (kidney) failure and hypocalcemia (calcium deficiency) as secondary complications
- hypercalcemia of malignancy
- syndrome of inappropriate antidiuretic hormone (SIADH)
- hyponatremia (low blood sodium)
- hypoglycemia (low blood sugar)
- adrenal failure
- lactic acidosis—the accumulation of lactic acid in body tissues

Hematologic emergencies include:

- febrile neutropenia
- hyperviscosity syndrome
- hyperleukocytosis

Structural or mechanical emergencies are classified according to the affected organ system:

- Cardiovascular emergencies include superior vena cava (SVC) syndrome, malignant pericardial effusion, and cardiac tamponade (the mechanical compression of the heart by fluid or blood).
- Neurologic emergencies include epidural spinal cord compression, increased intracranial pressure (ICP), and status epilepticus (prolonged or recurrent seizure activity).
- Respiratory emergencies include airway obstruction.
- Urologic emergencies include upper or lower urinary tract obstruction.
- Gastrointestinal emergencies include obstructions of the gastrointestinal tract.

Emergency side effects of **chemotherapy** include:

- extravasation injuries
- gastrointestinal emergencies such as severe dehydration
- inflammatory conditions including inflammation of the lungs (pneumonitis), pancreas (pancreatitis), urinary

bladder (hemorrhagic cystitis), or intestines (enterocolitis), and tissue death (necrosis)

Both cancer and its treatments put patients at risk for acute life-threatening infections by:

- bacteria
- fungi
- viruses
- parasites

Risk factors

Different types of cancer are risk factors for different oncologic emergencies:

- TLS is more common with hematologic malignancies and with bulky, rapidly growing, aggressive, and treatment-sensitive tumors. It is often associated with acute leukemias, such as ALL and acute myeloid leukemia (AML), and high-grade non-Hodgkin lymphomas such as Burkitt lymphoma.
- Hypercalcemia occurs with various cancers. It is most commonly associated with multiple myeloma and cancers of the lung, breast, and kidney. It can occur in children with acute lymphoblastic leukemia, non-Hodgkin lymphoma, neuroblastoma, and various other types of tumors.
- Hematologic emergencies involving the overproduction of certain types of blood cells are associated with acute leukemia.
- Hyperviscosity syndrome is most common in patients with Waldenstrom's macroglobulinemia, leukemia, or multiple myeloma.
- SVC syndrome is most often caused by lung cancer, but can also be caused by other chest tumors or by catheters.
- Most pericardial effusions develop from metastatic lung or breast cancer, but they also can be caused by malignant melanoma, leukemia, lymphoma, chemotherapy, or radiation therapy to the chest wall.
- Epidural spinal cord compression is most often associated with breast and lung cancers, but also occurs with renal and prostate cancers.
- Airway obstruction is the most common respiratory emergency in children with cancer and is associated with leukemia, lymphoma, Hodgkin disease, rhabdomyosarcoma, and neuroblastoma.

Any type of immunosuppression is a risk factor for **infection**. **Neutropenia** from leukemia, chemotherapy, or **radiation therapy** is a major risk factor for bacterial and fungal infections. Corticosteroid treatment, catheters, dysfunction or removal of the spleen, and various other procedures also increase the risk of infection.

Causes and symptoms

Among metabolic emergencies:

- TLS is caused by the rapid destruction of cancer cells upon the initiation of radiation therapy or chemotherapy. The rapid release into the bloodstream of the contents of large numbers of cancer cells overwhelms the ability of the body to maintain balances of uric acid, potassium, phosphates, and calcium. TLS usually develops within one to five days of treatment.
- Hypercalcemia of malignancy usually results from bone loss (resorption), which disrupts calcium regulation, causing a variety of symptoms including nausea, vomiting, constipation, progressive decline in mental function, renal failure, and coma.
- SIADH often is caused by the production of antidiuretic hormone by cancer cells. It also can be caused by certain chemotherapy drugs. Symptoms may include anorexia nervosa, nausea, muscle pain, headaches, and severe neurologic symptoms including seizures or coma.
- Hyponatremia usually results from water retention combined with normal or excessive administration of fluids. Some chemotherapy drugs interfere with water secretion, causing hyponatremia. Symptoms are primarily neurologic and can be life-threatening.
- Hypoglycemia is most often caused by tumors of the insulin-producing islet cells. Symptoms are neurologic.

Hematologic emergencies are caused by abnormal blood cell production—most often low production of a particular type of blood cell—or by hemorrhage and/or thrombosis (a clot in a blood vessel):

- Underproduction of blood cells is caused by disease infiltration of the bone marrow, bone marrow failure, or treatment, resulting in anemia (red blood cell deficiency), thrombocytopenia (decreased platelets), and neutropenia. Neutropenia is most often a side effect of chemotherapy. Low neutrophil counts leave patients vulnerable to infection.
- Hyperviscosity syndrome is caused by elevated levels of circulating serum immunoglobulins (antibodies) that coat the cells, causing increased blood viscosity, sludging of the blood, and decreased blood flow through the organs. Symptoms include spontaneous bleeding, neurologic defects, and vision changes.
- Symptoms of hyperleukocytosis are usually respiratory and neurologic.

Structural oncologic emergencies are caused by direct compression, obstruction, or displacement of tissues by cancer:

- The superior vena cava, the second largest vein in the body, returns blood from the upper part of the body to the atrium of the heart. SVC obstruction is caused by external compression or an internal clot. SVC compression leads to swelling or discoloration of the neck, head, face, or upper extremities. Other symptoms of SVC syndrome may include cough, hoarseness, chest pain, labored breathing, difficulty swallowing, and distension of the superficial veins in the chest wall, progressing to headache, confusion, altered vision, and loss of consciousness.
- Symptoms of pericardial effusions include difficult or labored breathing, especially when lying down, fatigue, heart palpitations, and dizziness. Other symptoms may include a pulse that weakens during inspiration, rapid heart rate, and distended neck veins. Pericardial effusion often goes undiagnosed in cancer patients.
- Cardiac tamponade is the inability of the heart ventricle to maintain cardiac output because of external pressure or an intrinsic mass.
- Epidural spinal cord compression is caused by a tumor that compresses the spinal cord, most often in the thoracic spine between the neck and the abdomen. Symptoms include new back pain and pain that worsens when lying down. Late neurologic signs include weakness, incontinence, and sensory defects. Epidural spinal cord compression can cause permanent neurologic impairment if treatment is delayed for even a few hours.
- Increased intracranial pressure (ICP) is associated with cerebral herniation, which can result from an expanding mass in the head or from an obstruction of cerebrospinal fluid circulation. Symptoms include impaired consciousness, abnormal eye movements, abnormal pupil size, nausea, vomiting, and a stiff neck.
- Status epilepticus can result from either mechanical or metabolic perturbation of the central nervous system from a tumor or from treatment.
- Symptoms of gastrointestinal obstruction may include cramping, abdominal pain, an abdominal mass, and currant-jelly stool.

Many chemotherapy agents, such as anthracyclines and vinca alkaloids, are irritants or blistering agents. Leakage of these agents onto the skin during infusion therapy can cause severe scarring and irreversible damage to joints. Symptoms of extravasation injuries include redness, swelling, and necrosis at the infusion site, usually within hours of chemotherapy.

Dehydration is a serious side effect of cancer treatment that is often overlooked. Up to 30% of cancer patients with delirium are dehydrated.

Severe constipation, characterized by hard stools every three to five days and abdominal pain, is commonly associated with narcotic medications, but also sometimes with neurotoxic chemotherapy agents.

Among inflammatory conditions:

- Noninfectious pneumonitis can be a complication of radiation therapy, chemotherapy, stem cell transplantation, or transfusions. Symptoms range from none to respiratory failure.
- Pancreatitis is a complication of some chemotherapies and systemic steroid treatment. The primary symptom is severe abdominal pain.
- Hemorrhagic cystitis is most often caused by cyclophosphamide and ifosfamide. It also is associated with pelvic irradiation and viral infections. Symptoms can occur anywhere from hours to years after treatment. Painful urination is the major symptom.

Infectious emergencies most often are caused by immunosuppression. The most common sources of bacterial infections are skin and gastrointestinal tract bacteria. Common causes of bacterial infectious emergencies in cancer patients include:

- enterobacteria
- *Staphylococcus* spp.
- *Streptococcus* spp.
- *Enterococcus* spp.
- *Pseudomonas aeruginosae*
- *Aeromonas hydrophila*
- *Bacillus* spp.
- *Corynebacteria* spp.
- *Haemophilus influenzae*
- *Neisseria meningitidis*
- *Salmonella* spp.
- *Escherichia coli*
- *Listeria monocytogenes*
- *Legionella* spp.
- *Nocardia* spp.
- *Clostridium difficile*
- *Mycobacterium tuberculosis*
- atypical mycobacteria

Fungal infections in cancer patients often are caused by:

- *Candida* spp.
- *Aspergillus* spp.
- *Fusarium* spp.
- *Cryptococcus neoformans*
- *Coccidioides immitis*
- Mucoraceae

Viral infections that can be emergencies in cancer patients include:

- herpes viruses
- influenza
- parainfluenza
- echovirus
- measles virus
- varicella
- respiratory syncytial virus (RSV)
- adenoviruses

Parasites that can cause infectious emergencies include:

- *Giardia lamblia*
- *Cryptosporidium* spp.
- *Toxoplasma gondii*
- *Strongyloides stercoralis*
- *Babesia microti*

Diagnosis

Examination

Oncologic emergencies are often diagnosed based on symptoms, the type of cancer, and the patient's treatments. Symptoms of bacterial infections include a temperature of at least 101°F (38.3°C).

Tests

There are a variety of tests used to diagnose oncologic emergencies:

- Tests for TLS include serum electrolytes, blood urea nitrogen (BUN), uric acid, serum potassium, phosphate, magnesium, calcium, creatinine, and lactic dehydrogenase (LDH) levels, and an electrocardiogram (ECG). Elevated levels of uric acid, potassium, phosphate, or LDH before the start of chemotherapy indicate that TLS is already present or impending.
- Laboratory testing for SIADH may reveal hyponatremia (low serum sodium levels), decreased serum osmolarity, and concentrated urine.
- High serum viscosity is indicative of hyperviscosity syndrome.
- SVC syndrome diagnosis may include microscopic examination of the sputum and/or chest fluid obtained via thoracentesis or needle aspiration.
- Hemorrhagic cystitis is suggested by leukocytes and erythrocytes (white and red blood cells) or clots in the urine.
- Infections are diagnosed by various blood tests and culturing of the skin, blood, and/or stool, a complete blood count, an absolute neutrophil count (ANC), BUN, serum creatinine, and transaminase measurements.

Procedures

Diagnostic procedures for many oncologic emergencies may include **x rays**, **magnetic resonance imaging** (MRI), **computed tomography** (CT) scans, ultrasound, and/or fluoroscopy:

- Although SVC syndrome is a clinical diagnosis, plain radiography, CT scans, and venography (radiography of the vein) are used to confirm the diagnosis. Bronchoscopy may be used to examine the bronchi.
- Pericardial effusions are diagnosed by echocardiography and fluid samples examined under the microscope.
- Epidural spinal cord compression may be diagnosed by radiography and MRI.
- Chest x rays are used to diagnose infections with respiratory symptoms.

Treatment

Traditional

Treatment of oncologic emergencies is initiated as soon as possible:

- Treatment for TLS includes inpatient monitoring, hyperhydration, urinary alkalinization with sodium bicarbonate, and hemodialysis. Hyperkalemia treatment may include removing potassium from IV fluids and administering sodium polystyrene resin and calcium gluconate. Treatment for hyperphosphatemia may include aluminum hydroxide.
- Hypercalcemia of malignancy is treated with aggressive rehydration and possibly hemodialysis.
- SIADH usually is treated immediately with fluid restriction and slow correction of serum sodium levels, as well as treatment of the underlying tumor.
- Hyponatremia is treated with saline administration and management of fluid volume.
- Hypoglycemia is treated with increased feeding and intravenous (IV) dextrose.
- Depressed bone marrow activity may be treated with transfusion of individual blood components. Severe anemia is treated with blood transfusions.
- Hyperviscosity syndrome is treated with plasmapheresis (removal of blood plasma), followed by targeted chemotherapy.
- Leukocytosis is addressed by anti-leukemic treatments to reduce peripheral leukocytes.
- SVC syndrome treatments include chemotherapy and radiation to reduce the tumor that is causing the

obstruction or intravenous stents to open the vein. The head of the patient's bed is elevated.

- Acute symptoms of pericardial effusion are treated with pericardiocentesis (surgical puncture of the pericardium to aspirate the fluid) or a pericardial window procedure. Chemotherapy, radiation, or sclerosis therapy can prevent fluid reaccumulation.
- Most patients with epidural spinal cord compression need radiation treatment or surgery and possibly chemotherapy.
- Gastrointestinal obstruction from external compression is treated with chemotherapy, surgery, radiation therapy, or a combination.
- Extravasation injuries require prompt diagnosis to avoid extensive skin damage. The infusion is halted and the excess drug is aspirated. Depending on the drug, ice or warm packs are applied. Pressure to the site is avoided.
- Dehydration is treated by fluid resuscitation.
- Urinary obstruction may require the removal of clots or placement of a catheter.
- Hemorrhagic cystitis is treated with hyperhydration, continuous bladder irrigation, platelet transfusion, and treatment of poor blood coagulation.

Drugs

Drug treatments for oncologic emergencies include:

- allopurinol (Zyloprim) or recombinant urate oxidase (Rasburicase) to lower uric acid levels, and diuretics, insulin, and dextrose for hyperkalemia of TLS
- furosemide (Lasix), intravenous bisphosphonates, glucocorticoids, calcitonin (Miacalcin), plicamycin (Mithracin), gallium nitrate (Ganite), pamidronate (Aredia), and zoledronic acid (Zometa) for hypercalcemia of malignancy
- furosemide for SIADH
- demeclocycline (Declomycin) for persistent hyponatremia
- corticosteroids and glucagon for hypoglycemia
- broad-spectrum antibiotics, possibly multiple antibiotics or vancomycin and antifungal agents, myeloid growth factors, granulocyte colony-stimulating factor (G-CSF), granulocyte-macrophage colony-stimulating factor (GM-CSF), and androgens for neutropenia
- diuretics, corticosteroids, thrombolytics, and anticoagulatants for superior vena cava syndrome
- dexamethasone (Cortastat) for neurologic symptoms of epidural spinal cord compression
- antidotes for extravasation injuries
- anti-vomiting and antidiarrheals for dehydration
- corticosteroids for noninfectious pneumonitis
- oxybutynin chloride (Ditropan) for relief of bladder spasms associated with hemorrhagic cystitis
- antibiotics for bacterial infections
- anti-fungal agents, especially amphotericin B, for fungal infections
- antiviral agents for viral infections

QUESTIONS TO ASK YOUR DOCTOR

- What type of oncologic emergency do I have?
- How is it related to my cancer?
- How will my emergency condition be treated?
- What is my prognosis?

Prognosis

If untreated or if treatment is delayed, most oncologic emergencies lead to severe impairment, irreversible damage, and possibly death. Untreated epidural **spinal cord compression** can result in permanent paraplegia. Prognoses for treated oncologic emergencies vary tremendously depending on the specific condition, the underlying cancer, and various other factors. **Hypercalcemia** of malignancy has a poor prognosis, with more than 50% of patients dying within 30 days of diagnosis. Patients with SVC syndrome usually have advanced disease and less than 10% survive for more than 30 months following treatment.

Prevention

Some oncologic emergencies can be foreseen and prevented. Infections may be prevented by prophylactic administration of **antibiotics** and antifungal agents in patients undergoing stem cell transplants and some chemotherapies. Prevention of TLS includes:

- identifying high-risk patients
- allopurinol or urate oxidase to lower uric acid levels
- alkalinization to inhibit the precipitation of uric acid crystals in the tubules of the kidneys
- limiting potassium and phosphorus intake
- hydration to maximize excretion of uric acid, potassium, and phosphate
- ECG monitoring before the start of chemotherapy

Resources

BOOKS

Daya, Mohamud, and Charles R. Thomas, eds. *Cancer Emergencies, Part 1*. Philadelphia: Saunders, 2009.

Dutcherand, Janice, and Peter Wiernik. *Hematologic and Oncologic Emergencies*. New York: McGraw-Hill, 2008.

Kaplan, Marcelle, ed. *Understanding and Managing Oncologic Emergencies: A Resource for Nurses*. Pittsburg, PA: Oncology Nursing Society, 2006.

PERIODICALS

Grafton, Eileen. "Detecting Oncological Emergencies.' *Australian Nursing Journal* 15, no. 9 (April 2008): 35.

Halfdanarson, T., W. Hogan, and T. Moynihan. "Oncologic Emergencies: Diagnosis and Treatment." *Mayo Clinic Proceedings* 81, no. 6 (2006): 835-848.

Higdon, Mark L., and Jennifer A. Higdon. "Treating Oncologic Emergencies." *American Family Physician* 74, no. 11 (December 1, 2006): 1873-1880.

OTHER

Ikeda, Alan K., et al. "Tumor Lysis Syndrome.' *eMedicine*. http://emedicine.medscape.com/article/989050-overview.

Krishnan, Koyamangalath, and Ahmad Hammad. "Tumor Lysis Syndrome.' *eMedicine*.http://emedicine.medscape.com/article/282171-overview.

Taylor, Douglas S., and Amanda S. Penny. "Oncologic Emergencies." *eMedicine*.http://emedicine.medscape com/article/990480-overview.

ORGANIZATIONS

American Cancer Society, 1599 Clifton Road NE, Atlanta, GA, 30329-4251, (800) ACS-2345, http://www.cancer.org.

National Cancer Institute, NCI Public Inquiries Office, 6116 Executive Boulevard, Room 3036A, Bethesda, MD, 20006, (800) 4-CANCER, http://www.cancer.gov.

Margaret Alic, PhD

Ondansetron *see* **Antiemetics**

Oophorectomy

Definition

Unilateral oophorectomy (also called an ovariectomy) is the surgical removal of an ovary. If one ovary is removed, a woman may continue to menstruate and have children. If both ovaries are removed, a procedure called a bilateral oophorectomy, menstruation stops and a woman loses the ability to have children.

Purpose

Oophorectomy is performed to:

- remove cancerous ovaries
- remove the source of estrogen that stimulates some cancers
- remove a large ovarian cyst
- excise an abscess
- treat endometriosis

In an oophorectomy, one or a portion of one ovary may be removed or both ovaries may be removed. When an oophorectomy is done to treat **ovarian cancer** or other spreading cancers, both ovaries are removed (called a bilateral oophorectomy). Removal of the ovaries and fallopian tubes is performed in about one-third of hysterectomies (surgical removal of the uterus), often to reduce the risk of ovarian **cancer**.

Oophorectomies are sometimes performed on premenopausal women who have estrogen-sensitive **breast cancer** in an effort to remove the main source of estrogen from their bodies. This procedure has become less common than it was in the 1990s. Today, **chemotherapy** drugs are available that alter the production of estrogen and **tamoxifen** blocks any of the effects any remaining estrogen may have on cancer cells.

Until the 1980s, women over age 40 having hysterectomies routinely had healthy ovaries and fallopian tubes removed at the same time. This operation is called a bilateral salpingo-oophorectomy. Many physicians reasoned that a woman over 40 was approaching menopause and soon her ovaries would stop secreting estrogen and releasing eggs. Removing the ovaries would eliminate the risk of ovarian cancer and only accelerate menopause by a few years.

In the 1990s, the thinking about routine oophorectomy began to change. The risk of ovarian cancer in women who have no family history of the disease is less than 1%. Meanwhile, removing the ovaries increases the risk of cardiovascular disease and accelerates osteoporosis unless a woman takes prescribed hormone replacements.

Under certain circumstances, oophorectomy may still be the treatment of choice to prevent breast and ovarian cancer in certain high-risk women. A study done at the University of Pennsylvania and released in 2000 showed that healthy women who carried the BRCA1 or BRCA2 genetic mutations that pre-disposed them to breast cancer had their risk of breast cancer drop from 80–19% when their ovaries were removed before age 40. Women between the ages of 40 and 50 showed less risk reduction, and there was no

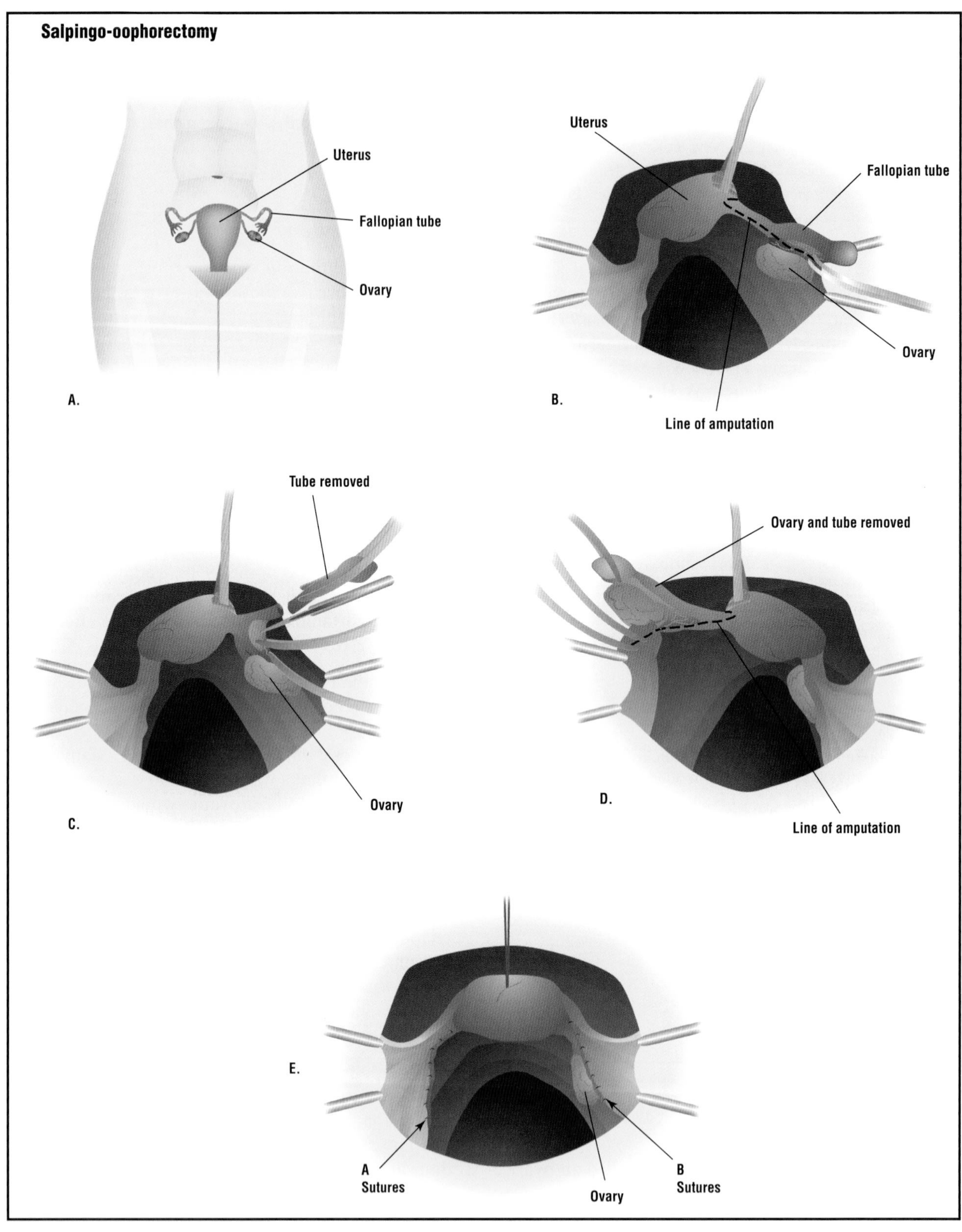

(Illustration by Argosy Publishing. Cengage Learning, Gale.)

significant reduction of breast cancer risk in women over age 50. A 2002 study showed that five years after being identified as carrying BRCA1 or BRCA2 genetic mutations, 94% of women who had received a bilateral salpingo-oophorectomy were cancer-free, compared to 79% of women who had not received surgery.

The value of ovary removal in preventing both breast and ovarian cancer has been documented. However, there are disagreements within the medical community about when and at what age this treatment should be offered. Preventative oophorectomy, also called prophylactic oophorectomy, is not always covered by insurance. One study conducted in 2000 at the University of California at San Francisco found that only 20% of insurers paid for preventive bilateral oophorectomy (PBO). Another 25% had a policy against paying for the operation, and the remaining 55% said that they would decide about payment on an individual basis.

Demographics

Overall, ovarian cancer accounts for only 4% of all cancers in women. But the lifetime risk for developing ovarian cancer in women who have mutations in BRCA1 is significantly increased over the general population and may cause an ovarian cancer risk of 30% by age 60. For women at increased risk, oophorectomy may be considered after the age of 35 if childbearing is complete.

Other factors that increase a woman's risk of developing ovarian cancer include age (most ovarian cancers occur after menopause), the number of menstrual periods a woman has had (affected by age of onset, pregnancy, breastfeeding, and oral contraceptive use), history of breast cancer, diet, and family history. The incidence of ovarian cancer is highest among Native Americans (17.5 cases per 100,000 population), white (15.8 per 100,000), Vietnamese (13.8 per 100,000), white Hispanic (12.1 per 100,000), and Hawaiian (11.8 per 100,000) women; it is lowest among Korean (7.0 per 100,000) and Chinese (9.3 per 100,000) women. African American women have an ovarian cancer incidence of 10.2 per 100,000 population.

Description

Oophorectomy is done under general or regional anesthesia. It is often performed through the same type of incision, either vertical or horizontal, as an abdominal hysterectomy. Horizontal incisions leave a less noticeable scar, but vertical incisions give the surgeon a better view of the abdominal cavity. After the incision is made, the abdominal muscles are stretched apart, not cut, so that the surgeon can see the ovaries. Then the ovaries, and often the fallopian tubes, are removed.

Oophorectomy can sometimes be done with a laparoscopic procedure. With this surgery, a tube containing a tiny lens and light source is inserted through a small incision in the navel. A camera can be attached that allows the surgeon to see the abdominal cavity on a video monitor. When the ovaries are detached, they are removed though a small incision at the top of the vagina. The ovaries can also be cut into smaller sections and removed.

The advantages of abdominal incision are that the ovaries can be removed even if a woman has many adhesions from previous surgery. The surgeon gets a good view of the abdominal cavity and can check the surrounding tissue for disease. A vertical abdominal incision is mandatory if cancer is suspected. The disadvantages are that bleeding is more likely to be a complication of this type of operation. The operation is more painful than a laparoscopic operation and the recovery period is longer. A woman can expect to be in the hospital two to five days and will need three to six weeks to return to normal activities.

Diagnosis/Preparation

Before surgery, the doctor will order blood and urine tests, and any additional tests such as ultrasound or **x rays** to help the surgeon visualize the woman's condition. The woman may also meet with the anesthesiologist to evaluate any special conditions that might affect the administration of anesthesia. A colon preparation may be done, if extensive surgery is anticipated.

KEY TERMS

Cyst—An abnormal sac containing fluid or semisolid material.

Endometriosis—A benign condition that occurs when cells from the lining of the uterus begin growing outside the uterus.

Fallopian tubes—Slender tubes that carry ova from the ovaries to the uterus.

Hysterectomy—Surgical removal of the uterus.

Osteoporosis—The excessive loss of calcium from the bones, causing the bones to become fragile and break easily.

On the evening before the operation, the woman should eat a light dinner, then take nothing by mouth, including water or other liquids, after midnight.

Aftercare

After surgery a woman will feel discomfort. The degree of discomfort varies and is generally greatest with abdominal incisions, because the abdominal muscles must be stretched out of the way so that the surgeon can reach the ovaries. In order to minimize the risk of postoperative **infection**, **antibiotics** will be given.

When both ovaries are removed, women who do not have cancer are started on hormone replacement therapy to ease the symptoms of menopause that occur because estrogen produced by the ovaries is no longer present. If even part of one ovary remains, it will produce enough estrogen that a woman will continue to menstruate, unless her uterus was removed in a hysterectomy. To help offset the higher risks of heart and bone disease after loss of the ovaries, women should get plenty of exercise, maintain a low-fat diet, and ensure intake of calcium is adequate.

Return to normal activities takes anywhere from two to six weeks, depending on the type of surgery. When women have cancer, chemotherapy or radiation are often given in addition to surgery. Some women have emotional trauma following an oophorectomy, and can benefit from counseling and support groups.

Risks

Oophorectomy is a relatively safe operation, although, like all major surgery, it does carry some risks. These include unanticipated reaction to anesthesia, internal bleeding, blood clots, accidental damage to other organs, and post-surgery infection.

Complications after an oophorectomy include changes in sex drive, hot flashes, and other symptoms of menopause if both ovaries are removed. Women who have both ovaries removed and who do not take estrogen replacement therapy run an increased risk for cardiovascular disease and osteoporosis. Women with a history of psychological and emotional problems before an oophorectomy are more likely to experience psychological difficulties after the operation.

Complications may arise if the surgeon finds that cancer has spread to other places in the abdomen. If the cancer cannot be removed by surgery, it must be treated with chemotherapy and radiation.

WHO PERFORMS THE PROCEDURE AND WHERE IS IT PERFORMED?

Oophorectomies are usually performed in a hospital operating room by a gynecologist, a medical doctor who has completed specialized training in the areas of women's general health, pregnancy, labor and childbirth, prenatal testing, and genetics.

QUESTIONS TO ASK THE DOCTOR

- Why is a oophorectomy being recommended?
- How will the procedure be performed?
- Will I have a remaining ovary (or portion of ovary)?
- What alternatives to oophorectomy are available to me?

Normal results

If the surgery is successful, the ovaries will be removed without complication, and the underlying problem resolved. In the case of cancer, all the cancer will be removed. A woman will become infertile following a bilateral oophorectomy.

Morbidity and mortality rates

Studies have shown that the complication rate following oophorectomy is essentially the same as that following hysterectomy. The rate of complications associated with hysterectomy differs by the procedure performed. Abdominal hysterectomy is associated with a higher rate of complications (9.3%), while the overall complication rate for vaginal hysterectomy is 5.3%, and 3.6% for laparoscopic vaginal hysterectomy. The risk of death is about one in every 1,000 women having a hysterectomy. The rates of some of the more commonly reported complications are:

- excessive bleeding (hemorrhaging): 1.8–3.4%
- fever or infection: 0.8–4.0%
- accidental injury to another organ or structure: 1.5–1.8%

Because of the cessation of hormone production that occurs with a bilateral oophorectomy, women who lose both ovaries also prematurely lose the protection these hormones provide against heart disease and osteoporosis. Women who have undergone bilateral oophorectomy are seven times more likely to develop coronary heart disease and much more likely to develop bone problems at an early age than are premenopausal women whose ovaries are intact.

Alternatives

Depending on the specific condition that warrants an oophorectomy, it may be possible to modify the surgery so at least a portion of one ovary remains, allowing the woman to avoid early menopause. In the case of prophylactic oophorectomy, drugs such as tamoxifen may be administered to block the effects that estrogen may have on cancer cells.

Resources

PERIODICALS

Kauff, N. D., J. M. Satagopan, M. E. Robson, et al. "Risk-Reducing Salpingo-oophorectomy in Women With a BRC1 or BRC2 Mutation." *New England Journal of Medicine* 346 (May 23, 2002): 1609–15.

ORGANIZATIONS

American Cancer Society. 1599 Clifton Road NE, Atlanta, GA 30329. (800) ACS-2345. http://www.cancer.org.

American College of Obstetricians and Gynecologists. 409 12th St., SW, PO Box 96920, Washington, DC 20090-6920. http://www.acog.org.

Cancer Information Service, National Cancer Institute. Building 31, Room 10A19, 9000 Rockville Pike, Bethesda, MD 20892. (800) 4-CANCER. http://www.nci.nih.gov/cancerinfo/index.html.

OTHER

"Ovarian Cancer: Detailed Guide." *American Cancer Society*. October 20, 2000 [cited March 14, 2009]. http://www.cancer.org/downloads/CRI/CRC_-_OVARIAN_CANCER.pdf.

"Removing Ovaries Lowers Risk for Women at High Risk of Breast, Ovarian Cancer." *ACS News Today* November 8, 2000. [cited May 13, 2009]. http://www.cancer.org.

Surveillance, Epidemiology, and End Results. "Racial/Ethnic Patterns of Cancer in the United States: Ovary." *National Cancer Institute*. 1996 [cited March 14, 2009]. <http://seer.cancer.gov/publications/ethnicity/ovary.pdf>.

Tish Davidson, A.M.
Stephanie Dionne Sherk

Opioids

Definition

Opioids are narcotic drugs that are generally prescribed to manage pain. The most commonly prescribed opioids are: buprenorphine, butorphanol, codeine, fentanyl, hydrocodone, hydromorphone, levorphanol, **meperidine**, methadone, morphine, nalbuphine, oxycodone, oxymorphone, pentazocine, and propoxyphene. These opioids are prescribed alone or in combination with aspirin or acetaminophen (Tylenol).

The most common brand names for these drugs are:

- Actiq
- Astramorph PF
- Buprenex
- Cotanal-65
- Darvon
- Demerol
- Dilaudid
- Dolophine
- Duragesic
- Duramorph
- Hydrostat IR
- Kadian
- Levo-Dromoran
- Methadose
- M S Contin
- MSIR
- MS/L
- MS/S
- Nubain
- Numorphan
- OMS
- Oramorph SR
- OxyContin
- PP-Cap
- Rescudose
- RMS Uniserts
- Roxanol
- Roxicodone
- Stadol
- Talwin

When combined with aspirin or acetaminophen, the most common brand names are:

- Allay
- Anexsia
- Anolor
- Bancap-HC
- Capital with Codeine
- Co-Gesic
- Damason-P
- Darvocet
- Darvon
- DHCplus
- Dolacet
- Dolagesic
- Duocet
- E-Lor
- Empirin with codeine
- Endocet
- Endodan
- EZ III
- Hycomed
- Hyco-Pap
- Hydrocet
- Hydrogesic
- HY-PHEN
- Lorcet
- Lortab
- Margesic
- Oncet
- Panacet
- Panasal
- Panlor
- Percocet
- Percodan
- Phenaphen with codeine
- Polygesic
- Propacet
- Propoxyphene Compound-65
- Pyregesic-C
- Roxicet
- Roxilox
- Roxiprin
- Stagesic
- Synalgos-DC
- Talacen
- Talwin compound
- T-Gesic
- Tylenol with codeine
- Tylox
- Ugesic
- Vanacet
- Vendone
- Vicodin
- Vicoprofen
- Wygesic
- Zydone

KEY TERMS

Central nervous system depressant—Any drug that tends to reduce the activity of the central nervous system. The major drug categories included in this classification are alcohol, anesthetics, antianxiety medications, antihistamines, antipsychotics, hypnotics, narcotics, sedatives, and tranquilizers.

Narcotic—Any drug that produces insensibility or stupor and/or generally causes effects similar to those caused by morphine.

Purpose

Opioids are primarily used to manage pain. Some narcotics are also used just prior to, or during, surgery to increase the effectiveness of certain anesthetics. Codeine and hydrocodone are used to relieve coughing. Methadone is used to help people control their dependence on heroine or other narcotics.

Description

Opioids act on the central nervous system (CNS) to relieve pain. Many of these drugs are habit-forming and physical dependence may lead to withdrawal side effects when the medication is stopped. Because of the potential habit-forming nature of these drugs, most prescriptions cannot be refilled and a new prescription must be obtained after each preceding prescription runs out.

Recommended dosage

Opioids may be taken either orally (in pill or liquid form), by injection (or as part of an intravenous [IV]. line), as an anal suppository, or as a patch attached to the skin. The dosage prescribed may vary widely depending on the patient, the **cancer** being treated, and whether or not other medications are also being taken.

A typical adult dosage for buprenorphine is 0.3 mg injected into a muscle or vein every six hours as necessary. For children between the ages of two and twelve years, the dosage is typically 0.002–0.006 mg per kilogram (2.2 pounds) of body weight.

A typical adult dosage for butorphanol is 1–4 mg injected into a muscle or 0.5–2 mg injected into a vein every four hours as necessary. For children between the ages of two and twelve years, the dosage is typically based on the body weight of the child.

A typical adult dosage for codeine is 15–60 mg taken orally or injected into a muscle or vein every four to six hours as necessary for pain. This dosage is decreased to 10–20 mg when codeine is used to control coughing.

Fentanyl is most often used to manage pain in cancer patients who are already receiving and are tolerant to other opioids. This drug is available as a lozenge and as a skin patch. It is not used for the treatment of pain caused by injury or surgery. The dosage of fentanyl is determined on an individual patient basis by that patient's oncologist.

A typical adult dosage for hydrocodone is 5–10 mg taken orally every four to six hours as necessary for pain, 5 mg to control coughing.

A typical adult dosage for hydromorphone is 1–2 mg injected into a muscle, 2–2.5 mg taken orally, or 3 mg taken as a suppository every three to six hours as necessary.

A typical adult dosage for levorphanol is 2–4 mg taken orally or injected into a vein every four hours as necessary.

A typical adult dosage for meperidine is 100 mg taken orally or injected into a muscle or vein every four hours as necessary.

A typical adult dosage for methadone is 5–20 mg as an oral solution, 2.5–10 mg as an oral tablet or injection, every four to eight hours as necessary for pain. When used for detoxification, methadone is initially given in a dose of 15–40 mg per day as an oral solution. This dose is then decreased until the patient no longer requires the medication. The injection form of methadone is only used for detoxification in patients who are unable to take the medication by mouth.

Morphine is most often used to manage severe, chronic pain in patients who have already been receiving other narcotic pain relievers. The starting dose of morphine is generally determined based on the dosages of prior narcotic pain relievers the patient had been receiving. A typical starting dose is 5–30 mg every four hours.

A typical adult dosage for nalbuphine is 10 mg injected into a muscle or vein every three to six hours as necessary.

A typical adult dosage for oxycodone is 5 mg taken orally every three to six hours, or 10–40 mg taken as a suppository three to four times per day as necessary.

A typical adult dosage for oxymorphone is 1–1.5 mg injected into a muscle every three to six hours, or 5 mg taken as a suppository every four to six hours as necessary.

A typical adult dosage for pentazocine is 50 mg taken orally, or 30 mg injected into a muscle or vein every three to four hours as necessary.

Propoxyphene comes in two salt forms: propoxyphene hydrochloride and propoxyphene napsylate. The typical adult dosage for propoxyphene hydrochloride is 65 mg taken orally every four hours with a maximum daily dosage of 390 mg. The typical adult dosage for propoxyphene napsylate is 100 mg taken orally every four hours with a maximum daily dosage of 600 mg.

Precautions

Opioids magnify the effects of alcohol and other central nervous system depressants, such as antihistamines, cold medicines, sedatives, tranquilizers, other prescription and over-the-counter pain medications, barbiturates, seizure medications, muscle relaxants, and certain anesthetics including some dental anesthetics. Alcohol and other central nervous system depressants should not be taken or consumed while opioids are being taken.

Opioids are powerful narcotics. These drugs can cause some people to feel drowsy, dizzy, or lightheaded. People taking opioids should not drive a car or operate machinery.

Opioids can be habit-forming. Patients who have been taking these types of medication for a period of several weeks should not stop taking this type of medication all at once. The dosage should be slowly tapered off to avoid potential withdrawal side effects.

Intentional or accidental overdose of any of the opioids can lead to unconsciousness, coma, or death. The signs of opioid overdose include confusion, difficulty speaking, seizures, severe nervousness or restlessness, severe dizziness, severe drowsiness, and/or slow or troubled breathing. These symptoms are increased by alcohol or other central nervous system depressants. Anyone who feels that he or she, or someone else, may have overdosed on opioids, or a combination of opioids and other central nervous system depressants, should seek emergency medical attention for that person at once.

Opioids can interfere with or exacerbate certain medical conditions. For these reasons, it is important that the prescribing physician is aware of any current case, or history of:

- alcohol abuse
- brain disease or head injury
- colitis
- drug dependency, particularly of narcotics
- emotional problems
- emphysema, asthma, or other chronic lung disease
- enlarged prostate
- gallstones or gallbladder disease
- heart disease
- kidney disease
- liver disease
- problems with urination
- seizures
- underactive thyroid

Side effects

The most common side effects of opioids include:

- constipation
- dizziness
- drowsiness
- itching
- nausea
- urine retention
- vomiting

Less common side effects of opioids include:

- abnormally fast or slow heartbeat
- blurred or double vision
- cold, clammy skin
- depression or other mood changes
- dry mouth
- fainting
- hallucinations
- hives
- loss of appetite
- nightmares or unusual dreams
- pinpoint pupils of the eyes
- redness or flushing of the face
- restlessness
- rigid muscles
- ringing or buzzing in the ears
- seizure
- severe drowsiness
- skin reaction at the site of injection
- stomach cramps or pain
- sweating
- trouble sleeping (insomnia)
- yellowing of the skin or whites of the eyes

Interactions

Opioids should not be taken in combination with any prescription drug, over-the-counter drug, or herbal remedy without prior consultation with a physician. It is particularly important that the prescribing physician be aware of the use of any of the following drugs:

- carbamazepine (Tegretol; antiepileptic)
- central nervous system depressants
- monoamine oxidase (MAO) inhibitors (a class of antidepressants) such as furazolidone, isocarboxazid, pargyline, phenelzine, procarbazine, or tranylcypromine
- Naltrexone (opioid antagonist)
- Rifampin (antituberculosis drug)
- tricyclic antidepressants such as amitriptyline, amoxapine, clomipramine, desipramine, doxepin, imipramine, nortiptyline, protriptyline, or trimipramine
- Zidovudine (antiviral against aids virus)
- any radiation therapy or chemotherapy medicines

Paul A. Johnson, Ed.M.

Opium tincture *see* **Antidiarrheal agents**

Oprelvekin

Definition

Oprelvekin, also known as Neumega, is a hematopoietic stimulant used as supportive care after myelosuppressive **chemotherapy** to combat thrombopenia.

Purpose

Oprelvekin is a prescription medication used following the administration of myelosuppressive chemotherapy drugs such as **azathioprine** and **mercaptopurine**. Myelosuppressive chemotherapy acts on bone marrow and causes a decrease in the amount of white blood cells (leukopenia) and platelets (thrombopenia). Oprelvekin

KEY TERMS

Growth factor—A body-produced substance that regulates cell division and cell survival. It can also be produced in a laboratory for use in biological therapy.

Hematopoietic—Related to the formation of blood cells.

Thrombopenia—Decreased number of platelets.

Papilledema—Swelling around the optic disk.

acts as a growth factor stimulating stem cells to proliferate. The result is an increase in the amount of platelets (or thrombocytes).

Description

Oprelvekin is a recombinant human interleukin. Further it is a synthetic version of the naturally occurring interleukin-11, which is produced by the cells of the bone marrow. It is a growth factor that stimulates the formation of platelets, which are necessary in the process of blood clot formation. Oprelvekin is therefore important in increasing platelet formation after treatment with **cancer** medications that cause **thrombocytopenia**.

The Food and Drug Administration approve oprelvekin for prevention of severe thrombocytopenia, which is observed after chemotherapy. Oprelvekin is in **clinical trials** for treatment support and therapy for acute myelocytic leukemia.

Recommended dosage

This drug is available by injection. The dose is different from person to person and is dependent on the patient's body weight. Generally, 50 mcg/kg is given once daily in either the abdomen, thigh or hip. This medication should be taken at the same time every day for best results. If a dosage of oprelvekin is missed, the patient should skip the missed dose and take the next dose at the scheduled time.

Precautions

Although oprelvekin is effective at increasing the number of platelets in patients following chemotherapy, patients should understand that there are a number of precautions that should be taken when their physician is prescribing oprelvekin.

If the patient has any existing medical problems, he or she should tell the doctor prior to beginning treatment with oprelvekin. Congestive heart failure may be worsened when taking oprelvekin as it causes increased water retention. Oprelvekin can also cause atrial arrhythmias that result in heart rhythm problems. It should also be used with caution in patients with preexisting papilledema or with tumors that involve the central nervous system.

Oprelvekin has not been studied in pregnant women, women who are nursing or children. However, animal testing has shown that oprelvekin can have negative effects on the fetus and can cause joint and tendon problems in children. It is eliminated primarily by the kidneys and should be used carefully in patients with renal impairment.

Side effects

Although oprelvekin is a synthetic version of a naturally occurring growth factor, there are side effects associated with taking it. The side effects should be weighed against the needed effects of this medication. Some side effects do not require medical attention and others do.

The following are side effects that do not require medical attention and could gradually go away as treatment progresses:

- red eyes
- weakness
- numb extremities such as the hands and feet
- skin reactions such as rash and discoloration

If patients encounter any of the following side effects, they should contact their physicians immediately:

- rapid heartbeat
- irregular heartbeat
- short breath
- white spots in the mouth or on the tongue
- swelling feet and legs
- bloody eye
- blurred vision
- heart rhythm problems

If the patient notices any other side effects not listed,a physician should be contacted immediately.

Interactions

There are no known interactions with oprelvekin.

Sally C. McFarlane-Parrott

Oral cancers

Definition

Cancer of the mouth or the oral cavity and the oropharynx is referred to as oral cancer.

Description

Oral cavity describes a broad array of parts within the mouth including the lips, lining on the lips and cheeks referred to as buccal mucosa, teeth, tongue, floor of the mouth under the tongue, hard palate (which is the firm bony top of the mouth), and the gums. The oropharynx includes the back of the tongue, the soft palate, and the tonsils (fleshy part on either side of the mouth). There are glands through out the oral cavity that produce saliva that keep the mouth moist, known as salivary glands. The secretions from these glands called saliva aid in digesting the food.

Under normal circumstances, the oral cavity and oropharynx are comprised of several types of tissues and cells, and tumors can develop from any of these cells. These tumors may either be benign (they do not spread to the adjoining tissues), or the tumor may invade other tissues of the body. Any potential growth of a benign tumor into a cancerous (malignant) tumor is referred to as a precancerous condition. Leukoplakia or erythroplakia, which are abnormal areas in the oral cavity, may develop in many of the oral cancers as the first stage. Leukoplakia is a white area that is a benign condition, but approximately 5% of leukoplakias develop into cancer. Erythroplakia is a red bumpy area that bleeds when scraped, and has the potential to develop into cancer within 10 years if not treated.

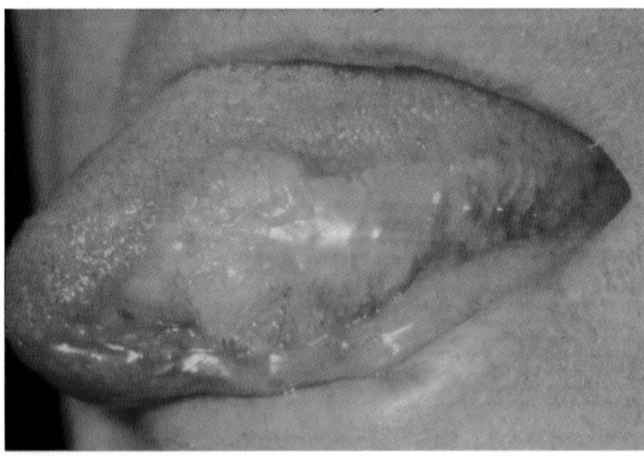

Close-up of large cancerous tumor on the tongue. *(Biophoto Associates, Science Source/Photo Researchers, Inc. Reproduced by permission.)*

KEY TERMS

Biopsy—Removal of a portion of tissue or cells for microscopic examination. Incisional biopsy is removal of only a sample tissue. Excisional biopsy is removal of entire tumor or lesion. Sample of tissue or fluid removed with a needle is fine-needle biopsy.

Lymph node—Bean-shaped mass of lymphatic tissue surrounded by connective tissue. These contain lymphocytes which are cells that helps in maintaining the immune system

Benign tumors are those that are not invasive and thus incapable of spreading. Examples of benign tumors of the oral cavity include keratocanthoma, leiomyoma, osteochondroma, neurofibroma, papilloma, schwannoma, and odontogenic tumors. These tumors are generally harmless and can be surgically removed. Recurrence of these tumors after surgical removal is very rare.

More than 90% of malignant tumors of the oral cavity and oropharynx are squamous cell **carcinoma** also referred to as squamous cell cancer. Squamous cells form the lining of the oral cavity and oropharynx and morphologically, they appear flat and scale-like. When the cancer cells appear just in the lining of the oral cavity, it marks the initial stages of the squamous cell cancer and is referred to as carcinoma in situ. Appearance of cancer cells on deeper layers of the oral cavity or oropharynx refers to invasive squamous cell cancer which is a more serious condition. Verrucous carcinomas are a type of squamous cell carcinoma that seldom metastasize but can spread to the adjoining tissues. Thus a surgeon might suggest removal of a wide area of surrounding tissues in addition to removing the cancerous tissue. The chances of developing a second cancer in the oral region (oral cavity or pharynx) at a later time during the life period is about 10-40%, thus necessitating thorough follow-up examinations. In addition, refraining from smoking and drinking will help to prevent the disease recurrence. Among other types of malignant tumors of the oral cavity are salivary gland cancers and **Hodgkin's disease**. The former affects the salivary glands present throughout the mucosal lining of the oral cavity and oropharynx. The latter is the cancer that develops in the lymphoid tissue of the tonsils and base of the tongue.

Demographics

The statistical survey on oral cancers reveals that more men are affected by the disease than women. The

QUESTIONS TO ASK THE DOCTOR

- What is oral cavity or oropharyngeal cancer?
- What is the extent of cancer spread beyond the primary site?
- What is the stage, and the severity of the stage?
- What are the treatment options available?
- What are the chances of survival,and the time frame of survival?
- What are the side of effects of treatment?
- What are the potential risks of specific treatments?
- How long will it take to recover from treatment?
- What are the chances of recurrence?
- What is the benefit of one treatment over the other in terms of recurrence?
- How to get ready for the treatment?
- Discuss the possibility of getting a second opinion.

American Cancer Society has estimated that about 35,720 new cases of oral cavity and pharyngeal cancers will be diagnosed in the United States in the year 2009. Of these, predictions are that 25,240 cases will occur in men and 10,480 in women. The estimates also suggest that about 7,600 Americans will die of cancer of the oral cavity or oropharynx in 2004. The incidence and the mortality rate have been directed toward a decreasing trend in the last 20 years. Studies on patient survival show that about 82% of patients diagnosed with oral cancer survive for more than a year, about 51% survive for five years and about 48% for 10 years.

Certain geographic differences affect the incidence of oral cavity cancers. Hungary and France show higher incidence of the disease as compared to the United States. However, the disease is much less common in Japan and Mexico suggesting that environmental factors do play a key role in the outcome of the disease.

About 15% of patients diagnosed with either oral or oropharynx cancer are more often known to develop cancer of the adjoining organs (or tissues) including larynx, oesophagus or lung. The chances of developing a second cancer in the oral region (oral cavity or pharynx) for survivors, at a later time during the life period is about 10–40%. Thus, a person once diagnosed with cancer of oral cavity has to undergo through follow up examinations for the rest of his or her life, even if cured completely. In addition, restraining from smoking tobacco and drinking alcohol will greatly facilitate in preventing the disease occurrence as tobacco use has been shown to be responsible for 90% of tumors of oral cavity in men and 60% among women.

Causes and symptoms

The major risk factors for oral and oropharyngeal cancers are smoking and **alcohol consumption**. These two factors account for 75% of all the oral cavity cancers reported in the United States. Smokeless tobacco (chew or spit tobacco) is yet another important cause for oral cancers. Each dip or chew of tobacco has been shown to contain five times more nicotine than one cigarette and 28 potential carcinogens. For lip cancer, exposure to sun may be one of the risk factors. Geographical factors and sexual differences also attribute to the risk factors of oral cancers. Men are twice as susceptible to oral cancers than women. While oral cancer is ranked sixth leading cancer among men in the United States, it is the fourth leading cancer in African American men. Age also seems to be a factor in the susceptibility of oral cancer. About 95% of oral cancer cases are diagnosed in people older than 45 years and the median age for diagnosis is 64 years. In addition to these factors, genetic predisposition may be one of the factors that should not be ignored in any type of cancer.

Many of the symptoms listed below may be of a less serious nature or related to other cancers. Common symptoms include:

- mouth sores that do not heal
- persistent pain in the mouth
- thickening in the mouth
- white or red patch on tongue, gums, tonsils or lining of the mouth
- sore throat
- difficulty in chewing or swallowing
- difficulty moving the jaw or tongue
- numbness of gums, tongue or any other area of the mouth
- swelling of the jaw
- loosening of the teeth
- voice changes
- weight loss
- feeling of lumpy mass in the neck

Any of the above symptoms that persists for more than a few weeks needs prompt medical attention.

Diagnosis

Routine screening or examination of oral cavity by a physician or a dentist is the key for early detection of oral and oropharyngeal cancers. Thorough self-examination is also highly recommended by physicians that may lead to an early diagnosis of abnormal growth in the oral cavity or neck. If any of the signs outlined above suggests the presence of oral cancer, the physician may recommend additional tests or procedures to confirm the diagnosis. These may be one or more of the following factors.

Head and neck examination

In addition to thorough physical examinations, physicians attach special attention to the neck and head area. Highly sophisticated fiberoptic scopes are used to view the oropharynx after inserting a tube through the mouth or nose. Because of the risk of additional cancers in patients with oral cancers, other parts of the head and neck including nose, larynx, lymph nodes are carefully examined. Depending on the parts examined, the procedures are termed as pharyngoscopy, **laryngoscopy** or nasopharyngoscopy.

Panendoscopy

Depending on the risk factors, the surgeon may suggest further examination of oral cavity, oropharynx, larynx, esophagus, trachea, and the bronchi. This overall examination called panendoscopy is done under general anesthesia to avoid discomfort to the patient and allow a thorough check-up of the neck and head regions. During this process, a **biopsy** of the suspected tissue is done to determine the severity of the cancer. The specimens used could be a scraping from the suspected area and smeared into a slide which is stained and viewed under the microscope. This technique is easy, inexpensive and offers information on the abnormal lesions. Incisional biopsy is the removal of a piece of small tissue from an area of the tumor. This is a relatively simple procedure and is performed either in the doctor's office or in the operating room depending upon the area of the tumor to be removed. The biopsy tissue samples are treated through various steps before the cells can be viewed under the microscope. Fine-needle aspiration (FNA) biopsy is the aspiration of fluid from a mass, lump or cyst in the neck. This would also include excisional biopsy. Depending upon the type of cells recognized in the aspiration, the pathologists can determine whether the cancer is related to neck or oral region or it has metastasized from a distant organ. FNA may also determine whether the neck mass is benign that resulted from any **infection** related to mouth or oropharynx.

Computed tomography (or Computer Axial tomography)

A sophisticated x-ray test that scans parts of body in cross-section. This procedure is carried out after administering a dye that can aid in locating abnormalities. This helps in judging the extent of cancer spread to lymph nodes, lower mandible and neck.

Magnetic resonance imaging (MRI)

This is used for evaluting soft tissue details such as the cancers of the tonsil and base of tongue and the procedure is governed by magnets and radio waves.

Panorex

This is a rotating x ray of upper and lower jawbones that determines changes that occur due to cancers in the oral cavity.

In addition to the imaging tests already noted, chest **x rays** help in checking for lung cancers in oral cancer patients with smoking habits. Barium swallow is a commonly performed series of x rays to assess the cancers of the digestive tract in patients with oral cancer. A radionulide bone scan may be suggested if there is concern that the cancer may have spread to the bones.

Other tests may include blood tests given to provide a complete blood analysis, including a determination of **anemia**, liver disease, kidney disease and RBC and WBC counts.

Treatment team

Cancer care team typically involves physician specialists to include, surgeon (oral or neck and head surgeon), a dentist (in cases of oral cancers), a medical oncologist and a radiation therapist.

Clinical staging, treatments, and prognosis

Clinical staging

TNM system of the American Joint Committee on Cancer has been followed in staging the cancer in which the size (T), spread to regional lymph nodes (N) and **Metastasis** to other organs (M) are classified.

T CLASSIFICATION.

- Tx: Information not known and thus tumor cannot be assessed.
- T0: No evidence of primary tumor.
- Tis: Carcinoma in situ which means the cancer has affected the epithelial cells lining the oral cavity or the oropharynx and the tumor is not deep.

- T1: Tumor 2 cm (1 cm equals 0.39 inches) or smaller.
- T2: Tumor larger than 2 cm but smaller than 4 cm.
- T3:Tumor larger than 4 cm.
- T4: Tumor of any size that invades adjacent structures like larynx, bone, connective tissues or muscles.

N CLASSIFICATION.

- Nx: Information not known, cannot be assessed.
- N0: No metastasis in the regional lymph node.
- N1: Metastasis in one lymph node on the same side of the primary tumor and smaller than 3cm.
- N2: Divided into 3 subgroups. N2a is metastasis in one lymph node larger than 3cm and smaller than 6cm. N2b is metastasis in multiple lymph nodes on the same side of tumor, none larger than 6cm. N2c denotes one or more lymph nodes, may or may not be on the side of primary tumor, none larger than 6 cm.
- N3: Metastasis in lymph node larger than 6cm.

M CLASSIFICATION.

- Mx: Distant metastasis cannot be assessed, information not known.
- M0: No distant metastasis.
- M1: Distant metastasis present.

STAGE GROUPING.

- Stage 0 (carcinoma in situ): Tis,N0,M0
- StageI: T1,N0,M0
- Stage II: T2,N0,M0
- Stage III: T3,N0,M0 or T1,N1,M0 or T2,N1,M0 or T3,N1,M0
- Stage IVA: T4,N0,M0 or T4,N1,M0 or Any T,N2,M0
- Stage IVB: Any T,N3,M0
- Stage IVC: Any T, any N,M1

Treatments

After the cancer is diagnosed and staged, the medical team dealing with the case will discuss the choice of treatment. This may be **chemotherapy** alone or in combination with **radiation therapy** or surgery. The treatment option is made depending upon the stage of the disease, the physical health of the patient, and after discussing the possible impact of the treatment on speech, swallowing, chewing, or general appearance.

SURGERY. Primary tumor resection involves removal of the entire tumor with some normal adjacent tissue surrounding the tumor to ensure that all of the residual cancerous mass is removed. Partial mandible resection is carried out in cases where the jaw bone is suspected to have been invaded but with no evidence from x ray results. Full mandible resection is performed when the x rays indicate jaw bone destruction.

Maxillectomy is the removal of the hard palate if that is affected. A special denture called a prosthesis can alter the defect caused in the hard palate resulting from the surgery. Moh's surgery involves removal of thin sections of lip tumors. Immediate examination of the sections for potential cancer cells allows the surgeons to decide whether or not the cancer is completely removed.

Laryngectomy is the surgical removal of larynx (voice box). This is done when there is risk of food entering the trachea and infecting the lungs, as a result of removal of tumors of tongue or oropharynx. By removing the larynx, the trachea is attached to the skin of the neck thus eliminating the risk of infecting the lung and potential **pneumonia**.

Neck dissection is a surgical procedure involving removal of lymph nodes in the neck that are known to contain cancer cells. The side effects of this surgery include numbness of the ear, difficulty in raising the arm above the head, discomfort to the lower lip—all of which are caused by different nerves involved in the surgery.

Tracheostomy is an incision made in the trachea to facilitate breathing for oral cancer patients who may develop considerable swelling following surgical removal of the tumor in oral cavity. This prevents any obstruction in the throat and allows easy breathing.

In addition to the those surgical procedures, dental extractions and removal of large tumors in oral cancer patients may need reconstructive surgeries which may vary from one patient to the other depending upon the site and size of the tumors.

RADIATION THERAPY. Use of high-energy rays to kill the cancer cells or reduce their growth is radiation therapy. It may be given as the only treatment of small tumors or given in combination with surgery to destroy deposits of cancer cells. Radiation is also suggested for relieving symptoms of cancer including difficulty in swallowing and bleeding. Radiation may be externally or internally administered. External radiation (also called external beam radiation therapy) delivers radiation to oral or oropharyngeal cancers from outside the body. Brachytherapy or internal radiation involves the surgical implant of metal rods that deliver radioactive materials in or near the cancer.

CHEMOTHERAPY. Chemotherapy involves administering of **anticancer drugs** parenterally or orally. Chemotherapy may be suggested in combination with radiation therapy to avoid surgery in some large tumors of head and neck region. Some studies reveal that chemotherapy is ideal for shrinking the size of the tumor before surgery or radiation therapy is initiated. This is termed neoadjuvant chemotherapy.

Treatment choices by stage and prognosis

Depending on the stage of cancer spread, different treatment options are recommended for oral cancer.

Stage 0: Surgical stripping or thin resection is suggested at this stage where the cancer has not become invasive. If there is repeated recurrence, radiation therapy is an option. More than 95% of the patients at this stage survive for long-term without the requirement of any surgery of their oral cavity.

Stages I and II: Surgery or radiation therapy is the choice of treatment depending on the location of the tumor in the oral cavity and oropharynx.

Stages III and IV: A combination therapy of either surgery and radiation or radiation and chemotherapy or all the three types of treatment may be required for these advanced stages of cancer. About 20–50% of patients undergoing a combination of surgery and radiation for stages III and IV oral cavity and oropharyngeal cancers have the chances of five-year disease-free survival.

Alternative and complementary therapies

Various alternative medications are being tried periodically. While choosing any alternative therapy, a thorough discussion of the advantages and disadvantages of the suggested therapy with the medical team is highly recommended.

In 2000, researchers demonstrated that Bowman-Birk inhibitor, a protein found in soybeans shrinks leukoplakia or the precancerous growth in the mouth. The study has pointed to a reduction in the size of the leukoplakia to a third or half of the original size when the protein is orally administered for a month. The studies also suggest that a combination of soybean intake and termination of smoking tobacco will have a cumulative effect in the shrinking of leukoplakia. However, a thorough investigations in a larger patient population is necessary to confirm the therapeutic utility of the soybean protein in oral cancer.

Coping with cancer treatment

Cancer of any type is a psychologically distressful journey from the time of diagnosis, treatment and recovery. Coping with the side effects of treatment both physically and emotionally is a challenge to the patient, the family and the medical team. Oral cancers are further complicated by the fact that surgery most often leads to disfigurement which may be devastating in a society where importance is attached to physical appearance. Reconstruction surgeries or facial prostheses may be psychologically helpful and the cancer care team may advise on this issue. Laryngectomy or removal of the voice box leaves the person without speech, and breathing through stoma (in the neck). A stoma cover helps in hiding the mucus that the stoma secretes and also serves as a filter in the absence of nose's natural filter. The odors from the stoma can be prevented by use of cologne, and by avoiding strongly scented foods such as garlic. Studies reveal that lack of normal speech has a serious impact on sexual activity in couples. In addition to laryngectomy, surgery on the jaw, plate or tongue can also disrupt speech. These problems need to be discussed with the cancer care team or contact organizations such as the American Cancer Society who could provide relevant information on coping with specific issues on oral cancers.

Side effects of chemotherapy such as **fatigue** and hair loss (**alopecia**) may affect the quality of life in a patient. A wig may be used for cosmetic purposes that can hide the hair loss. Studies have shown that patients may gradually regain their health after chemotherapy if they abstain from smoking and drinking.

Clinical trials

Evaluation of a potential treatment method for a disease on aselected patient population is called a clinical trial. Some of the ongoing **clinical trials** include:

- Paclitaxel and cisplatin for Stage III and IV of squamous cell carcinoma of the oral cavity following radiotherapy.
- Phase I study of intratumoral EGFR antisense DNA and DC chol liposomes in patients with advanced squamous cell carcinoma of oral cavity.
- Phase I immunotoxin therapy (PE38 immunotoxin) in treating patients with advanced lip and oral cavity cancer.
- Phase III megestrol acetate administration to patients undergoing cancer treatment for lip, oral cavity, and oropharyngeal cancers. This drug improves appetite and thus may prevent weight loss in cancer patients.
- Phase I combination of chemotherapy and radiation therapy in treating Stage III/IV lip, oral cavity, and oropharyngeal cancer. The drug tested is docetaxel. Resources regarding these clinical trials, as well as many others regarding oral cancers, including any recruiting of patients for the trial are available at http://www.clinical trials.gov, a service of the National Cancer Institute, National Institutes of Health.

Prevention

Oral cavity and **oropharyngeal cancer** patients are at risk for recurrences, or for developing secondary cancers in the head and neck area. Thus a close follow-up is mandatory in the first couple of years following the indicence. A thorough examination every month in the first year, and at least every three months during the following year, and each year thereafter is the recommended schedule to facilitate early detection, if any. Various chemopreventive drugs are being tested to prevent the occurrence of secondary tumors in the neck and head region. Vitamin A analog is one such chemopreventive drug under investigation that may help in suppressing the tumor formation.

Tobacco (smoking, chewing, spitting) and alcohol consumption are the major causes of oral and oropharyngeal cancers. Public knowledge regarding the risk factors of the oral cancers and the signs of early detection is limited. Only 25% of U.S. adults can detect early signs of abnormal oral cavity; and only 13% understand the implications of regular alcohol consumption in developing oral cancer. **Cancer prevention** and control programs are growing rapidly with screening services for high risk opulation, health promotion, education and intervention strategies. National Spit Tobacco Education Program (NSTEP), an initiative of Oral Health America, has been educating the public about dangers of spit tobacco and oral cancer.

Exposure to sun may cause **lip cancers**. Use of a lip balm will protect the lip from the sun rays. In addition, pipe smokers are more at risk for lip cancers.

Special concerns

Surgery for oral cancer treatment may affect normal speech and swallowing. A speech pathologist will educate, and suggest remedies for restoring speech and swallowing problems. In addition, a dietitian may be consulted for choosing the more palatable food in the advent of chewing and swallowing problems. In case of dryness, a saliva supplement can be recommended by a physician

Advances in **reconstructive surgery** of the mouth and lower face in the early 2000s have significantly improved patients' appearance and quality of life after treatment for oral cancer.

The side effects of cancer treatment will make the patient fatiqued. Giving ample time to recover will help improve energy for the long-term. **Smoking cessation** and elimination of alcohol, and maintaining a balanced diet with fruits, vegetables, and whole grain are key to returning to a normal life for patients suffering from oral cancers.

See also Cancer biology; Cancer genetics; Cigarettes.

Resources

BOOKS

Beers, Mark H., MD, and Robert Berkow, MD, editors. "Disorders of the Oral Region: Neoplasms." In *The Merck Manual of Diagnosis and Therapy*. Whitehouse Station, NJ: Merck Research Laboratories, 2007.

PERIODICALS

Oliver, R. J., P. Sloan, and M. N. Pemberton. "Oral Biopsies: Methods and Applications." *British Dental Journal* 196 (March 27, 2004): 329–333.

Palme, C. E., P. J. Gullane, and R. W. Gilbert. "Current Treatment Options in Squamous Cell Carcinoma of the Oral Cavity." *Surgical Oncology Clinics of North America* 13 (January 2004): 47–70.

van de Pol M., P. C. Levendag, R. R. de Bree, et al. "Radical Radiotherapy Compared with Surgery for Advanced Squamous Cell Carcinoma of the Base of Tongue." *Brachytherapy* 3 (February 2004): 78–86.

OTHER

American Cancer Society (ACS). *Cancer Facts & Figures 2004*.http://www.cancer.org/downloads/STT/CAFF_finalPWSecured.pdf.

"Chemical Found in Soybeans May Help Prevent Oral Cancer." *American Cancer Society*. [cited July 5, 2009]. http://www2.cancer.org/zine/index.cfm?fn = 001_122720001_0, ACS News Today.

"Oral and Oropharyngeal Cancers: Clinical Trials" *National Institutes of Health*. [cited July 5, 2009]. http://www.clinicaltrials.gov/ct/gui/action/find condition?.

"Oral Cancer." *National Cancer Institute*. Dec 2000. [cited July 5, 2009]. http://cancernet.nci.nih.gov/wyntk_pubs/oral.htm.

ORGANIZATIONS

American Academy of Facial Plastic and Reconstructive Surgery (AAFPRS). 310 South Henry Street, Alexandria, VA 22314. (703) 299-9291. http://www.facemd.org.

American Society of Plastic Surgeons (ASPS). 444 East Algonquin Road, Arlington Heights, IL 60005. (847) 228-9900. http://www.plasticsurgery.org.

Support for People with Oral and Head and Neck Cancer (SPOHNC). P.O. Box 53, Locust Valley, NY 11560-0053. (800) 377-0928. http://www.spohnc.org.

Kausalya Santhanam, Ph.D.
Rebecca J. Frey, Ph.D.

Orbital exenteration and Pelvic exenteration *see* **Exenteration**

Orchiectomy

Definition

Orchiectomy is a surgical procedure to remove one or both testes in men with prostate or **testicular cancer**. The procedure is sometimes called orchidectomy.

Purpose

In men who have **prostate cancer**, an orchiectomy, up until the 1990s, was considered the standard treatment. By removal of the testes, the influence of **testosterone**, the male hormone produced by the testes, is removed. Testosterone stimulates prostate **cancer** growth and progression of the disease.

Orchiectomy is done in men with testicular cancer to remove one or both testes that have cancer. By removing the cancerous testes, there will then be zero chance that the cancer can recur in the testes.

In children or in younger men, the surgeon may perform what is known as testis-sparing or testicular-sparing surgery, in which only the tumor is removed while the healthy testicular tissue is allowed to remain. According to one Canadian study of 51 boys between infancy and 16 years of age, testicular-sparing surgery is highly successful with regard to cancer control as well as tissue preservation.

Precautions

The orchiectomy operation is generally a very basic and safe operation. As in any surgery, some bleeding will be expected, so men should not be taking any medications like aspirin or ibuprofen that could decrease their blood's ability to clot.

Description

An orchiectomy usually takes place in a hospital setting, either in an outpatient surgery clinic or in the hospital itself. General presurgery procedures, such as blood work, are done a few days to a week before the procedure.

To ensure that a patient having an orchiectomy does not suffer any pain, anesthetic will be used during the procedure. Generally, two types of anesthetic are used during an orchiectomy: general anesthesia and epidural anesthesia. General anesthesia causes the patient to go into a sleeplike state. With epidural anesthesia, the patient is awake but is totally numb from the waist down and therefore cannot feel the operation.

Once the patient is adequately anesthetized, the surgeon will make a four-inch incision through the lower abdomen. After the incision in the lower abdomen is made, the surgeon will gently push the testicles up through the inguinal canal and out through the incision.

The orchiectomy operation generally takes only 45 minutes to an hour. Patients either stay overnight in

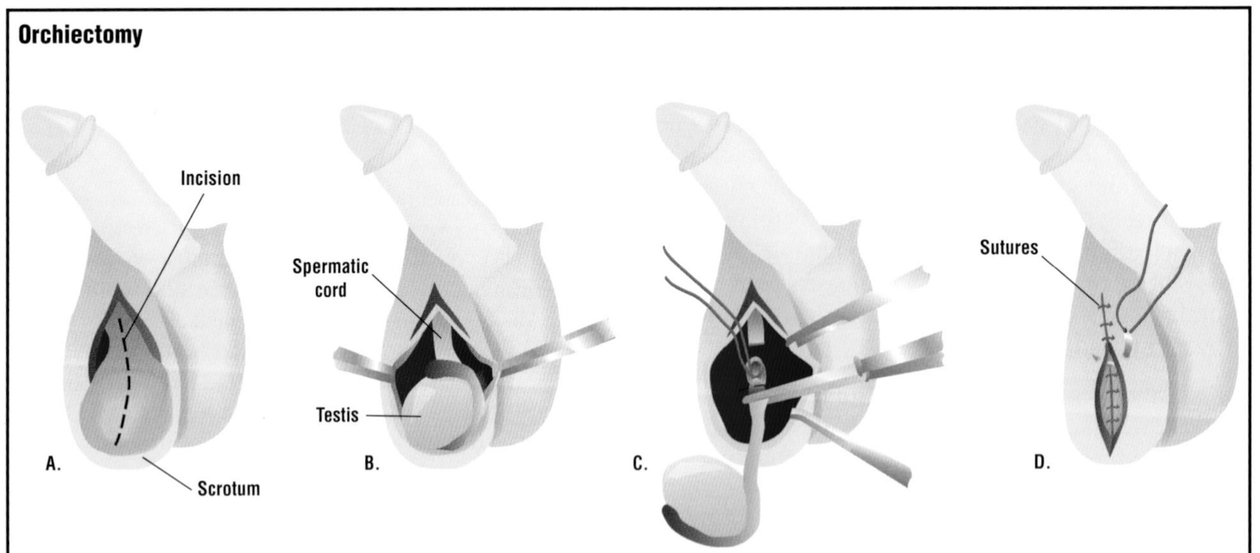

In an orchiectomy, the scrotum is cut open (A). Testicle covering is cut to expose the testis and spermatic cord (B). The cord is tied and cut, removing the testis (C), and the wound is repaired (D). *(Illustration by GGS Information Services. Cengage Learning, Gale.)*

KEY TERMS

Inguinal canal— A pair of internal openings that connect the abdominal cavity with the scrotum in the male fetus, allowing for the developing testes to descend into the scrotal sac.

Testes— The male sex organs that produce sperm and male sex hormones.

the hospital or are discharged from the hospital the same day if there appear to be no complications. Pain from the surgery is usually mild to moderate; narcotic pain medications can control the pain for most patients.

Preparation

There are no specific preparations for having an orchiectomy versus any other type of surgery. Blood will be taken before the surgery to check for infections or other contraindications to surgery. Patients are also advised not to take any medications such as aspirin or ibuprofen that may interfere with the blood's clotting ability.

Aftercare

For approximately two to four weeks or even longer, patients are advised not to participate in any strenuous physical activity. Pain in the scrotum and abdominal area may persist for days to weeks. The surgical wound site should be kept clean and dry. It should also be watched for any signs of **infection**, such as an increase in pain, unusual redness or swelling, or a foul-smelling discharge.

Risks

The risks of orchiectomy include such general surgical risks as pain, bleeding, and infection. In rare cases more serious complications could develop, including abscess formation and bladder damage.

Normal results

The goal of an orchiectomy is to remove the testicles without undue damage to any other organs or structures. For testicular cancer, the end result is to remove the cancerous testicle and cure the cancer. For prostate cancer, the end result is to remove the testicles to shut down the synthesis of testosterone, which is known to promote prostate cancer growth.

Abnormal results

Abnormal results of an orchiectomy can include incomplete removal of the testicles. In the case of both testicular cancer and prostate cancer, this could result in the progression of the cancer.

Resources

PERIODICALS

Chandak, P., A. Shah, A. Taghizadeh, et al. "Testis-Sparing Surgery for Benign and Malignant Testicular Tumours." *International Journal of Clinical Practice* 57 (December 2003): 912–913.

Garnick, Marc B., and Mario Eisenberger. "Hormonal Treatment of Prostate Cancer." *New England Journal of Medicine* 340 (1999): 812–4.

Jones, R. H., and P. A. Vasey. "Part I: Testicular Cancer—Management of Early Disease." *Lancet Oncology* 4 (December 2003): 730–737.

Metcalfe, P. D., H. Farivar-Mohseni, W. Farhat, et al. "Pediatric Testicular Tumors: Contemporary Incidence and Efficacy of Testicular Preserving Surgery." *Journal of Urology* 170 (December 2003): 2412–2416.

Schwenter, C., J. Oswald, H. Rogatsch, et al. "Stromal Testis Tumors in Infants. A Report of Two Cases." *Urology* 62 (December 2003): 1121.

OTHER

The TCRC Orchiectomy Page. [cited July 17, 2009]. http://www.acor.org/TCRC/orch.html.

ORGANIZATIONS

American Urological Association (AUA). 1000 Corporate Boulevard, Linthicum, MD 21090. (866) RING-AUA or (410) 689-3700. http://www.auanet.org.

Edward R. Rosick, D.O., M.P.H.
Rebecca J. Frey, Ph.D.

Oropharyngeal cancer

Definition

Oropharyngeal **cancer** is an uncontrolled growth of cells that begins in the oropharynx, the area at the back of the mouth.

Description

The oropharynx is the passageway at the back of the mouth. It connects the mouth to the esophagus (tube through which food passes) and to the pharynx (the channel for the flow of air into and out of the lungs). It takes its name from the way it ties the oral cavity (hence the oro) to the rest of the pharynx, one

KEY TERMS

Biopsy—Tissue sample is taken from body for examination.

Bronchi—Branches of the trachea that distribute air to the air sacs (alveoli) of the lungs.

Computed tomography (CT)—X rays are aimed at slices of the body (by rotating equipment) and results are assembled with a computer to give a three-dimensional picture of a structure.

Endoscope—Instrument designed to allow direct visual inspection of body cavities, a sort of microscope in a long access tube.

Fiberoptics—Cool, refracted (bounced) light passes (bounces) along extremely small diameter glass tubes. (Used to illuminate body cavities, such as the oropharynx, with high intensity, and almost heatless light.)

Larynx—Commonly known as the voice box, the place between the pharynx and the trachea where the vocal cords are located.

Magnetic resonance imaging (MRI)—Magnetic fields and radio frequency waves are used to take pictures of the inside of the body.

Salivary glands—Structures in the mouth that make and release (secrete) saliva that helps with digestion.

Tonsils—Lymph nodes in the throat that are partly encapsulated (enclosed). They are components of the lymphatic system that functions in immunity and removes the excess fluid around cells and returns it to cells.

Trachea—Tube ringed with cartilage that connects the larynx with the bronchi.

part of which extends toward the back of the nose (nasopharynx). The base of the tongue, the soft palate (the soft roof of the mouth, above the base of the tongue) and the tonsils are part of the oropharynx.

If the oropharynx is blocked or injured in any way, the condition presents a threat to life because it interferes with both eating and breathing. Thus, an obstruction caused by oropharyngeal cancer is in itself a problem. Oropharyngeal cancer also contributes to problems with chewing and talking because of the importance of the oropharynx in these activities. If the oropharyngeal cancer spreads to the bone, muscle, and soft tissue in the neck, there is a severe effect on the ability of the neck to support the head. In individuals with oropharyngeal cancer that has spread, surgical options might be limited.

QUESTIONS TO ASK THE DOCTOR

- In which stage is the cancer?
- What is the outlook for a patient with my profile?
- What are the side effects of the treatments that are recommended? Which treatment gives the best combination of survival and quality of life?
- Is there a clinical trial for which I am eligible?

Oropharyngeal cancer usually begins in the squamous cells of the epithelial tissue. The squamous cells are flat, and often layered. The epithelial tissue forms coverings for the surfaces of the body. Skin, for example, has an outer layer of epithelial tissue. Throughout the oropharynx there are some very small salivary glands and one of more of them sometimes becomes the site of tumor growth.

Many times cancer that begins in the oropharynx spreads to the base of the tongue. Oropharyngeal cancer can spread to the muscle and bone in the neck, and also to the soft tissue that fills the space around the muscle and bone.

Demographics

In the United States, about 4,000 cases of oropharyngeal cancer are diagnosed each year. Most of the cancer is found in people who are more than 50 years old. A history of tobacco or alcohol use, especially heavy use, is typically linked to the diagnosis. Men are three to five times more likely to be diagnosed than women.

Some benign tumors arise in the oropharynx. Although they are benign, many studies suggest the growths indicate the person is at greater risk for a malignant tumor growth in the future.

Causes and symptoms

The cause of oropharyngeal cancer is not known, but the risk factors for oropharyngeal cancer are understood. Three important lifestyle choices increase the chance a person will be diagnosed with cancer of the oropharynx. They are tobacco use, **alcohol consumption**, and certain sexual practices.

Anything that passes into the lungs or stomach through the nose and mouth must move through the oropharynx. (Air moves through the nasopharynx to reach the oropharynx.) Long periods of exposure to substances such as tobacco byproducts and alcohol somehow trigger cells to begin uncontrolled growth, cancer. About 90% of all cancer of the oropharynx starts in a squamous cell.

Since tobacco and alcohol come into direct contact with the squamous cells of the oropharynx as they move through the cavity, they might change the genetic material (DNA) of cells. If a cell cannot repair damage to DNA, a cancerous growth can begin.

A serious interaction occurs between tobacco and alcohol. Individuals who smoke and drink alcoholic beverages are at much greater risk for oropharyngeal cancer. They have as much as 30 times or 40 times the normal risk. The estimate is difficult to make because not all individuals diagnosed are accurate in the statements they make to physicians about their use of these substances. Patients often say they used less tobacco or less alcohol than they actually did.

Viral **infection** increases the risk of oropharyngeal cancer. So does reduced immunity, which is a condition that may be caused by viral infection. Individuals with human papilloma viruses, which are sexually transmitted, are known, to be at greater risk, particularly those infected by HPV-16. The virus increases a person's risk of cancer because it inactivates the TP53 gene, which regulates the cycle of cell division by keeping cells from dividing in an uncontrolled fashion. The specific sexual practices associated with an increased risk of oropharyngeal cancer include a high lifetime number of sexual partners, oral-gential sex, and oral-anal sex.

Marijuana seems to be linked with oropharyngeal cancer too. Vitamin A deficiency, or specifically, the absence of the carotene (from fruits and vegetables) that the body uses to make vitamin A, might also be a contributing factor.

Symptoms of oropharyngeal cancer include:

- difficulty swallowing
- difficulty chewing
- change in voice
- loss of weight
- lump in the throat
- lump in the neck

Diagnosis

Cells grow old and flake off regularly from epithelial tissues. The first step in diagnosing oropharyngeal cancer often makes use of the natural process. It is given the name exfoliative **cytology**. A physician scrapes cells from the part of the oropharynx where a cancer is suspected and smears them on a slide. The cells are then treated with chemicals so they can be studied with a microscope. If they do not appear normal, a **biopsy**, or a tissue sample from a deeper layer of cells, is taken for examination.

Different sorts of biopsies are used. An incision, or cut, is be made to obtain tissue. Or, a needle with a small diameter is inserted into the neck to obtain cells, especially if there is a lump in the neck.

Computed tomography (CT) and **magnetic resonance imaging** (MRI) scans are also used. They help determine whether the cancer has spread from the walls of the oropharynx. MRI offers a good way to examine the tonsils and the back of the tongue, which are soft tissues. CT is used as a way of studying the jaw, which is bone.

Many extremely specialized means of determining the condition of the oropharynx have been developed. One of them relies on the same sort of light wave technology that now powers much of the communications world, fiberoptics. A fiber (a bundle of glass fibers, actually) with a very small diameter is inserted in the oropharynx and the area is probed with light that is reflected on mirrors for interpretation. Lighting up the oropharynx with the high intensity, very low heat illumination of fiberoptics, a physician can get a good look at the cavity.

Another special way of getting a good look at the oropharynx involves studying it from within by inserting an endoscope into the oropharynx and then, weaving it through adjacent connecting structures. The structures include the trachea, the bronchi, the larynx and the esophagus. The patient is given an anesthetic, local or general, for this procedure. When several organs are examined at the same time, the procedure is called a panendoscopy. The tool used is generally named for the organ for which it is most closely designed. For example, there is a laryngoscope.

Because oropharyngeal cancer often spreads, bones near the oropharynx must be examined carefully. Some special types of equipment are used. A rotating x ray called panorex provides for close inspection of the jaw.

Oropharyngeal cancer also spreads to the esophagus, so physicians usually examine the esophagus when they diagnose oropharyngeal cancer. To do so, they ask the patient to drink a liquid containing barium, a chemical that can be seen on **x rays**. Then, they can x ray the esophagus and look for bulges or lumps that indicate cancer there.

Treatment team

Generally, physicians with special training in the organs of the throat take responsibility for the care of a patient with oropharyngeal cancer. They are called otolaryngologists or occasionally by a longer name, otorhinolaryngologists.

In abbreviation, otolaryngologists are usually labeled ENT (for Ear, Nose and Throat) specialists. An ENT specializing in cancer will probably lead the team. Some ENTs have a specialty in surgery. Some have a specialty in oncology. Some have a specialty in both.

Nurses, as well as a nutritionist, speech therapist and social worker will also be part of the team. Depending on the extent of the cancer when diagnosed, some surgery and treatments result in extensive changes in the throat, neck and jaw. The social worker, speech therapist and nutritionist are important in helping the patient cope with the changes caused by surgery and radiation treatment. If there is great alteration to the neck because of surgery, rehabilitation will also be part of the recovery process and a rehabilitation therapist will be added to the team.

The treatment team may also include a psychiatrist, as patients with oropharyngeal cancer have extremely high rates of **depression** compared with other cancer patients. A study carried out at Memorial Sloan-Kettering Cancer Center in New York reported in 2004 that as many as 57% of patients with oropharyngeal cancer suffer an episode of major depression, compared to 50% of **pancreatic cancer** patients, 46% of **breast cancer** patients, and 44% of lung cancer patients.

Clinical staging, treatments, and prognosis

Stage 0 indicates some cells with the potential to grow erratically are discovered. But the cells have not multiplied beyond the surface layer of the epithelial tissue of the oropharynx. Stage I describes a cancer less than approximately 2.5 cm (about one inch in diameter) that has not spread. Stage II describes a bigger cancer, up to about 5 cm. (about two inches), that has not spread.

Stage III oropharyngeal cancer is either larger than two inches or has spread to one lymph node. The lymph node is enlarged but not much larger than an inch.

In Stage IV, one or more of several things happens. There is either a spread of cancer to a site near the original site. Or, there is more than one lymph node with cancer. Or, the cancer has spread to other parts of the body, such as the larynx, the trachea, the bronchi, the esophagus, or even more distant points, such as the lungs.

The outlook for recovery from oropharyngeal cancer is better the earlier the stage in which the cancer is diagnosed. For stage I and stage II, surgical removal or **radiation therapy** of the affected area is sometimes all that is required to halt the cell growth. Decisions about which method to use depend on many factors. The tolerance a patient has for radiation or **chemotherapy**, and the size of the tumor are crucial to the decision process.

Surgical removal can interfere with speech, eating and breathing. So, if nonsurgical treatment is an option, it is a good one to try. The larger the tumor, the more urgent is its removal. Smaller tumors can be treated with radiation or chemotherapy to shrink them before surgery. Some smaller tumors can be removed completely with a carbon dioxide laser. In some cases, surgery might be avoided. For stage III cancer with lymph node involvement, the lymph nodes with the cancer are also removed.

Chemotherapy might be used at any stage, but it is particularly important for stage IV cancer. In some cases, chemotherapy is used before surgery, just as radiation is, to try to eliminate the cancer without cutting, or at least to make it smaller before it is cut out (excised). After surgery, radiation therapy and chemotherapy are both used to treat patients with stage IV oropharyngeal cancer, sometimes in combination. Treatments vary in Stage IV patients depending on the extent of the spread.

Some tumors are so large they cannot be completely removed by surgery. Often, the most promising treatment option for a person with such a tumor is a clinical trial. One technique that has had some success with recurrent or advanced oropharyngeal tumors is **radiofrequency ablation**. In radiofrequency ablation, the tumor is heated by the application of 90–150 watts of energy to an internal temperature of 60–110°C (140–230°F) for a period of five to 15 minutes.

Besides categories, or stages, that indicate how far the disease has progressed, there are many categories that are used to describe the kind, or grade, of tumor. The grades take into account such factors as the density of a tumor. Eventually, physicians hope information about tumor grade will make it possible to match treatment and condition very precisely.

Coping with cancer treatment

The patient should be an active member of the treatment team, listening to information and making decisions about which course of treatment to take. Premier cancer centers encourage such a role.

Prior to surgery, discuss the need for a way to communicate if speech is impaired after surgery. A pad and pencil might be all that are needed for a short interval. If there will be a long period of difficulty, the patient should be ready with other means, including special phone service.

A change in appearance after the removal of part of the oropharynx, whether part of the tongue or soft palate or some other portion, can lead to concerns about **body image**. Social interaction might suffer. A support group can help. Discussions with a social worker also can be beneficial.

If any part of the oropharynx is removed, speech therapy might be necessary to relearn how to make certain sounds. If the surgery requires the removal of some or all of the tongue, a person's speech will be greatly impaired.

Appetite might be affected before, during and after treatment. Before treatment, the presence of a tumor can interfere with chewing and swallowing food, and food might not seem as appealing as it once did. During treatment, particularly radiation treatment, the treated oropharynx will be sore and eating and breathing will be difficult, or impossible.

In some cases, a patient requires a feeding tube (inserted at the opening of the esophagus, through the mouth), a stomach tube (inserted directly in the stomach, if there is no access to the opening of the esophagus) or a breathing tube (inserted directly in the trachea) for some interval of time. The tubes bypass the normal entryways to the stomach and lungs. Liquid food is put directly into the esophagus or stomach. Air is taken directly into the trachea during breathing. The incision or cut in the trachea is called a tracheotomy and the opening in the neck around the trachea is a **tracheostomy**. Air that enters the trachea directly is not warmed or moistened, and the dry, cold air in the lungs can lead to respiratory complications. Attachments are now available that are positioned at the opening in the neck and filter and add moisture to the air entering the tracheal tube. Learning how to care for the tracheotomy and tracheostomy, how to keep the openings clean and what to do if the tube pops out, relieves anxiety and improves ease of breathing.

After treatment, a loss of sensation in the part of the oropharynx affected, or a loss of part of the tongue or the jaw, can reduce appetite. A nutritionist can help with supplements for people who experience significant **weight loss** and who do not have an appetite (**anorexia**).

Patients who are dependent on tobacco or alcohol products and want to reduce or eliminate their intake, will have to deal with the psychological effects of substance withdrawal in addition to the side-effects from treatment. A support group for tobacco or alcohol dependence might be considered, and joined before treatment begins.

Clinical trials

There are a number of **clinical trials** in progress. For example, the better researchers understand the nature of cancer cells, the better they are able to design drugs that attack only cancer cells. Or, in some cases, drugs that make it easier to kill cancer cells have also been designed.

The Cancer Information Service at the National Institutes of Health, Bethesda, Md., offers information about clinical trials that are looking for volunteers. The Service offers a toll-free number at 1-800-422-6237.

Prevention

Avoiding smoking, drinking alcohol, and having oral sex with a large number of partners are important in the prevention of oropharyngeal cancer. Including lots of fruits and vegetables in the diet is also an important step to preventing cancer. (Even though the importance of fruits and vegetables is not proven to prevent oropharyngeal cancer, overall fruits and vegetables are demonstrated cancer fighters.) Carotene, which the body uses to make vitamin A, seems to be important in the diet of people who are less likely to be diagnosed with oropharyngeal cancer. Any precaution that is taken to avoid contracting sexually transmitted diseases, such as the use of condoms, also offers protection from oropharyngeal cancer.

Special concerns

Growths sometimes develop in the oropharynx that are not cancerous. The benign tumors can be removed by surgery. They usually do not recur. The surgeon should be able to give a patient an accurate appraisal identifying the noncancerous growth, and whether it is likely to indicate future problems.

Oropharyngeal cancer frequently recurs in patients who have been treated for the condition. Thus, after treatment, patients must be examined monthly for one year. They also must be committed to telling their physician if they notice any changes. By the second year, examinations can be at two-month intervals; and then, three-month intervals by the third year and six-month intervals beyond that.

Mouthwash has been suspected as a cancer-causing agent for oropharyngeal cancer. Studies are not conclusive. One line of reasoning suggests alcohol-based mouthwashes add to the effects of alcohol consumed by heavy drinkers. Alcohol-based mouthwashes can be avoided.

See also Cigarettes; Oral cancer; Nasopharyngeal cancer; Smoking cessation.

Resources

BOOKS

Beers, Mark H., MD, and Robert Berkow, MD, editors. "Disorders of the Oral Region: Neoplasms." *The Merck Manual of Diagnosis and Therapy*. Whitehouse Station, NJ: Merck Research Laboratories, 2007.

PERIODICALS

Dai, M., G. M. Clifford, F. le Calvet, et al. "Human Papillomavirus Type 16 and TP53 Mutation in Oral Cancer: Matched Analysis of the IARC Multicenter Study." *Cancer Research* 64 (January 15, 2004): 468–471.

Massie, M. J. "Prevalence of Depression in Patients with Cancer." *Journal of the National Cancer Institute: Monographs* 32 (2004): 57–71.

Owen, R. P., C. E. Silver, T. S. Ravikumar, et al. "Techniques for Radiofrequency Ablation of Head and Neck Tumors." *Archives of Otolaryngology—Head and Neck Surgery* 130 (January 2004): 52–56.

Smith, E. M., J. M. Ritchie, K. F. Summersgill, et al. "Age, Sexual Behavior and Human Papillomavirus Infection in Oral Cavity and Oropharyngeal Cancers." *International Journal of Cancer* 108 (February 20, 2004): 766–772.

Villarreal Renedo, P. M., F. Monje Gil, L. M. Junquera Gutierrez, et al. "Treatment of Oral and Oropharyngeal Epidermoid Carcinomas by Means of CO2 Laser." *Medicina Oral* 9 (March-April 2004): 168–175.

OTHER

"Oral Cavity and Pharyngeal Cancer" Online text. American Cancer Society. [cited July 5, 2009]. http://www3.cancer.org.

ORGANIZATIONS

American Academy of Facial Plastic and Reconstructive Surgery (AAFPRS). 310 South Henry Street, Alexandria, VA 22314. (703) 299-9291. http://www.facemd.org.

American Society of Plastic Surgeons (ASPS). 444 East Algonquin Road, Arlington Heights, IL 60005. (847) 228-9900. http://www.plasticsurgery.org.

SPOHNC, Support for People with Oral and Head and Neck Cancer. P.O. Box 53, Locust Valley, NY 11560-0053. 800-377-0928.http://www.spohnc.org.

Diane M. Calabrese
Rebecca J. Frey, Ph.D.

Osteosarcoma

Definition

Osteosarcoma, also called osteogenic **sarcoma**, is a type of **cancer** that develops from bone. Osteosarcoma is destructive at its original area and is likely to spread to other parts of the body.

Description

Osteosarcoma is a malignant (cancerous) tumor that arises from bone itself, and is thus called a primary bone cancer. Primary bone cancers are relatively rare overall. Approximately 900 new cases of osteosarcoma occur in the United States every year.

Osteosarcoma occurs most frequently during childhood or adolescence. About 10% of cases of this disease develop between ages 10 and 30. The incidence of osteosarcoma rises again among people in their 60s.

Osteosarcoma may occur in any bone, but develops most commonly in long bones, particularly near the knee or in the upper arm. The cancer starts growing within a bone and forms an expanding, ball-like mass. The tumor eventually breaks through the surface of the bone and begins to invade adjoining structures such as muscles. If untreated, the disease usually appears elsewhere in the same limb and metastasizes to distant parts of the body, such as the lungs.

Causes and symptoms

There are numerous theories regarding the causes of osteosarcoma. Many cases occur during a time of rapid bone growth, as in teenagers or people with

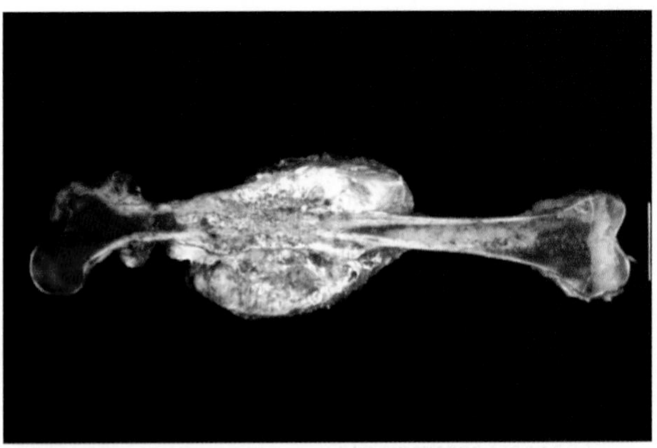

This excised specimen of a femur thigh bone shows the decaying and dryness caused by cancer. *((c) SPL/Photo Researchers, Inc. Reproduced by permission.)*

KEY TERMS

Alkaline phosphatase (Alk phos)—A body protein, measurable in the blood, that often appears in high amounts in patients with osteosarcoma. However, many other conditions also elevate the level of alkaline phosphatase.

Chemotherapy—A type of treatment for cancer that attempts to kill tumor cells with doses of powerful, often toxic, chemicals.

Grade—As a noun: a classification of the cancerous qualities of an individual tumor. A higher grade indicates a more serious disease than does a lower grade. As a verb: to classify the cancerous qualities of an individual tumor.

Malignant—Cancerous.

Metastasize—To spread to another part of the body.

Monoclonal antibody—A protein, produced in large quantities in a laboratory, designed to attack a specific target in the body.

Osteogenic—Creating bone.

Osteogenic sarcoma—Osteosarcoma.

Paget's disease—A non-cancerous disease marked by excessive growth of abnormal bone material.

Retinoblastoma—A cancerous tumor of the eye.

Stage—As a noun: the extent to which an individual cancer has spread. A higher stage indicates a more serious disease than does a lower stage. As a verb: to determine the extent to which an individual cancer has spread.

Tumor—An abnormal growth of cells in the body. Tumors may be benign (non-cancerous) or malignant.

Paget's disease. This suggests that the cancer may develop when the body loses its ability to control the multiplication of certain bone cells. Some cases of osteosarcoma are likely to have a genetic basis, and numerous genetic abnormalities have been found in patients with osteosarcoma. Osteosarcoma is also the most common second cancer to develop in survivors of **retinoblastoma**, a cancer of the eye that often has a genetic cause. Other cases arise in people who have been exposed to radiation, either accidentally or as part of a medical treatment.

The most common early symptoms of osteosarcoma are often vague. There may be pain or swelling at the site of the tumor, but these symptoms initially may not seem serious in a young, active person. Thus, the patient or medical personnel may attribute the symptoms to growing pains, or an injury from sports, for example, and the diagnosis may be delayed. Eventually, it is usually possible to feel a firm lump on the bone, and this lump will be uncomfortable to the touch.

Diagnosis

The complete diagnosis of osteosarcoma is a complicated process, requiring a variety of tests and the help of several types of medical specialists. Physicians must determine the stage of the cancer (the extent to which it has spread), and the grade of the cancer (the degree of cancerous qualities shown by its cells in a **biopsy** specimen). A higher grade or stage indicates a more serious disease than does a lower grade or stage.

Initial diagnosis begins with x-ray images of the affected area. These pictures will show a destructive growth within the bone, which is often described as having a "moth-eaten appearance". The patient then requires further imaging tests such as **computed tomography** (CT, CAT) or magnetic resonance (MR, MRI) scans of the tumor, a chest x-ray series or chest CT, and a nuclear medicine scan of the entire skeleton (bone scan). Blood tests, such as measurements of alkaline phosphatase (alk phos) provide additional information. These tests all help determine the stage of the cancer.

Finally, physicians require a biopsy sample of the diseased bone, obtained with a needle or by a surgical procedure, to be sure that the disease is truly cancer and to identify its grade. There are numerous tests, mostly involving examinations under the microscope, to perform on this biopsy specimen.

Treatments and prognosis

Before the 1980s, limb **amputation** was the standard treatment for osteosarcoma. Usually, however, the tumor had already spread elsewhere in the body and the patient eventually died of the disease. Overall results were dismal.

Newer medical developments make it possible to avoid amputation and yet treat many patients with osteosarcoma successfully. Patients almost always receive **chemotherapy** with more than one drug (multi-drug therapy) before surgery to shrink the original cancer and reduce the likelihood of spread to other areas. Techniques known as limb-sparing surgery often allow removal of the tumor while saving the rest of the extremity. Afterward, patients usually continue to receive chemotherapy, and may require bone grafts or prosthetic devices to replace parts of bones or joints that have been removed.

Future treatments under investigation include **monoclonal antibodies** that destroy specific cancer cells, techniques to slow cancer growth by controlling certain cellular genes, and bone-seeking substances that directly target areas of active bone growth.

Alternative and complementary therapies

Current treatments with chemotherapy and surgery offer a substantial improvement over past therapies. Radiation treatment has not been effective. Complementary and alternative medicine techniques may improve a patient's sense of well-being but will not cure this destructive type of cancer.

Prognosis

Prognosis for an individual patient reflects a complex balance among the extent to which the cancer has already spread at the time of diagnosis, the aggressiveness of the cells within the cancer, and the response to chemotherapy. Early detection is extremely important. The best chance of cure occurs when a tumor shows no sign of **metastasis** at the time of original surgery, is well-confined within a single bone and is completely removed, and responds well to chemotherapy. The five-year survival rate for osteosarcoma in a long bone of a limb is about 70%. All patients must be followed closely by a physician to watch for cancer recurrence.

Prevention

Prevention of osteosarcoma is difficult since doctors do not know the cause of most cases. Perhaps research eventually will make prevention possible. Early detection of the disease remains vital. Anyone with persistent pain in a bone or limb should report this to a physician. People with special risk factors including Paget's disease, exposure to significant amounts of radiation, or a family history of certain types of cancer must be especially vigilant.

Resources

PERIODICALS

Marina, Neyssa, et al. "Biology and Therapeutic Advances for Pediatric Osteosarcoma."*The Oncologist* 9 (2004): 422-41.

Wittig, James C., et al. "Osteosarcoma: A Multidisciplinary Approach to Diagnosis and Treatment."*American Family Physician* 65 (2002): 1123-32, 1135-6.

Kenneth J. Berniker, M.D.
Abigail V. Berniker, B.A.

Ovarian cystadenocarcinoma, Primary peritoneal carcinoma *see* **Ovarian cancer**

Ovarian cancer

Definition

Ovarian **cancer** is cancer of the ovaries, the egg-releasing and hormone-producing organs of the female reproductive tract. In ovarian cancer, malignant (cancerous) cells divide and multiply in an uncontrolled, abnormal fashion to form a tumor.

Demographics

Ovarian cancer can develop at any age, but is most likely to occur in women who are 50 years or older; most women are diagnosed after menopause. More than half the cases are among women who are over age 63. Industrialized countries have the highest incidence of ovarian cancer. Caucasian women, especially those of Ashkenazi Jewish descent, are at somewhat higher risk; African-American and Asian women are at a slightly lower risk.

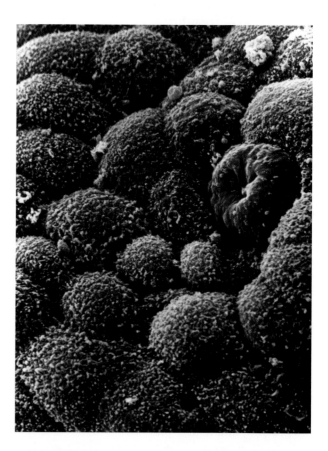

Colored scanning electron micrograph (SEM) of cancer cells in the ovary. These tumor cells are a variety of shapes and sizes, typical of the chaotic arrangement and growth of malignant cancer cells. *(© Quest, Science Source/Photo Researchers, Inc. Photo reproduced by permission.)*

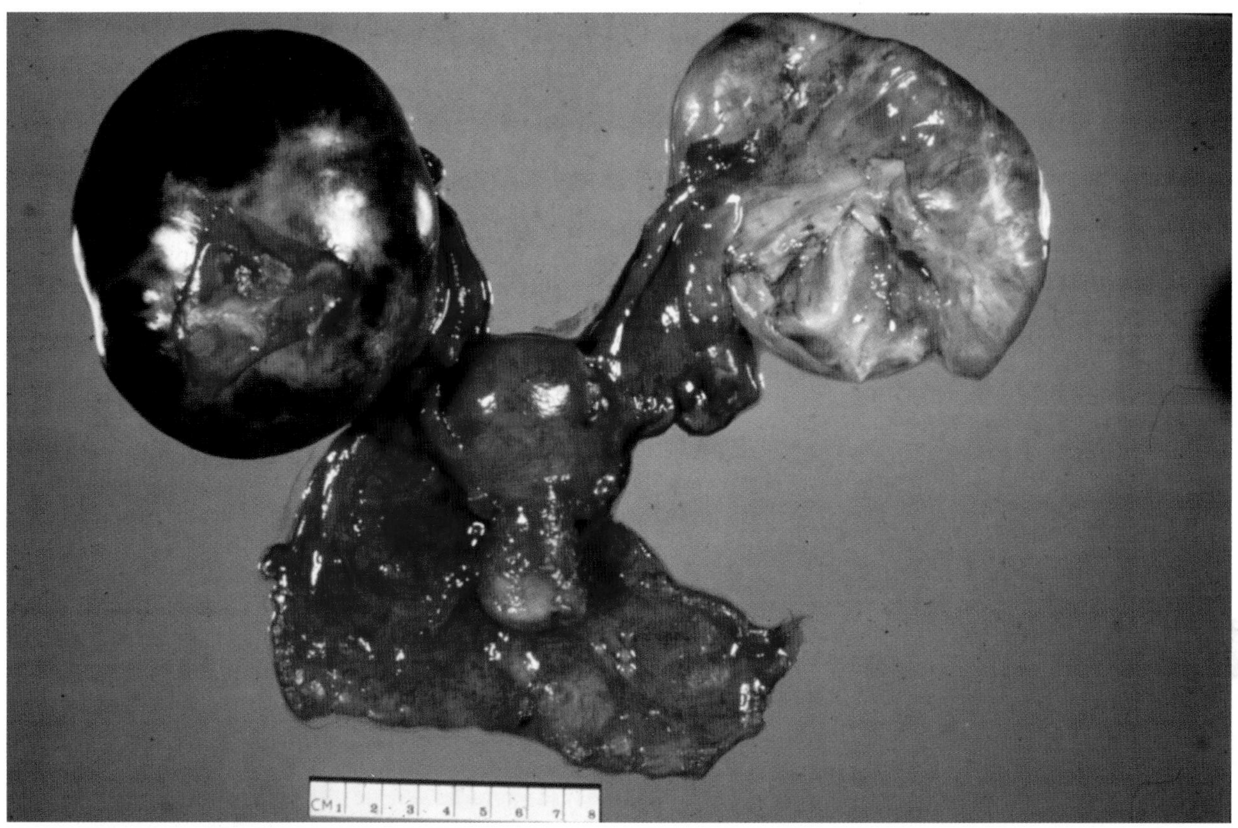

Excised female reproductive organs, showing a cancerous ovary (left, black). *(© St. Bartholomew's Hospital, Science Source/Photo Researchers, Inc. Reproduced by permission.)*

In 2009, ovarian cancer was the eighth most common cancer among women in the United States. It accounted for about 3.3% of all new cancers in American women. However, because of poor early detection, ovarian cancer is the fifth most common cause of cancer death among women. About one in 71 American women will develop ovarian cancer during her lifetime, and one in 95 will die from it. Rates are thought to be similar worldwide. The American Cancer Society estimated about 21,550 new cases of ovarian cancer would be diagnosed in the United States in 2009, and the cancer would cause about 14,600 deaths that year.

Description

The ovaries are small, almond-shaped organs located in the pelvic region, one on either side of the uterus. During a woman's childbearing years, the ovaries generally alternate to produce and release one egg each month as part of the normal menstrual cycle. The released egg is shunted into the adjacent Fallopian tube and moves downward to the uterus where, if fertilized, it will implant and develop into a fetus, and if unfertilized will be shed along with menstrual blood. The ovaries also secrete the female hormones estrogen and progesterone, which help regulate the menstrual cycle and pregnancy, as well as support the development of the secondary female sexual characteristics (i.e., breasts, body shape, and body hair). During pregnancy and when women take certain medications, mainly oral contraceptives, the ovaries do not produce eggs.

Types of ovarian tumors

The ovaries contain three main types of cells: epithelial cells, stromal cells, and germ cells. About 90% of all ovarian cancers develop from epithelial cells lining the surface of the ovaries. About 15% of tumors that develop from epithelial cells are considered low malignant potential (LMP) tumors. These tumors occur more often in younger women, are more likely to be diagnosed early, and thus have a better prognosis

.

Stromal cells are located inside the ovary and produce the hormones estrogen and progesterone. About 5% of ovarian cancers begin in the stromal cells.

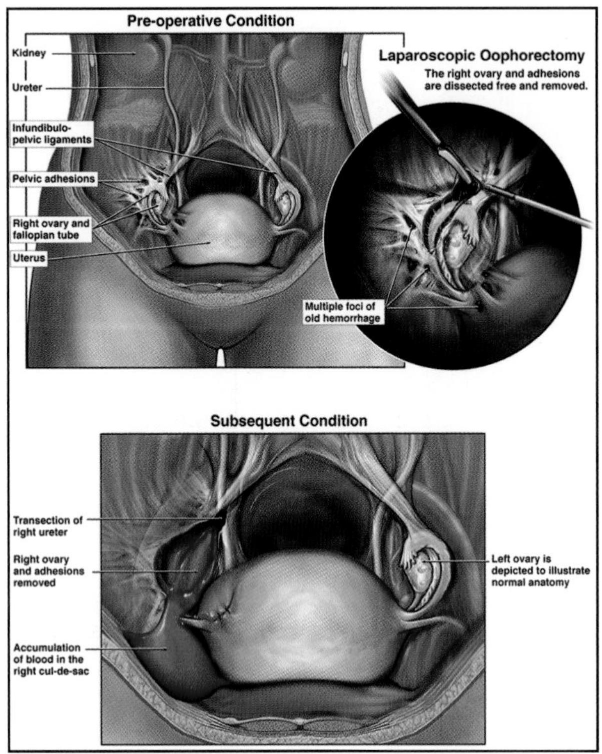

Ovarian surgery. *(Nucleus Medical Art, Inc. / Alamy. Reproduced by permission.)*

Germ cells also are located within the ovary. **Germ cell tumors** develop in the cells that would become eggs (ova). They account for about 2% of ovarian tumors. Many germ cell tumors are benign (noncancerous). These tumors often occur in teenaged girls and young women. The prognosis is good if they are found early, but as with other ovarian cancers, early detection is difficult.

Risk factors

Age is one of the greatest risk factors in developing ovarian cancer, with risk increasing after menopause. Another risk factor is a family or personal history of cancers of the female reproductive tract or breast that is caused by an inherited the genetic mutation BRCA1 or BRCA2. Not all women with BRCA1 or BRCA2 mutations will develop ovarian cancer. By age 70, a woman who has the BRCA1 mutation carries about a 40–60% risk of developing ovarian cancer. Women with the genetic mutation BRCA2 have a 15% risk of developing ovarian cancer. However, these gene mutations play a role only in about 5% of all ovarian cancer cases.

Early first menstruation (before age 12) and late menopause also seem to put women at a higher risk of ovarian cancer. The use of talcum powder in the genital area has been implicated in ovarian cancer in many studies. It may be because talc contains particles of asbestos, a known carcinogen. Female workers exposed to asbestos have a higher-than-normal risk of developing ovarian cancer. Genital deodorant sprays may also present an increased risk, however, not all studies have brought consistent results. Other risk factors include eating a diet high in saturated fats, treatment with androgens (male hormones), and never having been pregnant (nulliparity). Conversely, having been pregnant, breastfeeding, and using oral contraceptives decrease the risk of developing ovarian cancer.

Causes and symptoms

Cells in ovarian tissue normally divide and grow according to controls and instructions by proteins produced by various genes. If certain genes develop changes (mutations), instructions for cellular growth and division may go awry. Abnormal, uncontrolled cell growth may occur, causing cancer. Most of these genetic changes are not inherited. Instead, they are sporadic, still unexplained changes. Most ovarian cancers occur later in life after years of exposure to various environmental factors (e.g., the body's own hormones, asbestos exposure, or smoking) that may cause sporadic genetic alterations.

Ovarian cancer often is clled a silent killer because it produces few symptoms in its early stages. Most women are unaware they have the disease until it has progressed to advanced stages. Most early symptoms are vague and either abdominal or gastrointestinal in nature. These symptoms may not be properly diagnosed or may recognized as ovarian in nature only after a significant length of time had passed and ovarian cancer has advanced.

The following symptoms are warning signs of ovarian cancer, but these symptoms also can be due to many other causes. Symptoms that persist for two to three weeks or symptoms that are unusual for the particular woman should be evaluated by a doctor.

- digestive symptoms, such as gas, indigestion, constipation, or a feeling of fullness after a light meal
- bloating, distention or cramping
- abdominal or low-back discomfort
- pelvic pressure or frequent urination
- unexplained changes in bowel habits
- nausea or vomiting
- pain or swelling in the abdomen
- loss of appetite (anorexia)
- fatigue
- unexplained weight gain or loss
- pain during intercourse
- vaginal bleeding in post-menopausal women

Diagnosis

In the best-case scenario a woman is diagnosed with ovarian cancer while it is still contained in just one ovary. Early detection can bring five-year survival to about 93%. Advanced ovarian cancer is at stage III or stage IV, and it has already spread (metastasized) to other organs.) A physical examination and pelvic exam generally do not reveal early-stage ovarian cancer.

Tests

If ovarian cancer is suspected, several of the following tests and examinations will be necessary to make a definitive diagnosis.

- a complete medical history to assess all the risk factors
- a thorough bi-manual pelvic examination
- CA-125 assay
- one or more various imaging procedures
- a lower GI series, or barium enema
- diagnostic laparoscopy for definitive diagnosis

BI-MANUAL PELVIC EXAMINATION. The exam should include feeling the following organs for any abnormalities in shape or size: the ovaries, Fallopian tubes, uterus, vagina, bladder, and rectum. Because the ovaries are located deep within the pelvic area, it is unlikely that a manual exam will detect any abnormality while the cancer is still localized. However, a full examination provides the practitioner with a more complete picture. An enlarged ovary does not confirm cancer, as the ovary may be large because of a cyst or endometriosis. While women should have an annual Pap test to detect **cervical cancer**, this test is ineffective in detecting ovarian cancer.

CA-125 ASSAY. This is a blood test to determine the level of CA-125, a biomarker or tumor marker. A tumor marker is a measurable protein-based substance given off by the tumor. A series of CA-125 tests may be done to see if the amount of the marker in the blood is stable, increasing, or decreasing. A rising CA-125 level often indicates cancer, while a stable or declining value is more characteristic of a cyst. The CA-125 level should never be used alone to diagnose ovarian cancer. It can be normal in 50% of women with early-stage ovarian cancer. It is elevated in about 80% of women with late-stage ovarian cancer, but in 20% of cases is not elevated. In addition, this is a general biomarker and can be elevated because of a non-ovarian cancer, or from a non-malignant gynecologic conditions such as endometriosis or ectopic pregnancy. During menstruation the CA-125 level may be elevated, so the test is best done when the woman is not menstruating period.

IMAGING. Several different imaging techniques are used in evaluating ovarian cancer. Ultrasound uses high-frequency sound waves that create a visual pattern of echoes of the structures at which they are aimed. It often can distinguish between a fluid-filled structure such as a cyst and a solid structure, such as a tumor Ultrasound is painless and harmless; it is the same technique used to check a developing fetus in the womb. Ultrasound may be done externally through the abdomen and lower pelvic area, or with a transvaginal probe (**transvaginal ultrasound**).

Other painless imaging techniques are **computed tomography** (CT) and **magnetic resonance imaging** (MRI). Color Doppler analysis provides additional contrast and accuracy in distinguishing masses. These imaging techniques allow better visualization of the internal organs and can detect abnormalities without having to perform surgery.

LOWER GI SERIES. A lower GI series, or **barium enema**, uses a series of **x rays** to highlight the colon and rectum. To provide contrast, the patient drinks a chalky liquid containing barium. This test might be done to see if cancer has spread to these areas.

DIAGNOSTIC LAPAROSCOPY. This technique uses a thin hollow lighted instrument inserted through a small incision in abdomen to visualize the organs inside of the abdominal cavity. If the ovary is believed to be malignant, the entire ovary may be removed (**oophorectomy**) and its tissue sent for evaluation to the pathologist, even though only a small piece of the tissue is needed for evaluation. If cancer is present, great care must be taken not to cause the rupture of the malignant tumor, as this could spread cancer cells to adjacent organs. If the cancer is completely contained in the ovary, its removal also functions as the treatment. If the cancer has spread or is suspected to have spread, then a saline solution may be instilled into the cavity and then drawn out again. This technique is called peritoneal lavage. The aspirated fluid will be evaluated for the presence of cancer cells. If peritoneal fluid is present, called **ascites**, a sample of this will also be drawn and examined for malignant cells. If cancer cells are present in the peritoneum, then treatment will be directed at the abdominal cavity as well.

Treatment

Treatment is based on the stage of cancer at diagnosis and the woman's age.

Clinical staging

Staging is the term used to determine if the cancer is localized or has spread, and if so, how far and to where. Staging helps define the cancer and will determine the course of suggested treatment. Staging involves examining any tissue samples (biopsies) that have been taken from the ovary, nearby lymph nodes, and any structures where **metastasis** was suspected. This may include the diaphragm, lungs, stomach, intestines, and omentum (the tissue covering internal organs), and any fluid as described above.

The National Cancer Institute Stages uses the Tumor/Node/Metastasis (TNM) system for staging ovarian cancer. Other staging systems such as the International Federation of Gynecology and Obstetrics (FIGO) staging system also may be used. The TNM staging system is summarized as follows:

- Stage I: Cancer is confined to one or both ovaries.
- Stage II: Cancer is found in one or both ovaries and/or has spread to the uterus, Fallopian tubes, and/or other body parts within the pelvic cavity.
- Stage III: Cancer is found in one or both ovaries and has spread to lymph nodes or other body parts within the abdominal cavity, such as the surfaces of the liver or intestines.
- Stage IV: Cancer is found in one or both ovaries and has spread to other distant organs such as the lung.

Individual stages are further subdivided. Accurate staging is important in determining a treatment plan.

Surgery

Surgery is done to remove as much of the tumor as possible (called tissue debulking), usually followed by **chemotherapy** and/or radiation (adjuvant therapy) to target cancer cells that have remained in the body without jeopardizing the woman's health. This can be hard to achieve once the cancer has spread. Removal of the ovary is called oophorectomy, and removal of both ovaries is called bi-lateral oophorectomy. Unless it is very clear that the cancer has not spread, the Fallopian tubes are removed as well (salpingo-oophorectomy). Removal of the uterus is called hysterectomy.

If the woman is young and wishes to have children, all attempts will be made to spare the uterus. It is crucial that a woman discuss with her surgeon her childbearing plans before surgery. Ovarian cancer spreads easily and often spreads swiftly throughout the reproductive tract, so may be necessary to remove all reproductive organs as well as part of the lining of the peritoneum to provide the woman with the best possible chance of long-term survival. Fertility-sparing surgery can be successful if the ovarian cancer is diagnosed very early.

Side effects of the surgery will depend on the extent of the surgery, but may include pain and temporary difficulty with bladder and bowel function, as well as reaction to the loss of hormones produced by the organs removed. A hormone replacement patch may be applied to the woman's skin in the recovery room to help with the transition. An emotional side effect involve the feeling of loss stemming from the removal of reproductive organs.

Chemotherapy

Chemotherapy is used to target cells that have traveled to other organs, and throughout the body via the lymphatic system or the blood stream (metastasized). Chemotherapy drugs are designed to kill cancer cells, but they also harm to healthy cells. Chemotherapy may be administered through a vein in the arm (intravenous, IV), may be taken in tablet form (orally), and/or may be given through a thin tube called a catheter directly into the abdominal cavity (intraperitoneal). IV and oral chemotherapy drugs travel throughout the body; intraperitoneal chemotherapy is localized in the abdominal cavity.

Side effects of chemotherapy vary greatly depending on the drugs used. Currently, chemotherapy drugs are often used in combinations to treat advanced ovarian cancer, and usually the combination includes a platinum-based drug (such as **cisplatin**) with a taxol agent, such as paclitaxel. Some of the combinations used or being studied include: carboplatin/paclitaxel, cisplatin/paclitaxel, cisplatin/topotecan, and cisplatin/carboplatin. **Antineoplastic agents** such as topotecan (Hycamtin) or **gemcitabine** (Gemzar) that interfere with the ability of the tumor cells to reproduce also may be given. The goal of chemotherapy is to maximize effectiveness with minimum of side effects. Side effects include **nausea and vomiting**, **diarrhea**, decreased appetite and resulting **weight loss**, **fatigue**, headaches, loss of hair, and numbness and tingling (parethesia) in the hands or feet. Managing these side effects is an important part of cancer treatment.

After the full course of chemotherapy has been given, the surgeon may perform a "second look" surgery to examine the abdominal cavity again to evaluate the success of treatment.

Radiation

Radiation uses high-energy, highly focused x rays to target very specific areas of cancer. This is done using a machine that generates an external energy beam. Careful measurements are taken so that the targeted area can be as focused and small as possible. Another form of radiation uses a radioactive liquid that is administered into the abdominal cavity in the same fashion as intraperitoneal chemotherapy. Radiation usually is given on a daily Monday though Friday schedule and for several weeks. Radiation is not painful, but side effects can include skin damage at the area exposed to the external beam and extreme fatigue. Fatigue may hit suddenly around the third week of treatment and may take a while to resolve even after treatments have terminated. Other side effects may include **nausea**, **vomiting**, diarrhea, loss of appetite, weight loss, and urinary difficulties. For patients with incurable ovarian cancer, radiation may be used to shrink tumor masses to provide pain relief and improve quality of life (palliative care).

Following treatment, regular follow-up appointments will be scheduled to monitor for any long-term side effects, relapse, or metastases.

Clinical trials

Clinical trials are human research studies. Their goal is to evaluate the effectiveness of new ways to treat cancer. There are many different designs, and they target different aspects of care. For example, some may investigate the response of different chemotherapy drugs, while another study may compare different types of treatment/chemotherapy combinations.

Research studies often are designed to compare the effectiveness of a new treatment method against the standard method or the effectiveness of a drug against a placebo (an inert substance that would be expected to have no effect on the outcome). Since the research is experimental in nature, there are no guarantees about the outcome. New drugs being used may have harmful, unknown side effects. Some people participate to help further knowledge about their disease. For others, the study may provide a possible treatment that is not yet available otherwise. Although there is no cost to participate, participants have to meet certain criteria before being admitted into the study. It is important to fully understand one's role in the study, and weigh the potential risks versus benefits when deciding whether or not to participate. A list of clinical trials currently enrolling patients can be found at http://clinicaltrials.gov.

Alternative and complementary therapies

The term alternative therapy refers to therapy used instead of conventional treatment. By definition, these treatments have not been scientifically proven or investigated as thoroughly and by the same standards as conventional treatments. The terms complementary or integrative therapy denote practices used in conjunction with rather than instead of conventional treatment. Patients should inform their doctors of any alternative or complementary therapies being used or considered as some alternative and complementary therapies adversely affect the effectiveness of conventional treatments. Some common complementary and alternative medicine therapies include:

- prayer and faith healing
- meditation
- mind/body techniques such as support groups, visualization, guided imagery and hypnosis
- energy work such as Therapeutic Touch and Reiki
- acupuncture and traditional Chinese medicine
- body work such as yoga, massage, and t'ai chi
- vitamin, mineral, and/or herbal supplements
- special diets such as vegetarian, vegan, or macrobiotic

Mind/body techniques along with meditation, prayer, yoga, t'ai chi, and acupuncture have been shown to reduce stress levels, and the relaxation provided may help boost the body's immune system. The effectiveness of some other complementary and alternative treatments is being studied by the National Institutes of Health's National Center for Complementary and Alternative Medicine (NCCAM). For a current list of the research studies, recent results and publications, patients can visit the NCCAM web site at http://nccam.nih.gov or call (888) 644-6226.

Coping with cancer treatment

While the cancer may only be in part of the body, it is very much a full mind/body experience. Strategies for coping with the treatment need to address the entire range of the experience. Each woman will have different needs. She might want to create a personal support team of friends. They can provide support by:

- Finding helpful information in the library or on the Internet about clinical trials, new therapies or treatments, different treatment centers, etc.
- Providing transportation to and from appointments. A diagnosis of cancer can be overwhelming. In such a stressful and distracted state it is often hard to remember what a doctor has said, or even to remember the questions to be asked. Having a second set of ears during this stressful time can be helpful.
- Helping with household duties so that the woman can rest after treatments and have more energy to devote to her family.
- Assisting with childcare. Children are very much affected by a parent's cancer diagnosis, whether or not they have been fully informed of what is taking

QUESTIONS TO ASK YOUR DOCTOR

- What tests will be used to look for and diagnose my cancer?
- How should I prepare for the tests?
- What will take place during the test? Will it be painful? What can I do to decrease the pain?
- When will I learn the results?
- Once the results are in: What do these results mean?
- What type and stage is my cancer?
- What are my treatment options?
- Who will be involved in my care?
- Are there clinical trials that might benefit me?
- What changes in my ability to work or perform my daily functions should I expect during treatment?
- How long will my treatment last?
- What side effects should I expect from treatment?
- Are there any conventional or alternative therapies that can diminish side effects of treatments?
- During treatment will I need a caregiver or will I be able to care for myself?
- How soon after treatment will I be able to resume my regular activities?
- What is the plan for my follow-up care?

place. For a child to go to a friend's house can provide a sense of normalcy and security.

- Being available to participate in activities and conversations not centering on the cancer. While in the midst of cancer treatments, it is important to talk about non-cancer issues as well and to maintain social relationships and activities.

A woman may wish to join a support group of women with ovarian cancer. This group can provide the environment to talk about the diagnosis, the treatments, the side effects, and the impact the diagnosis has on her life with others who can empathize. If there is no support group nearby, she may be able to join one on the Internet. Support groups also may exist for caregivers and loved ones.

Prognosis

Prognosis for ovarian cancer depends largely on the stage at which it is first diagnosed. Stage I ovarian cancer has the best survival rate, although ovarian cancer is rarely diagnosed at this stage. The 2009 5-year survival rates for the four stages of ovarian cancer are: stage I, 92.8%; stage II, 78.6%; stage III, 50%; stage IV, 17.5%.

Prevention

Since the cause of ovarian cancer is not known, it is not possible to fully prevent the disease. However, there are ways to reduce one's risks of developing the disease.

Decrease ovulation

Pregnancy temporarily stops ovulation, and multiple pregnancies appear to further reduce the risk of ovarian cancer. The research is not clear as to whether the pregnancy must result in a term delivery to have full benefit. Women who breastfeed their children also appear to have a lower risk of developing the disease. Since oral contraceptives also suppress ovulation, women who take birth control pills have a lower incidence of ovarian cancer. It appears that the longer a woman takes oral contraceptives, the lower her risk for ovarian cancer. However, since oral contraceptives alter a woman's hormonal status, her risk for other hormonally related cancers may change. The woman should discuss the risks and benefits of oral contraceptives with her health care provider.

Genetic testing

Genetic testing is available that can help determine whether a woman who carries certain genes that increase her risk of breast and ovarian cancer. If the woman tests positive for a BRCA1 or BRCA2 mutation, then she may be able to consider having their ovaries removed as a preventative measure (prophylactic oophorectomy).

Surgery

Procedures such as tubal ligation (in which the Fallopian tubes are blocked or tied) and hysterectomy (in which the uterus is removed) appear to reduce the risk of ovarian cancer. However, any removal of the reproductive organs has surgical as well as hormonal side effects.

Screening

There are no definitive tests or screening procedures as of late 2009 to detect ovarian cancer in its early stages. Women at high risk should consult their physicians about possible regular screenings, which may include transvaginal ultrasound and a blood test for the CA-125 protein. The American Cancer Society recommends annual pelvic examinations for all women after age 40, in order to increase the chances of early detection of both cervical and ovarian cancer.

Early detection remains the key focal point in increasing survival rates for ovarian cancer because the more ovarian cancer has spread, the poorer the chance for survival past one or two years. As women and practitioners become more alert to vague early warning signs and seek out more accurate family histories, earlier awareness may begin to lead to earlier detection and improved survival rates.

Resources

BOOKS

Montz, F. J., Robert E. Bristow, and Paula J. Anastasia *A Guide to Survivorship for Women with Ovarian Cancer*. Baltimore, MD: Johns Hopkins Press, 2005.

OTHER

"Detailed Guide to Ovarian Cancer." American Cancer Society August 27, 2009 [September 26, 2009]. http://www.cancer.org/docroot/CRI/CRI_2_3x.asp?dt=33.

Garcia, Agustin. ldquo;Ovarian Cancer." eMedicine.com December 13, 2007 [September 26, 2009]. http://emedicine.medscape.com/article/255771-overview.

"OncoLink." Abramson cancer Center of the University of Pennsylvania 2009 [September 26, 2009]. http://www.oncolink.upenn.edu.

"Ovarian Cancer." MedlinePlus September 22, 2009 [September 26, 2009]. http://www.nlm.nih.gov/medlineplus/ovariancancer.html.

ORGANIZATIONS

American Cancer Society, 1599 Clifton Rd., NE, Atlanta, GA, 30329, (404) 320-3333, (800) ACS-2345, http://www.cancer.org.

Cancer Research and Prevention Foundation, 1600 Duke Street, Suite 500, Alexandria, VA, 22314, (703) 836-4412, (800) 227-2732, info@preventcancer.org, http://www.preventcancer.org.

Gynecologic Cancer Foundation, 230 W. Monroe, Suite 2528, Chicago, IL, 60606, (312) 578-1439, (800) 444-4441, (312) 578-9769, info@thegcf.org, http://www.wcn.org/gcf.

National Cancer Institute Public Inquires Office., 6116 Executive Boulevard, Room 3036A, Bethesda, MD, 20892-8322, (800) 4-CANCER. TTY (800) 332-8615, http://www.cancer.gov.

National Center for Complementary and Alternative Medicine Clearinghouse, PO Box 7923, Gaithersburg, MD, 20898, (301) 519-3153. TTY: (866) 464-3615<, (888) 644-6226, (866) 464-3616, info@nccam.nih.gov, http://nccam.nih.gov.

Ester Csapo Rastegari, R.N., B.S.N., Ed.M.
Tish Davidson, A.M.

Ovarian epithelial cancer

Definition

Ovarian epithelial **cancer** is a type of cancer that develops in the cells that line the surface of the ovaries.

Description

Part of the female reproductive system, the ovaries are a pair of almond-shaped organs that are located on either side of the uterus, just above the pelvic bone. The ovaries produce estrogen and progesterone, which are female hormones. At birth, each ovary contains thousands of eggs. During a woman's fertile years, one ripened egg (or sometimes more) is released each month into a fallopian tube. As the egg takes its journey toward the uterus, a sperm can fertilize it. When a baby is conceived, it stays in the uterus until birth. During the birth process, powerful muscles in the uterus help to push the baby out through the cervix and vagina.

When an ovarian cell becomes cancerous, it tends to multiply quickly, forming a growth (or tumor). The resulting tumor may interfere with the way the ovary normally functions, but not in every case. Sometimes the cancer cells break off from the tumor and spread contiguously, which means they spread to nearby organs, such as to other areas of the pelvis.

Demographics

Although **ovarian cancer** rates differ significantly from country to country, Europe has been recognized as having one of the highest incidence rates of ovarian cancer in the world. Having carefully studied the ovarian cancer trends of 28 European countries, Bray and colleagues reported in a 2004 article published by the *International Journal of Cancer* that European countries with the highest ovarian cancer rates in the past included the Nordic countries, Austria, Germany, and the United Kingdom, but current trends in these and other northern European countries showed a decline in ovarian cancer rates, especially with regard to mortality. However, the opposite was found to be true with regard to some of the southern and eastern European countries. In the Czech Republic and Hungry, there has been a drop in the mortality rates associated with ovarian cancer, but not a drop in the number of cases diagnosed. Bray a colleagues reported that "recent trends in ovarian cancer have led to a leveling of rates across various areas of the [European] continent, although a 2.5-fold variation was still observed in the late 1990s between the highest mortality rate of

KEY TERMS

Pap test—A procedure that involves taking cells from the cervix, which are examined under a microscope for signs of abnormality.

Peritoneum—The tissue that lines the abdomen.

QUESTIONS TO ASK YOUR DOCTOR

- What clinical trials do you recommend?
- Will I be able to have children?
- When will I be able to return to work?
- Are there any local cancer support groups?
- How will the treatment affect my sex life?
- Are there any medications that could alter the test or treatment results?
- What prescription and over-the-counter medications should be avoided during treatment?

9.3/100,000 in Denmark and the lowest one of 3.6 in Portugal."

The American Cancer Society estimates that 21,550 news cases of ovarian cancer will be diagnosed in the United States in 2009, resulting in approximately 14,600 deaths. Rarely seen in women under the age of 30, the risk of developing ovarian cancer increases with age. Nearly 90% of all the cases of ovarian cancer are ovarian epithelial cancer. Ranked fifth as the most frequent cause of cancer death in women, ovarian epithelial cancer most commonly occurs in women over the age of 65.

Causes and symptoms

The presence of mutations in the **BRCA1** and **BRCA2** genes increase a woman's risk of developing breast or ovarian cancer, including ovarian epithelial cancer. When these gene mutations are not present in woman who has ovarian epithelial cancer, it is difficult to identify the cause. Several factors may increase a woman's risk of developing ovarian epithelial cancer, such as having a close relative with the disease or a personal history of **breast cancer**.

There seems to be a connection between the development of ovarian epithelial cancer and the number of times a woman ovulates in her lifetime. Statistics show that a woman who ovulates less seems to have less risk. For example, a woman who has had a child may have a decreased risk of developing ovarian epithelial cancer, because she has had a nine-month break in ovulation. On the other hand, a woman who has used birth control pills may lessen her risk for the same reason, because she, too, has had a break in ovulation.

Ovarian epithelial cancer often produces no symptoms in its early stages; therefore, by the time it is discovered, the disease is often widespread. In addition, women often ignore the symptoms, because they don't identify them with anything serious. Some of the symptoms include:

- gas and indigestion
- bloating
- swelling of the abdomen
- constipation, nausea, and vomiting
- fullness or pressure in the pelvis
- abnormal bleeding from the vagina
- lower abdominal pain (such as cramps)

Diagnosis

A variety of tests and examinations are used to diagnose ovarian epithelial cancer.

Pelvic Exam

Many women are familiar with this exam and schedule one on a yearly basis along with a pap smear. The exam is usually performed by a gynecologist, but is also sometimes performed by a physician specializing in family or internal medicine. Many women think a Pap test will detect ovarian cancer, but, in truth, it is the pelvic examination that helps a physician diagnose ovarian epithelial cancer, whereas the Pap test is useful in detecting **cervical cancer**.

To perform a pelvic examination, the physician inserts one or two lubricated, gloved fingers of one hand into a woman's vagina while pressing down on her abdomen with the other hand. By touch, the physician examines the uterus and ovaries, checking for any abnormalities in shape, size, or position. This examination only takes a few minutes and is not painful, although some women may feel some pressure or minor discomfort. The patient should tell the physician immediately if any pain is experienced. As part of the examination, the physician will also insert a lubricated, gloved finger into the rectum to feel for lumps.

Ultrasound

Often referred to as a sonogram, ultrasound is a completely painless procedure performed by radiologist in which high-energy sound waves are bounced off internal organs.

Magnetic Resonance Imaging (MRI)

Although an expense test, an MRI is often covered by many insurance plans. Using a magnetic field and imaging waves, an MRI scans a specific portion of the body from any angle. Painless and noninvasive, MRI testing does not require the use of contrast dye. However, the MRI is an unnerving machine for anyone claustrophobic, because the machine surrounds almost the entire body. Claustrophobic patients should ask their physician to refer them to the nearest Open Air MRI facility. The open design of an Open Air MRI provides access from all four sides and allows patients to feel more comfortable during their exam.

Blood Test

A test that measures the level of CA 125 in the blood is often recommended if ovarian epithelial cancer is suspected. An increased level of CA 125 may be a sign that cancer is present in the body.

Barium Enema

Sometimes referred to as a lower GI, a liquid that contains barium is put into the rectum, which coats the gastrointestinal tract so that **x rays** can be taken. It is usually performed by an x-ray technician or radiologist and is considered by many people to be as unpleasant as a normal enema.

Intravenous Pyelogram (IVP)

The purpose of this test, which normally takes about 30 minutes to an hour, is to see if any abnormalities exist in the kidneys and bladder. An IVP is essentially a series of x rays. A contrast dye, which is injected into the patient's vein, enhances the x-ray images that are taken to see if there are any blockages.

The night before the exam, the patient will be asked to fast (not eat any food) and to take a mild laxative, such as a teaspoon of castor oil. Patients who suspect they might be pregnant should inform their physicians prior to having an IVP. Although it is often not necessary for patients to remove their clothing, they will often be asked to remove any jewelry that might interfere with the images.

An IVP itself is painless, although some patients experience **nausea** and/or a metallic taste in their mouth as the dye is being inserted. Both the nausea and metallic taste tend to go away as the patient's body gets used to the dye. Some patients develop hives, which is an allergic reaction to the dye. The radiologist, who performs the test, will have medication on hand to treat the hives. When the test is completed, the radiologist will examine the x rays and write up a report for the referring physician who will deliver the results to the patient.

Computerized Tomography (CT Scan)

A CT scan, also referred to as a CAT scan, is a procedure that takes a series of detailed pictures of the inside of the body and is considered one of the best tools available for studying abdominal tissue, especially with regard to the presence of a tumor.

Like an IVP, a contrast dye is injected into a vein to help the organs and surrounding tissue show up more clearly. In some cases, the contrast dye is swallowed by the patient rather than injected. A computer linked to an x-ray machine generates the pictures. The test is painless and generally takes about 30 minutes to an hour, depending on how many images are needed. Unlike the IVP, however, the x-ray technician or radiologist will not remain in the room while the x rays are being taken. The patient will be able to hear and speak to the person performing the test, which is either an x-ray technician or radiologist. Because of the radiation used to perform a CT scan, patients that suspect they are pregnant should tell their physicians prior to having the test. If the images show a tumor, many different specialists, such as a radiologist, oncologist, surgeon, and the referring physician, will often work together to arrive at a suitable course of treatment.

Biopsy

A physician may recommend that a **biopsy** be performed, which is a surgical procedure to remove tissue or cells from the surface of the ovary to see if they are cancerous.

Treatment team

The treatment team is comprised of physicians from a variety of medical specialties. For example, a patient diagnosed with ovarian epithelial cancer may have a treatment team that includes the patient's primary care physician and her gynecologist, as well as a radiologist, oncologist, surgeon, and **pain management** specialist. At-home caretakers are also part of the treatment team, providing important physical and emotional support to the patient. Physicians and patients that value a holistic approach to fighting cancer may add a variety of other advisors to the treatment team, such as psychologists, pastors, and alternative medicine specialists.

Clinical staging, treatments, and prognosis

Staging

After ovarian epithelial cancer has been diagnosed, it is classified as being in one of four stages based on whether the cancer cells have or have not spread within the ovaries or to other parts of the body. To determine the stage of the disease, the patient is placed under general anesthesia and a surgical procedure called a laparotomy is performed. By making an incision through the abdomen, the surgeon can inspect the ovaries and adjacent organs for cancer. A biopsy is often done at that time and the cells are viewed under a microscope by the surgeon who often specializes in oncology. If there are clear indications that cancerous tissue is present, the surgeon will usually remove it and any effected organs during the laparotomy. A tissue sample is also sent to a lab where a pathologist can further classify the sample and confirm the diagnosis. It can take several days to receive the pathologist's report.

The National Cancer Institute explains the four main stages of ovarian epithelial cancer as follows:

- Stage I: The cancer is present in one or both ovaries, but the cancer has not spread.
- Stage II: The cancer is present in one or both ovaries and has spread to the pelvis.
- Stage III: The cancer is present in one or both ovaries and has spread to other parts of the abdomen.
- Stage IV: The cancer is not only in one or both ovaries, but it has spread beyond the abdomen to other parts of the body.

All four stages have subcategories A, B, and C, which further indicate the characteristics and severity of the cancer within each stage. For example, according to the National Cancer Institute, in Stage IIIB, "The cancer has spread to the peritoneum but is 2 centimeters or smaller in diameter, whereas in Stage IIIC, the cancer has spread to the peritoneum and is larger than 2 centimeters and/or has spread to lymph nodes in the abdomen."

Treatment Options

Depending on the patient and the stage of the cancer, there are a variety of treatment options for patients with ovarian epithelial cancer. The three convention treatment options are surgery, **radiation therapy**, and **chemotherapy**. As the National Cancer Institute states, "Most patients have surgery to remove as much of the tumor as possible." Although ovarian epithelial cancer usually does not strike young women, it does pose a special concern for young women hoping to have a family. In the event that the disease is caught early enough, it might be possible to perform a unilateral salpingo-oophorectomy, which is the removal of only the involved ovary and fallopian tube, thereby giving the woman a chance to have children someday. However, in many cases, it is necessary to remove both ovaries, as well as the uterus, fallopian tubes, and nearby lymph glands. Sometimes it is even necessary to remove the omentum, which is a fold of the peritoneum.

Depending on the stage of cancer, radiation therapy may be recommended. There are generally two types of radiation therapy external radiation therapy, which comes from a machine outside of the body, and internal radiation therapy, such as implant radiation or brachytherapy. Chemotherapy is a commonly known cancer treatment that utilizes strong drugs to stop the growth of cancer cells. Chemotherapy is either given intravenously or orally; it often involves combination drug therapy. The administration and combination of chemotherapy drugs utilized is largely dependant on the extent of the cancer and the patient's medical profile.

Prognosis

The survival rate depends on a variety of factors, such as the patient's age and general health as well as the type and stage of tumor. When ovarian epithelial cancer is found early, the five-year survival rate is approximately 60–80%. However, because ovarian epithelial cancer is often found late in its development, the overall survival rate is 30–40%. In addition, ovarian epithelial cancer can recur after it has been treated.

Coping with cancer treatment

Patients having difficulty coping with the pain associated with cancer and chemotherapy might find it helpful to be referred to a physician who specializes in pain management or a pain clinic. Physicians specializing in the treatment of pain come from a variety of medical backgrounds, such as anesthesiology, obstetrics and gynecology, neurology, and surgery. Because of the complicated nature of cancer and cancer-related pain, ideally a pain management team should be formed that works with the patient's primary care physician, oncologist, and radiologist to provide comprehensive care to the patient.

Much has been written about coping with the physical side effects of cancer treatment; however, patients with ovarian epithelial cancer also face emotional challenges associated with their treatment. For example, women who are still in their reproductive years and need to have both ovaries removed must deal with an abrupt end to their reproductive choices. Women of all ages will have to deal with a variety of psychological issues, such as **body image** versus self-image. Some woman may need to be reminded, especially by family members and friends, that they are more than a collection of body parts. The spirit of their womanhood remains even if their ovaries do not.

It is important for cancer patients to understand that they are not alone. Support groups exist to help patients cope not only with the physical aspects of having cancer, but with the psychological ones as well. Patients should be encouraged to talk about their feelings. The positive support (both emotional and otherwise) provided by caregivers can help to improve a patient's quality of life. In addition, support groups on the Internet have made it possible for women, even those in rural or remote areas, to reach out to one another in ways that allow anonymity.

Clinical trials

Patients should ask their doctor if there are any **clinical trials** being conducted in their areas that they should consider joining. Clinical trials are conducted to improve current methods of treatment or to develop new treatments. Patients with cancer who participate in clinical trials may improve their chances of survival.

Prevention

Women with a strong family history of ovarian epithelial cancer should be sure to have regular pelvic examinations, because an early diagnosis increases the chance of survival. However, there really is no way to prevent ovarian epithelial cancer, other than to have both ovaries removed before cancer has had a chance to grow, which is an extremely controversial prevention method. Nonetheless, some women with a high risk of developing ovarian epithelial cancer who have had the chance to have a family have elected to have a prophylactic **oophorectomy**, which is the medical name for the procedure that refers to the removal of healthy ovaries. Women considering this procedure need to know that it isn't necessarily a guarantee against ovarian cancer.

Resources

BOOKS

Lema, Mark J., Day, Miles, Myers, David P., et al. Cancer Pain. In *Pain Medicine: A Comprehensive Review, edited by P. Prithvi Raj and Lee Ann Paradise* St. Louis, MO: Mosby, 2003, pp.110–118.

Northrup, C. *Women's Bodies, Women's Wisdom*. New York, NY: Bantam Books, 1994.

PERIODICALS

Amos, C. I., Struewing, J. P. "Genetic epidemiology of epithelial ovarian cancer. " *Cancer* 71 (1993): 566–572.

Piver, M. S., Jishi, M. F., Tsukada, Y., et al. "Primary peritoneal carcinoma after prophylactic oophorectomy in women with a family history of ovarian cancer. A report of the Gilda Radner Familial Ovarian Cancer Registry." *Cancer* 71 (1993): 2751–2755.

OTHER

American Cancer Society "Cancer Facts and Figures 2005." *American Cancer Society* 2005 American Cancer Society. [6 April 2009] http://www.cancer.org/.

Bray, Freddie, Loos, Anja Helena, Tognazzo, Sandro, La Vecchia, Carlo "Ovarian Cancer in Europe: Cross-sectional trends in incidence and mortality in 28 countries, 1953-2000." *International Journal of Cancer* October 25, 2004 [cited November 7, 2009]. <http://www3.interscience. wiley.com/>.

National Cancer Institute "Ovarian Epithelial Cancer (PDQ[R]): Treatment. " *National Cancer Institute* 2009 National Cancer Institute. [22 Nov. 2009] http://www.cancer.gov/.

ORGANIZATIONS

National Cancer Institute Public Inquiries Office. Suite 3036A, 6116 Executive Blvd., MSC 8322, Bethesda, MD 20892-8322. 800-4-CANCER. http://www.cancer.org/

Lee Ann Paradise

Oxycodone *see* **Opioids**

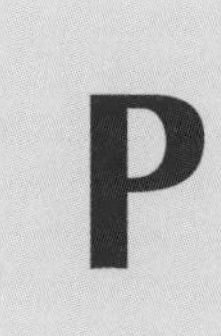

Paget's disease of the breast

Definition

Paget's disease of the breast is a rare type of **breast cancer** that is characterized by a red, scaly lesion on the nipple and surrounding tissue (areola).

Description

Paget's disease of the breast, also called mammary Paget's disease, is a rare breast condition that is often associated with underlying breast **cancer**. It is believed that Paget's disease of the breast occurs when invasive **carcinoma** or intraductal carcinoma (cancer of the milk ducts) spreads through the milk ducts to the nipple.

Although in most cases the underlying breast cancer is extensive, in 10% of the cases, cancer only affects the nipple and surrounding tissue. Rarely, there is no detectable underlying breast cancer. Paget's disease located elsewhere on the body (extramammary Paget's disease) is rarely associated with an underlying invasive cancer. This type of Paget's disease, most commonly found on and around the genitals, is believed to arise directly from the cells lining certain sweat gland ducts. Possibly, the few cases of mammary Paget's disease without an underlying breast cancer have a similar origin.

Paget's disease of the breast accounts for 2% of all breast cancers. On average, women are 62 years old and men are 69 years old at diagnosis. Breast cancer rarely occurs in men.

Causes and symptoms

The causes of Paget's disease of the breast are unknown. The most common signs and symptoms of Paget's disease include redness, scaling, and flaking on and around the nipple and areola. Other symptoms include **itching**, tingling, burning, oversensitivity, or pain. The lesion may bleed or weep and open sores (ulcers) may be present.

Diagnosis

A thorough breast examination would be performed. A breast mass can be felt (palpated) in about half of the women with Paget's disease. **Mammography** and **ultrasonography** should be conducted to look for cancer within the breast that cannot be felt.

The definitive diagnosis of Paget's disease is the presence of a certain cell type, called Paget's cells, in the skin of the nipple. A tissue sample may be easily obtained by touching a microscope slide to a weeping lesion or by scraping a scaly or crusted lesion gently with a microscope slide. Alternatively, a sample of the lesion may be obtained by cutting out a small piece of nipple tissue (**biopsy**). The biopsy would be performed with local anesthetic in the physician's office. If a mass was felt, a breast biopsy would be performed.

Treatments and prognosis

Treatments

The traditional treatment of Paget's disease of the breast is to surgically remove the breast (**mastectomy**). Conservative surgery, (nipple-areolar sacrificing **lumpectomy**) in which just the nipple, areola, and underlying tissue are removed, may be sufficient in some cases. The underarm (axillary) lymph nodes are rarely sampled or removed (lymphadenectomy), unless an underlying invasive cancer is a concern.

Radiation therapy may be used as adjuvant therapy to complement the surgical treatment, and if a lumpectomy is performed, radiation must be employed. Radiation therapy uses high-energy radiation from **x rays** and gamma rays to kill the cancer cells. The skin in the treated area may become red and dry, and **fatigue** is also a common side effect.

KEY TERMS

Areola—The darkened area that surrounds the nipple.

Diethylstilbestrol (DES)—A medication used between 1945 and 1970 to prevent miscarriage.

Extramammary Paget's disease—Paget's disease that is located anywhere on the body, excluding the breasts.

Luteal phase—That part of the menstrual cycle that begins after ovulation and ends at menstruation.

Mastectomy—Surgical removal of breast tissue. Mastectomy may be partial, when only some tissue is removed, or radical, when all breast tissue and adjacent tissues are removed.

Chemotherapy, also used as adjuvant therapy if an underlying invasive breast cancer is found, uses drugs to kill the cancer cells. The side effects of chemotherapy include stomach upset, **vomiting**, appetite loss (**anorexia**), hair loss (**alopecia**), mouth or vaginal sores, fatigue, menstrual cycle changes, premature menopause, and low white blood cell counts with an increased risk of **infection**.

Prognosis

As with other breast cancers, the prognosis of Paget's disease depends on the extent of the cancer and whether it has spread to the lymph nodes and other organs.

PAGET'S DISEASE ALONE. The survival rate of women with Paget's disease of the breast alone is 99.5%.

PAGET'S DISEASE WITH INVASIVE BREAST CANCER. The prognosis for Paget's disease and invasive cancer is based on the stage of the underlying breast cancer. Staging for breast cancer is as follows:

- Stage 1—The cancer is no larger than 2 cm (0.8 in) and no cancer cells are found in the lymph nodes.
- Stage 2—The cancer is between 2 cm and 5 cm, and the cancer has spread to the lymph nodes.
- Stage 3A—Tumor is larger than 5 cm (2 in) or is smaller than 5 cm, but has spread to the lymph nodes, which have grown into each other.
- Stage 3B—Cancer has spread to tissues near the breast, (local invasion), or to lymph nodes inside the chest wall, along the breastbone.

QUESTIONS TO ASK THE DOCTOR

- What type of cancer do I have?
- What stage of cancer do I have?
- What is the five-year survival rate for women with this type and stage of cancer?
- Has the cancer spread?
- What are my treatment options?
- How much breast tissue will you be removing?
- Where will the scars be?
- What will my breast look like after surgery?
- When can I have breast reconstruction?
- What are the risks and side effects of these treatments?
- What medications can I take to relieve treatment side effects?
- Are there any clinical studies underway that would be appropriate for me?
- What effective alternative or complementary treatments are available for this type of cancer?
- How debilitating is the treatment? Will I be able to continue working?
- Are there any local support groups for breast cancer patients?
- What is the chance that the cancer will recur?
- Is there anything I can do to prevent recurrence?
- How often will I have follow-up examinations?

- Stage 4—Cancer has spread to skin and lymph nodes beyond the axilla (regional lymph nodes) or to other organs of the body.

The prognosis depends on the type and stage of cancer. Over 80% of stage I patients are cured by current therapies. Stage II patients survive overall about 70% of the time, those with more extensive lymph nodal involvement doing worse than those with disease confined to the breast. About 40% of stage III patients survive five years, and about 20% of stage IV patients do so.

Alternative and complementary therapies

Although alternative and complementary therapies are used by many cancer patients, very few controlled studies on the effectiveness of such therapies exist. Mind-body techniques such as biofeedback, visualization, meditation, and yoga, have not shown any effect in reducing cancer but they can reduce stress and lessen some of the side effects of cancer treatments.

A few studies found an association between longer survival time and a diet high in beta-carotene and fruits. Acupuncture has been found to relieve chemotherapy-induced **nausea and vomiting** and reduce pain. In some studies, **mistletoe** has been shown to reduce tumor size, extend survival time, and enhance immune function. Other studies have failed to show a response to mistletoe treatment.

For more comprehensive information, the patient should consult the book on complementary and alternative medicine published by the American Cancer Society listed in the Resources section.

Prevention

There are no specific factors that increase a person's risk of developing Paget's disease. Men who are at an increased risk of developing breast cancer include those who have had radiation exposure and those with Klinefelter's syndrome. Women's risk factors for breast cancer include:

- a personal history of breast cancer
- a family history of breast cancer
- alterations in certain genes (e.g. BRCA1 and BRCA2)
- changes in breast tissue (e.g. lobular carcinoma in situ or atypical hyperplasia)
- long-term exposure to estrogen (e.g. early age at first menstruation or late menopause), and possibly use of hormone replacement therapy
- exposure to diethylstilbestrol (DES) before birth
- first pregnancy after 30 years of age
- alcohol consumption

Regularly scheduled screening mammograms are recommended for all women over the age of 40 years. Those with a significant family history (one or more first-degree relatives who have been treated for breast cancer), should start annual mammograms 10 years younger than the youngest relative was when she was diagnosed, but not earlier than 35. Monthly breast self examinations and yearly clinical breast examinations are recommended for all women. Daily exercise, totalling two to four hours a week, decreases a woman's risk of breast cancer by 50% to 75%. Women with a high risk of breast cancer may take the drug **tamoxifen**, which has been shown to reduce the occurrence (or recurrence) of breast cancer. Women at a very high risk may choose to have a mastectomy to prevent breast cancer (prophylactic mastectomy).

Special concerns

Of special concern to the young woman with breast cancer is the impact that treatment will have on her fertility and **body image**. **Depression** is common. There is ongoing research investigating whether timing breast cancer surgery to coincide with the luteal phase (after ovulation) of the menstrual cycle leads to an increased survival rate.

Resources

BOOKS

Bruss, Katherine, Christina Salter, and Esmeralda Galan, editors. *American Cancer Society's Guide to Complementary and Alternative Cancer Methods*. Atlanta: American Cancer Society, 2000.

Jatoi, Ismail, editor. *The Surgical Clinics of North America: Breast Cancer Management*. Philadelphia: W. B. Saunders Company, 1999.

Kronenberg, Fredi, Patricia Murphy, and Christine Wade. "Complementary/Alternative Therapies in Select Populations: Women." In *Complementary/Alternative Medicine: An Evidence- Based Approach*, edited by John Spencer and Joseph Jacobs. St. Louis: Mosby, 1999, pp.340-62.

Lemon, Henry. "Cancer of the Female Breast." In *Current Therapy in Cancer*, edited by John Foley, Julie Vose, and James Armitage. Philadelphia: W. B. Saunders Company, 1999, pp.109-15.

PERIODICALS

Lloyd, J., and A. M. Flanagan. "Mammary and Extra-mammary Paget's Disease." *Journal of Clinical Pathology* 53 (October 2000): 742-49.

ORGANIZATIONS

American Cancer Society. 1599 Clifton Road NE, Atlanta, GA 30329. (800) ACS-2345. http://www.cancer.org.

Cancer Research Institute, National Headquarters. 681 Fifth Ave., New York, NY 10022. (800) 992-2623. http://www.cancerresearch.org.

National Alliance of Breast Cancer Organizations. 9 East 37th St., 10th Floor, New York, NY 10016. (888) 806-2226. http://www.nabco.org.

National Institutes of Health. National Cancer Institute. 9000 Rockville Pike, Bethesda, MD 20982. Cancer Information Service: (800) 4-CANCER. <http://cancernet.nci.nih.gov>.

Y-Me Advocacy Program. 212 West Van Buren St., 5th Floor, Chicago, IL 60607. (312) 986-8338. http://www.y-me.org.

Belinda Rowland, Ph.D.

Pain management

Definition

Pain management in **cancer** care encompasses all the actions taken to keep people with cancer as free of pain as possible. It includes pharmacological, psychological, and spiritual approaches to prevent, reduce, or stop pain sensations.

Purpose

It is estimated that more than 800,000 new cases of cancer are diagnosed each year in the United States, and 430,000 cancer victims will die. Though recent figures are hopeful and suggest a decline in both the incidence of cancer and the number of people who die from it, studies have consistently shown that at least 70% of cancer patients in the advanced stage of the disease will experience significant pain. Pain is a localized sensation ranging from mild discomfort to an unbearable, excruciating experience. It is, in its origins, a protective mechanism, designed to alert the brain to injury or disease conditions. Unfortunately, when the cause of the pain is known, such as in diagnosed cancer, and treatment is initiated, pain can often continue.

Once the message of cancer has been received and interpreted by the brain, further pain can be counterproductive. Pain can have a negative impact on a person's quality of life, causing **depression** and impeding recovery. Unrelieved pain can become a syndrome in its own right and cause a downward spiral in a person's health and outlook. Proper pain management facilitates recovery, prevents additional health complications, and improves an individual's quality of life.

Several independent studies of the relief of pain have shown that pain is often under-treated by the medical profession. For this reason, in the spring and summer of 2000, the Joint Commission on Accreditation of Healthcare Organizations (JCAHO) and the American Pain Society (APS) developed standards for proper pain management.

Description

What is pain?

The treatment of pain has been a major endeavor since ancient times. By 400 B.C., the father of modern medicine, Hippocrates, had theorized that the brain, not the heart, was the controlling center of the body, and Greek anatomists had begun to identify various nerves and their purposes. The pain-relieving properties of opium were already known and were being utilized to stop suffering. Two thousand years ago, in China, acupuncture was being used to reduce pain.

Pain is the means by which the peripheral nervous system (PNS) warns the central nervous system (CNS) of injury or potential injury to the body. The CNS comprises the brain and spinal cord, and the PNS is composed of the nerves that stem from and lead into the CNS. PNS includes all nerves throughout the body except the brain and spinal cord.

A pain message is transmitted to the CNS by special PNS nerve cells called nociceptors. Nociceptors are distributed throughout the body and respond to different stimuli depending on their location. For example, nociceptors that extend from the skin are stimulated by sensations such as pressure, temperature, and chemical changes.

When a nociceptor is stimulated, neurotransmitters are released from cells. Neurotransmitters are chemicals found within the nervous system that facilitate nerve cell communication. The nociceptor transmits its signal to nerve cells within the spinal cord, which conveys the pain message to the thalamus, a specific region in the brain.

Once the brain has received and processed the pain message and coordinated an appropriate response, pain has served its purpose. The body uses natural pain killers, called endorphins, that are meant to derail further pain messages from the same source. However, these natural pain killers may not adequately dampen a continuing pain message. Also, depending on how the brain has processed the pain information, certain hormones, such as prostaglandins, may be released. These hormones enhance the

QUESTIONS TO ASK THE DOCTOR

- Does my type of cancer usually cause pain, and if so, how will the pain be treated?
- Does the radiation or chemotherapy that I may have cause pain?
- What are the side-effects of the medications you will order?
- What things can I do to help with my pain management?
- Does the pain necessarily mean that the cancer is getting worse?

KEY TERMS

Acute—A short-term pain in response to injury or other stimulus that resolves when the injury heals or the stimulus is removed.

Chemotherapy—The treatment of infections or malignant diseases by drugs that act selectively on the cause of the disorder, but which may have substantial side effects.

Chronic—Pain that endures beyond the term of an injury or painful stimulus. Also refers to cancer pain, pain from a chronic or degenerative disease, and pain from an unidentified cause.

CNS or central nervous system—The part of the nervous system that includes the brain and the spinal cord.

Hepatic capsule—The membranous bag enclosing the liver.

Iatrogenic—Resulting from the activity of the physician.

Metastasis—A secondary malignant tumor (one that has spread from a primary cancer to affect other parts of the body.

Neuropathy—Nerve damage.

Neurotransmitter—Chemicals within the nervous system that transmit information from or between nerve cells.

Nociceptor—A nerve cell capable of sensing pain and transmitting a pain signal.

Non-pharmacological—Therapy that does not involve drugs.

Palliative—Serving to relieve or alleviate the symptoms of a disease or disorder without curing the disease.

Pharmacological—Therapy that relies on drugs.

PNS or peripheral nervous system—Nerves that are outside of the brain and spinal cord.

Radiation—A treatment for cancer (and occasionally other diseases) by x rays or other sources of radioactivity, both of which produce ionizing radiation. The radiation, as it passes through diseased tissue, destroys or slows the development of abnormal cells.

Stimulus—A factor capable of eliciting a response in a nerve.

Virtual reality—The creation of a convincing environment by computer technology, displayed either on a computer screen or viewed through special stereoscopic goggles. Virtual reality is primarily a visual and auditory experience. It appears to be a useful approach to pain management in children.

pain message and play a role in immune system responses to injury, such as inflammation. Certain neurotransmitters, especially substance P and **calcitonin** gene-related peptide, actively enhance the pain message at the injury site and within the spinal cord.

It has been hypothesized that uninterrupted and unrelenting pain can induce changes in the spinal cord. In the past, intractable pain (pain that can't be managed or cured) has been treated by severing a nerve's connection to the CNS. However, the lack of any sensory information being relayed by that nerve can cause pain transmission in the spinal cord to go into overdrive, as evidenced by the phantom limb pain experienced by amputees. Evidence is accumulating that unrelenting pain or the complete lack of nerve signals increases the number of pain receptors in the spinal cord. Nerve cells in the spinal cord may also begin secreting pain-amplifying neurotransmitters independent of actual pain signals from the body. Immune chemicals, primarily cytokines, may play a prominent role in such changes.

What is cancer pain?

The majority of cancer pain results from a cancerous tumor pressing on organs, nerves, or bone. However, several studies by pain-pioneer Dr. John Bonica and others have shown that a predictable 78% of all cancer pain is indeed related to the disease, but an impressive 19% was found to be caused instead by treatment of the cancer. Three percent of all complaints of pain were unrelated to either the disease or treatment.

Cancer pain is generally divided into three categories:

- *Visceral pain*, usually caused by pressure resulting from the invasiveness of the tumor, expansion of the hepatic capsule, or injury caused by radiation or chemotherapy.
- *Somatic pain* often resulting from bone metastasis.
- *Neuropathic pain*, or pain caused by the pressure of a tumor on nerves, or the trauma to nerves resulting from either radiation, chemotherapy, or surgery.

Managing cancer pain

PHARMACOLOGICAL OPTIONS. General guidelines developed by the World Health Organization (WHO) for pain management apply to cancer pain management as well. These guidelines follow a three-step ladder approach:

- Mild pain is alleviated with acetominophen or nonsteroidal anti-inflammatory drugs (NSAIDs). NSAIDs and acetaminophen are available as over-the-counter and prescription medications, and are frequently the initial pharmacological treatment for pain. These drugs can also be used as adjuncts to the other drug therapies, which might require a doctor's prescription. NSAIDs include aspirin, ibuprofen (Motrin, Advil, Nuprin), naproxen sodium (Aleve), and ketoprofen (Orudis KT). These drugs are used to treat pain from inflammation and work by blocking production of pain-enhancing neurotransmitters, such as prostaglandins. Acetaminophen is also effective against pain, but its ability to reduce inflammation is limited. NSAIDs and acetaminophen are effective for most forms of acute (sharp, but of a short course) pain.
- Mild to moderate pain is eased with a milder opioid medication plus acetominophen or NSAIDs. Opioids are both actual opiate drugs such as morphine and codeine, and synthetic drugs based on the structure of opium. This drug class includes drugs such as oxycodone, methadone, and meperidine (Demerol). They provide pain relief by binding to specific opioid receptors in the brain and spinal cord, and thus block the perception of pain.
- Moderate to severe pain is treated with stronger opioid drugs plus acetominophen or NSAIDs. Morphine is sometimes referred to as the "Gold Standard" of palliative care as it is not expensive, can be given starting with smaller doses and gradually increased, and is highly effective over a long period of time. It can also be administered orally (by mouth), rectally, or by injection. A newer method of administering morphine involves a patient-controlled delivery system implanted in the covering of the spinal cord. Researchers in North Carolina reported in late 2003 that the new system not only provided more effective pain relief, but also lowered the patients' use of morphine and the complications associated with long-term use of morphine. In general, the development of implantable pumps has greatly improved pharmacological approaches to pain management.

Although antidepressant drugs were developed to treat depression, they are also effective in combating chronic headaches, cancer pain, and pain associated with nerve damage. Antidepressants shown to have analgesic (pain reducing) properties include **amitriptyline** (Elavil), trazodone (Desyrel), and imipramine (Tofranil). Anticonvulsant drugs share a similar background with antidepressants. Developed to treat epilepsy, anticonvulsants were found to relieve pain as well. Drugs such as **phenytoin** (Dilantin) and **carbamazepine** (Tegretol) are prescribed to treat the pain associated with nerve damage.

Close monitoring of the effects of pain medications is required in order to assure that adequate amounts of medication are given to produce the desired pain relief. When a person is comfortable with a certain dosage of medication, oncologists typically convert to a long-acting version of that medication. Transdermal fentanyl patches (Duragesic) are a common example of an long-acting opioid drug often used for cancer pain management. A patch containing the drug is applied to the skin where the drug is continuously absorbed by the body, usually for three days. Pumps are also available that provide an opioid medication upon demand when the person is experiencing pain. By pressing a button, they can release a set dose of medication into an intravenous solution or an implanted catheter. Another mode of administration involves implanted catheters that deliver pain medication directly to the spinal cord. Delivering drugs in this way can reduce side effects and increase the effectiveness of the drug. Research is underway to develop toxic substances that act selectively on nerve cells that carry pain messages to the brain, killing these selected cells, and thus stopping transmission of the pain message.

NON-PHARMACOLOGICAL OPTIONS. Pain treatment options that do not involve drugs are often used as adjuncts to, rather than replacements for, drug therapy. One of the benefits of non-drug therapies is that an individual can take a more active stance against pain. Relaxation techniques, such as yoga and meditation, are used to shift the focus of the brain away from the pain, decrease muscle tension, and reduce stress. Tension and stress can also be reduced through biofeedback, in which an individual consciously attempts to modify skin temperature, muscle tension, blood pressure, and heart rate. A group of researchers in New York reported in 2003 that the hypnotic-like approaches—particularly imagery, relaxation techniques, and hypnotic suggestion—appear to be more effective in managing pain than other behavioral approaches.

Participating in normal activities and exercising can also help control pain levels. Through physical therapy, an individual learns beneficial exercises for reducing stress, strengthening muscles, and staying fit.

Regular exercise has been linked to production of endorphins, the body's natural pain killers.

Acupuncture involves the insertion of small needles into the skin at key points. The acupuncturist will usually stimulate points on the ear when treating cancer pain. Acupressure uses these same key points, but involves applying pressure rather than inserting needles. Both of these methods may work by prompting the body to release endorphins. Applying heat or being massaged are very relaxing and help reduce stress. Transcutaneous electrical nerve stimulation (TENS) applies a small electric current to certain parts of nerves, potentially interrupting pain signals and inducing release of endorphins. To be effective, use of TENS should be medically supervised.

A new method for managing pain in children with cancer is virtual reality, which works by distracting the child's attention from the pain and accompanying anxiety. Virtual reality has been used successfully in the treatment of anxiety disorders, and shows great promise in treating children suffering from cancer pain. Larger-scale studies are under way.

Preparation

Assessment of cancer pain is absolutely essential to good pain management. Pain scales or questionnaires are sometimes used to attach an objective measure to a subjective experience. Objective measurements allow health care workers a better understanding of the pain being suffered by the patient. Pain has been called "the fifth vital sign," (temperature, pulse, respiration and blood pressure being the other four vital signs), by the Veterans Administration. Evaluation also includes physical examinations and diagnostic tests to determine underlying cause of the pain. Some evaluations require assessments from several viewpoints, including neurology, psychiatry and psychology, and physical therapy.

Risks

Owing to toxicity over the long term, even nonprescription drugs must be carefully monitored in chronic pain management. NSAIDs have the well-known side effect of causing gastrointestinal bleeding, and long-term use of acetaminophen has been linked to kidney and liver damage. Other drugs, especially narcotics, have side effects such as constipation, drowsiness, and **nausea**. Sedation can often be reduced by the timing of when medication is taken (such as at bedtime), and constipation can be reduced by increasing the amount of fruits, vegetables, and whole-grain foods in the diet, or by the use of **laxatives**, stool softeners, or even enemas. Serious side effects can also accompany antidepressants and anticonvulsants, which may discourage or prevent their use depending upon the circumstances. These side effects include mood swings, confusion, bone thinning, cataract formation, increased blood pressure, and other problems.

Non-pharmacological therapies carry little or no risks. However, it is advised that individuals recovering from serious illness or injury consult with their health care providers or physical therapists before making use of adjunct therapies. Invasive procedures carry risks similar to other surgical procedures, such as **infection**, reaction to anesthesia, iatrogenic injury (injury as a result of treatment), and heart failure.

A traditional concern about narcotics use has been the risk of promoting addiction or tolerance. As narcotic use continues over time, as in terminal cancer, the body becomes accustomed to the drug and adjusts normal functions to accommodate to its presence. Therefore, to elicit the same level of action, it is necessary to increase dosage over time. Tolerance can be defined as a gradual lessening of the effectiveness of an opioid drug from continued use.

Many studies involving cancer patients have indicated that proper dosage of narcotic medication does not create an addiction to it. A major concern for many cancer patients though, is that the medication will stop working for them. Evidence suggests this is not true. A simple increase in the dose will usually cause the medication to relieve pain again. One of the biggest dangers is abruptly stopping an opioid medication or reducing the dose, as the person can then go into withdrawal, a potentially serious medical condition characterized by agitation, rapid heart rate, profuse sweating and sleeplessness.

However, physical dependence is different from psychological addiction. Physical dependence is characterized by discomfort if drug administration suddenly stops, while psychological addiction is characterized by an overpowering craving for the drug for reasons other than pain relief. Psychological addiction is a very real and necessary concern in some instances, but it should not interfere with a genuine need for narcotic pain relief.

Normal results

Effective application of pain management techniques reduces or eliminates cancer pain. This treatment can improve an individual's quality of life and aid in recovery.

Perhaps the best measure of the results of pain management for cancer patients would be the fulfillment of the recently developed Bill of Rights for Cancer Pain. It is as follows:

- You have the right to be believed about the severity of your pain.
- You have the right to have your pain controlled.
- You have the right to have pain resulting from treatments and procedures prevented, or at least minimized.
- You have the right to be treated with respect at all times when you need medication; to not be treated like a drug abuser.

Resources

PERIODICALS

Alimi, D., C. Rubino, E. Pichard-Leandri, et al. "Analgesic Effect of Auricular Acupuncture for Cancer Pain: A Randomized, Blinded, Controlled Trial." *Journal of Clinical Oncology* 21 (November 15, 2003): 4120–4126.

Gershon, J., E. Zimand, R. Lemos, et al. "Use of Virtual Reality as a Distractor for Painful Procedures in a Patient with Pediatric Cancer: A Case Study." *Cyberpsychology and Behavior* 6 (December 2003): 657–661.

Mundy, E. A., K. N. DuHamel, and G. H. Montgomery. "The Efficacy of Behavioral Interventions for Cancer Treatment-Related Side Effects." *Seminars in Clinical Neuropsychiatry* 8 (October 2003): 253–275.

Perron, Vincent, MD, and Ronald S. Schonwetter, MD. "Assessment and Management of Pain in Palliative Care Patients." *Cancer Control: Journal of the Moffitt Cancer Center* 27 (January 2001).

Rauck, R. L., D. Cherry, M. F. Boyer, et al. "Long-Term Intrathecal Opioid Therapy with a Patient-Activated, Implanted Delivery System for the Treatment of Refractory Cancer Pain." *Journal of Pain* 4 (October 2003): 441–447.

Rosenthal, K. "Implantable Pumps Deliver Innovative Pain Management." *Nursing Management* 34 (December 2003): 46–49.

ORGANIZATIONS

American Chronic Pain Association. PO Box 850, Rocklin, CA 95677-0850. (916) 632-0922. <http://members.tripod.com/~widdy/acpa.html>.

American Pain Society. 4700 West Lake Ave., Glenview, IL 60025. (847) 375-4715. http://www.ampainsoc.org.

Cancer Care, Inc. "Bill of Rights for Cancer Pain." http://www.cancerpainrelief.com/cancerpain/guide/relief/content.htm.

National Cancer Institute. "Cancer Facts." [citedSeptember 26, 2000]. <http://cancer.gov>.

National Chronic Pain Outreach Association, Inc. PO Box 274, Millboro, VA 24460-9606. (540) 997-5004.

Julia Barrett
Joan Schonbeck, R.N.
Rebecca J. Frey, Ph.D.

Pamidronate *see* **Bisphosphonates**

Pancreatectomy

Definition

A pancreatectomy is the surgical removal of the pancreas. A pancreatectomy may be total, in which case the entire organ is removed, usually along with the spleen, gallbladder, common bile duct, and portions of the small intestine and stomach. A pancreatectomy may also be distal, meaning that only the body and tail of the pancreas are removed, leaving the head of the organ attached. When the duodenum is removed along with all or part of the pancreas, the procedure is called a pancreaticoduodenectomy, which surgeons sometimes refer to as "Whipple's procedure." Pancreaticoduodenectomies are increasingly used to treat a variety of malignant and benign diseases of the pancreas. This procedure often involves removal of the regional lymph nodes as well.

Purpose

A pancreatectomy is the most effective treatment for **cancer** of the pancreas, an abdominal organ that secretes digestive enzymes, insulin, and other hormones. The thickest part of the pancreas near the duodenum (a part of the small intestine) is called the head, the middle part is called the body, and the thinnest part adjacent to the spleen is called the tail.

While surgical removal of tumors in the pancreas is the preferred treatment, it is only possible in the 10–15% of patients who are diagnosed early enough for a potential cure. Patients who are considered suitable for surgery usually have small tumors in the head of the pancreas (close to the duodenum, or first part of the small intestine), have jaundice as their initial symptom, and have no evidence of metastatic disease (spread of cancer to other sites). The stage of the cancer will determine whether the pancreatectomy to be performed should be total or distal.

A partial pancreatectomy may be indicated when the pancreas has been severely injured by trauma, especially injury to the body and tail of the pancreas. While such surgery removes normal pancreatic tissue as well, the long-term consequences of this surgery are minimal, with virtually no effects on the production of insulin, digestive enzymes, and other hormones.

Chronic pancreatitis is another condition for which a pancreatectomy is occasionally performed. Chronic pancreatitis—or continuing inflammation of the pancreas that results in permanent damage to this organ—can develop from long-standing, recurring episodes of acute (periodic) pancreatitis. This painful

KEY TERMS

Chemotherapy—A cancer treatment that uses synthetic drugs to destroy the tumor either by inhibiting the growth of the cancerous cells or by killing the cancer cells.

Computed tomography (CT) scan—An imaging technique that creates a series of pictures of areas inside the body, taken from different angles. The pictures are created by a computer linked to an x-ray machine.

Endoscopic retrograde cholangiopancreatography (ERCP)—A procedure to x-ray the ducts (tubes) that carry bile from the liver to the gallbladder and from the gallbladder to the small intestine.

Laparoscopy—In this procedure, a laparoscope (a thin, lighted tube) is inserted through an incision in the abdominal wall to determine if the cancer is within the pancreas only or has spread to nearby tissues and if it can be removed by surgery later. Tissue samples may be removed for biopsy.

Magnetic resonance imaging (MRI)—A procedure in which a magnet linked to a computer is used to create detailed pictures of areas inside the body.

Pancreas—A large gland located on the back wall of the abdomen, extending from the duodenum (first part of the small intestine) to the spleen. The pancreas produces enzymes essential for digestion, and the hormones insulin and glucagon, which play a role in diabetes.

Pancreaticoduodenectomy—Removal of all or part of the pancreas along with the duodenum. Also known as "Whipple's procedure" or "Whipple's operation."

Pancreatitis—Inflammation of the pancreas, either acute (sudden and episodic) or chronic, usually caused by excessive alcohol intake or gallbladder disease.

Positron emission tomography (PET) scan—An imaging system that creates a picture showing the location of tumor cells in the body. A substance called radionuclide dye is injected into a vein, and the PET scanner rotates around the body to create the picture. Malignant tumor cells show up brighter in the picture because they are more active and take up more dye than normal cells.

Radiation therapy—A treatment using high energy radiation from x-ray machines, cobalt, radium, or other sources.

Ultrasonogram—A procedure where high-frequency sound waves that cannot be heard by human ears are bounced off internal organs and tissues. These sound waves produce a pattern of echoes which are then used by the computer to create sonograms, or pictures of areas inside the body.

condition usually results from alcohol abuse or the presence of gallstones. In most patients with the alcohol-induced disease, the pancreas is widely involved, therefore, surgical correction is almost impossible.

Description

A pancreatectomy can be performed through an open surgery technique, in which case one large incision is made, or it can be performed laparoscopically, in which case the surgeon makes four small incisions to insert tube-like surgical instruments. The abdomen is filled with gas, usually carbon dioxide, to help the surgeon view the abdominal cavity. A camera is inserted through one of the tubes and displays images on a monitor in the operating room. Other instruments are placed through the additional tubes. The laparoscopic approach allows the surgeon to work inside the patient's abdomen without making a large incision.

If the pancreatectomy is partial, the surgeon clamps and cuts the blood vessels, and the pancreas is stapled and divided for removal. If the disease affects the splenic artery or vein, the spleen is also removed.

If the pancreatectomy is total, the surgeon removes the entire pancreas and attached organs. He or she starts by dividing and detaching the end of the stomach. This part of the stomach leads to the small intestine, where the pancreas and bile duct both attach. In the next step, he removes the pancreas along with the connected section of the small intestine. The common bile duct and the gallbladder are also removed. To reconnect the intestinal tract, the stomach and the bile duct are then connected to the small intestine.

During a pancreatectomy procedure, several tubes are also inserted for postoperative care. To prevent tissue fluid from accumulating in the operated site, a temporary drain leading out of the body is inserted, as well as a gastrostomy or g-tube leading out of the stomach in order to help prevent **nausea and vomiting**. A jejunostomy or j-tube may also be inserted into the small intestine as a pathway for supplementary feeding.

Diagnosis/Preparation

Patients with symptoms of a pancreatic disorder undergo a number of tests before surgery is even considered. These can include **ultrasonography**, x-ray examinations, **computed tomography** scans (CT scan), and **endoscopic retrograde cholangiopancreatography** (ERCP), a specialized imaging technique to visualize the ducts that carry bile from the liver to the gallbladder. Tests may also include **angiography**, another imaging technique used to visualize the arteries feeding the pancreas, and needle aspiration **cytology**, in which cells are drawn from areas suspected to contain cancer. Such tests are required to establish a correct diagnosis for the pancreatic disorder and in the planning the surgery.

Since many patients with **pancreatic cancer** are undernourished, appropriate **nutritional support**, sometimes by tube feedings, may be required prior to surgery.

Some patients with pancreatic cancer deemed suitable for a pancreatectomy will also undergo **chemotherapy** and/or **radiation therapy**. This treatment is aimed at shrinking the tumor, which will improve the chances for successful surgical removal. Sometimes, patients who are not initially considered surgical candidates may respond so well to chemoradiation that surgical treatment becomes possible. Radiation therapy may also be applied during the surgery (intraoperatively) to improve the patient's chances of survival, but this treatment is not yet in routine use. Some studies have shown that intraoperative radiation therapy extends survival by several months.

Patients undergoing distal pancreatectomy that involves removal of the spleen may receive preoperative medication to decrease the risk of **infection**.

Aftercare

Pancreatectomy is major surgery. Therefore, extended hospitalization is usually required with an average hospital stay of two to three weeks.

Some pancreatic cancer patients may also receive combined chemotherapy and radiation therapy after surgery. This additional treatment has been clearly shown to enhance survival rates.

After surgery, patients experience pain in the abdomen and are prescribed pain medication. Follow-up exams are required to monitor the patient's recovery and remove implanted tubes.

A total pancreatectomy leads to a condition called pancreatic insufficiency, because food can no longer be normally processed with the enzymes normally produced by the pancreas. Insulin secretion is likewise no longer possible. These conditions are treated with pancreatic enzyme replacement therapy, which supplies digestive enzymes; and with insulin injections. In some case, distal pancreatectomies may also lead to pancreatic insufficiency, depending on the patient's general health condition before surgery and on the extent of pancreatic tissue removal.

Risks

There is a fairly high risk of complications associated with any pancreatectomy procedure. A recent Johns Hopkins study documented complications in 41% of cases. The most devastating complication is postoperative bleeding, which increases the mortality risk to 20–50%. In cases of postoperative bleeding, the patient may be returned to surgery to find the source of hemorrhage, or may undergo other procedures to stop the bleeding.

One of the most common complications from a pancreaticoduodenectomy is delayed gastric emptying, a condition in which food and liquids are slow to leave the stomach. This complication occurred in 19% of patients in the Johns Hopkins study. To manage this problem, many surgeons insert feeding tubes at the original operation site, through which nutrients can be fed directly into the patient's intestines. This procedure, called enteral nutrition, maintains the patient's nutrition if the stomach is slow to recover normal function. Certain medications, called promotility agents, can help move the nutritional contents through the gastrointestinal tract.

The other most common complication is pancreatic anastomotic leak. This is a leak in the connection that the surgeon makes between the remainder of the pancreas and the other structures in the abdomen. Most surgeons handle the potential for this problem by checking the connection during surgery.

Normal results

After a total pancreatectomy, the body loses the ability to secrete insulin, enzymes, and other substances; therefore, the patient has to take supplements for the rest of his or her life.

Patients usually resume normal activities within a month after surgery, although they are asked to avoid heavy lifting for six to eight weeks and not to drive as long as they take narcotic medication.

WHO PERFORMS THE PROCEDURE AND WHERE IS IT PERFORMED?

A pancreatectomy is performed by a surgeon trained in gastroenterology, the branch of medicine that deals with the diseases of the digestive tract. An anesthesiologist is responsible for administering anesthesia and the operation is performed in a hospital setting, with an oncologist on the treatment team if pancreatic cancer motivated the procedure.

When a pancreatectomy is performed for chronic pancreatitis, the majority of patients obtain some relief from pain. Some studies report that one-half to three-quarters of patients become free of pain.

Morbidity and mortality rates

The mortality rate for pancreatectomy has decreased in recent years to 5–10%, depending on the extent of the surgery and the experience of the surgeon. A study of 650 patients at Johns Hopkins Medical Institution, Baltimore, found that only nine patients, or 1.4%, died from complications related to surgery.

Unfortunately, pancreatic cancer is the most lethal form of gastrointestinal malignancy. However, for a highly selective group of patients, a pancreatectomy offers a chance for cure, especially when performed by experienced surgeons. The overall five-year survival rate for patients who undergo pancreatectomy for pancreatic cancer is about 10%; patients who undergo pancreaticoduodenectomy have a 4–5% survival at five years. The risk for tumor recurrence is thought to be unaffected by whether the patient undergoes a total pancreatectomy or a pancreaticoduodenectomy, but is increased when the tumor is larger than 1.2 in (3 cm) and the cancer has spread to the lymph nodes or surrounding tissue.

Alternatives

Depending on the medical condition, a pancreas transplantation may be considered as an alternative for some patients.

QUESTIONS TO ASK THE DOCTOR

- What do I need to do before surgery?
- What type of anesthesia will be used?
- How long will it take to recover from the surgery?
- When can I expect to return to work and/or resume normal activities?
- What are the risks associated with a pancreatectomy?
- How many pancreatectomies do you perform in a year?
- Will there be a scar?

Resources

BOOKS

Bastidas, J. Augusto, and John E. Niederhuber. "The Pancreas." In *Fundamentals of Surgery*. Edited by John E. Niederhuber. Stamford: Appleton & Lange, 1998.

Mayer, Robert J. "Pancreatic Cancer." In *Harrison's Principles of Internal Medicine*. Edited by Anthony S. Fauci, et al. New York: McGraw-Hill, 1997.

PERIODICALS

Cretolle, C., C. N. Fekete, D. Jan, et al. "Partial elective pancreatectomy is curative in focal form of permanent hyperinsulinemic hypoglycaemia in infancy: A report of 45 cases from 1983 to 2000." *Journal of Pediatric Surgery* 37 (February 2002): 155–158.

Lillemoe, K. D., S. Kaushal, J. L. Cameron, et al. "Distal pancreatectomy: indications and outcomes in 235 patients." *Annals of Surgery* 229 (May 1999): 698–700.

McAndrew, H. F., V. Smith, and L. Spitz. "Surgical complications of pancreatectomy for persistent hyperinsulinaemic hypoglycaemia of infancy." *Journal of Pediatric Surgery* 38 (January 2003): 13–16.

Patterson, E. J., M. Gagner, B. Salky, et al. "Laparoscopic pancreatic resection: single-institution experience of 19 patients." *Journal of the American College of Surgeons* 193 (September 2001): 281–287.

OTHER

NIH CancerNet: Pancreatic Cancer Homepage. [cited July 1, 2009]. http://www.cancer.gov/cancerinfo/types/pancreatic.

ORGANIZATIONS

American College of Gastroenterology. 4900 B South 31st St., Arlington, VA 22206. (703) 820-7400. http://www.acg.gi.org.

American Gastroenterological Association (AGA). 4930 Del Ray Avenue, Bethesda, MD 20814. (301) 654-2055. http://www.gastro.org.

National Cancer Institute (NCI). NCI Public Inquiries Office, Suite 3036A, 6116 Executive Boulevard, MSC8322 Bethesda, MD 20892-8322. (800) 422-6237. http://www.cancer.gov.

Caroline A. Helwick
Monique Laberge, Ph.D.

Pancreatic cancer

Definition

There are two types of **cancer** of the pancreas. **Endocrine pancreatic cancer** is a disease in which cancerous cells originate within the tissues of the pancreas that produce hormones. **Exocrine pancreatic cancer** is a disease in which cancerous cells originate within the tissues of the pancreas that produce digestive juices.

Demographics

Exocrine cancer

Although pancreatic cancer accounts for only 3% of all cancers, in 2000 it was the fourth frequent cause of cancer deaths. The American cancer Society estimated that in 2009, an estimated 42,470 new cases of pancreatic cancer will be diagnosed in the United States and 35,420 individuals will die from the disease. Pancreatic cancer is primarily a disease associated with advanced age, with 80% of cases occurring between the ages of 60 and 80. Men are more likely to develop this disease than women. Countries with the highest frequencies of pancreatic cancer include the United States, New Zealand, Western European nations, and Scandinavia. The lowest occurrences of the disease are reported in India, Kuwait, and Singapore. African Americans have the highest rate of pancreatic cancer of any ethnic group worldwide. Whether this difference is due to diet or environmental factors remains unclear.

Endocrine cancer

Endocrine cancer is rare, accounting for 3–10 cases per million individuals. Between one and four cases of insulinoma occur per million people per year, and 90% of these tumors are benign. They occur mostly in people between the ages of 30 and 50 and affect men and women equally. Less than three cases of gastrinoma per million people are diagnosed each year, but it is the most common functional islet cell tumor in patients with multiple endocrine tumors, a condition known as multiple endocrine neoplasia (MEN) syndrome. Vipoma and glucagonoma are even rarer and they occur more frequently in women. Somatostatinoma is exceedingly uncommon, and fewer than 100 cases have been reported worldwide. Nonfunctional islet cell cancers account for approximately one-third of all cancers of the endocrine pancreas, and the majority of these are malignant.

Description

The pancreas is a six- to eight-inch long, slipper-shaped gland located in the abdomen. It lies behind the stomach, within a loop formed by the small intestine. Other nearby organs include the gallbladder, spleen, and liver. The pancreas has a wide end (head), a narrow end (tail), and a middle section (body). A healthy pancreas is important for normal food digestion and plays a critical role in the body's metabolic processes.

The pancreas has two main functions, each performed by distinct types of tissue. The exocrine pancreas secretes fluids into an intricate system of channels or ducts, which are tubular structures that carry pancreatic juices to the small intestine where they are used for digestion. The endocrine tissue secretes substances that are circulated in the bloodstream. The exocrine pancreas makes up the vast majority of the gland; it produces pancreatic juices containing enzymes that help break down proteins and fatty food. The endocrine tissue of the pancreas makes up only 2% of the gland's total mass. It consists of small patches of cells that produce hormones (such as insulin) that control how the body stores and uses nutrients. These patches are called islets (islands) of Langerhans or islet cells and are interspersed evenly throughout the pancreas. Each islet contains approximately 1,000 endocrine cells and a dense network of capillaries (tiny blood vessels), which allows immediate entry of hormones into the circulatory system.

Pancreatic tumors are classified as either exocrine or endocrine tumors depending on which type of tissue they arise from within the gland. Endocrine tumors of the pancreas are very rare, accounting for only 5% of all pancreatic cancers. The majority of endocrine pancreatic tumors are functional adenocarcinomas that overproduce a specific hormone. There are several types of islet cells and each produces its own hormone or peptide (small protein molecule). Functional endocrine tumors are named after the hormone they secrete. Insulinoma is the most common tumor of the endocrine pancreas. Patients with this disease usually develop hypoglycemia due to increased insulin production that leads to abnormally low blood sugar levels. Gastrinoma, a disease in which gastrin (hormone that stimulates stomach acid production) is overproduced, causes multiple ulcers in the upper gastrointestinal (GI) tract. Gastrinoma was first described in patients with a rare form of severe peptic ulcer disease known as **Zollinger-Ellison syndrome** (ZES). The less common glucagonoma causes mild diabetes due to excess glucagon (hormone that stimulates glucose production) secretion. Other rare islet cell tumors include vipoma (vasoactive intestinal peptide) and somatostatinoma. Nonfunctional pancreatic endocrine tumors are not associated with an excess production of any hormone and can be difficult to distinguish from exocrine pancreatic cancer. Cancers of the endocrine pancreas are relatively slow-growing compared to the more common ductal adenocarcinomas of the exocrine pancreas.

Ninety-five percent of pancreatic cancers occur in tissues of the exocrine pancreas. Ductal adenocarcinomas arise in the cells that line the ducts of the exocrine pancreas and account for 80% to 90% of all tumors of the pancreas. Unless specified, nearly all reports on pancreatic cancer refer to ductal adenocarcinomas. Less common types of pancreatic exocrine tumors include acinar cell **carcinoma**, cystic tumors that are typically benign but may become cancerous, and papillary tumors that grow within the pancreatic ducts. Pancreatoblastoma is a very rare disease that primarily affects young children.

Two-thirds of pancreatic tumors occur in the head of the pancreas, and tumor growth in this area can lead to the obstruction of the nearby common bile duct that empties bile fluid into the small intestine. When bile cannot be passed into the intestine, patients may develop yellowing of the skin and eyes (jaundice) due to the buildup of bilirubin (a component of bile) in the bloodstream. Tumor blockage of bile or pancreatic ducts also may cause digestive problems since these fluids contain enzymes critical to the digestive process. Depending on their size, pancreatic tumors may cause abdominal pain by pressing on the surrounding nerves. Because of its location deep within the abdomen, pancreatic cancer often remains undetected until it has spread to other organs such as the liver or lung. Pancreatic cancer tends to spread rapidly to other organs, even when the primary (original) tumor is relatively small.

Risk factors

Although the exact cause for pancreatic cancer is not known, several risk factors have been shown to increase susceptibility to this particular cancer, the greatest of which is cigarette smoking. Approximately one-quarter of pancreatic cancer cases occur among smokers. People who have diabetes develop pancreatic cancer twice as often as non-diabetics. Numerous studies suggest that a family history of pancreatic cancer is another strong risk factor for developing the disease, particularly if two or more relatives in the immediate family have the disease. Other risk factors include chronic (long-term) inflammation of the pancreas (pancreatitis), diets high in fat, obesity, and occupational exposure to certain chemicals such as petroleum.

Causes and symptoms

The exact cause of most pancreatic cancers is unknown. Nevertheless, about 10% of cancers of the pancreas are attributable to specific gene mutations. These include:

- mutations in the BRCA2 gene, which also predisposes women to breast and ovarian cancer.
- mutations in the gene p16, which predisposes individuals to melanoma (aggressive skin cancer)
- mutations in the gene PRSS1, which predisposes individuals to pancreatitis
- mutations in multiple genes that predispose individuals to certain types of colorectal cancer
- mutations in gene STK1, which predisposes individuals to digestive tract cancers

There are no known causes of islet cell cancer, but a small percentage of cases occur due to hereditary syndromes such as MEN. This is a condition that frequently causes more than one tumor in several endocrine glands, such as the parathyroid and pituitary, in addition to the islet cells of the pancreas. Twenty-five percent of gastrinomas and less than 10% of insulinomas occur in MEN patients. Von Hippel-Lindau (VHL) syndrome is another genetic disorder that causes multiple tumors, and 10% to 15% of VHL patients will develop islet cell cancer.

Exocrine pancreatic cancer often does not produce symptoms until it reaches an advanced stage. Even then, many of the symptoms also can be caused by other diseases and disorders. Patients with exocrine pancreatic cancer may present with the following signs and symptoms:

- upper abdominal and/or back pain
- jaundice
- weight loss
- loss of appetite (anorexia)
- diarrhea
- weakness
- nausea

Symptoms of endocrine pancreatic vary among the different islet cell cancer types. Insulinoma causes repeated episodes of hypoglycemia (low blood sugar), sweating, and tremors, while patients with gastrinoma have inflammation of the esophagus, epigastric pain, multiple ulcers, and possibly **diarrhea**. Symptoms of glucagonoma include a distinctive skin rash, inflammation of the stomach, glucose intolerance, **weight loss**, weakness, and **anemia** (less common). Patients with vipoma have episodes of profuse, watery diarrhea, even after fasting. Somatostatinoma causes mild diabetes, diarrhea/steatorrhea (fatty stools), weight loss, and gallbladder disease. Nonfunctional endocrine tumors frequently produce the same symptoms as cancer of the exocrine pancreas such as abdominal pain, jaundice, and weight loss.

Diagnosis

Pancreatic cancer is difficult to diagnose, especially in the absence of symptoms, and there is no current screening method for early detection. The most sophisticated techniques available often do not detect very small tumors that are localized (have not begun to spread). At advanced stages where patients show symptoms, a number of tests may be performed to confirm diagnosis and to assess the stage of the disease. Approximately half of all pancreatic cancers are metastatic (have spread to other sites) at the time of diagnosis.

The first step in diagnosing pancreatic cancer is a thorough medical history and complete physical examination. The abdomen will be palpated to check for fluid accumulation, lumps, or masses. If there are signs of jaundice, blood tests will be performed to rule out the possibility of liver diseases such as hepatitis. Urine and stool tests may be performed as well.

Tests

Non-invasive imaging tools such as high-resolution contrast-enhanced spiral **computed tomography** (CT) scans and **magnetic resonance imaging** (MRI) can be used to produce detailed pictures of the internal organs. CT is the tool most often used to diagnose pancreatic cancer, as it allows the doctor to determine if the tumor can be removed by surgery or not. It is also useful in staging a tumor by showing the extent to which the tumor has spread. During a CT scan, patients receive an intravenous injection of a contrast dye so the organs can be visualized more clearly. MRI may be performed instead of CT if a patient has an allergy to the CT contrast dye. In some cases where the tumor is impinging on blood vessels or nearby ducts, MRI may be used to generate an image of the pancreatic ducts.

If the doctor suspects pancreatic cancer and no visible masses are seen with a CT scan, a patient may undergo a combination of invasive tests to confirm the presence of a pancreatic tumor. Endoscopic ultrasound (EUS) involves the use of an ultrasound probe at the end of a long, flexible tube that is passed down the patient's throat and into the stomach. This instrument can detect a tumor mass through high frequency sound waves and echoes. EUS can be accompanied by fine needle aspiration (FNA), where a long needle, guided by the ultrasound, is inserted into the tumor mass in order to take a **biopsy** sample. **Endoscopic retrograde cholangiopancreatography** (ERCP) is a technique often used in patients with severe jaundice because it enables the doctor to relieve blockage of the pancreatic ducts. The doctor, guided by endoscopy and **x rays**, inserts a small metal or plastic stent into the duct to keep it open. During ERCP, a biopsy can be done by collecting cells from the pancreas with a small brush. The cells are then examined under the microscope by a pathologist, who determines the presence of any cancerous cells.

In some cases, a biopsy may be performed during a type of surgery called **laparoscopy**, which is done under general anesthesia. Doctors insert a small camera and instruments into the abdomen after a minor incision is made. Tissue samples are removed for examination under the microscope. This procedure allows a doctor to determine the extent to which the disease has spread and decide if the tumor can be removed by further surgery.

An **angiography** is a type of test that studies the blood vessels in and around the pancreas. This test may be done before surgery so that the doctor can determine the extent to which the tumor invades and interacts with the blood vessels within the pancreas. The test requires local anesthesia and a catheter is inserted into the patient's upper thigh. A dye is then injected into blood vessels that lead into the pancreas, and x rays are taken.

Functional endocrine tumors can occur in multiple sites in the pancreas and are often small (less than 1 cm), making them difficult to diagnose. Nonfunctional tumors tend to be larger, which makes them difficult to distinguish from tumors of the exocrine pancreas. Methods such as computed tomography (CT) scan and magnetic resonance imaging (MRI) are used to take pictures of the internal organs and allow the doctor to determine whether a tumor is present. Somatostatin receptor scintigraphy is an imaging system used to localize endocrine tumors, especially gastrinomas and somatostatinomas. Endoscopic ultrasound (EUS) is a more sensitive technique that may be used if a CT scan fails to detect a tumor. Endocrine tumors usually have many blood vessels, so angiography may be useful in the doctor's assessment and staging of the tumor. Surgical exploration is sometimes necessary in order to locate very small tumors that occur in multiple sites. These techniques also help the doctor evaluate how far the tumor has spread. A biopsy can be taken to confirm diagnosis, but more often, doctors look at the size and local invasion of the tumor in order to plan a treatment strategy.

Treatment, exocrine cancer

Treatment of pancreatic cancer will depend on several factors, including the stage of the disease and the patient's age and overall health status. A combination of therapies is often employed in the treatment of this disease to improve the patient's chances for survival.

Clinical staging

After cancer of the pancreas has been diagnosed, doctors typically use a Tumor/Node/Metastasis (TNM) staging system to classify the tumor based on its size and the degree to which it has spread to other areas in the body. T indicates the size and local advancement of the primary tumor. Since cancers often invade the lymphatic system before spreading to other organs, regional lymph node involvement (N) is an important factor in staging. M indicates whether the tumor has metastasized (spread) to distant organs. In stage I, the tumor is localized to the pancreas and has not spread to surrounding lymph nodes or other organs. Stage II pancreatic cancer has spread to nearby organs such as the small intestine or bile duct, but not the surrounding lymph nodes. Stage III indicates lymph node involvement, whether the cancer has spread to nearby organs or not. Stage IVA pancreatic cancer has spread to organs near the pancreas such as the stomach, spleen, or colon. Stage IVB is a cancer that has spread to distant sites (liver, lung). If pancreatic cancer has been treated with success and then appears again in the pancreas or in other organs, it is referred to as recurrent disease.

Surgery

Three types of surgery are used in the treatment of pancreatic cancer, depending on what section of the pancreas the tumor is located in. A **Whipple procedure** removes the head of the pancreas, part of the small intestine and some of the surrounding tissues. This procedure is most common since the majority of pancreatic cancers occur in the head of the organ. A total **pancreatectomy** removes the entire pancreas and the organs around it. Distal pancreatectomy removes only the body and tail of the pancreas. **Chemotherapy** and radiation may precede surgery (neoadjuvant therapy) or follow surgery (adjuvant therapy). Surgery is also used to relieve symptoms of pancreatic cancer by draining fluids or bypassing obstructions. Side effects from surgery can include pain, weakness, **fatigue**, and digestive problems. Some patients may develop diabetes or malabsorption as a result of partial or total removal of the pancreas.

Radiation therapy

Radiation therapy is sometimes used to shrink a tumor before surgery or to remove remaining cancer cells after surgery. Radiation may also be used to relieve pain or digestive problems caused by the tumor if it cannot be removed by surgery. External radiation therapy refers to radiation applied externally to the abdomen using a beam of high-energy x rays. High-dose intraoperative radiation therapy is sometimes used during surgery on tumors that have spread to nearby organs. Internal radiation therapy refers to the use of small radioactive seeds implanted in the tumor tissue. The seeds emit radiation over time to kill tumor cells. Radiation treatment may cause side effects such as fatigue, tender or itchy skin, **nausea**, **vomiting**, and digestive problems.

Chemotherapy

Chemotherapeutic agents are powerful drugs that are used to kill cancer cells. They are classified according to the mechanism by which they induce cancer cell death. Multiple agents are often used to increase the chances of tumor cell death. **Gemcitabine** is the standard drug used to treat pancreatic cancers and can be used alone or in combination with other drugs, such as 5-fluorouracil (5-FU, or **fluorouracil**). Other drugs are being tested in combination with gemcitabine in several ongoing **clinical trials**, specifically **irinotecan** (CPT-11) and oxaliplatin. Chemotherapy may be administered orally or intravenously in a series of doses over several weeks. During treatment, patients may experience fatigue, nausea, vomiting, hair loss (**alopecia**), and mouth sores, depending on which drugs are used.

Biological Treatments

Numerous vaccine treatments are being developed in an effort to stimulate the body's immune system into attacking cancer cells. This is also referred to as immunotherapy. Another type of biological treatment involves using a targeted monoclonal antibody to inhibit the growth of cancer cells. The antibody is thought to bind to and neutralize a protein that contributes to the growth of the cancer cells. Investigational treatments such as these may be considered by patients with metastatic disease who would

QUESTIONS TO ASK YOUR DOCTOR

- What type of pancreatic cancer do I have?
- Do you have experience in treating this form of cancer?
- What is the standard course of treatment for my cancer at this stage?
- How long will the course of treatment take?
- What side effects will I experience?
- Am I at risk for developing other endocrine tumors?
- What can be done to relieve my abdominal pain?
- What should I do to prepare for surgery?
- Can you refer me to a nutritionist or dietician?
- Are there any alternative therapies you would recommend?
- Am I eligible to participate in a clinical trial?
- Will my health insurance cover costs associated with a clinical trial?
- Are there any support groups I can join?

like to participate in a clinical trial. Biological treatments typically cause flu-like symptoms (chills, **fever**, loss of appetite) during the treatment period.

Treatment, endocrine cancer

Clinical staging

The staging system for islet cell cancer is still evolving, but the tumors typically fall into three categories: cancers that arise in one location within the pancreas, cancers that arise in several locations within the pancreas, and cancers that have spread to nearby lymph nodes or to other organs in the body.

Combination treatment

Surgery is the only curative method for islet cell (endocrine) cancers, and studies have shown that an aggressive surgical approach can improve survival and alleviate symptoms of the disease. As with most forms of cancer, the earlier it is diagnosed, the greater the chance for survival. With the exception of insulinoma, the majority of islet cell tumors are malignant at the time of diagnosis, and more than half are metastatic. However, surgery and chemotherapy have been shown to improve the outcome of patients even if they have metastatic disease. Surgery may include partial or total removal of the pancreas, and in patients with gastrinoma, the stomach may be removed as well. **Streptozocin**, **doxorubicin**, and 5-fluorouracil (5-FU, or fluorouracil) are chemotherapeutic agents commonly used in the treatment of islet cell cancer. Patients may experience **nausea and vomiting**, as well as kidney toxicity, from streptozocin, and bone marrow suppression from doxorubicin. Hormone therapy is used to relieve the symptoms of functional tumors by inhibiting excess hormone production. Other techniques may be used to block blood flow to the liver in an attempt to kill the cancer cells that have spread there. Abdominal pain, nausea, vomiting, and fever may result from this type of treatment. Radiation has little if any role in the treatment of islet cell cancer.

Alternative

Acupuncture or hypnotherapy may be used in addition to standard therapies to help relieve the pain associated with pancreatic cancer. Because of the poor prognosis associated with pancreatic cancer, some patients may try special diets with vitamin supplements, certain exercise programs, or unconventional treatments not yet approved by the FDA. Patients should always inform their doctors of any alternative treatments they are using as they could interfere with standard therapies. As of 2000, the National Cancer Institute (NCI) was funding phase III clinical trials of a controversial treatment for pancreatic cancer that involves the use of supplemental pancreatic enzymes (to digest cancerous cells) and coffee enemas (to stimulate the liver to detoxify the cancer). These theories remain unproven and the study is widely criticized in the medical community. It remains to been seen whether this method of treatment has any advantage over the standard chemotherapeutic regimen in prolonging patient survival or improving quality of life.

Prognosis, exocrine cancer

Cancer of the pancreas is often fatal, and median survival from diagnosis is less than six months, while the overall five-year survival rate is 4%. The five-year survival rate by stage is as follows: stage IA, 37%; stage IB, 21%; stage IIA, 12%; stage IIB, 6%; stage III, 2percnt;; stage IV, 1%. These statistics demonstrate the aggressive nature of most pancreatic cancers and their tendency to recur. Pancreatic cancers tend to be resistant to radiation and chemotherapy and these modes of treatment are mainly used to relieve pain and tumor burden (palliative care).

Prognosis, endocrine cancer

Islet cell cancers overall have a more favorable prognosis than cancers of the exocrine pancreas, and the median survival from diagnosis is three-and-a-half years. This is mainly due to their slow-growing nature. Insulinomas have a five-year survival rate of 80% and gastrinomas have 65%. When malignant, islet cell cancers do not generally respond well to chemotherapy, and the treatment is mainly palliative. Most patients with **metastasis** do not survive five years. Islet cell cancer tends to spread to the surrounding lymph nodes, stomach, small intestine, and liver.

Prevention

Although the exact cause of pancreatic cancer is not known, there are certain risk factors that may increase a person's chances of developing the disease. Quitting smoking will certainly reduce the risk for pancreatic cancer and many other cancers. The American Cancer Society recommends a diet rich in fruits, vegetables, and dietary fiber in order to reduce the risk of pancreatic cancer. According to the National Cancer Institute, workers who are exposed to petroleum and other chemicals may be at greater risk for developing the disease and should follow their employer's safety precautions. People with a family history of pancreatic cancer are at greater risk than the general population, as a small percentage of pancreatic cancers are considered hereditary.

Special concerns

Pain control is probably the single greatest problem for patients with pancreatic cancer. As the cancer grows and spreads to other organs in the abdomen, it often presses on the surrounding network of nerves, which can cause considerable discomfort. In most cases, pain can be alleviated with analgesics or **opioids**. If medication is not enough, a doctor may inject alcohol into the abdominal nerve area to numb the pain. Surgical treatment of the affected nerves is also an option.

Pancreatic cancer patients frequently have difficulty maintaining their weight because food may not taste good or the pancreas is not releasing enough enzymes needed for digestion. Therefore, supplements of pancreatic enzymes may be helpful in restoring proper digestion. Other nutritional supplements may be given orally or intravenously in an effort to boost calorie intake. However, cachexia (severe muscle breakdown) caused by certain substances that the cancer produces, remains a significant problem to treat.

Patients with pancreatic cancer may experience anxiety and **depression** during their diagnosis and treatment. Statistics on the prognosis for the disease can be discouraging, however, there are many new treatments on the horizon that may significantly improve the outcome for this disease. Many patients find it helpful to join support groups where they can discuss their concerns with others who are also coping with the illness.

Resources

OTHER

"Detailed Guide: Pancreatic Cancer." American Cancer Society May 12. 2009 [September 26, 2009]. http://www.cancer.org/docroot/CRI/CRI_2_3x.asp?rnav=cridg&dt=34.

"Pancreatic Cancer." MedlinePlus September 22, 2009 [September 26, 2009]. http://www.nlm.nih.gov/medlineplus/pancreaticcancer.html.

ORGANIZATIONS

American Cancer Society, 1599 Clifton Rd., NE, Atlanta, GA, 30329, (404) 320-3333, (800) ACS-2345, http://www.cancer.org.

Cancer Research and Prevention Foundation, 1600 Duke Street, Suite 500, Alexandria, VA, 22314, (703) 836-4412, (800) 227-2732, info@preventcancer.org, http://www.preventcancer.org.

National Cancer Institute Public Inquires Office., 6116 Executive Boulevard, Room 3036A, Bethesda, MD, 20892-8322, (800) 4-CANCER. TTY (800) 332-8615, http://www.cancer.gov.

National Center for Complementary and Alternative Medicine Clearinghouse, PO Box 7923, Gaithersburg, MD, 20898, (301) 519-3153. TTY: (866) 464-3615<, (888) 644-6226, (866) 464-3616, info@nccam.nih.gov, http://nccam.nih.gov.

National Pancreas Foundation, 101 Federal Street, Suite 1900, Boston, MA, 02110, (617) 578-0382, (866) 726-2737, (617) 578-0383, http://www.pancreasfoundation.org.

Elizabeth Pulcini, M. Sc.
Tish Davidson, A.M.

Pancreatic cancer, endocrine

Definition

Endocrine **pancreatic cancer** is a disease in which cancerous cells originate within the tissues of the pancreas that produce hormones.

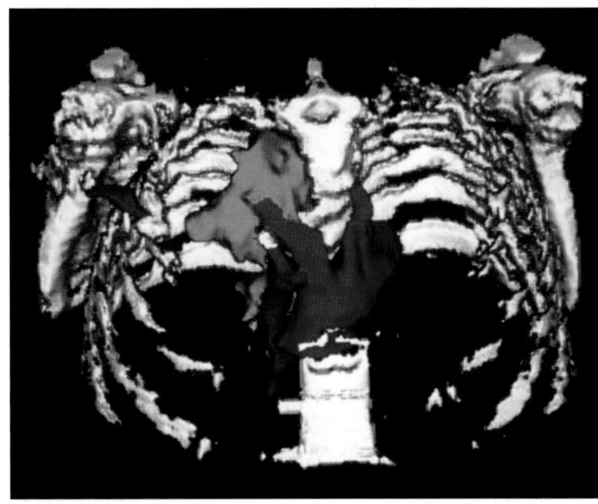

Colorized computed tomography (CT) scan showing the location of a cancerous tumor of the pancreas (green). *(Copyright Clinique Ste Catherine/CNRI, Science Source/Photo Researchers, Inc. Reproduced by permission.)*

KEY TERMS

Adenocarcinoma—A malignant tumor that arises within the tissues of a gland and retains its glandular structure.

Angiography—Diagnostic technique used to study blood vessels in a tumor.

Biopsy—Removal and microscopic examination of cells to determine whether they are cancerous.

Chemotherapy— Drug treatment administered to kill cancerous cells.

Endocrine—Refers to glands that secrete hormones circulated in the bloodstream.

Endoscopic ultrasonography (EUS)—Diagnostic imaging technique where an ultrasound probe is inserted down a patient's throat to determine if a tumor is present.

Gastrinoma—Tumor that arises from the gastrin-producing cells in the pancreas.

Insulinoma—Tumor that arises from the insulin-producing cells in the pancreas.

Islets of Langerhans—Clusters of cells in pancreas that make up the endocrine tissue.

Description

The pancreas is a six- to eight-inch long, slipper-shaped gland located in the abdomen. It lies behind the stomach, within a loop formed by the small intestine. Other nearby organs include the gallbladder, spleen, and liver. The pancreas has a wide end (head), a narrow end (tail), and a middle section (body). A healthy pancreas is important for normal food digestion and plays a critical role in the body's metabolic processes. The pancreas has two main functions, each performed by distinct types of tissue. The exocrine tissue secretes fluids into the other organs of the digestive system, while the endocrine tissue secretes substances that are circulated in the bloodstream. The exocrine pancreas makes up the vast majority of the gland; it produces pancreatic juices containing enzymes that help break down proteins and fatty food. The endocrine tissue of the pancreas makes up only 2% of the gland's total mass. It consists of small patches of cells that produce hormones (like insulin) that control how the body stores and uses nutrients. These patches are called islets (islands) of Langerhans or islet cells and are interspersed evenly throughout the pancreas. Each islet contains approximately 1,000 endocrine cells and a dense network of capillaries (tiny blood vessels), which allows immediate entry of hormones into the circulatory system.

Pancreatic tumors are classified as either exocrine or endocrine tumors depending on which type of tissue they arise from within the gland. Endocrine tumors of the pancreas are very rare, accounting for only 5% of all pancreatic cancers. The majority of endocrine pancreatic tumors are functional adenocarcinomas that overproduce a specific hormone. There are several types of islet cells and each produces its own hormone or peptide (small protein molecule). Functional endocrine tumors are named after the hormone they secrete. Insulinoma is the most common tumor of the endocrine pancreas. Patients with this disease usually develop hypoglycemia due to increased insulin production that leads to abnormally low blood sugar levels. Gastrinoma, a disease in which gastrin (hormone which stimulates stomach acid production) is overproduced, causes multiple ulcers in the upper gastrointestinal (GI) tract. Gastrinoma was first described in patients with a rare form of severe peptic ulcer disease known as **Zollinger-Ellison syndrome** (ZES). The less common glucagonoma causes mild diabetes due to excess glucagon (hormone which stimulates glucose production) secretion. Other rare islet cell tumors include vipoma (vasoactive intestinal peptide) and somatostatinoma. Nonfunctional pancreatic endocrine tumors are not associated with an excess production of any hormone and can be difficult to distinguish from **exocrine pancreatic cancer**. Cancers of the endocrine pancreas are relatively slow-growing compared to the more common ductal adenocarcinomas of the exocrine pancreas.

QUESTIONS TO ASK THE DOCTOR

- What type of islet cell cancer do I have?
- Do you have experience in treating this form of cancer?
- Is my tumor benign or malignant?
- What is my prognosis?
- Can my tumor be removed by surgery?
- What medication will I need to take?
- Am I at risk for developing other endocrine tumors?
- Is there a clinical trial I can participate in?
- Is there a support group available?

Demographics

Between one and four cases of insulinoma occur per million people per year, and 90% of these tumors are benign. They occur mostly between the ages of 50 and 60 and affect men and women equally. Less than three cases of gastrinoma per million people are diagnosed each year, but it is the most common functional islet cell tumor in patients with multiple endocrine tumors, a condition known as multiple endocrine neoplasia (MEN) syndrome. Vipoma and glucagonoma are even rarer and they occur more frequently in women. Somatostatinoma is exceedingly uncommon, and less than 100 cases have been reported worldwide. Nonfunctional islet cell cancers account for approximately one-third of all cancers of the endocrine pancreas, and the majority of these are malignant.

Causes and symptoms

There are no known causes of islet cell **cancer**, but a small percentage of cases occur due to hereditary syndromes such as MEN. This is a condition that frequently causes more than one tumor in several endocrine glands, such as the parathyroid and pituitary, in addition to the islet cells of the pancreas. Twenty-five percent of gastrinomas and less than 10% of insulinomas occur in MEN patients. Von Hippel-Lindau (VHL) syndrome is another genetic disorder that causes multiple tumors, and 10% to 15% of VHL patients will develop islet cell cancer.

Symptoms vary among the different islet cell cancer types. Insulinoma causes repeated episodes of hypoglycemia, sweating, and tremors, while patients with gastrinoma have inflammation of the esophagus, epigastric pain, multiple ulcers, and possibly **diarrhea**. Symptoms of glucagonoma include a distinctive skin rash, inflammation of the stomach, glucose intolerance, **weight loss**, weakness, and **anemia** (less common). Patients with vipoma have episodes of profuse, watery diarrhea, even after fasting. Somatostatinoma causes mild diabetes, diarrhea/steatorrhea (fatty stools), weight loss, and gallbladder disease. Nonfunctional endocrine tumors frequently produce the same symptoms as cancer of the exocrine pancreas such as abdominal pain, jaundice, and weight loss.

Diagnosis

A thorough physical exam is usually performed when a patient visits a doctor with the above symptoms; however, functional endocrine tumors of the pancreas tend to be small and are not detected by palpating the abdomen. Once other illnesses such as **infection** are ruled out, the doctor will order a series of blood and urine tests. The functional endocrine tumors can be identified through increased levels of hormone in the bloodstream.

Functional endocrine tumors can occur in multiple sites in the pancreas and are often small (less than 1 cm), making them difficult to diagnose. Nonfunctional tumors tend to be larger, which makes them difficult to distinguish from tumors of the exocrine pancreas. Methods such as **computed tomography** (CT) scan and **magnetic resonance imaging** (MRI) are used to take pictures of the internal organs and allow the doctor to determine whether a tumor is present. Somatostatin receptor scintigraphy (trade name OctreoScan) is an imaging system used to localize endocrine tumors, especially gastrinomas and somatostatinomas. Endoscopic ultrasound (EUS) is a more sensitive technique that may be used if a CT scan fails to detect a tumor. Endocrine tumors usually have many blood vessels, so **angiography** may be useful in the doctor's assessment and staging of the tumor. Surgical exploration is sometimes necessary in order to locate very small tumors that occur in multiple sites. These techniques also help the doctor evaluate how far the tumor has spread. A **biopsy** can be taken to confirm diagnosis, but more often, doctors look at the size and local invasion of the tumor in order to plan a treatment strategy.

Treatment team

Patients with islet cell cancer are cared for by a number of specialists from different disciplines. Medical oncologists, gastroenterologists, radiologists, and surgeons all interact with the patient to develop an appropriate treatment plan. Endocrinologists play an important role in helping patients with diabetes maintain steady blood sugar levels. Much of the treatment of islet cell cancer focuses on relieving symptoms of the tumor through medication that inhibits hormone overproduction. It is best for patients to work with doctors who are experienced in treating this rare form of cancer.

Clinical staging, treatments, and prognosis

Staging

The staging system for islet cell cancer is still evolving, but the tumors typically fall into three categories: cancers that arise in one location within the pancreas, cancers that arise in several locations within the pancreas, and cancers that have spread to nearby lymph nodes or to other organs in the body.

Treatments

Surgery is the only curative method for islet cell cancers, and studies have shown that an aggressive surgical approach can improve survival and alleviate symptoms of the disease. As with most forms of cancer, the earlier it is diagnosed, the greater the chance for survival. With the exception of insulinoma, the majority of islet cell tumors are malignant at the time of diagnosis, and more than half are metastatic. However, surgery and **chemotherapy** have been shown to improve the outcome of patients even if they have metastatic disease. Surgery may include partial or total removal of the pancreas, and in patients with gastrinoma, the stomach may be removed as well. **Streptozocin**, **doxorubicin**, and 5-fluorouracil (5-FU, or **fluorouracil**) are chemotherapeutic agents commonly used in the treatment of islet cell cancer. Patients may experience **nausea and vomiting**, as well as kidney toxicity, from streptozocin, and bone marrow suppression from doxorubicin. Hormone therapy is used to relieve the symptoms of functional tumors by inhibiting excess hormone production. Other techniques may be used to block blood flow to the liver in an attempt to kill the cancer cells that have spread there. Abdominal pain, **nausea**, **vomiting**, and **fever** may result from this type of treatment. Radiation has little if any role in the treatment of islet cell cancer.

Prognosis

Islet cell cancers overall have a more favorable prognosis than cancers of the exocrine pancreas, and the median survival from diagnosis is three-and-a-half years. This is mainly due to their slow-growing nature. Insulinomas have a five-year survival rate of 80% and gastrinomas have 65%. When malignant, islet cell cancers do not generally respond well to chemotherapy, and the treatment is mainly palliative. Most patients with **metastasis** do not survive five years. Islet cell cancer tends to spread to the surrounding lymph nodes, stomach, small intestine, and liver.

Coping with cancer treatment

Patients should discuss with their doctors any side effects they experience from treatment. Many drugs are available to relieve nausea and vomiting associated with cancer treatments and for combating **fatigue**. Insulin may be prescribed if patients develop diabetes as a result of partial or total removal of their pancreas. Special diets or fluids may be recommended if patients have more than one digestive organ removed. These patients may require intravenous feeding after surgery until they recover.

Clinical trials

Because this is such a rare disease, relatively few **clinical trials** are available to people with islet cell cancer. Most are investigating the efficacy of new chemotherapeutic drugs or combinations of drugs and biological therapies. R115777 is an agent being tested in combination with **trastuzumab (Herceptin)** for patients with advanced or metastatic **adenocarcinoma**. Two new drugs that are antineoplastons, A10 and AS2-1, are being examined together as a treatment regimen for patients with metastatic or incurable **neuroendocrine tumors**. Patients should ask their doctors whether they qualify for these or other clinical trials.

Prevention

There are no known risk factors associated with sporadic islet cell cancer. Therefore, it is not clear how to prevent its occurrence. Individuals with MEN syndrome or VHL, however, have a genetic predisposition to developing islet cell cancer should be screened regularly in an effort to catch the disease early.

Special concerns

Many patients find it helpful to join support groups after being diagnosed with cancer. Discussing the condition with others who are experiencing a similar situation may help to relieve anxiety and **depression**, which are often associated with cancer and its treatment. Medication may also be prescribed to alleviate depression. Patients should learn as much as they can about their illness and find out what their treatment options are. It is important for patients to remember that each cancer has unique characteristics and responds differently to treatment depending on those characteristics.

See also Carcinoid tumors, gastrointestinal; Chemoembolization; Complementary cancer therapies; Endocrine system tumors; Familial cancer syndromes; Pancreatic cancer, exocrine; Upper gastrointestinal endoscopy.

Resources

PERIODICALS

Anderson, M.A., et. al. "Endoscopic Ultrasound is Highly Accurate and Directs Management of Patients With Neuroendocrine Tumors of the Pancreas." *American Journal of Gastroenterology* 95, no. 9 (September 2000): 2271–7.

Hellman, Per, et. al. "Surgical Strategy for Large or Malignant Endocrine Pancreatic Tumors." *World Journal of Surgery* 24 (2000): 1353–60.

OTHER

"Islet Cell Carcinoma." *CancerNet PDQ*. May 2001. [cited July 19, 2009]. http://www.cancernet.nci.nih.gov.

Pancreatic Cancer Home Page Johns Hopkins Medical Institutions. [cited July 19, 2009]. http://www.path.jhu.edu/pancreas.

ORGANIZATIONS

National Cancer Institute. 9000 Rockville Pike, Bldg.31, Rm.10A16, Bethesda, MD, 20892 (800) 422-6237. http://www.nci.nih.gov.

National Familial Pancreas Tumor Registry. The Johns Hopkins Hospital. 600 North Wolfe St., Baltimore, MD 21287-6417. (410) 377-7450.

National Organization for Rare Disorders. 100 Route 37, PO Box 8923. New Fairfield, CT 06812. (203) 746-6518. http://www.nord-rdb.com/~orphan.

Elizabeth Pulcini, M.Sc.

Pancreatic cancer, exocrine

Definition

Exocrine **pancreatic cancer** is a disease in which cancerous cells originate within the tissues of the pancreas that produce digestive juices.

Description

The pancreas is a six- to eight-inch long, slipper-shaped gland located in the abdomen. It lies behind the stomach, within a loop formed by the small intestine. Other nearby organs include the gallbladder, spleen, and liver. The pancreas has a wide end (head), a narrow end (tail), and a middle section (body). A healthy pancreas is important for normal food digestion and also plays a critical role in the body's metabolic processes. The pancreas has two main functions, and each are performed by distinct types of tissue. The exocrine tissue makes up the vast majority of the gland and secretes fluids into the other organs of the digestive system. The endocrine tissue secretes hormones (like insulin) that are circulated in the bloodstream, and these substances control how the body stores and uses nutrients. The exocrine tissue of the pancreas produces pancreatic (digestive) juices. These juices contain several enzymes that help break down proteins and fatty foods. The exocrine pancreas forms an intricate system of channels or ducts, which are tubular structures that carry pancreatic juices to the small intestine where they are used for digestion.

Pancreatic tumors are classified as either exocrine or endocrine tumors depending on which type of tissue they arise from within the gland. Ninety-five percent of pancreatic cancers occur in the tissues of the exocrine pancreas. Ductal adenocarcinomas arise in the cells that line the ducts of the exocrine pancreas and account for 80–90% of all tumors of the pancreas. Unless specified, nearly all reports on pancreatic **cancer** refer to ductal adenocarcinomas. Less common types of pancreatic exocrine tumors include acinar cell **carcinoma**, cystic tumors that are typically benign but may become cancerous, and papillary tumors that grow within the pancreatic ducts. Pancreatoblastoma is a very rare disease that primarily affects young children. Two-thirds of pancreatic tumors occur in the head of the pancreas, and tumor growth in this area can lead to the obstruction of the nearby common bile duct that empties bile fluid into the small intestine. When bile cannot be passed into the intestine, patients may develop yellowing of the skin and eyes (jaundice) due to the buildup of bilirubin (a component of bile) in the bloodstream. Tumor blockage of bile or pancreatic ducts may also cause digestive problems since these fluids contain critical enzymes in the digestive process. Depending on their size, pancreatic tumors may cause abdominal pain by pressing on the surrounding nerves. Because of its location deep within the abdomen, pancreatic cancer often remains undetected until it has spread to other organs such as the liver or lung. Pancreatic cancer tends to rapidly spread to other organs, even when the primary (original) tumor is relatively small.

Demographics

Though pancreatic cancer accounts for only 3% of all cancers, it is the fifth most frequent cause of cancer deaths. In 2009, an estimated 42,470 new cases of pancreatic cancer will be diagnosed in the United States. Pancreatic cancer is primarily a disease

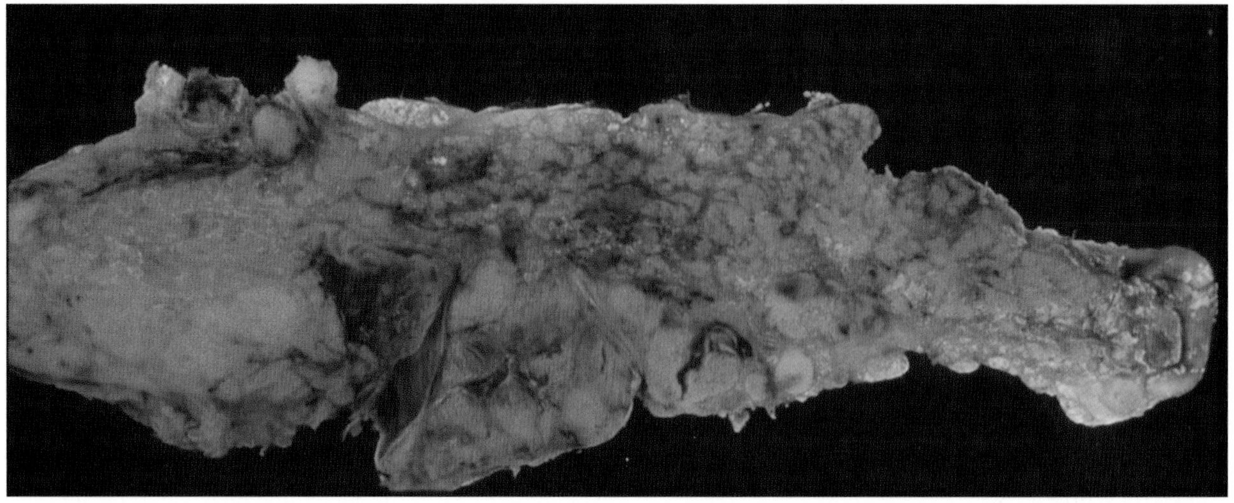

Carcinoma of the head of the pancreas. Tumors appear as gritty, gray, hard nodules, invading the adjacent gland. *(Copyright Biophoto Associates, Science Source/Photo Researchers, Inc. Reproduced by permission.)*

associated with advanced age, with 80% of cases occurring between the ages of 60 and 80. Men are almost twice as likely to develop this disease than women. Countries with the highest frequencies of pancreatic cancer include the U.S., New Zealand, Western European nations, and Scandinavia. The lowest occurrences of the disease are reported in India, Kuwait and Singapore. African Americans have the highest rate of pancreatic cancer of any ethnic group worldwide. Whether this difference is due to diet or environmental factors remains unclear.

Causes and symptoms

Although the exact cause for pancreatic cancer is not known, several risk factors have been shown to increase susceptibility to this particular cancer, the greatest of which is cigarette smoking. Approximately one-third of pancreatic cancer cases occur among smokers. People who have diabetes develop pancreatic cancer twice as often as non-diabetics. Numerous studies suggest that a family history of pancreatic cancer is another strong risk factor for developing the disease, particularly if two or more relatives in the immediate family have the disease. Other risk factors include chronic (long-term) inflammation of the pancreas (pancreatitis), diets high in fat, and occupational exposure to certain chemicals such as petroleum.

Pancreatic cancer often does not produce symptoms until it reaches an advanced stage. Patients may then present with the following signs and symptoms:

- upper abdominal and/or back pain
- jaundice
- weight loss
- loss of appetite (anorexia)
- diarrhea
- weakness
- nausea

These symptoms may also be caused by other illnesses; therefore, it is important to consult a doctor for an accurate diagnosis.

Diagnosis

Pancreatic cancer is difficult to diagnose, especially in the absence of symptoms, and there is no current screening method for early detection. The most sophisticated techniques available often do not detect very small tumors that are localized (have not begun to spread). At advanced stages where patients show symptoms, a number of tests may be performed to confirm diagnosis and to assess the stage of the disease. Approximately half of all pancreatic cancers are metastatic (have spread to other sites) at the time of diagnosis.

The first step in diagnosing pancreatic cancer is a thorough medical history and complete physical examination. The abdomen will be palpated to check for fluid accumulation, lumps, or masses. If there are signs of jaundice, blood tests will be performed to rule out the possibility of liver diseases such as hepatitis. Urine and stool tests may be performed as well.

Non-invasive imaging tools such as **computed tomography** (CT) scans and **magnetic resonance imaging** (MRI) can be used to produce detailed

KEY TERMS

Acinar cell(s)—Cells that comprise small sacs terminating the ducts of some exocrine glands.

Acinar cell carcinoma—A malignant tumor arising from the acinar cells of the pancreas.

Angiography—Diagnostic technique used to study blood vessels in a tumor.

Biopsy—Removal and microscopic examination of cells to determine whether they are cancerous.

Cancer vaccines—A treatment that uses the patient's immune system to attack cancer cells.

Chemotherapy— Drug treatment administered to kill cancerous cells.

Ductal adenocarcinoma—A malignant tumor arising from the duct cells within a gland.

Endoscopic retrograde cholangiopancreatography (ERCP)—Diagnostic technique used to obtain a biopsy. Also a surgical method of relieving biliary obstruction caused by a tumor.

Endoscopic ultrasonography (EUS)—Diagnostic imaging technique in which an ultrasound probe is inserted down a patient's throat to determine if a tumor is present.

Exocrine—Refers to glands which secrete their products through a duct.

Laparoscopic surgery—Minimally invasive surgery in which a camera and surgical instruments are inserted through a small incision.

Pancreatectomy—Partial or total surgical removal of the pancreas.

Radiation therapy—Use of radioisotopes to kill tumor cells. Applied externally through a beam of x rays, intraoperatively (during surgery), or deposited internally by implanting radioactive seeds in tumor tissue.

Whipple procedure—Surgical removal of the head of the pancreas, part of the small intestine, and some surrounding tissue.

pictures of the internal organs. CT is the tool most often used to diagnose pancreatic cancer, as it allows the doctor to determine if the tumor can be removed by surgery or not. It is also useful in staging a tumor by showing the extent to which the tumor has spread. During a CT scan, patients receive an intravenous injection of a contrast dye so the organs can be visualized more clearly. MRI may be performed instead of CT if a patient has an allergy to the CT contrast dye. In some cases where the tumor is impinging on blood vessels or nearby ducts, MRI may be used to generate an image of the pancreatic ducts.

QUESTIONS TO ASK THE DOCTOR

- What is my prognosis?
- What is the standard course of treatment for my cancer at this stage?
- How long will the course of treatment take?
- What side effects will I experience?
- What can be done to relieve my abdominal pain?
- What should I do to prepare for surgery?
- Can you refer me to a nutritionist or dietician?
- Are there any alternative therapies you would recommend?
- Am I eligible to participate in a clinical trial?
- Will my health insurance cover costs associated with a clinical trial?
- Are there any support groups I can join?

If the doctor suspects pancreatic cancer and no visible masses are seen with a CT scan, a patient may undergo a combination of invasive tests to confirm the presence of a pancreatic tumor. Endoscopic ultrasound (EUS) involves the use of an ultrasound probe at the end of a long, flexible tube that is passed down the patient's throat and into the stomach. This instrument can detect a tumor mass through high frequency sound waves and echoes. EUS can be accompanied by fine needle aspiration (FNA), where a long needle, guided by the ultrasound, is inserted into the tumor mass in order to take a **biopsy** sample. **Endoscopic retrograde cholangiopancreatography** (ERCP) is a technique often used in patients with severe jaundice because it enables the doctor to relieve blockage of the pancreatic ducts. The doctor, guided by endoscopy and **x rays**, inserts a small metal or plastic stent into the duct to keep it open. During ERCP, a biopsy can be done by collecting cells from the pancreas with a small brush. The cells are then examined under the microscope by a pathologist, who determines the presence of any cancerous cells.

In some cases, a biopsy may be performed during a type of surgery called **laparoscopy**, which is done under general anesthesia. Doctors insert a small camera and instruments into the abdomen after a minor incision is made. Tissue samples are removed for examination under the microscope. This procedure allows a doctor to determine the extent to which the disease has spread and decide if the tumor can be removed by further surgery.

An **angiography** is a type of test that studies the blood vessels in and around the pancreas. This test may be done before surgery so that the doctor can determine the extent to which the tumor invades and interacts with the blood vessels within the pancreas. The test requires local anesthesia and a catheter is inserted into the patient's upper thigh. A dye is then injected into blood vessels that lead into the pancreas, and x rays are taken.

As of April 2001, doctors at major cancer research institutions such as Memorial Sloan-Kettering Cancer Center in New York were investigating CT angiography, an imaging technique that is less invasive than angiography alone. CT angiography is similar to a standard CT scan, but allows doctors to take a series of pictures of the blood vessels that support tumor growth. A dye is injected as in a CT scan (but at rapid intervals) and no catheter or sedation is required. A computer generates 3D images from the pictures that are taken, and the information is gathered by the surgical team who will develop an appropriate strategy if the patient's disease can be operated on.

Treatment team

Pancreatic cancer is a complex disease that involves specialists from a variety of medical disciplines. Patients are likely to interact with medical oncologists, gastroenterologists, radiologists, and surgeons to develop a suitable treatment plan. Treatment plans vary depending on the stage of the disease and the overall health of the patient. Cancers of the pancreas frequently cause intense pain by pressing on the surrounding network of nerves in the abdomen; therefore, anesthesiologists who specialize in **pain management** may play a role in making a patient more comfortable. Obstruction of the intestine or bowel can also be a cause of pain, but is usually relieved through surgery. Patients receiving **chemotherapy** meet with oncologists who determine the dose schedule and oncology nurses who administer the chemotherapy. Patients who undergo partial or total removal of their pancreas may develop diabetes, and an endocrinologist will prescribe insulin or other medication to help them manage this condition. It is important for patients to get proper nutrition during any treatment for cancer. Patients may wish to consult a nutritionist or dietician to assist them (this may require oral replacement of digestive enzymes).

Clinical staging, treatments, and prognosis

Staging

After cancer of the pancreas has been diagnosed, doctors typically use a TNM staging system to classify the tumor based on its size and the degree to which it has spread to other areas in the body. T indicates the size and local advancement of the primary tumor. Since cancers often invade the lymphatic system before spreading to other organs, regional lymph node involvement (N) is an important factor in staging. M indicates whether the tumor has metastasized (spread) to distant organs. In stage I, the tumor is localized to the pancreas and has not spread to surrounding lymph nodes or other organs. Stage II pancreatic cancer has spread to nearby organs such as the small intestine or bile duct, but not the surrounding lymph nodes. Stage III indicates lymph node involvement, whether the cancer has spread to nearby organs or not. Stage IVA pancreatic cancer has spread to organs near the pancreas such as the stomach, spleen, or colon. Stage IVB is a cancer that has spread to distant sites (liver, lung). If pancreatic cancer has been treated with success and then appears again in the pancreas or in other organs, it is referred to as recurrent disease.

Treatments

Treatment of pancreatic cancer will depend on several factors, including the stage of the disease and the patient's age and overall health status. A combination of therapies is often employed in the treatment of this disease to improve the patient's chances for survival. Surgery is used whenever possible and is the only means by which cancer of the pancreas can be cured. However, less than 15% of pancreatic tumors can be removed by surgery. By the time the disease is diagnosed (usually at Stage III), therapies such as radiation and chemotherapy or both are used in addition to surgery to relieve a patient's symptoms and enhance quality of life. For patients with metastatic disease, chemotherapy and radiation are used mainly as palliative (pain-alleviating) treatments.

SURGERY. Three types of surgery are used in the treatment of pancreatic cancer, depending on what section of the pancreas the tumor is located in. A **Whipple procedure** removes the head of the pancreas, part of the small intestine and some of the surrounding tissues. This procedure is most common since the majority of pancreatic cancers occur in the head of the organ. A total **pancreatectomy** removes the entire pancreas and the organs around it. Distal pancreatectomy removes only the body and tail of the pancreas. Chemotherapy and radiation may precede surgery (neoadjuvant therapy) or follow surgery (adjuvant therapy). Surgery is also used to relieve symptoms of pancreatic cancer by draining fluids or bypassing obstructions. Side effects from surgery can include pain, weakness, **fatigue**, and digestive problems. Some patients may develop diabetes or malabsorption as a result of partial or total removal of the pancreas.

RADIATION THERAPY. **Radiation therapy** is sometimes used to shrink a tumor before surgery or to remove remaining cancer cells after surgery. Radiation may also be used to relieve pain or digestive problems caused by the tumor if it cannot be removed by surgery. External radiation therapy refers to radiation applied externally to the abdomen using a beam of high-energy x rays. High-dose intraoperative radiation therapy is sometimes used during surgery on tumors that have spread to nearby organs. Internal radiation therapy refers to the use of small radioactive seeds implanted in the tumor tissue. The seeds emit radiation over a period of time to kill tumor cells. Radiation treatment may cause side effects such as fatigue, tender or itchy skin, **nausea**, **vomiting**, and digestive problems.

CHEMOTHERAPY. Chemotherapeutic agents are powerful drugs that are used to kill cancer cells. They are classified according to the mechanism by which they induce cancer cell death. Multiple agents are often used to increase the chances of tumor cell death. **Gemcitabine** is the standard drug used to treat pancreatic cancers and can be used alone or in combination with other drugs, such as 5-fluorouracil (5-FU, or **fluorouracil**). Other drugs are being tested in combination with gemcitabine in several ongoing **clinical trials**, specifically **irinotecan** (CPT-11) and oxaliplatin. Chemotherapy may be administered orally or intravenously in a series of doses over several weeks. During treatment, patients may experience fatigue, nausea, vomiting, hair loss (**alopecia**), and mouth sores, depending on which drugs are used.

BIOLOGICAL TREATMENTS. Numerous vaccine treatments are being developed in an effort to stimulate the body's immune system into attacking cancer cells. This is also referred to as immunotherapy. Another type of biological treatment involves using a targeted monoclonal antibody to inhibit the growth of cancer cells. The antibody is thought to bind to and neutralize a protein that contributes to the growth of the cancer cells. Investigational treatments such as these may be considered by patients with metastatic disease who would like to participate in a clinical trial. Biological treatments typically cause flu-like symptoms (chills, **fever**, loss of appetite) during the treatment period.

Prognosis

Unfortunately, cancer of the pancreas is often fatal, and median survival from diagnosis is less than six months, while the five-year survival rate is 4%. This is mainly due to the lack of screening methods available for early detection of the disease. Yet, even when localized tumors can be removed by surgery, patient survival after five years is only 10–15%. These statistics demonstrate the aggressive nature of most pancreatic cancers and their tendency to recur. Pancreatic cancers tend to be resistant to radiation and chemotherapy and these modes of treatment are mainly used to relieve pain and tumor burden.

Alternative and complementary therapies

Acupuncture or hypnotherapy may be used in addition to standard therapies to help relieve the pain associated with pancreatic cancer. Because of the poor prognosis associated with pancreatic cancer, some patients may try special diets with vitamin supplements, certain exercise programs, or unconventional treatments not yet approved by the FDA. Patients should always inform their doctors of any alternative treatments they are using as they could interfere with standard therapies. As of 2000, the National Cancer Institute (NCI) was funding phase III clinical trials of a controversial treatment for pancreatic cancer that involves the use of supplemental pancreatic enzymes (to digest cancerous cells) and coffee enemas (to stimulate the liver to detoxify the cancer). These theories remain unproven and the study is widely criticized in the medical community. It remains to been seen whether this method of treatment has any advantage over the standard chemotherapeutic regimen in prolonging patient survival or improving quality of life.

Coping with cancer treatment

Patients should discuss with their doctors any side effects they experience from treatment. Many drugs are available to relieve **nausea and vomiting** associated with cancer treatments and for combating fatigue. Special diets or supplements, including pancreatic enzymes, may be recommended if patients are experiencing digestive problems. Insulin or other medication may be prescribed if patients develop diabetes as a result of partial or total removal of their pancreas.

Clinical trials

A large number of clinical trials are underway to assess the therapeutic effect of new chemotherapy regimens and several new immunotherapies. Gemcitabine is being tested in combination with irinotecan (CPT-11) in patients with metastatic pancreatic disease. Other agents under investigation are DX-8951f and R115777. Some drugs are being tested in combination with radiation therapy or with biological therapies. Two preliminary studies using the vaccine G17DT showed a significant improvement in the survival of patients with advanced pancreatic cancer. The monoclonal antibody **cetuximab** (IMC-C225) in combination with gemcitabine also showed positive preliminary results. There are trials available for patients with all stages of pancreatic cancer. Patients can find out which trials they are eligible for by talking with their doctors. Information about ongoing trials can be found at http://cancernet.nci.nih.gov/trialsrch.shtml. Many treatments given during clinical trials are considered experimental by **health insurance** companies and may not be covered by certain health plans. Patients should discuss their options with their doctors and health insurance providers.

Prevention

Although the exact cause of pancreatic cancer is not known, there are certain risk factors that may increase a person's chances of developing the disease. Quitting smoking will certainly reduce the risk for pancreatic cancer and many other cancers. The American Cancer Society recommends a diet rich in fruits, vegetables, and dietary fiber in order to reduce the risk of pancreatic cancer. According to the NCI, workers who are exposed to petroleum and other chemicals may be at greater risk for developing the disease and should follow their employer's safety precautions. People with a family history of pancreatic cancer are at greater risk than the general population, as a small percentage of pancreatic cancers are considered hereditary.

Special concerns

Pain control is probably the single greatest problem for patients with pancreatic cancer. As the cancer grows and spreads to other organs in the abdomen, it often presses on the surrounding network of nerves, which can cause considerable discomfort. In most cases, pain can be alleviated with analgesics or **opioids**. If medication is not enough, a doctor may inject alcohol into the abdominal nerve area to numb the pain. Surgical treatment of the affected nerves is also an option.

Pancreatic cancer patients frequently have difficulty maintaining their weight because food may not taste good or the pancreas is not releasing enough enzymes needed for digestion. Therefore, supplements of pancreatic enzymes may be helpful in restoring proper digestion. Other nutritional supplements may be given orally or intravenously in an effort to boost calorie intake. However, cachexia (severe muscle breakdown) caused by certain substances that the cancer produces, remains a significant problem to treat.

Patients with pancreatic cancer may experience anxiety and **depression** during their diagnosis and treatment. Statistics on the prognosis for the disease can be discouraging, however, there are many new treatments on the horizon that may significantly improve the outcome for this disease. Many patients find it helpful to join support groups where they can discuss their concerns with others who are also coping with the illness.

See also Cigarettes; Drug resistance; Gastrointestinal cancers; Immunologic therapies; Nutritional support; Pain management; Pancreatic cancer, endocrine; Smoking cessation.

Resources

BOOKS

Teeley, Peter, and Philip Bashe. *The Complete Cancer Survival Guide*. New York: Doubleday, 2000.

PERIODICALS

Bornman, P.C., and I.J. Beckingham. "ABC of Diseases of Liver, Pancreas, and Biliary System. Pancreatic Tumours." *British Medical Journal* 322, no. 7288 (March 24, 2001): 721–3.

Haut, E., A. Abbas, and A. Schuricht. "Pancreatic Cancer: The Role of the Primary Care Physican." *Consultant* 39, no. 12 (December 1999): 3329.

Parks, R.W., and O.J. Garden. "Ensuring Early Diagnosis in Pancreatic Cancer." *Practitioner* 244, no. 1609 (April 2000): 336–8, 340–1, 343.

OTHER

Johns Hopkins Medical Institutions. [cited July 20, 2009]. http://www.path.jhu.edu/pancreas.

Memorial Sloan-Kettering Cancer Center. Patient Information on Pancreatic Cancer. [cited July 20, 2009]. http://www.mskcc.org/patients_n_public/about_cancer_and_treatment/cancer_information_by_type/pancreatic_cancer/index.html.

University of Texas MD Anderson Cancer Center. Pancreatic Tumor Study Group. [cited July 20, 2009]. http://www.mdanderson.org/DEPARTMENTS/pancreatic/.

"What You Need To Know About Cancer of the Pancreas." National Cancer Institute. [cited July 20, 2009]. http://cancernet.nci.nih.gov/wyntk_pubs/pancreas.htm.

ORGANIZATIONS

CancerNet. National Cancer Institute, 9000 Rockville Pike, Bldg.31, Rm.10A16, Bethesda, Maryland, 20892. (800) 422-6237. http://wwwicic.nci.nih.gov.

Hirshberg Foundation for Pancreatic Cancer Research. 375 Homewood Rd., Los Angeles, CA 90049. (310) 472-6310. http://www.pancreatic.org.

National Pancreas Foundation. PO Box 935, Wexford, PA 15090-0935. http://www.pancreasfoundation.org.

Pancreatic Cancer Action Network. PO Box 1010, Torrance, CA 90505. (877) 272-6226. http://www.pancan.org.

Lata Cherath, Ph.D.
Elizabeth Pulcini, M.Sc.

Panitumumab

Definition

Panitumumab is an anti-cancer drug designed to treat colorectal **cancer**. Panitumumab inhibits tumor cellular signaling by antagonizing a signaling pathway effecting tumor cell development. The tumor cells panitumumab is used against have a receptor on their cell surface called the epidermal growth factor receptor (EGFR).

Purpose

Panitumumab is used to treat colorectal cancer that has high levels of the epidermal growth factor receptor. Panitumumab treats colorectal cancer that is metastatic (spread from other parts of the body) and has failed to respond to treatment with other drugs. Only colorectal cancer that has EGFR may be targeted by panitumumab. Patients in the **clinical trials** that evaluated panitumumab treatment were required to have immunohistochemical evidence (testing cancer cells viewed under a microscope) of EGFR expression.

Description

Panitumumab is manufactured by Amgen under the trade name Vectibix. Panitumumab is a type of monoclonal antibody used in the treatment of colorectal cancer. **Monoclonal antibodies** are produced in the laboratory as substances that can locate and bind to cancer cells to destroy them. Studies have shown that use of panitumumab increases progression-free survival compared to placebo. The term progression-free survival describes the length of time during and after treatment in which a patient is living with a disease that does not get worse. In a clinical trial designed to test out a cancer drug in human, progression-free survival is a way to measure how effective a treatment is.

Panitumumab specifically targets the EGFR expressed by cancer cells to prevent cancer cell growth and replication. The EGFR is a type of chemical receptor that sits on the outer membrane of both normal cells and cancer cells. Chemical receptors in the body activate a sequence of cellular events known as a chemical cascade or signaling pathway. It is these signaling pathways that are responsible for many normal body functions. Drugs or natural chemicals that bind to and activate the receptor signaling pathway are known as receptor agonists. Drugs that bind to the receptor and block them from creating a signaling pathway are known as receptor antagonists, because

KEY TERMS

Abscess—Pocket of infection present in body tissues.

Angiogenesis—Physiological process involving the growth of new blood vessels from pre-existing blood vessels, process used by some cancers to create their own blood supply.

B cell—Type of white blood cell that creates antibodies to fight infection.

Cytochrome P450— Enzymes present in the liver that metabolize drugs.

Epidermal growth factor—Natural body chemical involved in cellular processes of growth and development.

Epidermal growth factor receptor—Structure on the surface of cells that binds growth factors to allow them to effect growth via a chemical signaling cascade.

Metastasize—The process by which cancer spreads from its original site to other parts of the body.

Monoclonal antibody—Antibodies produced by one type of B cell that are all clones of the parent cell and so are identical.

Pulmonary thromboembolism—Formation in a blood vessel of a clot (thrombus) that breaks loose (embolus) and is carried by the blood stream to plug a vessel in the lungs.

Septic blood—Blood that is infected with bacteria to the point of illness, may be fatal.

they antagonize the effects of that receptor. EGFR are receptors that bind growth factors to create signaling cascades that are a natural part of cell development and necessary for normal cell growth. The agonist that normally binds to the EGFR is epidermal growth factor (EGF). When EGF binds to the EGFR, it initiates chemical signals that tell the cell how to grow and replicate. Some cancer cells have a mutated form of the EGFR that can be targeted by drugs that differentiate between the normal and mutated EGFR. Panitumumab antagonizes the mutant EGFR by binding and prevent the signaling pathway for growth from happening. Panitumumab mainly acts on cancer cells instead of normal cells because it targets the mutated form of the EGFR.

Panitumumab is a chimeric (fusion) mouse and human monoclonal antibody used to treat metastatic colorectal cancer and malignant head and neck cancer. Drugs like panitumumab are made in mice for experimental purposes but need to be humanized to eliminate or reduce the chance that patients will mount an immune reaction to the antibody when administered in therapy. Panitumumab binds to and blocks the EGFR to fight tumor cells, and in some cases has also been shown to be directly toxic to tumor cells. By blocking EGFR, panitumumab blocks the biological signal that promotes tumor growth and **metastasis**. The biological signal also promotes new blood vessel formation in the process of angiogenesis. Once a solid tumor reaches a certain size, it needs blood vessels in order for its cells to remain alive, and to continue to grow. Blood vessels that grow in tumors in the process called angiogenesis also contribute to its metastasis to other parts of the body. All of these components are critical to the ongoing survival of the tumor and blocked by panitumumab.

Recommended dosage

Panitumumab is administered intravenously. It is not given as a rapid infusion or as a bolus (one larger dose at one time). Panitumumab is given as an infusion over 60 minutes if the dose is less than or equal to a total of 1 g. Panitumumab is given as an infusion over 90 minutes if the dose is greater than a total of 1 g. The dose chosen for use depends on the weight of the patient and the response to treatment with regard to both the development of side effects and therapeutic effect. A typically used dosage for EGFR-expressing metastatic colorectal cancer that has not responded to other treatments is 6 mg/kg given as a 60 minute infusion every 14 days.

While panitumumab is not frequently associated with the development of adverse reactions to drug infusions, intravenous drugs often cause serious medical conditions upon infusion. The infusion rate of panitumumab is altered in the case of infusion reactions, based on the presence and severity level. If the infusion reaction is considered of mild or moderate degree the infusion rate is decreased by 50%. If the infusion reaction is considered severe therapy is discontinued permanently.

QUESTIONS TO ASK YOUR PHARMACIST

- How long will I need to take this drug before you can tell if it helps for me?
- How often do I have to have blood work and other laboratory tests done to check the effect the drug is having?
- Is this drug safe to take with the other drugs that I am currently taking?
- What side effects should I watch for? When should I call the doctor about them?
- Are there any clinical trials of this drug combined with other therapies that might benefit me?

Precautions

Panitumumab is a pregnancy category C drug, and is used during pregnancy only when medically necessary. A pregnancy category C drug is one for which studies done in animals have shown potential harm to a fetus but there is not sufficient data in humans. If the potential benefits for the patient outweigh the potential risks to the fetus, the drug may be used during pregnancy. However, panitumumab may cause harm or death of a fetus. Panitumumab is contraindicated for use during breastfeeding and cannot be used within 2 months of beginning breastfeeding. The safety and effectiveness of panitumumab has not been established in patients less than 18 years of age. Panitumumab may not be appropriate for use in patients with skin inflammation or infections, some types of lung disease, or septic blood.

Monoclonal antibody drugs have been associated with severe infusion reactions, such as breathing complications, heart attack, collapse of the blood vessels, shock, and death. Panitumumab has a very low rate of infusion reactions compared with other monoclonal antibody cancer drugs. In clinical trials infusion reactions only occurred in 4% of patients with only 1% severe. No fatalities were reported. However in patients who do develop infusion reactions the dosage may need to be decreased, infusion rate decreased, or therapy discontinued altogether.

Caution is used when dosing panitumumab due to toxic reactions. Skin related toxicity is commonly associated with panitumumab therapy. Toxicity may involve **itching**, redness and inflammation, rash, acne, peeling skin, inflammation of the inner lining of the mouth, and fissured skin. Skin reactions that are severe may develop into infections leading to septic blood and death. Eye toxicity involves inflammation and redness, tearing, and irritation. Many of these toxic reactions occur within the first 14 to 15 days of treatment and resolve approximately 84 days after the last dose.

Panitumumab is associated with risk of photosensitivity and severe sunburn. Excessive sun exposure should be avoided and protective measures such as sunscreen are advised. Panitumumab may cause severe imbalances in blood chemicals called electrolytes, especially for magnesium. Blood is monitored to check for signs of toxicity or abnormality. Panitumumab may also cause severe lung disease in some patients, including permanent fibrous changes to lung tissue that interfere with breathing capacity. Panitumumab therapy may not be appropriate for patients with existing skin abscesses, skin inflammation, or lung disease.

Side effects

Panitumumab is used when the medical benefit is judged to be greater than the risk of side effects. Commonly seen side effects include abdominal pain and cramping, constipation, **diarrhea**, peeling skin infections, **fatigue**, blood chemistry imbalances in magnesium and calcium, **nausea**, **vomiting**, itchy skin, rash, fissured painful skin, and sun sensitivity. Other side effects include acne, eye inflammation, cough, dehydration, dry skin, and mouth sores. Rarely panitumumab may cause lung disease, **fever**, septic blood, severely low pressure, and pulmonary thromboembolism. These side effects are most commonly seen with toxic doses of panitumumab and avoided during therapy.

Interactions

Panitumumab may cause multiple different potentially serious adverse effects. Use of panitumumab in the same time period as other drugs that cause similar medical problems may cause an additive effect. An additive effect is seen with the drug **bevacizumab**, increasing risk for skin related toxicity, severe diarrhea, and lung disease. Interactions may occur between panitumumab and the drug **erlotinib**, causing an increased risk of gastrointestinal perforation and toxicity. Combination of panitumumab and the drugs **fluorouracil** or **irinotecan** increases risk of severe diarrhea reactions.

Most medications are metabolized by a set of liver enzymes known as cytochrome P450 (CYP450). There are multiple subtypes of CYP450s, each responsible for metabolism of their own set of drugs. It is unknown which specific CYP450 subtypes metabolize panitumumab. However, other drugs that induce, or activate the CYP450 enzyme subtype that acts on panitumumab would increase the metabolism of panitumumab. This may result in lower levels of therapeutic panitumumab, thereby negatively effecting treatment. For this reason drugs that induce the panitumumab CYP450 subtype may interact with panitumumab, and any medications, herbs, or supplements taken during fertility treatment should be temporarily minimized if medically appropriate.

Resources

BOOKS

Goodman and Gilman's The Pharmacological Basis of Therapeutics, Eleventh Edition. McGraw Hill Medical Publishing Division, 2006.

Tarascon Pharmacopoeia Library Edition. Jones and Bartlett Publishers, 2009.

OTHER

Epocrates. *Panitumumab.* http://www.epocrates.com.

Medscape. *Panitumumab IV.* http://www.medscape.com.

RxList. *Panitumumab.* http://www.rxlist.com.

ORGANIZATIONS

National Cancer Institute. 6116 Executive Boulevard, Room 3036A, Bethesda, MD 20892-8322. (800)4-CANCER. http://www.cancer.gov.

FDA U.S. Food and Drug Administration. 10903 New Hampshire Ave, Silver Spring, MD 20993. (888)INFO-FDA. http://www.fda.gov.

Maria Basile, Ph.D.

Pap test

Definition

The Pap test is a procedure in which a physician scrapes cells from the cervix or vagina to check for cervical cancer, vaginal cancer, or abnormal changes that could lead to cancer. It often is called a Pap smear.

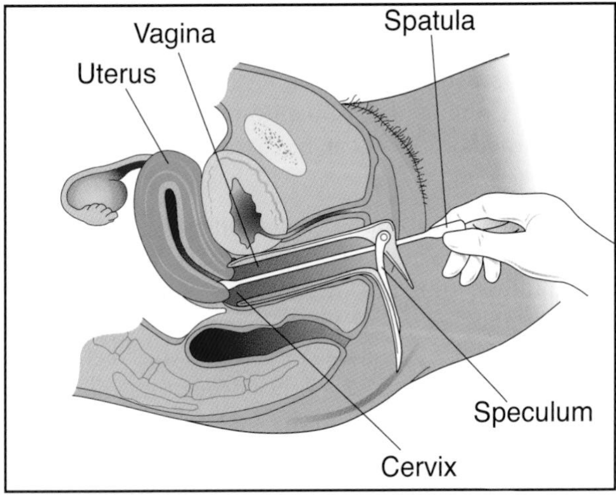

The Pap test is a procedure used to detect abnormal growth of cervical cells that may be a precursor to cancer of the cervix. It is administered by a physician who inserts a speculum into the vagina to open and separate the vaginal walls. A spatula is then inserted to scrape cells from the cervix. These cells are transferred onto glass slides for laboratory analysis. The Pap test may also identify vaginitis, some sexually transmitted diseases, and cancers of the uterus and ovaries. *(Illustration by Electronic Illustrators Group. Cengage Learning, Gale.)*

Purpose

The Pap test is used to detect abnormal growth of cervical cells at an early stage so that treatment can be started when the condition is easiest to treat. This microscopic analysis of cells can detect cervical cancer, precancerous changes, inflammation (vaginitis), infections, and some sexually transmitted diseases (STDs). The Pap test can occasionally detect endometrial (uterine) cancer or ovarian cancer, although it was not designed for this purpose.

Women should begin to have Pap tests at the age of 21 or within three years of becoming sexually active, whichever comes first. Young people are more likely to have multiple sex partners, which increases their risk of certain diseases that can cause cancer, such as human papillomavirus (HPV).

The American Cancer Society (ACS) updated its guidelines concerning Pap test frequency in late 2002. In brief, women should continue screening every year with regular Pap tests until age 30, every two years if using the liquid-based Pap test. Once a woman age 30 and older has had three normal results in a row, she may get screened every two to three years. A doctor may suggest more frequent screening if a woman has certain risk factors for cervical cancer. Women who have had total hysterectomies including the removal of the cervix do not need Pap tests unless the hysterectomy resulted from cervical cancer. Those over age 70 who have had three normal results generally do not need to continue having Pap tests under the new guidelines.

Women with certain risk factors should always have yearly tests. Those at highest risk for cervical cancer are women who started having sex before age 18, those with many sex partners (especially if they did not use condoms, which protect against STDs), those who have had STDs such as genital herpes or genital warts, and those who smoke. Women older than 40 may have the test yearly, if experiencing bleeding after menopause. Women who have had a positive test result in the past may need screening every six months. Women who have had cervical cancer or precancer should have regular Pap smears.

Other women also benefit from the Pap test. Women over age 65 account for 25% of all cases of cervical cancer and 41% of deaths from this disease. Women over age 65 who have never had a Pap smear benefit the most from a Pap smear. Even a woman who has had a hysterectomy (removal of the uterus) should continue to have regular Pap tests at the discretion of the woman and the provider. If the surgery was for cancer, she may need to be examined more often than once a year. (Some women have the cervix left in place after hysterectomy.) Finally, a pregnant woman should have a Pap test as part of her first prenatal examination.

The Pap test is a screening test. It identifies women who are at increased risk of cervical dysplasia (abnormal cells) or cervical cancer. Only an examination of the cervix with a special lighted instrument (colposcopy) and samples of cervical tissue (biopsies) can actually diagnose these problems.

Precautions

The Pap test is usually not done during the menstrual period because of the presence of blood cells. The best time is in the middle of the menstrual cycle.

Description

The Pap test is an extremely cost-effective and beneficial test. Cervical cancer used to be a leading cause of cancer deaths in American women, but widespread use of this diagnostic procedure reduced the death rate from this disease by 74% between 1955 and 1992. A 2003 study reported that the test reduces rates of invasive cervical cancer by as much as 94%. In 2003, the FDA approved a new screening test that combines DNA testing for the HPV type that causes the most

KEY TERMS

Carcinoma in situ—Malignant cells that are present only in the outer layer of the cervix.

Cervical intraepithelial neoplasia (CIN)—A term used to categorize degrees of dysplasia arising in the epithelium, or outer layer, of the cervix.

Dysplasia—Abnormal changes in cells.

Human papillomavirus (HPV)—The most common STD in the United States. Various types of HPV are known to cause cancer.

Neoplasia—Abnormal growth of cells, which may lead to a neoplasm, or tumor.

Squamous intraepithelial lesion (SIL)—A term used to categorize the severity of abnormal changes arising in the squamous, or outermost, layer of the cervix.

cases of cervical cancer with the standard Pap test, increasing its screening value.

The Pap test, sometimes called a cervical smear, is the microscopic examination of cells scraped from both the outer cervix and the cervical canal. (The cervix is the opening between the vagina and the uterus, or womb.) It is called the "Pap" test after its developer, Dr. George N. Papanicolaou. This simple procedure is performed during a gynecologic examination and is usually covered by insurance. For those with coverage, Medicare will pay for one screening Pap smear every three years.

During the pelvic examination, an instrument called a speculum is inserted into the vagina to open it. The doctor then uses a tiny brush, or a cotton-tipped swab and a small spatula to wipe loose cells off the cervix and to scrape them from the inside of the cervix. The cells are transferred or "smeared" onto glass slides, the slides are treated to stabilize the cells, and the slides are sent to a laboratory for microscopic examination. The entire procedure is usually painless and takes five to ten minutes at most.

The newer method called liquid-based cytology, or the liquid-based Pap test, involves spreading the cells more evenly on a slide after removing them from the sample. The liquid-based method prevents cells from drying out and becoming distorted. Studies show that liquid-based testing slightly improves cancer detection and greatly improves detection of precancers, but it costs more than the traditional Pap test. Trade names in 2003 for liquid-based Pap smears were ThinPrep and AutoCyte.

Preparation

The Pap test may show abnormal results when a woman is healthy or normal results in women with cervical abnormalities as much as 25% of the time. It may even miss up to 5% of cervical cancers. Some simple preparations may help to ensure that the results are reliable. Among the measures that may help increase test reliability are:

- Avoiding sexual intercourse for two days before the test.
- Not using douches for two or three days before the test.
- Avoiding using tampons, vaginal creams, or birth control foams or jellies for two to three days before the test.
- Scheduling the Pap smear when not menstruating. However, most women are not routinely advised to make any special preparations for a Pap test.

If possible, women may want to ensure that their test is performed by an experienced gynecologist, physician, or provider and sent to a reputable laboratory. The physician should be confident in the accuracy of the chosen lab.

Before the exam, the physician will take a complete sexual history to determine a woman's risk status for cervical cancer. Questions may include date and results of the last Pap test, any history of abnormal Pap tests, date of last menstrual period and any irregularity, use of hormones and birth control, family history of gynecologic disorders, and any vaginal symptoms. These topics are relevant to the interpretation of the Pap test, especially if any abnormalities are detected. Immediately before the Pap test, the woman should empty her bladder to avoid discomfort during the procedure.

Aftercare

Harmless cervical bleeding is possible immediately after the test; a woman may need to use a sanitary napkin. She should also be sure to comply with her doctor's orders for follow-up visits.

Risks

No appreciable health risks are associated with the Pap test. However, abnormal results (whether valid or due to technical error) can cause significant anxiety. Women may wish to have their sample double-checked, either by the same laboratory or by the

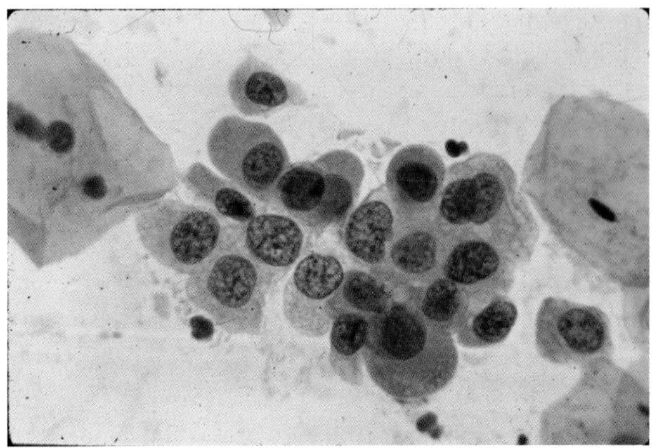

These malignant cells were taken from a woman's cervix during a Pap test. *(Photograph by Parviz M. Pour, Photo Cengage Learning, Gale.)*

new technique of computer-assisted rescreening. The Food and Drug Administration (FDA) has approved the use of AutoPap and PAPNET to doublecheck samples that have been examined by technologists. AutoPap may also be used to perform initial screening of slides, which are then checked by a technologist. Any abnormal Pap test should be followed by colposcopy, not by double checking the Pap test.

Normal results

Normal (negative) results from the laboratory exam mean that no atypical, dysplastic, or cancer cells were detected, and the cervix is normal.

Abnormal results

Terminology

Abnormal cells found on the Pap test may be described using two different grading systems. Although this can be confusing, the systems are quite similar. The "Bethesda" system is based on the term "squamous intraepithelial lesion" (SIL). Precancerous cells are classified as "atypical squamous cells of undetermined significance," "low-grade" SIL, or "high-grade" SIL. Low-grade SIL includes mild dysplasia (abnormal cell growth) and abnormalities caused by HPV; high-grade SIL includes moderate or severe dysplasia and carcinoma in situ (cancer that has not spread beyond the cervix).

Another term that may be used is "cervical intraepithelial neoplasia" (CIN). In this classification system, mild dysplasia is called CIN I, moderate is CIN II, and severe dysplasia or carcinoma in situ is CIN III.

Regardless of terminology, it is important to remember that an abnormal (positive) result does not necessarily indicate cancer. Results may be falsely abnormal after infection or irritation of the cervix. Up to 40% of mild dysplasia reverts to normal tissue without treatment, and only 1% of mild abnormalities ever develop into cancer.

Treatment

CHANGES OF UNKNOWN CAUSE. The most common abnormality found in Pap tests is atypical squamous cells of undetermined significance (ASCUS), which are found in 4% of all Pap tests. Sometimes these results are described further as either reactive or precancerous. Reactive changes suggest that the cervical cells are responding to inflammation, such as from a yeast infection. These women may be treated for infection and then undergo repeat Pap testing in three to six months. If those results are negative, no further treatment is necessary. This category may also include atypical "glandular" cells, which could imply a more severe type of cancer and requires repeat testing and further evaluation.

DYSPLASIA. The next most common finding (in about 25 of every 1,000 tests) is low-grade SIL, which includes mild dysplasia or CIN I and changes caused by HPV. Unlike cancer cells, these cells do not invade normal tissues. Women are most susceptible to cervical dysplasia between the ages of 25 and 35. Typically, dysplasia causes no symptoms, although women may experience abnormal vaginal bleeding. Because dysplasia is precancerous, it should be treated if it is moderate or severe.

Treatment of dysplasia depends on the degree of abnormality. In women with no other risk factors for cervical cancer, mild precancerous changes may be simply observed over time with repeat testing, perhaps every four to six months. This strategy works only if women are diligent about keeping later appointments. Premalignant cells may remain that way without causing cancer for five to ten years, and may never become malignant.

In women with positive results or risk factors, the gynecologist must perform colposcopy and biopsy. A colposcope is an instrument that looks like binoculars, with a light and a magnifier, used to view the cervix. Biopsy, or removal of a small piece of abnormal, cervical or vaginal tissue for analysis, is usually done at the same time.

High-grade SIL (found in three of every 50 Pap tests) includes moderate to severe dysplasia or carcinoma in situ (CIN II or III). After confirmation by colposcopy and biopsy, it must be removed or destroyed to prevent further growth. Several outpatient techniques are available: conization (removal of a cone-shaped piece of tissue), laser surgery, cryotherapy (freezing), or the "loop electrosurgical excision procedure." Cure rates are nearly 100% after prompt and appropriate treatment of carcinoma in situ. Of course, frequent checkups are then necessary.

CANCER. HPV, the most common STD in the United States, may be responsible for many cervical cancers. Cancer may be manifested by unusual vaginal bleeding or discharge, bowel and bladder problems, and pain. Women are at greatest risk of developing cervical cancer between the ages of 30 and 40 and between the ages of 50 and 60. Most new cancers are diagnosed in women between 50 and 55. Although the likelihood of developing this disease begins to level off for Caucasian women at the age of 45, it increases steadily for African-Americans for another 40 years. Biopsy is indicated when any abnormal growth is found on the cervix, even if the Pap test is negative.

Doctors have traditionally used radiation therapy and surgery to treat cervical cancer that has spread within the cervix or throughout the pelvis. In severe cases, postoperative radiation is administered to kill any remaining cancer cells, and chemotherapy may be used if cancer has spread to other organs. Recent studies have shown that giving chemotherapy and radiation at the same time improves a patient's chance of survival. The National Cancer Institute has urged physicians to strongly consider using both chemotherapy and radiation to treat patients with invasive cervical cancer. The survival rate at five years after treatment of early invasive cancer is 91%; rates are below 70% for more severe invasive cancer. That is why prevention, risk reduction, and frequent Pap tests are the best defense for a woman's gynecologic health.

Resources

PERIODICALS

"American Cancer Society Issues New Early Detection Guidelines." *Women's Health Weekly* December 19, 2002: 12.

"Get Ready to Take Cervical Cancer Screening to the Next Level: Newly Approved Human Papillomavirus Test Offers 2-in-1 Package."*Contraceptive Technology Update* June 2003: 61–64.

Kennedy, A.W. "What do you recommend for a patient with a Pap smear indicating atypical cells?" *Cleveland Clinic Journal of Medicine* 67, no. 9 (2000).

Law, Malcolm. "How Frequently Should Cervical Screening Be Conducted?" *Important Journal of Medical Screening* Winter 2003: 159–161.

"Patient info: Why you need a Pap test." *Patient Care* 33, no. 12 (1999).

"Topics in Women's Health—Contending with the Abnormal Pap test." *Patient Care* 33, no. 12 (1999).

OTHER

"Pap smear: Simple, life-saving test." [cited June 28, 2009]. http://www.mayohealth.org/home?id = HQ01177.

"Pap Smears: The simple test that can save your life." [cited June 28, 2009]. http://www.mayohealth.org/home?id = HQ01178.

ORGANIZATIONS

American Cancer Society. (800) ACS-2345. http://www.cancer.org/.

American College of Obstetricians and Gynecologists. 409 12th St. SW, PO Box 96920, Washington, DC 20090-6920. (202) 863-2518. http://www.acog.com.

National Cancer Institute, Office of Communications. 31 Center Dr., MSC 2580, Bethesda, MD 20892-2580. (800) 4-CANCER. http://cancernet.nci.nih.gov/.

Laura J. Ninger
Teresa G. Odle

Paracentesis

Definition

Also known as peritoneal tap or abdominal tap, paracentesis consists of drawing fluid from the abdomen through a needle.

Purpose

Although little or no fluid is present in the abdominal (peritoneal) cavity of a healthy man, more than half an ounce may accumulate at certain times during a woman's menstrual cycle. Any **cancer** that originates in or spreads to the abdomen can result in fluid accumulation (malignant **ascites**).

Doctors remove fluid (ascites) from the abdomen to analyze its composition and determine its origin, to relieve the pressure and discomfort it causes, and to check for signs of internal bleeding This procedure should be performed whenever an individual experiences sudden or worsening abdominal swelling or when ascites is accompanied by **fever**, abdominal pain, confusion, or coma.

Paracentesis in cancer patients

When performed on a patient who has been diagnosed with cancer, paracentesis helps doctors determine the extent (stage) of the disease and whether

QUESTIONS TO ASK THE DOCTOR

- How will paracentesis benefit me?
- Will I have to have this procedure more than once?
- How soon after this procedure can I resume my normal activities?
- Will paracentesis cure my problem?
- Will I require hospitalization?

conservative or radical treatment approaches would most effectively relieve symptoms or lengthen survival.

Precautions

Before undergoing paracentesis, a patient must make the doctor aware of any allergies, bleeding problems or use of anticoagulants, pregnancy, or possibility of pregnancy.

Description

Paracentesis is performed in a doctor's office or a hospital. The puncture site is cleansed and, if necessary, shaved. The patient may feel some stinging as a local anesthetic is administered, and pressure as the doctor inserts a special needle (tap needle) into the abdomen. Occasionally, guidance with CT or ultrasound may be used.

When paracentesis is performed for diagnostic purposes, less than an ounce of fluid is drawn from the patient's abdomen into a syringe. As much as 15 ounces may be needed to determine whether ascites contains cancer cells. When the purpose of the procedure is to relieve pressure or other symptoms, many quarts of ascites may be drained from the abdomen. Because removing large amounts of fluid in a short time can cause dizziness, lightheadedness, and a sudden drop in blood pressure, the doctor may drain fluid slowly enough that the patient's circulatory system has time to adapt.

Laboratory analysis of abdominal fluid can detect blood, cancer cells, **infection**, and elevated protein levels often associated with malignant ascites. Results of these tests can help doctors determine the most appropriate course of treatment for a particular patient.

KEY TERMS

Appendicitis—Inflammation of the appendix.

Cirrhosis—Scarring of the liver (from infection or tumor) resulting in liver dysfunction.

Lymphoma—Cancer of the lymph system.

Preparation

No special preparations are required before this procedure. Patients should ask their doctors about special preparation requirements, but usually may eat, drink and take medications normally prior to paracentesis.

Aftercare

After removing the tap needle, the doctor may use a stitch or two to close any incision made (to ease the needle's entry into the abdomen) and applies an adhesive dressing to the puncture site.

Risks

Paracentesis occasionally causes infection. There is also a slight chance of the tap needle puncturing the bladder, bowel, or blood vessels in the abdomen. If large amounts of ascites are removed, the patient may need to be hospitalized and given intravenous (IV) fluids to prevent or correct severe fluid, protein, or electrolyte imbalances. A patient who has undergone extensive paracentesis should be warned about the possibility of fainting (syncope) episodes.

Normal results

Paracentesis is designed to establish the cause of, or to relieve symptoms associated with, an abnormal accumulation of fluid in the abdomen.

Abnormal results

Laboratory tests of ascites may indicate the presence of:

- appendicitis
- cancer
- cirrhosis
- damaged bowel
- disease of the heart, kidneys, or pancreas
- infection

Ascites that contains cancer cells is usually bloody. Cloudy abdominal fluid has been found in patients with extensive intraabdominal lymphomas. Ascites will continue to accumulate until its cause is identified and eliminated. Some patients need to undergo paracentesis repeatedly.

Resources

BOOKS

Tierney, Lawrence J., et al., editors. *Current Medical Diagnosis & Treatment 2000*. New York: Lange Medical Books/McGraw-Hill, 2000.

Maureen Haggerty

Paranasal sinus cancer

Definition

Paranasal sinus **cancer** is a disease in which cancer (malignant) cells are found in the tissues of the paranasal sinuses—the four hollow pockets of bone surrounding the nasal cavity.

Description

The paranasal sinuses, which are arranged symmetrically around the nasal cavity, include the:

- frontal sinuses (in the forehead, directly above the nose)
- ethmoidal sinuses (on each side of the nasal cavity, just behind the upper part of the nose)
- maxillary sinuses (on each side of the nasal cavity, in the upper region of the cheek bones)
- sphenoidal sinuses (behind the ethmoidal sinuses, in the center of the skull)

The paranasal sinuses, which normally contain air, are lined by mucous membranes that moisten the air entering the nose. Because they contain air, the sinuses allow the voice to echo and resonate.

Because the paranasal sinus area lies in an anatomically complex region, tumors in the paranasal sinuses can invade a variety of structures—such as the orbit (the bony cavity protecting the eyeball), the brain, the optic nerves, and the carotid arterie–even before symptoms appear.

The pharynx (throat) is divided into three sections: the nasopharynx, oropharynx, and laryngopharynx. The nasopharynx is the area behind (posterior to) the nose. The oropharynx is the area posterior to the mouth. The laryngopharynx opens into the larynx and esophagus. Usually, cancers of the paranasal sinuses originate in the lining of the nasopharynx or oropharynx. In rare cases, melanomas—a type of cancer arising from dark pigment-producing cells called melanocytes—may appear in the naso- or oropharynx. There is also an area of specialized sensory epithelium (surface layer of cells) through which the terminal branches of the olfactory nerve enter the roof of the nasal cavity, which gives rise to a very rare malignant neoplasm (growth) known as an esthesioneuroblastoma, or olfactory **neuroblastoma**.

Infrequently, a cancer may arise from the muscles or the soft tissues of the paranasal sinus region; these lesions are called sarcomas. Occasionally, lesions called midline granulomas (a granular-type tumor usually from lymphoid or epithelioid cells) occur; these lesions arise in the nose or paranasal sinuses and spread to surrounding tissues. Also rare are

KEY TERMS

Adenopathy—Large or swollen lymph glands.

Adjuvant therapy—Treatment (such as chemotherapy, radiation therapy, or hormone therapy) given after the primary treatment to increase the chances of a cure.

Adenocarcinoma—Cancer that begins in cells that line certain internal organs and that have glandular (secretory) properties.

Angiogenesis inhibitor—A substance that prevents the growth of new blood vessels.

Antimetabolite—A chemical very similar to one required in normal biochemical reactions in cells; an antimetabolite can stop or slow down the reaction.

Antineoplaston—A substance isolated from normal human blood and urine and tested as a type of treatment for some tumors and AIDS. Treatment is considered experimental in 2001.

Epithelium—A thin layer of tissue that covers organs, glands, and other structures within the body.

Monoclonal antibody—Laboratory-produced substance that can locate and bind to cancer cells.

Nasal cavity—The cavity between the floor of the cranium and the roof of the mouth.

Neoplasm—Any new and abnormal formation of tissue, as a tumor or growth.

Radiotherapy—Radiation treatment (external or internal).

QUESTIONS TO ASK THE DOCTOR

- What kinds of treatments will I receive?
- What benefits can be expected from this therapy?
- What are the risks and side effects of these treatments?
- Will my treatments be covered by health insurance?
- What clinical trials are available for this type of cancer? Am I a candidate?
- Are there any complementary treatments that would benefit me?

slow-growing cancers called inverting papillomas (papillae are tiny, nipple-like protuberances).

Demographics

Malignant growths of the paranasal sinuses are uncommon in the general population. Paranasal sinus cancer represents 3% of all cancers in the upper aerodigestive tract (air and food passages) and less than 1% of all malignancies in the body. The incidence of paranasal sinus cancer is about one case per 100,000 people per year in the United States. Only about 200 new cases a year are diagnosed in the United States. The disease is more common in Asia Minor and China than in Western countries. The incidence of maxillary sinus cancer is highest in the South African Bantus and in Japan.

Paranasal sinus tumors occur about two to three times more frequently in men than women, and diagnosis usually occurs between the ages of 50 and 70. Cancers of the maxillary sinus are the most common of the paranasal sinus cancers, occurring in about 80% of individuals. Tumors of the ethmoidal sinuses are less common (about 20%), and tumors of the sphenoidal and frontal sinuses are rarest (less than 1%).

Squamous cell **carcinoma** (cancer that originates from squamous keratinocytes in the epidermis, the top layer of the skin) is the most frequent type of malignant tumor in the paranasal sinuses (about 80%). Adenocarcinomas (cancer that begins in cells that line certain internal organs and that have glandular, or secretory, properties) constitute 15%, and the remaining 5% are composed of all other types.

Causes and symptoms

Although the causes of paranasal sinus cancer are not known, several occupational groups have been found to have an increased risk of developing these tumors. These groups include leather and textile workers, nickel refiners, woodworkers, and manufacturers of isopropyl alcohol, chromium, and radium. Also, snuff and thorium dioxide (a radiological contrast agent) have been associated with an increased incidence of paranasal sinus cancer. It is unclear whether these factors cause cancer by direct **carcinogenesis** (cancer production) or by altering the normal nasal epithelial physiology.

Nickel workers primarily develop squamous cell carcinomas, which usually arise in the nasal cavity. Woodworkers, however, usually develop adenocarcinomas that usually arise in the ethmoidal sinuses. The incidence of adenocarinomas in these workers is 1,000 times higher than that of the general population. Tobacco and alcohol use have not been demonstrated conclusively as a causative factor in the development of paranasal sinus tumors. However, viral agents, especially the **human papilloma virus** (HPV), may also play a causative role.

In patients with cancer of the head and neck, the immune system is often not functioning properly. Malignant cells are not recognized as foreign, or when recognized, the immune system does not effectively destroy cancer cells. Causes of the failure of the immune system include severe malnutrition, substances in the tumor that deactivate the immune system, or a genetic predisposition.

The symptoms of paranasal sinus cancer vary with the type, location, and stage of cancer present. Symptoms typical of early lesions often resemble those of an upper respiratory tract **infection** and include nasal obstruction, facial pain, and thin, watery nasal discharge (rhinorrhea), which can at times be blood-tinged. The key factor that differentiates the symptoms of an upper respiratory infection from a malignant lesion, however, is the duration of the symptoms. An upper respiratory infection generally clears up or improves dramatically in several weeks with appropriate medical care, but symptoms associated with a malignancy persist.

The most common symptoms of paranasal sinus cancer include:

- persistently blocked nose
- feeling of recurrent "sinus infections"
- bleeding without apparent cause from the nose or the paranasal sinuses

- progressive pain and swelling of the upper region of the face or around the eyes
- closing up of one eye, blurred vision, or visual loss
- persistent pain in the forehead, the front of the skull, or over the cheekbones
- swelling in the roof of the mouth
- loosening of teeth, poorly fitting dentures, or bleeding from upper teeth sockets

Tumors in the nasal cavity and paranasal sinuses metastasize (spread) to the cervical lymph nodes (lymph nodes in the neck) in about 15% of individuals.

Diagnosis

There are several steps in establishing a diagnosis of paranasal sinus cancer. The first step is a thorough medical history, followed by a physical examination. The physical examination may reveal a lesion in the nose or a submucosal (below the mucous membrane) mass arising in an adjacent sinus.

After the history and physical examination, a series of tests are performed to determine the precise nature of the suspicious growth and the extent of its spread. These tests may include:

- Biopsy (the removal of a sample of tissue that appears to be suspicious) is performed after a lesion is identified. The tissue is studied under the pathologist's microscope.
- Computed tomography (CT) scan, which is a series of detailed pictures with thin cross-sectional slices taken radiologically through the body and interpreted with a computer.
- Nasoscopy, which utilizes an instrument called the nasoscope for examining the nasal cavity and the paranasal sinuses.
- Magnetic resonance imaging study (MRI), an imaging study that consists of detailed pictures, but instead of using x rays, a powerful magnet is used to polarize electrons inside the body to obtain images, which are then interpreted by a computer.
- Posterior rhinoscopy, in which the nasopharynx and the rear portion of the nose are examined using a light and a special mirror.

Although endoscopic techniques (visualizing the nasal cavity with an endoscope—a tube-like device to which an optical system is attached) have greatly improved the ability to examine the nasal cavities and the paranasal sinuses, radiographic studies are also necessary in completing the evaluation. The most important radiographic studies include CT and MRI scans, usually used in combination. The MRI scan has become the most essential radiographic test for accurate delineation of pretreatment tumor extent, and also for following up patients after treatment.

However, each scanning technique has its own advantages and limitations. The CT scan is preferred in evaluating the bony structures in the paranasal sinus area. The MRI better assesses soft-tissue differences, enabling not only the differentiation of tumor from inflammatory changes in the nose and sinuses, but also the determination of involvement of the soft tissues in, for example, the orbit, the brain, and the optic nerve.

Obtaining a **biopsy** is crucial to diagnosis. Endoscopic sinus surgery is widely used for obtaining tissue for biopsy. Combining endoscopic surgery with CT imaging, however, allows the surgeon access into small recesses of the nose and sinuses and along the base of the skull, making biopsy not only more accurate but also safer for the patient.

Treatment team

Patients with paranasal sinus cancer are usually treated by a team of specialists using a multifaceted approach. Each patient receives a treatment plan that is tailored to fit his or her requirements, specifically the patient's overall constitution, grade, and stage of disease. Usually, however, the treatment team includes:

- an otorhinolaryngologist (ear, nose, and throat specialist)
- an oncologist (cancer specialist)
- a radiotherapist (x-ray treatment specialist)

If extensive surgery is required, a plastic and reconstructive surgeon may also serve as part of the treatment team.

Clinical staging, treatments, and prognosis

Paranasal sinus cancer staging involves carefully establishing the degree of cancer spread. If the cancer has spread, it is also necessary to establish the extent of spread and organ involvement.

Cancer grading is a microscopic issue; the pathologist determines the degree of aggressiveness of the cancer. The term well-differentiated means less aggressive; the terms moderately differentiated, intermediately aggressive, and poorly differentiated mean more aggressive.

Both grading and staging help the physician establish the prognosis (degree of seriousness of the disease) and likely outcome.

Staging

Staging may involve additional imaging tests such as CT scan of the brain, abdominal ultrasound, bone scan, or chest x ray. Although no clear-cut staging protocol exists for the relatively uncommon cancers of the paranasal sinuses, the following practical staging exists for cancer of the maxillary sinuses, the most common cancer of this area:

- Stage I: The cancer is confined to the maxillary sinus, with no bony erosion or spread to the lymph nodes.
- Stage II: The cancer has begun to destroy the surrounding bones but without spread to the lymph nodes.
- Stage III: The cancer has spread no farther than the bones around the sinus and to one node on the same side of the neck, and is no greater than 3 cm (1.1 in) in size, or has spread to the cheek, the rear portion of the sinus, the eye socket, or the ethmoidal sinus (spread to lymph nodes on the same side of the neck may or may not be present).
- Stage IV: The cancer has spread to the eye, other sinuses, or tissues adjacent to the sinuses (spread to lymph nodes on the same side of the neck may or may not be present). The cancer may have spread within the sinus itself or to surrounding tissues, to lymph nodes in the neck on one or both sides, to any node larger than 6 cm (2.3 in), or to other parts of the body. Recurrent maxillary sinus cancer—either in the same location or in a different one after primary treatment has been completed—is also in this category.

Treatment options

The major treatment options for paranasal sinus cancer include:

- Surgery. May be necessary for the removal of a section of the nasal cavity or the paranasal sinus at any stage of the disease. Also, some lymph node dissection may be required in the neck, depending upon the staging and grading. May be combined with radiotherapy at any stage, depending on the type of cancer and its location.
- Radiotherapy. Also called radiation therapy, radiotherapy is sometimes used alone in stage I and II disease, or in combination with surgery in any stage of the disease. In the early stages of paranasal sinus cancer, radiotherapy is considered the alternative local therapy to surgery. Radiotherapy involves the use of high energy, penetrative rays to destroy cancer cells in the zone treated. Radiation therapy is also employed for palliation (control of symptoms) in patients with advanced cancer. Teletherapy (external radiation) is administered via a machine remote from the body while internal radiation (brachytherapy) is given by implanting a radioactive source into the cancerous tissues. Patients may or may not require both types of radiation. Radiotherapy usually takes just five to 10 minutes per day, five days a week for about six weeks, depending upon the type of radiation used.
- Chemotherapy. Usually reserved for stage III and IV disease. Besides local therapy, the best attempt to control cancer cells circulating in the body is by using systemic therapy (therapy that affects the entire body) in the form of injections or oral medications. This form of treatment, called chemotherapy, is given in cycles (each drug or combination of drugs is usually administered every three to four weeks). Chemotherapy may also be used in combination with surgery, radiotherapy, or both.

At the forefront of research into head and neck cancer, molecular biology and gene therapy are providing new insights into the basic mechanisms of cancer genesis and treatment. The detection of various oncogenes (genes that can induce tumor formation) in head and neck cancer is also progressing rapidly. Gene therapy trials, still in their infancy as of 2005, are also introducing genetic material to help the immune system recognize cancer cells.

Alternative and complementary therapies

Alternative and complementary therapies may also be used at any stage of the disease. Alternative treatments are treatments used instead of conventional treatments. Complementary therapies are used in addition to conventional treatments. Although not specifically used in treating paranasal sinus cancer, there is much anecdotal (nonscientific) evidence for a number of alternative cancer therapies. Some insurance plans cover complementary therapies, such as acupuncture.

The safest and most accepted of these complementary therapies include:

- acupuncture
- biofeedback
- diet that includes fresh fruit, vegetables, and whole grains
- massage
- meditation, prayer, or creative visualization
- vitamins (especially antioxidants A, E, and C), minerals, and herbs

The National Center for Alternative and Complementary and Alternative Medicine, part of the

National Institutes of Health, discusses some alternative and complementary cancer treatments on its web site http://www.nccam.nih.gov.

Prognosis

The high mortality rate and poor prognosis association with paranasal sinus cancer is related to late diagnosis. Most lesions (75%) are at an advanced stage at the time of definitive diagnosis. Surgical treatment alone may be sufficient for stage I or II lesions if adequate surgical margins are obtained. However, for advanced tumors, combined therapy with radical surgical excision and postoperative radiotherapy has been demonstrated to improve the five-year survival rate.

The primary cause of death is failure of local control. Most paranasal sinus cancers grow rapidly and invade nearby tissues but are slow to spread to distant sites. Thus, patients with advanced disease usually die from a local recurrence of the tumor, even after aggressive treatment.

Coping with cancer treatment

Cancer treatments such as radiotherapy and **chemotherapy** not only destroy cancer cells but also damage healthy tissue. The effects of radiation depend upon the dose of radiation, the size of the area radiated, and the number and size of each fraction. When doses are fractionated, the total dose of **radiation therapy** is divided into several smaller, equal doses delivered over a period of several days.

The most common side effect of radiotherapy is extreme **fatigue**. Although rest is encouraged, most radiotherapists advise patients to move around as much as possible. Another common side effect is radiation dermatitis—the skin covering the radiated area becomes red, dry, itchy, and may show signs of scaling. This skin problem is associated only with teletherapy (external radiation therapy).

Radiation also may cause **nausea and vomiting**, **diarrhea**, and urinary discomfort. There may also be a decrease in white blood cells, which are needed to fight infection. Usually the radiotherapist can suggest the drugs and diet necessary to alleviate these problems.

Chemotherapy drugs may cause a wide spectrum of side effects. The severity of these symptoms vary with each drug and with each individual. Some of the most common side effects of chemotherapy include:

- diarrhea
- hair loss (alopecia)
- hearing loss
- skin rashes
- tingling and numbness in the fingers and toes
- vomiting

Most of these side effects are treatable, temporary, and recede after therapy ends. However, the attitude of the patient is very important during cancer therapy. The better psychologically prepared the patient is for treatment, the better the chances of experiencing decreased side effects.

If extensive surgery is required, reconstruction and rehabilitation by specialized physicians can improve the patient's quality of life.

Clinical trials

As of 2009, 225 **clinical trials** involving paranasal sinus cancer were operating in the United States. Clinical trials can be located at the web site http://www.clinicaltrials.gov, a service of the National Institutes of Health and the National Library of Medicine.

Some of the new drugs under investigation for advanced, recurrent, or metastatic head and neck cancer—either alone, in combination, with concurrent radiotherapy, or with standard chemotherapy drugs such as **fluorouracil** (5-FU), paclitaxel, or cisplatin—include:

- A10 and AS2-1 (antineoplastons)
- Dimesna (chemoprotective agent)
- Fenretinide (retinoid, or vitamin A derivative)
- Filgrastim (G-CSF or granulocyte colony-stimulating factor; increases white blood cells)
- Flavopiridol (cyclin-dependent kinase [Cdk] inhibitor; kinases plays a role in cell cycle regulation and tumor formation)
- Gemcitabine (antimetabolite)
- ONYX-015 (genetically engineered cold virus)
- C225/cetuximab (monoclonal antibody)
- Oxaliplatin (platinum compound; chemotherapeutic agent)
- SU5416 (angiogenesis inhibitor)

Prevention

The causes of paranasal sinus cancer are unknown. However, avoiding environmental risk factors such as heavy smoking or drinking, or inhaling wood dust or other toxic substances (such as isopropyl alcohol, chromium, or radium) on a regular basis may decrease the chances of developing this form of cancer.

Special concerns

Although surgical treatment of squamous cell carcinoma of the head and neck offers the best chance for cure in many patients, the results of the surgery have often been extremely disfiguring and functionally debilitating. The changes in facial appearance and loss of ability to speak, swallow, and breathe normally can be devastating, both physically and psychologically.

If the anticipated surgical defect is large, often a reconstructive team will harvest tissue from a distant site in the body to use as a graft while the oncology team is removing the cancer. Initially, reconstructive teams were more concerned with simply closing the surgical defect and re-establishing a more natural form. Increasingly, the focus has been to re-establish normal function.

Resources

BOOKS

Abeloff, Martin D., James O. Armitage, Allen S. Licter, and John E. Niederhuber. "Paranasal Sinuses and Nose." In *Clinical Oncology*. 2nd ed. New York: Churchill Livingstone, 2000, pp. 1297-1299.

Harrison, Louis B., Roy B. Sessions, and Waun Ki Hong, editors. *Head and Neck Cancer: A Multidiscplinary Approach*. Philadelphia: Lippincott Williams & Wilkins, 1999.

PERIODICALS

Khuri, Fadlo, et al. "A Controlled Trial of Intratumor ONYX- 015, a Selectively Replicating Adenovirus, in Combination with Cisplatin and 5-Fluorouracil in Patients With Recurrent Head and Neck Cancer." *Nature Medicine*. 6 (August 2000): 879-885.

Lee, Misa M., et al. "Multimodality Therapy in Advanced Paranasal Sinus Carcinoma: Superior Long-Term Results." *Cancer Journal from Scientific American* 5 (August 1999): 219-223.

OTHER

Cancernet (List of organizations and web sites offering information and services for cancer patients and their families). http://www.cancernet.nci,nih.gov/cancerlinks.html.

http://cancersource.com (Cancer resources for patients and families).

http://www.clinicaltrials.gov. (List of clinical trials).

ORGANIZATIONS

American Cancer Society, 1599 Clifton Road, NE, Atlanta, GA 30329-4251. http://www.cancer.org. (800) ACS-2345.

National Cancer Institute. Public Inquiries Office, Building 31, Room 10A03, 31 Center Drive, MSC 2580, Bethesda, MD 20892-2580. http://www.nci.nih.gov. (800) 4-CANCER.

National Center for Complementary and Alternative Medicine (NCCAM), NCCAM Clearinghouse, P.O. Box 8218, Silver Springs, MD 20907-8218. http://www.nccam.nih.gov. (800) 644-6226.

Genevieve Slomski, Ph.D.

Paraneoplastic syndromes

Description

Paraneoplastic syndromes are rare disorders caused by substances that are secreted by a benign tumor, a malignant (cancerous) tumor, or a malignant tumor's metastases. The disturbances caused by paraneoplastic syndromes occur in body organs at sites that are distant or remote from the primary or metastatic tumors. Body systems that may be affected by paraneoplastic syndromes include neurological, endocrine, cutaneous, renal, hematologic, gastrointestinal, and other systems. The most common manifestations of paraneoplastic syndromes are cutaneous, neurologic, and endocrine disorders. An example of a cutaneous paraneoplastic disorder are telangiectasias, which can be caused by **breast cancer** and lymphomas. **Lambert-Eaton myasthenic syndrome** (LEMS, and also known as Eaton-Lambert syndrome) is a neurologic paraneoplastic syndrome that can be caused by a variety of tumors including **small cell lung cancer**, **lymphoma**, breast, colon and other cancers. **Syndrome of inappropriate antidiuretic hormone** (SIADH) is an endocrine paraneoplastic syndrome, which is seen in as many as 40% of patients diagnosed with small cell lung **cancer**.

Approximately 15% of patients already have a paraneoplastic disorder at the time of initial diagnosis with cancer. As many as 50% of all cancer patients will develop a paraneoplastic syndrome at some time during the course of their disease. Some clinicians categorize the **anorexia**, cachexia, and **fever** which occur as a result of cancer as metabolic paraneoplastic syndromes. Virtually all patients diagnosed with cancer are affected by at least one of these metabolic paraneoplastic syndromes.

Paraneoplastic syndromes can occur with any type of malignancy. However, they occur most frequently with lung cancer, specifically small-cell lung **carcinoma**. Other types of cancer that commonly cause paraneoplastic syndromes are breast cancer and **stomach cancer**. With the exception of **Wilms' tumor** and **neuroblastoma**, paraneoplastic syndromes do not usually occur in children diagnosed with cancer.

In general, paraneoplastic syndromes may be present in the patient before a diagnosis of cancer is made, or, as stated earlier, may be present at the time the patient is first diagnosed with cancer. Most paraneoplastic syndromes appear in the later stages of the disease. Frequently, the presence of a paraneoplastic syndrome is associated with a poor prognosis. Paraneoplastic syndromes are difficult to diagnose and are often misdiagnosed. Some paraneoplastic syndromes may be confused with metatastic disease or spread of the cancer. The presence of the syndrome may be the only indication that a patient has a malignancy or that a malignancy has recurred. Paraneoplastic syndromes may be useful as clinical indicators to evaluate the response of the primary cancer to the treatment. Resolution of the paraneoplastic syndrome can be correlated with tumor response to treatment. That is, if the paraneoplastic syndrome resolves, the tumor has usually responded to the treatment.

Causes

Paraneoplastic syndromes occur when the primary or original tumor secretes substances such as hormones, proteins, growth factors, cytokines, and antibodies. The substances are referred to as mediators. These mediators have effects at remote or distant body organs, which are termed target organs. Mediators interfere with communication between cells in the body. This miscommunication results in abnormal or increased activity of the cell's normal function. For example, a lung tumor may cause the paraneoplastic syndrome, ectopic **Cushing's syndrome**, which is the result of abnormal functioning of the pituitary gland located in the brain. In this example, the lung cancer is the primary tumor and the pituitary gland is the target organ. Ectopic Cushing's Syndrome is caused by overproduction of the mediator, adrenocorticotropic hormone (ACTH).

Treatment

There are usually two approaches taken in the treatment of paraneoplastic syndromes. The first step is treatment of the cancer that is causing the syndrome. This treatment can be surgery, administration of **chemotherapy**, biotherapy, **radiation therapy**, or a combination of these therapies. The next approach is to suppress the substance or mediator causing the paraneoplastic syndrome. Often treatment targeted to the underlying cancer and to the paraneoplastic syndrome occur at the same time. However, even with treatment, irreversible damage to the target organ can occur.

Selected Paraneoplastic Syndromes

SYNDROME OF INAPPROPRIATE ANTIDIURETIC HORMONE (SIADH). SIADH is a common paraneoplastic syndrome that affects the endocrine system. This syndrome is most often associated with small cell lung cancer; however, other cancers such as **brain tumors**, leukemia, lymphoma, colon, prostate, and **head and neck cancers** can lead to SIADH. SIADH is caused by the inappropriate production and secretion of arginine vasopressin or antidiuretic hormone (ADH) by tumor cells. Patients with SIADH may not have symptoms, especially in the early stages. When symptoms do occur they are usually related to hyponatremia, which leads to central nervous system toxicity if left untreated. Signs and symptoms associated with hyponatremia include **fatigue**, anorexia, headache, and mild alteration in mental status in early stages. If SIADH remains untreated, symptoms can progress to confusion, delirium, seizures, coma, and death. Treatment approaches for SIADH are to treat the underlying tumor and restriction of fluids. More severe cases may require the administration of medications.

LAMBERT-EATON MYASTHENIC SYNDROME. Lambert-Eaton myasthenic syndrome, also known as LEMS and Eaton-Lambert syndrome, has been associated with a number of cancers including small-cell lung cancer, lymphoma, breast, stomach, colon, and prostate cancers. Potential mediators associated with paraneoplastic LEMS are antibodies that interfere with release of acetylcholine at the neuromuscular junction. This interference prevents the flow of calcium, which results in decreased or absent impulse transmission to muscle. The disruption in muscular impulse transmission leads to mild symptoms including weakness in the legs and thighs, muscle aches, muscle stiffness, and muscle fatigue. Treatment of LEMS includes administration of **corticosteroids**, intravenous immunoglobulin, and plasmapheresis. Depending on the extent of damage, irreversible loss of function may occur even with treatment.

ECTOPIC CUSHING'S SYNDROME. Cushing's Syndrome is most often associated with small cell lung cancer, **ovarian cancer**, and medullary cancers of the thyroid. ACTH precursors are activated by tumor cells that results in overproduction of ACTH by the pituitary gland. Signs and symptoms of ectopic Cushing's Syndrome include hypertension, hyperglycemia, hypokalemia, edema, muscle weakness, and **weight loss**. The primary approach to treating ectopic

Cushing's Syndrome is to treat the underlying cancer. In early stages, surgery is the treatment of choice. However, surgery is not usually an option for patients diagnosed with small cell cancer of the lung. If the tumor is unable to be removed or controlled, or if the patient has severe symptoms, then treatment targeted to the syndrome is initiated. Medical therapy is usually focused on inhibiting cortisol production and involves the use of medications such as ketoconazole and **aminoglutethimide**.

Resources

OTHER

"10 Most Commonly Asked Questions about Paraneoplastic Syndromes." *Williams and Wilkins*. 1998. [cited June 27, 2009]. http://www.wwilkins.com/theneurologist/articles/paraneoplastic.html.

"Neoplastic and Paraneoplastic Syndromes." *Lung Cancer Online*. 1999-2001. Lung Cancer Online. [cited June 27, 2009]. http://www.lungcanceronline.org/syndrom.html.

Melinda Granger Oberleitner, R.N., D.N.S.

Parathyroid cancer

Definition

Parathyroid **cancer** is a rare, slow-growing tumor of a parathyroid gland in the neck.

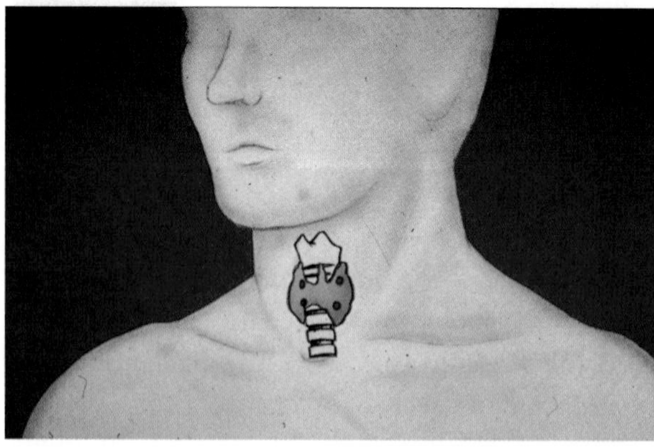

The parathyroid glands, embedded in the thyroid gland but separate from the thyroid in function, control calcium metabolism in the body by producing parathyroid hormone (PTH). Cancer of the parathyroid glands is rare. *(Photograph by Rick Hall. Custom Medical Stock Photo. Reproduced by permission.)*

Description

The four parathyroid glands in the human body are designated as the right superior, right inferior, left superior, and left inferior glands. They usually lay adjacent to the thyroid, but rarely can be found in the upper chest. The parathyroid glands secrete parathyroid hormone, which plays a central role in regulating calcium levels in the blood. In the condition called primary hyperparathyroidism, excess production of parathyroid hormone leads to abnormally high levels of calcium (**hypercalcemia**). Adenomas, or hyperplasia, of the parathyroid glands are responsible for about 99% of all cases of primary hyperparathyroidism. Parathyroid cancer accounts for the remaining 1%.

Parathyroid cancer is a slow-growing tumor that manifests itself mainly by production of parathyroid hormone.

Demographics

Only a few hundred cases of parathyroid cancer have been reported in medical literature. It is more common in Japan than in Western countries. No gender preference has been reported. The average age of the patient with parathyroid cancer is in the fifth decade.

Causes and symptoms

Unlike some cancers, there are no predisposing factors that have been found to clearly increase the risk for parathyroid cancer. There are some reported cases of parathyroid cancer arising in patients with adenomas or hyperplasia of the parathyroid.

Most parathyroid cancers are functioning tumors, in that they overproduce parathyroid hormone. Thus, the signs and symptoms of parathyroid cancer are chiefly related to hyperparathyroidism and the resultant hypercalcemia. Common complaints are weakness, **fatigue**, **weight loss**, **anorexia**, constipation, **nausea**, and **vomiting**. Patients may also report frequent urination and extreme thirst. Since excess parathyroid hormone causes bones to release too much calcium into the bloodstream, patients may experience **bone pain** and fractures. The extra calcium in the blood can be deposited in the kidneys, leading to the formation of painful kidney stones. Pancreatitis is another consequence of hypercalcemia. The levels of parathyroid hormone and calcium in patients with parathyroid cancer are usually dramatically elevated—much more so than in patients with benign causes of hyperparathyroidism.

Parathyroidectomy

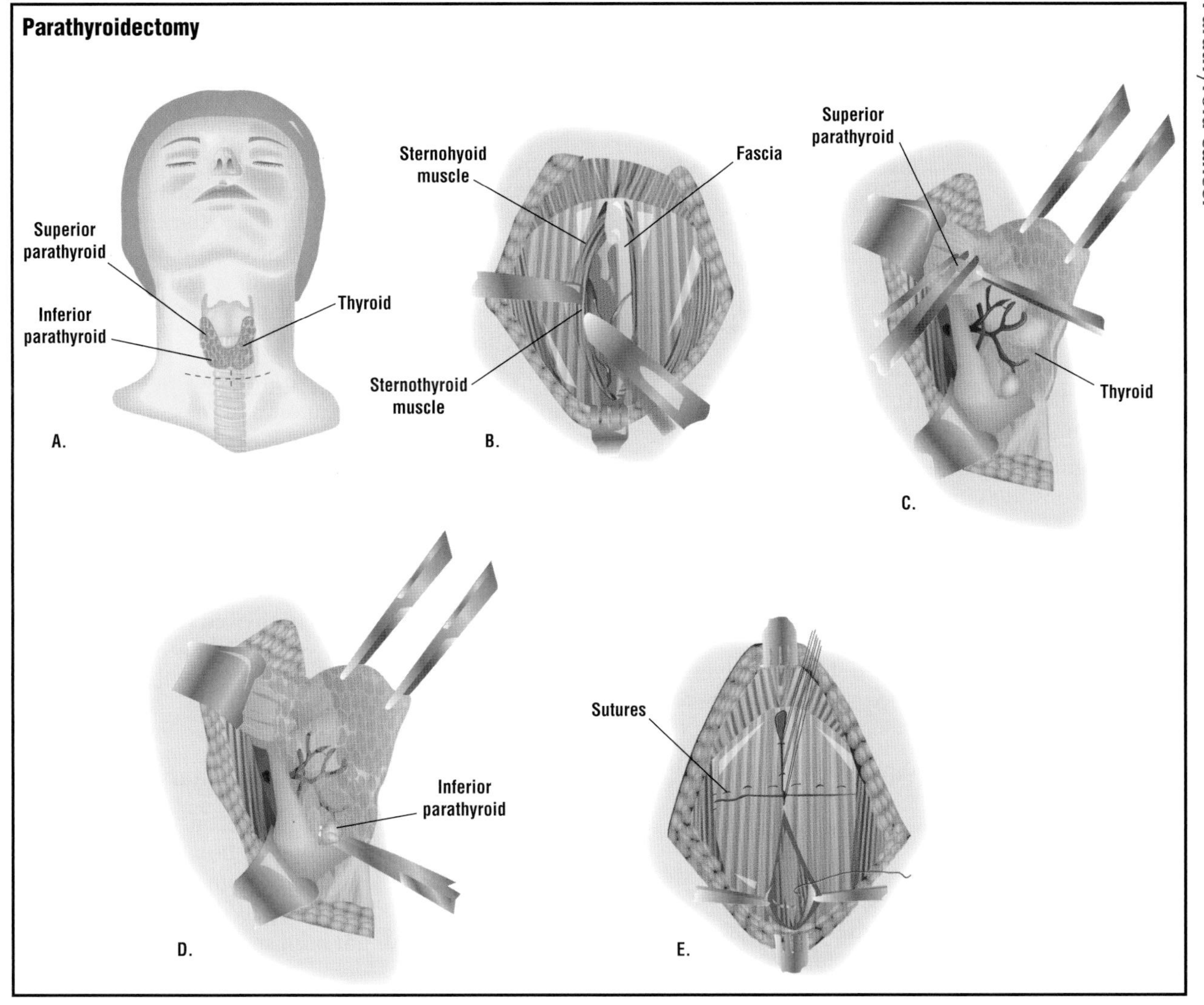

(Illustration by Argosy Publishing. Cengage Learning, Gale.)

Sometimes the parathyroid cancer is large enough to form a mass in the neck that can be easily felt. If the mass is large enough, it can impinge upon a nerve that controls the vocal cords, leading to hoarseness. In contrast, these features are uncommon in benign hyperparathyroidism.

Diagnosis

The diagnosis of parathyroid cancer can be difficult because it produces symptoms similar to those of benign hyperparathyroidism due to adenomas or hyperplasia. However, the symptoms of parathyroid cancer are generally more severe and the levels of parathyroid hormone and calcium are usually higher. The presence of a neck mass or hoarseness also suggests cancer. Beyond this, there are no biochemical or radiological tests that can definitively diagnose parathyroid cancer.

There are four general scenarios for the diagnosis of parathyroid cancer:

- Parathyroid cancer is suspected, based on symptoms and signs. Surgery is performed with the intent to remove the cancer.
- A patient with hyperparathyroidism undergoes surgery to remove one or more glands that are thought to contain an adenoma or hyperplasia. During surgery, it is discovered that the underlying lesion is most likely cancer.
- Similarly, a patient with hyperparathyroidism undergoes surgery to remove one or more glands that are thought to contain an adenoma or hyperplasia. After the surgery is complete, the resected specimen is found to contain cancer.

KEY TERMS

Adenoma—Benign tumor derived from glandular structures.

Biopsy—Obtaining a piece of tissue from a living being for diagnostic examination.

Computed tomography—A radiology test by which images of cross-sectional planes of the body are obtained.

Diuretic—A drug that promotes the excretion of urine.

Hyperplasia—Generalized overgrowth of a tissue or organ due to excess number of cells.

Magnetic resonance imaging—A radiology test that reconstructs images of the body based on magnetic fields.

Pancreatitis—Inflammation of the pancreas.

Peptic ulcer—Distinct erosions of the inner layer of the stomach or small intestine.

Scintigraphy—A radiology test that involves injection and detection of radioactive substances to create images of body parts.

Ultrasound—A radiology test utilizing high-frequency sound waves.

- When symptoms of hyperparathyroidism reappear after surgery, it should raise the suspicion of an incompletely treated parathyroid cancer. This cancer may be localized to the neck or may have spread to distant organs. Several imaging tests can be helpful in this situation. Scintigraphy and ultrasound are useful in detecting recurrent tumors in the neck. Computed tomography (CT scan) and magnetic resonance imaging (MRI) can detect cancer at distant organs, such as the lungs or liver. Sometimes, careful biopsy of a suspected tumor may confirm the diagnosis of cancer.

Clinical staging, treatments, and prognosis

Parathyroid cancer begins in the parathyroid gland and extends to adjacent structures. Late in the course of the disease, it spreads to lymph nodes and ultimately to the lungs and liver.

The best treatment for parathyroid cancer is surgical removal of the cancerous gland. In order to assure complete resection of the cancer, part of the thyroid gland, nearby lymph nodes, and other adherent tissue must be removed with the specimen. Cancer that has spread to distant organs should be removed if possible.

Surgical cure is not possible if the cancer has spread too widely. Therapy then becomes focused on controlling hypercalcemia. General measures include infusing saline solution intravenously to restore lost fluid and to encourage urinary excretion of calcium. Diuretics are drugs that further stimulate urinary excretion of calcium. **Bisphosphonates** and **plicamycin** both inhibit the release of calcium from the bone. Other agents, such as **gallium nitrate**, have shown promise in the treatment of hypercalcemia associated with parathyroid cancer. However, further studies must be conducted to confirm their effectiveness and safety.

The prognosis of parathyroid cancer depends upon the stage of the cancer and the completeness of the surgical resection. If the cancer is detected early and completely removed, cure is possible, but the cancer has been reported to recur up to 20 years after surgery. Cure is unlikely after recurrence. Even so, survival can be signficantly extended by surgery aimed at removing as much recurrent or distant cancer as possible. In general, parathyroid cancer grows and spreads slowly, so that oversecretion of parathyroid hormone is more clinically evident than the actual growth of the cancer.

Alternative and complementary therapies

There have been a few cases in which **radiation therapy** or **chemotherapy** have been reported to partially control the growth and symptoms of parathyroid cancer. In the majority of patients, these interventions have not been successful.

Resources

BOOKS

Macdonald, John S., D. Haller, I.R. McDougall, et al. "Endocrine System." In *Abeloff: Clinical Oncology*, edited by Martin D. Abeloff, 2nd ed. New York: Churchill Livingstone, 2000, pp.1360–97.

Kevin O. Hwang, M.D.

PC-SPES

Definition

PC-SPES is an herbal mixture of eight botanical compounds adapted from traditional Chinese medicine that is used to treat **prostate cancer**, particularly the forms that do not respond to anti-androgen (hormone) therapy.

As PC-SPES is considered an alternative treatment for **cancer**, the National Center for Complementary and Alternative Medicine (NCCAM) began to conduct four separate **clinical trials** of the compound in the early 2000s. These studies were put on hold in June 2002, after the Food and Drug Administration (FDA) determined that samples of PC-SPES were contaminated with "undeclared prescription drug ingredients that could cause serious health effects if not taken under medical supervision." The California distributors of the product voluntarily recalled it, and closed their business at the end of 2002.

Because the early trials of PC-SPES gave promising results, NCCAM is interested in funding newer studies of the product, but will not do so until a fully standardized and uncontaminated product using the original formulation becomes available.

Purpose

PC-SPES is an herbal remedy that has been marketed as an over-the-counter drug for the treatment of prostate cancer. Anecdotal evidence of greatly reduced prostate-specific antigen (PSA) levels in patients taking this preparation prompted more formal testing of its effect. Laboratory studies show that PC-SPES has the ability to slow growth of both hormone-sensitive and hormone-insensitive prostate cancer cell lines in the test tube. Studies done with mice that have been implanted with prostate cancer cells indicate that the treatment triggers apoptosis (programmed cell death) in the artificially created hormone-insensitive tumors.

PC-SPES was shown in three clinical studies to reduce the serum prostate-specific antigen (PSA) levels in the overwhelming majority of patients suffering from prostate cancer that is unresponsive to androgen therapy. The treatment also reduces prostate acid phosphatase (PAP) levels, an enzyme often elevated with hormone-resistant disease. Treatment with the mixture has been shown to decrease pain, decrease narcotic use, and increase perceived quality of life. Researchers noted bone scan improvements, indicating a reduction in the size of cancer metastases to the bone. The majority of the work with this treatment has been done with patients having advanced disease, characterized by elevated PSA values and Gleason tumor scores.

According to one Japanese study, PC-SPES also shows promise in treating Leukemia.

Description

PC-SPES is a mixture of eight herbs used in Chinese medicine: *Ganoderma lucidum*, *Scutellaria baicalensis*, *Rabdosia rubescens*, *Isatis indigotica*, *Dendranthema morifolium*, *Seronoa repens* (**saw palmetto**), *Panax pseudoginseng*, and *Glycyrrhiza uralensis* (licorice). The "PC" portion of the name stands for prostate cancer, while SPES is Latin for "hope." It has been commercially available since 1996. Manufacturers claim it stimulates the immune system and has anti-tumor activity. The mixture appears to act like estrogen against the tumors, and the side effects are very similar for the two therapies. Yet an analysis using liquid chromatography shows that diethylstilbestrol (DES), estrone, or estradiol are all absent. Additionally, some patients who did not respond to traditional estrogen therapy and alkylating agents did respond to PC-SPES, suggesting the mechanism may be unique from that used by DES or **estramustine** (nitrogen mustard, an alkylating agent). Researchers plan a clinical trial that will directly compare the action of DES and PC-SPES in an effort to compare and contrast the two treatment methods.

Recommended dosage

In the clinical trials, PC-SPES was given either in a dosage of nine tablets per day, three before each mealtime or six tablets a day, three before breakfast and three before dinner. As there was essentially no

KEY TERMS

Alkylating agent—A chemical that alters the composition of the genetic material of rapidly dividing cells, such as cancer cells, causing selective cell death; used as a chemotherapeutic agent to treat prostate cancer.

Androgen—Hormones responsible for male characteristics that can be necessary for growth of prostate tumors; blocking the action of androgens can treat prostate cancer.

Apoptosis—An innate process of a cell that brings about its death at the end of the cell's useful lifetime; when malfunctioning can cause cancer.

Gleason grading system—A method of predicting the tendency of a tumor in the prostate to metastasize based on how similar the tumor is to normal prostate tissue; the higher the number the greater the predicted tendency of the tumor to metastasize.

Prostate-specific antigen (PSA)—A protein produced by the cells of the prostate that can be elevated in patients suffering from prostate cancer, abbreviated PSA.

difference in the anti-tumor effect for the studies, six tablets a day might be a recommended starting dosage.

With herbal medications, such as PC-SPES, potency of herb per tablet and recommended dosage may vary from manufacturer to manufacturer.

Precautions

As PC-SPES has been used only in relatively small clinical trials, the full spectrum of precautions has yet to be determined. The clinical trials required taking the tablets on an empty stomach. Furthermore, despite the small sample size, experience does suggest that patients with known heart disease or stroke tendencies should take this medicine with caution, as it might aggravate these conditions.

Side effects

The side effects for PC-SPES are relatively mild and include, from most frequent to least frequent, nipple tenderness, **nausea and vomiting**, **diarrhea**, **fatigue**, gynecomastia (swelling of the male breast), leg cramps or swelling, angina, increased hot flashes, and blood clots. The incidence of angina occurred in a patient with pre-existing coronary disease and was treated by altered heart medications and a reduction in PC-SPES administered.

Interactions

There have been no studies of drug interactions between PC-SPES and other medications. The lack of information about potential adverse interactions suggests caution in adding PC-SPES to other more traditional treatment methods for prostate cancer.

Resources

PERIODICALS

Ikezoe, T., S. Chen, T. Saito, et al. "PC-SPES Decreases Proliferation and Induces Differentiation and Apoptosis of Human Acute Myeloid Leukemia Cells." *International Journal of Oncology* 23 (October 2003): 1203–1211.

Ikezoe, T., S. S. Chen, Y. Yang, et al. "PC-SPES: Molecular Mechanism to Induce Apoptosis and Down-Regulate Expression of PSA in LNCaP Human Prostate Cancer Cells." *International Journal of Oncology* 23 (November 2003): 1461–1470.

OTHER

FDA MedWatch Safety Alert for PC-SPES, SPES, updated September 20, 2002. http://www.fda.gov/medwatch/SAFETY/2002/safety02.htm#spes.

National Center for Complementary and Alternative Medicine (NCCAM). *Recall of PC-SPES and SPES Dietary Supplements*. NCCAM Publication No. D149, September 2002. <http://nccam.nih.gov/health/alerts/spes/index.htm>.

ORGANIZATIONS

National Center for Complementary and Alternative Medicine (NCCAM) Clearinghouse. P. O. Box 7923, Gaithersburg, MD 20898. (888) 644-6226. <http://nccam.nih.gov>.

United States Food and Drug Administration (FDA). 5600 Fishers Lane, Rockville, MD 20857-0001. (888) INFO-FDA (463-6332). http://www.fda.gov.

Michelle Johnson, M.S., J.D.
Rebecca J. Frey, Ph.D.

Pegaspargase

Definition

Pegaspargase (also known as PEG-L-asparaginase and Oncaspar) is a medicine used to stop growth of **cancer** and formation of new cancer cells.

Purpose

Pegaspargase is used as part of induction regimen for the treatment of **acute lymphocytic leukemia** (ALL) in children who developed an allergy to **asparaginase**.

Description

Pegaspargase is a slightly changed version of the native form of asparaginase (*E. coli* asparaginase) that is linked to polyethylene glycol (PEG) molecule. This medicine was made available in 1994 under the brand name Oncaspar. It is more expensive than the native form and is mainly used in patients who developed an allergy to the native form. The advantage of pegaspargase over asparaginase is that it is less likely to cause an allergic reaction and has a longer duration in the body and can be given less frequently. Pegaspargase kills cancer cells by depleting a certain amino acid in the blood (L-asparagine), which is needed for survival and growth of tumor cells in patients with acute lymphocytic leukemia. Fortunately, normal cells can make their own L-asparagine and are not dependent on L-asparagine from the blood for survival.

Pegaspargase is mainly given in combination with other drugs **vincristine** (a vinca alkaloid anticancer drug) and steroids (either prednisone or **dexamethasone**). Other **chemotherapy** medicines are added to

KEY TERMS

Acute lymphocytic leukemia (ALL)—This is the most common cancer in children. Patients with ALL can present with fever, weakness, fatigue, pallor, unusual bleeding and easy bruising, pinpoint dots on the skin, large lymph nodes, and large liver and spleen. ALL in children has a much better prognosis than in adults, with over 90% of children going into remission and an over 80% cure rate with chemotherapy.

Induction therapy—The first stage in treatment of ALL. The purpose of this stage is to quickly cause remission of the disease. The combination of vincristine, asparaginase, and steroids make up the foundation of induction regimen.

Nonsteroidal anti-inflammatory drugs (NSAIDS)—Drugs such as ibuprofen (Advil, Motrin) and naproxen (Aleve) that reduce pain, fever, and inflammation.

this regimen if a patient is at a high risk for disease recurrence.

Recommended dosage

Adults and children with body surface area greater than 0.6 square meters

In induction chemotherapy for acute lymphocytic leukemia, doses vary between different chemotherapy protocols. The usual dose is 2500 international units (IU) per square meter of body surface area given every 14 days.

Children with body surface area less than 0.6 square meters

In induction chemotherapy for acute lymphocytic leukemia, the usual dose is 82.5 IU per kg given every 14 days.

Administration

This medicine can be given directly into the muscle (intramuscular) or into the vein (intravenous). Intramuscular injection of pegaspargase is preferred over the intravenous route because of lower risk of liver disease, blood clotting problems, stomach, and kidney problems. When used intramuscularly, it must be administered as deep injection into a large muscle. When given intravenously, it must be infused over one to two hours. Patients will be monitored closely by a physician for 30 to 60 minutes.

Precautions

The use of this medication should be avoided in patients with active pancreatitis (inflammation of the pancreas) or history of pancreatitis and in patients who have had a serious allergic reaction to pegaspargase in the past.

Pegaspargase should only be administered in a hospital, and a patient will need to be observed by a physician for the first hour.

This medication can lower the body's ability to fight infections. Patients should avoid contact with any individuals that may have a cold, flu, or other **infection**.

Pegaspargase should be used with caution in the following populations:

- People with gout (it may increase uric acid levels and worsen gout).
- People with diabetes (it may increase blood sugar).
- Breast-feeding mothers (it is not known if asparaginase crosses into breast milk).
- Women who are pregnant or may become pregnant (unless benefits to the mother outweigh the risks to the baby).

Patients should contact a doctor immediately if any of these symptoms develop:

- fever, chills, sore throat
- chest pain or heart palpitations
- yellowing of the skin or eyes
- puffy face, skin rash, trouble breathing, joint pain
- drowsiness, confusion, hallucinations, convulsions
- unusual bleeding or bruising
- stomach pain with nausea and vomiting, and loss of appetite (anorexia)

A physician will be doing blood tests before starting therapy and during therapy to monitor complete blood count, blood sugar, pancreas, kidney, and liver functions.

Side effects

Pegaspargase is a very potent medicine that can cause serious side effects. An allergic reaction with skin rash, **itching**, joint pain, puffy face, and difficulty breathing is a side effect that happens very quickly after the drug is injected. The allergic reaction to pegaspargase is less common than with asparaginase. The severe type of this allergic reaction (anaphylaxis) can result in death. Other common side effects include **nausea**, **vomiting**, **diarrhea**, loss of appetite, stomach cramps, yellowing of the eyes or skin, swelling of hands or feet, and pain at the injection site. Less frequent side effects include high blood sugar, chest pain, heart palpitations, headache, chills, **night sweats**, convulsions, decreased kidney function, increased blood clotting, mouth sores, and decreased body's ability to fight infections. Usually the side effects of pegaspargase are more severe in adults than in children.

Interactions

Pegaspargase can decrease effectiveness of **methotrexate** (an antimetabolite, or compound that prevents the synthesis and utilization of normal cellular metabolite, anticancer drug) in killing cancer cells when given right before and together with methotrexate. The use of these two medicines together should be avoided.

Pegaspargase can decrease breakdown and increase toxicity of **cyclophosphamide** (a DNA alkylating anticancer drug).

Risk of liver disease may be increased in patients getting both pegaspargase and **mercaptopurine** (a purine analog antimetabolite anticancer drug).

This medicine can increase blood sugar, especially when given with steroids.

Pegaspargase should be given after vincristine instead of before or with vincristine because it can increase the risk of numbing, tingling, and pain in hands and feet.

People taking blood thinners (**warfarin**, **heparin**, or its derivatives), aspirin, and non-steroidal anti-inflammatory drugs (ibuprofen, naproxen) may be at an increased risk of bleeding. A physician and a pharmacist must be informed about any prescription or over-the-counter medications the patient is taking.

Olga Bessmertny, Pharm.D.

PEG-L-asparaginase *see* **Pegaspargase**

Pemetrexed

Definition

Pemetrexed is an anticancer drug that is used to treat malignant pleural **mesothelioma** and **non-small cell lung cancer**.

KEY TERMS

Cisplatin—An anticancer drug that is used together with pemetrexed to treat MPM.

Docetaxel—An anticancer drug, belonging to the drug family called mitotic inhibitors, that was the standard treatment for recurrent NSCLC prior to pemetrexed.

Folic acid, folate—A member of the vitamin B complex that is a required cell nutrient.

Malignant pleural mesothelioma, MPM—A cancer of the mesothelium that lines the chest cavity; caused by exposure to asbestos.

Multitargeted anti-folate, MTA—A drug that targets various folate-dependent enzymes.

Non-small cell lung cancer, NSCLC—The most common type of lung cancer; includes squamous cell carcinoma, adenocarcinoma, and large cell carcinoma.

Orphan drug—A drug that treats a rare condition; such drugs receive special treatment by the FDA under the Orphan Drug Act.

Vitamin B_{12}—Cobalamin; a protein complex of animal origin that is required for the formation of red blood cells.

White blood cells (WBC)—Blood cells, including lymphocytes, neutrophils, eosinophils, marcrophages, and mast cells, that are produced in the bone marrow and help the body fight infection and disease.

Purpose

Malignant pleural mesothelioma (MPM) is a rare type of **cancer** of the mesothelium (the lining of the chest cavity around the lungs and the abdomen). About 2,000–2,500 new cases of MPM are diagnosed in the United States annually. Twice that many cases occur in Europe. MPM usually is caused by exposure to asbestos. Inhaled asbestos fibers attach to the outer lining of the lung and the chest wall, causing tumor growth. The disease takes years to develop after asbestos exposure. Symptoms of MPM usually are not apparent or are misdiagnosed until after the disease is well-advanced and difficult to treat with surgery or **radiation therapy**. Average survival time is nine to 13 months after diagnosis. Pemetrexed is used for patients with MPM that cannot be treated surgically.

Lung cancer—usually caused by smoking—is the most common cause of cancer death in the United

States. Almost 174,000 people develop lung cancer each year and more than 160,000 die from it annually. Non-small cell lung cancer (NSCLC) accounts for about 80% of all lung cancers and includes squamous cell **carcinoma**, **adenocarcinoma**, and large cell carcinoma. Pemetrexed is used to treat stage III or IV NSCLC in patients whose cancer has recurred following **chemotherapy** and is advancing or has spread (metastasized). Pemetrexed does not improve rates of survival over the standard second-line treatment drug **docetaxel** but has fewer side effects and thus may improve the quality of life. Neither drug cures recurrent lung cancer.

Description

During the 1980s a new class of drugs called multi-targeted anti-folates (MTA) were developed. These drugs limited the ability of cancer cells to obtain **folic acid**, a member of the B-vitamin complex that is required for cell growth and reproduction. However, these drugs were considered too toxic to use until pemetrexed was discovered by a Princeton University biochemist in the 1990s.

Pemetrexed disodium heptahydrate (Alimta), manufactured by Eli Lilly, was approved by the U.S. Food and Drug Administration (FDA) in February of 2004 for use in combination with the anticancer drug **cisplatin** to treat MPM. Pemetrexed, also known as LY231514, was the first drug for treating this type of cancer and, as an orphan drug for a rare disease, received priority review from the FDA. The Orphan Drug Act granted Eli Lilly seven years of exclusive marketing. In August of 2004 the FDA approved pemetrexed for the treatment of NSCLC.

Pemetrexed is a member of a large group of chemotherapy drugs known as antineoplastics or antimetabolites; it sometimes is referred to as an antifolate antineoplastic agent. It inhibits three folate-dependent enzymes that mesothelioma and lung cancer cells need for the synthesis of the nucleotides that make up DNA and RNA. Fast growing cancer cells have a much higher requirement for nucleotides than normal cells.

Effectiveness

The effectiveness of pemetrexed for treating MPM was established in a single clinical trial with 448 patients, comparing combined treatment with pemetrexed and cisplatin to treatment with cisplatin alone. Patients receiving the combined treatment lived three months longer than those receiving cisplatin alone—12 months versus nine months. Patients also had improved lung function. Tumors shrank in 41% of the patients treated with the combined drugs, compared with 17% of those treated with cisplatin alone.

In an earlier clinical trial pemetrexed combined with the chemotherapy drug **carboplatin**, which is similar to cisplatin, increased the average survival time of mesothelioma patients to 15 months and some patients were still alive after nearly three years. More than two-thirds of the treated patients had reduced pain and improvement in other symptoms. Tumors shrank in almost one-third of the patients.

In a clinical trial of 571 patients with recurrent NSCLC, those treated with either pemetrexed or docetaxel had a one-year survival rate of 30%; however, those receiving pemetrexed were significantly less likely to experience the following:

- fever
- infections
- hospitalizations
- hair loss
- numbness in the arms and legs

Recommended dosage

Pemetrexed is supplied as a sterile powder in single-dose vials of 500 mg pemetrexed and 500 mg mannitol. Pemetrexed is given in a single 10-minute intravenous infusion, once every three weeks. The dose depends on body size and may be adjusted or delayed depending on the patient's blood counts, kidney and liver function, and general condition.

For treating MPM, cisplatin is infused for two hours, beginning about 30 minutes after the end of pemetrexed infusion. As much fluid as possible is taken before and after treatment with cisplatin to keep the kidneys functioning properly. Intravenous fluids usually are given during cisplatin infusion.

Since pemetrexed interferes with both folic acid and vitamin B_{12}, these nutrients are always taken as supplements to prevent severe side effects. Folic acid—350–1,000 micrograms—is taken every day for at least five out of seven days prior to pemetrexed treatment. It is continued daily until 21 days after the final treatment. Folic acid is available over-the-counter as well as in many multivitamins. Vitamin B_{12} is injected during the week before the first pemetrexed treatment and once every nine weeks during treatment.

Patients also take a corticosteroid such as **dexamethasone** twice a day for three days, beginning the day before pemetrexed infusion, to lower the risk of skin reactions.

Precautions

Pemetrexed causes birth defects if administered to a woman during the conception period or during pregnancy or to a man near the time of conception. Birth control must be used by patients while they receive pemetrexed treatment. Women should not breastfeed while being treated with pemetrexed. Like many other chemotherapy drugs, pemetrexed may cause sterility.

Medical conditions that may interfere with the use of pemetrexed include the following:

- chicken pox or exposure to chicken pox
- gout
- heart disease
- congestive heart failure
- shingles
- kidney stones or kidney disease
- liver disease
- third space fluid (extra body fluid such as ascites in the stomach area or pleural effusion in the lungs and chest)
- other types of cancer

Other precautions during pemetrexed treatment include avoiding the following:

- touching the eyes or inside of the nose without first washing the hands
- cuts or bleeding
- contact sports, bruising, or injury

It is important to avoid vaccinations during and after pemetrexed treatment. It also is important to avoid contact with those who have taken oral polio vaccine within the past several months. A protective face mask that covers the nose and mouth may be used if contact is unavoidable. If possible, people with any **infection** should be avoided.

Side effects

Pemetrexed has fewer side effects than many **anticancer drugs**; however, the most common side effects are as follows:

- anemia (low red blood cell count) that may cause fatigue, paleness, or shortness of breath
- a temporary decline in white blood cells, particularly during the first 10–14 days after each treatment
- a decline in blood platelets
- nausea and vomiting
- diarrhea
- constipation
- loss of appetite
- weight loss
- heartburn
- dry mouth
- redness or sores in the mouth or throat or on the lips a few days after treatment
- rash or itching between treatments
- wrinkled or peeling skin
- burning, tingling, numbness, or pain in the extremities
- muscle aches, cramping, stiffness, or pain
- joint swelling or pain
- difficult or rapid breathing
- pain or burning in the throat
- difficult or painful swallowing
- stuffy or runny nose
- sunken eyes
- irritability
- mood swings or depression
- lightheadedness or dizziness
- confusion
- insomnia
- difficulty concentrating
- hair loss
- increased heart rate
- decreased urination
- severe weakness and fatigue for a few days after treatment
- liver problems, as indicated by fluctuating liver function blood tests

Blood counts are taken before and after each pemetrexed treatment. Rare side effects of pemetrexed include a severe allergic reaction or blood clots.

Pemetrexed suppresses production of blood cells by the bone marrow and decreases the white blood cell count. Symptoms of infection caused by decreased white blood cells include the following:

- fever above 100.5°F (38°C)
- chills
- cough
- hoarseness
- lower back or side pain
- difficult or painful urination

Pemetrexed can reduce blood platelets, thereby increasing the risk of the following:

- unusual bleeding or bruising
- nosebleeds
- bleeding gums when teeth are being cleaned

- black, tarry stools
- tiny red spots on the skin
- blood in the urine or stool

Other serious side effects of pemetrexed can include:

- swollen glands
- increased thirst
- swelling of the eyes, face, fingers, or lower legs
- pain in the chest, groin, or legs, especially in the calves
- sudden severe headaches
- sudden changes in vision
- sudden slurred speech
- fast or irregular breathing
- chest tightness or wheezing
- increased blood pressure
- loss of coordination
- fainting or loss of consciousness
- weight gain

Interactions

Known interactions of pemetrexed with other drugs include:

- oral contraceptives
- vitamins and herbal supplements
- nonsteroidal anti-inflammatory drugs (NSAIDs), including aspirin, ibuprofen such as Motrin, naproxen such as Aleve, celecoxib (Celebrex), rofecoxib (Vioxx)

Margaret Alic, Ph.D.

Penile cancer

Definition

Penile **cancer** is the growth of malignant cells on the external skin and in the tissues of the penis.

Demographics

Penile cancer is a rare form of cancer that develops in about one out of 100,000 men per year in the United States. According to the American Cancer society, about 0.2% of cancers in men in the United States are penile cancers. Penile cancer is more common in other parts of the world, particularly Africa and South

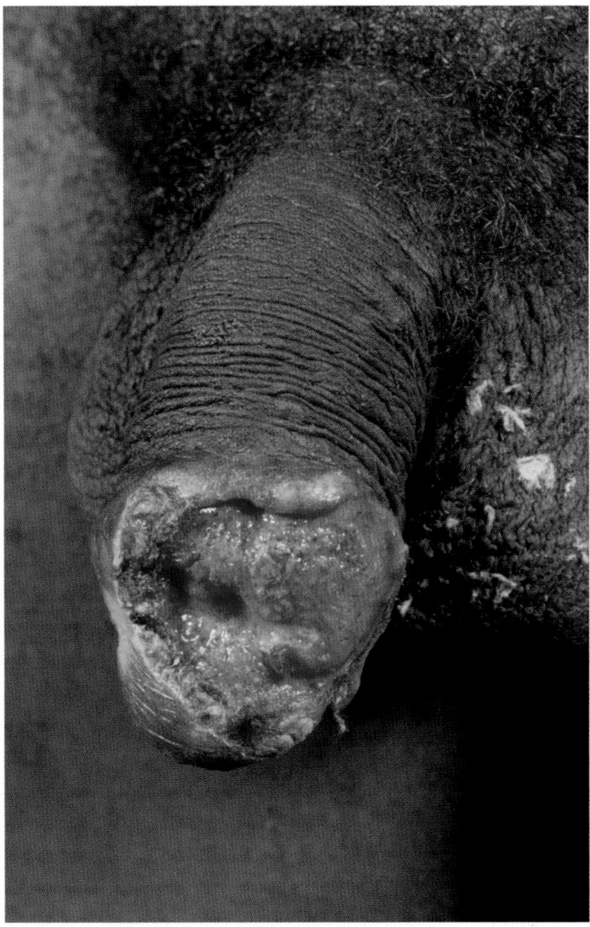

Carcinoma of penis. *(Custom Medical Stock Photo. Reproduced by permission.)*

America. The American Cancer Society reports that up to 10% of cancer in men in these areas is penile caner. In Uganda, penile cancer is the most common form of cancer for men. Penile cancer occurs more commonly in men over age 65; nearly two-thirds of men diagnosed with penile cancer are over age 65.

Description

Penile cancer is a disease in which cancerous cells appear on the penis. If left untreated, this cancer can grow and spread from the penis to the lymph nodes in the groin and eventually to other parts of the body.

Risk factors

The risk factors for penile cancer are not known with any certainty. It is believed that being circumcised as an infant reduces the risk of penile cancer. Being circumcised as an adult is not believed to reduce this risk. Many scientists also believe that human papillomavirus (HPV) **infection** increases the risk of penile cancer. Smoking increases the risk of all cancers, and men who smoke have been found to be 4 times more likely to be diagnosed with penile cancer than men who do not smoke.

Causes and symptoms

The cause of penile cancer is unknown. The most common symptoms of penile cancer are:

- a tender spot, an open sore, or a wart-like lump on the penis.
- unusual liquid discharges from the penis.
- pain or bleeding in the genital area.

Diagnosis

In order to diagnose penile cancer, the doctor examines the patient's penis for lumps or other abnormalities. A tissue sample (**biopsy**) may be ordered to distinguish cancerous cells from syphilis and penile warts. If the results confirm a diagnosis of cancer, additional tests are done to determine whether the disease has spread to other parts of the body.

Treatment

A doctor who specializes in the genitourinary tract (urologist) is usually the first point of contact for the patient and makes the diagnosis of penile cancer. Once a diagnosis of cancer is made, a specialist in cancer (oncologist) will become involved to determine the stage of the cancer and recommend appropriate treatments.

Medical side effects of treatment include constipation, **fatigue**, and sleep disorders. These effects may be managed through a combination of diet and environment as well as supplemental drug treatments. The patient should seek support resources for the psychological effects that treatment for penile cancer may cause, such as **depression**, decreased **sexuality**, anxiety, and feelings of grief.

Traditional

In Stage I penile cancer, malignant cells are found only on the surface of the head (glans) and on the foreskin of the penis. If the cancer is limited to the foreskin, treatment may involve wide local excision and circumcision. Wide local excision is a form of surgery that removes only cancer cells and a small amount of normal tissue adjacent to them. Circumcision is removal of the foreskin.

If the Stage I cancer is only on the glans, treatment may involve the use of a **fluorouracil** cream (Adrucil, Efudex), and/or microsurgery. Microsurgery removes cancerous tissue and the smallest possible amount of normal tissue. During microsurgery, the doctor uses a special instrument that provides a comprehensive view of the area where cancer cells are located and makes it possible to determine that all malignant cells have been removed.

In Stage II, the penile cancer has spread to the surface of the glans, tissues beneath the surface, and the shaft of the penis. The treatment recommended may be **amputation** of all or part of the penis (total or partial penectomy). If the disease is diagnosed early enough, surgeons are often able to preserve enough of the organ for urination and sexual activity. Treatment may also include microsurgery and external **radiation therapy**, in which a machine provides radiation to the affected area. Laser surgery is an experimental treatment for Stage II cancers. Laser surgery uses an intense precisely focused beam of light to dissolve or burn away cancer cells.

In Stage III, malignant cells have spread to lymph nodes in the groin, where they cause swelling. The recommended treatment may include amputation of the penis and removal of the lymph nodes on both sides. Radiation therapy may also be suggested. More advanced disease requires systemic treatments using drugs (**chemotherapy**). In chemotherapy, medicines are administered intravenously or taken by mouth. These drugs enter the bloodstream and kill cancer cells that have spread to any part of the body.

In Stage IV, the disease has spread throughout the penis and lymph nodes in the groin, or has traveled to other parts of the body. Treatments are similar to that for Stage III cancer.

Recurrent penile cancer is disease that recurs in the penis or develops in another part of the body after treatment has eradicated the original cancer cells.

In addition to the treatments previously described, biological therapy is another treatment that is currently being studied. Biological therapy is a type of treatment that is sometimes called biological response modifier (BRM) therapy. It uses natural or artificial substances to boost, focus, or reinforce the body's disease-fighting resources.

Alternative and complementary therapies

The term alternative therapy refers to therapy used instead of conventional treatment. By definition, these treatments have not been scientifically proven or investigated as thoroughly and by the same standards as conventional treatments. The terms complementary or integrative therapy denote practices used in

QUESTIONS TO ASK YOUR DOCTOR

- Is there a local support group you can refer me to?
- Can I continue to have sexual relations normally?
- Will I be able to maintain regular urinary tract functioning?

conjunction with rather than instead of conventional treatment. Patients should inform their doctors of any alternative or complementary therapies being used or considered as some alternative and complementary therapies adversely affect the effectiveness of conventional treatments. Some common complementary and alternative medicine therapies include:

- prayer and faith healing
- meditation
- mind/body techniques such as support groups, visualization, guided imagery and hypnosis
- energy work such as Therapeutic Touch and Reiki
- acupuncture and traditional Chinese medicine
- body work such as yoga, massage, and t'ai chi
- vitamin, mineral, and/or herbal supplements
- special diets such as vegetarian, vegan, or macrobiotic

Prognosis

Cure rates are high for cancers diagnosed in Stage I or II, but much lower for Stages III and IV, by which time cancer cells have spread to the lymph nodes. Prognosis depends on the type of cancer, the stage of the cancer, and locations to which the cancer has spread.

Prevention

There is no certain way to prevent penile cancer. However, taking actions that reduce the risk factors for penile cancer is an important step. Quitting smoking can reduce the risk of cancer, as well as many other diseases and conditions. Circumcising male infants may help reduce the risk of penile cancer. Taking steps that reduce the risk of contracting HPV, such as having protected sex, may also help to prevent penile cancer.

Resources

BOOKS

Miller, Kenneth D., ed. *Medical and Psychosocial Care of the Cancer Survivor*. Sudbury, MA: Jones and Bartlett, 2010.

Judd, Sandra, J., ed. *Men's Health Concerns Sourcebook*, 3rd ed. Detroit: Omnigraphics, 2009.

Raghavan, Derek, et al., eds. *Textbook of Uncommon Cancer*, 3rd ed. Hoboken, NJ: Wiley, 2006.

PERIODICALS

Buellen, Kathryn, et al. "Exploring Men's Experiences of Penile Cancer Surgery to Improve Rehabilitation." *Nursing Times* (March 31, 2009): 20-24.

Hegarty, Paul K., et al. "Contemporary Management of Penile Cancer." *BJU International*, (September 2008): 928-932.

ORGANIZATIONS

American Cancer Society, (800) ACS-2345, www.cancer.org.

National Cancer Institute, 6116 Executive Boulevard Room 3036A, Bathesda, MD, 20892-8322, (800) 4-CANCER (800-422-6237), www.cancer.gov.

Maureen Haggerty
Tish Davidson, A.M.

Pentamidine *see* **Antibiotics**

Pentostatin

Definition

Pentostatin is an anticancer (antineoplastic) agent belonging to the class of drugs called antimetabolites (compounds that prevent the synthesis and utilization of normal cellular metabolite). It is a natural product isolated from *Streptomyces antibioticus*. It also acts as a suppressor of the immune system. It is available under the brand name Nipent. Other common names for pentostatin include 2'-deoxycoformycin and 2'DCF.

Purpose

Pentostatin is primarily used to treat a particular type of **cancer** of the blood called **hairy cell leukemia**. It is also used in the treatment of low-grade lymphomas. **Clinical trials** are underway to determine the effectiveness of pentostatin in fighting **cutaneous T-cell lymphoma** (CTCL), **chronic lymphocytic leukemia** (CLL), non-Hodgkin's lymphomas (NHL), and prolymphocytic leukemia.

KEY TERMS

Antineoplastic—A drug that prevents the growth of a neoplasm by interfering with the maturation or proliferation of the cells of the neoplasm.

Hairy cell leukemia—A rare form of cancer in which hairy cells grow out of control in the blood, liver, and spleen.

Lymphoma—A malignant tumor of the lymphatic system.

Neoplasm—New abnormal growth of tissue.

Description

Pentostatin chemically interferes with the synthesis of genetic material (DNA and RNA) of cancer cells, which prevents these cells from being able to reproduce and continue the growth of the cancer.

Recommended dosage

Pentostatin may be taken only as an injection. It is generally given once every two weeks. A typical dosage is 4 mg per square meter of body surface area. However, the dosage prescribed can vary widely depending on the patient, the cancer being treated, and whether or not other medications are also being taken.

Precautions

Pentostatin should be taken on an empty stomach. If stomach irritation occurs, it should be taken with small amounts of food or milk. Pentostatin should always be taken with plenty of fluids.

Pentostatin can cause an allergic reaction in some people. Patients with a prior allergic reaction to pentostatin should not take pentostatin.

Pentostatin can cause serious birth defects if either the man or the woman is taking this drug at the time of conception or if the woman is taking this drug during pregnancy.

Because pentostatin is easily passed from mother to child through breast milk, breast feeding is not recommended while pentostatin is being taken.

Pentostatin suppresses the immune system and interferes with the normal functioning of certain organs and tissues. For these reasons, it is important that the prescribing physician is aware of any of the following pre-existing medical conditions:

- a current case of, or recent exposure to, chicken pox
- herpes zoster (shingles)
- a current case, or history of, gout or kidney stones
- all current infections
- kidney disease.
- liver disease

Also, because pentostatin is such a potent immunosuppressant, patients taking this drug must exercise extreme caution to avoid contracting any new infections. They should do their best to:

- avoid any person with any type of infection
- avoid bleeding injuries, including those caused by brushing or flossing the teeth
- avoid contact of the hands with the eyes or nasal passages (inside of the nose) unless the hands have just been washed and have not touched anything else since this washing
- avoid contact sports or any other activity that could cause a bruising or bleeding injury

Side effects

The most common side effects of pentostatin are cough, extreme **fatigue**, increased susceptibility to **infection**, loss of appetite (**anorexia**), skin rash or **itching**, **nausea**, temporary hair loss (**alopecia**), **vomiting**, and **weight loss**.

Less common side effects include anxiety or nervousness; changes in vision; nosebleed; sores in the mouth or on lips; sore, red eyes; trouble sleeping (insomnia); numbness or tingling in the hands and/or feet; and swelling in the feet or lower legs.

A doctor should be consulted immediately if the patient experiences shortness of breath, chest or abdominal pain, persistent cough, **fever** and chills, pain in the lower back or sides, painful or difficult urination, unusual bleeding or bruising, blood in the urine or stool, or tiny red dots on the skin.

Interactions

Pentostatin should not be taken in combination with any prescription drug, over-the-counter drug, or herbal remedy without prior consultation with a physician. It is particularly important that the prescribing physician be aware of the use of any of the following drugs or any **radiation therapy** or **chemotherapy** medicine:

- amphotericin B
- antithyroid agents
- azathioprine

- chloramphenicol
- colchicine
- flucytosine
- fludarabine
- ganciclovir
- interferon
- plicamycin
- probenecid
- sulfinpyrazone
- vidarabine
- zidovudine

Paul A. Johnson, Ed.M.

Percutaneous transhepatic cholangiography

Definition

Percutaneous transhepatic cholangiography (PTHC) is an x-ray test used to identify obstructions either in the liver or bile ducts that slow or stop the flow of bile from the liver to the digestive system.

Purpose

Because the liver and bile ducts are not normally seen on **x rays**, the doctor injects the liver with a special dye that will show up on the resulting picture. This dye distributes evenly to fill the whole liver drainage system. If the dye does not distribute evenly, this is indicative of a blockage, which may caused by a gallstone or a tumor in the liver, bile ducts, or pancreas.

Precautions

Patients should report allergic reactions to:

- anesthetics
- dyes used in medical tests
- iodine
- shellfish

PTHC should not be performed on anyone who has cholangitis (inflammation of the bile duct), massive **ascites**, a severe allergy to iodine, or a serious uncorrectable or uncontrollable bleeding disorder. Patients who have diabetes should inform their doctors.

KEY TERMS

Ascites—Abnormal accumulation of fluid in the abdomen.

Bile ducts—Tubes that carry bile, a thick yellowish-green fluid that is made by the liver, stored in the gallbladder, and helps the body digest fats.

Cholangitis—Inflammation of the bile duct.

Fluoroscope—An x-ray machine that projects images of organs.

Granulomatous disease—Characterized by growth of tiny blood vessels and connective tissue.

Jaundice—Disease that causes bile to accumulate in the blood, causing the skin and whites of the eyes to turn yellow. Obstructive jaundice is caused by blockage of bile ducts, while non-obstructive jaundice is caused by disease or infection of the liver.

Description

PTHC is performed in a hospital, doctor's office, or outpatient surgical or x-ray facility. The patient lies on a movable x-ray table and is given a local anesthetic. The patient will be told to hold his or her breath, and a doctor, nurse, or laboratory technician will inject a special dye into the liver as the patient exhales.

The patient may feel a twinge when the needle penetrates the liver, a pressure or fullness, or brief discomfort in the upper right side of the back. Hands and feet may become numb during the 30-60 minute procedure.

The x-ray table will be rotated several times during the test, and the patient helped to assume a variety of positions. A special x-ray machine called a fluoroscope will track the dye's movement through the bile ducts and show whether the fluid is moving freely or if its passage is obstructed.

PTHC costs about $1,600. The test may have to be repeated if the patient moves while x rays are being taken.

Preparation

An intravenous antibiotic may be given every four to six hours during the 24 hours before the test. The patient will be told to fast overnight. Having an empty stomach is a safety measure in case of complications, such as bleeding, that might require emergency repair surgery. Medications such as aspirin, or non-steroidal anti-inflammatory drugs that thin the blood, should be stopped for some three to seven days prior to taking the PRHC test. Patients may also be given a sedative a few minutes before the test begins.

Aftercare

A nurse will monitor the patient's vital signs and watch for:

- itching
- flushing
- nausea and vomiting
- sweating
- excessive flow of saliva
- possible serious allergic reactions to contrast dye

The patient should stay in bed for at least six hours after the test, lying on the right side to prevent bleeding from the injection site. The patient may resume normal eating habits and gradually resume normal activities. The doctor should be informed right away if pain develops in the right abdomen or shoulder or in case of **fever**, dizziness, or a change in stool color to black or red.

Risks

Septicemia (blood poisoning) and bile peritonitis (a potentially fatal **infection** or inflammation of the membrane covering the walls of the abdomen) are rare but serious complications of this procedure. Dye occasionally leaks from the liver into the abdomen, and there is a slight risk of bleeding or infection.

Normal results

Normal x rays show dye evenly distributed throughout the bile ducts. Obesity, gas, and failure to fast can affect test results.

Abnormal results

Enlargement of bile ducts may indicate:

- obstructive or non-obstructive jaundice
- cholelithiasis (gallstones)
- hepatitis (inflammation of the liver)
- cirrhosis (chronic liver disease)
- granulomatous disease
- pancreatic cancer
- bile duct or gallbladder cancers

Resources

BOOKS

Komaroff, A. L. *The Harvard Medical School Family Health Guide*. New York: Simon & Schuster, 1999.

PERIODICALS

Cieszanowski, A., et al. "Imaging techniques in Patients with Biliary Obstruction." *Medical Science Monitor* 6 (November-December 2000): 1197-202.

OTHER

"Percutaneous Transhepatic Cholangiography." http://207.25.144.143/health/Library/medtests/.

"Percutaneous Transhepatic Cholangiography (PTHC)." http://www.uhs.org/frames/health/test/test3554.htm.

"Test Universe Site: Percutaneous Transhepatic Cholangiography." http://www.testuniverse.com/mdx/MDX-3055.html.

Maureen Haggerty

Pericardial effusion

Definition

A pericardial effusion is a fluid collection that develops between the pericardium, the lining of the heart, and the heart itself. Pericardial effusions can be found in up to 20% of **cancer** patients at autopsy, but of those, only about 30% would have had symptoms from their effusions.

Description

Most of the organs of the body are covered by thin membranes. The membrane that surrounds the heart is called the pericardium. Normally, only a few milliliters of fluid sit between the pericardium and the muscle of the heart. Any larger, abnormal collection of fluid in that space is called a pericardial effusion.

A pericardial effusion can interfere with the normal contraction and expansion of the heart muscle, which decreases the heart's ability to pump blood effectively. A large or rapidly developing effusion can cause a condition called cardiac tamponade. Tamponade is a medical emergency and can be fatal if not diagnosed and treated promptly. Symptoms of tamponade include shortness of breath, rapid pulse, cough, and chest discomfort. As tamponade progresses, low blood pressure and shock develop and cardiac arrest can follow.

A smaller or more slowly developing pericardial effusion also causes chest discomfort. Other

KEY TERMS

Pericardium—The thin membrane that surrounds the heart.

Sclerosing agents—Drugs that are instilled into parts of the body to deliberately induce scarring.

Tamponade—A medical emergency in which fluid or other substances between the pericardium and heart muscle compress the heart muscle and interfere with the normal pumping of blood.

Thoracoscopy—Chest surgery done with the guidance of special video cameras that permit the surgeon to see inside the chest.

symptoms, such as shortness or breath, difficulty swallowing, hoarseness or hiccups result from pressure from the enlarged, fluid-filled pericardium pressing against nearby organs. Although chronic or smaller effusions are not emergencies, they do cause discomfort and can become more serious.

The diagnosis of pericardial effusion is made on the basis of patient history, physical examination and appropriate laboratory studies. Heart sounds can be muffled, the veins in the neck engorged and the pulse rapid. A chest x ray shows enlargement of the silhouette of the heart. An echocardiogram or cardiac ultrasound will show the fluid surrounding the heart, as will CT and MRI scans.

Causes

A pericardial effusion in a cancer patient is caused either by the disease itself or by the treatment for the disease.

Many cancers can metastasize or spread to the pericardium or the heart itself. They include:

- lung
- breast
- thyroid
- esophagus
- kidney
- pancreas
- endometrium
- larynx
- cervix
- stomach
- mouth
- liver
- ovary
- colon
- prostate
- leukemia
- melanoma
- lymphoma
- sarcoma
- myeloma

The presence of the cancerous cells on the pericardium is an irritant and causes a reactive fluid buildup, much as a blister forms under the skin due to irritation. Some cancers cause less fluid buildup, instead thickening the pericardium and making it less elastic. This can also cause symptoms of tamponade.

Another cause of pericardial effusion in a cancer patient is previous **radiation therapy** to the chest, especially in the case of lung cancer or **lymphoma**. While such effusions are less likely to produce tamponade, it is possible.

Many of the drugs that are used to treat cancer can cause pericardial disease and can thus potentially cause pericardial effusions. Some of the chemotherapeutic drugs that can affect the pericardium are **cytarabine**, **fluorouracil**, **cyclophosphamide**, **doxorubicin** and **daunorubicin**. Granulocyte-macrophage colony-stimulating factor (**sargramostim**), often given to help increase the population of white blood cells during intensive **chemotherapy**, is also a pericardial irritant.

Other causes of pericardial effusions are heart failure, liver disease, and kidney disease. Any of these can also affect cancer patients.

Treatments

Treatment of pericardial effusion depends on the presence or absence of cardiac tamponade. Tamponade is a medical emergency and symptoms such as cyanosis, a blue tinge to the lips and skin, shock, or a change in mental status require urgent drainage of the fluid. This drainage is accomplished with a procedure called **pericardiocentesis**, in which a needle is inserted into the pericardial space and the fluid withdrawn into a large syringe. Chronic effusions can be drained electively, and some need not be drained at all. If a patient's prognosis is poor and the pericardial effusion is not compromising the function of the heart, the risks of a drainage procedure may outweigh its benefits and the effusion may be left alone. Effusions caused by lymphoma often resolve after aggressive chemotherapy and need no further treatment.

Elective drainage of a pericardial effusion is done by one of several surgical procedures. The surgeon might open the chest, make a small incision under the bottom of the breastbone, or use a video-assisted technique called **thoracoscopy**. In addition to permitting drainage of the pericardial fluid, these procedures permit the surgeon to take a pericardial **biopsy**, which can confirm the diagnosis of metastatic cancer.

Sometimes a catheter is placed in the pericardium and connected to an external drainage system to collect any fluid that might reaccumulate.

Occasionally, sclerosing agents—drugs that cause scarring—are infused into the pericardium through a catheter. These agents, such as tetracycline, minocycline or **bleomycin**, irritate the pericardium, causing it to thicken and adhere to the heart muscle. This scarring prevents the further accumulation of fluid. Some malignant pericardial effusions resolve after the instillation of chemotherapeutic drugs such as **thiotepa** or platinum directly into the pericardial cavity. Others resolve after radiation therapy directed at the pericardium.

Alternative and complementary therapies

No complementary or alternative treatments are aimed specifically at treating pericardial effusions, but practitioners of acupressure and acupuncture designate a pressure point for the pericardium at two and a half finger breadths above the wrist crease on the inner aspect of the arm. Acupressure and acupuncture do offer some relief of symptoms to those suffering from shortness of breath and might offer benefit to those with pericardial effusions.

See also Pericardiocentesis.

Resources

BOOKS

Moore, Katen, and Libby Schmais. *Living Well with Cancer: A Nurse Tells You Everything You Need to Know About Managing the Side Effects of Your Treatment.* New York: Putnam Publishing Group, 2001.

PERIODICALS

Bastian, A., et. al. " Pericardiocentesis: Differential Aspects of a Common Procedure." *Intensive Care Medicine* 26, no. 5 (May 2000): 572-6.

Brigden, M. L. "Hematologic and Oncologic Emergencies. Doing the Most Good in the Least Time." *Postgraduate Medicine* 109, no. 3 (March 2001): 143-6, 151-4, 157-8.

Gibbs, C. R., R. D. Watson, S.P. Singh, and G.Y. Lip. "Management of Pericardial Effusion by Drainage: A Survey of 10 Years' Experience in a City Centre General Hospital Serving a Multiracial Population." *Postgraduate Medicine Journal* 76, no. 902 (December 2000): 809-13.

OTHER

Heart Center Online Home Page [cited June 6, 2009]. http://www.heartcenteronline.com/. This web site serves cardiologists and their patients and has sections on pericardiocentesis, pericarditis and tamponade.

Marianne Vahey, M.D.

Pericardiocentesis

Definition

Pericardiocentesis is a therapeutic and diagnostic procedure in which fluid is removed from the pericardium, the sac that surrounds the heart.

Purpose

The pericardium normally contains only a few milliliters (less than a teaspoon) of fluid to cushion the heart. Many illnesses cause larger volumes of fluid, called pericardial effusions, to develop. Spread of **cancer** to the pericardium is a frequent cause of pericardial effusions. If an effusion is too large, pressure develops within the sac that can interfere with the normal pumping action of the heart. Should that interference become severe, a life-threatening condition called cardiac tamponade can develop, which can lead to shock or death.

Pericardiocentesis is a procedure to remove that fluid, which allows the heart to pump normally again. The fluid is analyzed for the presence of cancer cells or microorganisms. If cardiac tamponade is present, pericardiocentesis must be done on an urgent basis. If tamponade is not present, an elective surgical pericardial drainage procedure can be scheduled.

Precautions

The presence of tamponade is a medical emergency and requires urgent treatment. The blood pressure can be low and breathing compromised. Fluids and intravenous medications might be needed to raise the blood pressure until the pericardiocentesis can be performed.

Description

When possible, pericardiocentesis is performed in the cardiac catheterization laboratory of the hospital, but it can be done at the bedside or in the emergency department. The patient lies on his or her back with the head elevated at about 45 degrees. The skin is

QUESTIONS TO ASK THE DOCTOR

- What is a pericardiocentesis?
- Why do I need this procedure?
- What are the risks?
- What are the risks of not having a pericardiocentesis?
- What sort of anesthesia will I have?
- What do you expect to find?
- What can I expect after the test?
- How long will I need to stay in the hospital?

KEY TERMS

Pericardium—The thin membrane that surrounds the heart.

Sclerosing agents—Drugs that are instilled into parts of the body to deliberately induce scarring.

Tamponade—A medical emergency in which fluid or other substances between the pericardium and heart muscle compress the heart muscle and interfere with the normal pumping of blood.

Thoracoscopy—Chest surgery done with the guidance of special video cameras that permit the surgeon to see inside the chest.

sterilized and local anesthetic given. A long needle attached to a large sterile syringe is inserted under the breastbone into the pericardium. If available, an echocardiogram or cardiac ultrasound is done to guide the physician to the pericardium. Once the needle is in the pericardium, the doctor withdraws the pericardial fluid into the syringe. The fluid can then be tested for cancer cells. If the volume of the fluid is large or likely to reaccumulate, a catheter or drain is placed with one end in the pericardial space and the other outside the chest, attached to a collecting bag. This can stay in place for several days, until there is no more fluid to drain. After withdrawing either the needle or the catheter, the doctor will apply direct pressure to the site.

If a pericardiocentesis is unsuccessful at draining the **pericardial effusion**, other procedures are available such as percutaneous balloon pericardiotomy, in which a balloon-tipped catheter is inserted through the skin and then used to puncture a hole in the pericardium. This is a painful procedure and should be done under anesthesia. The pericardial fluid is allowed to drain into the chest cavity, into the pleural space, the area between the pleura, the membranes that line the lungs, and the lungs themselves. The pleural space can accommodate more fluid than the pericardium without significant discomfort.

Alternatively, if emergent pericardiocentesis is unsuccessful, the patient can be taken to the operating room for a surgical procedure that will drain the fluid. These elective surgical procedures are similar to pericardiocentesis; however, for open surgical procedures, image guidance is not necessary. These are typically performed under general anesthesia. These procedures present the surgeon with the opportunity to perform a **biopsy** of the pericardium, to confirm the suspicion that the patient's cancer has metastasized there. The operation can also be performed as a thoracoscopic procedure.

Finally, if necessary, a pericardiectomy, sometimes called a pericardial stripping, can be performed. This is a surgical procedure to remove the pericardium and is reserved for the most refractory cases. Pericardiectomy tends to carry more risk than other procedures.

Preparation

For a scheduled pericardiocentesis, a patient will take nothing by mouth for several hours before the procedure. The patient will undergo preoperative blood tests, an electrocardiogram, and an echocardiogram or ultrasound of the heart.

Aftercare

Most patients are admitted to an intensive care unit for monitoring after a pericardial drainage procedure. Frequent checks of blood pressure and pulse will be done, and the neck veins will be examined for bulging. Such bulging might indicate a bleeding complication. If a drain has been placed, the fluid collected will be measured, and the site checked for signs of bleeding or **infection**. Most patients spend several days in the hospital after pericardial drainage, but a few who do not have drains placed can go home the next day.

Risks

There is about a 5% risk of complications with a pericardiocentesis. These risks include:

- cardiac arrest
- myocardial infarction or heart attack
- abnormal heart rhythms

- laceration or puncture of the heart muscle
- laceration of the coronary arteries
- laceration of the lungs
- laceration of the stomach, colon or liver
- air embolism, in which a pocket of air becomes trapped in a blood vessel, blocking blood flow

When a pericardial effusion is caused by the presence of cancer cells, there is also a risk that the fluid might reaccumulate. Injecting irritants into the pericardial sac can initiate scarring of the pericardium. This causes it to adhere to the surface of the heart and prevents fluid from collecting there again. The irritating or sclerosing agents that are instilled into the pericardial space through a catheter include tetracycline, minocycline, and **bleomycin**. The injection of these drugs into the pericardium can cause pain. Sometimes, the simple presence of a drainage catheter will introduce the desired scarring, and this method is preferred, when possible, to the use of the irritant drugs.

Normal results

The most important result is the relief of tamponade or other symptoms of heart failure from excess pericardial fluid. The blood pressure should return to normal, chest pain should be relieved, and breathing should become easier.

The fluid will be analyzed. Normal pericardial fluid is clear, has no cancer cells, no evidence of infection, and fewer than 1,000 white blood cells.

Abnormal results

On rare occasions, the pressure changes surrounding the heart that occur after pericardial drainage can cause temporary worsening of symptoms. This is called pericardial shock.

The most likely cause of a pericardial effusion in a person with cancer is spread of cancer to the pericardium. Thus, the fluid might, upon analysis, contain cancerous cells, high levels of protein, and many white blood cells. This can make the fluid thick and viscous. If the pericardial biopsy is performed, as can be done with a surgical drainage procedure, that biopsy might also reveal the presence of cancer cells.

Resources

BOOKS

Moore, Katen, and Libby Schmais. *Living Well with Cancer: A Nurse Tells You Everything You Need to Know About Managing the Side Effects of Your Treatment*. New York: Putnam Publishing Group, 2001.

PERIODICALS

Bastian A., A. Meissner, M. Lins, E. G. Seigel, F. Moller, and R. Simon. "Pericardiocentesis: Differential Aspects of a Common Procedure." *Intensive Care Medicine* May 2000: 572–76.

Brigden, M. L. "Hematologic and Oncologic Emergencies: Doing the Most Good in the Least Time." *Postgraduate Medicine* March 2001: 143–46, 151–54, 157–58.

Gibbs, C. R., R. D. Watson, S. P. Singh, and G. Y. Lip. "Management of Pericardial Effusion by Drainage: A Survey of 10 Years' Experience in a City Centre General Hospital Serving a Multiracial Population." *Postgraduate Medicine Journal* December 2000: 809–13.

OTHER

Heart Center Online Home Page. http://www.heartcenteronline.com/.

Marianne Vahey, M.D.

Peritoneovenous shunt

Definition

A peritoneovenous shunt (PVS) is a device that is inserted surgically into the body to create a passage between the peritoneum (abdominal cavity) and the jugular vein to treat refractory cases of peritoneal **ascites**. Ascites is a condition in which an excessive amount of fluid builds up within the abdominal cavity.

Purpose

The abnormal build-up of fluid in the spaces found between the tissues and organs of the abdominal cavity is a common symptom of liver disease such as cirrhosis of the liver, but approximately 10% of the diagnosed cases occur as a side effect of several types of cancers, such as ovarian, gastric, exocrine pancreatic, and colorectal cancers, and **lymphoma**. This condition is known as ascites and it causes pain and discomfort in patients. When doctors can not treat advanced ascites with medication, they recommend an operation such as the PVS procedure as a means to empty the abdomen of the accumulated fluid.

The ascites that results from **cancer** contains high levels of proteins. It occurs because of functional imbalances in the cells of the organs affected by the cancer and because the walls of the capillaries containing the normal abdominal fluid start leaking. Depending on the type of cancer, there may also be a decrease in the ability of the lymphatic system of the body to absorb fluids.

QUESTIONS TO ASK THE DOCTOR

- What are the benefits of PVS for my condition?
- Why is medication not possible?
- What complications are possible?
- What happens if the PVS device gets blocked?
- How experienced is the surgeon with PVS surgery?

Precautions

The PVS procedure is restricted to patients with livers that function normally. Additionally, the required veins must be healthy so as to allow the insertion of the shunt device. The PVS insertion is not performed in the following cases:

- patients having undergone previous extensive abdominal surgery
- patients diagnosed with bacterial peritonitis
- patients with diseased veins in the esophagus
- patients with heart disease
- patients with a diseased major organ

In cases of ascites due to cancer (malignant ascites), there is a concern that the use of a PVS could enhance the spread of the cancer. In evaluating a cancer patient as a candidate for a PVS, the risk of cancer spread must be balanced against pain/discomfort relief, quality of life issues, and the expected survival period.

Description

The most common PVS device is the LeVeen shunt, used since the 1970s to relieve ascites due to liver disease and since the 1980s for cancer-related ascites. It consists of a plastic or silicon rubber tube fitted with a pressure-activated one-way polypropylene valve that connects the peritoneal space where the fluid is collecting to a large vein located in the neck called the jugular vein. The tube enters the jugular vein and terminates in another large vein called the superior vena cava that returns blood to the heart. Thus, the fluid goes from the abdominal cavity to the venous blood circulatory system and is then eliminated by the kidneys. The function of the one-way valve is to prevent blood from flowing back into the peritoneal space.

KEY TERMS

Abdomen—The part of the body which lies between the diaphragm and the rim of the pelvis.

Circulatory system—The circulatory system consists of the heart and blood vessels. It serves as the body's transportation system.

Esophagus—The part of the digestive tract that brings food from the mouth to the stomach.

Jugular veins—Large veins returning the blood from the head to the heart into two branches (external and internal) located on each side of the neck.

Lymph—Colorless liquid that carries the white blood cells in the lymphatic vessels.

Lymphatic system—A subsystem of the circulatory system, it consists of lymphatic fluid, lymphatic vessels, and lymphatic tissues (lymph nodes, tonsils, spleen, and thymus). It returns excess fluid to the blood and defends the body against disease.

Peritoneum—Smooth membrane which lines the cavity of the abdomen and which surrounds the viscera (large interior organs) forming a nearly closed bag.

Peritonitis—Inflammation of the peritoneum.

Vena cava—Very large veins. There are two vena cava in the body. The superior vena cava returns blood from the upper limbs, head, and neck to the heart and the inferior vena cava returns blood from the lower limbs to the heart.

The PVS is inserted under the skin of the chest under local or general anesthesia, depending on the general health condition of the patient.

An alternative option to treat ascites due to cirrhosis is to use a transjugular intrahepatic portosystemic shunt (TIPS). This is also a tube that is passed through the skin of the neck and into the jugular vein but it is pushed all the way through the liver and into the portal vein, which drains into the liver. It thus creates a shunt of blood across the liver in an attempt to reduce pressure and fluid formation.

Preparation

Abdominal **computed tomography** (CT) scans are used to determine the extent of the ascites. Lab tests are usually performed to determine if the excess abdominal fluid is infected and other **imaging studies** such as ultrasound may be performed to assess the general condition of the veins selected for insertion of the PVS tube. For the operation, the patient is usually injected with a mild sedative and local anesthetic. The surgeon uses a puncture needle to create the opening required for insertion of the PVS device so as to avoid surgical incisions which take longer to heal.

Aftercare

Antibiotics are usually prescribed for approximately four days after surgery. Any **fever** or chills that the patient experiences should be reported to the doctor without delay.

Risks

Complications following PVS insertion are very common and include **infection**, leakage of fluid, fluid build-up in the lungs, problems with blood coagulation, heart failure and blockage of the PVS device.

Normal results

The PVS insertion is considered successful when the abdominal fluid build-up gradually disappears after the operation.

Abnormal results

The most common complication resulting from PVS insertion is obstruction of the valve or tube, which can be due to a blood clot or to scar tissue forming around the shunt and eventually blocking it. This complication occurs in approximately 60% of cases during the first year of follow-up.

Resources

BOOKS

Grannis, F. W, et al. "Fluid Complications." In *Cancer Management: A Multidisciplinary Approach*. Melville, NY: Publisher Research & Representation, Inc., 2000.

Monique Laberge, Ph.D.

PET scan *see* **Positron emission tomography**

Peutz-Jeghers syndrome

Definition

Peutz-Jeghers syndrome (PJS) is a rare familial **cancer** syndrome that causes intestinal polyps, skin freckling, and an increased risk for cancer.

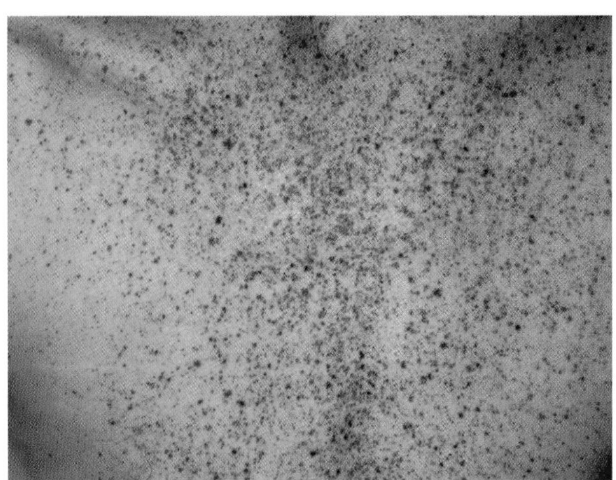

The unusual skin freckling of Peutz-Jeghers syndrome. Here, the freckles are shown on the chest. *(Custom Medical Stock Photo. Reproduced by permission.)*

Description

Peutz-Jeghers syndrome affects both males and females. The characteristic, or pathognomonic, features of PJS are unusual skin freckling and multiple polyps of the small intestine. The skin freckles, which are bluish to brown to black in color, can be found on the lips, inside the mouth, around the eyes, on the hands and feet, and on the genitals. The freckles are called benign hyperpigmented macules and do not become cancerous. The polyps in PJS are called hamartomatous polyps, and are found in the small intestine, small bowel, stomach, colon, and sometimes in the nose or bladder. Hamartomatous polyps are usually benign (not cancerous), but occasionally become malignant (cancerous). Dozens to thousands of hamartomatous polyps may develop. A person with PJS with benign hamartomatous polyps can have abdominal pain, blood in the stool, or complications such as colon obstruction or intussusception (a condition in which one portion of the intestine telescopes into another). Surgery may be required to remove the affected part of the colon. A person with PJS is at increased risk for cancer of the colon, small intestine, stomach and pancreas. Women with PJS are also at increased risk for breast and **cervical cancer**, and a specific type of benign ovarian tumor called SCTAT (sex cord tumors with annular tubules). Men with PJS are also at increased risk for benign testicular tumors.

Diagnosis

The diagnosis of Peutz-Jehgers syndrome can be made clinically in a person with the characteristic freckles and at least two hamartomatous polyps. A

KEY TERMS

Gynecomastia—Overdevelopment of the mammary glands in males; male breast development.

Intussusception— The folding of one segment of the intestine into another segment of the intestine.

Pathognomonic—Characteristic of a disease; a pattern of symptoms not found in any other condition.

Polyp—A mushroom-like growth that may be a precursor to cancer.

pathologist needs to confirm that the polyps are hamartomatous instead of another type of polyp. If a person has a family history of PJS, the diagnosis can be made in a person who has either freckles or hamartomatous polyps. When someone is the first person in his/her family to be diagnosed with PJS, it is important for all first-degree relatives to be carefully examined for clinical signs of PJS. About half of all persons with PJS will have family members with symptoms of PJS. Symptoms can vary between families and between members of the same family. Some family members may just have freckling and others may have more serious medical problems such as bowel obstruction or cancer diagnosis. The freckles in PJS usually appear in childhood and fade as a person gets older, so it may be necessary to look at childhood photos in an adult who is being examined for signs of PJS.

Risks

Hamartomatous polyps may be diagnosed from early childhood to later in adulthood. On average, a person with PJS develops polyps by his or her early 20s. The lifetime risk for cancer is greatly increased over the general population, and cancer may occur at an earlier age. Early and regular screening is important to try to detect any cancers at an early stage. The benign ovarian tumors in women with PJS may cause early and irregular menstruation. The benign testicular tumors in men may cause earlier growth spurts and gynecomastia (development of the male breasts).

Causes

PJS is a genetic disease caused by a mutation of a tumor suppressor gene called LBK1 (or STK11) on chromosome 19. The exact function of LBK1 is unknown at this time. PJS is inherited as an autosomal dominant condition, which means that a person with PJS has a 50% chance of passing it on to each of his or her children. Screening and/or **genetic testing** of family members can help sort out who has PJS or who is at risk for developing PJS. Identification of a person with PJS in a family may result in other family members with more mild symptoms being diagnosed, and then receiving appropriate screening and medical care.

Genetic Testing

Fifty percent of people clinically diagnosed with PJS will have a mutation in the LBK1/STK11 gene detected in the lab. The other half will not have a detectable mutation at that time, but may have other PJS-causing genetic mutations discovered in the future. In families where a mutation is known, family members can be tested for the same mutation. A person who tests positive for the family mutation will be diagnosed with PJS (even if he or she does not currently show signs of PJS), will need to have the recommended screening evaluations, and is able to pass on the mutation to his or her children. A person who tests negative for a known family mutation will be spared from screening, and his or her children will not be at risk for PJS. When the mutation cannot be found in a family, genetic testing is not useful, and all persons at risk for inheriting PJS will need to have screening for PJS throughout their life spans.

Screening and treatment

Regular medical examinations and special screening tests are needed in people with PJS. The age at which screening begins and the frequency of the tests is best determined by a physician familiar with PJS. Screening schedules depend on symptoms and family history. **Colonoscopy**, used to search for polyps in the colon, usually begins in adolescence. **X rays** and/or **upper gastrointestinal endoscopy** are used to screen for polyps in the stomach and small intestine. The goal of screening is to remove polyps before they cause symptoms or become cancerous. Surgery may be necessary. Females with PJS need to have annual gynecologic examinations by age 18, and breast **mammography** starting between the ages of 25 and 35. Males with PJS need to have annual testicular examinations. If a person with PJS develops cancer, it is treated as it would be in the general population.

See also Cancer genetics; Familial cancer syndromes.

Resources

PERIODICALS

Genetic Alliance. 4301 Connecticut Ave. NW, Suite 404, Washington, DC, 20008-2304. (202) 966-5557. http://www.geneticalliance.org. Support, education, and advocacy.

McGarrity, T., et al. "Peutz-Jeghers Syndrome." *The American Journal of Gastroenterology* 95 (2000): 596–604.

Network for Peutz-Jeghers Syndrome and Juvenile Polyposis Syndrome. http://www.epigenetic.org/~pjs/homepage.html. Online support group, list of physicians interested in PJS, research studies, and a mutation database.

Wang, J., et al. "Germline Mutations of the LKB1 (STK11) Gene in Peutz-Jeghers Patients." *Journal of Medical Genetics* 36 (1999): 365–8.

Westerman, A.M., and J.H.P. Wilson. "Peutz-Jeghers Syndrome: Risks of a Hereditary Condition." *Scandanavian Journal of Gastroenterology* 34, Supplement 230 (1999): 64–70.

Laura L. Stein, M.S., C.G.C

Pharyngectomy

Definition

A pharyngectomy is the total or partial surgical removal of the pharynx, the cavity at the back of the mouth that opens into the esophagus at its lower end. The pharynx is cone-shaped, has an average length of about 3 in (76 mm), and is lined with mucous membrane.

Purpose

A pharyngectomy procedure is performed to treat cancers of the pharynx that include:

- Throat cancer. Throat cancer occurs when cells in the pharynx or larynx (voice box) begin to divide abnormally and out of control. A total or partial pharyngectomy is usually performed for cancers of the hypopharynx (last part of the throat), in which all or part of the hypopharynx is removed.
- Hypopharyngeal carcinoma (HPC). A carcinoma is a form of cancerous tumor that may develop in the pharynx or adjacent locations and for which surgery may be indicated.

Description

Whether a pharyngectomy is performed in total or with only partial removal of the pharnyx depends on the localized amount of **cancer** found. The procedure may also involve removal of the larynx, in which case it is called a laryngopharyngectomy. Well-localized, early stage HPC tumors can be amenable to a partial pharyngectomy or a laryngopharyngectomy, but laryngopharyngectomy is more commonly performed for more advanced cancers. It can be total, involving removal of the entire larynx, or partial and may also involve removal of part of the esophagus (esophagectomy). Patients undergoing laryngopharyngectomy will lose some speaking ability and require special techniques or reconstructive procedures to regain the use of their voice.

Following a total or partial pharyngectomy, the surgeon may also need to reconstruct the throat so that the patient can swallow. A tracheotomy is used when the tumor is too large to remove. In this procedure, a hole is made in the neck to bypass the tumor and allow the patient to breathe.

For this type of surgery, patient positioning requires access to the lower part of the neck for the surgeon. This is conveniently achieved by placing the patient on a table fitted with a head holder, allowing the head to be bent back but well supported.

If a laryngopharyngectomy is performed, the surgeon starts with a curved horizontal neck skin incision. The **laryngectomy** incision is usually made from the breastbone to the lower most of the laryngeal cartilages, such that a 1–2 in (2.54–5.08 cm) bridge of skin is preserved. Once the incision is deepened, flaps are elevated until the larynx is exposed. The anterior jugular veins and strap muscles are left undisturbed. The sternocleidomastoid muscle is then identified. The layer of cervical fibrous tissue is cut (incised) longitudinally from the hyoid (the bony arch that supports the tongue) above to the clavicle (collarbone) below. Part of the hyoid is then divided, which allows the surgeon to enter the loose compartment bounded by the sternomastoid muscle and carotid sheath (which covers the carotid artery) and by the pharynx and larynx in the neck. The pharyngectomy incisions and laryngeal removal are performed, and a view of the pharynx is then possible. Using scissors, the surgeon performs bilateral (on both sides), direct cuts, separating the pharynx from the larynx. If a preliminary tracheotomy has not been performed, the oral endotracheal tube is withdrawn from the tracheal stump and a new, cuffed, flexible tube inserted for connection to new anesthesia tubing. The wound is thoroughly irrigated (flushed); all clots are removed; and the wound is closed. The pharyngeal wall is closed in two layers. The muscle layer closure always tightens the opening to some extent and is usually left undone at points where narrowing may be excessive. In fact, studies show that a mucosal (inner layer) closure alone is sufficient for proper healing.

Diagnosis/preparation

The initial physical examination for a pharyngectomy usually includes examination of the neck, mouth, pharynx, and larynx. A neurologic examination is sometimes also performed. **Laryngoscopy** is the examination of choice, performed with a long-handled mirror, or with a lighted tube called a laryngoscope. A local anesthetic might be used to ease discomfort. A MRI of the oral cavity and neck may also be performed.

If the physician suspects throat cancer, a **biopsy** will be performed—this involves removing tissue for examination in the laboratory under a microscope. Throat cancer can only be confirmed through a biopsy or using fine needle aspiration (FNA). The physician also may use an imaging test called a **computed tomography** (CT) scan. This is a special type of x ray that provides images of the body from different angles, allowing a cross-sectional view. A CT-scan can help to find the location of a tumor, to judge whether or not a tumor can be removed surgically, and to determine the cancer's stage of development.

Before surgery, the patient is also examined for nutritional assessment and supplementation, and careful staging of cancer, while surgical airway management is planned with the anesthesiologist such that a common agreement is reached with the surgeon concerning the timing of tracheotomy and intubation. The anesthesiologist may elect to use an orotracheal (through the mouth and trachea) tube with anesthetic, which can be removed if a subsequent tracheotomy is planned.

Aftercare

After undergoing a pharyngectomy, special attention is given to the patient's pulmonary function and fluid/nutritional balance, as well as to local wound conditions in the neck, thorax, and abdomen. Regular postoperative checks of calcium, magnesium, and phosphorus levels are necessary; supplementation with calcium, magnesium, and 1,25-dihydroxycholecalciferol is usually required. A patient may be unable to take in enough food to maintain adequate nutrition and experience difficulty eating (dysphagia). Sometimes it may be necessary to have a feeding tube placed through the skin and muscle of the abdomen directly into the stomach to provide extra nutrition. This procedure is called a gastrostomy.

Reconstructive surgery is also required to rebuild the throat after a pharyngectomy in order to help the patient with swallowing after the operation. Reconstructive surgeries represent a great challenge because of the complex properties of the tissues lining the throat and underlying muscle that are so vital to the proper functioning of this region. The primary goal is to re-establish the conduit connecting the oral cavity to the esophagus and thus retaining the continuity of the alimentary tract. Two main techniques are used:

- Myocutaneous flaps. Sometimes a muscle and area of skin may be rotated from an area close to the throat, such as the chest (pectoralis major flap), to reconstruct the throat.
- Free flaps. With the advances of microvascular surgery (sewing together small blood vessels under a microscope), surgeons have many more options to reconstruct the area of the throat affected by a pharyngectomy. Tissues from other areas of the patient's body such as a piece of intestine or a piece of arm muscle can be used to replace parts of the throat.

WHO PERFORMS THE PROCEDURE AND WHERE IS IT PERFORMED?

A pharyngectomy is major surgery performed by a surgeon trained in otolaryngology. An anesthesiologist is responsible for administering anesthesia and the operation is performed in a hospital setting. Otolaryngology is the oldest medical specialty in the United States. Otolaryngologists are physicians trained in the medical and surgical management and treatment of patients with diseases and disorders of the ear, nose, throat (ENT), and related structures of the head and neck. They are commonly referred to as ENT physicians.

With cancer involved in pharyngectomy procedures, the otolaryngologist surgeon usually works with radiation and medical oncologists in a treatment team approach.

Risks

Potential risks associated with a pharyngectomy include those associated with any head and neck surgery, such as excessive bleeding, wound **infection**, wound slough, fistula (abnormal opening between organs or to the outside of the body), and, in rare cases, blood vessel rupture. Specifically, the surgery is associated with the following risks:

- Drain failure. Drains unable to hold a vacuum represent a serious threat to the surgical wound.
- Hematoma. Although rare, blood clot formation requires prompt intervention to avoid pressure separation of the pharyngeal repair and compression of the upper windpipe.

QUESTIONS TO ASK THE DOCTOR

- How will the surgery affect my ability to swallow and to eat?
- What type of anesthesia will be used?
- How long will it take to recover from the surgery?
- When can I expect to return to work and/or resume normal activities?
- To what extent will my ability to speak be affected?
- What are the risks associated with a pharyngectomy?
- How many pharyngectomies do you perform in a year?

- Infection. A subcutaneous infection after total pharyngectomy is recognized by increasing redness and swelling of the skin flaps at the third to fifth postoperative day. Associated odor, fever, and elevated white blood cell count will occur.
- Pharyngocutaneous fistula. Patients with poor preoperative nutritional status are at significant risk for fistula development.
- Narrowing. More common at the lower, esophageal end of the pharyngeal reconstruction than in the upper end, where the recipient lumen of the pharynx is wider.
- Functional swallowing problems. Dysphagia is also a risk which depends on the extent of the pharyngectomy.

Normal results

Oral intake is usually started on the seventh postoperative day, depending on whether the patient has had preoperative **radiation therapy**, in which case it may be delayed. Mechanical voice devices are sometimes useful in the early, post-operative phase, until the pharyngeal wall heals. Results are considered normal if there is no re-occurrence of the cancer at a later stage.

Morbidity and mortality rates

Smokers are at high risk of throat cancer. According to the Harvard Medical School, throat cancer also is associated closely with other cancers: 15% of throat-cancer patients also are diagnosed with cancer of the mouth, esophagus, or lung. Another 10–20% of throat-cancer patients develop these other cancers later. Other people at risk include those who drink a lot of alcohol, especially if they also smoke. Vitamin A deficiency and certain types of human papillomavirus (HPV) infection also have been associated with an increased risk of throat cancer.

Surgical treatment for hypopharyngeal carcinomas is difficult as most patients are diagnosed with advanced disease, and five-year disease specific survival is only 30%. Cure rates have been the highest with surgical resection followed by postoperative radiotherapy. Immediate reconstruction can be accomplished with regional and free tissue transfers. These techniques have greatly reduced morbidity, and allow most patients to successfully resume an oral diet.

Resources

BOOKS

Orlando, R. C., ed. *Esophagus and Pharynx*. London: Churchill Livingstone, 1997.

Pitman, K. T., J. L. Weissman, and J. T. Johnson. *The Parapharyngeal Space: Diagnosis and Management of Commonly Encountered Entities (Continuing Education Program (American Academy of Otolaryngology–Head and Neck Surgery Foundation).)* Alexandria, VA: American Academy of Otolaryngology, 1998.

Shin, L.M., L. M. Ross, and K. Bellenir, eds. *Ear, Nose, and Throat Disorders Sourcebook: Basic Information About Disorders of the Ears, Nose, Sinus Cavities, Pharynx, and Larynx Including Ear Infections, Tinnitus, Vestibular Disorders*. Holmes, PA: Omnigraphics Inc., 1998.

PERIODICALS

Chang, D. W., C. Hussussian, J. S. Lewin, et al. "Analysis of pharyngocutaneous fistula following free jejunal transfer for total laryngopharyngectomy." *Plastic and Reconstructive Surgery* 109 (April 2002): 1522–1527.

Ibrahim, H. Z., M. S. Moir, and W. W. Fee. "Nasophar yngectomy after failure of 2 courses of radiation therapy." *Archives of Otolaryngology - Head & Neck Surgery* 128 (October 2002): 1196–1197.

Iwai, H., H. Tsuji, T. Tachikawa, et al. "Neoglottic formation from posterior pharyngeal wall conserved in surgery for hypopharyngeal cancer." *Auris Nasus Larynx* 29 (April 2002): 153–157.

ORGANIZATIONS

American Academy of Otolaryngology. One Prince Street, Alexandria, VA 22314-3357. (703) 836-4444. http://www.entnet.org/.

American Cancer Society (ACS). 1599 Clifton Rd. NE, Atlanta, GA 30329-4251. (800) 227-2345. http://www.cancer.org.

OTHER

"Throat Cancer." Harvard Medical School. [cited May 31,2009] http://www.intelihealth.com/IH/ihtIH/WSIHW000/8987/29425/211361.html?d=dmtHealthAZ.

"Treatment of Laryngeal and Hypopharyngeal Cancers." American Cancer Society. [cited May 31, 2009]. http://www.cancer.org/docroot/CRI/content/CRI_2_2_4X_Treatment_of_laryngeal_and_hypopharyngeal_cancers_23.asp?sitearea=.

Monique Laberge, Ph.D.

Phenytoin

Definition

Phenytoin is an anticonvulsant, a drug that acts to prevent seizures. In the United States, phenytoin is sold under the brand name Dilantin.

KEY TERMS

Anticonvulsant—A type of medication given to prevent seizures. Phenytoin is an anticonvulsant.

Bipolar disorder—A mood disorder in which the patient experiences both periods of mania and periods of depression.

Epilepsy—Disorder of the nervous system that causes seizures.

Lymph system—a part of the immune system that includes lymph nodes and tissue.

Mania—The phase of bipolar disorder in which the patient is easily excited, hyperactive, agitated, and unrealistically cheerful. Phenytoin appears to be a useful treatment for mania.

Purpose

Phenytoin helps prevent some types of seizure activity. It is often used to aid in controlling nerve pain associated with some cancers and **cancer** treatments. Nerve pain causes a burning, tingling sensation. Phenytoin also may be ordered to control a rapid or irregular heart rate. Phenytoin may be given to stop uncontrolled seizures. It may be used during brain surgery to prevent seizure activity. In 2003 a group of researchers in California reported that phenytoin is effective in controlling the acute mania associated with bipolar disorder. Additional uses are under study.

Description

Phenytoin works on areas of the brain to limit electrical discharges and stabilize cellular activity. Like many drugs that control seizures, it also has proven helpful in managing nerve pain.

Recommended dosage

The dose ordered depends on blood levels of the drug determined during routine monitoring. For pain, doctors usually order 200–500 mg per day, either at bedtime or in divided doses. Patients usually start on a low dose. Depending on the patient's response and drug blood levels, the dose may be increased. For seizures, patients are usually started at 100 mg, three times per day. Blood is drawn to check the level of phenytoin in seven to 10 days. The dose is adjusted accordingly. The doctor may prescribe a dose based on an older person's weight. A child's dose also is based on his or her weight.

It is very important that this drug be used exactly as directed. This medication should be taken at the same time every day. Patients should take a missed dose as soon as it is noted. But patients should not take two doses within four hours of each other. This medication should be stored in a dry place, not in the bathroom.

Precautions

Patients should not suddenly stop taking this medication. The abrupt withdrawal of phenytoin could trigger seizures. Patients should not crush or break extended-release drugs. Chewable tablets should be chewed before swallowing. Other pills should be swallowed whole. Older adults may be more prone to adverse effects than younger people. Patients should not change brands without approval of the doctor.

Phenytoin should not be taken by patients who are allergic to this drug. People with slow heart rates, certain other heart conditions, or a flaking, open skin condition also should not take it. Phenytoin may be used cautiously for patients with asthma, allergies, limited kidney or liver function, heart disease, and blood disorders. It also should be used with caution in those with alcoholism, diabetes mellitus, lupus, poor thyroid function, or porphyria, a rare metabolic disorder. Pregnant women should discuss the risks and benefits of this medication with the doctor. It has been associated with birth defects and possibly cancer in children born to women taking the drug; one study done in 2003 suggests that phenytoin interferes with the normal development of the baby's blood circulation. Expectant mothers who are taking it to prevent seizures should not abruptly stop the drug. Those using it for pain control should discuss its continued use with the doctor. Patients on this drug should not breast feed.

Side effects

Drowsiness is a common side effect of phenytoin. Patients should exercise caution when driving or operating machinery. Alcohol may increase drowsiness. Patients should not consume alcoholic beverages while taking this drug. Other, less frequent effects related to the central nervous system include an unsteady gait, slurred speech, confusion, and dizziness. Patients may experience **depression**, difficulty sleeping, nervousness, irritability, tremors, and numbness. Twitching, headache, mental-health problems including psychotic episodes, and more seizure activity may occur. This medication may also cause **nausea and vomiting**, stomach upset, **diarrhea**, constipation, and swollen gum tissue. Side effects also include a rash, hair loss (**alopecia**) or excessive hair growth, vision changes, uncontrolled eye movements, and inflammation of the surface of the eye. Patients may develop chest pain, swelling, **fever**, increase in weight, enlarged lips, or joint or muscle pain. Patients should practice good dental hygiene to decrease the risk of gum disease. With the doctor's approval, it may be taken with food to decrease stomach upset.

Phenytoin may produce changes in the normal makeup of the blood, including high blood sugar levels and **anemia**. It may trigger disorders of the lymphatic system and cause liver damage. If the liver is not able to properly break down phenytoin, it can produce toxic effects, even at small doses. Doctors typically assess kidney and liver function prior to ordering it. The tests are repeated at regular intervals. Patients should notify the doctor promptly of any side effects. If a skin rash develops, the doctor will instruct the patient how to taper off and stop the drug.

Interactions

Many drugs interact with phenytoin and may increase or decrease its blood levels. Phenytoin may alter the effectiveness of other drugs. The list of interactions is long and varied. Drugs that interfere with phenytoin include anticoagulants (blood thinners), sulfa and other **antibiotics**, antifungal agents, drugs used to treat ulcers, methadone, antidepressants, and disulfiram, which is used to treat alcoholism. It also interacts with **corticosteroids**, estrogen hormones, birth control pills and injections, drugs to treat hypoglycemia, asthma drugs, such other anticonvulsants as **carbamazepine**, lidocaine, heart medications, Parkinson's disease drugs, anti-inflammatory drugs, narcotic pain relievers, and **anticancer drugs**. Additionally, taking phenytoin with certain antidepressants may cause seizures in some patients.

Phenytoin has also been reported to interact with certain herbs, including evening primrose (*Oenothera biennis*), gingko (*Gingko biloba*), wormwood (*Artemisia pontica*), and an Ayurvedic preparation known as Shankapulshpi. Patients should always tell their doctors about any herbal preparations they may be taking as well as other prescription medications.

Alcohol ingestion can interfere with maintaining proper blood levels of phenytoin. Patients should not drink alcoholic beverages while taking this medication, as phenytoin can accumulate to toxic levels in the body of noncompliant patients. Antacids and calcium can lower the effectiveness of phenytoin. These drugs should be taken two to three hours apart from phenytoin. Tube feeding may decrease the amount of phenytoin absorbed. Patients should not give tube feedings for two hours before and after taking this drug. Patients should talk to the doctor before taking **folic acid**. It may interfere with this drug.

Resources

PERIODICALS

Akula, R., S. Hasan, R. Pipalla, and C. Ferguson. "Noncompliance Leading to Drug Accumulation Resulting in Phenytoin Toxicity." *Journal of the National Medical Association* 95 (December 2003): 1201–1203.

Gatzonis, S. D., E. Angelopoulos, P. Sarigiannis, et al. "Acute Psychosis Due to Treatment with Phenytoin in a Nonepileptic Patient." *Epilepsy and Behavior* 4 (December 2003): 771–772.

Lyon, H. M., L. B. Holmes, and T. Huang. "Multiple Congenital Anomalies Associated with In Utero Exposure of Phenytoin: Possible Hypoxic Ischemic Mechanism?" *Birth Defects Research, Part A: Clinical and Molecular Teratology* 67 (December 2003): 993–996.

Misra, U. K., J. Kalita, and C. Rathore. "Phenytoin and Carbamazepine Cross-Reactivity: Report of a Case and Review of Literature." *Postgraduate Medical Journal* 79 (December 2003): 703–704.

Wang, P. W., T. A. Ketter, O. V. Becker, and C. Nowakowska. "New Anticonvulsant Medication Uses in Bipolar Disorder." *CNS Spectrums* 8 (December 2003): 930–2, 941–7.

ORGANIZATIONS

United States Food and Drug Administration (FDA). 5600 Fishers Lane, Rockville, MD 20857-0001. (888) INFO-FDA (463-6332). http://www.fda.gov.

Debra Wood, R.N.
Rebecca J. Frey, Ph.D.

Pheochromocytoma

Definition

Pheochromocytoma is a tumor of special cells (called chromaffin cells), most often found in the middle of the adrenal gland.

Description

Because pheochromocytomas arise from chromaffin cells, they are occasionally called chromaffin tumors. Most (90%) are benign tumors so they do not spread to other parts of the body. However, these tumors can cause many problems and if they are not treated and can result in death.

Pheochromocytomas can be found anywhere chromaffin cells are found. They may be found in the heart and in the area around the bladder, but most (90%) are found in the adrenal glands. Every individual has two adrenal glands that are located above the kidneys in the back of the abdomen. Each adrenal gland is made up of two parts: the outer part (called the adrenal cortex) and the inner part (called the adrenal medulla). Pheochromocytomas are found in the adrenal medulla. The adrenal medulla normally secretes two substances, or hormones, called norepinephrine and epinephrine. These two substances, when considered together, are known as adrenaline. Adrenaline is released from the adrenal gland, enters the bloodstream and helps to regulate many things in the body including blood pressure and heart rate. Pheochromocytomas cause the adrenal medulla to secrete too much adrenaline, which in turn causes high blood pressure. The high blood pressure usually causes the other symptoms of the disease.

Demographics

Pheochromocytomas are rare tumors. They have been reported in babies as young as five days old as well as adults as old as 92 years old. Although they can be found at any time during life, they usually occur in adults between 30-40 years of age. Pheochromocytomas are somewhat more common in women than in men.

Causes and symptoms

The cause of most pheochromocytomas is not known. A small minority (about 10–20%) of pheochromocytomas arise because a person has an inherited susceptibility to them. Inherited pheochromocytomas are associated with four separate syndromes: Multiple Endocrine Neoplasia, type 2A (MEN2A), Multiple Endocrine Neoplasia, type 2B (MEN2B), **von Hippel-Lindau disease** (VHL), and Neurofibromatosis type 1 (NF1).

Individuals with pheochromocytomas as part of any of these four syndromes usually have other medical conditions, as well. People with MEN2A often have **cancer** (usually **thyroid cancer**) and other hormonal problems. Individuals with MEN2B can also have cancer and hormonal problems, but also have other abnormal physical features. Both MEN2A and MEN2B are due to genetic alterations or mutations in a gene called RET, found at chromosome 10q11.2. Individuals with VHL often have other benign tumors of the central nervous system and pancreas, and can sometimes have renal cell cancer. This syndrome is caused by a mutation in the VHL gene, found at chromosome 3p25-26. Individuals with NF1 often have neurofibromas (benign tumors of the peripheral nervous system). NF1 is caused by mutations in the NF1 gene, found at chromosome 17q11.

All of these disorders are inherited in an autosomal dominant inheritance pattern. With autosomal dominant inheritance, men and women are equally likely to inherit the syndrome. In addition, children of individuals with the disease are at 50% risk of inheriting it. **Genetic testing** is available for these four syndromes (MEN2A, MEN2B, VHL and NF1) but, due to the complexity, genetic counseling should be considered before testing.

Most people (90%) with pheochromocytoma have hypertension, or high blood pressure. The other symptoms of the disease are extremely variable. These symptoms usually occur in episodes (or attacks) called paroxysms and include:

- headaches
- excess sweating
- racing heart
- rapid breathing
- anxiety/nervousness

KEY TERMS

Adrenal medulla—The central core of the adrenal gland.

Laparoscope—An instrument used to examine body cavities during certain types of surgery; for example, surgeries to remove fibroid tumors, or gall bladders, are often removed through the navel rather than cutting into the body.

Paroxysm—A sudden attack of symptoms.

- nervous shaking
- pain in the lower chest or upper abdomen
- nausea
- heat intolerance

The episodes can occur as often as 25 times a day or, as infrequently as once every few months. They can last a few minutes, several hours or days. Usually, the attacks occur several times a week and last for about 15 minutes. After the episode is over, the person feels exhausted and fatigued.

Between the attacks, people with pheochromocytoma can experience the following:

- increased sweating
- cold hands and feet
- weight loss
- constipation

Diagnosis

If a pheochromocytoma is suspected, urine and/or a blood tests are usually recommended. A test called "24-hour urinary catacholamines and metanephrines" will be done. This test is designed to look for adrenaline and the break-down products of adrenaline. Since the body gets rid of these hormones in the urine, those testing will need to collect their urine for 24 hours. The laboratory will determine whether or not the levels of hormones are too high. This test is very good at making the diagnosis of pheochromocytoma. Another test called "serum catacholamines" measures the level of adrenaline compounds in the blood. It is not as sensitive as the 24-hour urine test, but can still provide some key information if it shows that the level of adrenaline compounds is too high.

One of the difficulties with these tests is that a person needs to have an attack of symptoms either during the 24-hour urine collection time period or shortly before the blood is drawn for a serum test to ensure the test's accuracy. If a person did not have an episode during that time, the test can be a "false negative." If a doctor suspects the patient has gotten a "false negative" test, additional tests called "pharmacologic tests" can be ordered. During these tests, a specific drug is given to the patient (usually through an IV) and the levels of hormones are monitored from the patient's blood. These types of tests are only done rarely.

Once a person has been diagnosed with a pheochromocytoma, he or she will undergo tests to identify exactly where in the body the tumor is located. The imaging techniques used are usually **computed tomography** scan (CT scan) and **magnetic resonance imaging** (MRI). A CT scan creates pictures of the interior of the body from computer-analyzed differences in **x rays** passing through the body. CT scans are performed at a hospital or clinic and take only a few minutes. An MRI is a computerized scanning method that creates pictures of the interior of the body using radio waves and a magnet. An MRI is usually performed at a hospital and takes about 30 minutes.

Treatment team

A pheochromocytoma will usually be treated by an internist (general medical doctor) an anesthesiologist (doctor who administers anesthesia for surgery) and a specialized surgeon (doctor who removes the tumor from the body). If the tumor is found to be malignant, a radiation oncologist (doctor who specializes in radiation treatment for cancer) and medical oncologist (doctor who specializes in **chemotherapy** treatment for cancer) may be consulted.

Clinical staging, treatments and prognosis

Once a pheochromocytoma is found, more tests will be done to see if the tumor is benign (not cancer) or malignant (cancer). If the tumor is malignant, tests will be done to see how far the cancer has spread. There is no accepted staging system for pheochromocytoma; but an observation of the tumor could provide one of these four indications:

- Localized benign pheochromocytoma means that the tumor is found only in one area, is not cancer, and cannot spread to other tissues of the body.
- Regional pheochromocytoma means that the tumor is malignant and has spread to the lymph nodes around the original cancer. Lymph nodes are small structures that are found all over the body that make and store infection-fighting cells.
- Metastatic pheochromocytoma means that the tumor is malignant and has spread to other, more distant parts of the body.
- Recurrent pheochromocytoma means that a malignant tumor that was removed has come back.

Treatment in all cases begins with surgical removal of the tumor. Before surgery, medications such as alpha-adrenergic blockers are given to block the effect of the hormones and normalize blood pressure. These medications are usually started seven to 10 days prior to surgery. The surgery of choice is laparoscopic laparotomy, which is a minimally invasive outpatient procedure performed under general or local anesthesia. A small incision is made in the abdomen, the laparoscope is inserted and the tumor is removed. The patient can usually return to normal activities within two weeks. If a laparoscopic laparotomy cannot be done, a traditional laparotomy will be performed. This is a more invasive surgery done under spinal or general anesthesia and requires five to seven days in the hospital. Usually patients are able to return to normal activities after four weeks. After surgery, blood and urine tests will be done to make sure hormone levels return to normal. If the hormone levels are still above normal, it may mean that some tumor tissue was not removed. If not all tumor can be removed (as in malignant pheochromocytoma, for example) drugs will be given to control high blood pressure.

If a pheochromocytoma is malignant, **radiation therapy** and/or chemotherapy may be used. Radiation therapy uses high-energy x rays to kill cancer cells and shrink tumors. Because there is no evidence that radiation therapy is effective in the treatment of malignant pheochromocytoma, it is not often used for treatment. However, it is useful in the treatment of painful bone metastases if the tumor has spread to the bones. Chemotherapy uses drugs to kill cancer cells. Like radiation therapy, it has not been shown to be effective in the treatment of malignant pheochromocytoma. Chemotherapy, therefore, is only used in rare instances.

Untreated pheochromocytoma can be fatal due to complications of the high blood pressure. In the vast majority of cases, when the tumor is surgically removed, pheochromocytoma is cured. In the minority of cases (10%) where pheochromocytoma is malignant, prognosis depends on how far the cancer has spread, and the patient's age and general health. The overall median five-year survival from the initial time of surgery and diagnosis is approximately 43%.

Coping with cancer treatment

If laparascopic laparotomy is done and no further treatment is necessary, patients usually return to normal activity within two weeks. If more extensive surgery is performed, normal activity is delayed for a few weeks and can be emotionally difficult. In rare cases where radiation and/or chemotherapy are needed, coping can be very difficult. Consultation with physicians, nurses, social workers, and psychologists may be beneficial.

Prevention

Unfortunately, little is known about environmental and other causes of pheochromocytoma. Some of the tumors are due to inherited predisposition. Because of these factors, pheochromocytoma cannot be prevented.

Special concerns

Pheochromocytoma in children

Pheochromocytoma is rare in children, but occurs most commonly between the ages of eight and 14 years. Diagnosis of pheochromocytoma can be more difficult at this age, because other **childhood cancers** (e.g. **neuroblastoma**) can also elevate adrenaline compounds in the body. Pheochromocytomas in children are more likely to be bilateral (on both the left and right sides of the body) and outside the adrenal glands. For this reason, transabdominal surgery is usually performed to remove the tumor.

Pheochromocytoma in pregnancy

Although rare, pheochromocytoma in pregnancy can be very dangerous. Because x rays are to be avoided in pregnancy, MRI and/or ultrasound is used to locate the tumor. Alpha-adrenergic blocking agents to reduce blood pressure are given to the woman as soon as the diagnosis is made. If the woman is in the first two trimesters of pregnancy, most often the tumor is removed. In the third trimester, the woman usually remains on alpha-adrenergic blocking agents until a cesarean section can be safely performed.

See also Multiple endocrine neoplasia syndromes; von Recklinghausen's neurofibromatosis.

Resources

BOOKS

Goldfien, Alan. "Adrenal Medulla." In *Basic and Clinical Endocrinology*, edited by Francis Greenspan and David Gardner. New York: Lange Medical Books/McGraw-Hill, 2001, pp. 399–421.

Keiser, Harry R. "Pheochromocytoma and Related Tumors.". In *Endocrinology*, edited by Leslie J DeGroot and J. Larry Jameson, 4th ed. New York: W.B. Saunders Company, 2001, pp1862–1883.

PERIODICALS

Barzon, Luisa, and Marco Boscaro. "Diagnosis and Management of Adrenal Incidentaloma." In *The Journal of Urology* 163 (February 2000): 398–407.

Young, William F. "Management Approaches to Adrenal Incidentaloma". *Endocrinology and Metabolism Clinics of North America* 29 (March 2000): 159–185.

OTHER

"Pheochromocytoma" *National Cancer Institute CancerWeb.* [cited June 29, 2009]. http://www.graylab.ac.uk/cancernet/202494.html.

Lori De Milto
Kristen Mahoney Shannon, M.S., C.G.C.

Pheresis

Definition

Pheresis is a blood purification process that consists of:

- drawing blood,
- separating red cells, plasma, platelets, and cryoprecipitated antihemophilic factor,
- isolating the blood component needed to diagnose a suspected abnormality or treat a known disease,
- and returning the remaining blood to the donor.

Purpose

Because most of the blood is returned to the donor, pheresis enables an individual to donate more of a specific component. The two main types of pheresis are removal of platelets (plateletpheresis) and removal of plasma (plasmapheresis).

Plateletpheresis

Cancer and cancer treatments can deplete the body's supply of platelets, the colorless particles that stick to the lining of blood vessels and make it possible for blood to clot. Patients who have leukemia or aplastic **anemia**, are receiving **chemotherapy**, or undergoing **bone marrow transplantation** need platelets donated by healthy volunteers to prevent potentially fatal bleeding problems.

Plasmapheresis

Also known as therapeutic plasma exchange, plasmapheresis removes cells from the straw-colored liquid portion of the blood, which contains clotting factors, infection-fighting antibodies, and other proteins. Plasma regulates blood pressure and maintains the body's mineral balance.

Frozen immediately after collection and thawed when needed for transfusion, fresh frozen plasma is sometimes given to control **disseminated intravascular coagulation** (DIC). A particular problem for cancer patients, this rare condition causes large numbers of blood clots to form, then dissolve.

Leukapheresis

Also known as apheresis, leukapheresis may be used to treat certain leukemia and to collect cells for autologous stem cell transplant. Performed before chemotherapy is administered, leukapheresis increases the treatment's impact by reducing the number of cancer cells in the bloodstream and permitting the medication to circulate more freely.

QUESTIONS TO ASK THE DOCTOR

- If I make a pheresis donation, can I still donate whole blood?
- What should I do if I change my mind about making a pheresis donation?
- What should I do if I make a pheresis donation and later realize my blood might not be safe?
- How can I find out if I could be a pheresis donor?
- Can I make a pheresis donation for myself, a friend, or a member of my family?

Precautions

The American Red Cross will not accept blood or blood products from anyone who is:

- less than 17 years old
- not in good health
- taking antibiotics or insulin
- unable to meet other requirements established to ensure the safety of donated blood

In general, cancer survivors who were treated surgically or with radiation and have been cancer-free for at least five years may donate blood. Because of the remote danger of contracting cancer as the result of a transfusion, blood donations are not accepted from cancer survivors who have been treated with chemotherapy or hormonal therapy or diagnosed with leukemia or **lymphoma**.

The Food and Drug Administration (FDA) requires every blood donor to provide a detailed health history and have a physical examination. All donated blood is tested for babesiosis, bacterial infections, Chagas disease, human immunodeficiency virus (HIV), Lyme disease, malaria, syphilis, and viral hepatitis.

Description

Throughout the procedure, which lasts between 90 minutes and three hours, the pheresis donor relaxes in a specially contoured chair and watches movies or listens to music. A flexible tube inserted into the donor's arm slowly draws blood into a sophisticated machine (centrifuge) which separates the various

KEY TERMS

Babesiosis—Infection transmitted by the bite of a tick and characterized by fever, headache, nausea, and muscle pain.

Blood typing—Technique for determining compatibility between donated blood products and transfusion recipients.

Chagas disease—Acute or chronic infection caused by the bite of a tick and characterized by fever, swollen glands, rapid heartbeat, and other symptoms.

blood components, collects whichever component is being donated, and returns the remaining blood through a vein in the donor's other arm. Each pheresis donation is typed and designated for a specific patient.

Inserting the needle can cause mild, momentary discomfort. Some pheresis donors feel a slight tingling around the lips and nose, but this sensation disappears as soon as the procedure is completed.

Plasmapheresis and plateletpheresis can be performed in a hospital or blood collection center. Leukapheresis should be performed in a hospital where bone marrow transplantation is frequently performed.

Preparation

Before undergoing pheresis, a donor should get a good night's sleep, eat a well-balanced meal, and drink plenty of caffeine-free liquids. A donor should not take aspirin within 72 hours or ibuprofen within 24 hours before undergoing plateletpheresis, because these medications would make the platelets less beneficial to the patient receiving the transfusion. The donor's physician will determine whether any other medications should be discontinued in preparation for the procedure.

Aftercare

A pheresis donor may feel tired for a few hours and should not plan on driving home after the procedure. Although the donor may resume normal activities right away, heavy lifting or strenuous exercise should be avoided until the following day.

Resources

OTHER

"Adult Chronic Leukemia." American Cancer Society. [cited June 28, 2009]. http://www3.cancer.org.

"All About Blood." American Red Cross. [cited June 28, 2009]. http://www.redcross.org/al/alabama/all.htm.

American Cancer Society. *Hodgkin's disease* [cited June 28, 2009]. http://www3.cancer.org.

"Blood Product Donation and Transfusion." American Cancer Society. [cited June 28, 2009]. http://www3.cancer.org.

"Pheresis—A Different Donation." American Red Cross. [cited June 28, 2009]. http://www.redcross.org/pa/nepablood/rc/pheresis/pheresis.html.

Maureen Haggerty

Photodynamic therapy

Definition

Photodynamic therapy (PDT) is a form of nonsurgical **cancer** treatment available since the early 1990s that combines a photosensitizing medication with exposure to a laser or other specific light wavelength to kill cancer cells. It can be used before or after surgery and other forms of cancer treatment. In some cases, PDT can even be administered during surgery to kill any cancer cells that were not removed by excision.

Purpose

Photodynamic therapy is still evolving, both in terms of the types of cancer it is approved to treat and the specific drugs that are used. PDT with a drug called **porfimer sodium** (Photofrin) was first approved as a treatment for **esophageal cancer** in 1995. The Food and Drug Administration (FDA) then extended its approval of this drug to cover **non-small cell lung cancer** in 1998. As of the early 2000s, the FDA has also approved porfimer sodium for the treatment of tumors located in the bronchi of the lungs and for palliative treatment of advanced cancers of the esophagus. Some cancer centers in the United States administer PDT with porfimer sodium for the treatment of certain types of **skin cancer** (squamous cell **carcinoma**, **basal cell carcinoma**, and Bowen's disease), recurrences of **breast cancer** following **mastectomy**, colorectal cancer, and cancers of the vulva and cervix, but these applications of PDT are still considered experimental.

In December 1999, the FDA approved a compound called aminolevulinic acid (ALA or Levulan Kerastick) for the treatment of actinic keratosis, a precancerous skin disorder caused by sun exposure. Experimental uses of ALA, as of the early 2000s,

QUESTIONS TO ASK YOUR DOCTOR

- Is photodynamic therapy a possible treatment option for my cancer?
- Are you experienced in treating patients with PDT?
- Should I consider enrolling in a clinical trial of a new PDT drug?

include treatment of **mycosis fungoides** and cancerous tumors on the surface of the skin.

Porfimer sodium and ALA are the only photosensitizing agents approved by the FDA for use in the United States as of 2005; however, several newer drugs for PDT are being tested in cancer centers in the United States and Europe. The most important of these will be described below.

In addition to cancer therapy, PDT is used to treat such conditions as wet macular degeneration, an eye disorder that can lead to blindness, as well as such benign skin conditions as psoriasis, acne, and skin disorders caused by the **human papilloma virus**. In addition, PDT is under investigation as a possible treatment for certain forms of coronary artery disease.

Precautions

Precautions for porfimer sodium (Photofrin):

- Porfimer sodium cannot be used in patients who are allergic to hematoporphyrin, a blood pigment used to make the drug.
- It cannot be used in pregnant or nursing women because its safety during pregnancy or lactation has not been established.
- It cannot be used to treat children.
- Lung tumors treated with Photofrin must be located in an airway where the doctor can reach them with a brochoscope.
- Photofrin cannot be used to treat tumors in the esophagus or bronchi that are beginning to break into the patient's windpipe or a major blood vessel. The drug should also be used cautiously in treating bronchial tumors that could block the airway if they develop inflammation following PDT.
- Patients who are receiving radiotherapy should not have PDT with porfimer sodium until four weeks after their last radiation treatment. They should also not be treated with radiotherapy until two to four weeks after a PDT treatment.

KEY TERMS

Actinic keratosis (plural, keratoses)—A type of precancerous skin growth with a scaly or bumpy surface caused by overexposure to the sun.

Barrett's esophagus—A precancerous condition of the esophagus that may develop as a complication of gastroesophageal reflux disease (GERD).

Bronchi (singular, bronchus)—The larger air passages inside the lungs.

Fiberoptics—Bundles of specially treated glass or plastic fibers that intensify light from a light source by internal reflection. Fiberoptics can be attached to lasers for use in PDT.

Free radicals—Molecules that contain at least one unpaired electron. They are highly reactive and can destroy cells by disrupting their normal biological processes. Free radicals are released during PDT and help to kill tumor cells.

Hematoporphyrin—A dark reddish-purple pigment found in blood. A purified form of hematoporphyrin is used to make porfimer sodium.

Nanometer—A measurement of length equal to 10^{-9} meters, or one billionth of a meter. It is used as a unit of measurement for light waves.

Orphan drug—A drug that treats a rare disease—"rare disease" being defined by the Food and Drug Association as one affecting fewer than 200,000 Americans. The category of orphan drug includes experimental as well as approved medications. Some photosensitizing drugs used in Europe are considered orphan drugs in the United States.

Palliative—Referring to treatment used to relieve the symptoms of a disease or disorder rather than to cure it.

Singlet oxygen—A highly reactive form of the oxygen molecule (O_2) formed during PDT that helps to destroy cancer cells by attacking their cell membranes.

Precautions for aminolevulinic acid (ALA):

- Patients being treated with ALA must protect their skin from exposure to sunlight or bright indoor light in the short time period between application of the drug to the skin and the PDT treatment.
- ALA should be used cautiously in pregnant women or nursing mothers.
- If a second treatment is necessary, it should not be done before eight weeks after the first treatment.

Description

How PDT works

Photodynamic therapy is based on a series of chemical reactions involving a specific wavelength of visible light, a photosensitizing drug, and oxygen. There is no standard wavelength of light, light source, exposure period, or method of administering the medication that covers all forms of PDT. Most photosensitizing drugs are given intravenously, but some are applied to the skin or taken by mouth. Photosensitizers given by injection are activated by light in the red portion of the visible light spectrum, around 630–700 nanometers (nm; a nanometer is a measure of length, one billionth of a meter), while those applied to the skin are usually activated by blue light.

In general, cancerous tumors inside the body need more concentrated doses of light than abnormal growths on the body surface. Lasers are usually used to deliver highly concentrated light at one specific wavelength, while light sources that provide a larger area of illumination, such as light-emitting diodes (LEDs), are more efficient for treating skin tumors.

In contrast to their uses in surgery, lasers are not used in PDT to remove tissue or seal blood vessels with heat; rather they are used to start a chemical reaction. As a result, they do not become hot enough to burn tissue. The burning or stinging sensation that some patients experience during PDT is caused by the release of oxygen stimulating nearby nerve endings rather than heat from the laser itself.

Lasers can be attached to fiberoptics for treating tumors inside the body. Fiberoptics are thin strands of plastic or glass with special optical properties that can be threaded through a bronchoscope or endoscope, which are special tubes that allow the doctor to see into the patient's lungs or esophagus. Light from the laser is then transmitted along the special fibers to the tumor, thus allowing the doctor to activate the photosensitizing medication in a very small area of tissue without damaging normal tissue nearby.

PDT is a two-step form of therapy. First, the photosensitizing medication is injected into a vein or applied to the skin several days or hours before the scheduled treatment. The drug is absorbed by all body tissues but remains in cancer cells longer than in normal cells because the cancer cells are multiplying faster. After the medication has had time to collect in the malignant cells, the doctor directs a light source of the proper wavelength on the targeted area. When the light source strikes tissue containing the photosensitizing medication in the presence of oxygen, the medication is activated and produces free radicals and a highly reactive form of oxygen called singlet oxygen. The free radicals and singlet oxygen interact with the cell membranes of the cancer cells to destroy the energy-producing structures inside the cancer cells. In addition to killing the cancer cells directly, PDT works by closing blood vessels inside the tumor, thereby shutting off its supply of nutrients, and by stimulating the immune system to produce interleukins (nonantibody proteins) and other substances that attack the cancer.

Photosensitizing drugs

PORFIMER SODIUM. Porfimer sodium, or Photofrin, was the first medication used for PDT. It is a purified derivative of hematoporphyrin, a dark reddish-purple pigment found in blood. Photofrin is activated by red light at a wavelength of 630 nm; one disadvantage of this short wavelength is that it cannot penetrate tissue deeper than about a third of an inch, thus making Photofrin unsuitable for treating tumors that lie deep beneath the surface. The light used to activate Photofrin is usually generated by a laser.

Porfimer sodium has several other disadvantages for PDT: It is a complex chemical mixture that tends to break down over time; it has limited ability to penetrate tissue; and it takes four to six weeks to be cleared from the skin, thus leaving patients susceptible to a photosensitivity reaction for a long period of time after their PDT treatment. A photosensitivity reaction occurs when sensitized skin is exposed to sunlight or other bright light and is characterized by redness, swelling, and blistering of the exposed skin. As a result of Photofrin's disadvantages, researchers have been studying other photosensitizers with the following characteristics:

- They are single compounds rather than mixtures of chemicals.
- They are more effective in absorbing the red region of the visible light spectrum.
- They are more selective in targeting malignant tissue.
- They are more efficient in generating singlet oxygen.

AMINOLEVULINIC ACID. Aminolevulinic acid, or ALA, is a short-lived photosensitizer that is applied to the skin as a 5–20% oil-in-water mixture. It is activated by either a special blue light illuminator or by light at 630–635 nm.

SECOND-GENERATION PHOTOSENSITIZERS. Newer photosensitizing agents that are being used in **clinical trials** include:

- HPPH (2-[1-hexyloethyl]-2-devinyl-pyropheophorbide-a; brand name Photochlor). HPPH is a photosensitizer that is activated by light more efficiently than Photofrin. In addition, patients treated with HPPH do not have the long-term photosensitivity reactions associated with Photofrin. HPPH has been used experimentally since 2003 at the Roswell Park Cancer Institute in Buffalo, New York, to treat esophageal cancer, Barrett's esophagus, basal cell carcinoma, and recurrent breast cancer following mastectomy. It is also undergoing clinical trials in schools of veterinary medicine as a possible treatment for cancers in cats and dogs. Like Photofrin, HPPH is given intravenously.
- Verteporfin (also known as BPD-MA [benzoporphyrin derivative monoacid ring A]; brand name Visudyne). Verteporfin is a second-generation photosensitizer used primarily to treat eye disorders, including age-related macular degeneration, other abnormal formations of blood vessels within the eye, and histoplasmosis (an eye infection caused by a fungus). Verteporfin is also being investigated as a possible treatment for skin cancer and psoriasis.
- Temoporfin (Meta-tetra hydroxyphenyl chlorin; brand name Foscan). Temoporfin is a chlorin-type photosensitizer developed in the United Kingdom. It was approved by the European Union in 2001 for the treatment of head and neck cancers and certain types of lung cancer, but is categorized as an orphan drug in the United States. The FDA lists temoporfin as an orphan drug for the palliative treatment of inoperable head and neck cancers.
- Motexafin lutetium (brand name Lu-Tex). Lu-Tex is an injectable dye that has been used in clinical trials to treat malignant melanoma. It has a high degree of selectivity for cancer cells. It also shows promise as a treatment for recurrent breast cancer and atherosclerosis.

Clinical trials

Although the National Cancer Institute (NCI) is not conducting trials of new PDT drugs, there are several cancer centers in the United States and Canada that are investigating Photochlor and other second-generation photosensitizers.

Preparation

PDT for skin conditions

A patient receiving PDT for skin cancer or a precancerous skin disorder will have ALA applied to the affected area three to six hours before the scheduled treatment. The skin may or may not be covered with a dressing. The patient does not need to fast or make any other special preparations. If the affected area of skin is on the face, the patient may be given goggles to wear to protect the eyes from the blue light used to activate the drug.

PDT for internal cancers

The photosensitizing agents used for PDT or palliative treatment of esophageal or lung cancers are given by injection, usually two to three days before treatment. The patient may return home after the injection, but must avoid sunlight and bright light indoors before the light treatment. The patient does not need to fast or discontinue other medications, but should cover the windows and skylights in his or her home before receiving the light treatment to prevent exposure to bright light after returning home.

Patients undergoing PDT for esophageal or lung cancers are given a local or general anesthetic before the doctor inserts the bronchoscope or endoscope. They may also be given a mild tranquilizer to relieve anxiety.

Aftercare

Aftercare following PDT with porfimer sodium involves four to six weeks of protection from sunlight and other sources of bright light, including tanning lamps or the examination lamps found in doctors' and dentists' offices. During this period, the patient should wear dark glasses: long-sleeved shirts of light-colored, and tightly woven fabric; long pants or slacks; and a wide-brimmed hat to protect the skin and eyes outdoors for at least 30 days after treatment. Sunscreen creams and lotions do not provide enough protection. It is best to run necessary errands after sundown or ask someone else in the household to drive the car. Women should not use helmet-type hair dryers or hand-held dryers on a high setting, as the drug remains in the scalp for several weeks and may cause burns if exposed to high heat. Exposure to low levels of indoor light is necessary, however, in order to break down the Photofrin remaining in the skin. After 30 days, the doctor will give the patient instructions on testing the skin for any remaining sensitivity to light.

Patients who have received PDT for cancers in the lining of the bronchi must return two days after the treatment for a follow-up **bronchoscopy**, in which the doctor will remove dead tumor cells and other pieces of tissue from the treated area. This follow-up procedure is necessary to prevent inflammation and possible blockage of the patient's airway. Treated tumor sites require between four and eight weeks for complete healing.

Patients who receive PDT with ALA do not need to take special precautions regarding sun exposure after treatment because the drug is short-lived. The treated skin will usually form a crust or scale for several days before healing completely.

Risks

Porfimer sodium

Risks of PDT with porfimer sodium include photosensitivity reactions if the patient fails to observe the guidelines for aftercare; chest pain or a burning sensation in the chest or throat; difficulty swallowing; **itching**; the formation of ulcers or scar tissue; and discomfort in the eyes when exposed to sunlight, bright lights, or car headlights. Breast cancer and lung cancer patients who have severe chest pain after PDT can be given medications to control the pain.

Aminolevulinic acid

Some patients experience a stinging or burning sensation in the skin during the blue light treatment, but this usually goes away as soon as the light is turned off. Some patients also report temporary swelling or redness of the skin in the treated areas, or minor changes in the pigmentation of their skin.

Normal results

Normal results of PDT of the esophagus or the lining of the bronchi are shrinkage of the tumor and destruction of cancer cells. Normal results of palliative treatment for cancer of the esophagus are sufficient shrinkage of the tumor to allow the patient to swallow again.

Normal results for PDT of the skin include shrinkage and destruction of the tumor, although large skin tumors may require a second treatment for complete removal.

Abnormal results

Abnormal results include allergic reactions to the photosensitizing medication or failure of the tumor to respond to PDT.

See also Esophageal cancer; Porfimer sodium.

Resources

BOOKS

"Esophageal Tumors." In *The Merck Manual of Diagnosis and Therapy*, edited by Mark H. Beers, MD, and Robert Berkow, MD. Whitehouse Station, NJ: Merck Research Laboratories, 2007.

PERIODICALS

Bellnier, David A., William R. Greco, Gregory M. Loewen, et al. "Population Pharmacokinetics of the Photodynamic Therapy Agent 2-[1-Hexyloethyl]-2-devinyl-Pyropheophorbide-a in Cancer Patients." *Cancer Research* 63 (April 15, 2003): 1806–1813.

Dimofte, A., T. C. Zhu, S. M. Hahn, and R. A. Lustig. "In vivo Light Dosimetry for Motexafin Lutetium-Mediated PDT of Recurrent Breast Cancer." *Lasers in Surgery and Medicine* 31 (2002): 305–312.

Fulton, James Jr., MD, PhD. "Actinic Keratosis." *eMedicine*, 12 November 2003. http://www.emedicine.com/derm/topic9.htm.

Patti, Marco, MD, and Robert Li, MD. "Esophageal Cancer." *eMedicine*, 14 June 2004. http://www.emedicine.com/med/topic741.htm.

Suthamjariya, Kittisak, MD, and Charles R. Taylor, MD. "Photodynamic Therapy for the Dermatologist." *eMedicine*, 20 August 2002. http://www.emedicine.com/erm/topic636.htm.

OTHER

American Cancer Society (ACS), Making Treatment Decisions. *What Is Photodynamic Therapy?*. http://www.cancer.org/docroot/ETO/content/ETO_1_4X_What_Is_Photodynamic_Therapy_.asp.

Food and Drug Administration (FDA). *FDA Talk Paper* T03-60, 4 August 2003. "FDA Approves Photofrin for Treatment of Pre-Cancerous Lesions in Barrett's Esophagus." http://www.fda.gov/bbs/topics/ANSWERS/2003/ANS01246.html.

Guyton, Kate Z., PhD, Ellen Richmond, MS, and Ernest T. Hawk, MD. (National Cancer Institute and the National Institute of Diabetes and Digestive and Kidney Diseases) *Report of the Barrett's Esophagus Working Group*. Bethesda, MD: NCI, 2001.

National Cancer Institute (NCI). *Cancer Facts: Photodynamic Therapy for Cancer: Questions and Answers*. Bethesda, MD: NCI, 2004. <http://cis.nci.nih.gov/fact/7_7.htm>.

National Cancer Institute (NCI). *Oropharyngeal Cancer (PDQ®): Treatment*. http://www.cancer.gov/cancertopics/pdq/treatment/oropharyngeal/healthprofessional.

Roswell Park Cancer Institute. *Photodynamic Therapy (PDT) Center*. Buffalo, NY: Roswell Park Cancer Institute, 2005. http://www.roswellpark.org/document_187_620.html.

Rebecca Frey, Ph.D.

PICC lines *see* **Vascular access**

Pilocarpine

Definition

Pilocarpine is a medicine used to treat **xerostomia**, or dryness of the mouth, caused by a decrease in saliva production following radiation or due to **Sjögren's syndrome**, a disorder of the immune system characterized by the failure of the exocrine glands.

KEY TERMS

Exocrine—Referring to a gland that secretes outward by way of a duct.

Sialogogue—A medication given to increase the flow of saliva. Pilocarpine may be used as a sialogogue.

Xerostomia—The medical term for dry mouth.

Pilocarpine is also known as pilocarpine hydrochloride or Salagen.

Purpose

Pilocarpine is used to treat side effects arising from radiation treatment for **head and neck cancers**. It alleviates dryness of the mouth and throat and aids in chewing, tasting, and swallowing. It may also be given to treat dryness of the eyes resulting from **cancer** treatment.

Pilocarpine is also used in the form of eye drops or eye gel to treat glaucoma; it works by lowering the pressure of the fluid inside the eye.

Description

Pilocarpine is a naturally occurring substance found in the leaflets of *Pilocarpus jaborandi*, a South American shrub.

Pilocarpine works by stimulating the function of the exocrine glands, including the glands that produce saliva, sweat, tears, and digestive secretions. It also stimulates smooth muscles, such as those found in the bronchus, gallbladder, bile ducts, and intestinal and urinary tracts.

Pilocarpine was approved by the U.S. Food and Drug Administration as a sialogogue, or medication to increase the flow of saliva, in 1994. Pilocarpine was effective in relieving xerostomia symptoms after twelve weeks in over half the patients studied; however, the medication may not work for everyone.

Recommended dosage

Pilocarpine is taken orally. It is available in round white tablets containing 5 mg. Different patients may require different dosages of the drug. The usual dose for adults is five milligrams taken three times a day. If necessary, the physician may increase the dosage to 10 mg, three times a day. Since increasing the dose increases the likelihood of side effects, the lowest dose that is effective should be used for treatment.

Pilocarpine begins to act 20 minutes after ingestion. It will continue to act for three to five hours, with the maximum effect taking place one hour after ingestion. Twelve weeks of regular use may be required for an improvement of symptoms.

If a dose is missed, it should be taken as soon as possible; however, if it is almost time for the next dose, only the next dose should be taken.

Precautions

Patients may wish to take this medication with a meal to avoid stomach upset; however, pilocarpine will have reduced effectiveness if it is taken with a meal that is high in fat. Patients should drink plenty of water to avoid dehydration due to increased sweating. Alcohol and antihistamines should not be used while taking pilocarpine. Due to the possibility of visual disturbances or dizziness, people using this medication should avoid driving or operating machinery, particularly at night. Patients should continue to see a dentist regularly during treatment even though symptoms may be improved, since xerostomia may increase the likelihood of tooth decay and other dental problems.

Studies have not been done to test the safety of pilocarpine use in pregnant or nursing women; very high doses of the drug may cause birth defects in animals. Studies have also not been done to test the use of pilocarpine by children.

Pilocarpine should not be taken by people who are sensitive to it or who have uncontrolled asthma, or such eye problems as inflammation of the iris or angle-closure glaucoma. It should be used with caution by people with breathing problems, gallbladder disease, kidney problems, peptic ulcer, psychological disturbances, retinal disease, or heart or blood vessel disease.

Side effects

The most common side effect of pilocarpine use is increased sweating. Other less common side effects are as follows: **nausea and vomiting**, irritated nose, chills, flushing, frequent urination, dizziness, weakness, headache, difficulty with digestion, increased tear production, **diarrhea**, bloating, abdominal pain, and visual problems.

Symptoms of overdose include irregular heartbeat, chest pain, fainting, confusion, stomach cramps or pain, and trouble breathing. Unusually severe or continuing side effects such as diarrhea, headache, weakness, trembling, visual difficulties, **nausea**, and **vomiting** may also indicate overdose.

Interactions

Pilocarpine may interact with other medications, reducing or increasing their effects or, sometimes, increasing the side effects of the other medications.

Pilocarpine may also be less effective as a result of interaction with other medications. The following drugs may cause interactions:

- amantadine
- anticholinergics
- antidepressants
- antidyskinetics
- antihistamines
- antimyasthenics
- antipsychotics
- beta-adrenergic blocking agents
- bethanecol
- buclizine
- carbamazepine
- cyclizine
- cyclobenzaprine
- disopyramide
- flavoxate
- glaucoma medications
- ipratropium
- meclizine
- methylphenidate
- orphenadrine
- oxybutynin
- physostigmine
- procainamide
- promethazine
- quinidine

Pilocarpine may also interact with alcohol, cocaine, and marijuana.

Resources

BOOKS

Beers, Mark H., MD, and Robert Berkow, MD, editors. "Dentistry in Medicine." In *The Merck Manual of Diagnosis and Therapy*. Whitehouse Station, NJ: Merck Research Laboratories, 2007.

PERIODICALS

Bruce, S. D. "Radiation-Induced Xerostomia: How Dry Is Your Patient?" *Clinical Journal of Oncology Nursing* 8 (February 2004): 61–67.

Gorsky, M., J. B. Epstein, J. Parry, et al. "The Efficacy of Pilocarpine and Bethanechol upon Saliva Production in Cancer Patients with Hyposalivation Following Radiation Therapy." *Oral Surgery, Oral Medicine, Oral Pathology, Oral Radiology, and Endodontics* 97 (February 2004): 190–195.

Racquel Baert, M.Sc.
Rebecca J. Frey, Ph.D.

Pineoblastoma

Definition

A pineoblastoma is an aggressive primary brain tumor that develops in the pineal body (sometimes called the epiphysis cerebri or pineal gland), which is a small cone-shaped organ located in the midbrain. The pineal body secretes melatonin, a hormone that regulates moods and the sleep-wake cycle in humans. Pineoblastomas are also known as pinealoblastomas.

Description

Pineoblastomas are rapidly growing tumors, and thereby distinguished from pineocytomas, which grow relatively slowly. They are defined by the World Health Organization (WHO) as primitive neuroectodermal tumors (PNETs) in the pineal gland; the word *primitive* in this context means that these tumors are composed of cells that have not yet separated into more specialized types of cells. The word *neuroectodermal* means that these tumors develop out of a layer of cells in the embryo that eventually gives rise to the baby's nervous system.

Pineoblastomas are considered highly malignant. They may invade nearby areas of brain tissue as well as spread into the cerebrospinal fluid, although they rarely metastasize to other parts of the body. In addition, pineoblastomas sometimes cause bleeding into the ventricles of the brain. The child's radiologist may be able to see areas of dying tissue in the brain when **imaging studies** are performed.

Demographics

Pineoblastomas are extremely rare, accounting for only 0.5–2% of childhood tumors of the central nervous system (CNS). About 2200 children below the age of 15 are diagnosed with malignant tumors of the brain and spinal cord each year in the United States; between 10 and 40 of these children will be diagnosed with pineoblastomas.

KEY TERMS

Blastoma—An abnormal growth of embryonic cells. A pineoblastoma is a blastoma that develops in the pineal body.

Endocrinologist—A doctor who specializes in diagnosing and treating disorders that affect the balance of hormones in the body or the organs that produce these hormones.

Melatonin—A hormone that regulates moods and the sleep-wake cycle in humans. It is produced by the pineal body.

Pineal body—A small cone-shaped endocrine gland attached to the roof of the third ventricle of the brain. The pineal body, which is also known as the pineal gland or epiphysis, secretes melatonin.

Pineocytoma—A slower-growing tumor of the pineal body found more commonly in adults.

Primary brain tumor—A tumor that starts in the brain, as distinct from a metastatic tumor that begins elsewhere in the body and spreads to the brain. A pineoblastoma is one type of primary brain tumor.

Primitive—Simple or undifferentiated. Pineoblastomas are classified as primitive tumors because they arise from cells that have not yet separated into groups of more specialized cells.

Shunt—A tube inserted by a surgeon to relieve pressure on the brain from blocked cerebrospinal fluid. The tube allows the fluid to bypass the tumor that is blocking its flow.

Ventricle—One of the small cavities located within the brain. The pineal body is attached to the roof of the third ventricle.

It is difficult to evaluate the statistical significance of racial or gender differences in such a small group; however, the available evidence from American **cancer** registries suggests that these cancers occur more frequently in Caucasian children than in African Americans, and more frequently in males than in females.

Pineoblastomas occur almost exclusively in younger children, with very few cases reported in adolescents or adults. The slower-growing pineocytomas, by contrast, are most likely to develop in adults between the ages of 25 and 35.

Causes and symptoms

The cause of pineoblastomas is unknown, but may be associated with gene mutations. A group of British radiologists reported in 2004 that the chances of survival in children diagnosed with pineoblastoma who had inherited a mutation of the **retinoblastoma** (RB) gene are much lower than the chances of children who did not inherit the RB mutation. The researchers suggested that this mutation may cause pineoblastomas as well as reduce or inhibit their response to therapy.

The symptoms of a pineoblastoma result from blockage of the flow of cerebrospinal fluid and increased pressure on the brain. Depending on the size of the tumor, symptoms may include the following:

- headache
- double vision
- nausea and vomiting
- weakness or loss of sensation on one side of the body
- seizures
- developmental delays or failure to thrive (in younger children)
- lowered energy level or unusual need for sleep
- personality changes
- unexplained changes in weight or appetite

Parents should note, however, that these symptoms are not unique to pineoblastomas; they may be produced by other types of **brain tumors**, head trauma, meningitis, migraine headaches, or several other medical conditions. In any event, a child with these symptoms should be seen by a doctor at once.

Diagnosis

The diagnosis of a pineoblastoma begins with a review of the child's medical history and a thorough physical examination. The child may be given several vision tests if he or she is seeing double or having other visual disturbances. The child's doctor will then order both laboratory tests and imaging studies. The laboratory tests are done to rule out such diseases as meningitis and to see whether the child's liver and other organs are functioning normally. The imaging studies are performed to determine the extent of the cancer and to assign the child to a risk group.

Unless surgical removal of the tumor is considered too risky, a neurosurgeon will perform what is known as an open **biopsy** to confirm the diagnosis of pineoblastoma. He or she will remove a small piece of the tumor for examination by a pathologist.

Laboratory tests

Standard laboratory tests for children with brain tumors include a complete blood count (CBC),

QUESTIONS TO ASK YOUR DOCTOR

- Which risk group has my child been assigned to?
- What treatments would you recommend for a child in that group, and why would you recommend them?
- Is my child eligible for any current clinical trials for children with pineoblastoma?
- Would you recommend any of the treatments currently considered experimental?
- What is my child's life expectancy? What can I do to make the remaining time as pain-free and enjoyable as possible?

electrolyte analysis, tests of kidney, liver, and thyroid function, and tests that determine whether the child has been recently exposed to certain viruses. In addition, a **lumbar puncture** will be performed to look for cancer cells in the child's spinal fluid.

Imaging tests

Imaging tests for pineoblastomas include the following:

- Magnetic resonance imaging (MRIs).
- Computed tomography (CT) scan. Doctors usually order MRIs and CT scans that cover the full length of the spinal column as well as the brain, because pineoblastomas are more likely than other PNETs to spread into the cerebrospinal fluid.
- Chest x ray.
- Bone scan. This test is necessary to determine whether the tumor has spread beyond the central nervous system.

Treatment team

Since the 1960s, most children diagnosed with brain tumors have been treated in specialized children's cancer centers. A child with pineoblastoma will usually have a pediatric oncologist as his or her primary doctor, along with one or more specialists. These specialists may include a neurosurgeon, pathologist, neuroradiologist, radiation oncologist, medical oncologist, endocrinologist, nutritionist, physical therapit or rehabilitation specialist, and psychologist or psychiatrist. The team will also include social workers, clergy, and other professionals to help the parents cope with the stresses of their child's illness and treatments.

Clinical staging, treatments, and prognosis

Staging

Pineoblastomas are not staged in the same way as cancers elsewhere in the body. Instead, children with these tumors are divided as of the early 2000s into two risk groups, average risk and poor risk. Assignment to these groups is based on the following factors:

- child's age
- size and location of the tumor
- whether the tumor has spread to other parts of the central nervous system
- whether the tumor has spread beyond the CNS to other parts of the body

Average-risk children are those older than three years, with most or all of the tumor removed by surgery and no evidence that the cancer has spread beyond the pineal body. Poor-risk children are those who are younger than three years, whose cancer was located near the center of the brain or could not be removed completely by surgery, and whose cancer has spread to or beyond other parts of the CNS. The risk of recurrence is higher for children in the poor risk group.

Treatments

Treatments for pineoblastoma depend on the child's age and his or her risk group. Children younger than three years are not usually given **radiation therapy** because it can affect growth and normal brain development; they are usually treated with surgery to remove as much of the tumor as possible, followed by **chemotherapy** if they are considered poor-risk patients. The drugs most commonly used to treat PNETs include **lomustine**, **cisplatin**, **carboplatin**, and **vincristine**.

In addition to removing the tumor, the surgeon may also place a shunt to reduce pressure on the child's brain if the tumor is blocking the flow of cerebrospinal fluid. The shunt is a plastic tube with one end placed within the third ventricle of the brain. The rest of the shunt is routed under the skin of the head, neck, and chest with the other end placed in the abdomen or near the heart. Shunts are used very conservatively in children with pineoblastomas, however, because there have been reports of these tumors spreading into the abdomen via the shunt.

Children three years and older are treated with surgery first, followed by radiation treatment of the entire brain and spinal cord. Those considered poor risks may also be given chemotherapy. Recurrent pineoblastomas are treated with further surgery and an additional course of chemotherapy.

Treatments for pineoblastoma that are considered experimental as of 2005 include the following:

- Gamma knife surgery (GKS). One group of neurosurgeons in Florida has reported good results in treating children with tumors in the pineal body with GKS. The advantages of GKS include more complete tumor removal and quicker recovery for the patient.
- Gene therapy.
- High-dose chemotherapy.
- Photodynamic therapy.
- Stem cell and bone marrow transplantation.
- Newer drugs: Irinotecan, tipifarnib, lapatinib, ixabepilone, cilengitide, and tariquidar.

Prognosis

The prognosis for children with pineoblastomas depends largely on their risk group. In general, however, these tumors have a poorer prognosis than other types of brain tumors, in part because of the difficulty of removing the complete tumor due to the location of the pineal body deep within the brain. The overall five-year survival rate of children with pineoblastoma is reported to be 50–%, but is much lower in children younger than three years and in older children who do not respond to radiation therapy.

Recurrent pineoblastomas are almost always fatal; there are no effective therapies for recurrent PNETs, as of the early 2000s.

Alternative and complementary therapies

Some complementary therapies that are reported to help children with pineoblastomas include pet therapy, humor therapy, and music therapy. All of these can be pleasurable for the child as well as relaxing. Ginger or peppermint may help to relieve the **nausea and vomiting** associated with chemotherapy.

Coping with cancer treatment

Children can be given additional medications to treat **nausea** and other side effects of chemotherapy. With regard to homesickness and other emotional reactions to being away from home, children's cancer centers have social workers and child psychologists who can educate the child's family about the cancer as well as help the child deal with separation issues.

The side effects of radiation therapy in children with brain tumors may include the formation of dead tissue at the site of the tumor. This formation is known as radiation necrosis. It occurs in about 5% of children who receive radiation therapy and may require surgical removal. Radiation necrosis, however, is not as serious as recurrence of the tumor.

Children who have difficulty speaking after brain surgery, or who experience physical weakness, difficulty walking, visual impairment, or other sensory problems, are given physical therapy and/or speech therapy on either an inpatient or outpatient basis.

Clinical trials

Because pineoblastomas are so rare, the American Cancer Society recommends that children diagnosed with these tumors be enrolled in an appropriate clinical trial. As of early 2009, there are about 54 **clinical trials** in the United States for children with pineoblastomas and other PNETs. Some of these trials involve gene testing to improve diagnosis of children with brain tumors, while others are exploring various combinations of chemotherapy (including new agents), **photodynamic therapy**, stem cell transplantation, and **bone marrow transplantation** as treatments for pineoblastomas.

Special concerns

Children diagnosed with pineoblastomas, like children with other long-term illnesses, may develop emotional problems in reaction to restrictions on their activities, uncomfortable treatments, or being treated in a cancer center away from home. These children may withdraw from others, become angry or bitter, or feel inappropriately guilty about their illness. It is important to reassure the child that he or she did not cause the cancer or deserve it as a punishment for being "bad." Parents may benefit from consulting a child psychiatrist about these and other emotional problems.

Another special concern is the task of explaining the child's illness and treatments to other family members and friends in ways that they can understand. Members of the child's treatment team can be helpful in providing simplified descriptions for siblings or schoolmates.

A third area of concern with **childhood cancers** is the parents' relationships with their other children and with each other. Siblings may resent the amount of time and attention given to the child with cancer, or they may fear that they too will develop a brain tumor. Support groups for families of children with cancer can help by sharing strategies for coping with these problems as well as allowing members to express anxiety and other painful feelings in a safe setting.

See also Brain tumors; Supratentorial primitive neuroectodermal tumors.

Resources

BOOKS

American Brain Tumor Association (ABTA). *A Primer of Brain Tumors*. Des Plaines, IL: ABTA, 2004. The entire book can be downloaded free of charge as one large PDF file from the ABTA website.

"Intracranial Neoplasms (Brain Tumors)." Section 14, Chapter 177 in *The Merck Manual of Diagnosis and Therapy*, edited by Mark H. Beers, MD, and Robert Berkow, MD. Whitehouse Station, NJ: Merck Research Laboratories, 2004.

Pelletier, Kenneth R., MD. *The Best Alternative Medicine*. New York: Simon & Schuster, 2002.

PERIODICALS

Amendola, B. E., A. Wolf, S. R. Coy, et al. "Pineal Tumors: Analysis of Treatment Results in 20 Patients." *Journal of Neurosurgery* 102 (January 2005) (Supplement): 175–179.

Bruce, J. N., and A. T. Ogden. "Surgical Strategies for Treating Patients with Pineal Region Tumors." *Journal of Neurooncology* 69 (August-September 2004): 221–236.

MacDonald, Tobey, MD. "Medulloblastoma." *eMedicine*, 29 July 2004. http://www.emedicine.com/ped/topic1396.htm.

Plowman, P. N., B. Pizer, and J. E. Kingston. "Pineal Parenchymal Tumours: II. On the Aggressive Behaviour of Pineoblastoma in Patients with an Inherited Mutation of the RB1 Gene." *Clinical Oncology (Royal College of Radiology) 16 (June 2004): 244–247.*

Young, Guy, MD, Jeffrey A. Toretsky, MD, Andrew B. Campbell, MD, and Allen E. Eskenazi, MD. "Recognition of Common Childhood Malignancies." *American Family Physician* 61 (April 1, 2000): 2144–2154.

OTHER

American Academy of Child and Adolescent Psychiatry (AACAP). *The Child with a Long-Term Illness*. AACAP Facts for Families #19. Washington, DC: AACAP, 1999.

American Cancer Society (ACS), Cancer Reference Information. *Brain and Spinal Cord Tumors in Children*. http://documents.cancer.org/144.00/144.00.pdf.

ORGANIZATIONS

American Academy of Child and Adolescent Psychiatry. 3615 Wisconsin Avenue, NW, Washington, DC 20016-3007. (202) 966-7300. Fax: (202) 966-2891. http://www.aacap.org.

American Brain Tumor Association (ABTA). 2720 River Road, Des Plaines, IL 60018. (800) 886-2282 or (847) 827-9910. http://www.abta.org. This independent nonprofit association supports research as well as providing patient and family education materials.

CureSearch Children's Oncology Group (COG) Research Operations Center. 440 East Huntington Drive, P. O. Box 60012, Arcadia, CA 91066-6012. CureSearch is a joint effort of two organizations, the Children's Oncology Group (COG) and the National Childhood Cancer Foundation (NCCF). The COG conducts research and clinical trials while the NCCF conducts fundraising and advocacy initiatives.

Rebecca Frey, Ph.D.

Pituitary tumors

Definition

Pituitary tumors are abnormal growths in the pituitary gland.

Description

Located in the brain, the pituitary gland is often referred to as the "master gland" of the body. This is because it makes and releases (secretes) at least nine distinct hormones (including oxytocin, antidiuretic hormone [ADH], prolactin, thyroid-stimulating hormone [TSH], adrenocorticotropic hormone [ACTH], follicle-stimulating hormone [FSH], luteinizing hormone [LH], and human growth hormone [HGH]) that regulate the activities of several other endocrine glands and influence a number of physiological processes including growth, sexual development and functioning, and the fluid balance of the body. The pituitary is divided into two parts: front (anterior) and rear (posterior). Each half of the pituitary gland secretes specific hormones. Tumors in the anterior part are common and are usually noncancerous (benign). Tumors rarely develop in the posterior portion. Between 10% and 15% of all tumors in the skull are pituitary tumors, which makes them the third most common type of brain tumor.

Virtually all pituitary tumors arise from a single cell which, for unknown reasons, has grown out of control. Tumors that have originated from a single cell are called monoclonal. Some tumors secrete hormones normally made by the pituitary gland. Because the tumor cells are uncontrolled, they secrete large amounts of hormones. As a result, hormone imbalance occurs. The symptoms caused by the hormone imbalance are often the first sign of a pituitary tumor.

There are several different types of pituitary tumors. Pituitary adenomas (adenomas are tumors that grow

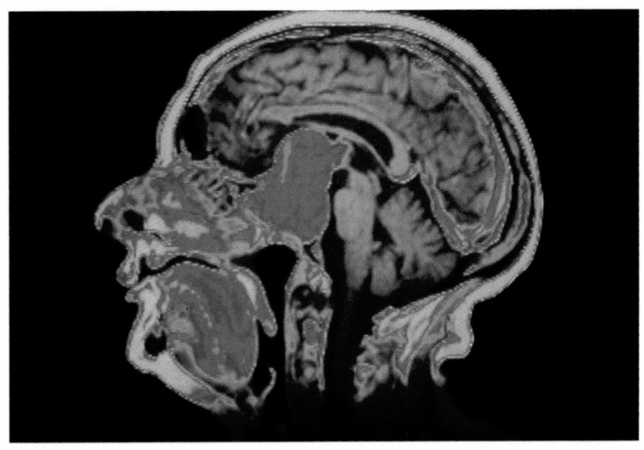

This colored magnetic resonance imaging (MRI) scan of a sagittal section of the brain reveals a large pituitary tumor (pink mass in center) located to the left of the brainstem. *(© SPL/Photo Researchers, Inc. Reproduced by permission.)*

KEY TERMS

Adenoma—A tumor that is derived from glandular tissue.

Agonist—A drug that increases the effectiveness of another drug or chemical.

Benign—A term used to describe a noncancerous growth.

Carney complex—A genetic disorder characterized by myxomas, spotty pigmentation of the skin and mucous membranes, and endocrine overactivity.

Dopamine—A neurotransmitter that is a chemical messenger in the brain.

Hormone—A chemical that is produced and released by one organ to regulate the function of another organ.

Invasive—A descriptive term for tumors that spread to nearby structures.

McCune-Albright syndrome—A genetic disorder that includes bone, endocrine, and skin abnormalities. Some individuals with this syndrome show the effects of excessive secretion of pituitary growth hormone.

Multiple endocrine neoplasia syndrome type I—An inherited disorder that affects the endocrine glands. The pituitary gland becomes overactive in about one-sixth of the individuals with this syndrome.

Nelson's syndrome—An endocrine disorder characterized by increase secretion of ACTH and melanocyte stimulating hormone by the pituitary gland.

from gland tissues) are the most common type. Most pituitary adenomas are benign, although they may spread to nearby tissues. Pituitary adenomas can be further classified based on which, if any, hormones are secreted by the tumor. Thirty-five percent of pituitary adenomas do not secrete hormones, 27% secrete prolactin (prolactinomas), and 21% secrete growth hormone. The remaining pituitary adenomas secrete sex hormones (6%), thyroid hormones (1%), or adrenal (adrenocorticotropic) hormones (8%). Plurihormonal adenomas secrete more than one type of hormone. Tumors that secrete adrenocorticotropic hormone cause **Cushing's syndrome** and Nelson's syndrome.

Craniopharyngiomas are benign tumors that originate in tissues next to the pituitary gland. Technically speaking, they are not pituitary tumors although they affect the pituitary gland. They are extremely difficult to remove and radiation does not stop craniopharyngiomas from spreading throughout the pituitary gland. Craniopharyngiomas account for less than 5% of all **brain tumors**.

Pituitary **carcinoma** is a very rare condition. Fewer than 100 cases have ever been reported. It is usually diagnosed when a pituitary tumor, which was believed to be an **adenoma**, spreads (metastasizes) to distant organs. These pituitary tumors may or may not release hormones. Because pituitary carcinoma is often diagnosed late, it has a high death rate.

Demographics

Pituitary tumors occur more frequently in women than in men. They usually develop between the ages of 30 and 40. Half of all craniopharyngiomas occur in children, with symptoms most often appearing between the ages of five and ten.

Causes and symptoms

The cause of pituitary tumors is not known. Most pituitary tumors presumably result from changes to the DNA of one cell, leading to uncontrolled cell growth. The genetic defects, multiple endocrine neoplasia syndrome type I (MEN I or Wermer's syndrome), McCune-Albright syndrome, and the Carney complex, are associated with pituitary tumors. However, these defects account for only a small percentage of the cases of pituitary tumors. Also, a pituitary tumor may result from the spread (**metastasis**) of **cancer** from another site. **Breast cancer** in women and lung cancer in men are the most common cancers to spread to the pituitary

QUESTIONS TO ASK THE DOCTOR

- Is my tumor cancerous? Is it invasive?
- What are my treatment options?
- What are the risks and side effects of these treatments?
- Is surgery really necessary?
- Which surgical approach will you use?
- How experienced are you at performing pituitary surgery?
- How will I feel immediately following surgery?
- Will I need to take medication for the rest of my life?
- How long will it take for my symptoms to go away?
- Will I be able to have children?
- Is it safe to become pregnant while taking this medication?
- How will pregnancy affect my tumor?
- What medications can I take to relieve treatment side effects?
- Are there any clinical studies underway that would be appropriate for me?
- What is the chance that the tumor will recur?
- How will recurrence be detected?
- How often will I have follow-up examinations?

gland. Other cancers that spread to the pituitary gland include **kidney cancer**, **prostate cancer**, **melanoma**, and **gastrointestinal cancers**.

Symptoms related to tumor location, size, and pressure on neighboring structures include:

- persistent headache on one or both sides, or in the center of the forehead
- blurred or double vision; loss of side (peripheral) vision
- drooping eyelid (ptosis) caused by pressure on nerves leading to the eye
- numb feeling on the face
- dementia
- drowsiness
- enlarged head
- eating excessive (hyperphagia) or abnormally small (hypophagia) amounts of food
- seizures

The specific symptoms associated with hormone-secreting tumors will vary depending on which hormones are being over-produced. Symptoms related to hormonal imbalance include:

- excessive sweating
- loss of appetite
- loss of interest in sex
- inability to tolerate cold temperatures
- nausea
- menstrual problems
- excessive thirst
- frequent urination
- dry skin
- constipation
- premature or delayed puberty
- delayed growth in children
- milk secretion in the absence of pregnancy or breast feeding (galactorrhea)
- reduced strength
- mood alterations (depression, anxiety, unstable emotions)
- muscle pain
- low blood sugar (sudden occurrence of shakiness and sweating)

Patients who have sudden pituitary failure caused by bleeding or tissue death (pituitary apoplexy also known as Sheehan's syndrome) may experience very severe headaches, confusion, loss of sight, and drowsiness. This condition is considered an emergency.

Tumors that secrete growth hormone cause a condition called acromegaly. This long-term condition is characterized by enlargement of the nose, ears, jaws, toes, and fingers. Joint pain, blood sugar imbalances, high blood pressure, carpal tunnel syndrome, and airway blockages can result.

Diagnosis

As many as 40% of all pituitary tumors do not release excessive quantities of hormones into the blood. Known as clinically nonfunctioning, these tumors are difficult to distinguish from tumors that produce similar symptoms. They may grow to be quite large before they are diagnosed.

The diagnosis of pituitary tumors is based on:

- the patient's own observations and medical history
- physical examination
- laboratory studies of the patient's blood and brain/spinal fluid (cerebrospinal fluid)

- x rays of the skull and other studies that provide images of the inside of the brain (CT, MRI)
- vision tests
- urinalysis

Treatment team

The treatment team for pituitary tumors may include a neuroendocrinologist, endocrinologist, neurosurgeon, oncologist, radiation oncologist, nurse oncologist, psychiatrist, psychological counselor, and social worker.

Clinical staging, treatments, and prognosis

Clinical staging

Because most pituitary tumors are benign, there is no clinical staging system.

Treatments

Treatment is determined by the type of tumor, the type of hormone being released, and whether or not the tumor has invaded tissues next to the pituitary gland. The goals of treatment are to normalize hormone levels and reduce the size of (or remove) the tumor. Treatment options include surgery, radiation, and/or medication. Some pituitary tumors stabilize without treatment. Small tumors that are not causing significant symptoms may be watched only.

Surgery is usually used to remove all or part of a tumor within the gland or the area surrounding it. Surgery may be combined with **radiation therapy** to treat tumors that extend beyond the pituitary gland. A neurosurgeon will operate immediately to remove the tumor or pituitary gland (hypophysectomy) of a patient whose vision is deteriorating rapidly. Approximately 96% of the surgeries are performed through the nose (transsphenoidal). If the tumor is large, the skull may be opened (**craniotomy**) for tumor removal. Removal or destruction of the pituitary gland requires life-long hormone replacement therapy. The most common complications of surgery are leakage of cerebrospinal fluid through the nose and inflammation of the membranes that surround the brain and spinal column (meningitis).

Radiation therapy is not as effective as surgery and is usually reserved for tumors that have not responded to other treatments and those that recur. Radioactive pellets can be implanted in the brain to treat the tumor. Selected patients are treated with proton beam radiosurgery that uses high energy particles in the form of a high energy beam to destroy an overactive pituitary gland. **Fatigue**, upset stomach, **diarrhea**, and **nausea** are common complaints of patients having radiation therapy. Radiation therapy to the brain can damage certain brain tissues.

Dopamine agonists, drugs that increase the effect of the brain chemical dopamine, are effective in treating tumors that release hormones. These drugs can reduce symptoms caused by a pituitary tumor and reduce the size of the tumor. Commonly used dopamine agonists include bromocriptine, pergolide, and cabergoline. Cabergoline is the most effective and produces fewer side effects than the other two drugs. Side effects associated with dopamine agonists include nausea, **vomiting**, and light-headedness when rising (postural hypotension). Acromegaly may be treated with somatostatin and other drugs derived from somatostatin (analogues). Tumors, and the symptoms they are causing, return when drug use is stopped. Patients should wear medical identification tags identifying their condition and the hormonal replacement medicines they take.

The common treatments for specific pituitary tumors are:

- Prolactin-secreting adenoma. Prolactinomas are treated with a dopamine agonist. Surgical treatment is used if the drug fails or causes intolerable side effects.
- Gonadotropin-secreting adenoma. Small tumors are not treated unless they are causing symptoms. Large tumors and small tumors that are causing symptoms are treated surgically. Radiation therapy may be used.
- Adrenocorticotropic hormone-secreting adenoma. Surgery is the treatment of choice. Medications that prevent adrenal hormone production or radiation therapy may be used if surgery fails.
- Growth hormone-secreting adenoma. Surgery is the treatment of choice. Medications (dopamine agonists, somatostatins) or radiation therapy may be used.
- Thyroid stimulating hormone-secreting adenoma. Surgery, with or without radiation therapy, is the treatment of choice. Although somatostatin treatment may reduce hormone levels, it fails to shrink the tumor.
- Nonsecreting adenoma. Surgery is the treatment of choice. In general, medications are not effective for this type of tumor. Radiation therapy may be used to prevent tumor recurrence.
- Pituitary carcinoma. Carcinoma is treated with standard cancer radiation therapy and chemotherapy.
- Craniopharyngiomas. These tumors are difficult to treat. Due to the nature of craniopharyngiomas, surgery is often incomplete and needs to be complemented by radiation therapy.

Prognosis

Pituitary tumors are usually curable. Pituitary adenomas that secrete adrenocorticotropic hormone are frequently persistent and have a high rate of recurrence. Approximately 5% of pituitary adenomas invade nearby tissues and grow to large sizes, making them more difficult to treat and subject to frequent recurrences. Metastasis of most pituitary tumors is very rare. However, pituitary carcinomas can metastasize and are associated with a poor prognosis.

Alternative and complementary therapies

Alternative and complementary therapies have not been shown to be effective in treating pituitary tumors. For more comprehensive information, the patient should consult the book on complementary and alternative medicine published by the American Cancer Society listed in the Resources section.

Coping with cancer treatment

The patient should consult his or her treatment team regarding any side effects or complications of treatment. Patients may want to consult a psychotherapist and/or join a support group to deal with the emotional consequences of cancer and its treatment.

Clinical trials

There are two active **clinical trials** studying pituitary tumors are studying the safety and effectiveness of antineoplastons. Study #BRI-BT-9 is open to patients with serious or life-threatening brain tumors. Study #BRI-NE-2 is open to patients who have metastatic or incurable **neuroendocrine tumors**. The National Cancer Institute web site has information on these and other studies. Patients should consult with their treatment teams to determine if they are candidates for these or any other ongoing studies.

Special concerns

Long-term low levels of sex hormones (hypogonadism) can have negative effects on bone density and the cardiovascular system. The effect a pituitary tumor has on fertility is a concern for both men and women. Women taking medications to treat pituitary tumors need to question their physicians regarding the potential effect the medications may have on an unborn baby.

See also Mutliple endocrine neoplasia syndromes.

Resources

BOOKS

Bruss, Katherine, Christina Salter, and Esmeralda Galan, editors.*American Cancer Society's Guide to Complementary and Alternative Cancer Methods*. Atlanta: American Cancer Society, 2000.

DeAngelis, Lisa, and Jerome Posner. "Cancer of the Central Nervous System and Pituitary Gland." In *Clinical Oncology*, edited by Raymond Lenhard, Robert Osteen, and Ted Gansler. Atlanta: American Cancer Society, 2004, pp.653–703.

Krisht, Ali, and George Tindall, editors. *Pituitary Disorders: Comprehensive Management*. . Baltimore: Lippincott Williams & Wilkins, 1999.

Molitch, Mark, editor. *Endocrinology and Metabolism Clinics of North America: Advances in Pituitary Tumor Therapy*. Philadelphia: W.B. Saunders Company, 1999.

PERIODICALS

Wardlaw, Fred, P. Wardlaw, and S. Wardlaw. "Diagnosis and Treatment of Pituitary Tumors." *The Journal of Clinical Endocrinology & Metabolism* 84 (November 1999): 3859- 66.

ORGANIZATIONS

American Brain Tumor Association. 2770 River Road, Des Plaines, IL 60018. (800) 886-2289. http://www.abta.org.

American Cancer Society. 1599 Clifton Road NE, Atlanta, GA 30329. (800) ACS-2345. http://www.cancer.org.

Brain Tumor Information Services. Box 405, Room J341, University of Chicago Hospitals, 5841 S. Maryland Avenue, Chicago, IL 60637. (312) 684-1400.

Cancer Research Institute, National Headquarters. 681 Fifth Ave., New York, NY 10022. (800) 992-2623. http://www.cancerresearch.org.

National Institutes of Health. National Cancer Institute. 9000 Rockville Pike, Bethesda, MD 20982. Cancer Information Service: (800) 4-CANCER. http://cancernet.nci.nih.gov.

Maureen Haggerty
Belinda Rowland, Ph.D.

Plasma cell dyscrasias, or plasma cell neoplasms *see* **Multiple myeloma; Waldenstrom's macroglobulinemia**

Plasmacytoma *see* **Multiple myeloma**

Plasmapheresis *see* **Pheresis**

Plerixafor

Definition

Plerixafor (Mozobil) is a hematopoietic stem cell mobilizing drug manufactured by Genzyme Corporation. It is used in combination with granulocyte-colony stimulating factor (G-CSF) to increase the number of hematopoietic stem cells in the bloodstream as part of treatment for non-Hodgkin's **lymphoma** and **multiple myeloma**.

KEY TERMS

Apheresis—The practice of removing blood from an individual and separating out certain components, returning the blood to the individual and storing the separated component in order to later transfuse them back into the same individual (autologous transplantation).

Autologous transplantation—Transplantation in which the individual's own stem cells or bone marrow are removed and then transplanted back into the individual later. Autologous transplantation removes the risk of rejection of the transplanted material.

Granulocyte-colony stimulating factor (G-CFS)—A genetically produced form of a naturally occurring hormone that stimulates the production of infection-fighting white blood cells called granulocytes in the bone marrow. Chemotherapy drugs often kill these cells. Increasing the production of granulocytes can help to offset the effects of chemotherapy.

Hematopoietic stem cells—Cells that have the potential to differentiate into red blood cells, white blood cells, or platelets.

Leukocytes—Also called white blood cells, leukocytes fight infection and boost the immune system.

Lymphoma—A type of cancer that originates in the cells of the lymphatic system (lymph nodes, thymus, spleen, adenoids, tonsils and bone marrow). It is one of the four major types of cancer.

Multiple myeloma—Cancer of the plasma cells of the bone marrow.

Orphan drug status—An orphan drug is one that provides a significant benefit in treating a rare disease. Generally these drugs are not financially worthwhile for drug companies to produce despite their benefit to patients. If a drug is given orphan drug status in the United States or European Union, it may be receive fast-track approval or extra research money, making it more economically viable for manufacturers.

Platelet—A small, disk-shaped cell in the blood that has an important role in blood clotting. Platelets form the initial plug at the rupture site of a blood vessel.

Pregnancy category—A system of classifying drugs according to their established risks for use during pregnancy. Category A: Controlled human studies have demonstrated no fetal risk. Category B: Animal studies indicate no fetal risk, but no human studies; or adverse effects in animals, but not in well-controlled human studies. Category C: No adequate human or animal studies; or adverse fetal effects in animal studies, but no available human data. Category D: Evidence of fetal risk, but benefits outweigh risks. Category X: Evidence of fetal risk. Risks outweigh any benefits.

Purpose

High doses of **chemotherapy** drugs kill large numbers of healthy blood cells as well as killing cancerous (malignant) cells. To function well, the body needs to replace these healthy cells. Hematopoietic stem cells are undifferentiated cells that can become red blood cells that carry oxygen and remove wastes throughout the body, white blood cells that help fight **infection**, or platelets, which help the blood to clot. Plerixafor, when used in combination with G-CSF, stimulates the body to release hematopoietic stem cells from the bone marrow into the bloodstream. These stem cells can then be harvested through a process called apheresis.

Apheresis works by removing the blood from an individual and passing it through special filters that remove the desired component, in this case the hematopoietic stem cells, and then returning the blood to the individual. The hematopoietic stem cells are stored and later can be re-infused into the individual after high doses of chemotherapy. This process is called an autologous peripheral blood stem cell transplantation. The transfused stem cells settle into the bone marrow and begin differentiating into new blood cells. For an autologous peripheral blood stem cell transplantation to be successful, many millions of hematopoietic stem cells must be collected. Treatment with the combination of plerixafor and G-CSF stimulates the bone marrow to release these cells into blood stream and substantially reduces number of days and apheresis sessions needed to collect enough for successful transplantation.

Description

Plerixafor injection, sold under the brand name Mozobil, is a sterile, preservative-free clear liquid that is intended for injection under the skin (subcutaneous injection). The Food and Drug Administration approved the drug for use in the United States on

December 15, 2008. Application for approval in the European Union is underway, but has not been completed as of early October 2009. As of October 2009, plerixafor has been granted orphan drug status in the United States and Mexico. Plerixafor continues to be tested in **clinical trials** in the United States for use against other cancers and in combination with other therapies. A list of clinical trials currently enrolling volunteers can be found at <http://www.clinicaltrials.gov>.

Recommended dosage

Plerixafor comes in single-use vials that should be stored at room temperature. First the patient receives G-CSF once daily for four days. Following that, plerixafor is injected under the skin 11 hours before apheresis is to begin. Dosage is based on body weight, with a recommended dose of 0.24 mg/kg body weight and may be repeated for up to four consecutive days. There is no data on overdosage.

Plerixafor is removed from the body by the kidney. The recommended dosage for individuals with moderate to severe kidney (renal) impairment is reduced to 0.16 mg/kg body weight, not to exceed 27 mg/day. There are no other special recommendations for dosage.

The safety and effectiveness of this drug in children has not been established.

Precautions

The following precautions should be observed.

- Plerixafor should not be used in patients with leukemia because it may mobilize leukemia cells for release from bone marrow.
- A decrease in the number of blood platelets (thrombocytopenia) may reduce the ability of the blood to clot. An increase in the number of leukocytes also may occur. Blood count should be monitored.
- An increased number of tumor cells may be released from the bone marrow as a result of G-CSF/plerixafor stimulation. Some of these tumor cells may be unintentionally collected along with the hematopoietic stem cells harvested for transfusion. The effect of re-infusing these tumor cells is unknown.
- This drug may cause enlargement and rupture of the spleen. Symptoms of spleen enlargement should be evaluated promptly.
- Individuals with renal failure should receive reduced dosage (see recommended dosage above).

QUESTIONS TO ASK YOUR DOCTOR OR PHARMACIST

- Why do you believe the benefits outweigh the risks of using this drug?
- Is this drug safe to take with the other drugs that I am currently taking?
- What side effects should I watch for? When should I call the doctor about them?
- Are there any clinical trials of this drug combined with other therapies that might benefit me?

Pregnant or breastfeeding women

Plerixafor is a pregnancy category D drug. Woman who are pregnant or who might become pregnant should not use plerixafor. It is not known whether the drug is excreted in breast milk. Women taking this drug who are or who want to breast feed should discuss the risks and benefits with their doctor and err on the side of caution, as there is the potential for this drug to cause serious adverse effects on nursing infants.

Side effects

The most serious side effects seen in clinical trials were the potential for tumor cell mobilization in leukemia patients, increased leukocytes and decreased platelets in the blood, and enlargement of the spleen.

Side effects that occurred in more than 10% of individuals given plerixafor during clinical trials included:

- diarrhea
- nausea and vomiting
- fatigue
- reactions at the injection site
- headache
- joint pain (arthralgia)
- dizziness

Interactions

As of October 2009, plerixafor was not known to interact with any drugs, herbs, or supplements. Individuals should check with their oncologist for changes in this information as more people are treated with plerixafor and information about the drug is collected.

Resources

OTHER

Pazdur, Richard. FDA Approval for Plerixafor, National Cancer Institute. December 16, 2008 [October 4, 2009]. http://www.cancer.gov/cancertopics/druginfo/fda-plerixafor

Bone Marrow Transplantation and Peripheral Blood Stem Cell Transplantation. National Cancer Institute October 29, 2008 [October 4, 2009].

ORGANIZATIONS

American Cancer Society, 1599 Clifton Rd., NE, Atlanta, GA, 30329, (404) 320-3333, (800) ACS-2345, http://www.cancer.org.

National Cancer Institute Public Inquires Office., 6116 Executive Boulevard, Room 3036A, Bethesda, MD, 20892-8322, (800) 4-CANCER. TTY (800) 332-8615, http://www.cancer.gov.

Leukemia & Lymphoma Society, 1311 Mamaroneck Avenue, Suite 310 , White Plains, NY, 10605, (800) 955-4572, http://www.leukemia-lymphoma.org.

Tish Davidson, A.M.

Pleural fluid analysis *see* **Thoracentesis**

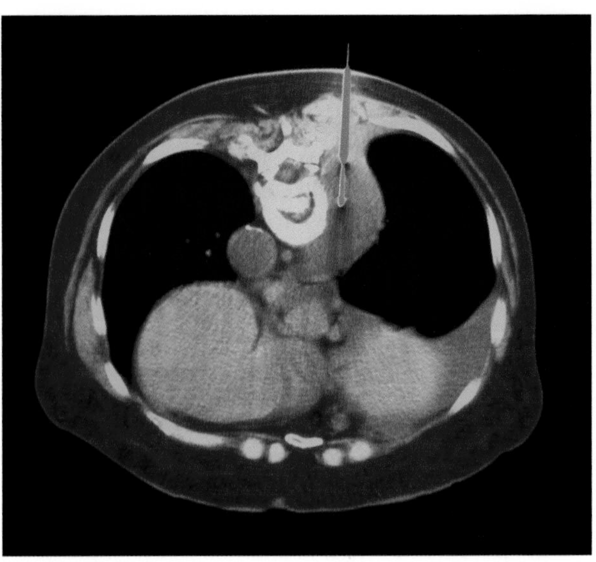

Colored computed tomography (CT) scan of an axial section through the chest, showing a lung biopsy being taken by bronchoscope. The front of the chest is at the top, and the heart is at the lower center (appearing orange). The bronchoscope (blue) has penetrated the back of the patient and has entered a tumor (orange). At the tip of the bronchoscope is a biopsy needle. *(© Mehau Kulyk, Science Source/Photo Researchers, Inc. Photo reproduced by permission.)*

Pleural biopsy

Definition

The pleura is the membrane that lines the lungs and chest cavity. A pleural **biopsy** is the removal of pleural tissue for examination and eventual diagnosis.

Purpose

Pleural biopsy is performed to differentiate between benign (noncancerous) and malignant (cancerous) disease, to diagnose viral, fungal, or parasitic diseases, and to identify a condition called collagen vascular disease of the pleura. It is also ordered when a chest x ray indicates a pleural-based tumor, reaction, or thickening of the pleura.

Precautions

Because pleural biopsy—especially open pleural biopsy—is an invasive procedure, it is not recommended for patients with severe bleeding disorders.

Description

Pleural biopsy is usually ordered when pleural fluid obtained by another procedure called **thoracentesis** (aspiration of pleural fluid) suggests **infection**, signs of **cancer**, or tuberculosis. However, the procedure is most successful in diagnosing pleural tuberculosis (with a sensitivity up to 75%) rather than pleural malignancy (40–50% sensitivity).

The procedure most often performed for pleural biopsy is called a percutaneous (passage through the skin by needle puncture) needle biopsy or closed needle biopsy. This procedure can only sample the outer pleural membrane (parietal pleura), and the size of the tissue sample obtained is relatively small.

Although the biopsy needle itself remains in the pleura for less than one minute, the procedure takes 30–45 minutes. This type of biopsy is usually performed by a physician at bedside if the patient is hospitalized or in an outpatient setting under local anesthesia.

The actual procedure begins with the patient in a sitting position, shoulders and arms elevated and supported. The skin overlying the biopsy site is anesthetized and a small incision is made to allow insertion of the biopsy needle. This needle is inserted with a cannula (a plastic or metal tube) until fluid is removed. Then the inner needle is removed and a trocar (an instrument for withdrawing fluid from a cavity) is inserted to obtain the actual biopsy specimen. As

KEY TERMS

Aspiration—Drawing out of fluid from a cavity by suction.

Endotracheal—Placed within the trachea, also known as the windpipe.

Pulmonary—Pertaining to the lungs.

QUESTIONS TO ASK THE DOCTOR

- What is the purpose of this test?
- Is the test dangerous?
- How do I prepare for the test?
- How long will the test take?
- How soon will I get my test results?

many as three separate specimens are taken from different sites during the procedure. These specimens are then placed into a fixative solution and sent to the laboratory for tissue (histologic) examination.

Although used less frequently than the closed needle biopsy, an open pleural biopsy may be performed surgically, in the operating room, when a larger tissue sample is required. The incision is larger than that required for a closed needle biopsy, and an endotracheal tube is inserted through the windpipe to assure proper breathing during the procedure. The procedure takes two to three hours, is more invasive, and requires general anesthesia and hospitalization for one or more days. Open biopsy is sometimes performed when there is no **pleural effusion** (an accumulation of fluid between the pleural layers) or when a direct view of the pleura and lungs is required.

Another procedure, called **thoracoscopy**, involves pleural biopsy under direct visualization through a thoracoscope. This procedure is highly accurate (sensitivity as high as 91%) in diagnosing both benign and malignant pleural disease. As in open needle biopsy, however, it requires general anesthesia and is usually used only after other diagnostic procedures fail.

Preparation

Preparations for this procedure vary, depending on the type of procedure requested. Closed needle biopsy requires little or no preparation. Open pleural biopsy, which is performed in a hospital, requires fasting (no solids or liquids) for eight to 12 hours before the procedure because the stomach must be empty before general anesthesia is administered.

Aftercare

Potential complications of this procedure include bleeding or injury to the lung, or a condition called pneumothorax, in which air enters the pleural cavity (the space between the two layers of pleura lining the lungs and the chest wall). Because of these possibilities, a chest x ray is always performed after the procedure (closed or open biopsy). Also, it is important for the patient is to report any shortness of breath and for the nurses to note any signs of bleeding, decreased blood pressure, or increased pulse rate during the recovery period.

Risks

Risks for this procedure include respiratory distress on the side of the biopsy, as well as bleeding, possible shoulder pain, infection, pneumothorax (immediate), or **pneumonia** (delayed). Risk increases with stress, obesity, smoking, chronic illness, and the use of some medications (such as insulin, tranquilizers, and antihypertensives).

Normal results

Normal findings indicate no evidence of any pathologic or disease conditions in the pleural cavity.

Abnormal results

Abnormal findings include tumors called neoplasms (any new or abnormal growth) that can be either benign or malignant. Pleural tumors are divided into two categories: primary (**mesothelioma**), or metastatic (spreading to the pleural cavity from a site elsewhere in the body). These tumors are often associated with pleural effusion, which itself may be caused by pneumonia, heart failure, cancer, or blood clot in the lungs (pulmonary embolism).

Other causes of abnormal findings include viral, fungal, or parasitic infections, and tuberculosis.

Resources

BOOKS

Fischbach, Frances Talaska. *A Manual of Laboratory and Diagnostic Tests*. 6th ed. Philadelphia: Lippincott Williams & Wilkins, 2000.

PERIODICALS

Baumann, Michael H. "Closed Needle Pleural Biopsy: A Necessary Tool?" *Pulmonary Perspectives*. [cited June

28, 2005]. http://www.chest.org/publications/Pulmonary Perspectives/vol17n4a.html.

Peek, Giles, Sameh Morcos, and Graham Cooper. "The Pleural Cavity." *British Medical Journal*. 320 (May 2000): 1318–1321.

ORGANIZATIONS

Alliance for Lung Cancer Advocacy, Support, and Education. P.O. Box 849, Vancouver, WA 98666. 800–298–2436. http://www.alcase.org.

American Cancer Society. 1599 Clifton Rd. NE, Atlanta, GA 30329. 800–ACS–2345 http://www.cancer.org.

American College of Chest Physicians. 3300 Dundee Road, Northbrook, IL 60062–2348. 847–498–1400. http://www.chestnet.org.

American Lung Association. 1740 Broadway, New York, NY 10019–4374. 800–LUNG–USA (800–586–4872) http://www.lungusa.org.

Janis O. Flores

Pleural effusion

Description

Pleural effusion is the accumulation of fluid in the pleural space. The pleural space is the region between the outer surface of each lung (visceral pleurae) and the membrane that surrounds each lung (parietal pleurae). Under normal conditions, the pleurae are kept wet with pleural fluid to allow movement of the lungs within the chest. The pleural fluid comes from cells that make up the pleurae. Pleural fluid is continuously being produced and removed, a process that is precisely controlled by many factors. **Cancer** can interfere with this delicate balance within the pleural space causing fluid to accumulate.

Cancer is responsible for 40% of all pleural effusions, which are then called malignant pleural effusions. Pleural effusion is the first symptom of cancer for up to 50% of the patients. Thirty-five percent of the cases of malignant pleural effusion are caused by lung cancer, 23% by **breast cancer**, and 10% by **lymphoma**.

Chest **x rays** and **computed tomography** scans may be performed to diagnose pleural effusion. **Thoracentesis**, the removal of pleural fluid through a long needle, is usually performed for diagnostic purposes. Fluid removed by thoracentesis will be sent to the lab to be thoroughly evaluated. **Thoracoscopy**, in which a wand-like lighted camera (endoscope) is inserted through the chest, may be conducted to diagnose pleural effusion. During thoracoscopy, samples (**biopsy**) of pleura may be taken.

Pleural effusion can hinder the normal function of the lungs. Symptoms of pleural effusion include chest pain, chest heaviness, breathing difficulties, and a dry cough. Patients with malignant pleural effusions tend to be weak and have a short-span life expectancy. The prognosis depends on the type of cancer. Sixty-five percent of patients with malignant pleural effusions die within three months and 80% die within six months. However, patients with pleural effusion related to breast cancer have a longer life expectancy.

Causes

Malignant pleural effusions are most often associated with lymphomas, leukemia, breast cancer, gastrointestinal cancer, lung cancer, and **ovarian cancer**. For the majority of patients, pleural effusion occurs in the lung on the same side as the cancer. For one third of the patients, pleural effusion occurs in both lungs.

Pleural effusion in cancer patients can be caused by several different conditions. Blockage of the lymphatic system, a series of channels for drainage of body fluids, interferes with the removal of pleural fluid. Blockage of the veins of the lungs increases the pressure at the pleurae which causes fluid accumulation. Cancerous cells may seed onto pleurae and cause inflammation which increases fluid in the pleural space. High numbers of cancerous cells may collect in the pleural space (tumor cell suspensions) which causes extra fluid to be released. Accumulation of fluid in the abdominal cavity may cross over to the pleural space.

Treatments

Management of pleural effusion strives to relieve symptoms and improve quality of life. Cure is not always possible. The treatment method depends on the patient's age, prognosis, and location of the first tumor. Treatment for patients with pleural effusion who are asymptomatic (do not have symptoms) consists solely of observation.

Treatment options for pleural effusion include:

- Thoracentesis. Removal of the excess pleural fluid often relieves the symptoms of pleural effusion. However, effusion usually recurs within a few days. Repeat thoracentesis is not recommended, unless the patient has end-stage disease.
- Tube thoracostomy. A tube is inserted through the chest and into the pleural space to drain pleural fluid. When used alone, recurrence is very common.
- Indwelling pleural catheters. A thin flexible tube (catheter) is placed between the pleural cavity and

the chest skin to allow drainage of pleural fluid. This method allows for continual drainage of pleural fluid without much pain.

- Pleurodesis. After tube thoracostomy, one of any number of chemicals (sclerosing agents) is put into the pleural space to cause the visceral and parietal pleurae to stick together. Chemical pleurodesis is considered to be the treatment of choice for patients with malignant pleural effusion.
- Pleurectomy. Surgical removal of the parietal pleura through an incision in the chest wall (thoracotomy) is nearly 100% effective. Pleurectomy is not routinely performed and is reserved for patients for whom other treatments have failed. To be eligible for pleurectomy, the patient must have a long life expectancy and be able to tolerate major surgery.
- Pleuroperitoneal shunt. This procedure places a rubber tube between the pleural space and the abdominal cavity. A pump is used to move excess fluid out of the pleural space and into the abdominal cavity, where it would be absorbed. The patient must press the pump for several minutes four times daily. Although not frequently used, this is an effective treatment for cases that failed tube thoracostomy and pleurodesis.
- External radiation. Patients who have pleural effusion caused by blockage of a lymph duct may be treated by radiation therapy. External radiation therapy is successful for patients with pleural effusion related to lymphoma.
- Supportive care. Patients with end-stage cancer may not receive treatment for pleural effusion. Pain medications and oxygen therapy can be provided to keep the patient comfortable.

Belinda Rowland, Ph.D.

Pleurodesis

Definition

Pleurodesis is the adherence of the outer surface of a lung to the membrane surrounding that lung, which is performed to treat the buildup of fluid around the lung.

Purpose

The pleural space is the region between the outer surface of each lung (visceral pleurae) and the membrane that surrounds each lung (parietal pleurae). Under normal conditions, the pleurae are kept wet with pleural fluid to allow movement of the lungs within the chest. **Pleural effusion**, the accumulation of fluid in the pleural space, is most commonly caused by **cancer**. Pleurodesis causes the pleurae to stick together, thereby eliminating the pleural space and preventing fluid accumulation. Chemical pleurodesis is considered to be the standard of care for patients with malignant pleural effusion.

KEY TERMS

Pleural effusion—The abnormal buildup of fluid within the pleural space.

Pleural space—The space between the outer surface of each lung and the membrane that surrounds each lung.

Sclerosant—A chemical that causes the membranes of the pleural space to stick together.

Description

Before pleurodesis is conducted, all pleural fluid must be removed. This is achieved by inserting a chest tube through the skin and into the pleural space (thoracostomy). Insertion of the chest tube is carried out in the hospital. The patient is awake during the procedure. The skin is sterilized and a local pain killer is injected into the skin and underlying tissue. A small cut is made into the skin and a tube is placed into the pleural space. Fluid is withdrawn and the tube remains in place until all pleural fluid is drained, which usually takes two to five days. After the chest tube is inserted, the patient may either remain in the hospital or be allowed to return home with instructions on how to care for the tube. A chest x ray may be taken to ensure that all the fluid has been drained.

Pleurodesis is achieved by putting one of any number of chemicals (sclerosing agents or sclerosants) into the pleural space. The sclerosant irritates the pleurae which results in inflammation (pleuritis) and causes the pleurae to stick together. The patient is given a narcotic pain reliever and lidocaine, a local pain killer, is added to the sclerosant. A variety of different chemicals are used as sclerosing agents. There is no one sclerosant that is more effective or safer than the others. Commonly used sclerosants and their success rates are:

- Talc: 90–96%
- Nitrogen mustard: 52%

QUESTIONS TO ASK THE DOCTOR

- Will I be hospitalized the entire time?
- How long will I be hospitalized?
- Is it possible to do this on an outpatient basis?
- How uncomfortable is the chest tube?
- Will I be given pain medication as needed?
- Will having a chest tube limit my movements in any way?
- Will I be confined to bed?
- Which sclerosant will you be using?
- Why are you using this sclerosant?
- What are the side effects of this sclerosant?
- What is the success rate associated with this sclerosant?
- How painful is the pleurodesis process?

- Doxycycline: 90%
- Bleomycin: 84%
- Quinacrine: 70% to 90%

After the sclerosant has been put through the chest tube, the tube is closed. The patient may be asked to change position every 15 minutes for a two-hour time period. This was believed to be necessary to achieve an even distribution of sclerosant in the pleural space. However, recent evidence suggests that the sclerosant spreads throughout the pleural space immediately. Afterward, the chest tube is reopened and the sclerosant is sucked out of the pleural space. The tube remains in place for several days to allow all fluid to drain. Once drainage slows down, the chest tube is removed and the wound edges stitched (sutured) back together.

Aftercare

The patient should keep the wound from the chest tube clean and dry until it heals. Also, the patient should watch for signs of wound **infection** such as redness, swelling, and/or drainage, and be alert to symptoms indicating that the effusion recurred.

Risks

Complications of pleurodesis are uncommon and include infection, bleeding, acute respiratory distress syndrome, collapsed lung (pneumothorax), and respiratory failure. In addition, other complications may be specific for each sclerosant. Talc and doxycycline can cause **fever** and pain. Quinacrine can cause low blood pressure, fever, and hallucination. **Bleomycin** can cause fever, pain, and **nausea**. Severe respiratory complications can be fatal.

Normal results

Tube thoracostomy with pleurodesis is the most effective method to treat malignant pleural effusion. Successful pleurodesis prevents the recurrence of pleural effusion which relieves symptoms thereby improving quality of life.

Abnormal results

If drainage of sclerosant from the chest tube exceeds approximately one cup, the pleurodesis was unsuccessful and needs to be repeated. Pleurodesis may fail because of:

- trapped lung, in which the lung is enclosed in scar or tumor tissue
- formation of isolated pockets (loculation) within the pleural space
- loss of lung flexibility (elasticity)
- production of large amounts of pleural fluid
- extensive spread (metastasis) of pleural cancer
- improper positioning of the tube
- blockage or kinking of the tube

Resources

BOOKS

Baciewicz, Frank. "Malignant Pleural Effusion." In *Lung Cancer: Principles and Practice*, edited by Harvey Pass, James Mitchell, David Johnson, Andrew Turrisi, and John Mina. Philadelphia: Lippincott Williams & Wilkins, 2000, pp.1027–1037.

Schrump, David, and Dao Nguyen. "Malignant Pleural and Pericardial Effusions." In *Cancer: Principles & Practice of Oncology*, edited by DeVita, Vincent, Samuel Hellman, and Steven Rosenberg. Philadelphia: Lippincott Williams & Wilkins, 2001, pp.2729–44.

Works, Claire, and Mary Maxwell. "Malignant Effusions and Edemas." In *Cancer Nursing: Principles and Practice*, edited by Connie Yarbro, Michelle Goodman, Margaret Frogge, and Susan Groenwald. Boston: Jones and Bartlett Publishers, 2000, pp.813–830.

PERIODICALS

Colice, Gene, and Jeffrey Rubins. "Practical Management of Pleural Effusions: When and How Should Fluid Accumulations be Drained?" *Postgraduate Medicine* 105 (June 1999): 67–77.

Erasmus, Jeremy, Philip Goodman, and Edward Patz. "Management of Malignant Pleural Effusions and Pneumothorax." *Radiologic Clinics of North America: Interventional Chest Radiology* 38 (March 2000): 375–83.

Belinda Rowland, Ph.D.

Plicamycin

Definition

Plicamycin is an antibiotic also known as mithramycin; it is sold under the trade name Mithracin. The medicine kills **cancer** cells. It may be used to treat cancer of the testicles. In addition, it may be used as treatment for **hypercalcemia**. Hypercalcemia is a condition characterized by high levels of calcium in the blood.

Purpose

Plicamycin is a drug used to treat **testicular cancer** in patients who are not good candidates for either surgery or x-ray therapy. It was first approved for this use by the Food and Drug Administration (FDA) in May 1970.

Plicamycin is also used to treat hypercalcemia. Many patients with hypercalcemia also have elevated levels of calcium in the urine. As treatment for this condition, plicamycin may not be a doctor's first choice. The reason for this is that plicamycin may cause serious side effects. Newer medicines, known as **bisphosphonates**, can effectively resolve hypercalcemia and these have fewer side effects. However, some patients cannot tolerate bisphosphonates. These patients may be given plicamycin.

Description

Plicamycin is produced by a bacterium known as *Streptomyces argillaceus*. It interacts chemically with the DNA in cells and so interferes with the production of RNA. It is thought that plicamycin also works by making tumor cells more sensitive to **tumor necrosis factor** (TNF), a nonantibody protein secreted by cells in the immune system that kills tumor cells. Plicamycin lowers levels of calcium in the blood by affecting the formation of new bone cells and interfering with the activities of certain hormones.

A new form of plicamycin, mithramycin SK, was developed at the University of Kentucky in 2003 from a genetically modified form of *S. argillaceus*. Mithramycin SK is a more effective antitumor drug than the original plicamycin.

Recommended dosage

For testicular cancer, some doctors give 25 micrograms per kilograms of body weight every two to four days to start. However, if the patient has kidney or liver problems, these doctors may give 12.5 micrograms per kilogram instead. Others administer 25 to 30 micrograms per kilograms of body weight every eight to ten days. Others may give as much as 50 micrograms per kilogram of body weight per dose for approximately eight doses every other day.

For high levels of calcium in the blood and urine, 15 to 25 micrograms per kilogram of body weight may be given every day for three or four days. Following this, additional medication may be required approximately once a week.

KEY TERMS

Hypercalcemia—A condition characterized by high levels of calcium in the blood.

Precautions

This medication is often not given to patients with problems with blood clotting or with the bone marrow. Plicamycin should not be given to pregnant women, nursing mothers, or children younger than 15 years of age. The medicine should be used with caution in patients with liver or kidney problems. To lessen side effects to the digestive tract, the medicine may be administered over the course of four to six hours. Additional precautions should be followed to minimize the chances that the medicine will cause blistering.

Since people taking plicamycin are at increased risk of developing an **infection** and of having bleeding problems, they should avoid people who do have an infection. In addition, they should wash their hands before touching the inside of their mouth, their eyes, or their nose. Also, they should not take aspirin or over-the-counter preparations containing aspirin. In addition, they should attempt not to cause bleeding, for example when they brush and floss their teeth or when they shave.

Doctors should carefully monitor blood counts, liver function, and kidney function for patients given more than one dose of plicamycin.

Certain precautions should be followed by all patients. For example, plicamycin probably should not be taken by anyone who is living is a household with someone who has recently received oral polio vaccine, as there is a risk of transmission of the polio virus. The person receiving plicamycin should wear a face mask if she or he is going to be in close proximity to anyone who has recently received the oral polio vaccine for an extended period. In addition, **vaccines** containing live organisms should not be given to anyone who is taking plicamycin or anyone who recently took plicamycin.

Side effects

The side effects of plicamycin include a tendency for abnormal bleeding. There may be low levels of calcium, potassium, and phosphorous in the blood, as well as other blood problems. The face may become flushed. Kidney or liver problems may develop. If bleeding does occur there may be damage to the surrounding skin.

Other side effects may include **diarrhea**, loss of appetite (**anorexia**), **nausea and vomiting**, and soreness of the mouth. Muscle cramps and abdominal cramps may develop, although these are likely to disappear as the body gets used to the medication. Uncommon side effects include pain, soreness at the injection side, **fever**, weakness, headache, depressed mood, **fatigue**, and drowsiness.

The side effects of this medicine tend to increase as the dose of the medicine exceeds 30 micrograms per kilogram.

It is important to notify the doctor if any of the following symptoms of plicamycin overdose appear: **vomiting** of blood; yellow eyes or skin; bloody, or black, tarry stools; swelling of the face or redness of the face; skin rash; or the appearance of tiny red spots on the skin.

Resources

BOOKS

Beers, Mark H., MD, and Robert Berkow, MD, editors. "Calcium Metabolism." Section 2, Chapter 12 In *The Merck Manual of Diagnosis and Therapy*. Whitehouse Station, NJ: Merck Research Laboratories, 2002.

Beers, Mark H., MD, and Robert Berkow, MD, editors. "Testicular Cancer." Section 17, Chapter 233 in *The Merck Manual of Diagnosis and Therapy*. Whitehouse Station, NJ: Merck Research Laboratories, 2002.

Karch, A. M. *Lippincott's Nursing Drug Guide*. Springhouse, PA: Lippincott Williams & Wilkins, 2003.

PERIODICALS

Duverger, V., A. M. Murphy, D. Sheehan, et al. "The Anticancer Drug Mithramycin A Sensitises Tumour Cells to Apoptosis Induced by Tumour Necrosis Factor (TNF)." *British Journal of Cancer* 90 (May 17, 2004): 2025–2031.

Remsing, L. L., A. M. Gonzalez, M. Nur-e-Alam, et al. "Mithramycin SK, A Novel Antitumor Drug with Improved Therapeutic Index, Mithramycin SA, and Demycarosyl-Mithramycin SK: Three New Products Generated in the Mithramycin Producer *Streptomyces argillaceus* through Combinatorial Biosynthesis." *Journal of the American Chemical Society* 125 (May 14, 2003): 5745–5753.

ORGANIZATIONS

American Society of Health-System Pharmacists (ASHP). 7272 Wisconsin Avenue, Bethesda, MD 20814. (301) 657-3000. http://www.ashp.org.

United States Food and Drug Administration (FDA). 5600 Fishers Lane, Rockville, MD 20857-0001. (888) INFO-FDA. http://www.fda.gov.

Bob Kirsch
Rebecca J. Frey, Ph.D.

Ploidy analysis

Definition

Ploidy analysis is a test that measures the amount of DNA in tumor cells. It is also called DNA ploidy analysis.

Purpose

DNA ploidy analysis is used in addition to the traditional grading system as another way to evaluate how malignant a tumor might be. The advantage of this test is that it provides a numeric, and therefore objective, evaluation of how aggressive the **cancer** might be. Because this test was relatively new in 2001, and the significance of information gained by this test was not completely understood, this test had not yet replaced traditional systems of **tumor grading**. It would be used only to supplement those tests in order to give the doctor as much information about the nature of the tumor as possible. Doctors may also use this test to help predict how a tumor may respond to the planned therapy.

Precautions

This test requires a certain sample size in order to be performed; the specimens acquired in some biopsies may not provide enough material to run the test. It is also important in this test that only tumor material is used to create the population of cells which are analyzed, as any healthy tissue included can significantly affect the results. Interpretation of the numeric results of this test is still somewhat controversial. There is no commonly accepted system for interpreting the results; in addition, the results of the test can vary greatly from one part of a tumor to another.

QUESTIONS TO ASK THE DOCTOR

- Why did you order this test? What are you hoping it will tell us?
- What do the results mean?
- How much faith should I put in these results?
- Am I taking any medications that could influence the results of this test?
- Will my insurance company pay for this test?

KEY TERMS

Aneuploid—Any number of chromosomes except the normal two sets.

Diploid—Two sets of 23 chromosomes. The normal amount in a human cell.

Ploidy—The number of sets of 23 chromosomes a human cell has.

Tetraploid—Four sets of chromosomes. The normal amount in a human cell that is about to divide to form two new cells.

The way the test should be used for optimum results in the management of cancer patients remained questionable due to many unexplored issues, and results due to the lack of data accumulated so early into its history. Although research has shown that in general, patients whose tumors have lots of cells with abnormal amounts of DNA have shorter survival times, the results of the test have not, for the most part, been that successful in predicting how an individual patient will do.

Description

Ploidy analysis is performed on a sample of the tumor to determine how many of the cells have the normal amount of DNA and how many have more or less than the normal amount (called aneuploid). Cancerous cells are rapidly dividing cells. When cells divide there is a period before the actual division during which the cells have twice the normal amount of DNA. Tumors with higher proportions of aneuploid cells are generally considered to be more aggressive tumors.

Taking a sample of a tumor is called a **biopsy**. How and where that is done depends on where the tumor is located. Tissue from the surface of body cavities like the mouth or the vagina can be easily sampled from a simple scraping, in a doctor's office. For some types of tumors (such as in **breast cancer**) it is possible to extract enough cells with a needle and syringe. Often, however, a surgical biopsy will need to be performed in the hospital. The tissue removed will be taken to a laboratory and analyzed.

Preparation

Patient preparation for the collection of a tumor sample through biopsy will vary depending on the site of the tumor. Most biopsies call for little that the patient will need to do. For biopsies of internal organs the patient may need to avoid eating after midnight before the test, in case a complication occurs and surgery may be necessary. Patients should try not be fearful of the collection of the sample. Doctors will make the procedure as painless as possible by using appropriate anesthetic.

Aftercare

There can be a little soreness at the biopsy site for a few days following the procedure; acetominophen or another over-the-counter painkiller can be used if the patient feels a need for pain relief. If the site becomes swollen, red, or hot to the touch it may be infected and the patient should contact a physician.

Risks

The risks involved in this test are only the risks inherent in having a biopsy. Since this procedure uses tissue obtained through a biopsy already being performed for the purpose of grading the tumor, there are no additional risks to the patients involved as a result of the test. This test can also be performed on stored biopsy tissues that were obtained at some previous time.

Normal results

Normal cells, most of the time, have two sets of 23 chromosomes, one from each parent, for a total of 46 chromosomes. Normal cells contain four sets–or 92 total chromosomes–for a very brief time right before they divide. Normal tissues have a largely homogenous population of cells containing 46 chromosomes, with a very small percentage of dividing cells that contain 92.

Abnormal results

Tumors have lots of cells that are in the process of reproducing, so tumor tissues typically have a significant population of cells, containing four sets of chromosomes, that are about to divide, in addition to the large population of normal cells containing two sets of chromosomes. Tumor cells can also contain numerous other variations of normal. Any tissue comprised of significant numbers of cells that have anything but two sets of chromosomes would be considered abnormal.

See also DNA flow cytometry.

Resources

BOOKS

Freeman, J. Stuart, editor. *Cancer, Principles and Practice of Oncology*. Philadelphia: Lippincott, Williams & Wilkins, 2001.

OTHER

"DNA Ploidy 101." In *Prostate. Org*. [cited June 29, 2005]. http://www.prostate.org/.

Wendy Wippel, M.S.

Pneumonectomy

Definition

Pneumonectomy is the surgical removal of a lung.

Purpose

Pneumonectomy is most often used to treat lung **cancer** when less radical surgery cannot achieve satisfactory results. It also may be the most appropriate treatment for a tumor that is located near the center of the lung and that affects the pulmonary artery or veins, which transport blood between the heart and lungs. For the treatment of cancer, pneumonectomy may be combined with **chemotherapy** or **radiation therapy**. Pneumonectomy may also be the treatment of choice when traumatic chest injury has damaged the main air passage (bronchus) or the lung's major blood vessels so severely that they cannot be repaired. A form of this procedure known as extrapleural pneumonectomy is often used to treat malignant **mesothelioma**.

Precautions

Before scheduling a pneumonectomy, the surgeon reviews the patient's medical and surgical history and orders a number of tests to determine how successful the surgery is likely to be.

Blood tests, a bone scan, and **computed tomography** (CT) scans of the head and abdomen reveal whether the cancer has spread beyond the lungs. **Positron emission tomography** scanning (PET) is also used to help "stage" the disease. Cardiac screening indicates how well the patient's heart will tolerate the procedure, and extensive pulmonary testing (breathing tests and quantitative ventilation/perfusion scans) predicts whether the remaining lung will be able to compensate for the body's diminished breathing capacity.

Because extrapleural pneumonectomy is such an invasive operation, the patient must have no serious illness other than the cancer the surgery is designed to treat.

QUESTIONS TO ASK THE DOCTOR

- Why is it necessary to remove the whole lung?
- Why might I also need chemotherapy or radiation therapy?
- What should I do to prepare for this operation?
- How long will I have to stay in the hospital?
- Why is recovery such a slow process?

Description

Traditional pneumonectomy removes only the diseased lung. A more complex surgery generally performed in specialized medical centers, extrapleural pneumonectomy also removes:

- a section of the membrane (pericardium) covering the heart
- a portion of the muscular partition (diaphragm) that separates the chest and abdomen
- the membrane (parietal pleura) that lines the affected side of the chest cavity

General anesthesia is given to a patient undergoing either of these procedures. An intravenous (IV) line inserted into one arm supplies fluids and medication throughout the operation, which usually lasts between one and three hours; extrapleural pneumonectomies may last up to six hours.

The surgeon begins the operation by cutting a large opening on the side of the chest where the diseased lung is located. This posterolateral **thoracotomy** incision extends from below the shoulder blade, around the side of the patient's body, and along the curvature of the ribs at the front of the chest. Sometimes removing part of the fifth rib gives the surgeon a clearer view of the lung and makes it easier to remove the diseased organ.

KEY TERMS

Bronchopleural fistula—An abnormal connection between an air passage and the membrane that covers the lungs.

Empyema—Accumulation of pus in the lung cavity, usually as a result of infection.

Pleural space—A small space between the two layers of the membrane that covers the lungs and lines the inner surface of the chest.

Pulmonary embolism—Blockage of a pulmonary artery by a blood clot or foreign matter.

A surgeon performing a traditional pneumonectomy then:

- deflates (collapses) the diseased lung
- ties off the lung's major blood vessels to prevent bleeding into the chest cavity
- clamps the main bronchus to prevent fluid from entering the air passage
- cuts through the bronchus
- removes the lung
- staples or sutures the end of the bronchus that has been cut
- makes sure that air is not escaping from the bronchus
- inserts a temporary drainage tube between the layers of the pleura (pleural space) to draw air, fluid, and blood from the surgical cavity
- closes the chest incision

Besides removing the diseased lung, a surgeon performing an extrapleural pneumonectomy:

- cuts the pleura away from the chest wall
- removes parts of the pericardium and diaphragm on the affected side of the chest
- substitutes sterile synthetic patches for the tissue that has been removed
- closes the incision

Preparation

A patient who smokes must stop as soon as the disease is diagnosed.

A patient who takes aspirin or any other other blood-thinning medication must stop taking the medication about a week before the scheduled surgery, and patients may not eat or drink anything after midnight on the day of the operation.

Aftercare

Chest tubes drain fluid from the incision and a respirator helps the patient breathe for at least 24 hours after the operation. The patient may be fed and medicated intravenously. If no complications arise, the patient is transferred from the surgical intensive care unit (ICU) to a regular hospital room within one to two days.

A traditional pneumonectomy patient will probably be discharged within 10 days. A patient who has had an extrapleural pneumonectomy is likely to remain in the hospital between 10 and 12 days after the operation. While the patient is hospitalized, care focuses on:

- relieving pain
- monitoring to ensure that concentrations of oxygen in the blood do not become dangerously low (hypoexemia)
- encouraging the patient to walk in order to prevent formation of blood clots
- encouraging the patient to cough productively in order to clear accumulated lung secretions. If the patient cannot cough productively, the doctor uses a flexible tube (bronchoscope) to remove lung secretions and fluids (**bronchoscopy**).

Recovery is usually a slow process, with the remaining lung gradually taking on the tasks of the lung that has been removed and the patient gradually resuming normal, non-strenuous activities. Within eight weeks, a pneumonectomy patient who does not experience postoperative problems may be well enough to return to a job that is not physically demanding, but 60% of all pneumonectomy patients continue to experience marked shortness of breath six months after having surgery.

Risks

In the United States, the immediate survival rate from the surgery for patients who have had the left lung removed is between 96% and 98%. Due to the greater risk of complications involving the stump of the cut bronchus in the right lung, between 88% and 90% of patients survive removal of this organ.

Between 40% and 60% of pneumonectomy patients experience such short-term postoperative difficulties as:

- prolonged need for a mechanical respirator

- abnormal heart rate (cardiac arrhythmia), heart attack (myocardial infarction), or other heart problems
- pneumonia
- infection at the site of the incision
- a blood clot in the remaining lung (pulmonary embolism)
- an abnormal connection between the stump of the cut bronchus and the pleural space due to a leak in the bronchus stump (bronchopleural fistula)
- accumulation of pus in the pleural space (empyema)
- kidney or other organ failure

Over time, the chest's remaining organs may move toward the space created by the surgery. This condition is called postpneumonectomy syndrome, and a surgeon can correct it by inserting a fluid-filled prosthesis into the space the diseased lung occupied.

Normal results

The doctor will probably advise the patient to refrain from strenuous activities for a few weeks after the operation. Ribs that were cut during surgery will remain sore for some time.

A patient whose lungs have been weakened by noncancerous diseases like emphysema or chronic bronchitis may experience long-term shortness of breath as a result of this surgery.

Abnormal results

A patient who experiences a **fever**, chest pain, persistent cough, or shortness of breath, or whose incision bleeds or becomes inflamed, should notify his or her doctor immediately.

Resources

BOOKS

Pass, H., D. Johnson, et al. *Lung Cancer: Principles and Practice*. 2nd ed. Philadelphia: Lippincott Williams & Wilkins, 2000.

OTHER

ACS Cancer Resource Center. [cited July 17, 2005]. <http://www3.cancer.org/cancerinfo>.

"Pneumonectomy." [cited July 17, 2005]. http://www.intelihealth.com.

Maureen Haggerty

Pneumonia

Description

One of the most common pulmonary complications affecting **cancer** patients, pneumonia is a potentially life-threatening inflammation of one or both lungs.

Causes

Serious side effects in cancer patients most often occur in the lungs and may indicate that the cancer is progressing or that the patient has developed a new problem. Both cancer and the therapies used to treat it can injure the lungs or weaken the immune system in ways that make cancer patients especially susceptible to the bacteria, fungi, viruses, and other organisms that cause pneumonia.

Tumors and infections can block the patient's airway or limit the lungs' ability to rid themselves of fluid and other accumulated secretions that make breathing difficult. Other factors that increase a cancer patient's risk of developing pneumonia include:

- radiation therapy
- chemotherapy
- surgery
- depressed white blood cell count (neutropenia)
- antibiotics
- steroids
- malnutrition
- limited mobility
- splenectomy-immune system deficits

The risk of developing pneumonia is greatest for a cancer patient who has one or more additional health problems.

Treatments

Pneumonia in cancer patients must be treated promptly in order to speed recovery and prevent complications that could arise if the inflammation were allowed to linger. Treatment always includes bed rest and coughing to expel phlegm and other fluids from the lungs (productive cough). To determine which course of treatment would be most appropriate, a doctor considers when symptoms first appeared, what pattern the illness has followed, and whether cancer or its treatments have diminished the patient's infection-fighting ability (**immune response**).

A doctor generally prescribes broad-spectrum oral **antibiotics** if:

- the patient has had a fever for less than a week
- pneumonia has not spread beyond the lung area where it originated
- the patient's cancer is responding to treatment
- the patient is otherwise in good health

The doctor uses a flexible tube (bronchoscope) to examine the lungs and airway (**bronchoscopy**) for inflammation, swelling, obstruction, and other abnormalities and washes the lungs (bronchoalveolar lavage) with a mucus-dissolving solution if:

- pneumonia is extensive, aggressive, or severe
- antibiotics don't clear the infection
- the patient is very ill

The doctor may also remove a small piece of lung tissue (transbronchial **biopsy**) for microscopic examination and cultures, and prescribe medication to combat fungal and viral organisms that might be responsible for the patient's symptoms. If the patient's condition continues to worsen, the doctor may remove additional lung tissue (thoracic needle biopsy or open **lung biopsy**) for microscopic analysis and cultures.

Alternative and complementary therapies

Non-medical treatments will not cure pneumonia but may relieve symptoms and make the patient more comfortable. All of these therapies require the treating doctor's approval.

ACCUPUNCTURE. Accupuncture may relieve congestion and reduce **fatigue**.

ESSENTIAL OILS. Added to a warm bath or vaporizer, essential oils of eucalyptus (*Eucalyptus globus*), lavender (*Lavandula officinalis*), or pine (*Abies sibirica*) can create a fragrant steam that helps the patient breathe more easily. Because steam inhalations can irritate the lungs, individuals who have asthma should not use them.

POSTURAL DRAINAGE. A strenuous exercise that can help clear phlegm from the lungs, postural drainage should be practiced only with a doctor's approval and in the presence of a person who can provide support for a patient who becomes tired or weak.

Leaning over the side of the bed with forearms braced on the floor, the patient coughs up phlegm and spits it into a container. If the patient cannot cough productively enough to dislodge phlegm, the support person can help clear lung secretions by pounding gently on the patient's upper back. Postural drainage should be performed three times a day. Each session should last between five and 15 minutes, unless the patient tires or weakens sooner.

MASSAGE. After the patient's **fever** has broken, gently massaging the upper back may relieve congestion and encourage productive cough.

HERBAL REMEDIES. Homemade cough medicines (expectorants) containing licorice (*Glycyrrhiza glabra*), black cherry (*Prunus serotina*) bark, raw onions, honey, and other natural ingredients can relieve congestion and encourage productive cough. Because natural substances can be poisonous, they should be used only with a doctor's approval and according to label directions.

Eating raw garlic (*Allium sativum*) or taking garlic supplements is believed to strengthen the immune system. Echinacea, brewed as tea or taken in liquid or capsule form, may help some patients recover more quickly.

VITAMINS. Zinc supplements and large doses of **Vitamins** A, C, and E may strengthen the patient's immune system. Because large doses of some vitamins can cause **diarrhea** and other serious side effects, they should not be taken without a doctor's approval. Additionally, large doses of vitamins and herbal remedies may interfere with the primary cancer treatment programs. Approval from the treating doctor is imperative.

Resources

BOOKS

Ito, James, MD. "Infectious Complications." In *Cancer Management: A Multidisciplinary Approach*, edited by R. Pazdur, et al., 4th ed. New York: PRR Inc., 2000.

Stockdale-Wooley, R., and L. Norton. "Pulmonary Function." In *Handbook of Oncology Nursing*, edited by B. Johnson and J. Gross, 3rd ed. Sudbury, MA: Jones and Bartlett Publishers, 2001.

OTHER

"American Lung Association Fact Sheet." [cited July 3, 2005]. http://www.lungusa.org/diseases/pneumonia_factsheet.html.

Maureen Haggerty

Polyomavirus hominis type 1 (BK virus) infection

Definition

Infection with polyomavirus hominis type 1—commonly called BK virus or BKV—is ubiquitous in human populations. This pathogen normally causes problems only in immunocompromised individuals, primarily organ transplant recipients. However a possible association between BKV and various cancers is the subject of ongoing research.

Demographics

The vast majority of people become infected with BKV in early childhood, usually between the ages of four and five. Between 65% and 90% of all people are thought to be infected with BKV by the age of ten. The virus is found in humans throughout the world, except in a few very isolated communities. One study published in 2009 found that 92% of 451 control subjects had antibodies against BKV. Another 2009 study found that that 82% of healthy blood donors tested positive for BKV.

BKV infection usually becomes symptomatic only in patients with suppressed immune systems. It has been estimated that the virus causes polyomavirus-associated nephropathy (PVAN) in 1–10% of kidney transplant recipients. Other researchers have estimated that up to 10% of kidney transplants fail because of BKV infection. Following the first identification of BKV in 1971, there were very few additional reports until 1995, when it was identified in about 1% of kidney transplant recipients. By 2001 the incidence had risen to 5% of kidney transplant recipients. BKV infection can be a serious problem for other transplant recipients as well. A 2009 study found that 42% of lung transplant recipients excreted BKV in their urine, an indication of active infection.

There have been occasional reports of reactivated BKV infection and viral shedding in the urine of patients who are not immunosuppressed. There also have been reports of PVAN arising in non-transplanted kidneys.

Description

As a so-called "emerging virus," there remains a great deal to be learned about BKV. It was first isolated in 1971 from the urine of a Sudanese kidney transplant patient who was suffering from acute kidney failure and ureteral stenosis (constriction of the ureters—the ducts that carry urine from the kidney to the bladder). The virus was named with the patient's initials, B.K. There are two known species of polyoma virus that infect humans: BK (hominis 1) and JC (hominis 2). In healthy people BKV establishes a lifelong subclinical or latent infection, primarily in the kidneys and urinary tract. BKV replicates (reproduces itself) in the nuclei of proximal tubular cells of the human kidney and the daughter viruses then spread to other cells.

Organ transplant recipients are treated with drugs that suppress their immune systems to prevent rejection of the transplanted organs. This immunosuppression can allow BKV to reactivate, causing severe disease in the kidney (nephropathy) and/or urinary bladder. In addition to reactivation of latent virus, transplant patients can contract a primary BKV infection from the donor kidney or blood transfusions. Severe BKV nephritis (inflammation) or other PVAN is a major cause of graft loss in kidney transplant recipients.

BKV has emerged as a major pathogen in bone marrow transplant recipients. It is associated with late-onset hemorrhagic cystitis (inflammation and bleeding of the urinary bladder), a rare but serious complication of **bone marrow transplantation** in children. BKV also can cause hemorrhagic cystitis in HIV/AIDS patients and kidney disease in other organ transplant recipients, such as liver transplant patients.

It has been known for some time that BKV, as well as some other primate polyomaviruses, can cause tumors in experimental animals. Infection of rodents with BKV often results in tumor formation. BKV DNA encodes two oncoproteins, large tumor (T) antigen and small tumor (t) antigen. When these oncoproteins are co-expressed (produced) along with activated oncogenes (human genes that have the potential to cause **cancer**), cultured human cells can be transformed into cancer cells. Specifically, BKV large T antigen appears to interact with the human tumor suppressor gene p53 to deregulate the control of cell growth.

BKV gene sequences and proteins have been found in a variety of human tumors. It has been suggested that BKV is associated with the development of:

- bladder cancers, especially in transplant patients
- urinary tract cancer
- chronic lymphocytic leukemia
- neuroblastomas, the most common malignancy in infants
- brain cancer
- colorectal cancer
- prostate cancer

Although BKV has been detected in both normal and abnormal prostate cells, large T antigen is detected much more frequently in cancerous prostates than in normal prostates. One suggestion is that BKV interferes with tumor suppression by p53 in the early stages of cancer development. Nevertheless, as of 2009 no clear relationship has been established between BKV infection and any human cancer.

Risk factors

The primary risk factor for active BKV infection is immune system suppression due either to immunosuppressive drugs administered to transplant recipients or to diseases such as HIV/AIDS.

Causes and symptoms

Most people become infected with BKV in early childhood and perhaps even before birth. BKV is shed in saliva and may be transmissible through oral fluids. BKV can also be detected in 18% of stool samples from healthy adults and 46% of stool samples from hospitalized children. This suggests that BKV may be present in the gastrointestinal tract as well as the kidneys and that it may be transmitted through feces. Initial infection with BKV rarely causes symptoms. When they do occur, symptoms are a mild **fever** or similar to those of a respiratory flu infection.

Symptoms of active BKV infection include:

- fever
- kidney problems or renal failure following an organ transplant
- interstitial nephritis following a kidney transplant
- narrowed ureters following a kidney transplant
- hemorrhagic cystitis following bone marrow transplantation

The major symptom of hemorrhagic cystitis is painful urination. Symptoms of kidney disease may include:

- changes in urine or patterns of urination
- swelling in the legs, ankles, feet, face, and/or hands from the failure of the kidneys to remove excess fluid
- fatigue due to anemia
- skin rash or itching from the buildup of waste products in the blood
- a metallic taste in the mouth and bad breath
- nausea and vomiting
- shortness of breath
- chills
- dizziness and difficulty concentrating
- pain in the back or leg

Diagnosis

Examination

A complete medical history and physical examination will be performed.

QUESTIONS TO ASK YOUR DOCTOR

- How will you determine if my infection is caused by BKV?
- What treatments are available?
- What is my prognosis?
- Is my BKV infection likely to cause cancer?

Tests

The presence of BKV in the urine or blood serum indicates an active BKV infection.

Procedures

Diagnosis of PVAN requires a renal biopsy—the removal of a small amount of tissue from the kidney. The pathologist examines the tissue cells for changes that indicate polyomavirus activity. Immunohistochemical techniques are used to confirm infection with BKV.

Treatment

Traditional

The primary treatment for active BKV infection is the reduction of immunosuppressive therapy in transplant recipients. Following renal graft loss to PVAN, retransplantation is an option.

Drugs

BKV infection may be treated with the antiviral drugs vidarabine and cidofovir and the anti-inflammatory drug leflunomide.

Prognosis

Untreated PVAN has a poor prognosis. The more advanced the kidney damage at the time of diagnosis, the poorer the prognosis. Although antiviral drugs have been used successfully to treat BKV infection, organ failure is common in BKV-infected transplant patients. In one study BKV infection was associated with poorer survival among lung transplant patients.

Prevention

There is no known prevention for BKV infection. However it is recommended that kidney transplant recipients be screened for the presence of BKV prior to the onset of kidney disease.

Resources

BOOKS

Ahsan, Nasimul. *Polyomaviruses and Human Diseases.* New York: Springer Science, 2006.

PERIODICALS

Abend, J. R., M. Jiang, and M. J. Imperiale. "BK Virus and Human Cancer: Innocent Until Proven Guilty." *Seminars in Cancer Biology* 19, no. 4 (August 2009): 252-260.

Egli, Adrian, et al. "Prevalence of Polyoma Virus BK and JC Infection and Replication in 400 Healthy Blood Donors.' *Journal of Infectious Diseases* 199, no. 6 (March 15, 2009): 837-846.

OTHER

"Infection After Kidney Transplantation." *National Kidney Foundation*.http://www.kidney.org/professionals/kls/pdf/cme/mono_immuno_infect.pdf.

"Polyomaviruses." *MicrobiologyBytes*.http://www.microbiologybytes.com/virology/Polyomaviruses.html.

"Polyomaviruses.' *virology-online*.. http://virology-online.com/viruses/polyomaviruses.htm.

ORGANIZATIONS

National Institute of Diabetes and Digestive and Kidney Diseases (NIDDK), Building 31, Room 9A06, 31 Center Drive, MSC 2560, Bethesda, MD, 20892-2560, (301) 496-3583, http://www2.niddk.nih.gov.

National Kidney Foundation, Inc., 30 East 33rd Street, New York, NY, 10016, (212) 889-2210, (800) 622-9010, (212) 689-9261, http://www.kidney.org.

Margaret Alic, Ph.D.

Porfimer sodium

Definition

Porfimer sodium (trade name Photofrin) is a photosensitizing agent that belongs to a group of medicines known as antineoplastics. Porfimer sodium is sometimes called a hematoporphyrin derivative.

Purpose

Porfimer is used in a treatment called **photodynamic therapy** (PDT). This form of **cancer** treatment is for patients presenting with obstructing esophageal and endobronchial non-small cell lung cancers (NSCLC) and early stage radiologically occult endobronchial cancer. As of the early 2000s, PDT is considered an experimental treatment for cancer of the esophagus. In 2003, however, the Food and Drug Administration (FDA) added **Barrett's esophagus** to the list of conditions for which Photofrin is an approved treatment. Some patients with Barrett's esophagus develop precancerous lesions that respond well to treatment with porfimer sodium.

As of 2004, PDT is being studied as a treatment for **breast cancer** that has progressed to the chest wall. Of one group of 14 patients, nine demonstrated a complete response to PDT.

Another new development is the use of porfimer sodium to treat cancers in the abdominal cavity and the brain. A group of researchers in Boston have used a needle to insert a small-diameter quartz optical fiber that transmits laser light to the pancreas, liver, and spleen to activate the Photofrin. A second team in Salt Lake City has used a new light-delivery device based on light-emitting diode (LED) technology to administer PDT to patients with recurrent **brain tumors**.

KEY TERMS

Antineoplastic—An agent that inhibits or prevents the maturation and proliferation of malignant cells.

Free radicals—Highly reactive molecules that act as agents of tissue damage.

Necrosis—The sum of all the morphological changes that indicate cell death.

Oncologist—A physician who specializes in the diagnosis and treatment of cancer patients.

Photodynamic therapy—Cancer treatment that uses the interaction between laser light and an agent that makes cells more sensitive to light.

Photosensitizing agents—Ultraviolet or sunlight-activated drugs used in the treatment of certain cancer types.

Porphyrins—Pigments found in the body that have an active affinity for metals.

Radiologically occult—Radiologically unapparent or undefined.

Description

The FDA granted its original approval to porfimer sodium in December 1995. Porfimer is a chemical mixture of up to eight porphyrin units. The freeze-dried compound exists as a dark red to reddish-brown cake or powder and is typically reconstituted with 5% dextrose or 0.9% sodium chloride. Porfimer sodium's antitumor effects are dependent upon its activation by a specific wavelength of light that results in the subsequent release of highly toxic oxygen-free radicals.

Additionally, PDT using porfimer produces a significant decrease in blood flow to the treatment area that enhances necrosis in certain tumor cells. Clinical test results suggest that use of porfimer sodium for the palliative management of **esophageal cancer**, and NSCLC yields a statistically significant improvement after a single course of therapy. Porfimer sodium and the associated laser treatment have not been formally tested in conjunction with other photosensitizing compounds. However, it may be speculated that an increase in the photosensitive reaction would result.

Recommended dosage

The dose of porfimer sodium will vary among patients. The oncologist will make a final dose determination based on a number of factors, including body weight. An appropriate starting regimen for adults would be:

- 2mg porfimer per kg of body weight injected into a vein.
- Approximately 48 hours post injection, tumor illumination with a laser light source set at 630nm wavelength.
- Two to three days post tumor illumination, the physician will remove the destroyed cancer cells.
- If prescribed, a second laser treatment may be given 96–120 hours after the initial porfimer injection followed by subsequent removal of destroyed cancer cells.
- Patients may receive a second dose of porfimer at a minimum of 30 days from the initial treatment for up to three cycles, each 30 days apart.

Precautions

All patients who have received PDT must avoid exposure of the skin and eyes to direct sunlight and bright indoor lighting for a minimum of 30 days. In July 2000, the FDA added the following to patient information labeling of Photofrin: "Some patients may remain photosensitive for up to 90 days or more." Sensitivity is produced from the residual porfimer that has not cleared the patient's system; therefore, ambient indoor lighting will help to gradually quench the photosensitive effect. Intermittent exposure trials of a small patch of skin to direct sunlight should be conducted in 10-minute segments beginning 30 days after PDT, and before returning to normal outdoor activities. If no photosensitive reaction (redness, edema, blistering) is apparent 24 hours after exposure, cautious and gradually increased exposure may continue. If the test results are positive, patients should continue precautions for an additional two weeks before repeating the exposure test. Over-the-counter sunscreens are of no use because the photo activation of porfimer occurs in the visible light range. Patient eye sensitivity should be guarded for a minimum of 30 days by wearing dark sunglasses that allow for no greater than 4% of available white light to pass through the lenses. PDT treatment scheduling before or after **radiation therapy** should be properly spaced to avoid any cumulative inflammatory response from one treatment regimen to the next. A two- to four-week recovery phase between treatment types is recommended. Careful monitoring of endobronchial lesion patients is required to reduce the risk of respiratory distress caused by necrotic tissue obstructing the airway. These patients are also at risk from bleeding problems associated with erosion into a major blood vessel. As with all **antineoplastic agents**, pregnancy should be avoided. If the patient is pregnant, PDT should only be used if the potential benefits outweigh the risks to the fetus.

Side effects

Side effects are associated with all antineoplastic drugs, and patients should be instructed to discuss any concerns. Side effects produced with porfimer that may engender patient concern, but do not typically require medical attention, may include mild **diarrhea** or constipation, mild **nausea and vomiting**, blistering, redness or swelling of the skin, difficulty sleeping, weakness, and vision changes. These conditions usually subside as the body adjusts to the porfimer. Side effects associated with porfimer sodium that do require immediate medical attention include:

- shortness of breath or trouble breathing
- fast or irregular heartbeat
- high or low blood pressure
- spitting blood
- severe stomach, abdominal, or chest pain
- chills or fever
- dizziness or fainting
- coughing or wheezing
- unusual weight gain
- excessive fatigue or weakness
- swelling in the face, feet, neck, or lower legs
- white patches in the mouth
- tightness in the chest
- yellow coloration of the eyes or skin

Interactions

There have been no formal interaction studies between porfimer and other drugs. One may speculate on the possible synergistic effects of porfimer in conjunction with other photosensitizing agents, such as phenothiazines, chlorpropramide, **demeclocycline**, doxycycline, and tetracycline. Animal research studies suggest certain compounds decrease the effectiveness of porfimer used in PDT. These inhibitors include drug compounds such as dimethyl sulfoxide (DMSO) and ethanol that act by inhibiting the formation of free radicals. Other drug groups, such as thromboxane A_2 inhibitors, inhibit by decreasing clotting, vasoconstriction, or platelet aggregation. Other pre-clinical trial data suggests a decrease in porfimer efficacy in PDT in response to glucocorticoids hormones, calcium channel blockers, and prostagladin synthesis inhibitors. As with any course of treatment, patients should first notify their doctors of any medications they are taking.

Resources

BOOKS

Beers, Mark H., MD, and Robert Berkow, MD, editors. "Tumors of the Gastrointestinal Tract." Section 3, Chapter 34 In *The Merck Manual of Diagnosis and Therapy*. Whitehouse Station, NJ: Merck Research Laboratories, 2004.

PERIODICALS

Chan, H. H., N. S. Nishioka, M. Mino, et al. "EUS-Guided Photodynamic Therapy of the Pancreas: A Pilot Study." *Gastrointestinal Endoscopy* 59 (January 2004): 95–99.

Cuenca, R. E., R. R. Allison, C. Sibata, and G. H. Downie. "Breast Cancer with Chest Wall Progression: Treatment with Photodynamic Therapy." *Annals of Surgical Oncology* 11 (March 2004): 322–327.

Schmidt, M. H., G. A. Meyer, K. W. Reichert, et al. "Evaluation of Photodynamic Therapy Near Functional Brain Tissue in Patients with Recurrent Brain Tumors." *Journal of Neurooncology* 67 (March-April 2004): 201–207.

OTHER

FDA Medwatch, July 2000. http://www.fda.gov/medwatch/safety/2000/jul00.htm#photof.

Food and Drug Administration, Center for Drug Evaluation and Research (CDER).*CDER Report to the Nation: 2003*. http://www.fda.gov/cder/reports/rtn/2003/rtn2003-1.HTM.

ORGANIZATIONS

United States Food and Drug Administration (FDA). 5600 Fishers Lane, Rockville, MD 20857-0001. (888) INFO-FDA. http://www.fda.gov.

Jane Taylor-Jones, MS
Rebecca J. Frey, Ph.D.

Positron emission tomography

Definition

Positron emission tomography (PET) is a highly specialized imaging technique using short-lived radiolabeled substances to produce powerful images of the body's biological function.

Purpose

Besides being used to investigate the metabolism of normal organs, PET has also become the technique of choice to investigate various neurological diseases and disorders, including stroke, epilepsy, Alzheimer's disease, Parkinson's disease, and Huntington's disease. Various psychiatric disorders, such as schizophrenia, **depression**, obsessive-compulsive disorder, attention-deficit/hyperactivity disorder, and Tourette syndrome, are also imaged by PET.

PET is especially useful in the context of **cancer** because it can detect metastatic tumors that may not be visualized by other imaging techniques. It is also being increasingly used not only as a cancer diagnostic tool, but also to help physicians design the most beneficial therapies. For example, it may be used to assess response to **chemotherapy**. PET imaging is very accurate in differentiating malignant from benign cell growths, and in assessing the spread of malignant tumors. PET is also used to detect recurrent **brain tumors** and cancers of the lung, colon, breast, lymph nodes, skin, and other organs.

Precautions

In some cases, patients may be allergic to the radioactive agents used for PET. A patient with known allergies should discuss this with his or her specialist before undergoing the PET scan.

Description

PET is used in conjunction with compounds that closely resemble a natural substance used by the body, such as a simple sugar (e.g. glucose), labeled with a radioactive atom and injected into the patient. These compounds (radionuclides or **radiopharmaceuticals**) emit particles called positrons. As positrons emitted from the radionuclides encounter electrons in the body, they produce high-energy photons (gamma rays) that can be recorded as a signal by detectors surrounding the body. The radionuclides move through the body and accumulate in the organs targeted for examination. A computer collects the distribution of radioactivity and reassembles them into actual images.

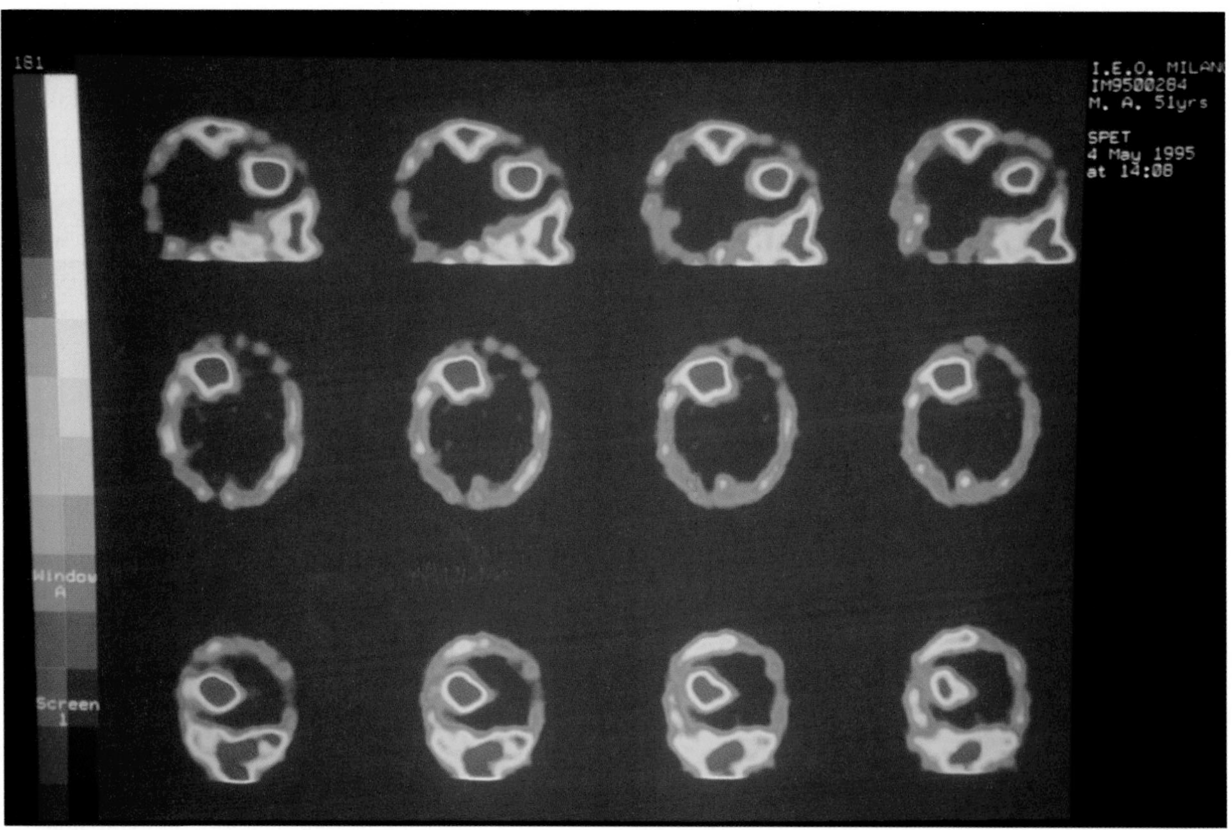

Positron emission tomography (PET) images of an oncology patient's brain. PET imaging can be used to differentiate between malignant and benign cell growths, assess the spread of malignant tumors, and detect recurrent brain tumors. *(Custom Medical Stock Photo. Reproduced by permission.)*

QUESTIONS TO ASK THE DOCTOR

- How many PET scans will I have to undergo?
- Are there any risks associated with the radiopharmaceuticals that will be injected?
- How reliable are PET scans for my type of cancer?

By further defining a lesion seen on other imaging modalities, PET may enhance assessment of tumors exceedingly well. This is because of its operating principle. The radiolabeled sugars injected into the patient will be used by all body cells, but more sugar will be used by cells that have an increased metabolism. Cancer cells are highly metabolic, meaning that they use more sugar than healthy nearby cells, and they are easily seen on the PET scan. PET images thus show the chemical functioning of an organ or tissue, unlike x ray, **computed tomography**, or **magnetic resonance imaging**, which show only body structure.

Preparation

The radiopharmaceutical is given by intravenous injection or inhaled as a gas a few minutes before the PET procedure. How it is administered depends on the radiopharmaceutical used and which one is selected depends on what organ or body part is being scanned. During the scan, the patient lies comfortably; the only discomfort involved may be the pinprick of a needle used to inject the radiopharmaceutical.

Aftercare

No special aftercare measures are indicated for PET.

Risks

Some of radioactive compounds used for PET scanning can persist for a long time in the body. Even though only a small amount is injected each time, the long half-lives of these compounds can limit the

KEY TERMS

Benign growth—A noncancerous cell growth that does not metastasize and does not recur after treatment or removal.

Cancer screening—A procedure designed to detect cancer even though a person has no symptoms, usually performed using an imaging technique.

CT scan—An imaging technique that uses a computer to combine multiple x-ray images into a two-dimensional cross-sectional image.

Electron—One of the small particles that make up an atom. An electron has the same mass and amount of charge as a positron, but the electron has a negative charge.

Gamma ray—A high-energy photon, emitted by radioactive substances.

Half-life—The time required for half of the atoms in a radioactive substance to disintegrate.

Malignant growth— A cell growth or tumor that becomes progressively worse and that can metastasize elsewhere in the body.

Metabolism—The sum of all physical and chemical processes occurring in the body to maintain its integrity and also the transformations by which energy is made available for its uses.

MRI—A special imaging technique used to image internal parts of the body, especially soft tissues.

Photon—A light particle.

Positron—One of the small particles that make up an atom. A positron has the same mass and amount of charge as an electron, but the positron has a positive charge.

number of times a patient can be scanned. However, PET is a relatively safe procedure. PET scans using radioactive fluorine result in patients receiving exposures comparable to (or less than) those from other medical procedures, such as the taking of **x rays**. Other scanning radiopharmaceuticals—for instance, 6-F-dopa or radioactive water—normally cause even less exposure.

Normal results

The PET scan of a healthy organ or body part will yield images without contrasting regions, because the radiolabeled sugar will have been metabolised at the same rate.

Abnormal results

The PET scan of a diseased organ or body part however, will yield images showing contrasting regions, because the radiolabeled sugar will not have been metabolized at the same rate by the healthy and diseased cells.

See also Imaging studies; Nuclear medicine scans.

Resources

BOOKS

von Schulthess, G.K., editor. *Clinical Positron Emission Tomography*. Philadelphia: Lippincott, Williams & Wilkins, 1999.

PERIODICALS

Anderson, H., and P. Price. "What Does Positron Emission Tomography Offer Oncology?" *European Journal of Cancer* 36 (October 2000): 2028–35.

Arulampalam, T. H., D.C. Costa, M. Loizidou, D. Visvikis, P.J. Ell, and I.Taylor. "Positron Emission Tomography and Colorectal Cancer." *British Journal of Surgery* 88 (February 2001): 176–89.

Roelcke, U., and K.L. Leenders. "PET in Neuro-oncology." *Journal of Cancer Research and Clinical Oncology* 127 (January 2001): 2–8.

Lisa Christenson
Monique Laberge, Ph.D.

Prednimustine

Definition

Prednimustine is one of a group of antineoplastic (antitumor) drugs known as alkylating agents. As of mid-2001, it is an investigational drug.

Purpose

Prednimustine has been used in the treatment of **chronic lymphocytic leukemia**, non-Hodgkin's lymphomas, and other malignant conditions including **breast cancer**.

Description

Prednimustine is one of a group of drugs based on the mustard gas used as a weapon in World War I. Like many antineoplastic (antitumor) therapies, prednimustine acts by killing quickly growing cells. Since cancerous cells are generally growing faster than normal cells, drugs that kill quickly growing cells generally affect tumors more than normal cells. However, some normal

KEY TERMS

Investigational drug—A drug that has not been approved for marketing by the FDA. These drugs are generally available to patients through participation in research studies.

cells, such as white blood cells and platelets, also grow quickly and can be severely affected by antineoplastic drugs. Antitumor therapies create a situation in which the drug is racing to kill the tumor before it causes irreparable damage to normal tissues. The ideal situation is one in which the growth of the tumor is severely affected, but the growth of normal cells is unaffected. However, not every situation is ideal. Some patients taking antitumor drugs may have to discontinue treatment due to the severity of the drug's side effects.

Prednimustine probably kills rapidly growing cells by modifying cell's DNA with a chemical structure called an alkyl group. Thus, it is included in the group of alkylating agents. Prednimustine is a combination of two drugs joined together: **chlorambucil** (an alkylating agent) and methylprednisolone (a steroid).

Prednimustine is an investigational drug in the United States. This means that the FDA has not approved this drug for marketing in the U.S., as of mid-2001. Generally, **investigational drugs** are made available through participation in research studies.

Many drugs have toxic side effects, some of which are difficult to detect. **Clinical trials** are used to determine the side effects, drug interactions, and precautions for medicines, as well as their efficacy. Successful completion of multi-step clinical trials results in FDA approval of a drug. Many drugs that are used in clinical trials never gain FDA approval, however, possibly because of severe side effects which outweigh the benefits of the medication, or because the medication does not perform the function for which it was tested. Final approval of a drug is also expensive. Some drugs may not receive the financial support necessary to achieve final approval.

Recommended dosage

Since prednimustine is investigational, there is no recommended dosage. Various dosing schedules have been reported in the literature for different cancers.

Precautions

Patients who take this drug should avoid pregnancy, since this drug may cause fetal abnormalities.

Side effects

In the published reports of prednimustine use, the most common side effect is **myelosuppression**, the damage to white blood cells and platelets. Such damage may result in **infection** and bleeding, respectively. Steroid side effects, such as fluid retention and high glucose, have also been reported.

Interactions

As of mid-2001, information on the interactions of prednimustine is not available.

See also Chlorambucil.

Michael Zuck, Ph.D.

Prednisone *see* **Corticosteroids**

Pregnancy and cancer

Definition

For the most part, **cancer** that strikes during a pregnancy is unrelated to the pregnancy. The exception is choriocarcinoma. This cancer is only found in pregnancy.

Description

Pregnancy can be a joyous time for a woman, but when cancer is diagnosed, a tremendous dilemma can arise, both for the woman and for her health care providers. Cancer is not common in pregnancy, and is rarely the cause of maternal mortality. However, in any pregnancy there are always two patients to consider—the mother and the fetus. When a pregnant woman has cancer, the health of the mother may be pitted against the well-being of the fetus. For women who do not have regular medical visits, pregnancy may be a time for regular prenatal visits. For them, screenings done in pregnancy may serve as an opportunity to detect a hidden cancer.

Interestingly, pregnancy also has some protective effects against **breast cancer**. Studies have firmly established that early full-time pregnancy helps lower risk for breast cancer for a woman's lifetime.

Choriocarcinoma arises from embryonic fetal tissue called the chorion and chorionic villi. It may be associated with a molar pregnancy, an ectopic pregnancy, and may even develop after the delivery of a

KEY TERMS

Cesarean section—This procedure to deliver a baby involves an incision made through the abdominal wall and into the uterus to extract the baby.

Colposcopy—During a colposcopy a practitioner uses a special lighted instrument with magnification lenses (called a colposcope) to clearly visualize and examine the vagina and cervix. This procedure may be done when a Pap smear has come back showing suspicious or abnormal cells. If an area of the vagina or cervix looks suspicious in any way the practitioner may take a sample of tissue, called a biopsy, for further review by a pathologist.

Ectopic pregnancy—A pregnancy that occurs outside the uterus, most commonly in a fallopian tube. Early detection is important to avoid potential rupture of the fallopian tube as the fetus grows.

Hydatiform mole—A hydatiform mole is characterized by a larger-than-normal-for-dates uterus, vaginal bleeding, and the presence of multiple cysts stemming from the degeneration of chorionic villi, the early fetal tissue that imbedded into the uterine lining with placental and embryo implantation.

Interdisciplinary team—A group of health care providers from a variety of specialties that meet as a team to address the various needs of a patient. For a woman with cancer, the team may consist of an obstetrician, gynecologic oncologist, radiologist, neonatologist, social worker, nurse specialists, as well as others specific to the needs of a particular patient.

Microcephaly—Microcephaly is a congenital anomaly in which the head is small in proportion to the body. The brain is also underdeveloped, and there is some mental retardation.

Molar pregnancy—A molar pregnancy may be either complete or partial. In a partial mole, there may be a fetal sac, and even initial fetal heart tones. However, the fetus has multiple anomalies, does not grow properly, and eventually dies. When vaginal bleeding occurs the molar pregnancy is discovered, and needs to be evacuated to avoid retention of the tissue. In a complete mole, the ovum is fertilized but contains no genetic material. The embryo is unable to survive for very long. Complete evacuation of the uterus in necessary to avoid the development of choriocarcinoma.

Teratogenic—A substance or process affecting normal fetal development, leading to congenital malformations. Teratogens include alcohol, certain medications, and radiation.

normal fetus. It may be referred to as gestational trophoblastic disease (GTD), or gestational trophoblastic tumor. A non-malignant form is a hydatiform mole, but the tissue can become cancerous. Vaginal bleeding and high beta human chorionic gonadotropin (hCG) levels characterize the condition.

Ultrasound is effective in evaluating the mass to establish the presence or absence of a fetus and of a fetal heartbeat. The tissue must be evacuated and sent to pathology for evaluation. If cancerous cells are found, **chemotherapy** is begun. Chemotherapy has been shown to be extremely effective in treating choriocarcinoma. If left untreated, choriocarcinoma readily metastasizes, or spreads to other organs.

Incidence of GTD rises with maternal age. Women who desire future pregnancies should discuss this as part of the treatment plan to ensure fertility-sparing choices. Some women normally have high hCG levels. If they have some abnormal vaginal bleeding they can be incorrectly diagnosed as having choriocarcinoma if they have a high hCG level without other evidence of a pregnancy. Before undergoing chemotherapy or surgery, women should have a urine pregnancy test done as well, and/or have blood hCG tests done that are able to discriminate between various forms of hCG. Some laboratory hCG tests have a high false-positive rate, and are not designed to screen for hCG that is associated with cancer.

The most common cancers occurring during pregnancy, in descending order are:

- Cervical cancer. About 0.5 to 5.0% of cervical cancers occur in pregnant women, and about one-third of women are under 35 when given the diagnosis. Survival rates for pregnant versus non-pregnant women are similar. It is safe to have a Pap smear during a prenatal visit. Suspicious findings may lead to a colposcopy and biopsy. There may be increased bleeding from the biopsy site in the pregnant woman. If cervical cancer is found, the stage of cancer and trimester of pregnancy will determine if immediate surgery is needed or if treatment can be postponed until the fetus matures. With cervical cancer a cesarean delivery will be recommended, perhaps before full term of 40 weeks if the fetus' lungs are sufficiently mature.

QUESTIONS TO ASK THE DOCTOR

- What type and stage is my cancer?
- If I were not pregnant how would you treat it?
- Since I am pregnant, how do you suggest treating it?
- What is the expected effect on my baby from the treatment?
- What is my prognosis?
- What part of the treatment can safely wait until after I deliver?
- What side effects can I expect from the treatment?
- What are the risks to me from this treatment?
- How will these treatments be managed?
- What long-term effects will my treatment have on my child?
- What alternative treatments are available to help me?
- Which members of my team are experienced in cancer and pregnancy?

- Breast cancer. Breast cancer occurs in about one out of every 3,000 pregnancies. As in non-pregnant women, infiltrating ductal carcinoma is the most prevalent type. When determining the type and stage, the tumor also will be evaluated for being estrogen receptor positive or negative (ER-positive, ER-negative). Pregnancy hormones accelerate the growth of ER-positive tumors. Pregnancy has less of an impact on ER-negative tumors. The pregnancy hormones can alter the test results and increase the number of false negatives of hormone receptor testing. Because of the normal breast changes in pregnancy, it is more difficult to detect a lump when pregnant, so diagnosis may be delayed while the tumor continues to grow. Pregnancy also increases the density of the breast and makes mammography less sensitive. Ultrasound can be used to differentiate between a fluid-filled lump and a solid tumor. About 67% of pregnant women with breast cancer have positive lymph nodes versus 38% of non-pregnant women. Studies indicate that about 47% of pregnant women with positive lymph nodes reach five-year survival versus 59% of non-pregnant women with positive nodes. For lactating women, some of the signs of mastitis are similar to the signs of inflammatory breast cancer. The diagnosis of cancer may be delayed because of the confusion. Some studies indicate that if an abscess is drained from a breast with mastitis, a sample should be sent to pathology. Pregnant women may experience bleeding from any procedures done on the breast due to increased vascularity.
- Melanoma. The average age for malignant melanoma is 45. About 30–40% of cases appear during the childbearing years. About 8% of women are pregnant at the time of diagnosis. During pregnancy the thickness of the lesion is greater, and nodal metastases more frequently occur. If there has been nodal metastasis, survival may be less than three years. Melanoma also can spread to the placenta and to the fetus. However, prognosis for the pregnant woman is greater if she carries to term (66.5% survival at five years), than if the pregnancy is terminated following diagnosis (33.5% survival at five years). Because most lesions appear on the extremities, treatment may begin during the pregnancy.
- Hodgkin's disease. Hodgkin's occurs about one in six thousand pregnancies. The average age for a diagnosis of Hodgkin's is 30. However, the prognosis for the pregnant woman is about the same as for a non-pregnant woman. Signs such as fever, night sweats, and unexplained weight loss indicate a higher stage of disease. A nodal biopsy can safely be done during pregnancy, but pregnancy can alter the test results. Treatment may include a short course of chemotherapy and radiation to the affected nodal area if the fetus can be adequately shielded. If this cannot be done safely, radiation may wait until after delivery. Nodal sclerosis is a common subtype of Hodgkin's and is frequently seen in adolescents and young adults. Non-Hodgkin's lymphoma is usually seen after the childbearing years.
- Ovarian cancer is extremely rare during pregnancy; only 1:10,000 to 1:100,000 full term deliveries are cases of this cancer. It is usually low grade and low stage (Stage 1) cancer. Germ cell malignancies are the most common form of ovarian cancer in young women. Germ cell cancer can grow very rapidly, so immediate chemotherapy will be discussed. During pregnancy alpha-fetoprotein levels are tested to check if the fetus may have a neural tube defect. However, this same test is used in the non-pregnant woman as a screening for germ cell cancer. Older women are more prone to epithelial and low malignancy potential ovarian cancers. It may be the prenatal ultrasound that first alerts a woman to her having ovarian cancer. The cancer tumor marker CA-125 is unreliable in pregnancy, as the levels go up during this time. Ovarian tumors may undergo torsion, or twisting, creating extreme pain that may

be mistaken for appendicitis or an ectopic pregnancy if gestation is still early.

- Colorectal cancer is the third most common cancer in women, with 67,000 cases in 1999. About 10% of cases occur in patients under the age of 40; only about 2% of cases occur under the age of 30. Early occurrence is linked with high risk. There may be a delay in diagnosis, as some of the symptoms of colorectal cancer overlap symptoms seen in pregnancy. Because of the delay, a higher degree of disease may present at diagnosis. Women considering pregnancy should request screening prior to becoming pregnant. Signs of colorectal cancer include: nausea, abdominal bloating, backache, rectal bleeding, pain, and a change in bowel habits.
- Leukemia is quite rare during pregnancy, occurring in one out of 75,000 pregnancies. During pregnancy, acute myelocytic leukemia is usually the form seen. If treatment is begun right away, the prognosis for the pregnant woman is similar to that of the non-pregnant woman. Complete remission rates are also similar. Untreated, the disease can be rapidly fatal. The woman with leukemia is at greater risk for miscarriage, fetal growth retardation, prematurity and stillbirth.

Causes

As women delay their childbearing years into their forties and even fifties, an increase of cancer during pregnancy is occurring. This is due to the overlap of childbearing with the usual times of occurrence of certain cancers. The exact cause of most cancers is not yet known. However, estrogen is known to play a role in the development of endometrial and ovarian cancers. Research has shown that smoking increases the risk of developing **cervical cancer**, as well as other cancers.

Special concerns

Decisions need to be made about commencing treatment, or delaying treatment until after the pregnancy is finished. Accurate staging of the tumor will be critical. The woman will be asked if the pregnancy is desired. If not, and if the gestation is less than 24 weeks, therapeutic abortion may be considered. Depending on the type and stage of the cancer, a delay in treatment might not affect the mother's prognosis. Fetal lung maturity may be monitored, so that a safe early delivery can be planned. As the fetus nears term, there is a significant decrease in morbidity and mortality for every extra two weeks it remains in utero.

A pregnant woman with cancer has a great need for an interdisciplinary team of experienced practitioners. Oncologists who have experience with treatment during pregnancy may be able to offer more choices for treating the cancer while maintaining a viable pregnancy. Practitioners also need experience in managing the treatment side effects in a safe way for the fetus. For example, corticosteroid use can increase the incidence of cleft palate, and affect maternal glucose intolerance.

Pregnant women should not take any over-the-counter medication, including herbal supplements, without first consulting their obstetrical provider. Medications and supplements considered safe for a non-pregnant woman may have harmful effects on the fetus.

Treatments

Cancer treatment usually involves some combination of surgery, radiation and chemotherapy. During the first trimester, or the first 12 weeks of gestation, the fetus' organs are developing and are very susceptible to teratogenic substances (substances that affect normal fetal development). When treatment is undertaken, it is most commonly in the second trimester, when early fetal development has already taken place.

When contemplating surgery during pregnancy, the risks for both mother and fetus must be considered. Abdominal surgery poses the greatest risk to the pregnancy, however some women can successfully have an ovary removed and still bring a healthy fetus to term. The removal of the ovary needs to take place after the first trimester, once the placenta has taken over the progesterone hormone production of the corpus luteum. General anesthesia is often chosen for surgery. The safest time for surgery is during the second trimester, but the risk of preterm labor, intrauterine growth retardation, and fetal death still exists. **Mastectomy** is often recommended for the treatment of breast cancer during pregnancy, although breast-conserving surgery may also be an option.

In the first 10 days following conception, radiation may kill the fetus, or may have no effect at all. From 10 days to 14 weeks, a fetus exposed to radiation is at risk for:

- intrauterine growth retardation
- central nervous system (CNS) abnormalities
- microcephaly
- severe mental retardation
- eye anomalies

From eight weeks until term, the fetus is still at risk for CNS abnormalities and milder forms of microcephaly and mental retardation from radiation. If the mother receives high doses of radiation, intrauterine death may occur. Because of the scarcity of research data, the *threshold dose* is unknown. **Childhood cancers**, other cancers later in life, and cancer appearing in later generations are also of concern. Research evaluating the outcome of the children of pregnant women exposed to the atomic bomb in Japan indicates the effects of radiation exposure may show up even five generations later.

When deciding on chemotherapy during pregnancy, several factors are considered:

- which chemotherapy drugs are effective for the woman's particular type of cancer, and of these which are safe for the developing fetus
- the stage of fetal development
- how long the chemotherapy will be administered
- how often it will be administered
- whether the chemotherapeutic agent crosses the placental barrier to the fetus

There are also maternal factors to consider. During pregnancy a woman's blood volume and cardiac output increase, which affects the drugs' concentration levels. If the woman has hyponatremia, this increases the drug concentration in her system. Maternal obesity can affect lipid-soluble drugs. As with radiation, the fetus is most susceptible during the first trimester. Congenital malformations and miscarriage are the most common consequences.

Fortunately, some chemotherapy drugs seem to be well tolerated by the fetus during the second and third trimesters. These drugs include **fluorouracil**, **doxorubicin** (Adriamycin), **bleomycin**, **vinblastine**, **dacarbazine**, and **cyclophosphamide**. Even so, the fetus is at risk for low birthweight, miscarriage, and premature birth. Chemotherapy is rarely administered near term. Treatment at this point may be delayed until after delivery, and during this time period the placenta is less able to effectively excrete the drug(s). Drugs that may not harm the fetus *in utero* may be harmful if consumed via the breast milk. For this reason, breastfeeding is usually discouraged. **Methotrexate** is known to be teratogenic and so is not given in pregnancy. **Daunorubicin** and **cytarabine** are teratogenic in the first trimester. There is not enough known about paclitaxel and pregnancy to consider its use. Of additional concern for the pregnant woman receiving treatment for cancer is the effects on the fetus of any medications that may be used to deal with treatment side effects.

Alternative and complementary therapies

A pregnant woman has many limitations on taking medications during pregnancy in order to protect the fetus. Medication that would ordinarily be available to deal with the side effects of cancer treatment may be harmful to the fetus. A helpful resource on the patient's interdisciplinary team is a practitioner with experience in the safe use of complementary therapies for cancer during pregnancy. Mind/body techniques such as guided imagery and meditation can help decrease some of the stress of this time. Acupuncture has been shown to be effective in dealing with the **nausea** associated with chemotherapy. Support groups can also be a great source of strength and information.

See also Fertility issues.

Resources

BOOKS

Runowicz, Carolyn D., Jeanne A. Petrek, and Ted S. Gansler. *American Cancer Society: Women and Cancer.* New York: Villard Books/Random House, 1999.

Teeley, Peter, and Philip Bashe. *The Complete Cancer Survival Guide.* New York: Doubleday, 2000.

PERIODICALS

"Pregnancy Has a Protective Effect Against Breast Cancer." *Medical Devices & Surgical Technology Week* March 28, 2004: 40.

Rotmensch, S., and L. Cole. "False Diagnosis and Needless Therapy of Presumed Malignant Disease in Women With False-positive Human Chorionic Gonadotropin Concentrations." *Lancet* February 26, 2000: 712–5.

ORGANIZATIONS

The American Cancer Society. (800) ACS-2345. http://www.cancer.org.

Cancer Research Institute. 681 Fifth Ave., New York, NY 10022. (800) 992-2623. http://www.cancerresearch.org.

The Gilda Radner Familial Ovarian Cancer Registry. Roswell Park Cancer Institute, Elm and Carlton Streets, Buffalo, NY 14263-0001. (800) 682-7426. http://www.ovariancancer.com.

National Cancer Institute. Building 31, Room 10A31, 31 Center Dr., MSC 2580, Bethesda, MD 20892-2580. (301) 435-3848. http://www.nci.nih.gov.

National Cancer Institute Cancer Trials Web Site. <http://cancertrials.nci.nih.gov/system>. http://www.cancertrials.com.

National Center for Complementary and Alternative Medicine. NCCAM Clearinghouse, PO Box 8218, Silver Spring, MD 20907-8218. (888) 644-6226. <http://nccam.nih.gov>.

Oncolink at the University of Pennsylvania. http://www.oncolink.upenn.edu.

Women's Cancer Network. c/o Gynecologic Cancer Foundation, 401 N. Michigan Ave., Chicago, IL 60611. (312) 644-6610. http://www.wcn.org.

Esther Csapo Rastegari, R.N., B.S.N., Ed.M.
Teresa G. Odle

Primary site

Definition

The area in which a **cancer** originates in the body. Once cancer spreads (metastasizes), the new tumors are called secondary tumors, or metastases.

Kate Kretschmann

Procarbazine

Definition

Procarbazine is an anticancer agent that kills **cancer** cells, also known by the brand name Matulane. It has received approval by the Food and Drug Administration (FDA) for the treatment of advanced **Hodgkin's disease** in combination with other **anticancer drugs**.

Purpose

Procarbazine is used in the treatment of various cancers, although the best established usage is with Hodgkin's disease. Other cancers in which procarbazine is sometimes used include other lymphomas, **brain tumors**, **skin cancer**, lung cancer, and **multiple myeloma**.

Description

Procarbazine is a cytotoxic drug, which means that it kills cancer cells. Procarbazine works by interfering with way the DNA and RNA in cells produce proteins by binding to it in the cells.

Recommended dosage

Procarbazine is often given at a dose of 60 to 100 mg per square meter of body surface area for ten to fourteen days of each course of therapy. In addition, patients who have had pre-existing problems with liver, kidney, or bone marrow function may receive reduced doses.

KEY TERMS

Cytotoxic drug—An anticancer drug that acts by killing or preventing the division of cells.

DNA (deoxyribonucleic acid)—An acid found in all living cells that contains tiny bits of genetic information.

Platelets—Components of the blood involved in clotting.

RNA (ribonucleic acid)—The tiny substances that transmit messages in the DNA to other elements in the cell.

Precautions

While on therapy with procarbazine, patients should not drink alcohol because it may interact with the drug to cause a flushed and hot sensation. Certain foods such as chocolate, fava beans, imported beer, Chianti wines, and ripe cheeses (camembert, cheddar, emmenthaler, stilton), caviar, pickled herring, fermented sausages (bologna, pepperoni, salami, summer sausage), should be avoided as they may cause a dangerous increase in blood pressure if eaten while receiving procarbazine.

Side effects

A carefully monitored side effect of procarbazine is a decrease in the white blood cells that fight **infection** and the platelet cells that prevent bleeding. The most severe side effect is **nausea and vomiting**. Patients should adhere to the antiemetic regimen prescribed for them to prevent this side effect. There may be neurologic side effects such as confusion, sleepiness, **depression**, nightmares, agitation, and nervousness. Patients may have reproductive dysfunction.

Interactions

Procarbazine has numerous drug interactions. Therefore, it is important that patients alert their physicians to all medications they are taking (prescription, over-the-counter, or herbal) prior to starting treatment with procarbazine or any other drug.

Bob Kirsch

Prochlorperazine *see* **Antiemetics**

Promethazine *see* **Antiemetics**

Prostate cancer

Definition

Prostate **cancer** is a disease in which cells in the prostate gland become abnormal and start to grow uncontrollably, forming tumors.

Description

Prostate cancer is a malignancy of one of the major male sex glands. Along with the testicles and the seminal vesicles, the prostate secretes the fluid that makes up semen. The prostate is about the size of a walnut and lies just behind the urinary bladder. A tumor in the prostate interferes with proper control of the bladder and normal sexual functioning. Often the first symptom of prostate cancer is difficulty in urinating. However, because a very common, non-cancerous condition of the prostate, benign prostatic hyperplasia (BPH), also causes the same problem, difficulty in urination is not necessarily due to cancer.

Cancerous cells within the prostate itself are generally not deadly on their own. However, as the tumor grows, some of the cells break off and spread to other parts of the body through the lymph or the blood, a process known as **metastasis**. The most common sites for prostate cancer to metastasize are the seminal vesicles, the lymph nodes, the lungs, and various bones around the hips and the pelvic region. The effects of these new tumors are what can cause death.

Demographics

Prostate cancer is the most commonly diagnosed malignancy among adult males in Western countries.

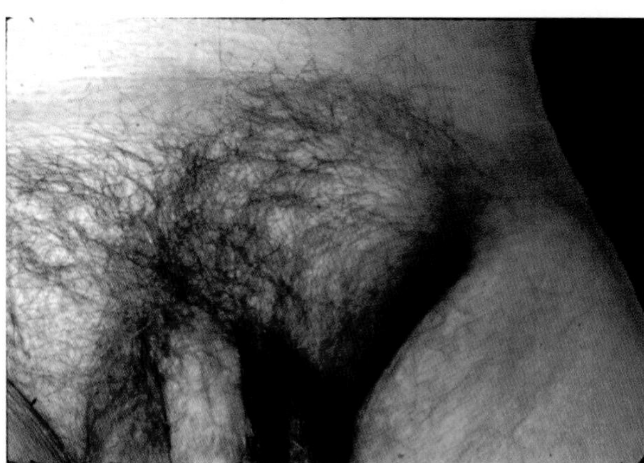

This patient's prostate cancer has metastasized, swelling the lymph nodes in the left groin. *(Photograph by Dr. P. Marazzi. Photo Researchers, Inc. Reproduced by permission.)*

Although prostate cancer is often very slow growing, it can be aggressive, especially in younger men. Given its slow growing nature, many men with the disease die of other causes rather than from the cancer itself.

Prostate cancer affects African-American men twice as often as white men; the mortality rate among African-Americans is also two times higher. African-Americans have the highest rate of prostate cancer of any world population group.

Causes and symptoms

The precise cause of prostate cancer is not known. However, there are several known risk factors for disease including age over 55, African-American heritage, a family history of the disease, occupational exposure to cadmium or rubber, and a high-fat diet. Men with high plasma **testosterone** levels may also have an increased risk for developing prostate cancer.

Frequently, prostate cancer has no symptoms and the disease is diagnosed when the patient goes for a routine screening examination. However, when the tumor is big or the cancer has spread to the nearby tissues, the following symptoms may be seen:

- weak or interrupted flow of the urine
- frequent urination (especially at night)
- difficulty starting urination
- inability to urinate
- pain or burning sensation when urinating
- blood in the urine
- persistent pain in lower back, hips, or thighs (bone pain)
- painful ejaculation

Diagnosis

Prostate cancer is curable when detected early. Yet the early stages of prostate cancer are often asymptomatic, so the disease often goes undetected until the patient has a routine physical examination. Diagnosis of prostate cancer can be made using some or all of the following tests.

Digital rectal examination (DRE)

In order to perform this test, the doctor puts a gloved and lubricated finger (digit) into the rectum to feel for any lumps in the prostate. The rectum lies just behind the prostate gland, and a majority of prostate tumors begin in the posterior region of the prostate. If the doctor does detect an abnormality, he or she may order more tests in order to confirm these findings.

KEY TERMS

Antiandrogen—A substance that blocks the action of androgens, the hormones responsible for male characteristics. Used to treat prostate cancers that require male hormones for growth.

Benign Prostate Hyperplasia (BPH)—A non-cancerous swelling of the prostate.

Brachytherapy—A method of treating cancers, such as prostate cancer, involving the implantation near the tumor of radioactive seeds.

Gleason Grading System—A method of predicting the tendency of a tumor in the prostate to metastasize based on how similar the tumor is to normal prostate tissue.

Granulocyte/macrophage colony stimulating factor (GM-CSF)—Also known as sargramostim, a substance produced by cells of the immune system that stimulates the attack upon foreign cells. Used to treat prostate cancers as a genetically engineered component of a vaccine that stimulates the body to attack prostate tissue.

Histopathology—The study of diseased tissues at a minute (microscopic) level.

Luteinizing hormone releasing hormone (LHRH) agonist—A substance that blocks the action of LHRH, a hormone that stimulates the production of testosterone (a male hormone) in men. Used to treat prostate cancers that require testosterone for growth.

Orchiectomy—Surgical removal of the testes that eliminates the production of testosterone to treat prostate cancer.

Prostate-Specific Antigen—A protein made by the cells of the prostate that is increased by both BPH and prostate cancer.

Radical Prostatectomy—Surgical removal of the entire prostate, a common method of treating prostate cancer.

Transurethral resection of the prostate (TURP)—Surgical removal of a portion of the prostate through the urethra, a method of treating the symptoms of an enlarged prostate, whether from BPH or cancer.

Blood tests

Blood tests are used to measure the amounts of certain protein markers, such as prostate-specific antigen (PSA), found circulating in the blood. The cells lining the prostate generally make this protein and a small amount can be detected normally in the bloodstream. In contrast, prostate cancers produce a lot of this protein, significantly raising the circulating levels. A finding of a PSA level higher than normal for the patient's age group therefore suggests that cancer is present.

Transrectal ultrasound

A small probe is placed in the rectum and sound waves are released from the probe. These sound waves bounce off the prostate tissue and an image is created. Since normal prostate tissue and prostate tumors reflect the sound waves differently, the test is an efficient and accurate way to detect tumors. Though the insertion of the probe into the rectum may be slightly uncomfortable, the procedure is generally painless and only takes 20 minutes.

Prostate biopsy

If cancer is suspected from the results of any of the above tests, the doctor will remove a small piece of prostate tissue with a hollow needle. This sample is then checked under the microscope for the presence of cancerous cells. Prostate **biopsy** is the most definitive diagnostic tool for prostate cancer, and this procedure is done quickly and with little pain or discomfort.

Prostate cancer can also be diagnosed based on the examination of the tissue removed during a transurethral resection of the prostate (TURP). This procedure is performed to help alleviate the symptoms of BPH, a benign enlargement of the prostate. Like a biopsy, this is a definitive diagnostic method for prostate cancer.

X rays and imaging techniques

A chest x ray may be ordered to determine whether the cancer has spread to the lungs. Imaging techniques (such as **computed tomography** (CT) scans and **magnetic resonance imaging** (MRI)), where a computer is used to generate a detailed picture of the prostate and areas nearby, may be done to get a clearer view of the internal organs. A bone scan may be used to check whether the cancer has spread to the bone.

Treatment team

Prostate cancer is often treated by a team of specialists including a urologist (who may or may not

QUESTIONS TO ASK THE DOCTOR

- How do my age, general health, and other medical conditions affect my treatment choices?
- What are the T, N, and M stages of my cancer and how do they influence my treatment options?
- How do the Gleason score of my cancer and my blood prostate-specific antigen (PSA) level predict my outlook for survival and affect treatment options?
- What are the likely side effects of each proposed therapy and how will they affect my quality of life?
- What can be done to help manage the side effects of treatment?

perform surgery), a surgeon (if surgical treatment is used and it is not performed by the urologist), a medical oncologist, and, if **radiation therapy** is used, a radiation oncologist.

Clinical staging, treatments, and prognosis

Once cancer is detected during the microscopic examination of the prostate tissue during a biopsy or TURP, doctors will determine two different numerical scores that will help define the patient's treatment and prognosis.

Tumor grading

Initially, the pathologist will grade the tumor based on his or her examination of the biopsy tissue. The pathologist scores the appearance of the biopsy sample using the Gleason system. This system uses a scale of one to five based on the sample's similarity or dissimilarity to normal prostate tissue. If the tissue is very similar to normal tissue, it is still well differentiated and given a low grading number, such as one or two. As the tissue becomes more and more abnormal (less and less differentiated), the grading number increases, up to five. Less differentiated tissue is considered more aggressive and more likely to be the source of metastases.

The Gleason grading system is best predictive of the prognosis of a patient if the pathologist gives two scores to a particular sample—a primary and a secondary pattern. The two numbers are then added together and that is the Gleason score reported to the patient. Thus, the lowest Gleason score available is two (a primary and secondary pattern score of one each). A typical Gleason score is five (which can be a primary score of two and a secondary score of three or visa-versa). The highest score available is 10, with a pure pattern of very undifferentiated tissue, that is, of grade five. The higher the score, the more abnormal behavior of the tissue, the greater the chance for metastases, and the more serious the prognosis after surgical treatment. A study found that the 10 year cancer survival rate without evidence of disease for grade two, three, and four cancers is 94% of patients. The rate is 91% for grade five cancers, 78% for grade six, 46% for grade seven, and 23% for grade eight, nine, and ten cancers.

Cancer staging

The second numeric score determined by the doctor will be the stage of the cancer, which takes into account the grade of the tumor determined by the pathologist. Based on the recommendations of the American Joint Committee on Cancer (AJCC), two kinds of data are used for staging prostate cancer. Clinical data is based on the external symptoms of the cancer, while histopathological data is based on surgical removal of the prostate and examination of its tissues. Clinical data is most useful to make treatment decisions, while pathological data is the best predictor of prognosis. For this reason, the staging of prostate cancer takes into account both clinical and histopathologic information. Specifically, doctors look at tumor size (T), lymph node involvement (N), the presence of visceral (internal organ) involvement (metastasis = M), and the grade of the tumor (G).

The classification of tumor as T1 means the cancer that is confined to the prostate gland and the tumor that is too small to be felt during a DRE. T1 tumors are often found after examination of tissue removed during a TURP. The T1 definition is subdivided into those cancers that show less than 5% cancerous cells in the tissue sample (T1a) or more than 5% cancerous cells in the tissue sample (T1b). T1c means that the biopsy was performed based on an elevated PSA result. The second tumor classification is T2, where the tumor is large enough to be felt during the DRE. T2a indicates that only the left or the right side of the gland is involved, while T2b means both sides of the prostate gland has tumor.

With a T3 tumor, the cancer has spread to the connective tissue near the prostate (T3a) or to the seminal vesicles as well (T3b). T4 indicates that cancer has spread within the pelvis to tissue next to the prostate such as the bladder's sphincter, the rectum, or the wall of the pelvis. Prostate cancer tends to spread next into the regional lymph nodes of the pelvis, indicated as N1. Prostate cancer is said to be at the M1 stage when it has metastasized outside the pelvis in distant lymph nodes (M1a), bone (M1b) or organs such as the liver or the brain (M1c). Pain, **weight loss**, and **fatigue** often accompany the M1 stage.

The grade of the tumor (G) can be assessed during a biopsy, TURP surgery, or after removal of the prostate. There are three grades recognized: G1, G2, and G3, indicating the tumor is well, moderately, or poorly differentiated, respectively. The G, LN, M descriptions are combined with the T definition to determine the stage of the prostate cancer.

- Stage I prostate cancer comprises patients who are T1a, N0, M0, G1.
- Stage II includes a variety of condition combinations including T1a, N0, M0, G2, 3 or 4; T1b, N0, M0, Any G; T1c, N0, M0, Any G; T1, N0, M0, Any G or T2, N0, M0, Any G.
- Stage III prostate cancer occurs when conditions are T3, N0, M0, any G.
- Stage IV is T4, N0, M0, any G; any T, N1, M0, any G; or any T, any N, M1, Any G.

Prognosis

The prognosis for cancers at Stages I and II is very good. For men treated with stage I or stage II disease, over 95% are alive after five years. Although the cancers of Stage III are more advanced, the five-year prognosis is still good, with 70% of men diagnosed at this stage still living. The spread of the cancer into the pelvis (T4), lymph (N1), or distant locations (M1) are very significant events, as the five-year survival rate drops to 30% for Stage IV.

Treatment options

The doctor and the patient will decide on the treatment mode after considering many factors. For example, the patient's age, the stage of the disease, his general health, and the presence of any co-existing illnesses have to be considered. In addition, the patient's personal preferences and the risks and benefits of each treatment protocol are also taken into account before any decision is made.

SURGERY. For stage I and stage II prostate cancer, surgery is the most common method of treatment because it theoretically offers the chance of completely removing the cancer from the body. Radical **prostatectomy** involves complete removal of the prostate. The surgery can be done using a perineal approach, where the incision is made between the scrotum and the anus, or using a retropubic approach, where the incision is made in the lower abdomen. Perineal approach is also known as nerve-sparing prostatectomy, as it is thought to reduce the effect on the nerves and thus reduce the side effects of impotence and **incontinence**. However, the retropubic approach allows for the simultaneous removal of the pelvic lymph nodes, which can give important pathological information about the tumor spread.

The drawback to surgical treatment for early prostate cancer is the significant risk of side effects that impact the quality of life of the patient. Even using nerve-sparing techniques, studies by the National Cancer Institute (NCI) found that 60% to 80% of men treated with radical prostatectomy reported themselves as impotent (unable to achieve an erection sufficient for sexual intercourse) two years after surgery. This side effect can be sometimes countered by prescribing sildenafil citrate (Viagra). Furthermore, 8% to 10% of patients were incontinent in that time span. Despite the side effects, the majority of men were reported as satisfied with their treatment choice. Additionally, there is some evidence that the skill and the experience of the surgeon are central factors in the ultimate side effects seen.

A second method of surgical treatment of prostate cancer is cryosurgery, or **cryotherapy**. Guided by ultrasound, surgeons insert up to eight cryoprobes through the skin and into close proximity with the tumor. Liquid nitrogen (temperature of -320.8 degrees F, or -196 C) is circulated through the probe, freezing the tumor tissue. In prostate surgery, a warming tube is also used to keep the urethra from freezing. Patients currently spend a day or two in the hospital following the surgery, but it could be an outpatient procedure in the near future. Recovery time is about one week. Side effects have been reduced in recent years, although impotence still affects almost all who have had cryosurgery for prostate cancer. Cryosurgery is considered a good alternative for those too old or sick to have traditional surgery or radiation treatments or when these more traditional treatments are unsuccessful. There is limited amount of information about the long-term efficacy of this treatment for prostate cancer.

RADIATION THERAPY. Radiation therapy involves the use of high-energy **x rays** to kill cancer cells or to shrink tumors. It can be used instead of surgery for stage I and II cancer. The radiation can either be administered from a machine outside the body (external beam radiation), or small radioactive pellets can be implanted in the prostate gland in the area surrounding the tumor, called brachytherapy or interstitial implantation. Pellets containing radioactive iodine (I-125), palladium (Pd 103), or iridium (Ir 192) can be implanted on an outpatient basis, where they remain permanently. The radioactive effect of the seeds last only about a year.

The side effects of radiation can include inflammation of the bladder, rectum, and small intestine as well as disorders of blood clotting (coagulopathies). Impotence and incontinence are often delayed side effects of the treatment. A study indicated that bowel control problems were more likely after radiation therapy when compared to surgery, but impotence and incontinence were more likely after surgical treatment. Long-term results with radiation therapy are dependent on stage. A review of almost 1,000 patients treated with megavoltage irradiation showed 10-year survival rates to be significantly different by T-stage: T1 (79%), T2 (66%), T3 (55%), and T4 (22%). There does not appear to be a large difference in survival between external beam or interstitial treatments.

HORMONE THERAPY. Hormone therapy is commonly used when the cancer is in an advanced stage and has spread to other parts of the body, such as stage III or stage IV. Prostate cells need the male hormone testosterone to grow. Decreasing the levels of this hormone or inhibiting its activity will cause the cancer to shrink. Hormone levels can be decreased in several ways. **Orchiectomy** is a surgical procedure that involves complete removal of the testicles, leading to a decrease in the levels of testosterone. Another method tricks the body by administering the female hormone estrogen. When estrogen is given, the body senses the presence of a sex hormone and stops making the male hormone testosterone. However, there are some unpleasant side effects to hormone therapy. Men may have "hot flashes," enlargement and tenderness of the breasts, or impotence and loss of sexual desire, as well as blood clots, heart attacks, and strokes, depending on the dose of estrogen. Another side effect is osteoporosis, or loss of bone mass leading to brittle and easily fractured bones.

WATCHFUL WAITING. Watchful waiting means no immediate treatment is recommended, but doctors keep the patient under careful observation. This is often done using periodic PSA tests. This option is generally used in older patients when the tumor is not very aggressive and the patients have other, more life-threatening, illnesses. Prostate cancer in older men tends to be slow-growing. Therefore, the risk of the patient dying from prostate cancer, rather than from other causes, is relatively small.

Alternative and complementary therapies

Alternative treatments that have been found helpful in coping with the emotional stress associated with prostate cancer include meditation, guided imagery, and relaxation techniques. Acupuncture is effective in relieving pain in some patients.

A variety of herbal products have been used to treat prostate cancer, including various compounds used in traditional Chinese medicine as well as single agents like Reishi mushrooms (*Ganoderma lucidum*). One herbal compound that was under investigation by the National Center for Complementary and Alternative Medicine (NCCAM) as a possible treatment for prostate cancer was **PC-SPES**, a mixture of eight herbs adapted from traditional Chinese medicine. In the summer of 2002, however, NCCAM put its studies of PC-SPES on hold when the Food and Drug Administration (FDA) determined that samples of the product were contaminated with undeclared prescription drug ingredients. PC-SPES was withdrawn from the American market in late 2002.

Coping with cancer treatment

The treatment process for prostate cancer can be a physically and emotionally exhausting time. Here are six general suggestions that can help make the process easier. Patients should:

- put their faith and trust in their doctors once a treatment course has been chosen
- remember that a patient is never without power and rights during the course of treatment
- put practical affairs in order
- closely monitor each step of the treatment
- keep close family and friends informed and delegate responsibilities as necessary
- work to make visits pleasant and comfortable
- be careful to eat, sleep, exercise, and conduct daily activities in a healthy manner

Clinical trials

Patients with extraprostatic disease are suitable candidates for **clinical trials**. One trial is the testing of a vaccine (GVAX) that causes the body to mount an **immune response** against all prostate cells. As the prostate is a nonessential organ, the destruction of the normal cells with the tumor cells is not a problem. The vaccine was made using cancer cells from a tumor that had been genetically engineered to express granulocyte/macrophage colony-stimulating factor (GM-CSF), a potent activator of the entire immune system. The additional protein jumpstarted the immune response against the prostate cells upon vaccination and resulted in anti-tumor immune response.

Other trials for prostate cancer include evaluation of combination therapies, such as postoperative radiation delivery, use of cytotoxic agents, and hormonal treatment using luteinizing hormone-releasing hormone (LHRH) agonists and/or **antiandrogens** to shut down the growth of the hormone-dependent tumors. Other drugs that are being tested as of 2003 are chemoprotective agents like **amifostine** (Ethyol), which are given to prostate cancer patients to counteract the harmful side effects of radiation treatment.

Prevention

Because the cause of the cancer is not known, there is no definite way to prevent prostate cancer. Given its common occurrence and the low cost of screening, the American Cancer Society (ACS) and the National Comprehensive Cancer Network (NCCN) recommends that all men over age 40 have an annual rectal exam and that men have an annual PSA test beginning at age 50. African-American men and men with a family history of prostate cancer, who have a higher than average risk, should begin annual PSA testing even earlier, starting at age 45.

However, mandatory screening for prostate cancer is controversial. Because the cancer is so slow growing, and the side effects of the treatment can have significant impact on patient quality of life, some medical organizations question the wisdom of yearly exams. Some organizations have even noted that the effect of screening is discovering the cancer at an early stage when it may never grow to have any outward effect on the patient during his lifetime. Nevertheless, the NCI reports that the current aggressive screening methods have achieved a reduction in the death rate of prostate cancer of about 2.3% for African-Americans and about 4.6% for Caucasians since the mid-1990s, with a 20% increase in overall survival rate during that period.

A low-fat diet may slow the progression of prostate cancer. To reduce the risk or progression of prostate cancer, the American Cancer Society recommends a diet rich in fruits, vegetables and dietary fiber, and low in red meat and saturated fats.

Special concerns

The availability of an early detection system for prostate cancer with the development of the PSA serum test has complicated the treatment of this disease. Early detection of an often slow-growing cancer, where treatment can significantly impact the quality of life of the patient, can be complicated. Long-term studies are currently in progress that should provide the first real quantitative information about the relative efficacy of the different treatment options, the actual occurrence of side effects, and the comparative benefits of watchful waiting treatment compared with more aggressive action.

Resources

BOOKS

Beers, Mark H., MD, and Robert Berkow, MD, editors. "Prostate Cancer." Section 17, Chapter 233 In *The Merck Manual of Diagnosis and Therapy*. Whitehouse Station, NJ: Merck Research Laboratories, 2004.

Carroll, Peter R., et al. "Cancer of the Prostate." In *Cancer Principles and Practice of Oncology*, edited by Devita, Vincent T., et al. Philadelphia: Lippincott Williams & Wilkins, 2001.

Wainrib, Barbara R., and Sandra Haber. *Men, Women, and Prostate Cancer*. Oakland, CA: New Harbinger Productions, Inc., 2000.

PERIODICALS

Alimi, D., C. Rubino, E. Pichard-Leandri, et al. "Analgesic Effect of Auricular Acupuncture for Cancer Pain: A Randomized, Blinded, Controlled Trial." *Journal of Clinical Oncology* 21 (November 15, 2003): 4120–4126.

Chang, S. S. "Exploring the Effects of Luteinizing Hormone-Releasing Hormone Agonist Therapy on Bone Health: Implications in the Management of Prostate Cancer." *Urology* 62 (December 22, 2003): 29–35.

de la Fouchardiere, C., A. Flechon, and J. P. Droz. "Coagulopathy in Prostate Cancer." *Netherlands Journal of Medicine* 61 (November 2003): 347–354.

Dziuk, T., and N. Senzer. "Feasibility of Amifostine Administration in Conjunction with High-Dose Rate Brachytherapy." *Seminars in Oncology* 30 (December 2003): 49–57.

Hsieh, K., and P. C. Albertsen. "Populations at High Risk for Prostate Cancer." *Urological Clinics of North America* 30 (November 2003): 669–676.

Linares, L. A., and D. Echols. "Amifostine and External Beam Radiation Therapy and/or High-Dose Rate Brachytherapy in the Treatment of Localized Prostate Carcinoma: Preliminary Results of a Phase II Trial." *Seminars in Oncology* 30 (December 2003): 58–62.

Sliva, D. "*Ganoderma lucidum* (Reishi) in Cancer Treatment." *Integrative Cancer Therapies* 2 (December 2003): 358–364.

Spetz, A. C., E. L. Zetterlund, E. Varenhorst, and M. Hammar. "Incidence and Management of Hot Flashes in Prostate Cancer." *Journal of Supportive Oncology* 1 (November-December 2003): 263–273.

Wilson, S. S., and E. D. Crawford. "Prostate Cancer Update." *Minerva Urologica e Nefrologica* 55 (December 2003): 199–204.

OTHER

FDA MedWatch Safety Alert for PC-SPES, SPES, updated September 20, 2002. http://www.fda.gov/medwatch/SAFETY/2002/safety02.htm#spes.

National Center for Complementary and Alternative Medicine (NCCAM). *Recall of PC-SPES and SPES Dietary Supplements.* NCCAM Publication No. D149, September 2002. <http://nccam.nih.gov/health/alerts/spes/index.htm>.

ORGANIZATIONS

The Association for the Cure of Cancer of the Prostate (CaPCure). 1250 Fourth St., Suite 360, Santa Monica, CA 90401. (800) 757-CURE. http://www.capcure.org.

National Cancer Institute. Building 31, Room 10A31 31 Center Drive, MSC 2580, Bethesda, MD 20892-2580. (800) 4-CANCER. <http://cancernet.nci.nih.gov>.

National Center for Complementary and Alternative Medicine (NCCAM) Clearinghouse. P. O. Box 7923, Gaithersburg, MD 20898. (888) 644-6226. <http://nccam.nih.gov>.

Lata Cherath, Ph.D.
Michelle Johnson, M.S., J.D.
Rebecca J. Frey, Ph.D.

Prostatectomy

Definition

Prostatectomy is surgical removal of part of the prostate gland (transurethral resection, a procedure performed to relieve urinary symptoms caused by benign enlargement), or all of the prostate (radical prostatectomy, the curative surgery most often used to treat **prostate cancer**).

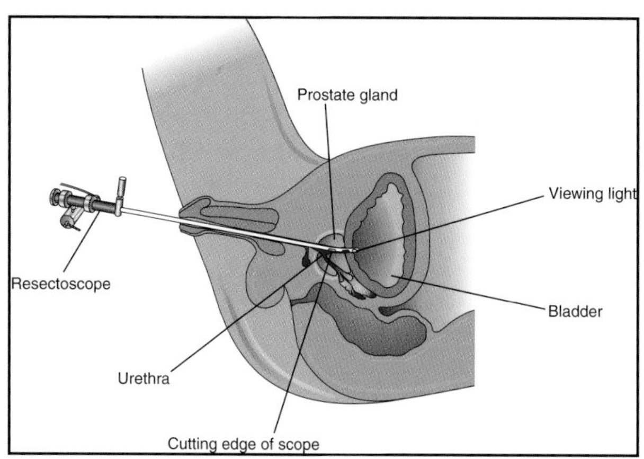

An illustration of a resectoscope inserted through penis in a prostatectomy. *(Illustration by Electronic Illustrators Group. Reproduced by permission.)*

Purpose

Benign disease

When men reach their mid-40s, the prostate gland begins to enlarge. This condition, benign prostatic hyperplasia (BPH) is present in more than half of men in their 60s and as many as 90% of those over 90. Because the prostate surrounds the urethra, the tube leading urine from the bladder out of the body, the enlarging prostate narrows this passage and makes urination difficult. The bladder does not empty completely each time a man urinates, and, as a result, he must urinate with greater frequency, night and day. In time, the bladder can overfill, and urine escapes from the urethra, resulting in **incontinence**. An operation called transurethral resection of the prostate (TURP) relieves symptoms of BPH by removing the prostate tissue that is blocking the urethra. No incision is needed. Instead a tube (retroscope) is passed through the penis to the level of the prostate, and tissue is either removed or destroyed, so that urine can freely pass from the body.

Malignant disease

Prostate **cancer** is the single most common form of non-skin cancer in the United States and the most common cancer in men over 50. Half of men over 70 and almost all men over the age of 90 have prostate cancer, and the American Cancer Society estimates that 198,000 new cases will be diagnosed in a given year. This condition does not always require surgery. In fact, many elderly men adopt a policy of "watchful waiting," especially if their cancer is growing slowly. Younger men often elect to have their prostate gland totally removed along with the cancer it contains—an operation called radical prostatectomy. The two main types of this surgery, radical retropubic prostatectomy and radical perineal prostatectomy, are performed only on patients whose cancer is limited to the prostate. If cancer has broken out of the capsule surrounding the prostate gland and spread in the area or to distant sites, removing the prostate will not prevent the remaining cancer from growing and spreading throughout the body.

Precautions

Potential complications of TURP include bleeding, **infection**, and reactions to general or regional anesthesia. About one man in five will need to have the operation again within 10 years.

Open (incisional) prostatectomy for cancer should not be done if the cancer has spread beyond the prostate,

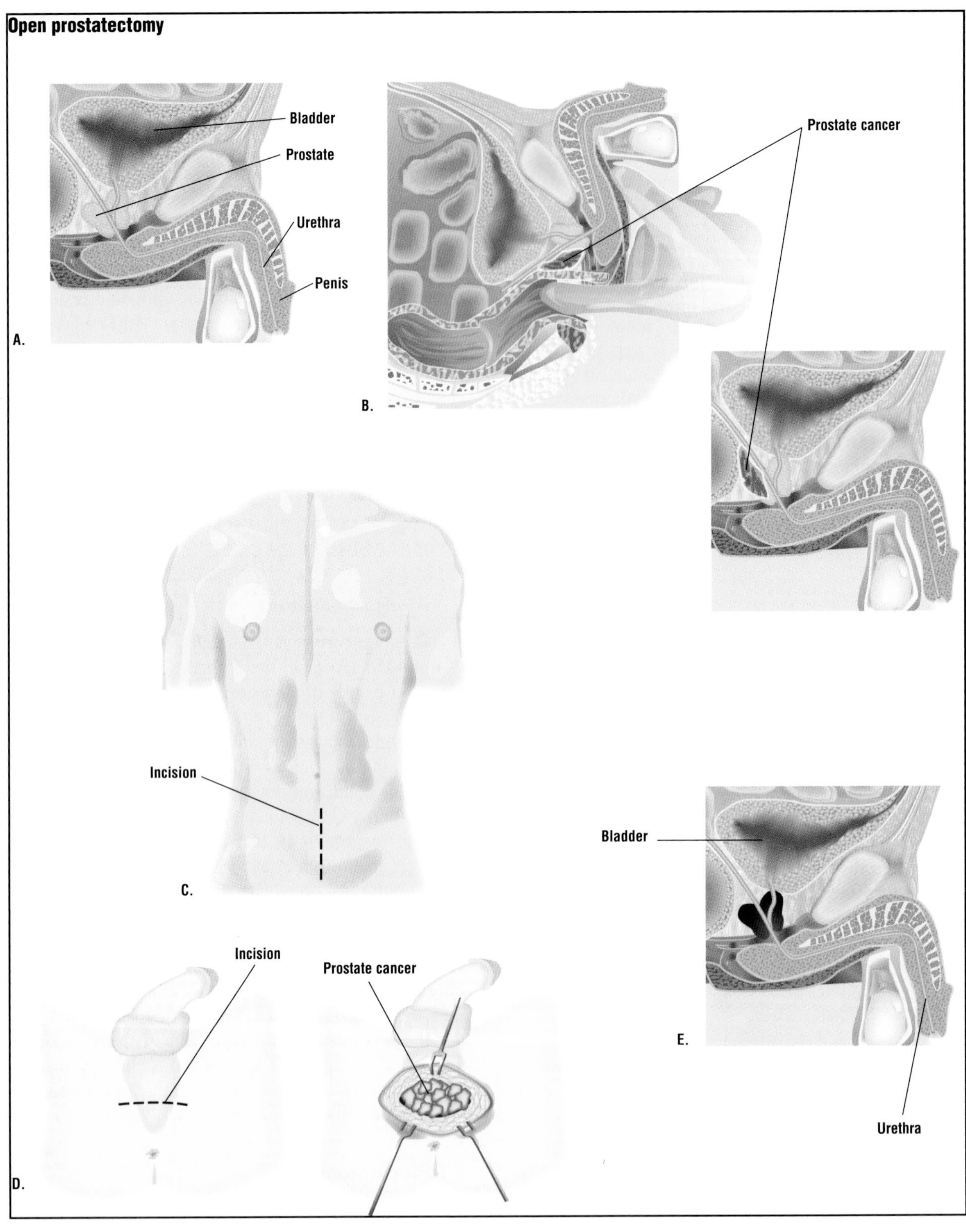

(Illustration by Argosy Publishing. Reproduced by permission of The Gale Group.)

KEY TERMS

BPH—Benign prostatic hypertrophy, a very common noncancerous cause of prostatic enlargement in older men.

Catheter—A tube that is placed through the urethra into the bladder in order to provide free drainage of urine and blood following either TUR or open prostatectomy.

Cryosurgery—In prostatectomy, the use of a very low-temperature probe to freeze and thereby destroy prostatic tissue.

Impotence—The inability to achieve and sustain penile erections.

Incontinence—The inability to retain urine in the bladder until a person is ready to urinate voluntarily.

Prostate gland—The gland surrounding the male urethra just below the base of the bladder. It secretes a fluid that constitutes a major portion of the semen.

Urethra—The tube running from the bladder to the tip of the penis that provides a passage for eliminating urine from the body.

as serious side effects may occur without the benefit of removing all the cancer. If the bladder is retaining urine, it is necessary to insert a catheter before starting surgery. Patients should be in the best possible general condition before radical prostatectomy. Before surgery, the bladder is inspected using an instrument called a cystoscope to help determine the best surgical technique to use, and to rule out other local problems.

Description

TURP

This procedure does not require an abdominal incision. With the patient under either general or spinal anesthesia, a cutting instrument or heated wire loop is inserted to remove as much prostate tissue as possible and seal blood vessels. The excised tissue is washed into the bladder, then flushed out at the end of the operation. A catheter is left in the bladder for one to five days to drain urine and blood. Advanced laser technology enables surgeons to safely and effectively burn off excess prostate tissue blocking the bladder opening with fewer of the early and late complications associated with other forms of prostate surgery. This procedure can be performed on an outpatient basis, but urinary symptoms do not improve until swelling subsides several weeks after surgery.

Radical prostatectomy

RADICAL RETROPUBIC PROSTATECTOMY. This is a useful approach if the prostate is very large, or cancer is suspected. With the patient under general or spinal anesthesia or an epidural, a horizontal incision is made in the center of the lower abdomen. Some surgeons begin the operation by removing pelvic lymph nodes to determine whether cancer has invaded them, but recent findings suggest there is no need to sample them in patients whose likelihood of lymph node metastases is less than 18%. A doctor who removes the lymph nodes for examination will not continue the operation if they contain cancer cells, because the surgery will not cure the patient. Other surgeons remove the prostate gland before examining the lymph nodes. A tube (catheter) inserted into the penis to drain fluid from the body is left in place for 14–21 days.

Originally, this operation also removed a thin rim of bladder tissue in the area of the urethral sphincter—a muscular structure that keeps urine from escaping from the bladder. In addition, the nerves supplying the penis often were damaged, and many men found themselves impotent (unable to achieve erections) after prostatectomy. A newer surgical method called potency-sparing radical prostatectomy preserves sexual potency in 75% of patients and fewer than 5% become incontinent following this procedure.

RADICAL PERINEAL PROSTATECTOMY. This procedure is just as curative as radical retropubic prostatectomy but is performed less often because it does not allow the surgeon to spare the nerves associated with erection or, because the incision is made above the rectum and below the scrotum, to remove lymph nodes. Radical perineal prostatectomy is sometimes used when the cancer is limited to the prostate and there is no need to spare nerves or when the patient's health might be compromised by the longer procedure. The perineal operation is less invasive than retropubic prostatectomy. Some parts of the prostate can be seen better, and blood loss is limited. The absence of an abdominal incision allows patients to recover more rapidly. Many urologic surgeons have not been trained to perform this procedure. Radical prostatectomy procedures last one to four hours, with radical perineal prostatectomy taking less time than radical retropubic prostatectomy. The patient remains in the hospital three to five days following surgery and can return to work in three to five weeks. Ongoing research indicates that laparoscopic radical prostatectomy may be as effective as open surgery in treatment of early-stage disease.

Cryosurgery

Also called **cryotherapy** or **cryoablation**, this minimally invasive procedure uses very low temperatures to freeze and destroy cancer cells in and around the prostate gland. A catheter circulates warm fluid through the urethra to protect it from the cold. When used in connection with ultrasound imaging, cryosurgery permits very precise tissue destruction. Traditionally used only in patients whose cancer had not responded to radiation, but now approved by Medicare as a primary treatment for prostate cancer, cryosurgery can safely be performed on older men, on patients who are not in good enough general health to undergo radical prostatectomy, or to treat recurrent disease. Recent studies have shown that total cryosurgery, which destroys the prostate, is at least as effective as radical prostatectomy without the trauma of major surgery.

Preparation

As with any type of major surgery done under general anesthesia, the patient should be in optimal condition. Most patients having prostatectomy are in the age range when cardiovascular problems are frequent, making it especially important to be sure that the heart is beating strongly, and that the patient is not retaining too much fluid. Because long-standing prostate disease may cause kidney problems from urine "backing up," it also is necessary to be sure that the kidneys are working properly. If not, a period of catheter drainage may be necessary before doing the surgery.

Aftercare

Following TURP, a catheter is placed in the bladder to drain urine and remains in place for two to three days. A solution is used to irrigate the bladder and urethra until the urine is clear of blood, usually within 48 hours after surgery. Whether **antibiotics** should be routinely given remains an open question. Catheter drainage also is used after open prostatectomy. The bladder is irrigated only if blood clots block the flow of urine through the catheter. Patients are given intravenous fluids for the first 24 hours, to ensure good urine flow. Patients resting in bed for long periods are prone to blood clots in their legs (which can pass to the lungs and cause serious breathing problems). This can be prevented by elastic stockings and by periodically exercising the patient's legs. The patient remains in the hospital one to two days following surgery and can return to work in one to two weeks.

Risks

The complications and side effects that may occur during and after prostatectomy include:

- Excessive bleeding, which in rare cases may require blood transfusion.
- Incontinence when, during retropubic prostatectomy, the muscular valve (sphincter) that keeps urine in the bladder is damaged. Less common today, when care is taken not to injure the sphincter.
- Impotence, occurring when nerves to the penis are injured during the retropubic operation. Today's "nerve-sparing" technique has drastically cut down on this problem.
- Some patients who receive a large volume of irrigating fluid after TURP develop high blood pressure, vomiting, trouble with their vision, and mental confusion. This condition is caused by a low salt level in the blood, and is reversed by giving salt solution.
- A permanent narrowing of the urethra called a stricture occasionally develops when the urethra is damaged during TURP.
- There is about a 34% chance that the cancer will recur within 10 years of the procedure. In addition, about 25% of patients experience what is known as biochemical recurrence, which means that the level of prostate-specific antigen (PSA) in the patient's blood serum begins to rise rapidly. Recurrence of the tumor or biochemical recurrence can be treated with radiation therapy or androgen deprivation therapy.

Normal results

In patients with BPH who have the TURP operation, urination should become much easier and less frequent, and dribbling or incontinence should cease. In patients having radical prostatectomy for cancer, a successful operation will remove the tumor and prevent its spread to other areas of the body (**metastasis**). If examination of lymph nodes shows that cancer already had spread beyond the prostate at the time of surgery, other measures are available to control the tumor.

Technology

Responding to spoken instructions, a specially engineered robot has assisted in more than 500 operations to remove the prostate glands of cancer patients. Used by surgeons in the United States and Europe, the AESOP system is the first surgical robot approved by the Food and Drug Administration (FDA). By positioning a slender optical tube (endoscope) that is passed through the patient's body, the robotic arm allows the surgeon to view the minimally invasive surgery on a video monitor and use both hands to improve surgical precision and results while minimizing side effects. Patients spend about 12 hours in the hospital and return to work within two days.

Research

Early findings released by the Prostate Cancer Outcomes Study (PCOS) confirm that radical prostatectomy results in significant sexual dysfunction and some loss of urinary control. Initiated by the National Cancer Institute (NCI) in 1994, PCOS is the first systematic evaluation of how primary cancer treatments affect patients' quality of life.

Resources

BOOKS

Beers, Mark H., MD, and Robert Berkow, MD, editors. "Prostate Cancer." Section 17, Chapter 233 In *The Merck Manual of Diagnosis and Therapy*. Whitehouse Station, NJ: Merck Research Laboratories, 2002.

Marks, Sheldon. *Prostate Vancer: A Family Guide to Diagnosis, Treatment and Survival*. Cambridge, MA: Fisher Books, 2000.

Wainrib, Barbara, et al. *Men, Women, and Prostate Cancer: A Medical and Psychological Guide for Women and the Men they Love*. Oakland, CA: New Harbinger Publications, 2000.

PERIODICALS

Augustin, H., and P. G. Hammerer. "Disease Recurrence After Radical Prostatectomy. Contemporary Diagnostic and Therapeutical Strategies." *Minerva Urologica e Nefrologica* 55 (December 2003): 251–261.

Gomella, L. G., I. Zeltser, and R. K. Valicenti. "Use of Neoadjuvant and Adjuvant Therapy to Prevent or Delay Recurrence of Prostate Cancer in Patients Undergoing Surgical Treatment for Prostate Cancer." *Urology* 62, Supplement 1 (December 29, 2003): 46–54.

Nelson, J. B., and H. Lepor. "Prostate Cancer: Radical Prostatectomy." *Urologic Clinics of North America* 30 (November 2003): 703–723.

Zimmerman, R. A., and D. G. Culkin. "Clinical Strategies in the Management of Biochemical Recurrence after Radical Prostatectomy." *Clinical Prostate Cancer* 2 (December 2003): 160–166.

ORGANIZATIONS

Cancer Research Institute. 681 Fifth Ave., New York, NY 10022. (800) 99CANCER. http://www.cancerresearch.org.

National Prostate Cancer Coalition. 1156 15th St., NW, Washington, DC 20005. (202) 463-9455. www.4npcc.org.

Prostate Health Council. American Foundation for Urologic Disease. 1128 N. Charles St., Baltimore, MD 21201-5559. (800) 828-7866. http://www.afud.org.

David A. Cramer, M.D.
Rebecca J. Frey, Ph.D.

Protein electrophoresis

Definition

Protein electrophoresis is a technique used to separate the different component proteins (fractions) in a mixture of proteins, such as a blood sample, on the basis of differences in how the components move through a fluid-filled matrix under the influence of an applied electric field.

Purpose

Protein electrophoresis is a **screening test** used to evaluate, diagnose, and monitor a variety of diseases and conditions through examination of the amounts and types of protein in a blood, urine, or cerebrospinal fluid (CSF) specimen.

Precautions

Certain other diagnostic tests or prescription medications can affect the protein electrophoresis results. The administration of a contrast dye used in some other tests may falsely elevate apparent protein levels. Drugs that can alter results include aspirin, bicarbonates, chlorpromazine (Thorazine), **corticosteroids**, isoniazid (INH), and neomycin (Mycifradin). The total serum protein concentration may also be affected by changes in the patient's posture or by the use of a tourniquet during the drawing of blood.

Because there is less protein in urine and CSF samples than in blood, these samples often must be concentrated before analysis. The added sample handling can lead to contamination and erroneous results. In collection of a CSF specimen, it is important that the sample not be contaminated with blood proteins that would invalidate the CSF protein measurements.

Description

Proteins—long chains of connected amino acids—are biologically important building-block chemicals that contain the elements carbon, hydrogen, nitrogen, and oxygen. Some proteins also contain sulfur, phosphorus, iron, iodine, selenium, or other trace elements. There are 22 amino acids commonly found in all proteins. The human body is capable of producing fourteen of these amino acids; the remaining eight are called essential amino acids, and must be obtained from food. Proteins are found in muscles, blood, skin, hair, nails, and the internal organs and tissues. Enzymes and antibodies are proteins, and many hormones are proteinlike. Electrophoresis is one of a variety of techniques that can be used to fractionate

KEY TERMS

Acute-phase proteins—Proteins produced during the acute-phase response, a set of physiological changes that occur in response to biologic stress such as trauma or sepsis.

Albumin—A blood protein produced in the liver that helps to regulate water distribution in the body.

Antibodies—Immunoglobulin protein molecules produced by B cells during the immune response. Each antibody recognizes an individual antigen to trigger immune defenses.

Antigen—Foreign body that triggers immune response.

Bence-Jones protein—The Ig light chain, part of an immunoglobulin, that is detected by urine protein electrophoresis in the case of multiple myeloma.

Complement—A group of complex proteins of the beta-globulin type in the blood that bind to antibodies during anaphylaxis. In the complement cascade, each complement interacts with another in a pattern that causes fluid build-up in cells, leading to lysis (cell destruction).

Electrophoresis—A technique used to separate the proteins in a biological sample on the basis of differences in how the components move through a fluid-filled matrix under the influence of an applied electric field.

Globulins—A group of proteins in blood plasma whose levels can be measured by electrophoresis in order to diagnose or monitor a variety of serious illnesses.

Hemolysis—Also called hematolysis, the breakage of red blood cells and concomitant liberation of hemoglobin.

Lumbar puncture—Also called spinal tap, a procedure for the withdrawal of spinal fluid from the lumbar region of the spinal cord for diagnosis, or for injection of a dye for imaging, or for administering medication or an anesthetic.

Paraprotein—A paraprotein is an immunoglobulin produced by a clone of identical B cells.

Protein—Proteins, such as enzymes and antibodies, are biologically important molecules made of long chains of connected amino acids that contain the elements carbon, hydrogen, nitrogen, and oxygen. Certain proteins may also contain sulfur, phosphorus, iron, iodine, selenium, or other trace elements.

(separate) protein mixtures into individual component proteins.

The serum protein electrophoresis test requires a blood sample drawn by venipuncture (having blood drawn from a vein) performed in the doctor's office or on site at a medical laboratory. The urine protein electrophoresis test requires either an early morning urine sample or a 24-hour urine sample, according to the physician's request. A CSF specimen must be collected by **lumbar puncture** (spinal tap), generally performed by a physician as an outpatient procedure in a hospital. Because of risks associated with the lumbar-puncture procedure, the patient must sign a consent form, and should be prepared to remain for six to eight hours under observation.

Preparation

It is usually not necessary for the patient to restrict food or fluids before blood is drawn for a serum protein electrophoresis test; a four-hour fast is requested before drawing blood for lipoprotein testing. For protein electrophoresis on all types of samples, any factors that might affect test results, such as whether the patient is taking any medications, should be noted.

Aftercare

After a blood sample is drawn, a small bandage may be applied to the puncture site, and the patient may be cautioned about the possibility of fainting or of lightheadedness. Following lumbar puncture for the collection of CSF, the patient must be kept lying flat in the hospital under observation for at least six to eight hours.

Risks

Risks posed by the venipuncture are minimal but may include slight bleeding from the puncture site, the development of a small bruise at the puncture site, or both. Other risks include fainting or lightheadedness after the sample is drawn. Lumbar puncture can lead to leakage of CSF from the puncture site, headache, **infection**, symptoms of meningitis, **nausea**, **vomiting**, or difficulty urinating. Rarely, pre-existing intracranial pressure can lead to brain herniation, resulting in brain damage or death.

Normal results

Blood proteins

Serum protein electrophoresis is used to determine the total serum protein concentration, which is an indication of the patient's hydration state: dehydration leads to high total serum protein concentration. Further, the levels of different blood proteins rise or fall in response to such disorders as **cancer** and associated protein-wasting syndromes, immune-system disorders, liver dysfunction, impaired nutrition, and chronic fluid-retaining conditions. The different types of blood proteins are separated into fractions of five distinct classes: albumin, $alpha_1$-globulins, $alpha_2$-globulins, beta-globulins, and gamma-globulins (immunoglobulins). In addition to standard protein electrophoresis, **immunoelectrophoresis** may be used to assess the blood levels of specific immunoglobulins. Immunoelectrophoresis is usually ordered when the serum protein electrophoresis test shows an unusually high amount of protein in the gamma-globulin fraction.

ALBUMIN. Albumin, which is produced in the liver, is the most abundant blood protein. It makes a major contribution to the regulation of water movement between the tissues and the bloodstream. Albumin binds calcium, thyroid hormones, fatty acids, and many drugs, keeping them in the blood circulation and preventing them from being filtered out by the kidneys. Albumin levels can play a role in the effectiveness and toxicity of therapeutic drugs and in drug interactions.

GLOBULINS. Serum globulins are separated in protein electrophoresis as four main fractions: $alpha_1$-, $alpha_2$-, beta-, and gamma-globulins.

- The major $alpha_1$-globulin is $alpha_1$-antitrypsin, produced by the lungs and liver. $Alpha_1$-antitrypsin deficiency is a marker of an inherited disorder characterized by an increased risk of emphysema.
- $Alpha_2$-globulins include serum haptoglobin, $alpha_2$-macroglobulin, and ceruloplasmin. Haptoglobin binds to hemoglobin, released from damaged red blood cells during hemolysis, to prevent its excretion by the kidneys. $Alpha_2$-macroglobulin accounts for about one third of the $alpha_2$-globulin fraction. Ceruloplasmin is involved in the storage and transport of copper and iron in the body.
- Beta-globulins include transferrin, low-density lipoproteins (LDL), and complement components. Transferrin transports dietary iron to the liver, spleen, and bone marrow. Low-density lipoprotein is the major carriers of cholesterol in the blood. Complement is a system of blood proteins involved in inflammatory response.
- The gamma-globulin fraction contains the immunoglobulins, a family of proteins that function as antibodies. Antibodies, in response to infection, allergic reactions, and organ transplants, recognize and bind foreign bodies, or antigens, to facilitate their destruction by the immune system. The immune response is regulated by a large number of antigen-specific gamma-globulins that fall into five main classes called IgG, IgA, IgM, IgB, and IgE. When the serum protein electrophoresis test demonstrates a significant deviation from the normal gamma-globulin levels, a supplemental test, immunoelectrophoresis, should be ordered to identify the specific globulin(s) involved.

The following serum protein electrophoresis reference values are representative; some variation among laboratories and specific methods is to be expected. (1 gm = approximately 0.02 pt and 1 dl = approximately 0.33 fluid oz.)

- Total protein: 6.4–8.3 g/dL
- Albumin: 3.5–5.0 g/dL
- $Alpha_1$-globulin: 0.1–0.3 g/dL
- $Alpha_2$ globulin: 0.6–1.0 g/dL
- Beta-globulin: 0.7–1.2 g/dL
- Gamma-globulin: 0.7–1.6 g/dL

Urinary proteins

Protein electrophoresis is performed on urine samples to classify disorders that cause protein loss via the kidneys. In urine, normally no globulins and less than 0.050 g/dL albumin are present.

Cerebrospinal fluid (CSF) proteins

In CSF, the total protein concentration is normally 0.015–0.045 g/dL, with gamma-globulin accounting for 3% to 12%. The main use of CSF protein electrophoresis testing is in the diagnosis of central nervous tumors and multiple sclerosis.

Abnormal results

Deviations in serum protein levels from reference levels are considered in conjunction with symptoms and results from other diagnostic procedures.

Albumin levels are increased in dehydration and decreased in malnutrition, pregnancy, liver disease, inflammatory diseases, and protein-losing states such as malabsorption syndrome and certain kidney disorders. Low serum albumin levels can indicate disease and can influence analysis of thyroid hormones and calcium.

Alpha$_1$-globulins are increased in inflammatory diseases and decreased or absent in juvenile pulmonary emphysema, a hereditary disease.

Alpha$_2$-globulins are increased in acute and chronic inflammation and nephrotic syndrome. Decreased values may indicate hemolysis (the release of hemoglobin from red blood cells). Low haptoglobin can indicate tumor **metastasis**, severe **sepsis**, or chronic liver disease. The concentration of macroglobulin is increased during nephrosis. Ceruloplasmin concentration is increased during pregnancy and decreased in Wilson's disease, a rare inherited condition that leads to accumulation of copper in the liver.

Beta-globulin levels are increased in **multiple myeloma** and also in conditions of high cholesterol (hypercholesterolemia), such as in atherosclerosis, and in iron deficiency **anemia**. Levels are decreased in coagulation disorders.

Gamma-globulin levels are increased in multiple **myeloma**. The levels are increased as well in chronic inflammatory disease and autoimmune conditions such as rheumatoid arthritis and systemic lupus erythematosus, cirrhosis, and acute and chronic infection. The gamma-globulins are decreased in leukemia, in a variety of genetic immune disorders, and in secondary immune deficiency related to steroid use or to severe infection. Immunoglobulin deficiency due to inherited disorders can range from partial or complete loss of a single immunoglobulin class to complete absence of all immunoglobulins.

Finding an individual (oligoclonal) band in the gamma fraction of the electrophoresis result indicates the presence of a paraprotein. Type IgG or IgA paraproteins associated with multiple myeloma may be found by serum protein electrophoresis testing; however, the tumor may also produce only Ig light chains that are removed from the blood by the kidneys. This Ig light chain (also known as the Bence-Jones protein) is detected by urine protein electrophoresis and is found nearly exclusively in patients with multiple myeloma.

In urine samples, abnormal results other than the presence of the Bence-Jones protein indicate disruption of kidney function or acute inflammation. Hemoglobin and myoglobin are found in the urine of patients with infection or hemolysis.

An increase in total protein concentration in the CSF is often found with central nervous system (CNS) tumors and in meningitis.

Resources

BOOKS

Marshall, W.J. *Clinical Chemistry*. 4th ed. Edinburgh, London, New York, Philadelphia, St. Louis, and Toronto: Mosby, 2000.

OTHER

HealthWide Website. 2000 Healthwide.com, Inc. http://www.healthwide.com/ency.

Patricia L. Bounds, Ph.D.

Proteomics

Definition

Proteomics is the systematic study of all of the proteins in a cell, tissue, or organism.

Description

The term proteome was coined in 1994 to describe all of the proteins in a given cell, tissue, or organism. Proteomes are extremely complex and differ among individuals, cell types, and within the same cell depending on cell activity, stimuli, and disease. There are estimated to be between one and ten million different proteins in the human body. Relatively few of these proteins have been identified.

Proteomics is being developed for use in **cancer** diagnosis and treatment. A protein pattern or array from blood or a cancer cell eventually may be the primary means of diagnosing cancer. Although significant advances have been made in clinical studies, as of 2005, proteomics was not yet available in clinical settings.

Proteomics technology for cancer diagnosis and treatment identifies biomarkers—proteins and protein patterns in blood, urine, and tissue that can be used to detect:

- early cancers
- treatment response
- the likelihood of relapse after treatment

It is expected that proteomics will be used to:

- develop better cancer treatments
- predict the effects of various treatments
- develop individualized therapies for each patient

Proteomics has led to the identification of many biomarker proteins and the discovery of many new proteins in the blood. Proteomics has been used to

KEY TERMS

Biomarker—A distinctive biological indicator of a condition or process.

Biopsy—The removal of a small piece of tissue for examination.

Laser capture microdissection microscope—An instrument that uses low-energy laser beams and special transfer film to lift single cells from a tissue.

Mass spectroscopy, MS—A technique that separates mixtures of substances on the basis of molecular weight and electrical charge.

Mass-to-charge ratio, m/z—The ratio of the molecular mass of a substance to its electrical charge; used for protein separation by MS.

Phosphorylation—The enzymatic addition of a phosphate group to a protein.

Prostate specific antigen, PSA—A biomarker used as a preliminary screen for prostate cancer.

Protein array—The pattern of proteins in blood, tissue, or a cell as determined by MS.

Proteome—The collection of all of the proteins in a cell, tissue, or organism.

identify hundreds of proteins in the ovary, prostate, breast, and esophagus that increase or decrease as cells begin to grow abnormally.

Procedures

Progress in proteomics has been made possible by the development of new technologies including:

- high-resolution mass spectrometry (MS) that can sort out thousands of proteins and protein fragments on the basis of their molecular weight and electrical charge
- sophisticated artificial intelligence computer programs that can learn to identify the specific patterns of a few proteins present in a huge protein array
- laser capture microdissection microscopes that use low-energy laser beams and special transfer film to lift single cells from a tissue, to collect and analyze all of the proteins in the cell by (MS) and computer technology

A mass spectrometer consists of:

- an ionization source that removes electrons from (ionizes) the proteins and protein fragments in a sample so that they all have a positive charge
- a mass analyzer that measures the mass-to-charge ratio (m/z) of the ionized (charged) proteins and fragments, as gases under a vacuum
- a detector that determines the number of ions present at each m/z value

The result is a mass spectrum or chart with a series of spikes or peaks, each representing a charged protein fragment from the sample. The height of each peak represents the amount of that particular protein or fragment that is present in the sample. The size of the peaks and the distance between them is the protein pattern or array of the entire sample. Each spectrum may have more than 15,000 data points—one for every protein and protein fragment—with their molecular weight and intensity values reflecting their relative abundance in the sample.

Computers rapidly analyze the MS data searching for subtle differences among multiple protein patterns and for proteins that might serve as biomarkers. Once potential biomarkers are identified, the computer is trained to sort through the patterns of thousands of proteins for the few small protein biomarkers that can distinguish between cancer and control samples or between cancer protein patterns before and after treatment.

MS-based proteomic analysis is very fast. The entire process—from collecting a few drops of blood to the spectral analysis—can occur in less than one minute. Extremely small amounts of protein can be detected and hundreds of samples can be analyzed sequentially.

Laser capture microdissection microscopes enable scientists to use tissue removed from a patient by a **biopsy** to isolate pure samples of normal cells, precancerous cells, and tumor cells from a single tissue of a single patient. Analysis of the protein patterns from these cells enable researchers to study:

- patterns that may predict early-stage cancer
- how a particular treatment affects the network of proteins in a cell
- early signs of cancer drug toxicity
- mechanisms of drug resistance
- means for reducing side effects of treatment
- changes in protein patterns during tumor recurrence It may be possible to predict from the protein patterns which patients are likely to have an early toxic response to a treatment, so that doses can be lowered or a different treatment can be chosen

Initially, researchers are concentrating on ovarian and prostate cancers, which usually are not detected in early stages when the cancer is progressing without symptoms. By using proteomics for early detection, tumors may be treated before they spread (metastasize) to other parts of the body. Scientists also are studying the most common, solid human tumors including breast, colon, lung, and pancreatic cancers.

Cancers

Ovarian cancer

More than 80% of ovarian cancers are not diagnosed until they have reached an advanced stage when the five-year-survival rate is 20% or less. However in the 20% of women whose **ovarian cancer** is diagnosed at an early stage, the prognosis is excellent, with a five-year-survival rate of over 95%.

In 2002 researchers used MS-based proteomics to examine the protein patterns in blood serum, obtained with a finger prick, from 50 patients with stage-I ovarian cancer and 66 controls who were either healthy or had a benign (non-cancerous) condition such as ovarian cysts, fibroids, endometriosis, or general inflammatory disease. Such conditions are much more common than ovarian cancer but may have symptoms that suggest the possibility of cancer. Out of the complex patterns of tens of thousands of serum proteins, the computer identified a specific combination of five proteins that could distinguish between the cancer patients and the controls. Using this identified sub-pattern, all of the cancer patients tested positive—a 100% sensitivity. Among the controls, 5% were false positives demonstrating a specificity of 95%.

In 2004, using higher-resolution MS, a different protein pattern, and a larger group of patients and controls, researchers were able to achieve 100% sensitivity and specificity for diagnosing ovarian cancer. However validation of the procedure on a large clinical sample is needed before a commercial test becomes available. These clinical studies are being carried out in high-risk clinics, in which many women are considering prophylactic oophorectomies—removal of the ovaries—to prevent ovarian cancer, because they have a family history of the disease or carry mutations in the BRCA genes that greatly increase their risk for breast and ovarian cancers.

As of 2005, a clinical trial also was underway comparing proteomics with standard CA-125 blood tests that use a single protein as a biomarker for ovarian cancer. The blood protein CA-125 may be elevated in women with benign conditions as well as ovarian cancer. Another ongoing clinical trial is attempting to use proteomics to predict the early recurrence of ovarian cancer.

The small low-level proteins that have proven useful for the proteomics of ovarian cancer have been found to accumulate on large carrier blood proteins such as albumin. Scientists have found that by extracting the carrier-protein fraction of the blood they can obtain much higher quantities of these biomarkers.

Prostate cancer

Prostate specific antigen (PSA) levels are used as a preliminary screen for **prostate cancer**. However 70–75% of men who undergo biopsies because of abnormal PSA levels do not have cancer. It has been difficult to rule-out cancer without a biopsy in patients with slightly elevated PSA levels (4–10 nanograms per ml). MS-based proteomics of the blood proteins in 167 patients with prostate cancer, 77 patients with benign prostate hyperplasia, and 82 healthy males correctly classified 96% of the samples as either prostate cancer or non-cancer including benign prostate hyperplasia. Most of the cancers were correctly identified and the specificity was 71%, meaning that were a number of false positives. The test was effective in men with normal, slightly elevated, and high PSA levels. Thus proteomics may prove useful for choosing whether to perform a biopsy and may reduce the incidence of unnecessary biopsies.

Molecules called phosphates commonly are added to or removed from proteins to change their activity or function. Specific changes in phosphorylated proteins—those with attached phosphates—are believed to be important for prostate cancer progression. Researchers are studying whether changes in phosphorylation, as detected by MS-based proteomics, can be used as biomarkers for diagnosing the progression of prostate and other cancers.

Breast cancer

Proteomic studies on **breast cancer** have found a combination of three blood proteins that may be useful for discriminating between women with breast cancer, women with benign breast disease, and healthy women. About 70–80% of breast cancers originate in the mammary ducts—the thin tubes that lead to the nipples. Nipple aspirate fluid from these ducts has a higher concentration of breast-specific proteins than blood. Possible tumor-marker proteins from this fluid are being studied by proteomics.

A 2003 proteomics study successfully identified fluctuating levels of specific active proteins inside breast and ovarian tumor cells. This may help determine early in treatment whether a particular drug is effective in a given patient.

About 25–30% of women with breast cancer have high levels of the protein Her-2/neu on the surfaces of their cancer cells. The cancer drug **Herceptin** is an antibody that attaches to Her-2/neu and prevents the protein from promoting cancer cell growth. Ongoing proteomics studies are monitoring key signaling systems in cells that may be influenced by Herceptin and other cancer drugs that target specific molecules. Proteomics has been used to measure the levels of active and inactive signaling proteins in isolated cancer cells obtained from tumor biopsies before and at various times after drug treatment. It has been found that breast cancer patients with a poor prognosis have more of the active form of the protein AKT that promotes cell survival. Herceptin lowers this AKT levels, promoting tumor cell death.

Other cancers

A 2004 proteomics study found a protein pattern that may predict which people with familial adenomatous polyposis (FAP)—an inherited condition that often leads to colon cancer—will respond to the preventive drug celecoxib. Protein patterns from patients before and after drug treatment distinguished between those in which celecoxib decreased the number of colon polyps that are characteristic of FAB and those who did not respond to the drug. One particular protein peak appeared only in patterns from non-responsive patients. A few protein peaks changed significantly in all patients following treatment with celecoxib.

Scientists are searching for blood protein patterns that may predict a person's risk for prostate cancer, **pancreatic cancer**, and **melanoma**. Protein patterns have been found in tumor tissue from lung and bladder cancers that may be able to discriminate between cancerous and healthy tissues.

As of 2005 proteomics **clinical trials** were testing blood protein patterns to:

- determine the response to radiation therapy in patients with localized prostate cancer and identify patients who might benefit from aggressive treatment
- predict the development of non-small cell lung cancer in patients with suspicious lung abnormalities
- determine whether a patient has a type of lymphoma known as mycosis fungoides/cutaneous T-cell lymphoma
- predict whether patients with psoriasis or cutaneous T-cell lymphoma will remain in remission.

See also ; .

Resources

BOOKS

Baxevanis, Andreas D., and B. F. Francis Ouellette, editors. *Bioinformatics: A Practical Guide to the Analysis of Genes and Proteins.* 3rd ed. Hoboken, NJ: John Wiley, 2005.

Clark, David P. *Molecular Biology*. Boston: Elsevier Academic Press, 2005.

Fuchs, Jurgen, and Maurizio Podda, editors. *Encyclopedia of Medical Genomics and Proteomics*. New York: Dekker, 2005.

PERIODICALS

Aebersold, R., and M. Mann. 'Mass Spectrometry-Based Proteomics.' *Nature* 422 (2003): 198–207.

Petricoin, E. F., et al. 'Use of Proteomic Patterns in Serum to Identify Ovarian Cancer.' *Lancet* 369 (2002): 772–7.

Rosenblatt, Kevin P., et al. 'Serum Proteomics in Cancer Diagnosis and Management. *Annual Review of Medicine* 55 (2004): 97.

Zhu, W., et al. 'Detection of Cancer-Specific Markers Amid Massive Mass Spectral Data.' *Proceedings of the National Academy of Sciences* 100 (2003): 14666–71.

OTHER

"NCI-CCR Initiatives: Proteomics." Center for Cancer Research, National Cancer Institute. [cited March 30, 2005]. <http://ccr.cancer.gov/initiatives/Proteomics.asp>.

NCI Press Office Staff. 'Proteomics: Research for the 21st Century." *BenchMarks* 2, no. 2. February 7, 2002. National Cancer Institute. [cited March 30, 2005]. http://www.cancer.gov/newscenter/benchmarks-vol2-issue2.

"Protein Patterns in Blood May Predict Prostate Cancer Diagnosis." *News*. October 15, 2002. National Cancer Institute. [cited March 30, 2005]. http://www.cancer.gov/newscenter/ProstateProteomics.

"Protein Patterns May Identify Ovarian Cancer." *News*. February 7, 2002. National Cancer Institute. [cited March 30, 2005]. http://www.cancer.gov/newscenter/proteomics07feb02.

"Proteomics Shows Promise in Colon Cancer Chemoprevention Study." *News*. April 15, 2004. National Cancer Institute. [cited March 30, 2005]. http://www.cancer.-gov/newscenter/doc.aspx?viewid=07A5FF5E-E140-4D80-9C94-F7DD9FA67C8F.

"Proteomics Research Aids Cancer Diagnosis and Treatment." *News*. April 9, 2003. National Cancer Institute. [cited March 30, 2005]. http://www.cancer.gov/newscenter/pressreleases/aacrproteomics.

"Questions and Answers: Proteomics and Cancer." *News*. April 30, 2004. National Cancer Institute. [cited March 30, 2005]. http://www.cancer.gov/newscenter/pressreleases/proteomicsQandA.

Understanding Cancer Series: Molecular Diagnostics. January 28, 2005. National Cancer Institute. [cited March 30, 2005]. http://www.cancer.gov/cancertopics/understandingcancer/moleculardiagnostics/allpages.

ORGANIZATIONS

American Cancer Society. PO Box 102454, Atlanta, GA 30368-2454. 800-ACS-2345. http://www.cancer.org. Information, research, and patient support.

Proteomics Program, Center for Cancer Research, National Cancer Institute. Public Inquiries Office, Suite 30361, 6116 Executive Blvd., MSC-8322, Bethesda, MD 20892-8322. 301-451-4347. <http://ccr.nci.nih.gov/initiatives/proteomics.asp>. Research and clinical trials on proteomics.

Margaret Alic, Ph.D.

Pruritis *see* **Itching**

Psycho-oncology

Definition

Psycho-oncology is a broad-based approach to **cancer** therapy that treats the emotional, social, and spiritual distress which often accompanies cancer. According to Dr. Jimmie Holland, the founder of psycho-oncology, the field has two major emphases. The first is the study of cancer patients' psychological reactions to their illness at all stages of its course; the second is analysis of the emotional, spiritual, social, and behavioral factors that influence the risk of developing cancer and long-term survival following treatment. Some psycho-oncologists consider their field a subspecialty of psychiatry while others emphasize its multidisciplinary aspects. In addition to psychiatrists, departments of psycho-oncology in major cancer centers may include nurses, surgeons, bioethicists, social workers, psychologists, clergy, palliative care specialists, and volunteers.

Description

Psycho-oncology is a relatively new addition to the care of cancer patients. It began in the mid-1970s when Dr. Holland returned to the practice of psychiatry after her children were in school. Married to an oncologist, she had noted that her husband's colleagues focused on the physical effects of the **anticancer drugs** they were giving their patients to the point of failing to take the patients' thoughts and emotions into account. To some extent this oversight was part of the medical culture of the 1950s and 1960s; at that time cancer carried a stigma because it had low rates of survival. Many doctors were taught in medical school to withhold a diagnosis of cancer from the patient on the grounds that the disease was virtually a death sentence and the truth would be unbearable. Such highly regarded newspapers as the *New York Times* even refused to print the words "breast cancer" when the founders of the Reach to Recovery program first wanted to insert notices of their meetings.

In the 1970s, however, this attitude of shame and secrecy was reversed, partly because of the patients' rights movement, but also because newer and more effective treatments for cancer came into use and the number of long-term survivors of cancer increased. In 1977 Dr. Holland started the first full-time psychiatric service in a cancer research center in order to study and treat the emotional and psychological crises experienced by cancer patients. She conducted some of the earliest research studies of the emotional impact of cancer on patients and their families.

In the early 2000s, psycho-oncology has become an accepted part of cancer treatment, with departments of psycho-oncology established in most major cancer centers in Canada and the United States. The field has its own journal, *Psycho-Oncology*, as well as national and international societies for interested professionals.

KEY TERMS

Bioethics—A field of study concerned with the moral and spiritual implications of medical research and treatments.

Distress—In general, any acute feeling of pain, anxiety, or sadness; in the context of psycho-oncology, any unpleasant emotion that interferes with a cancer patient's ability to cope with symptoms and treatment.

New Age thought—A general term for a set of beliefs that became popular in the 1970s but had been previously associated with the occult, secret doctrines and teachings, or paranormal phenomena. New Age writers commonly believe that the mind can control the body; some believe that this control includes disease processes.

Oncology—The medical specialty that deals with the development, diagnosis, and treatment of cancer.

Visualization—A technique for forming mental images or pictures of the healing process as a way of strengthening the immune system and/or fighting such disease agents as cancer cells or the AIDS virus.

Special concerns

Special concerns in psycho-oncology include the feelings of guilt or anxiety expressed by many cancer patients that they cannot adopt or maintain the positive attitudes that some people believe are essential to

QUESTIONS TO ASK YOUR DOCTOR

- How do you feel about my use of complementary or alternative therapies as part of my treatment program? Are there any that you would advise against?
- What reading materials or other resources would you recommend so that I can help myself cope with my symptoms and the side effects of cancer treatment?
- Where do you fit my emotional, psychological, and spiritual concerns into my treatment regimen?

fighting cancer. Such patients feel burdened by the notion—sometimes voiced by family members—that their literal survival depends on visualizations (usually visualizations of their immune system combating the cancer) or otherwise acting cheerful and upbeat. In addition, some extreme forms of New Age thought lead some people to "blame the victim" that is, to say such things to cancer patients as, "You must have subconsciously wanted to develop this cancer," or, "It's your bad karma—you must have done something bad in a previous existence to deserve this disease." Psycho-oncologists, however, do not regard mental attitudes toward cancer as the sole factor affecting long-term survival, and they do not insist that patients adopt a one-size-fits-all approach to coping with cancer. Dr. Holland's list of recommendations for coping with cancer emphasizes flexibility, as she urges patients to:

- Use coping techniques or patterns that have helped them in the past in dealing with the stresses of life. For example, someone who has been helped by talking through their problems with trusted friends or family members should not suddenly start to keep their problems to themselves in coping with cancer.
- Take the "one-day-at-a-time" approach in dealing with the symptoms and other problems that cancer brings with it. This approach, which is sometimes called "chunking it down," helps by keeping large-scale worries about the long-term future manageable.
- Seek out a doctor with whom they feel comfortable. A doctor/patient relationship based on trust and mutual respect makes it easier to ask appropriate questions and to be a full participant in treatment planning.
- Continue to draw on religious or spiritual beliefs and practices that have been helpful in the past. Patients who do not consider themselves religious or spiritual may still find comfort in activities that they found meaningful or inspiring, such as the performing arts or nature walks.
- Keep a notebook for recording dates of treatments, medication side effects, laboratory test results, x-ray findings, etc. This record can be valuable in monitoring or evaluating one's emotional ups and downs as well as changes in physical health.
- Keep a journal or diary for expressing feelings and emotional reactions. This record also may be useful in providing perspective.

Psycho-oncologists may also help patients deal with the increasing complexity of cancer therapy, as many patients have treatment teams consisting of several physicians in different subspecialties as well as social workers, nurses, clergy, and other professionals. Some patients experience the sheer number of caregivers involved in their treatment as an additional source of stress.

Treatments

Psycho-oncologists emphasize the importance of treating cancer patients as individuals with unique patterns of emotional responses to the disease as well as unique physical responses to medical and surgical treatments. Consequently, psycho-oncologists tailor their treatment to the needs and concerns of each patient. As of the early 2000s, psycho-oncologists may provide one or more of the following treatments for or services to cancer patients:

- individual psychotherapy or counseling
- leading support groups for patients and family members
- crisis intervention
- medication management
- strategies for dealing with pain and other physical symptoms of cancer
- monitoring the patient's emotional distress level
- referrals to a pastoral counselor in the patient's faith tradition

Many psycho-oncologists use a pain scale, "distress thermometer," or self-administered questionnaires as a way of identifying the patient's specific areas of concern as well as monitoring his or her levels of distress at various points in the treatment process. Some commonly used questionnaires are the Mental Adjustment to Cancer (MAC) scale, first published in the United Kingdom in 1987; the Brief Symptom Inventory (BSI); and the Distress Management Screening Measure (DMSM), a newer scale that was tested in the United States in 2003–2004. Sample questions from these self-administered measures, as well as explanations of the treatments offered to cancer patients at different levels of emotional distress, can be found in *Distress*, a 32-page booklet available free of charge from the American Cancer Society and the National Comprehensive Cancer Network (NCCN).

Psycho-oncologists may also provide specialized counseling in the areas of death and bereavement or sex therapy if they have the appropriate training, or they may refer patients with these needs to qualified counselors in those fields.

Alternative and complementary therapies

Most psycho-oncologists support patients' use of complementary and alternative (CAM) therapies provided that they do not interfere with the patient's surgery, **chemotherapy**, or other mainstream treatments. Dr. Larry Dossey, a well-known expert in the field of alternative medicine, thinks that cancer patients are drawn to CAM treatments because they address questions about the larger meaning of illness that many patients have. He says, "The immense popularity of alternative therapies . . . may be due in large measure to the fact that they help people find meaning in their lives when they need it most." Significantly, several studies of cancer patients who have integrated CAM approaches into their treatment regimens have *not* found that these patients are more distressed or more likely to develop psychiatric disorders than patients who rely on conventional treatments alone.

As of 2005, the National Cancer Institute (NCI) and the National Center for Complementary and Alternative Medicine (NCCAM) are jointly funding **clinical trials** of several complementary and alternative treatments for cancer. Present trials include studies of yoga, Reiki, acupuncture, massage therapy (for cancer-related **fatigue**), hyperbaric oxygen therapy, **mistletoe** extract, and pancreatic enzyme therapy (for **pancreatic cancer**). Details of these clinical trials are available on the NCCAM website.

New trends in research in psycho-oncology

Areas of particular concern to psycho-oncologists in the early 2000s include cultural differences that affect people's patterns of coping with cancer, and the long-term psychological effects of being a cancer survivor. With regard to the first, recent European studies suggest that English-speaking patients and patients from southern Europe have different styles of coping with cancer diagnosis and treatment even though both groups have similar percentages of highly distressed patients. With regard to survivorship, the Behavioral Research Center of the American Cancer Society is conducting a long-term study of cancer survivors' quality of life, with a special focus on their psychological adjustment and family relationships, to be completed in 2015.

See also Depression; Posttraumatic stress disorder.

Resources

BOOKS

Dossey, Larry, MD. *Healing Beyond the Body: Medicine and the Infinite Reach of the Mind.* Boston and London: Shambhala, 2001.

Holland, Jimmie, MD, and Sheldon Lewis. *The Human Side of Cancer: Living with Hope, Coping with Uncertainty.* New York: HarperCollins Publishers, 2000.

PERIODICALS

Davidson, R., L. Geoghegan, L. McLaughlin, and R. Woodward. "Psychological Characteristics of Cancer Patients Who Use Complementary Therapies." *Psycho-Oncology* 14 (June 10, 2004): 187–195.

Hoffman, B. M, M. A. Zevon, M. C. D'Arrigo, and T. B. Cecchini. "Screening for Distress in Cancer Patients: The NCCN Rapid-Screening Measure." *Psycho-Oncology* 13 (November 2004): 792–799.

Holland, Jimmie C., MD. "Psychological Care of Patients: Psycho-Oncology's Contribution." *Journal of Clinical Oncology* 21 (December 2003): 253S–265S. This article was originally given as the American Cancer Society Award Lecture at the annual meeting of the American Society of Clinical Oncology in May 2003.

Patenaude, A. F., and M. J. Kupst. "Psychosocial Functioning in Pediatric Cancer." *Journal of Pediatric Psychology* 30 (January-February 2005): 9–27.

Sunga, Annette, MD, Margaret Eberl, MD, Kevin C. Oeffinger, MD, et al. "Care of Cancer Survivors." *American Family Physician* 71 (February 15, 2005): 699–706.

OTHER

American Cancer Society (ACS) and National Comprehensive Cancer Network (NCCN). *Distress: Treatment Guidelines for Patients*, Version I. Jenkintown, PA: NCCN, 2004.

National Cancer Institute (NCI) and National Center for Complementary and Alternative Medicine (NCCAM). *Cancer Facts: Complementary and Alternative Medicine.* Bethesda, MD: NCCAM, 2004. <http://cis.nci.nih/gov/fact?9_14.htm>.

ORGANIZATIONS

American Psychosocial Oncology Society (APOS). 2365 Hunters Way, Charlottesville, VA 22911. (434) 293-5350. http://www.apos-society.org.

Behavioral Research Center, American Cancer Society. 1599 Clifton Road NE, Atlanta, GA 30329. (800) 758-0227 or (404) 329-7772. http://www.cancer.org.

National Comprehensive Cancer Network (NCCN). 500 Old York Road, Suite 250, Jenkintown, PA 19046. (215) 690-0300. http://www.nccn.org. The NCCN is a consortium of 19 major cancer centers in the United States.

Rebecca Frey, Ph.D.

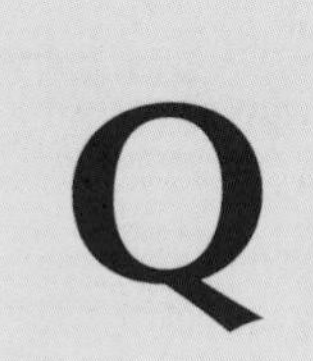

Quadrantectomy

Definition

Quadrantectomy is a surgical procedure in which a "quadrant" (approximately one-fourth) of the breast, including tissue surrounding a cancerous tumor, is removed. It is also called a partial or segmental **mastectomy**.

Purpose

Quadrantectomy is a type of breast-conserving surgery used as a treatment for **breast cancer**. Prior to the advent of breast-conserving surgeries, total mastectomy (complete removal of the breast) was considered the standard surgical treatment for breast **cancer**. Procedures such as quadrantectomy and **lumpectomy** (removing the tissue directly surrounding the tumor) have allowed doctors to treat cancer without sacrificing the entire affected breast.

Demographics

The American Cancer Society estimates that approximately 211,300 new cases of breast cancer are diagnosed annually in the United States, and 39,800 women die as a result of the disease. Approximately one in eight women will develop breast cancer at some point in her life. The risk of developing breast cancer increases with age: women ages 30–40 have a one in 252 chance; ages 40–50 have a one in 68 chance; ages 50–60 have a one in 35 chance; and ages 60–70 have a one in 27 chance.

In the 1990s, the incidence of breast cancer was higher among white women (113.1 cases per 100,000 women) than African American women (100.3 per 100,000). The death rate associated with breast cancer, however, was higher among African American women (29.6 per 100,000) than Caucasian women (22.2 per 100,000). Rates were lower among Hispanic women (14.2 per 100,000), Native American women (12.0), and Asian women (11.2 per 100,000).

Description

The patient is usually placed under general anesthesia for the duration of the procedure. In some instances, a local anesthetic may be administered with sedation to help the patient relax.

During quadrantectomy, a margin of normal breast tissue, skin, and muscle lining is removed around the periphery of the tumor. This decreases the risk of any abnormal cells being left behind and spreading locally or to other parts of the body (a process called **metastasis**). The amount removed is generally about one-fourth of the size of the breast (hence, the "quadrant" in quadrantectomy). The remaining tissue is then reconstructed to minimize any cosmetic defects, and then sutured closed. Temporary drains may be placed through the skin to remove excess fluid from the surgical site.

Some patients may have the lymph nodes removed from under the arm (called the axillary lymph nodes) on the same side as the tumor. Lymph nodes are small, oval- or bean-shaped masses found throughout the body that act as filters against foreign materials and cancer cells. If cancer cells break away from their **primary site** of growth, they can travel to and begin to grow in the lymph nodes first, before traveling to other parts of the body. Removal of the lymph nodes is therefore a method of determining if a cancer has begun to spread. To remove the nodes, a second incision is made in the area of the armpit and the fat pad that contains the lymph nodes is removed. The tissue is then sent to a pathologist, who extracts the lymph nodes from the fatty tissue and examines them for the presence of cancer cells.

Diagnosis/Preparation

Breast tumors may be found during self-examination or an examination by a health care professional. In other cases, they are visualized during a routine mammogram. Symptoms such as breast pain, changes in breast size or shape, redness, dimpling, or irritation may be an indication that medical attention is warranted.

Prior to surgery, the patient is instructed to refrain from eating or drinking after midnight on the night before the operation. The physician will tell the patient what will take place during and after surgery, as well as expected outcomes and potential complications of the procedure.

Aftercare

The patient may return home the same day or remain in the hospital for one to two days after the procedure. Discharge instructions will include how to care for the incision and drains, what activities to restrict (i.e., driving and heavy lifting), and how to manage postoperative pain. Patients are often instructed to wear a well-fitting support bra for at least a week following surgery. A follow-up appointment to remove stitches and drains is usually scheduled 10–14 days after surgery.

If lymph nodes are removed, specific steps should be taken to minimize the risk of developing lymphedema of the arm, a condition in which excess fluid is not properly drained from body tissues, resulting in chronic swelling. This swelling can sometimes become severe enough to interfere with daily activity. Prior to being discharged, the patient will learn how to care for the arm, and how to avoid **infection**. She will also be told to avoid sunburn, refrain from heavy lifting, and to be careful not to wear tight jewelry and elastic bands.

Most patients undergo **radiation therapy** as part of their complete treatment plan. The radiation usually begins immediately or soon after quadrantectomy, and involves a schedule of five days of treatment a week for five to six weeks. Other treatments, such as **chemotherapy** or hormone therapy, may also be prescribed depending on the size and stage of the patient's cancer.

Risks

Risks associated with the surgical removal of breast tissue include bleeding, infection, breast asymmetry, changes in sensation, reaction to the anesthesia, and unexpected scarring.

Some of the risks associated with removal of the lymph nodes include excessive bleeding, infection, pain, excessive swelling, and damage to nerves during surgery. Nerve damage may be temporary or permanent, and may result in weakness, numbness, tingling, and drooping. Lymphedema is also a risk whenever lymph nodes have been removed; it may occur immediately following surgery or months to years later.

WHO PERFORMS THE PROCEDURE AND WHERE IS IT PERFORMED?

Quandrantectomy is usually performed by a general surgeon, breast surgeon, or surgical oncologist. Radiation therapy is administered by a radiation oncologist, and chemotherapy by a medical oncologist. The surgical procedure is frequently done in a hospital setting (especially if lymph nodes are to be removed at the same time), but specialized outpatient facilities are sometimes preferred.

QUESTIONS TO ASK THE DOCTOR

- Why is quadrantectomy recommended?
- What methods of anesthesia and pain relief will be used?
- Where will the incision be located, and how much tissue will be removed?
- Will a lymph node dissection be performed?
- Is sentinel node biopsy appropriate in this case?
- Is postsurgical radiation therapy recommended?

Normal results

Most patients will not experience recurrences of the cancer following a treatment plan of quadrantectomy and radiation therapy. One study followed patients for a period of 20 years after breast-conserving surgery, and found that only 9% experienced recurrence of the cancer.

Morbidity and mortality rates

Following removal of the axillary lymph nodes, there is approximately a 10% risk of lymphedema and a 20% risk of abnormal skin sensations. Approximately 17% of women undergoing breast-conserving surgery have a poor cosmetic result (e.g., asymmetry or distortion of shape). The risk of complications associated with general anesthesia is less than 1%.

Alternatives

A full mastectomy, in which the entire affected breast is removed, is one alternative to quadrantectomy. A **simple mastectomy** removes the entire breast, while a radical mastectomy removes the entire breast plus parts of the chest muscle wall and the lymph nodes. In terms of recurrence and survival rates, breast-conserving surgery has been shown to be equally effective as mastectomy in treating breast cancer.

A new technique that may eliminate the need for removing many axillary lymph nodes is called sentinel node **biopsy**. When lymph fluid moves out of a region, the "sentinel" lymph node is the first node it reaches. The theory behind **sentinel lymph node biopsy** is that if cancer is not present in the sentinel node, it is unlikely to have spread to other nearby nodes. This procedure may allow individuals with early stage cancers to avoid the complications associated with partial or radical removal of lymph nodes if there is little or no chance that cancer has spread to them.

Resources

BOOKS

Iglehart, J. Dirk and Carolyn M. Kaelin. "Diseases of the Breast" (Chapter 30). In *Sabiston Textbook of Surgery*. Philadelphia: W. B. Saunders Company, 2001.

PERIODICALS

Apantaku, Leila. "Breast-Conserving Surgery for Breast Cancer." *American Family Physician* 66, no. 12 (December 15, 2002): 2271-8.

Sainsbury, J. R., T. J. Anderson, and D. A. L. Morgan. "Breast Cancer." *British Medical Journal* 321 (September 23, 2000): 745-50.

Veronesi, U., N. Cascinelli, L. Mariani, et al. "More Long-Term Data for Breast-Conserving Surgery." *New England Journal of Medicine* 347, no. 16 (October17, 2002): 1227-32.

ORGANIZATIONS

American Cancer Society. 1599 Clifton Rd. NE, Atlanta, GA 30329-4251. (800) 227-2345. http://www.cancer.org.

Society of Surgical Oncology. 85 W. Algonquin Rd., Suite 550, Arlington Heights, IL 60005. (847) 427-1400. http://www.surgonc.org.

OTHER

"All About Cancer: Detailed Guide." *American Cancer Society*. 2003 [cited April 9, 2003] http://www.cancer.org/docroot/CRI/CRI_2_3.asp.

Stephanie Dionne Sherk

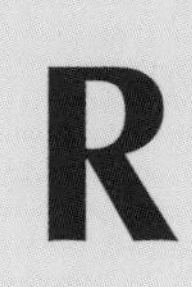

Radiation dermatitis

Definition

Radiation dermatitis, also called radiodermatitis or radiation-induced dermatitis, is injury to the skin from radiation, most often from **radiation therapy** for treating **cancer**.

Demographics

The most common radiation-induced injuries are to the skin. Up to 95% of cancer patients treated with radiation therapy develop some degree of radiation dermatitis. It is estimated that more than 90% of women treated with radiation for **breast cancer** develop radiation dermatitis. Most often the dermatitis is mild to moderate (grades 1–2). However about 20–25% of patients undergoing radiotherapy for locally advanced **head and neck cancers** experience severe radiation dermatitis.

Description

Radiation dermatitis has been associated with radiation exposure since the discovery of **x rays** in 1895. Now used almost exclusively for the treatment of cancer, in the past radiation therapy was used to treat a variety of conditions including acne, eczema, excessive hair growth, and ringworm, frequently resulting in radiation dermatitis. In the past when x-ray machines and other radiation sources were less well-shielded, chronic radiation dermatitis frequently occurred among radiologists and technicians who were constantly exposed to ionizing radiation.

Although radiation dermatitis is common after any radiation treatment, it is particular common after breast cancer treatment. Radiation dermatitis can occur immediately upon treatment or not develop until months after treatment is concluded. It can be very painful and it is not uncommon for breast cancer patients to temporarily halt radiation therapy because of the pain from dermatitis. Both the pain and disfigurement from radiation dermatitis can adversely affect quality of life. Radiation dermatitis can also give rise to basal cell and squamous cell carcinomas, the most common types of **non-melanoma skin cancer**.

There are several types of radiation dermatitis:

- Acute radiation dermatitis is a reddening of the skin called erythema, which can occur up to 24 hours after treatment with an "erythema dose" to the skin, defined as 2 gray (Gy) or more of ionizing radiation. It can occur with the very first radiation treatment.
- Chronic radiation dermatitis occurs from exposure to lower doses of radiation over a longer period, with varying degrees of damage to the skin and underlying layers. Chronic dermatitis becomes apparent after a latent period lasting from several months to decades.
- Eosinophilic, polymorphic, and pruritic (itching) eruption is a radiation dermatitis that occurs most often in women receiving internal cobalt radiotherapy for cancer.
- A radiation recall reaction is radiation dermatitis that occurs on a previously irradiated area of skin following the administration of a chemotherapy drug. It can occur months or years after radiation treatment.

Risk factors

The risk of radiation dermatitis depends on the type of cancer and the radiation regime. The risk of severe radiation dermatitis depends on:

- the total radiation dose
- the dose per treatment
- the total duration of treatment
- the type of radiation beam and its energy
- the surface area of skin exposed to radiation

Other factors also increase the risk for radiation dermatitis. Smoking and previous or concurrent

chemotherapy both increase the risk. There is some evidence that genetic factors play a role in the development of acute radiation dermatitis following radiotherapy for breast cancer.

Causes and symptoms

Although radiation dermatitis is almost always caused by radiation therapy for treating cancer, it can have other causes:

- Radiation dermatitis can be caused by fluoroscopy, a technique which is used in an increasing number of diagnostic procedures. Fluoroscopy-induced radiation dermatitis usually appears within 7–14 days of exposure and may be acute or chronic. However the onset of symptoms is unpredictable and it can develop months or years after radiation exposure.
- Very rarely, deep radiation sensitizes the skin in such a way that subsequent exposure to x rays triggers acute radiation dermatitis.
- Occupational whole-body radiation exposure exceeding 100 REM (radiation-equivalent-man) can cause radiation dermatitis.

Skin irradiation has complex effects involving direct tissue injury and the recruitment of inflammatory immune system cells to the damaged sites. Several different types of skin cells and vascular components may be damaged. With severe radiation dermatitis there is massive cell death. Tissue healing is reduced or prevented by the successive radiation doses used in many radiotherapy regimes.

Radiation dermatitis usually occurs within a few weeks to 90 days after the start of radiation therapy, depending on the intensity of the dose and the sensitivity of the patient's tissue. Transient erythema may redden the skin within hours of the initial radiation. Within 10–14 days the erythema may become persistent. As the cumulative radiation dose increases, damage to the basal cell layer in the deeper epidermis of the skin and injury to the oil (sebaceous) and sweat glands causes the skin to become dry. During the third to sixth week of therapy, skin cells start peeling off in scales, a process called desquamation. These scales can be dry or moist.

Symptoms of acute radiation dermatitis include:

- red patches of inflamed itchy skin
- blistering of the skin
- hair loss
- decreased sweating
- dry desquamation
- wet desquamation
- swelling (edema)
- ulcerations
- bleeding
- skin cell death

These acute symptoms can cause considerable pain, limit daily activities, and may even interrupt or delay radiation treatment. Severe acute dermatitis leads to more severe late complications. These late complications can include hypopigmentation or hyperpigmentation of the skin resulting from damage to melanocytes (the cells that produce skin color), atrophy of the skin, and abnormally dilated capillaries.

Chronic radiation dermatitis usually occurs after second- or third-degree acute radiation dermatitis, but may not become apparent until years after radiotherapy. Symptoms include:

- loss of hair follicles
- development of hard atrophied plaques that are often whitish or yellowish
- increased collagen (the fibrous protein of connective tissue)
- damage to the elastic fibers of the dermis (an inner layer of skin)
- fragility of the outer skin
- patchy discoloration of the skin
- ulcers that do not heal well
- overgrowth of horny tissue (keratosis)
- cancer

Diagnosis

Examination

A history of radiation exposure and physical examination are the primary tools for diagnosing radiation dermatitis.

Procedures

Various histological and immunological methods may be used to analyze a skin **biopsy** sample to diagnose radiation dermatitis. The results vary depending on the length of time that has elapsed since the radiation exposure. Although chronic radiation dermatitis usually is readily identified, it is much more difficult to distinguish subacute radiation dermatitis from other skin conditions.

Grading

A number of different systems have been developed for grading radiation dermatitis. The National Cancer Institute's toxicity grading is as follows:

- grade 1: faint erythema or dry desquamation
- grade 2: moderate to brisk erythema; patchy moist desquamation, mostly confined to skin folds and creases; moderate swelling
- grade 3: moist desquamation beyond skin folds and creases; bleeding induced by minor trauma or abrasion
- grade 4: skin necrosis or ulceration throughout the dermis; spontaneous bleeding from involved site
- grade 5: death

Treatment

Traditional

The aim of radiation dermatitis treatment is to relieve discomfort and pain, avoid further trauma, and restore skin integrity, if possible. In addition to topical creams and lotions, treatments include:

- reducing the radiation dose
- non-adherent dressings
- surgical removal of damaged tissue (debridement)
- chemical peels or chemoexfoliation methods

Drugs

There are a wide range of prescription and over-the-counter products that are used to both prevent and treat radiation dermatitis, although there is little or no evidence for the effectiveness of most of these products. Softening agents (emollients) and hydrating or hydrophilic lotions are generally used for the early stages of radiation dermatitis.

Trolamine ointment is one of the most widely used treatments. A 2006 study found that trolamine did not reduce the incidence or grade of radiation dermatitis in head and neck cancer patients. Biafine is a topical emulsion containing trolamine and sodium alginate. Studies have indicated that patients find Biafine soothing. It may enhance healing by recruiting macrophages (immune system cells) to affected areas and providing a protective barrier against environmental contaminants, reducing the risk of secondary **infection**.

Other topical skin and mucous membrane agents used to treat radiation dermatitis include:

- fluorouracil (Efudex, Fluoroplex, Carac)
- VitE-Allant-MannPly-Hyalr Acid
- Radiplex
- MimyX cream
- Xclair cream

More severe radiation dermatitis is treated by topical and intralesional corticosteroid administration. Evidence indicates that preventative and ongoing use of a topical corticosteroid or a dexpanthenol-containing emollient ameliorates but does not prevent radiation dermatitis.

Alternative

Various alternative commercial treatments are available for radiation dermatitis. A recent French study found that women who were treated with radiation following surgery for breast cancer suffered less skin irritation if they applied calendula (*Calendula officialis* L., marigold) ointment to the irradiated area than if they used trolamine ointment. In the study of 254 women, 41% of those treated with calendula had moderate to severe radiation dermatitis, compared with 63% of those treated with trolamine. The women treated with calendula also reported less severe pain than those who used trolamine; however 30% found the calendula difficult to apply. Only 5% of users found trolamine difficult to apply.

Reports in the 1930s of the beneficial effects of aloe vera gel on skin damaged by radiation exposure led its widespread use in topical skin products. Although it is still sometimes recommended for radiation dermatitis, scientific evidence suggests that aloe gel is not beneficial.

Home remedies

Home remedies for treating radiation dermatitis include:

- bathing
- applying saline compresses to alleviate discomfort
- avoiding shaving the affected area

Prognosis

Severe acute radiation dermatitis often leads to a severe chronic condition and eventually may lead to cancer. Without treatment, radiation dermatitis can cause the discontinuation or delay of subsequent radiation therapy sessions.

Prevention

Ointments applied at least twice a day beginning with the first radiation treatment and continuing throughout radiation therapy may help prevent more serious dermatitis. A recent study suggested that exposing women to low-energy non-thermal light-

QUESTIONS TO ASK YOUR DOCTOR

- Is my radiation dermatitis likely to get worse as my radiation treatments continue?
- Is there anything I can do to prevent radiation dermatitis?
- What treatment do you recommend?
- Should I delay my radiation therapy?

emitting diode (LED) photomodulation following radiotherapy for breast cancer can significantly reduce painful skin reactions and may reduce the need for postponing radiation treatments.

Resources

PERIODICALS

"A Fresh Look at Post-Procedural Wound Care & Radiation Dermatitis.' *Dermatology Times* 29, no. 6 (June 2008): S1-7.

McQuestion, M. "Evidence-Based Skin Care Management in Radiation Therapy.' *Seminars in Oncology Nursing* 22, no. 3 (August 2006): 163-173..

"Radiation Dermatitis; Radiation Dermatitis in Head and Neck Cancer Patients Not Improved by Trolamine.' *Science Letter* (July 18, 2006): 1126.

OTHER

Bernier, J., et al. "Consensus Guidelines for the Management of Radiation Dermatitis and Coexisting Acne-Like Rash in Patients Receiving Radiotherapy Plus EGFR Inhibitors for the Treatment of Squamous Cell Carcinoma." *Annals of Oncology*. http://www.medscape.com/viewarticle/573362

"Calendula Ointment May Help Radiation-Related Skin Pain." *National Cancer Institute*. http://www.cancer.gov/clinicaltrials/results/calendula0504

Henry, Michelle F., et al. "Fluoroscopy-Induced Chronic Radiation Dermatitis: A Report of Three Cases." *Dermatology Online Journal*. http://www.medscape.com/viewarticle/588730

National Research Standard Collaboration. "Calendula (Calendula officinalis L.)." *MedlinePlus*. http://www.nlm.nih.gov/medlineplus/druginfo/natural/patient-calendula.html

ORGANIZATIONS

American Academy of Dermatology, PO Box 4014, Schaumburg, IL, 60168, (847) 240-1280, (866) 503-SKIN (7546), (847) 240-1859, http://www.aad.org.

National Cancer Institute, NCI Public Inquiries Office, 6116 Executive Boulevard, Room 3036A, Bethesda, MD, 20006, (800) 4-CANCER, http://www.cancer.gov.

Margaret Alic, PhD

Radiation therapy

Definition

Radiation therapy, sometimes called radiotherapy, x-ray therapy radiation treatment, cobalt therapy, electron beam therapy, or irradiation uses high energy, penetrating waves or particles such as **x rays**, gamma rays, proton rays, or neutron rays to destroy **cancer** cells or keep them from reproducing.

Purpose

The purpose of radiation therapy is to kill or damage cancer cells. Radiation therapy is a common form of cancer therapy. It is used in more than half of all cancer cases. Radiation therapy can be used:

- alone to kill cancer
- before surgery to shrink a tumor and make it easier to remove
- during surgery to kill cancer cells that may remain in surrounding tissue after the surgery (called intraoperative radiation)
- after surgery to kill cancer cells remaining in the body
- to shrink an inoperable tumor in order to reduce pain and improve quality of life
- in combination with chemotherapy

For some kinds of cancers such as early-stage **Hodgkin's disease**, non-Hodgkin's lymphomas, and certain types of prostate or brain cancer, radiation therapy alone may cure the disease. In other cases, radiation therapy used in conjunction with surgery, **chemotherapy**, or both, increases survival rates over any of these therapies used alone.

Precautions

Radiation therapy does not make the person having the treatments radioactive. In almost all cases, the benefits of this therapy outweigh the risks. However radiation therapy can have has serious consequences, so anyone contemplating it should be sure to understand why the treatment team believes it is the best possible treatment option for their cancer. Radiation therapy is often not appropriate for pregnant women, because the radiation can damage the cells of the developing baby. Women who think they might be pregnant should discuss this with their doctor.

Description

Radiation therapy is a local treatment. It is painless. The radiation only acts on the part of the body

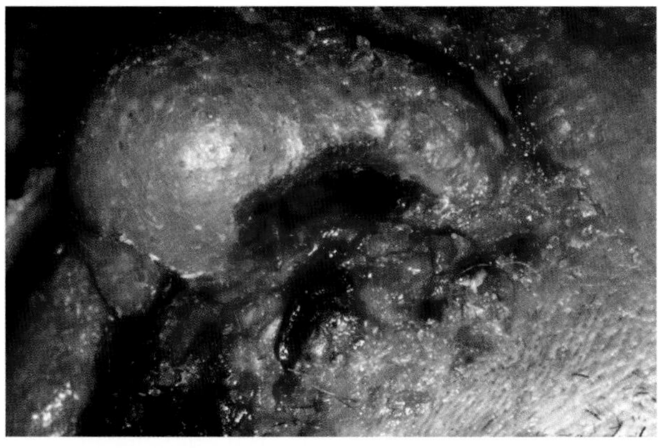

(Copyright Dr. P. Marrazzi, Science Source/Photo Researchers, Inc. Reproduced by permission.)

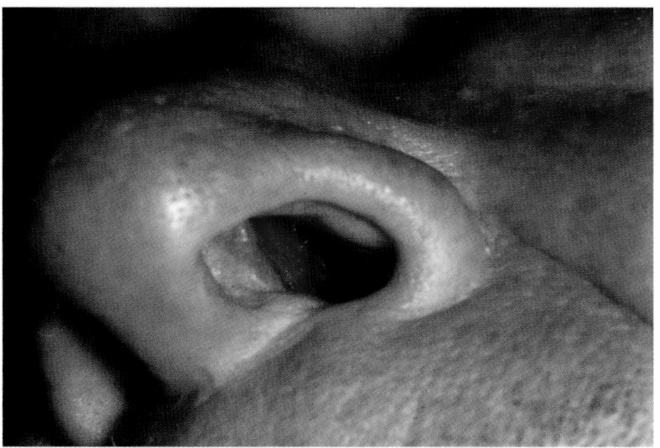

Two weeks after (l) and six months after (r) radiation therapy to treat squamous cell carcinoma inside the left nostril. *(Copyright Dr. P. Marazzi, Science Source/Photo Researchers, Inc. Reproduced by permission.)*

that is exposed to the radiation. This is very different from chemotherapy in which drugs circulate throughout the whole body. There are two main types of radiation therapy. In external radiation therapy a beam of radiation is directed from outside the body at the cancer. In internal radiation therapy, called brachytherapy or implant therapy, a source of radioactivity is surgically placed inside the body near the cancer.

How radiation therapy works

The protein that carries the code controlling most activities in the cell is called deoxyribonucleic acid or DNA. When a cell divides, its DNA must also double and divide. High-energy radiation kills cells by damaging their DNA. This blocks their ability to grow and increase in number.

KEY TERMS

Anemia—Insufficient red blood cells in the body.

Antibody—Protein molecule that recognizes and binds specifically to a foreign substance in the body in order to eliminate it.

Chemotherapy—Injecting drugs into the body where they circulate and kill cancer cells.

Computed tomography (CT or CAT) scan—Using X rays taken from many angles and computer modeling, CT scans help locate and size tumors and provide information on whether they can be surgically removed.

Fractionation—A procedure for dividing a dose of radiation into smaller treatment doses.

Gamma rays—Short wavelength, high energy electromagnetic radiation emitted by radioactive substances.

Hodgkin's disease—Cancer of the lymphatic system, characterized by lymph node enlargement and the presence of a large polyploid cells called Reed-Sternberg cells.

Magnetic resonance imaging (MRI)—MRI uses magnets and radio waves to create detailed cross-sectional pictures of the interior of the body.

Stereotactic—Characterized by precise positioning in space. When applied to radiosurgery, stereotactic refers to a system of three-dimensional coordinates for locating the target site.

One of the characteristics of cancer cells is that they grow and divide faster than normal cells. This makes them particularly vulnerable to radiation. Radiation also damages normal cells, but because normal cells are growing more slowly, they are better able to repair radiation damage than are cancer cells. In order to give normal cells time to heal and reduce side effects, radiation treatments are often given in small doses over a six- or seven-week period.

External radiation therapy

External radiation therapy is the most common kind of radiation therapy. It is usually done during outpatient visits to a hospital clinic and is usually covered by insurance.

Once a doctor called a radiation oncologist determines the proper dose of radiation for a particular cancer, the dose is divided into smaller doses called fractions. One fraction is usually given each day, five

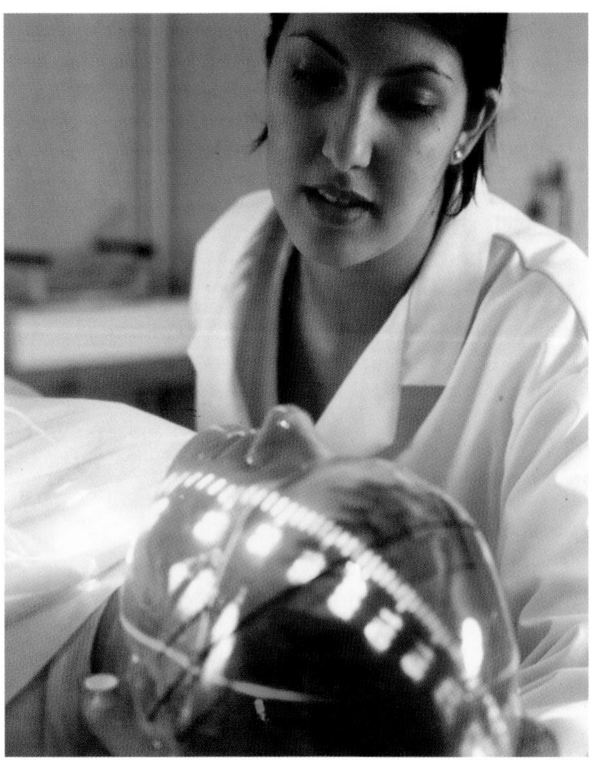

Radiographer prepares a patient for radiation therapy. She is aiming laser cross-hairs onto the site of a brain tumor. The patient's head is protected and held in place by a plastic mask. *(Copyright Simon Fraser, Science Source/Photo Researchers, Inc. Photo reproduced by permission.)*

days a week for six to seven weeks. However, each radiation plan is individualized depending on the type and location of the cancer and what other treatments are also being used. The actual administration of the therapy usually takes about half an hour daily, although radiation is only administered for one to five minutes at each session. It is important to attend every scheduled treatment to get the most benefit from radiation therapy.

Recently, trials have begun to determine if there are ways to deliver radiation fractions so that they kill more cancer cells or have fewer side effects. Some trials use smaller doses given more often. Up-to-date information on voluntary participation in **clinical trials** and where they are being held is available by entering the search term "radiation therapy" at the following web sites:

- National Cancer Institute: <http://cancertrials.nci.nih.gov> or (800) 4-CANCER
- National Institutes of Health Clinical Trials: <http://clinicaltrials.gov>
- Center Watch: A Clinical Trials Listing: <http://www.centerwatch.com>

The type of machines used to administer external radiation therapy and the material that provides the radiation vary depending on the type and location of the cancer. Generally, the patient puts on a hospital gown and lies down or sits in a special chair. Parts of the body not receiving radiation are covered with special shields that block the rays. A technician then directs a beam of radiation to a pre-determined spot on the body where the cancer is located. The patient must stay still during the administration of the radiation so that no other parts of the body are affected. As an extra precaution in some treatments, special molds are made to make sure the body is in the same position for each treatment. However, the treatment itself is painless, like having a bone x-rayed.

Internal radiation therapy

Internal radiation therapy is called brachytherapy, implant therapy, interstitial radiation, or intracavitary radiation. With internal radiation therapy, a bit of radioactive material is sealed in an implant (sometimes called a seed or capsule). The implant is then placed very close to the cancer. The advantage of internal radiation therapy is that it concentrates the radiation near the cancer and lessens the chance of damage to normal cells. Many different types of radioactive materials can be used in the implant, including cesium, iridium, iodine, phosphorus, and palladium.

How the implant is put near the cancer depends on the size and location of the cancer. Internal radiation therapy is used for some cancers of the head, neck, thyroid, breast, female reproductive system, and prostate. Most people will have the radioactive capsule implanted by a surgeon while under either general or local anesthesia at a hospital or surgical clinic.

Patients receiving internal radiation therapy do become temporarily radioactive. They must remain in the hospital during the time that the implant stays in place. The length of time is determined by the type of cancer and the dose of radioactivity to be delivered. During the time the implant is in place, the patient will have to stay in bed and remain reasonably still.

While the implant is in place, the patient's contact with other people will be limited. Health care workers will make their visits as brief as possible to avoid exposure to radiation, and visitors, especially children and pregnant women, will be limited.

The implant usually can be removed in a simple procedure without an anesthetic. As soon as the implant is out of the body, the patient is no longer radioactive, and restrictions on being with other people are lifted. Generally people can return to a level of activity that feels comfortable to them as soon as the implant is removed. Occasionally the site of the implant is sore for some time afterwards. This discomfort may limit specific activities.

In some cases, an implant is left permanently inside the body. People who have permanent implants need to stay in the hospital and away from other people for the first few days. Gradually the radioactivity of the implant decreases, and it is safe to be around other people.

Radioimmunotherapy

Radioimmunotherapy is a promising way to treat cancer that has spread (metastasized) to multiple locations throughout the body. Antibodies are immune system proteins that specifically recognize and bind to only one type of cell. They can be designed to bind only with a certain type of cancer cell. To carry out radioimmunotherapy, antibodies with the ability to bind specifically to a patient's cancer cells are attached to radioactive material and injected into the patient's bloodstream. When these man-made antibodies find a cancer cell, they bind to it. Then the radiation kills the cancer cell. This process is still experimental, but because it can be used to selectively attack only cancer cells, it holds promise for eliminating cancers that have spread beyond the primary tumor.

Radiation used to treat cancer

PHOTON RADIATION. Early radiation therapy used x rays like those used to take pictures of bones, or gamma rays. X rays and gamma rays are high-energy rays composed of massless particles of energy (like light) called photons. The distinction between the two is that gamma rays originate from the decay of radioactive substances (like radium and cobalt-60), while x rays are generated by devices that excite electrons (such as cathode ray tubes and linear accelerators). These high-energy rays act on cells by disrupting the electrons of atoms within the molecules inside cells, disrupting cell functions, and, most importantly, by stopping their ability to divide and make new cells.

PARTICLE RADIATION. Particle radiation is radiation delivered by particles that have mass. Proton therapy has been used since the early 1990s. Proton rays consist of protons, a type of positively charged atomic particle, rather than photons, which have neither mass nor charge. Like x rays and gamma rays, proton rays disrupt cellular activity. The advantage of using proton rays is that they can be shaped to conform to the irregular shape of the tumor more precisely than x rays and gamma rays. They allow delivery of higher radiation doses to tumors without increasing damage to the surrounding tissue.

Neutron therapy is another type of particle radiation. Neutron rays are very high-energy rays. They are composed of neutrons, which are particles with mass but no charge. The type of damage they cause to cells is much less likely to be repaired than that caused by x rays, gamma rays, or proton rays.

Neutron therapy can treat larger tumors than conventional radiation therapy. Conventional radiation therapy depends on the presence of oxygen to work. The center of large tumors lack sufficient oxygen to be susceptible to damage from conventional radiation. Neutron radiation works in the absence of oxygen, making it especially effective for the treatment of inoperable **salivary gland tumors**, bone cancers, and some kinds of advanced cancers of the pancreas, bladder, lung, prostate, and uterus.

Recent advances in radiation therapy

A newer mode of treating brain cancers with radiation therapy is known as stereotactic radiosurgery. As of the early 2000s, this approach is limited to treating cancers of the head and neck because only these parts of the body can be held completely still throughout the procedure. Stereotactic radiosurgery allows the doctor to deliver a single high-level dose of precisely directed radiation to the tumor without damaging nearby healthy brain tissue. The treatment is planned with the help of three-dimensional computer-aided analysis of CT and MRI scans. The patient's head and neck are held steady in a skeletal fixation device during the actual treatment. Stereotactic radiosurgery can be used in addition to standard surgery to treat a recurrent brain tumor, or in place of surgery if the tumor cannot be reached by standard surgical techniques.

Two major forms of stereotactic radiosurgery are in use as of 2003. The gamma knife is a stationary machine that is most useful for small tumors, blood vessels, or similar targets. Because it does not move, it can deliver a small, highly localized and precise beam of radiation. Gamma knife treatment is done all at once in a single hospital stay. The second type of radiosurgery uses a movable linear accelerator-based machine that is preferred for larger tumors. This treatment is delivered in several small doses given over several weeks. Radiosurgery that is performed with divided doses is known as fractionated radiosurgery. The total dose of radiation is higher with a linear accelerator-based machine than with gamma knife treatment.

Another advance in intraoperative radiotherapy (IORT) is the introduction of mobile devices that allow the surgeon to use radiotherapy in early-stage disease and to operate in locations where it would be difficult to transport the patient during surgery for radiation treatment. Mobile IORT units have been used successfully as of 2003 in treating early-stage **breast cancer** and **rectal cancer**.

Radiation sensitizers are another recent innovation in radiation therapy. Sensitizers are medications that are given to make cancer cells easier to kill by radiation than normal calls. **Gemcitabine** (Gemzar) is one of the drugs most commonly used for this purpose.

Preparation

Before radiation therapy, the size and location of the patient's tumor are determined very precisely using **magnetic resonance imaging** (MRI) and/or **computed tomography** scans (CT scans). The correct radiation dose, the number of sessions, the interval between sessions, and the method of application are calculated by a radiation oncologist based on the tumor type, its size, and the sensitivity of the nearby tissues.

The patient's skin is marked with a semi-permanent ink to help the radiation technologist achieve correct positioning for each treatment. Molds may be built to hold tissues in exactly the right place each time.

Aftercare

Many patients experience skin burn, **fatigue**, **nausea**, and **vomiting** after radiation therapy regardless of where the radiation is applied. After treatment, the skin around the site of the treatment may also become sore. Affected skin should be kept clean and can be treated like sunburn, with skin lotion or vitamin A and D ointment. Patients should avoid perfume and scented skin products and protect affected areas from the sun.

Nausea and vomiting are most likely to occur when the radiation dose is high or if the abdomen or another part of the digestive tract is irradiated. Sometimes nausea and vomiting occur after radiation to other regions, but in these cases the symptoms usually disappear within a few hours after treatment. Nausea and vomiting can be treated with antacids, Compazine, Tigan, or Zofran.

Fatigue frequently starts after the second week of therapy and may continue until about two weeks after the therapy is finished. Patients may need to limit their activities, take naps, and get extra sleep at night.

Patients should see their oncologist (cancer doctor) at least once within the first few weeks after their final radiation treatment. They should also see an oncologist every six to twelve months for the rest of their lives so they can be checked to see if the tumor has reappeared or spread.

Risks

Radiation therapy can cause **anemia**, nausea, vomiting, **diarrhea**, hair loss (**alopecia**), skin burn, sterility, and rarely death. However, the benefits of radiation therapy almost always exceed the risks. Patients should discuss the risks with their doctor and get a second opinion about their treatment plan.

Normal results

The outcome of radiation treatment varies depending on the type, location, and stage of the cancer. For some cancers such as Hodgkin's disease, about 75% of the patients are cured. **Prostate cancer** also responds well to radiation therapy. Radiation to painful bony metastases is usually a dramatically effective form of pain control. Other cancers may be less sensitive to the benefits of radiation.

Resources

BOOKS

Cukier, Daniel, and Virginia McCullough. *Coping with Radiation Therapy*. Los Angeles: Lowell House, 2001.

PERIODICALS

Goer, D. A., C. W. Musslewhite, and D. M. Jablons. "Potential of Mobile Intraoperative Radiotherapy Technology." *Surgical Oncology Clinics of North America* 12 (October 2003): 943–954.

Lawrence, T. S. "Radiation Sensitizers and Targeted Therapies." *Oncology (Huntington)* 17 (December 2003): 23–28.

Merrick, H. W. IIIrd, L. L. Gunderson, and F. A. Calvo. "Future Directions in Intraoperative Radiation Therapy." *Surgical Oncology Clinics of North America* 12 (October 2003): 1099–1105.

Nag, S., and K. S. Hu. "Intraoperative High-Dose-Rate Brachytherapy." *Surgical Oncology Clinics of North America* 12 (October 2003): 1079–1097.

Witt, M. E., M. Haas, M. A. Marrinan, and C. N. Brown. "Understanding Stereotactic Radiosurgery for Intracranial Tumors, Seed Implants for Prostate Cancer, and Intravascular Brachytherapy for Cardiac Restenosis." *Cancer Nursing* 26 (December 2003): 494–502.

OTHER

Radiation Therapy and You. A Guide to Self-Help During Treatment. National Cancer Institute CancerNet Information Service. <http://cancernet.nci.nih.gov>.

ORGANIZATIONS

American Cancer Society. 1599 Clifton Rd. NE, Atlanta GA 30329-4251. (800) ACS-2345. http://www.cancer.org.

International Radiosurgery Support Association (IRSA). 3005 Hoffman Street, Harrisburg, PA 17110. (717) 260-9808. www.irsa.org.

National Association for Proton Therapy. 7910 Woodmont Ave., Suite 1303, Bethesda, MD 20814. (301) 913-9360. http://www.proton-therapy.org/Default.htm.

Rebecca J. Frey, PhD

Radical neck dissection

Definition

Radical neck dissection is an operation used to remove cancerous tissue in the head and neck.

Purpose

The purpose of radical neck dissection is to remove lymph nodes and other structures in the head and neck that are likely or proven to be malignant. Variations on neck dissections exist depending on the extent of the **cancer**. A radical neck dissection removes the most tissue. It is done when the cancer has spread widely in the neck. A modified neck dissection removes less tissue, and a selective neck dissection even less.

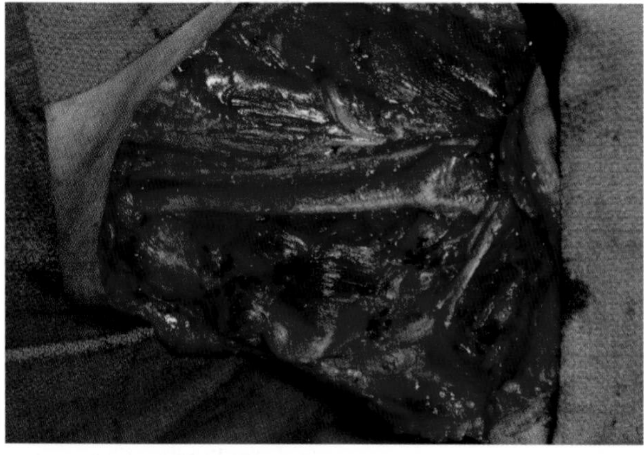

A radical neck surgery in progress. *(Custom Medical Stock Photo. Reproduced by permission.)*

KEY TERMS

Barium swallow—Barium is used to coat the throat in order to take x-ray pictures of the tissues lining the throat.

Computed tomography (CT or CAT) scan—Using x rays taken from many angles and computer modeling, CT scans help size and locate tumors and provide information on whether they can be surgically removed.

Lymphatic system—Primary defense against infection in the body. The tissues, organs, and channels (similar to veins) that produce, store, and transport lymph and white blood cells to fight infection.

Lymph nodes—Small, bean-shaped collections of tissue found in lymph vessels. They produce cells and proteins that fight infection and filter lymph. Nodes are sometimes called lymph glands.

Magnetic resonance imaging (MRI)—MRI uses magnets and radio waves to create detailed cross-sectional pictures of the interior of the body.

Malignant—Cancerous. Cells tend to reproduce without normal controls on growth and form tumors or invade other tissues.

Metastasize—Spread of cells from the original site of the cancer to other parts of the body where secondary tumors are formed.

Precautions

This operation should not be done if cancer has metastasized (spread) beyond the head and neck, or if the cancer has invaded the bones of the cervical vertebrae (the first seven vertebrae of the spinal column) or the skull. In these cases, the surgery will not effectively contain the cancer.

Description

Cancers of the head and neck (sometimes inaccurately called throat cancer) often spread to nearby tissues and into the lymph nodes. Removing these structures is one way of controlling the cancer.

Of the six hundred lymph nodes in the body, about 200 are in the neck. Only a small number of these are removed during a neck dissection. In addition, other structures such as muscles, veins, and nerves may be removed during a radical neck dissection. These include the sternocleidomastoid muscle (one of the muscles that functions to flex the head),

QUESTIONS TO ASK THE DOCTOR

- What tests will you do to determine if my cancer has spread?
- Which parts of my neck will be removed?
- How will a radical neck dissection affect my daily activities after recovery?
- What is the likelihood that all my cancer can be removed with a radical neck dissection?
- Are the lymph nodes on one or both sides of my neck involved?
- What will my appearance be like after surgery?
- How will my speech and breathing be affected?

internal jugular (neck) vein, submandibular gland (one of the salivary glands), and the spinal accessory nerve (a nerve that helps control speech, swallowing and certain movements of the head and neck). The goal is always to remove all the cancer but to save as many components surrounding the nodes as possible.

Radical neck dissections are done in a hospital under general anesthesia by a head and neck surgeon. An incision is made in the neck, and the skin is pulled back to reveal the muscles and lymph nodes. The surgeon is guided in what to remove by tests done prior to surgery and by examination of the size and texture of the lymph nodes.

Preparation

Radical neck dissection is a major operation. Extensive tests are done before the operation to try to determine where and how far the cancer has spread. These may include lymph node biopsies, CT (**computed tomography**) scans, **magnetic resonance imaging** (MRI) scans, and barium swallows. In addition, standard pre-operative blood and liver function tests are performed, and the patient will meet with an anesthesiologist before the operation. The patient should tell the anesthesiologist about all drug allergies and all medication (prescription, non-prescription, or herbal) that he or she is taking.

Aftercare

A person who has had a radical neck dissection will stay in the hospital several days after the operation, and sometimes longer if surgery to remove the primary tumor was done at the same time. Drains are inserted under the skin to remove the fluid that accumulates in the neck area. Once the drains are removed and the incision appears to be healing well, patients are usually discharged from the hospital, but will require follow-up doctor visits. Depending on how many structures are removed, a person who has had a radical neck dissection may require physical therapy to regain use of the arm and shoulder.

Risks

The greatest risk in a radical neck dissection is damage to the nerves, muscles, and veins in the neck. Nerve damage can result in numbness (either temporary or permanent) to different regions on the neck and loss of function (temporary or permanent) to parts of the neck, throat, and shoulder. The more extensive the neck dissection, the more function the patient is likely to lose. As a result, it is common following radical neck dissection for a person to have stooped shoulders, limited ability to lift the arm, and limited head and neck rotation and flexion due to the removal of nerves and muscles. Other risks are the same as for all major surgery: potential bleeding, **infection**, and allergic reaction to anesthesia.

Normal results

Normal lymph nodes are small and show no cancerous cells under the microscope.

Abnormal results

Abnormal lymph nodes may be enlarged and show malignant cells when examined under the microscope.

Resources

OTHER

The Voice Center at Eastern Virginia Medical School. (February 17, 2001). [cited June 7, 2001]. http://www.voice-center.com.

ORGANIZATIONS

American Cancer Society. National Headquarters, 1599 Clifton Road NE, Atlanta, GA 30329. (800) ACS-2345). http://www.cancer.org.

Cancer Information Service. National Cancer Institute, Building 31, Room 10A19, 9000 Rockville Pike, Bethesda, MD 20892. (800) 4-CANCER. http://www.nci.nih.gov/cancerinfo/index.html.

John Thomas Lohr
Tish Davidson, A.M.

Radiofrequency ablation

Definition

Radiofrequency ablation is a treatment that uses radio waves to create heat and directs the heat though a needle probe at **cancer** cells to destroy tumors.

Purpose

Radiofrequncy ablation (RFA) is minimally invasive, meaning it involves having to enter the body, but not as severely as major surgery. Because of this and its ability to create heat in a specific location, RFA is a good treatment choice for patients with many types of cancer. RFA also has proven to be an excellent alternative for many patients who have not been able to receive surgery or other cancer therapy, or who have tried other cancer treatments that have failed. For example, some patients cannot have surgery because they have heart or lung conditions that make a long procedure under general anesthesia risky. In other cases, the type, characteristics, or location of the cancer make RFA a better option. The treatment is used not only to help treat cancer, but to ease pain in cancer patients, treat tumors that recur, and to treat some conditions other than cancer.

Liver tumors

One of the cancers treated most by RFA is cancer of the liver. In many cases, removing the tumor with surgery would not leave enough healthy tissue for the liver to still function. Liver tumors that spread (metastasize) from cancers that started somewhere else in the body also are good candidates for RFA. If a patient has several tumors spread out across the liver, surgeons cannot operate. RFA can eliminate the smaller tumors and a surgeon can follow up by operating on the larger tumor if necessary. In some cases, a previous attempt to treat the tumor, such as with **chemotherapy**, has failed and RFA is the next option. RFA also might be used to treat a tumor that has recurred.

Lung tumors

Some patients with lung cancer also are too ill to have conventional surgery or want to avoid the long recovery and possible complications of surgery. RFA once was thought useful only for early, small lung cancers. But research released in 2004 showed that it safely and effectively treated advanced lung cancer as well. The technique also may be used to treat cancer spread to the lung (lung metastases). Physicians also may use RFA to remove most of a tumor that is too large to remove with surgery. The process of making the tumor smaller is called debulking.

> **QUESTIONS TO ASK YOUR DOCTOR**
>
> - Why is radiofrequency ablation the best alternative for my cancer?
> - What are the risks involved in the treatment?
> - How many of these procedures have you performed?

Kidney tumors

Many patients with kidney tumors have surgery, but some patients only have one kidney, making RFA the preferred treatment, since it helps spare the only kidney. As with other organs, RFA is an excellent alternative for patients who have conditions that might prevent them from having surgery or for whom recovery from surgery would be difficult. RFA for kidney (renal) cancer is an excellent choice for patients with more than one tumor, if the tumors are smaller than about 4 to 5 cm.

Bone cancer and pain

When cancer spreads to the bones, it can become very painful. Usually, RFA for bone cancer is not used to treat the cancer, but to relieve the pain associated with it. Physicians also may use RFA to relieve pain associated with other cancers by shrinking a tumor that is causing pain, particularly when the tumor has not responded to other treatments or cannot be reached or treated with surgery. This may be referred to as palliation or palliative care.

Other cancers

Researchers continue to find new uses for RFA to treat a number of cancers. For example, a 2004 report showed that RFA could assist with **lumpectomy** for **breast cancer** by giving the patient a cancer-free area around the site where the tumor is removed. RFA also improved cosmetic results. RFA is considered safe, predictable, and cheap when compared to many other treatments.

Precautions

RFA is safe for most patients, and generally can be used in place of surgery for patients who cannot

KEY TERMS

Lumpectomy—Removal of a breast tumor (by surgery) with a limited amount of surrounding breast tissue.

Metastasize—To spread to distant sites. This is the term used when cancer from one organ or site moves to another area of the body and causes cancer in another area or organ.

Percutaneous—Through the skin.

Recur, recurrence—Cancer that happens again after time has passed.

withstand longer surgical procedures, complications, and recovery times. Still, physicians will discuss the benefits and risks of RFA with patients in advance. The procedure usually will require some anesthesia. A medical history and blood tests may rule out some patients or require them to adjust certain medications. Also, some tumors or cancers are not considered treatable with RFA. The number and size of tumors that can be treated in a particular organ may be limited.

Description

Radiofrequency refers to the radio waves, or form of electromagnetic energy, produced by an electrical generator used in the RFA. Electromagnetic energy already is present in the natural environment, as in visible light, microwaves, and radio waves. The energy from radiofrequency is safer than that from **x rays** because it is absorbed by living tissue as simple heat, which does not change the structure of the cells.

The patient lies on a table in an examination or surgical suite and becomes a sort of electrical circuit through which the radio waves pass. Grounding pads are placed on the patient's back or thighs. Most RFA procedures today are performed by an interventional radiologist. An interventional radiologist is a medical doctor who specializes in performing medical procedures that involved radiology to diagnose and treat disease. The radiologist usually uses ultrasound, but sometimes **computed tomography** (CT) or **magnetic resonance imaging** (MRI) equipment and video monitors during the procedure to guide the way to the tumor.

Most interventional radiologists guide the small needle or probe that holds the current through the patient's skin and directly into the tumor. This is called the percutaneous method and will make for an easier recovery. Sometimes, a single needle electrode is used; at other times, one straight needle contains many curved needles that retract inside the main probe until its tip is positioned within the tumor. Once the physician has positioned the tumor, the electrodes can open up like an umbrella to deliver heat to a larger area.

The heat can be controlled by the physician. At temperatures above 113 degrees Fahrenheit, RFA "cooks" the tumor. During the procedure, the radiologist is using real-time imaging (ultrasound, CT, or MRI) to locate the cancerous tumor and guide the needle probe. A small needle can accurately heat a precise area. If a tumor is large, the radiologist may have to guide and reposition the probe several times to destroy the entire tumor. After destroying the tumor, the physician also will use the probe to heat and destroy a small margin or rim of healthy tissue around the cancerous tumor. This helps ensure that no single cancerous cell is left behind that can regrow. After the treatment is completed, a small bandage is placed over the probe insertion site. Each RFA treatment takes 15 to 30 minutes, but the entire procedure can take longer, depending on the number of tumors, tumor size, and location. For instance, the interventional radiologist may have to reposition the probe several times for one liver mass, then turn to a second smaller mass, for a total procedure time of 90 minutes. Some procedures can take up to three hours. RFA procedures are performed in hospitals, imaging centers, and physician offices. Most are done on an outpatient basis.

Some pain can be associated with RFA, even with the percutaneous method. Most physicians will insert an intravenous (IV) line in the patient through which they will give anesthesia that makes the patient drowsy, but not completely out. This is often called "conscious sedation." In complex procedures, general anesthesia may be required with an anesthesiologist or nurse anesthetist present and monitoring the patient's vital signs. Sometimes, the physician uses a laparascope to introduce the probe. Although **laparoscopy** requires a tiny incision, it still is considered surgery. Some surgeons also use RFA on patients as part of general surgery. RFA sometimes is called radiofrequency thermal ablation.

Preparation

Before the RFA procedure, patients may have blood drawn for routine blood tests. The physician, nurse, or scheduler will provide preparation instructions that will include concerns about eating or drinking before the procedure. These instructions will depend on the type of anesthesia planned. Normally, patients will be told not to eat or drink eight hours (or after midnight) before the RFA procedure. Certain medications may need to be changed or stopped before the procedure. For example, blood thinners and aspirin may interfere with the procedure. A patient should reveal all current medications to the interventional radiologist or surgeon and follow preparation instructions.

Aftercare

The treatment team will move the patient to a recovery room following the procedure to allow anesthesia to wear off and to receive pain medication as needed. Some patients also have **nausea** and will receive medications and instructions for nausea and pain care before leaving the facility. Patients will have to remain in bed for the first few hours following the procedure, but seldom have to stay overnight from RFA. However, those having the procedure through surgery will require some hospital stay.

Once they return home, patients will be instructed to drink plenty of fluid and to take a prescription narcotic such as Percocet for the first day or two if pain continues. The physician likely will instruct patients not to drive a car or make important decisions for 24 hours after the procedure because of anesthesia effects. Excessive physical activity also is discouraged. However, most patients can resume normal diet, physical activity, and sexual activity within a few days of RFA.

Risks

The risks associated with radiofrequency ablation are relatively minor compared to those associated with many other cancer treatments, particularly surgery. However, no procedure is risk-free. Although rare, there is a risk of serious injury if the needle makes a hole (perforates) a nearby organ. If this happens, the patient may require surgery to repair the injury. There also is a minor risk of **infection** at the site where the probe is inserted. Patients may experience bruising or bleeding. Another possible complication from RFA to the lungs is air or gas in the chest cavity (pneumothorax), which may require a chest tube for a few days to drain the air. Finally, RFA is a complicated procedure and should be performed only by a physician trained specifically to do the procedure. Most interventional radiologists have extensive experience in these and similar procedures, but patients can check with accrediting societies, local medical societies and their primary care physicians and ask questions of the physician who will perform the procedure.

Normal results

Results vary, depending on the location, type, and size of tumor. Normally, scar tissue replaces the tumor cells destroyed by RFA and shrinks over a period of time. Patients should have no pain from the procedure after a few days.

Abnormal results

If pain continues for more than a few days, the patient should contact the physician. Some patients also develop flu-like symptoms and **fever** following RFA that can last for a few weeks. Bleeding after RFA has been reported. If it continues and is severe, the patient may have to return for an additional RFA procedure or surgery to control the bleeding. Sometimes, cancer recurs following RFA because tumors are so tiny they cannot be seen. Some patients will need another RFA procedure in the future.

Resources

PERIODICALS

"Breast Cancer Study Examines New Radiofrequency Ablation Assisted Lumpectomy." *Medical Devices & Surgical Technology Week* (Dec. 12, 2004):34.

"CIGNA HealthCare Will Cover Radiofrequency Ablation Liver Treatment."*Drug Week* (Oct. 15, 2004):403.

Livraghi, Tito, et al. "Treatment of Focal Liver Tumors With Percutaneous Radiofrequency Ablation: Complications Encountered in a Multicenter Study. "*Drug Week* (Feb. 2003):441–451.

"Lung Cancer Survival Statistics Reported in Trial Using Radiofrequency Ablation."*Cancer Weekly* (Dec. 28, 2004):151.

Patti, Jay W., Ziv Neeman, and Bradford J. Wood. "Radiofrequency Ablation for Cancer-associated Pain." *The Journal of Pain* (Dec. 2002):471–473.

"Radiofrequency Ablation Safe and Feasible for Eradicating Lung Tumors." *Clinical Oncology Week* (Aug. 23, 2004):49.

OTHER

ARRS: Radiofrequency Ablation Effective in Treating Advanced Lung Cancer. Web site news release. Doctor's Guide Publishing Ltd. American Roentgen Ray Society, 2003. http://www.docguide.com/news.

Percutaneous Radiofrequency Ablation. Web page. National Institutes of Health, Warren Grant Magnuson Clinical Center, 2001. http://www.nih.gov.

Radiofrequency Ablation of Liver Tumors. Web page. Radiological Society of North America, 2005. http://www.radiologyinfo.org/content/interventional/rf_ablation.htm.

Radiofrequency Ablation of Lung Tumors. Web page. Radiological Society of North America, 2005. http://www.radiologyinfo.org/content/interventional/rfalung.htm.

Treatments. Web page. Society of Interventional Radiology, 2003. http://www.sirweb.org/patPub/cancerTreatments.html.

ORGANIZATIONS

Society of Interventional Radiology. 10201 Lee Highway, Suite 500, Fairfax, VA 22030. 703-691-1805. http://www.sirweb.org.

Teresa G. Odle

Radionuclide bone scan *see* **Nuclear medicine scans**

Radionuclide imaging *see* **Nuclear medicine scans**

Radiopharmaceuticals

Definition

Radiopharmaceuticals are radioactive substances that may be used to treat **cancer**.

Purpose

The common radiopharmaceuticals that are used in cancer treatment include:

- Chromic phosphate P 32 for the treatment of lung, ovarian, uterine, and prostate cancers
- Sodium iodide I 131 for treating certain types of thyroid cancer
- Strontium chloride Sr 89 for treating cancerous bone tissue
- Samarium Sm 153 lexidronam for treating cancerous bone tissue
- Sodium phosphate P 32 for treating cancerous bone tissue and other types of cancers.

Description

Radiopharmaceuticals used in cancer treatment are small, simple substances, containing a radioactive isotope or form of an element. They are targeted to specific areas of the body where cancer is present. Radiation emitted from the isotope kills cancer cells. These isotopes have short half-lives, meaning that most of the radiation is gone within a few days or weeks.

KEY TERMS

Half-life—Length of time for the decay of one half of the radiation in a sample of a given radioactive isotope.

Isotopes—Forms of a chemical element that have the same number of protons (atomic number) but different numbers of neutrons and different atomic weights.

Lymph nodes—Small round glands, located throughout the body, that remove foreign organisms and debris from the lymphatic fluid.

Metastasis—Spread of cancer from its point of origin to other parts of the body, such as the bone.

Millicurie—Unit for measuring radioactivity; one millicurie is the quantity of a radioactive isotope that undergoes 3.7×10^7 disintegrations per second.

Platelet—Blood component that aids in clotting.

Thyroid—Gland on each side of the trachea (windpipe) that secretes hormones to regulate metabolism and growth.

Chromic phosphate P 32 and sodium iodide I 131

Chromic phosphate P 32 is a salt of chromium and phosphoric acid, containing a radioactive form of the element phosphorous, ^{32}P. Its brand name is Phosphocol P 32. Chromic phosphate P 32 is used to treat fluid accumulations that can result from lung, ovarian, or uterine cancers. It is 50-80% effective in stopping fluid leakage from these organs. Chromic phosphate P 32 also is used to kill cancer cells that remain following surgery for uterine cancer. It may be used to treat ovarian or prostate cancers directly. The use of chromic phosphate P 32 is not combined with external beam radiation, but may be used in conjunction with **chemotherapy**.

Sodium iodide I 131, also called radioactive iodine or radioiodide, is a salt of sodium and a radioactive form of the element iodine, ^{131}I. Sodium iodide I 131 is taken up by the thyroid gland, which absorbs most of the iodine in the body. Sodium iodide I 131 can destroy the thyroid gland, with only minor effects on other parts of the body. It is used following surgery for **thyroid cancer** to destroy any remaining cancerous thyroid tissue, or to destroy thyroid cancer that has spread (metastasized) to lymph nodes or other tissues. Sodium iodide I 131 is a standard treatment for differentiated thyroid cancer that has spread to the neck and other parts of the body. Its use improves the survival rate for such patients. It is not clear whether radioiodide is beneficial for small cancers of the thyroid that have not metastasized to other tissues.

Bone metastasis

Several radiopharmaceuticals are used to treat cancerous tissue in the bone, particularly from **prostate cancer**. Most prostate cancer metastasizes to the bone and often this is the cause of death. When injected into a vein these radiopharmaceuticals accumulate in cancerous bone tissue and give off radiation that kills cancer cells and relieves pain in the majority of patients. These treatments are most effective for cancer that has metastasized to multiple bones. Sometimes these radiopharmaceuticals are used in conjunction with external beam radiation that is directed at the most painful areas.

Strontium chloride Sr 89 (strontium-89) is the most common radiopharmaceutical for treating bone cancer or prostate cancer that has metastasized to the bone. It is a salt of chlorine and a radioactive isotope of strontium, ^{89}Sr. Its brand name is Metastron. Men with advanced prostate cancer who are responding to chemotherapy appear to have a better chance of survival if bone metastases is treated with strontium-89 every six weeks in conjunction with a chemotherapy drug.

Samarium SM 153 lexidronam is a radioactive form of samarium, ^{153}Sm. The element is inside a small molecule called lexidronam. The brand name for samarium SM 153 lexidronam is Quadramet. It is used primarily to treat prostate cancer that has metastasized to the bone.

Sodium phosphate P 32 is a salt of sodium and phosphoric acid containing a radioactive form of the element phosphorous, ^{32}P. It is used primarily for breast and prostate cancers that have metastasized to the bone. It also may be used to treat other types of cancer.

Two other radioactive isotopes, rhenium 86 and rhenium 188, sometimes are used to treat bone **metastasis** from prostate cancer.

Recommended dosage

Dosages of radiopharmaceuticals vary with the individual and the type of treatment. Dosages of radioactive materials are expressed in units called millicuries.

Chromic phosphate P 32 is a suspension that is delivered through a catheter, or tube, inserted into the sac surrounding the lungs, or into the abdominal or pelvic cavities. The usual dosage is 15-20 millicuries for abdominal administration and 10 millicuries for administration to the lung sac. Chromic phosphate P 32 also may be injected into the ovaries or prostate.

Sodium Iodide I 131 is taken by mouth as a capsule or a solution. The usual dose for treating thyroid cancer is 30-200 millicuries, depending on age and body size. Doses may be repeated. Treatment usually requires two to three days of hospitalization. For this therapy to be effective there must be high levels of thyroid-stimulating hormone (TSH, or thyrotropin) in the blood. This hormone can be injected prior to treatment.

Strontium-89 is injected into a vein. The usual dosage is 4 millicuries, depending on age, body size, and blood cell counts. Repeated doses may be required.

The usual dosage of samarium Sm 153 lexidronam is 1 millicurie per kg (0.45 millicurie per lb) of body weight, injected slowly into a vein. Repeated doses may be necessary. Because samarium Sm 153 lexidronam may accumulate in the bladder, it is important to drink plenty of liquid prior to treatment and to urinate often after treatment. This reduces the irradiation of the bladder.

The dosage of sodium phosphate P 32 depends on age, body size, blood cell counts, and the type of treatment. The usual dosages range from 1–5 millicuries. Repeated doses may be required.

Precautions

Some individuals may have an allergic reaction to strontium-89, samarium SM 153 lexidronam, or sodium phosphate P 32.

Radiopharmaceuticals usually are not recommended for use during pregnancy. It is recommended that women do not become pregnant for a year after treatment with sodium iodide I 131. Breast-feeding is not possible during treatment with radiopharmaceuticals.

Precautions before treatment with sodium iodide I 131

Foods containing iodine, such as iodized salt, seafoods, cabbage, kale, or turnips, should be avoided for several weeks prior to treatment with sodium iodide I 131. The iodine in these foods will be taken up by the thyroid, thereby reducing the amount of radioiodide that can be taken up. Radiopaque agents containing iodine sometimes are used to improve imaging on an x ray. A recent x-ray exam that included such an agent may interfere with the ability of the thyroid to take up radioiodide.

Diarrhea or **vomiting** may cause sodium iodide I 131 to be lost from the body, resulting in less effective treatment and the risk of outside contamination. Kidney disease may prevent the excretion of radioiodide, increasing the risk of side effects from the drug.

Precautions after treatment with radiopharmaceuticals

Strontium-89, samarium Sm 153 lexidronam, and large total doses of sodium iodide I 131 may temporarily lower the number of white blood cells, which are necessary for fighting infections. The number of blood platelets (important for blood clotting) also may be lowered. Precautions for reducing the risk of **infection** and bleeding include:

- avoiding people with infections
- seeking medical help at the first sign of infection or unusual bleeding
- using care when cleaning teeth
- avoiding touching the eyes or inside of the nose
- avoiding cuts and injuries

It is important to drink plenty of liquids and to urinate often after treatment with sodium iodide I 131. This flushes the radioiodide from the body. To reduce the risk of contaminating the environment or other people, the following procedures should be followed for 48–96 hours after treatment is sodium iodide I 131:

- avoiding kissing and sex
- avoiding the handling of another person's eating utensils, etc.
- avoiding close contact with others, especially pregnant women
- washing the tub and sink after each use
- washing hands after using or cleaning the toilet
- using separate washcloths and towels
- washing clothes, bed linens, and dishes separately
- flushing the toilet twice after each use

Strontium-89 and samarium Sm 153 lexidronam also are excreted in the urine. To prevent radioactive contamination, special measures should be followed for one week after receiving strontium-89 and for 12 hours after receiving samarium Sm 153 lexidronam:

- using a toilet rather than a urinal
- flushing the toilet several times after each use
- wiping up and flushing any spilled urine or blood
- washing hands after using or cleaning a toilet
- washing soiled clothes and bed linens separately from other laundry.

Individuals with bladder control problems must take special measures following treatment to prevent contamination with radioactive urine.

Side effects

The more common side effects of chromic phosphate P 32 may include:

- loss of appetite (anorexia)
- abdominal cramps
- diarrhea
- nausea and vomiting
- weakness or fatigue

Less common but serious side effects of chromic phosphate P 32 may include:

- severe abdominal pain
- severe nausea and vomiting
- fever
- chills
- dry cough
- sore throat
- chest pain
- difficulty breathing
- bleeding or bruising

Side effects of treatment with sodium iodide I 131 are rare and temporary. However, they may include:

- loss of taste
- dry mouth (xerostomia)
- stomach irritation
- nausea and vomiting
- tenderness in the salivary glands or neck

Large total doses of radioiodine may cause infertility in men.

Flushing and transient increased **bone pain** are among the more common side effects of strontium-89.

Less common side effects of samarium Sm 153 lexidronam include:

- irregular heartbeat
- temporary increase in bone pain
- nausea and vomiting

Signs of infection due to low white blood cell counts after treatment with strontium-89, samarium Sm 153 lexidronam, or sodium iodide I 131 include:

- fever or chills
- cough or hoarseness
- lower back or side pain
- painful or difficult urination

Signs of low platelet count after treatment with strontium-89, samarium Sm 153 lexidronam, or sodium iodide I 131 include:

- bleeding or bruising
- black, tar-like stools
- blood in urine or stools
- tiny red spots on the skin

Side effects are rare with sodium phosphate P 32. However, for patients treated with sodium phosphate P 32 for bone pain, side effects may include:

- diarrhea
- fever
- nausea and vomiting

Anemia (low red blood cell count) or a decrease in the white blood cell count also are possible.

Since children and older adults are particularly sensitive to radiation, they may experience more side effects during and after treatment with radiopharmaceuticals.

Interactions

Radiation therapy or **anticancer drugs** may increase the harmful effects of strontium-89 and samarium SM 153 lexidronam on the bone marrow. Medicines containing calcium may prevent strontium-89 from being taken up by bone tissue. Etidronate (Didronel, one of the so-called **bisphosphonates** that may be used to prevent or treat osteoporosis) may prevent samarium Sm 153 lexidronam from working effectively.

Margaret Alic, Ph.D.

Raloxifene

Definition

Raloxifene is a synthetic called an antiestrogen. It mimics the action of estrogen on the bones, but blocks the effects of estrogen on breast and uterine tissues.

Purpose

Raloxifene is a hormone therapy drug that protects against bone loss (osteoporosis) in postmenopausal women. During large studies of raloxifene's effectiveness against osteoporosis, researchers discovered that women taking the drug developed fewer breast cancers than women taking the placebo. Therefore, it is being considered as a drug used to fight **breast cancer**.

KEY TERMS

Anticoagulant—An agent preventing the coagulation (clotting) of blood.

Apoptosis—A type of cell death where cells are induced to commit suicide.

Double-blind study—A study where neither the participant nor the physician know who has received the drug in question.

Granulosa cells—Cells that form the wall of the ovarian follicle.

Oncogene—A gene whose presence can cause cancer; these genes usually arise through mutation of a normal gene.

Ovarian follicle—Several layers of cells that surround a maturing egg in the ovary.

Thromboembolism—A blood clot that blocks a blood vessel in the cardiovascular system.

Description

In 1997 the United States Food and Drug Administration (FDA) approved raloxifene for use against bone loss (osteoporosis) in postmenopausal women. As of 2001, raloxifene (Evista) was being tested as a hormone therapy drug to reduce the risk and fight breast **cancer** in postmenopausal women. As of 2003, raloxifene was only approved for use in postmenopausal women. However, studies were looking at its effects in preventing cancer in all women and in lowering risk of fractures in women with osteopenia.

Raloxifene belongs to a family of compounds called **antiestrogens**. Antiestrogens are used in cancer therapy to inhibit the effects of estrogen on target tissues. Estrogen is a steroid hormone secreted by granulosa cells of a maturing follicle within the female ovary. Depending on the target tissue, estrogen can stimulate the growth of female reproductive organs and breast tissue, play a role in the female menstrual cycle, and protect against bone loss by binding to estrogen receptors on the outside of cells within the target tissue. Antiestrogens act selectively against the effects of estrogen on target cells in a variety of ways, thus they are called selective estrogen receptor modulators (SERMs).

Raloxifene selectively inhibits the effects of estrogen on breast tissue and uterine tissue, while selectively mimicking the effects of estrogen on bone (by increasing bone mineral density). Its effects on breast and uterine tissue are thought to make raloxifene an excellent therapeutic agent against breast cancer and uterine cancer. Although researchers are unclear on exactly how raloxifene kills cancer cells, it is known to compete with estrogen by binding to estrogen receptors, therefore limiting the effects of estrogen on breast and uterine tissue. Raloxifene also may be involved in other anti-tumor activities affecting oncogene expression, promotion of apoptosis, and growth factor secretion.

In 2000 the STAR (Study of **Tamoxifen** and Raloxifene) study began. The purpose of this double-blind study was to evaluate the use of tamoxifen (another type of SERM) and raloxifene over a five year period in 22,000 postmenopausal women 35 years or older who are at high risk for developing breast cancer. The study will evaluate both the effectiveness and degree of side effects to determine which drug is most beneficial.

Recommended dosage

Recommended dose for cancer treatment will emerge as **clinical trials** enter their final phases. Most studies, including the STAR trial, are using a total of 60 milligrams of raloxifene administered either once or twice (morning and night) each day with notable success. If a dosage is missed, patients should not double the next dosage. Instead, they should go back to their regular schedule and contact their doctor.

Precautions

Although raloxifene is only approved for use by women past the child bearing years, researchers emphasize that it is not recommended for women who are pregnant or breast feeding. In test animals, raloxifene caused birth defects and miscarriages. Although it is not known whether raloxifene is present in breast milk, it is possible that its presence may be toxic to infants. Further, this drug is not recommended for use in children.

Patients at risk for the formation of thromboembolisms should use raloxifene with caution. Raloxifene can cause a higher risk of developing blood clots. Additionally, women experiencing liver disease will have a higher level of raloxifene in their blood system.

Side effects

Although raloxifene is usually well tolerated by patients, there are some side effects. Commonly reported side effects include mild **nausea**, **vomiting**, hot flashes, weight gain, **bone pain**, and hair thinning, which are not severe enough to stop therapy. Most of the side effect information regarding raloxifene comes from studies using it to counter osteoporosis where patients have not needed to take it over a long period of time. When studied for anticancer properties, raloxifene needs to be taken over a longer period of time. Since raloxifene's anticancer properties still are under investigation, researchers are not completely aware of all of the long term and potentially serious side effects. Researchers are aware that women taking raloxifene are three times more likely to develop thromboembolisms than women not taking raloxifene.

Interactions

The usefulness of raloxifene can be diminished if patients also are on estrogen supplements (such as Premarin, Estrace, Estratab, Climara, or Vivelle) and cholesterol-lowering cholestyramines (such as Questran). Cholestyramines decrease the absorption of raloxifene into the blood, while estrogen supplements increase the amount of estrogen competing with raloxifene for binding sites on target cells' estrogen receptors.

Raloxifene interferes with the anticoagulant effect of **warfarin** with severe consequences and even death. Patients using warfarin should make sure their physician is aware prior to commencing treatment with raloxifene.

See also Toremifene.

Resources

PERIODICALS

Jancin, Bruce. "Breast Cancer Prevention Could be Next for Raloxifene." *Family Practice News* March 15, 2003: 32.

"Raloxifene Staunches the Risk for New Vertebral Fractures in Osteopenic Women." *Women's Health Weekly* November 20, 2003: 3.

Sally C. McFarlane-Parrott
Teresa G. Odle

Ranitidine *see* **Histamine 2 antagonists**

Receptor analysis

Definition

Receptor analysis is a diagnostic test that determines an important biological characteristic of the cells in a tumor—their response to normal growth factors.

KEY TERMS

Anti-estrogen —A drug, for example tamoxifen, that prevents the hormone estrogen from influencing the behavior of specific types of cells.

Biopsy—A piece of tissue removed for diagnostic examination.

Receptors—Molecules, usually found on the surface of a cell, that are required for cells to be influenced by hormones and other growth factors.

QUESTIONS TO ASK THE DOCTOR

- What fraction of the cells in my tumor has normal receptors?
- Do the results of the receptor assay on the biopsy of my tumor make me a candidate for anti-estrogen treatment?
- How do the results of the receptor assays on my tumor influence your decision as to my treatment and prognosis?

Purpose

The goal of receptor analysis is to reveal whether the **cancer** cells in a tumor have specific molecules, termed receptors, on the cell surface. This test is routinely performed for **breast cancer**, as well as other tumors. Information as to the presence of these specific receptors can play a role in deciding the best course of treatment for a particular patient.

Precautions

Because this test is performed on a piece of tissue that has already been removed during a surgical or diagnostic procedure, it does not require any precautionary measures on behalf of the patient.

Description

The cancer cells found in tumors or in the blood of leukemia patients can differ in many ways, and to varying degrees from the corresponding cells in normal tissues and blood. In some respects, cancer treatment depends upon the differences in behavior between tumor and normal cells. For example, tumor cells often grow faster than normal (non-cancerous) cells. The changes that occur as normal cells become cancerous are progressive. As a tumor develops the cells generally become less similar to normal cells and behave in a biologically different way. Some cancer treatments make use of the ways that cancer cells in a tumor can be like cells in the normal surrounding tissue.

One the most fundamental ways in which the early stages of some cancers resemble healthy tissue is that the growth of the cells in the tumor responds to some of the same factors that control the growth of normal tissues. The most common example of this is the response of breast cancer cells to estrogen. During the normal menstrual cycle, the mammary glands respond to changes in the levels of two hormones, estrogen and progesterone. In many cases, the growth of breast cancer tumor cells also responds to the presence or absence of estrogen. The response of both normal and tumor cells to these hormones depends upon presence of molecules termed estrogen and progesterone receptors. If cells in a breast tumor have these receptors, it is possible to inhibit the growth of the cancer cells by preventing estrogen from stimulating their growth. This is generally accomplished through the use of anti-estrogen drugs such as **tamoxifen**.

Receptor analysis usually involves a special technique, called immunocytochemistry, to examine a small piece of the tumor tissue. A tissue section, a slice of the tumor, is placed on a glass microscope slide. These tissue sections, which are very similar to those used in the initial diagnosis of the patient's breast cancer, are incubated with antibody preparations that will react with estrogen and progesterone receptors. Special reagents that lead to a chemical reaction where these antibodies are bound produce a visible color in cells that have hormone receptors. A pathologist then looks at the section with a microscope to determine the percentage of tumor cells that are receptor-positive. This information can be used to decide whether a woman with breast cancer should be treated with anti-estrogens. In addition, the presence of estrogen receptors is itself an accepted prognostic indicator. Tumors that have high levels of estrogen receptors are generally less aggressive. Taken together with information as to the patient's age, the size and grade of the tumor, and whether or not there is lymph node involvement, it is possible for a doctor to have some idea as to the likelihood the patient will remain disease-free after initial treatment.

Estrogen receptor analysis was an important and generally accepted part of managing breast cancer. More recently, assays for other cell surface receptors have been explored and introduced for the management of breast and other cancers. Examples of these include androgen receptors in **prostate cancer** and epidermal growth factor receptor (EGFR) in a variety of cancers. In 2001 the most prominent example of a receptor assay, other than estrogen receptor analysis, was testing for a cell surface molecule designated HER2. Patients whose tumors express higher than normal amounts of HER2 are believed to have worse prognoses. However, these patients may be treated with a specific reagent, a monoclonal antibody, which is targeted toward the HER2 protein. Analysis for HER2 can be performed in a similar way to estrogen receptor immunocytochemical assays, currently marketed as the HercepTest, or by using a different type of test that directly examines the gene for HER2. Treatment with the monoclonal antibody to HER2 can improve the survival of patients who express higher-than-normal levels of HER2 in their tumor cells

Risks

This test is performed on a piece of tissue that has been removed during the initial surgery or diagnostic procedure used to establish the nature of the tumor. It does not require any new surgery on the patient and, so, does not entail any risk to the patient.

Results

Receptor assays measure molecules that play normal and essential roles in the natural function of various tissues. Abnormal results depend upon the particular tissue and the type of cancer involved. The presence of the appropriate receptor, for example estrogen receptors in breast tumors, may be indicative that the cancer can be treated with compounds that can inhibit the growth of the cells that make up the tumor. In other cases, receptor assays may enable a doctor to know the origin of a tumor. That is, sometimes it is not possible for a pathologist to examine a **biopsy** and be certain what type of cancer a tumor represents. Knowing the identity of the receptors found on the tumor cells may then provide important information for establishing the diagnosis and best course of treatment for such patients.

Resources

PERIODICALS

Chang J., et al. "Prediction of Clinical Outcome from Primary Tamoxifen by Expression of Biologic Markers in Breast Cancer Patients." *Clinical Cancer Research* 6 (2000): 616–21.

Slamon, D., et al. "Use of Chemotherapy Plus a Monoclonal Antibody Against HER-2 for Metastatic Breast Cancer that Overexpresses HER 2." *New England Journal of Medicine* 344 (March 2001): 783–92.

OTHER

"HercepTest Frequently Asked Questions." *DAKO Corporation*. [cited July 24, 2001]. http://www.dakousa.com/herinfo/hctfaqs.htm.

Warren Maltzman, Ph.D.

Reconstructive surgery

Definition

Reconstructive surgery is a type of plastic surgery performed to reshape abnormal structures of the body to improve function and appearance. Reconstructive surgery is different from cosmetic surgery, which is performed to reshape normal structures of the body to improve a patient's appearance and self-esteem.

Purpose

The goals of reconstructive surgery are to reshape abnormal structures of the body, to improve function, and/or to allow a person to have a more normal appearance. Abnormal structures of the body that are corrected during reconstructive surgery may be the result of birth defects, developmental abnormalities, trauma or injury, **infection**, tumors, or disease. The three most commonly performed reconstructive surgeries in the United States are tumor ablation (removal) and reconstruction, hand surgery, and **breast reconstruction**.

Precautions

Reconstructive surgery should not be performed on patients who are not healthy enough to withstand a surgical procedure performed under general anesthetic. People with severe diabetes, an autoimmune disorder such as AIDS, or a suppressed immune system should not undergo reconstructive surgery. This type of surgery is also contraindicated in patients with a history of excessive smoking, obesity, poor wound healing, abnormal scarring and/or a bleeding disorder. Women who are pregnant should not undergo reconstructive surgeries.

Patients who have received recent irradiation treatments (generally within the last three to six months) should not undergo surgical procedures involving these

QUESTIONS TO ASK THE DOCTOR

- What are alternatives to this surgical procedure?
- What will the scars look like and can I expect them to decrease over time?
- How many reconstructions have you performed previously and may I see examples of the results or talk to former patients?
- Will this procedure be covered by my insurance?
- How long will the pre-operation waiting period, the hospital stay, and the recovery procedure be?

tissues. Recently irradiated tissue is highly prone to infection and has poorer wound healing.

In some cases, after tumor removal surgeries, it is necessary to monitor the affected tissue for redevelopment of the tumor. Patients requiring this type of postoperative surveillance should not undergo further reconstructive surgeries since these surgeries could obscure the results of imaging techniques (x ray, **computed tomography**, or **magnetic resonance imaging**) used to monitor tumor recurrence.

Patients with an allergy to collagen, beef, or beef products should not receive collagen injections.

Description

The most commonly performed reconstructive surgeries of **cancer** patients are breast reconstruction, laceration repair, scar revision, and tumor removal.

Breast reconstruction

Breast reconstruction surgeries can be performed as part of the procedure to remove the breast (immediate **mastectomy**). They may also be performed as a separate procedure after recuperation from a mastectomy (delayed). There are two types of breast reconstruction: autogenous free flap reconstruction and breast implants.

Autogenous free flap reconstructions use tissue from another part of the body to form the reconstructed breast. This category of breast reconstruction includes the techniques called TRAM (transverse rectus abdominis myocutaneous), LD (latissimus dorsi), VRAM (vertical rectus abdominis myocutaneous), and DIEP (deep inferior epigastric perforator) flaps. These names refer to the location from which the tissue for reconstruction is taken. As of 2001 TRAM, in which tissue is taken from the abdominal region, is the most common breast reconstruction procedure in the United States. As of 2004, DIEP is preferred when the reconstruction involves both breasts.

KEY TERMS

Cosmetic surgery—A form of plastic surgery that is performed to alter normal tissue to improve the appearance of that tissue.

Flap surgery—A procedure in which a portion of living tissue is moved from one part of a patient's body to another to restore shape and/or function to the targeted location.

Plastic surgery—A type of surgery that is performed to alter the physical characteristics of a patient. This medical discipline is subdivided into cosmetic surgery and reconstructive surgery.

Reconstructive surgery—A form of plastic surgery that is performed to repair or reshape abnormally formed tissue to improve the form and/or function of that tissue.

Scar revision—A surgical procedure that attempts to diminish the physical appearance of a scar. This procedure is also used to add flexibility and range of motion to joints and muscles that were previously hindered by a particular scar.

Breast implants involve the placement of an artificial object in the body to simulate the shape and size of the natural breast. The implant is most commonly a saline (salt water) or silicone-filled bag. Because of the health problems reported by many women after silicone breast implants, this technique is no longer as widespread as it once was, particularly for reconstructive surgeries.

A technique that is still in the experimental stage is breast tissue engineering, which seeks to use a relatively small amount of the patient's own adipose (fatty) tissue to create a larger volume of material that could be used to reconstruct the breast. As of 2004 one of the limitations on breast reconstruction is the need to use fairly large amounts of adipose tissue from the patient's body.

Breast reconstruction usually involves more than one operation; in fact the average number of secondary procedures required is four for reconstruction of one breast and 5.5 for reconstruction of both breasts. The factors that complicate breast reconstruction include delaying the reconstruction after the mastectomy; the need for **radiation therapy**; and the presence of other risk factors affecting the patient's health.

Laceration repair

Laceration repair includes the repair of large wounds caused by the removal of large tumors or tumors associated with the skin. It also includes the surgical repair of wounds that fail to heal or heal improperly. Laceration repair can be subdivided into four general categories: direct closure, skin grafts, tissue expansion, and flap surgery.

Direct closure (stitches) is usually only performed on wounds that are not very deep beneath the surface of the skin and that have straight edges of skin on either side of the wound. The primary goal in direct closure is to provide a permanent closure of the wound with a minimum of scarring.

Skin grafts are used for wounds that are wide and difficult or impossible to close directly. This technique involves removing healthy skin from a location on the patient (the donor site) and using it to cover the wound site. The skin will grow back at the donor site but often leaves a color mismatch. The donor site is chosen to best match the color of the skin needed in the graft area.

Tissue expansion is used to grow extra skin by stretching skin near the site that will require the skin. A small inflatable balloon is placed under the skin next to the area where the skin will be removed. Over time, this balloon is slowly filled with salt water until the skin has grown to the required size. The surgical procedure that involves the loss of skin is then performed and closed with the extra skin that was formed during the tissue expansion process. The major advantage associated with tissue expansion is that the skin grown in this way remains connected to its original blood and nerve supply, so the risk of loss of sensation in the area of the wound is greatly diminished. Also, the scars that result from tissue expansion are generally less noticeable than those from skin grafts or skin flaps. A final advantage of this method is the near perfect match in color provided by this skin.

Flap surgery involves taking a section of living tissue, with its blood supply, from one part of the patient and moving it to the area where it is needed. In most flap surgeries, one end of the flap remains attached to its original blood supply so that it continues to be nourished as it grows to heal the wound. In cases where the flap is completely removed and transplanted to another part of the body, the surgery involves the reconnection of all the tiny blood vessels of the flap tissue to the blood vessels of the new location (microsurgery). Flap surgery has the advantage of being able to restore both form and function to areas of the body that have lost skin, fat, muscle, and/or skeletal support. The most commonly performed flap surgeries are the autogenous breast reconstructions discussed above. But, this procedure is used throughout the body with a great amount of success.

Scar revisions

Many cancer patients have scarring that results from their particular form of cancer or from the number or severity of surgical procedures or radiation that they have undergone. In some of these cases, surgeries to minimize or reshape the scar, or scars, may be undertaken. Most physicians will recommend that a scar be allowed to heal for at least one year prior to a recommendation of scar revision. But, in extreme cases of loss of mobility, increased sensitivity, or inflamed and irritable scars that do not respond to topical steroid creams, this timetable may be shortened.

Unless proof of the scar contributing to a medical condition or a decrease in physical function can be shown, scar revision surgery is considered by most insurance companies to be a cosmetic surgery that is not covered as an insurance benefit. The most common reason for scar revision to be classified as a reconstructive rather than a cosmetic procedure is a loss of mobility of muscles or joints caused by the scar.

The most common procedure for scar revision is called Z-plasty. In this procedure, the old scar is removed and the two sides of the wound are cut into a z-shape that is designed to follow the natural lines and contours of the surrounding skin. This z-shaped wound is then closed with stitches. Other scar revision procedures include skin grafts and flap surgeries. Z-plasty is the least likely of these procedures to be covered by insurance.

Tumor removal

The surgical procedure used to remove a tumor will be chosen by the surgeon based on the type and size of the tumor. Other factors influencing the surgical technique chosen for tumor removal include: the location of the tumor within the body; the potential for recurrence of the tumor at this, or another, location in the body; and, the stage of development of both the tumor itself and the underlying cancer.

Skin cancers are generally removed by a cutting out (excision) of the cancerous portion of skin, with the wound closed by stitches or left to heal on its own.

In cases of large or spreading skin cancers, major surgery involving skin grafts or flap surgeries may be required. For skin cancers in the facial area, Moh's surgery with primary or flap closure may be performed.

Preparation

The preparation for a reconstructive surgery depends on the type of surgery that is to be performed. Some reconstructive surgeries can be performed on an outpatient basis. These procedures require only a local anesthetic and very little patient preparation other than counseling about the risks, possible achievable outcomes, and alternatives to the surgery. Other reconstructive surgeries are considered major operations. These require hospitalization, a general anesthetic, and much more extensive counseling and discussion of possible alternatives.

Prescription medications that may interfere with the performance of reconstructive surgery should be discontinued approximately two weeks prior to surgery, unless the surgeon advises otherwise. These medications include any medicines that may interfere with the anesthetic or that may increase bleeding. Over-the-counter medications, such as aspirin and **nonsteroidal anti-inflammatory drugs** (NSAIDs), should not be taken for at least one week prior to surgery unless approved by the doctor who will be performing the surgery. Patients undergoing surgeries that require a general anesthetic will be asked not to eat after midnight prior to the surgery and not to drink at least eight hours prior to surgery. The purpose of this is to ensure that the stomach is empty while the patient is unconscious. Otherwise, the stomach contents could end up in the lungs, causing complications with the surgery or the recovery.

For procedures involving skin flaps, the patient may be asked to donate blood for possible use in a later transfusion.

In the case of tissue expansion procedures, the amount of time that will be required for the expansion of the tissue depends on the amount of tissue that must be grown to ensure an adequate closure of the wound. This may take a matter of days or several weeks.

Psychological and emotional preparation is important in reconstructive surgery to manage patient expectations. The patient should not expect cosmetically perfect results. Complete understanding of the limitations, as well as the benefits, of this surgery is necessary for a successful outcome.

Aftercare

The aftercare of a patient who has undergone a reconstructive surgery depends on the surgery, the overall health of the patient, and the wound care process. Some outpatient procedures require little aftercare other than a follow-up examination to determine the success of the procedure. Other procedures may require an extended hospitalization followed by extensive physical therapy. Smoking should be avoided, as it may cause delayed wound healing and higher risk of complications, including infection.

Procedures involving skin flaps or grafts require careful monitoring in the first days after surgery to ensure that proper blood circulation is taking place. Bandages and drainage tubes will remain in place for at least a day.

Scars may remain reddened and raised for a month or longer and may cause **itching**. Many people find that inflammation or severe itching from post-surgical scars is lessened, or completely eliminated, by topical treatments with vitamin E or steroidal creams.

After tumor removal, many patients require follow-up treatments and medical imaging to ensure that the tumor is not redeveloping.

Risks

The risks associated with all reconstructive surgeries are infection, bleeding, an unsightly scar, improper wound closure, and adverse reactions to anesthesia. Complications associated with flap reconstruction of the breasts include unusual firmness of the fatty tissue (fat necrosis), partial flap loss, fluid collection beneath the flap site, and muscle weakness (including abdominal hernias) at the donor site. For breast implants, complications include the formation of fibrous tissue around an implant, rupture or leakage of the implant, or movement of the implant from its intended location.

Normal results

The normal result of a reconstructive surgery is a patient who has an improved ability to function and/or an improved **body image** as a result of the surgery. A normal result also depends on the patient's realistic goals and expectations. The patient should understand that the feeling and appearance of the reconstructed area will be improved, not fully restored, to an unaffected state.

Abnormal results

An abnormal result of a reconstructive surgery is a patient who suffers long-lasting health complications as a result of the surgery. Another abnormal result is a patient who suffers a degradation in the ability to function and/or has a loss of self-confidence caused by the loss of sensation or scarring that may accompany such procedures.

See also Breast cancer.

Resources

BOOKS

Kimberly, Henry A., and Penny Heckaman. *The Plastic Surgery Sourcebook*. Lincolnwood: NTC/ Contemporary Publishing, 1999.

PERIODICALS

Cordeiro, P. G., A. L. Pusic, J. J. Disa, et al. "Irradiation after Immediate Tissue Expander/Implant Breast Reconstruction: Outcomes, Complications, Aesthetic Results, and Satisfaction among 156 Patients." *Plastic and Reconstructive Surgery* 113 (March 2004): 877–881.

Guerra, A. B., S. E. Metzinger, R. S. Bidros, et al. "Bilateral Breast Reconstruction with the Deep Inferior Epigastric Perforator (DIEP) Flap: An Experience with 280 Flaps." *Annals of Plastic Surgery* 52 (March 2004): 246–252.

Losken, A., G. W. Carlson, M. B. Schoemann, et al. "Factors That Influence the Completion of Breast Reconstruction." *Annals of Plastic Surgery* 52 (March 2004): 258–261.

Patrick, C. W. "Breast Tissue Engineering." *Annual Review of Biomedical Engineering* 6 (2004): 109–130.

OTHER

Breast Reconstruction. [cited July 23, 2001]. http://www.vanhosp.bc.ca/html/women_breast.html.

ORGANIZATIONS

American Academy of Facial Plastic and Reconstructive Surgery (AAFPRS). 310 South Henry Street, Alexandria, VA 22314. (703) 299-9291. www.facemd.org.

American Society of Plastic Surgeons Plastic Surgery Educational Foundation. 444 E. Algonquin Rd., Arlington Heights, IL 60005. (888) 4-PLASTIC. http://www.plasticsurgery.org.

Foundation for Reconstructive Plastic Surgery. http://www.frps.org.

Paul A. Johnson, Ed.M.
Rebecca J. Frey, PhD

Rectal cancer

Definition

The rectum is the portion of the large bowel that lies in the pelvis, terminating at the anus. **Cancer** of the rectum is the disease characterized by the development of malignant cells in the lining or epithelium of the rectum. Malignant cells have changed such that they lose normal control mechanisms governing growth. These cells may invade surrounding local tissue or they may spread throughout the body and invade other organ systems.

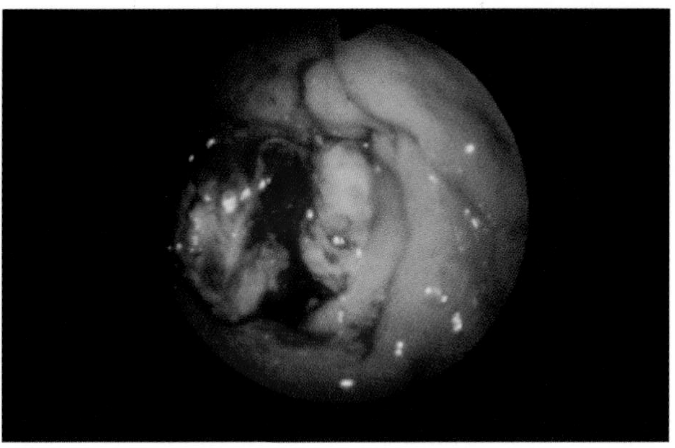

Rectal cancer seen through an endoscope. *(Custom Medical Stock Photo. Reproduced by permission.)*

Description

The rectum is the continuation of the colon (part of the large bowel) after it leaves the abdomen and descends into the pelvis. It is divided into equal thirds: the upper, mid, and lower rectum.

The pelvis and other organs in the pelvis form boundaries to the rectum. Behind, or posterior to the rectum is the sacrum (the lowest portion of the spine, closest to the pelvis). Laterally, on the sides, the rectum is bounded by soft tissue and bone. In front, the rectum is bounded by different organs in the male and female. In the male, the bladder and prostate are present. In the female, the vagina, uterus, and ovaries are present.

The upper rectum receives its blood supply from branches of the inferior mesenteric artery from the abdomen. The lower rectum has blood vessels entering from the sides of the pelvis. Lymph, a protein-rich fluid that bathes the cells of the body, is transported in small channels known as lymphatics. These channels run with the blood supply of the rectum. Lymph nodes are small filters through which the lymph flows on its way back to the blood stream. Cancer spreads elsewhere in the body by invading the lymph and vascular systems.

When a cell or cells lining the rectum become malignant, they first grow locally and may invade partially or totally through the wall of the rectum.

KEY TERMS

Adenocarcinoma—Cancer beginning in epithelial cells that line certain organs and have secretory properties.

Adjuvant therapy—Treatment involving radiation, chemotherapy (drug treatment), hormone therapy, or a combination of all three given after the primary treatment for the possibility of residual microscopic disease.

Anastomosis—Surgical re-connection of the ends of the bowel after removal of a portion of the bowel.

Anemia—The condition caused by too few circulating red blood cells, often manifested in part by fatigue.

Carcinogens—Substances in the environment that cause cancer, presumably by inducing mutations, with prolonged exposure.

Defecation—The act of having a bowel movement.

Epithelium—Cells composing the lining of an organ.

Lymphatics—Channels that are conduits for lymph.

Lymph nodes—Cellular filters through which lymphatics flow.

Malignant—Cells that have been altered such that they have lost normal control mechanisms and are capable of local invasion and spreading to other areas of the body.

Metastasis—Site of invasive tumor growth that originated from a malignancy elsewhere in the body.

Mutation—A change in the genetic makeup of a cell that may occur spontaneously or be environmentally induced.

Occult blood—Presence of blood that cannot be appreciated visually.

Polyps—Localized growths of the epithelium that can be benign, pre-cancerous, or harbor malignancy.

Resect—To remove surgically.

Sacrum—Posterior bony wall of the pelvis.

Systemic—Referring to throughout the body.

The tumor here may invade surrounding tissue or the organs that bound it, a process known as local invasion. In this process, the tumor penetrates and may invade the lymphatics or the capillaries locally and gain access to the circulation in this way. As the malignant cells work their way to other areas of the body, they again become locally invasive in the new area to which they have spread. These tumor deposits, originating in the primary tumor in the rectum, are then known as **metastasis**. If metastases are found in the regional lymph nodes, they are known as regional metastases. If they are distant from the primary tumor, they are known as distant metastases. The patient with distant metastases may have widespread disease, also referred to as systemic disease. Thus the cancer originating in the rectum begins locally and, given time, may become systemic.

By the time the primary tumor is originally detected, it is usually larger than one centimeter (about 3/8 inch) in size and has over one million cells. This amount of growth is estimated to take about three to seven years. Each time the cells double in number, the size of the tumor quadruples. Thus like most cancers, the part that is identified clinically is later in the progression than would be desired. Screening becomes a very important endeavor to aid in earlier detection of this disease.

Passage of red blood with the stool, (noticeable bleeding with defecation), is much more common in rectal cancer than that originating in the colon because the tumor is much closer to the anus. Other symptoms (constipation and/ or **diarrhea**) are caused by obstruction and, less often, by local invasion of the tumor into pelvic organs or the sacrum. When the tumor has spread to distant sites, these metastases may cause dysfunction of the organ they have spread to. Distant metastasis usually occurs in the liver, less often to the lung(s), and rarely to the brain.

Demographics

There are about 40,870 cases of rectal cancer diagnosed per year in the United States. Together, colon and rectal cancers account for 10% of cancers in men and 11% of cancers in women. It is the second most common site-specific cancer affecting both men and women. Nearly 49,920 people died from colon and rectal cancer in the United States in 2009. In recent years the incidence of this disease is decreasing very slightly, as has the mortality rate. It is difficult to tell if the decrease in mortality reflects earlier diagnosis, less death related to the actual treatment of the disease, or a combination of both factors.

Cancer of the rectum is felt to arise sporadically in about 80% of those who develop the disease. About 20% of cases probably arise from genetic predisposition; some people have a family history of rectal cancer occurring in a first-degree relative. Development of rectal cancer at an early age suggests a genetically transmitted form of the disease as opposed to the sporadic form.

Causes and symptoms

Causes of rectal cancer are probably environmental in sporadic cases (80%), and genetic in the heredity-predisposed (20%) cases. Since malignant cells have a changed genetic makeup, this means that in 80% of cases, the environment spontaneously induces change. Those born with a genetic predisposition are either destined to get the cancer, or it will take less environmental exposure to induce the cancer. Exposure to agents in the environment that may induce mutation is the process of **carcinogenesis** and is caused by agents known as carcinogens. Specific carcinogens have been difficult to identify; dietary factors, however, seem to be involved.

Rectal cancer is more common in industrialized nations. Dietary factors may be the reason. Diets high in fat, red meat, total calories, and alcohol seem to add to increased risk. Diets high in fiber are associated with a decreased risk. High-fiber diets may be related to less exposure of the rectal epithelium to carcinogens from the environment as the transit time through the bowel is faster with a high-fiber diet than with a low-fiber diet.

Age plays a definite role in rectal cancer risk. Rectal cancer is rare before age 40. This incidence increases substantially after age 50 and doubles with each succeeding decade.

There also is a slight increase of risk for rectal cancer in the individual who smokes.

Patients who suffer from an inflammatory disease of the colon known as ulcerative colitis are also at increased risk.

On chromosome 5 is the APC gene associated with familial adenomatous polyposis (FAP) syndrome. There are multiple mutations that occur at this site, yet they all cause a defect in tumor suppression that results in early and frequent development of **colon cancer**. This is transmitted to 50% of offspring and each of those affected will develop colon or rectal cancer, usually at an early age. Another syndrome, hereditary non-polyposis colon cancer (HNPCC), is related to mutations in any of four genes responsible for DNA mismatch repair. In patients with colon or rectal cancer, the p53 gene is mutated 70% of the time. When the p53 gene is mutated and ineffective, cells with damaged DNA escape repair or destruction, allowing the damaged cell to multiply. Continued replication of the damaged DNA may lead to tumor development. Though these syndromes (FAP and HNPCC) have a very high incidence of colon or rectal cancer, family history without the syndromes is also a substantial risk factor. When considering first-degree relatives, history of one with colon or rectal cancer raises the baseline risk from 2% to 6%; the presence of a second raises the risk to 17%.

The development of polyps of the colon or rectum commonly precedes the development of rectal cancer. Polyps are growths of the rectal lining. They can be unrelated to cancer, pre-cancerous, or malignant. Polyps, when identified, are removed for diagnosis. If the polyp, or polyps, are benign, the patient should undergo careful surveillance for the development of more polyps or the development of colon or rectal cancer.

Symptoms of rectal cancer most often result from the local presence of the tumor and its capacity to invade surrounding pelvic structure:

- bright red blood present with stool
- abdominal distention (stretching from internal pressure) bloating, inability to have a bowel movement
- narrowing of the stool, so-called ribbon stools
- pelvic pain
- unexplained weight loss
- persistent chronic fatigue
- rarely, urinary infection or passage of air in urine in males (late symptom)
- rarely, passage of feces through vagina in females(late symptom)

If the tumor is large and obstructing the rectum, the patient will not be evacuating stool normally and will get bloated and have abdominal discomfort. The tumor itself may bleed and, since it is near the anus, the patient may see bright red blood on the surface of the stool. Blood alone (without stool) may also be passed. Thus, hemorrhoids are often incorrectly blamed for bleeding, delaying the diagnosis. If **anemia** develops, which is rare, the patient will experience chronic **fatigue**. If the tumor invades the bladder in the male or the vagina in the female, stool will get where it doesn't belong and cause **infection** or discharge. (This condition is also rare.) Patients with widespread disease lose weight secondary to the chronic illness.

Diagnosis

Screening evaluation of the colon and rectum are accomplished together. Screening involves physical exam, simple laboratory tests, and the visualization of the lining of the rectum and colon. **X rays** (indirect visualization) and endoscopy (direct visualization) are used to visualize the organs' lining.

The physical examination involves the performance of a digital rectal exam (DRE). At the time of this exam, the physician checks the stool on the examining glove with a chemical to see if any occult (invisible), blood is present. At home, after having a bowel movement, the patient is asked to swipe a sample of stool obtained with a small stick on a card. After three such specimens are on the card, the card is then easily chemically tested for occult blood. These exams are accomplished as an easy part of a routine yearly physical exam.

Proteins are sometimes produced by cancers and these may be elevated in the patient's blood. When this occurs the protein produced is known as a tumor marker. There is a tumor marker for cancer of the colon and rectum; it is known as carcinoembryonic antigen, (CEA). Unfortunately, this may be made by other adenocarcinomas as well, or it may not be produced by a particular colon or rectal cancer. Therefore, screening by chemical analysis for CEA has not been helpful. CEA has been helpful in patients treated for colon or rectal cancer if their tumor makes the protein. It is used in a follow-up role, not a screening role.

Direct visualization of the lining of the rectum is accomplished using a scope or endoscope. The physician introduces the instrument into the rectum and is able to see the epithelium of the rectum directly. A simple rigid tubular scope may be used to see the rectal epithelium; however, screening of the colon is done at the same time. The lower colon may be visualized using a fiberoptic flexible scope in a procedure known as flexible **sigmoidoscopy**. When the entire colon is visualized, the procedure is known as total **colonoscopy**. Each type of endoscopy requires pre-procedure preparation (evacuation) of the rectum and colon.

The American Cancer Society has recommended the following screening protocol for colon and rectal cancers those over age 50:

- yearly fecal occult blood test
- flexible sigmoidoscopy at age 50
- flexible sigmoidoscopy repeated every 5 years
- double contrast barium enema every five years
- colonoscopy every 10 years

If there are predisposing factors such as positive family history, history of polyps, or a familial syndrome, screening evaluations should start sooner.

Evaluation of patients with symptoms

When patients visit their physician because they are experiencing symptoms that could possibly be related to colon or rectal cancer, the entire colon and rectum must be visualized. Even if a rectal lesion is identified, the entire colon must be screened to rule out a syndromous polyp or cancer of the colon. The combination of a flexible sigmoidoscopy and double contrast **barium enema** may be performed, but the much-preferred evaluation of the entire colon and rectum is that of complete colonoscopy. Colonoscopy allows direct visualization, photography, as well as the opportunity to obtain a **biopsy**, (a sample of tissue), of any abnormality visualized. If, for technical reasons the entire colon is not visualized endoscopically, a double contrast barium enema should complement the colonoscopy. A patient who is identified to have a problem in one area of the colon or rectum is at greater risk to have a similar problem in another area of the colon or rectum. Therefore the entire colon and rectum need to be visualized during the evaluation.

The diagnosis of rectal cancer is actually made by the performance of a biopsy of any abnormal lesion in the rectum. Many rectal cancers are within reach of the examiner's finger. Identifying how close to the anus the cancer has developed is important in planning the treatment. Another characteristic ascertained by exam is whether the tumor is mobile or fixed to surrounding structure. Again, this will have implications related to primary treatment. As a general rule, it is easier to identify and adequately obtain tissue for evaluation in the rectum as opposed to the colon. This is because the lesion is closer to the anus.

If the patient has advanced disease, areas where the tumor has spread, such as the liver, may require biopsy. Such biopsies are usually obtained using a special needle under local anesthesia.

Once a diagnosis of rectal cancer has been established by biopsy, in addition to the physical exam, an **endorectal ultrasound** will be performed to assess the extent of the disease. For rectal cancer, endorectal ultrasound is the most preferred method for staging both depth of tumor penetration and local lymph node status. Endorectal ultrasound:

- differentiates areas of invasion within large rectal adenomas that may appear benign
- determines the depth of tumor penetration into the rectal wall
- determines the extent of regional lymph node invasion, thereby determining the metastatic status
- can be combined with other tests (chest x rays and computed tomography scans, or CT scans) to determine the extent of cancer spread to distant organs, such as the liver and/or the lungs

The resulting rectal cancer staging allows physicians to determine the need for— and order of— radiation, surgery, and **chemotherapy**. In 2003, it was reported that **magnetic resonance imaging** (MRI) also may be useful in staging rectal cancer. MRI may help physicians determine if a tumor can be resected and what the risk of cancer recurrence will be.

Treatment team

Surgery, radiation treatment and chemotherapy are used in the therapy of cancer of the rectum. The extent of the primary tumor dictates whether surgery or radiation will be utilized first. When surgery is the primary local therapy, radiation often has an adjunctive role in helping to prevent local recurrence. Chemotherapy may be used as an adjunct also to decrease recurrence and improve overall survival. Thus, teamwork is required utilizing the skills of the surgeon and the radiation and medical oncologists.

Clinical staging, treatments, and prognosis

Once the diagnosis has been confirmed by biopsy and the endorectal ultrasound has been performed, the clinical stage of the cancer is assigned. The treating physicians use staging to plan the specific treatment protocol for the patient. In addition, the stage of the cancer at the time of presentation gives a statistical likelihood of the treatment outcome (prognosis).

Clinical staging

Rectal cancer first invades locally and then progresses to spread to regional lymph nodes or to other organs. Stage is derived using the characteristics of the primary tumor, its depth of penetration through the rectum, local invasion into pelvic structure, and the presence or absence of regional or distant metastases. A CT scan of the pelvis is helpful in staging because tumor invasion into the sacrum or pelvic sidewalls may mean surgical therapy is not initially possible. On this basis, clinical staging is used to begin treatment. The pathologic stage is defined when the results of analyzing the surgical specimen are available (typically stage I and II).

Rectal cancer is assigned stages I through IV, based on the following general criteria:

- Stage I: the tumor is confined to the epithelium (layer of cells covering the surface) or has not penetrated through the first layer of muscle in the rectal wall.
- Stage II: the tumor has penetrated through to the outer wall of the rectum or has gone through it, possibly invading other local tissue or organs.
- Stage III: Any depth or size of tumor associated with regional lymph node involvement.
- Stage IV: any of previous criteria associated with distant metastasis.

Treatments

SURGERY. Surgical resection remains the mainstay of therapy in the treatment of rectal cancer. Stage I, II, and even suspected stage III disease are treated by surgical removal of the involved section of the rectum (resection) along with the complete vascular and lymphatic supply. However, because of the improvement in staging methods (principally endorectal ultrasound), many rectal cancers are now selected for presurgical treatment with radiation and, often, chemotherapy. The use of chemotherapy prior to surgery is known as neoadjuvant chemotherapy, and, in rectal cancer, neoadjuvant chemotherapy is used primarily for Stage II and Stage III rectal cancers. Following neoadjuvant treatment, the remaining tumor (often only a scar) is resected. In some cases, such neoadjuvant treatment avoids the need for permanent **colostomy** by major tumor shrinkage prior to surgery. Following surgery, chemotherapy is completed.

In other patients, surgical therapy alone (some small Stage I lesions) is followed by additional radiation and chemotherapy is selected. In a small group of patients with small, Stage I lesions, endoluminal radiation alone is performed as a curative treatment.

When determining primary treatment for rectal cancer, the surgeon's ability to reconnect the ends of the rectum must be considered. The pelvis is a confining space that makes surgical reconnection more difficult to do safely when the tumor is in the lower rectum. The upper rectum does not usually present a substantial problem to the surgeon restoring bowel continuity after the cancer has been removed. Mid-rectal tumors, especially in males where the pelvis is usually smaller than a woman's, may present technical difficulties in hooking the proximal bowel to the remaining rectum. Technical advances in stapling instrumentation have largely overcome these difficulties. If the anastomosis (hook-up) leaks postoperatively, infection can occur. In the past, this was a major cause of complications in resection of rectal cancers. Today, utilizing the stapling instrumentation, a hook-up at the time of original surgery, is much safer. If the surgeon feels that the hook-up is compromised or may leak, a colostomy may be performed. A colostomy is performed by bringing the colon through the abdominal wall and sewing it to the skin. In these cases the stool is diverted away from the hook-up, allowing it to heal and preventing the infectious complications associated with leak. Later, when the hook-up has completely healed, the colostomy can be taken down and bowel continuity restored.

Stapling devices have allowed the surgeon to get closer to the anus and still allow the technical performance of a hook-up, but there are limits. It is generally felt that there should be at least three centimeters of normal rectum below the tumor or the risk of recurrence locally will be excessive. In addition, if there is no residual native rectum, the patient will not have normal sensation or control and will have problems with uncontrollable soilage, (**incontinence**). For these reasons, patients presenting with low rectal tumors may undergo total removal of the rectum and anus. This procedure is known as an abdominal-perineal resection. A permanent colostomy is performed in the lower left abdomen.

RADIATION. As mentioned, for many late stage II or stage III tumors, **radiation therapy** can shrink the tumor prior to surgery. The other roles for radiation therapy are as an aid to surgical therapy in locally advanced disease that has been removed, and in the treatment of certain distant metastases. Especially when utilized in combination with chemotherapy, radiation used postoperatively has been shown to reduce the risk of local recurrence in the pelvis by 46% and death rates by 29%. Such combined therapy is recommended in patients with locally advanced primary tumors that have been removed surgically. Radiation has been helpful in treating effects of distant metastases, particularly in the brain. In very few cases, radiation alone may be the curative treatment for rectal cancer.

CHEMOTHERAPY. Adjuvant chemotherapy, (treating the patient who has no evidence of residual disease but who is at high risk for recurrence), is considered in patients whose tumors deeply penetrate or locally invade (late stage II and stage III). If the tumor was not locally advanced, this form of chemotherapeutic adjuvant therapy may be recommended without radiation. This therapy is identical to that of colon cancer and leads to similar results. Standard therapy is treatment with 5-fluorouracil (5-FU, or **fluorouracil**) combined with **leucovorin** for a period of six to twelve months. 5-FU is an antimetabolite and leucovorin improves the response rate. Another agent, **levamisole** (which seems to stimulate the immune system) may be substituted for leucovorin. These protocols reduce the rate of recurrence by about 15% and reduce mortality by about 10%. The regimens have some toxicity but usually are tolerated fairly well.

Similar chemotherapy is administered for stage IV disease or if a cancer progresses and metastasis develops. Results show response rates of about 20%. A response is a temporary regression of the cancer in response to the chemotherapy. Unfortunately, these patients eventually succumb to the disease. **Clinical trials** have now shown that the results can be improved with the addition of another agent to this regimen. **Irinotecan** does not seem to increase toxicity but has improved response rates to 39%, added two to three months to disease-free survival, and prolonged overall survival by a little more than two months.

Prognosis

Prognosis is the long-term outlook or survival after therapy. Overall, about 50% of patients treated for colon and rectal cancer survive the disease. As expected, the survival rates are dependent upon the stage of the cancer at the time of diagnosis, making early detection crucial.

About 15% of patients present with stage I disease, or are diagnosed with Stage I disease when they initially visit a doctor, and 85-90% survive. Stage II represents 20-30% of cases and 65-75% survive; 30-40% comprise the stage III presentation, of which 55% survive. The remaining 20-25% present with stage IV disease and are rarely cured.

Alternative and complementary therapies

Most alternative therapies have not been studied in clinical trials. Large doses of **vitamins**, fiber, and green tea are among therapies tried. A 2003 report on a large Harvard University study showed that people who took multivitamins for at least 15 years had a 34% reduction in risk of rectal cancer. Before initiating any alternative therapies, the patient should consult his or her physician to be sure that these therapies do not complicate or interfere with the recommended therapy.

Coping with cancer treatment

For those with familial syndromes causing colon cancer, genetic counseling may be appropriate. Psychological counseling may help anyone having trouble coping with a potentially fatal disease. Local cancer support groups are often identified by contacting local hospitals or the American Cancer Society.

The Colon Cancer Alliance offers online support at the following web page: http://www.ccalliance.org/connect/support.html.

Clinical trials

Clinical trials are scientific studies in which new therapies are compared to current standards in an effort to identify therapies that offer better results.

Agents being tested for efficacy in patients with advanced disease include oxaliplatin and CPT-11. Please see reference below for current information available from the National Cancer Institute regarding these clinical trials.

Prevention

There is not an absolute method for preventing colon or rectal cancer. An individual can lessen risk or identify the precursors of colon and rectal cancer. The patient with a familial history can enter screening and surveillance programs earlier than the general population. High-fiber diets and vitamins, avoiding obesity, and staying active lessen the risk. In fact, a 2003 report said that vigorous exercise (to the point of sweating or feeling out of breath) lowered risk of rectal cancer by nearly 40% compared to those who exercised less. Avoiding **cigarettes** and alcohol may be helpful. By controlling these environmental factors, an individual can lessen risk and to this degree prevent the disease.

By undergoing appropriate screening when uncontrollable genetic risk factors have been identified, an individual may be rewarded by the identification of benign polyps that can be treated as opposed to having these growths degenerate into a malignancy.

Special concerns

Polyps are growths of the epithelium of the colon. They may be completely benign, pre-malignant, or cancerous. The association of colon and rectal cancers in patients with certain types of polyps is that many polyps begin as a benign growth and later acquire malignant characteristics. There are two types of polyps; pedunculated and sessile. This terminology comes from their appearance; those that are pedunculated are on a stalk like a mushroom and the sessile polyps are broad based and have no stalk. Unless a pedunculated polyp gets large, malignant potential is very small. This type may also be easily removed at endoscopy. The sessile polyp is also known as a villous **adenoma**, as many as one-third of these harbor a malignancy. Therefore, the villous adenoma is considered premalignant. Sessile polyps may or may not be easily managed with the colonoscope and may need surgical removal because of their pre-malignant nature.

Polyps commonly present with occult blood in the stool. Since they are associated with the development of cancer, patients who have developed polyps need to enter a program of careful surveillance.

Elderly or debilitated patients with rectal cancers that seem localized may be treated by local destruction of the tumor through the anus. If the tumor is amenable to local resection or destruction by laser or cautery through the anus, the patient may be treated this way. This select group of patients may not be able to tolerate the standard therapy. Local control becomes the main issue while avoiding high-risk surgery and the inherent complications.

Resources

BOOKS

Abelhoff, Martin, MD, James O. Armitage MD, Allen S. Lichter MD, and John E. Niederhuber MD. *Clinical Oncology Library*. Philadelphia: Churchill Livingstone, 1999.

Jorde, Lynn B., PhD, John C. Carey MD, Michael J. Bamshad MD, and Raymond L. White, PhD. *Medical Genetics*. 2nd ed. St. Louis: Mosby, 1999.

PERIODICALS

"Colon Cancer; Facts to Know." *NWHRC Health Center* December 15, 2003.

"Endoscopy and MRI Are Important in Staging Rectal Cancer." *Clinical Oncology Week* October 6, 2003: 56.

Greenlee, Robert T., PhD, MPH, Mary Beth Hill-Harmon, MSPH, Taylor Murray, and Michael Thun, MD, MS. "Cancer Statistics 2001." *CA: A Cancer Journal for Clinicians* 51, no. 1 (January-February 2001).

Saltz, Leonard, et al. "Irinotecan plus Fluorouracil and Leucovorin for Metastatic Colorectal Cancer." *The New England Journal of Medicine* 343, no. 13 (September 28, 2000).

Splete, Heidi. "Multivitamins May Lower Risk of Rectal Cancer: Drops 34% at 15 Years." *Family Practice News* December 1, 2003: 33.

"Vigourous Physical Activity May Reduce the Risk of Rectal Cancer." *Environmental Nutrition* October 2003: 8.

OTHER

Colon Cancer Alliance.http://www.ccalliance.org.

National Cancer Institute Clinical Trials. <cancertrials.nci.nih.gov>.

ORGANIZATIONS

American Cancer Society. (800) ACS-2345. http://www.cancer.org.

Cancer Information Service of the NCI. (1-800-4-CANCER). <http://wwwicic.nci.nih.gov>.

Richard A. McCartney, M.D.
Teresa G. Odle

Rectal resection

Definition

A rectal resection is the surgical removal of a portion of the rectum.

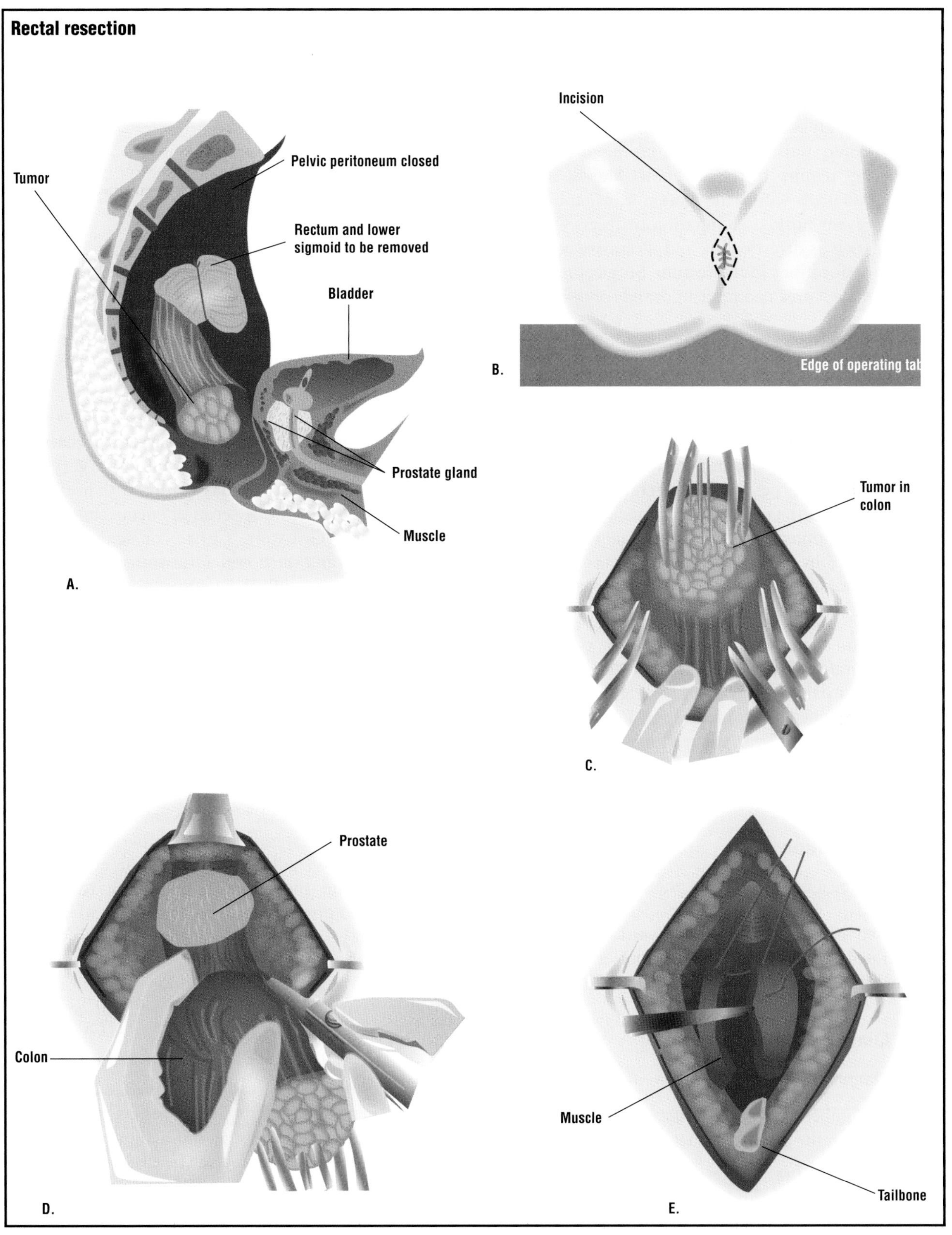

A tumor in the rectum or lower colon can be removed by a rectal resection (A). An incision is made around the patient's anus (B). The tumor is pulled down through the incision (C). An attached area of the colon is also removed (D). The area is repaired, leaving an opening for bowel functioning (E). *(Illustration by GGS Information Services. Cengage Learning, Gale.)*

Purpose

Rectal resections repair damage to the rectum caused by diseases of the lower digestive tract, such as **cancer**, diverticulitis, and inflammatory bowel disease (ulcerative colitis and Crohn's disease). Injury, obstruction, and ischemia (compromised blood supply) may require rectal resection. Masses and scar tissue can grow within the rectum, causing blockages that prevent normal elimination of feces. Other diseases, such as diverticulitis and ulcerative colitis, can cause perforations in the rectum. Surgical removal of the damaged area can return normal rectal function.

Demographics

Colorectal cancer affects 140,000 people annually, causing 60,000 deaths. Incidence of the disease in 2001 differed among ethnic groups, with Hispanics having 10.2 cases per 100,000 people and African Americans having 22.8 cases per 100,000. **Rectal cancer** incidence is a portion of the total colorectal incidence rate. Surgery is the optimal treatment for rectal cancer, resulting in cure in 45% of patients. Recurrence due to surgical failure is low, from 4–8%, when the procedure is meticulously performed.

Crohn's disease and ulcerative colitis, both chronic inflammatory diseases of the colon, each affect approximately 500,000 young adults. Surgery is recommended when medication fails patients with ulcerative colitis. Nearly three-fourths of all Crohn's patients will require surgery to remove a diseased section of the intestine or rectum.

Description

During a rectal resection, the surgeon removes the diseased or perforated portion of the rectum. If the diseased or damaged section is not very large, the separated ends are reattached. Such a procedure is called rectal anastomosis.

Diagnosis/Preparation

Diagnostic tests

A number of tests identify masses and perforations within the intestinal tract.

- A lower GI (gastrointestinal) series is a series of x rays of the colon and rectum that can help identify ulcers, cysts, polyps, diverticuli (pouches in the intestine), and cancer. The patient is given a barium enema to coat the intestinal tract, making disease easier to see on the x rays.
- Flexible sigmoidoscopy involves insertion of a sigmoidoscope, a flexible tube with a miniature camera, into the rectum to examine the lining of the rectum and the sigmoid colon, the last third of the intestinal tract. The sigmoidoscope can also remove polyps or tissue for biopsy.
- A colonoscopy is similar to the flexible sigmoidoscopy, except the flexible tube examines the entire intestinal tract.
- Magnetic resonance imaging (MRI), used both prior to and during surgery, allows physicians to determine the precise margins for the resection, so that all of the diseased tissue can be removed. This also identifies patients who could most benefit from adjuvant therapy such as chemotherapy or radiation.

Preoperative preparation

To cleanse the bowel, the patient may be placed on a restricted diet for several days before surgery, then placed on a liquid diet the day before, with nothing by mouth after midnight. A series of enemas and/or oral preparations (GoLytely, Colyte, or senna) may be ordered to empty the bowel. Oral anti-infectives (neomycin, erythromycin, or kanamycin sulfate) may be ordered to decrease bacteria in the intestine and help prevent post-operative **infection**. The operation can be done with an abdominal incision (laparotomy) or using minimally invasive techniques with small tubes to allow insertion of the operating instruments (**laparoscopy**).

Aftercare

Postoperative care involves monitoring blood pressure, pulse, respiration, and temperature. Breathing tends to be shallow because of the effect of the anesthesia and the patient's reluctance to breathe deeply due to discomfort around the surgical incision. The patient is taught how to support the incision during deep breathing and coughing, and given pain medication as necessary. Fluid intake and output is measured, and the wound is observed for color and drainage.

Fluids and electrolytes are given intravenously until the patient's diet can be resumed, starting with liquids, then adding solids. The patient is helped out of bed the evening of the surgery and allowed to sit in a chair. Most patients are discharged in two to four days.

Risks

Rectal resection has potential risks similar those of other major surgeries. Complications usually occur

WHO PERFORMS THE PROCEDURE AND WHERE IS IT PERFORMED?

Rectal resections are performed by general surgeons and colorectal surgeons as in-patient surgeries under general anesthesia.

while the patient is in the hospital and the patient's general health prior to surgery will be an indication of the risk potential. Patients with heart problems and stressed immune systems are of special concern. Both during and following the procedure, the physician and nursing staff will monitor the patient for:

- excessive bleeding
- wound infection
- thrombophlebitis (inflammation and blood clot in the veins in the legs
- pneumonia
- pulmonary embolism (blood clot or air bubble in the lungs' blood supply)
- cardiac stress due to allergic reaction to the general anaesthetic

Symptoms that the patient should report, especially after discharge, include:

- increased pain, swelling, redness, drainage, or bleeding in the surgical area
- flu-like symptoms such as headache, muscle aches, dizziness, or fever
- increased abdominal pain or swelling, constipation, nausea or vomiting, or black, tarry stools

Normal results

Complete healing is expected without complications. The recovery rate varies, depending on the patient's overall health prior to surgery. Typically, full recovery takes six to eight weeks.

Morbidity and mortality rates

Mortality has decreased from nearly 28% to under 6%, through the use of prophylactic **antibiotics** before and after surgery.

Alternatives

If the section of the rectum to be removed is very large, the rectum may not be able to be reattached. Under those circumstances, a **colostomy** would be preformed. The distal end of the rectum would be closed and left to atrophy. The proximal end would be brought through an opening in the abdomen to create an opening, a stoma, for feces to be removed from the body.

QUESTIONS TO ASK THE DOCTOR

- Am I a good candidate for laparoscopic surgery?
- What kinds of preoperative tests will be required?
- What medications will be given for pain relief after the surgery?
- What will I need to do to prepare for surgery?
- What will my recovery time be and what restrictions will I have?

Resources

BOOKS

Johnston, Lorraine. *Colon & Rectal Cancer: A Comprehensive Guide for Patients and Families*. Sebastopol, CA: O'Reilly, 2000.

Levin, Bernard. *American Cancer Society Colorectal Cancer*. New York: Villard, 1999.

PERIODICALS

Beets-Tan, R. G. H., et al. "Accuracy of Maganetic Resonance Imaging in Prediction of Tumour-free Resection Margin in Rectal Cancer Surgery." *The Lancet* 357 (February 17, 2001): 497.

Walling, Anne D. "Follow-up After Resection for Colorectal Cancer Saves Lives. (Tips from Other Journals)." *American Family Physician* 66 (August 1, 2002): 485.

ORGANIZATIONS

American Board of Colon and Rectal Surgery (ABCRS). 20600 Eureka Road, Suite 713, Taylor, MI 48180. (734) 282-9400. http://www.fascrs.org.

Mayo Clinic. 200 First St. S.W., Rochester, MN 55905. (507) 284-2511. http://www.mayoclinic.org.

Janie Franz

Renal pelvis tumors

Definition

Renal pelvis tumors are rare kidney cancers appearing in a specific part of the kidney known as the pelvis of the kidney.

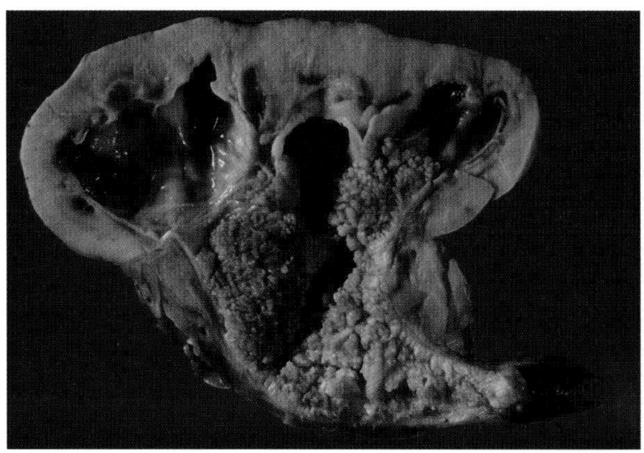

Transitional-cell carcinoma of the renal pelvis fills. *(Copyright Biophoto Associates, Science Source/Photo Researchers, Inc. Reproduced by permission.)*

KEY TERMS

Balkan nephropathy—A rare inherited kidney disorder that is associated with increased risk of developing renal pelvis tumors.

Cystoscopy—A medical procedure involving the use of a medical instrument that permits the physician to look directly at portions of the urinary tract.

Pyelography—A type of x-ray procedure applied to a portion of the urinary tract, of which the kidneys form part.

Renal—Having to do with the kidneys.

Renal papillary necrosis—A medical condition affecting the kidney and that increases a person's risk of developing a tumor of the renal pelvis.

Renal pelvis—That portion of the collecting system of the kidney that empties into the ureter.

Ureteroscopy—A diagnostic procedure that increases the diagnostic accuracy of the examination of possible renal pelvis tumors. Ureteroscopy may cause damage to some portion of the urinary tract. Therefore, ureteroscopy is usually reserved for those patients for whom unanswered questions remain after conventional diagnostic approaches have been completed.

Urography—A type of x-ray procedure applied to a portion of the urinary tract, of which the kidneys form part.

Description

The word "renal" means having to do with the kidneys. A part of each kidney in the human body is called the renal pelvis. The renal pelvis in each kidney is the portion of the collecting system that empties into the ureters (tubes that carry urine from the kidneys to the bladder).

Renal pelvis tumors usually appear after an earlier condition called renal papillary necrosis has already developed. The tumors may be composed of any one of several different types of cells. Most commonly, these tumors are of a type of cell known as a **transitional cell carcinoma**.

A transitional cell is intermediate between the flat squamous cell and the tall columnar cell. It is restricted to the epithelium (cellular lining) of the urinary bladder, ureters, and the renal pelvis. Transitional cell carcinomas have a wide range in their gross appearance depending on their locations. Some of these carcinomas are flat in appearance, some are papillary (small elevation), and others are in the shape of a node. Under the microscope, however, most of these carcinomas have a papillary-like look. There are three generally recognized grades of transitional cell **carcinoma**. The grade of the carcinoma is determined by particular characteristics found in the cells of the tumor. Transitional cell carcinoma typically affects the mucosa (the moist tissue layer that lines hollow organs or the cavity of the body) in the areas where it originates— in this case, the kidney.

Demographics

Because statistics on these tumors are gathered with statistics on other kidney tumors, little information specific to tumors of the pelvic area of the kidney, as opposed to other areas of the kidney, is available. These tumors are relatively uncommon, however; they account for no more than 5% of cancers of the kidney and upper urinary tract. This percentage would indicate that 1785 Americans (1104 men and 684 women) were diagnosed with **cancer** of the renal pelvis in 2004 and 624 patients (394 men and 230 women) died of the disease. Renal pelvis cancers are more common in men than in women, as the statistics indicate, and appear most commonly in persons over the age of 65.

Causes and symptoms

The causes of renal cell cancer are not completely understood as of the early 2000s, but are thought to be related to the excretion of irritating substances in the urine. The appearance of renal pelvis tumors is often associated with a history of cigarette smoking and the overuse of certain pain medicines, as well as with a history of either kidney stones or **bladder cancer**.

QUESTIONS TO ASK THE DOCTOR

- How can I obtain supportive care so I come through this not only alive but with my family and emotional life intact?
- What sort of benefit and what sort of side effects might each of the available treatment options bring?
- Would you please inform me about treatment options and let me tell you about the priorities in my life so I can participate in forming a treatment plan?
- What is my prognosis?
- What are the chances, after I have completed treatment, that cancer may return? How frequently should I be checked so we can defeat any cancer that appears in the future?

People who have worked in the rubber, paint, dye, printing, textile, and plastic industries and been exposed to certain chemicals are also at increased risk for this type of cancer. The risk is elevated, as well, for people with a rare kidney condition called Balkan nephropathy. This condition is more likely to affect people from Romania, Greece, Bulgaria, Serbia, Croatia, Bosnia-Herzegovina, and other countries included in the former Yugoslavia.

Approximately four out of five patients have symptoms of blood in the urine at the time of diagnosis. Approximately one out of three patients experiences pain in the side or lower back. Other frequent symptoms include urinary frequency or urgency, unintentional **weight loss**, brown or rusty-colored urine, and **fatigue**. Some patients may have no symptoms, while others may feel generally ill, visit the doctor for this general complaint, and have the cancer diagnosed at that time.

Diagnosis

Either urography or pyelography may be used to diagnose renal pelvis tumors. Both urography and pyelography are types of x-ray procedures that may be used to visualize portions of the urinary tract. The kidneys are part of the urinary tract. If urography is used, it is usually followed by **cystoscopy**. Cystoscopy involves the use of a medical instrument that permits the physician to look directly at portions of the urinary tract.

A newer technique is called ureteroscopy. Performing ureteroscopy increases the diagnostic accuracy doctors are able to attain. However, there is a risk that ureteroscopy may cause damage to some portion of the urinary tract. Therefore, ureteroscopy is usually reserved for those patients for whom unanswered questions remain after conventional diagnostic approaches have been completed.

The doctor may also order an x ray of the chest, a bone scan, and liver function tests to see whether the cancer has spread.

Clinical staging, treatments, and prognosis

Clinical staging

Tumor stage and grade provide important information on how an individual patient's renal pelvis tumor(s) will be treated and on the patient's prognosis. The primary tumor is staged on the basis of whether it remains superficial or has settled into the kidney. Patients with more superficial tumors have the best prognosis. However, even these patients may develop new tumors later.

Another factor important in determining treatment and prognosis is to determine the type and character of the individual cells that make up the tumor. Cells with a well-differentiated structure are associated with longer patient survival than cells with poorly differentiated structure.

Treatments

Surgery constitutes standard treatment for renal pelvis tumors. The surgical procedure is called a radical nephroureterectomy, and may involve the removal of a portion of the bladder as well. Some surgeons have attempted to perform part of the procedure through an endoscope rather than the standard open surgery, but early reports indicate that the rate of cancer recurrence is higher with endoscopic surgery.

Some patients should not receive surgical treatment for this cancer. Other patients should undergo a relatively more limited surgical procedure than the standard procedure—one in which less of the kidney is removed. Those who should be approached in the more limited way may include patients with only one single kidney, patients with cancer of both kidneys, and patients with Balkan nephropathy. In addition, patients who are in generally poor health may not be good candidates for surgery or may receive a limited surgical procedure.

Of course, patients with a single tumor comprised of well-differentiated cells are likely to have a better long-term outcome following a limited surgical procedure than are patients with several tumors comprised of poorly differentiated cells. It should be understood, however, that more limited procedures may involve a greater likelihood that the cancer will return.

Patients with Balkan nephropathy usually benefit from receiving the more limited procedure. These patients are at pre-existing risk of kidney failure because of the Balkan nephropathy; thus, the more of their kidneys preserved, the better for their future overall medical outcomes.

Some surgical procedures used for renal pelvis tumors are performed using a medical device that moves along the body channels used by urine. The use of this device in the treatment of renal pelvis tumors is, however, limited to extremely small tumors.

X-ray therapy may be used following a surgical procedure for renal pelvis tumors. In particular, it may be used if there is any evidence that tumor cells have affected any of the surrounding organs or if they are appearing in the lymph nodes. In addition, x-ray therapy may be recommended for patients who are at a higher-than-average risk for reappearance of cancer, for example, patients who are heavy smokers. Some authorities believe that additional studies are needed to clarify the effects of x-ray therapy for these patients.

Patients who experience pain related to renal pelvis tumors may receive x-ray treatment to control pain. Such treatment may be very effective. Patients with such pain may also benefit from **chemotherapy**.

The patient with advanced renal pelvis cancer does not receive treatment that attempts to cure the disease. Rather, the treatment is palliative—it is used in an attempt to make the patient feel better and to improve the patient's quality of life. **Cisplatin** used alone has been shown to be an effective chemotherapy medicine in this situation.

It may, however, be preferable to use combination chemotherapy rather than cisplatin alone for patients with advanced disease, as a recent study demonstrated. The combination chemotherapy used in this study is the so-called M-VAC regimen, which consists of **methotrexate**, **vinblastine**, Adriamycin (**doxorubicin**), and cisplatin. This combination of medicines permitted patients both to live for a longer time without return of cancer and to live for a longer time overall.

Another combination of chemotherapy medicines studied for patients with advanced disease is the so-called CMV, which consists of cisplatin, methotrexate, and vinblastine.

It is important to examine the side effects that may accompany chemotherapy in these patients. Some of these side effects are severe, and a small percentage of patients treated using this modality die. Both the M-VAC and the CMV regimens help approximately half of patients and give some patients additional months of life.

Other newer medicines that have been tried as chemotherapy for patients with renal pelvis tumors and advanced disease are paclitaxel (Taxol) and **gemcitabine** (Gemzar). In 2005, it was questionable whether the use of either one of these medicines as single-drug chemotherapy produces superior results to the M-VAC or CMV regimens.

Prognosis

In terms of patient survival, almost all patients with superficial tumors composed of relatively well-differentiated cells live more than five years. In contrast, patients with poorly differentiated (abnormal in maturity and function) tumors that have invaded deep into the kidney and transplanted cells to other parts of the body may live only one year or less.

Approximately two out of five patients given limited surgical treatment for renal pelvis tumors will have new tumors develop. Therefore, it is important that these patients receive careful and regular follow-up. Some authorities recommend examinations for new tumors of and near the renal pelvis at three-, six-, nine-, twelve-, eighteen, and twenty-four months following surgery, and annually afterwards.

Coping with cancer treatment

Cancer patients need supportive care to help them come through the treatment period with physical and emotional strength in tact. Many patients experience feelings of **depression**, anxiety, and fatigue, and many experience **nausea**, **vomiting**, and other side effects during treatment. Studies have shown that these can be managed effectively if the patient discusses these issues with the treating physician.

Prevention

Smoking cessation is the most important step. In addition, persons working in the rubber, paint, dye, printing, textile, and plastic industries might speak with their doctor about whether they are at elevated risk of developing this cancer.

Resources

BOOKS

Beers, Mark H., MD, and Robert Berkow, MD, editors. "Cancer of the Renal Pelvis and Ureter." Section 17, Chapter 233 In*The Merck Manual of Diagnosis and Therapy*. Whitehouse Station, NJ: Merck Research Laboratories, 2002.

Braunwald, Eugene, et al. *Harrison's Principles of Internal Medicine*. 15th ed. New York: McGraw-Hill, 2001.

Haskell, Charles M. *Cancer Treatment*. 5th ed. Philadelphia: W. B. Saunders, 2001.

Pazdur, Richard, et al. *Cancer Management: A Multidisciplinary Approach: Medical, Surgical, & Radiation Oncology*. 4th ed. Melville, NY: PRR, 2000.

PERIODICALS

Bamias, A., Ch. Deliveliotis, G. Fountzilas, et al. "Adjuvant Chemotherapy with Paclitaxel and Carboplatin in Patients with Advanced Carcinoma of the Upper Urinary Tract: A Study by the Hellenic Cooperative Oncology Group." *Journal of Clinical Oncology* 22 (June 1, 2004): 2150–2154.

Saika, T., J. Nishiguchi, T. Tsushima, et al. "Comparative Study of Ureteral Stripping Versus Open Ureterectomy for Nephroureterectomy in Patients with Transitional Carcinoma of the Renal Pelvis." *Urology* 63 (May 2004): 848–852.

OTHER

American Cancer Society (ACS). *Cancer Facts & Figures 2004*.http://www.cancer.org/downloads/STT/CAFF_finalPWSecured.pdf.

ORGANIZATIONS

American Urological Association (AUA). 1000 Corporate Boulevard, Linthicum, MD 21090. (866) 746-4282 or (410) 689-3700. http://www.auanet.org.

Bob Kirsch
Rebecca J. Frey, PhD

Renal cell carcinoma *see* **Kidney cancer, renal cell**

Retinoblastoma

Definition

Retinoblastoma is a malignant tumor of the retina that occurs predominantly in young children.

Description

The eye has three layers, the sclera, the choroid, and the retina. The sclera is the outer protective white coating of the eye. The choroid is the middle layer and contains blood vessels that nourish the eye. The front portion of the choroid is colored and is called the iris. The opening in the iris is called the pupil. The pupil is responsible for allowing light into the eye and usually appears black. When the pupil is exposed to bright light it contracts (closes), and when it is exposed to low light conditions it dilates (opens) so that the appropriate amount of light enters the eye. Light that enters through the pupil hits the lens of the eye. The lens then focuses the light onto the retina, the innermost of the three layers. The job of the retina is to transform the light into information that can be transmitted to the optic nerve, which will transmit this information to the brain. It is through this process that people are able to see the world around them.

Occasionally a tumor, called a retinoblastoma, will develop in the retina of the eye. Usually this tumor forms in young children but it can occasionally

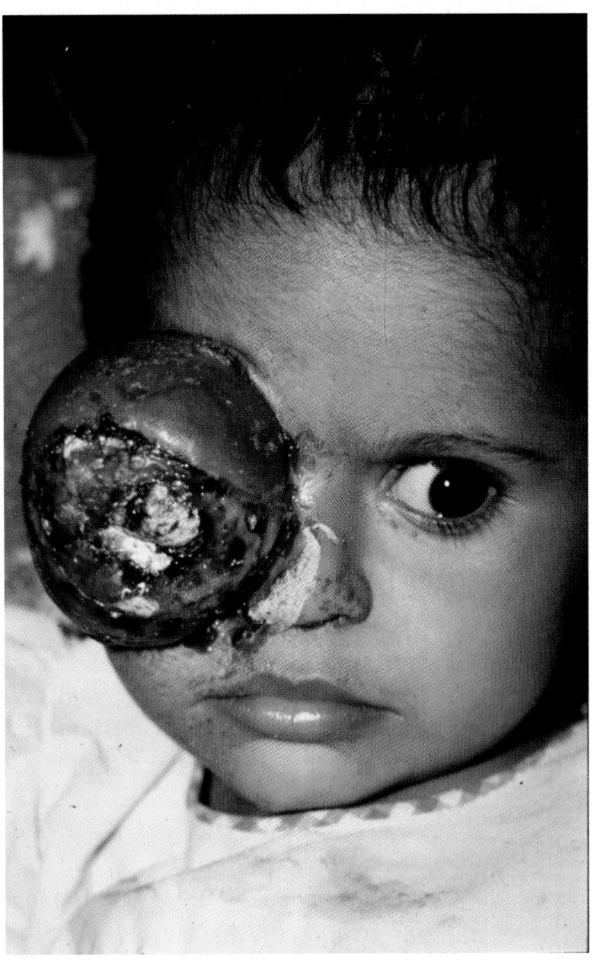

This child's right eye is completely covered with a retinoblastoma tumor. *(Custom Medical Stock Photo. Reproduced by permission.)*

KEY TERMS

Amniocentesis—Prenatal testing performed at 16 to 20 weeks of pregnancy that involves inserting a needle through the abdomen of a pregnant mother and obtaining a small sample of fluid from the amniotic sack, which contains the fetus. Often is used to obtain a sample of the fetus' cells for biochemical or DNA testing.

Benign tumor—An abnormal proliferation of cells that does not spread to other parts of the body.

Bilateral—Affecting both eyes.

Brachytherapy—Cancer treatment that involves the application of radioactive material to the site of the tumor.

Chorionic villus sampling (CVS)—Prenatal testing performed at 10 to 12 weeks of pregnancy, which involves inserting a catheter through the vagina of a pregnant mother or inserting a needle through the abdomen of the mother and obtaining a sample of placenta. Often is used to obtain a sample of the fetus' cells for biochemical or DNA testing.

Chromosome—A microscopic structure found within each cell of the body, made of a complex of proteins and DNA.

Cryotherapy—Cancer treatment in which the tumor is destroyed by exposure to intense cold.

DNA (deoxyribonucleic acid)—The hereditary material that makes up genes; influences the development and functioning of the body.

DNA testing—Testing for a change or changes in a gene or genes.

Enucleation—Surgical removal of the eye.

Equator—Imaginary line encircling the eyeball and dividing the eye into a front and back half.

Extraocular retinoblastoma—Cancer that has spread from the eye to other parts of the body.

Gene—A building block of inheritance, made up of a compound called DNA (deoxyribonucleic acid) and containing the instructions for the production of a particular protein. Each gene is found in a specific location on a chromosome.

Intraocular retinoblastoma—Cancer that is limited to the eye and has not spread to other parts of the body.

Malignant tumor—An abnormal proliferation of cells that can spread to other sites.

Multifocal—More than one tumor present.

Oncologist—A physician specializing in the diagnosis and treatment of cancer

Ophthalmologist—Physician specializing in the diseases of the eye.

Optic nerve—The part of the eye which contains nerve fibers that transmit signals from the eye to the brain.

Photocoagulation—Cancer treatment in which the tumor is destroyed by an intense beam of laser light.

Prenatal testing—Testing for a disease such as a genetic condition in an unborn baby.

Protein—A substance produced by a gene that is involved in creating the traits of the human body, such as hair and eye color, or is involved in controlling the basic functions of the human body, such as control of the cell cycle.

Retina—The light-sensitive layer of the eye that receives images and sends them to the brain.

Scotoma—An area of lost or depressed vision within the visual field surrounded by an area of normal vision. Survivors of retinoblastoma frequently develop scotomas.

Somatic cells—All the cells of the body with the exception of the egg and sperm cells.

Tumor—A growth of tissue resulting from the uncontrolled proliferation of cells.

Tumor-suppressor gene—Gene involved in controlling normal cell growth and preventing cancer.

Unifocal—Only one tumor present in one eye.

Unilateral—Affecting only one eye.

Vitreous—The transparent gel that fills the back part of the eye.

Vitreous seeding—When small pieces of tumor have broken off and are floating around the vitreous.

occur in adults. Most people with retinoblastoma develop only one tumor (unifocal) in only one eye (unilateral). Some, however, develop multiple tumors (multifocal) in one or both eyes. When retinoblastoma occurs independently in both eyes, it is then called bilateral retinoblastoma.

Occasionally, children with retinoblastoma develop trilateral retinoblastoma. Trilateral retinoblastoma results from the development of an independent brain tumor that often forms in a part of the brain called the pineal gland. In order for retinoblastoma to be classified as trilateral, the tumor must have developed

QUESTIONS TO ASK THE DOCTOR

- What form and stage of retinoblastoma does my child have? Has the cancer spread beyond the eye?
- Was this an inherited disease? Should other family members be tested?
- What are the chances of maintaining my child's sight? What treatment options are appropriate for this?
- Are there support groups in the area to help my family cope with this diagnosis?

independently and not as the result of the spread of the retinal **cancer**. The prognosis for trilateral retinoblastoma is quite poor.

The retinal tumor which characterizes retinoblastoma is malignant, meaning that it can metastasize (spread) to other parts of the eye and eventually other parts of the body. In most cases, however, retinoblastoma is diagnosed before it spreads past the eye to other parts of the body (intraocular) and the prognosis is quite good. The prognosis is poorer if the cancer has spread beyond the eye (extraocular).

Retinoblastoma can be inherited or can arise spontaneously. Approximately 40% of people with retinoblastoma have an inherited form of the condition and approximately 60% have a sporadic (not inherited) form. Individuals with multiple independent tumors, bilateral retinoblastoma, or trilateral retinoblastoma are more likely to be affected with the inherited form of retinoblastoma.

Demographics

Approximately 1 in 15,000 to 1 in 30,000 infants in Western countries are born with retinoblastoma, making it the most common childhood eye cancer. It is, however, a relatively rare childhood cancer and accounts for approximately 3% of **childhood cancers**. The American Academy of Ophthalmology estimates that 300–350 cases of retinoblastoma occur in the United States each year.

Retinoblastoma is found mainly in children under the age of five but can occasionally be seen in older children and adults. Retinoblastoma is found in individuals of all ethnic backgrounds and is found equally frequently in males and females. The incidence of bilaterial retinoblastoma in the United States is thought to be slightly higher among black children than among either Caucasian or Asian American children.

Causes and symptoms

Causes

Retinoblastoma is caused by changes in or absence of a gene called RB1. RB1 is located on chromosome 13q14. Cells of the body, with the exception of the egg and sperm cells, contain 23 pairs of chromosomes. All of the cells of the body excluding the egg and the sperm cells are called the somatic cells. The somatic cells contain two of each chromosome 13 and therefore two copies of the RB1 gene. Each egg and sperm cell contains only one copy of chromosome 13 and therefore only contains one copy of the RB1 gene.

RB1 produces a tumor suppressor protein that normally helps to regulate the cell cycle of cells such as those of the retina. A normal cell of the retina goes through a growth cycle during which it produces new cells. Genes such as tumor suppressor genes tightly regulate this growth cycle.

Cells that lose control of their cell cycle and replicate out of control are called cancer cells. These undergo many cell divisions, often at a quicker rate than normal cells, and do not have a limited lifespan. A group of adjacent cancer cells can form a mass called a tumor. Malignant (cancerous) tumors can spread to other parts of the body. A malignant tumor of the retina (retinoblastoma) can result when just one retinal cell loses control of it cell cycle and replicates out of control.

Normally the tumor suppressor protein produced by RB1 prevents a retinal cell from becoming cancerous. Each RB1 gene produces tumor suppressor protein. Only one functioning RB1 gene in a retinal cell is necessary to prevent the cell from becoming cancerous. If both RB1 genes in a retinal cell become nonfunctional, then a retinal cell can become cancerous and retinoblastoma can result. An RB1 gene is nonfunctional when it is changed or missing (deleted) and no longer produces normal tumor suppressor protein.

Approximately 40% of people with retinoblastoma have inherited a nonfunctional or deleted RB1 gene from either their mother or father. Therefore, they have a changed/deleted RB1 gene in every somatic cell. A person with an inherited missing or non-functional RB1 gene will develop a retinal tumor if the remaining RB1 gene becomes changed or deleted in a retinal cell. The remaining RB1 gene can become nonfunctional when exposed to environmental triggers such as chemicals and radiation. In most cases, however, the triggers are unknown. Approximately 90% of people who inherit a changed or missing RB1 gene will develop retinoblastoma.

People with an inherited form of retinoblastoma are more likely to have a tumor in both eyes (bilateral) and are more likely to have more than one independent tumor (multifocal) in one or both eyes. The average age of onset for the inherited form of retinoblastoma is one year, which is earlier than the sporadic form of retinoblastoma. Although most people with the inherited form of retinoblastoma develop bilateral tumors, approximately 15% of people with a tumor in only one eye (unilateral) are affected with an inherited form of retinoblastoma.

A person with an inherited missing or non-functional RB1 gene has a 50% chance of passing on this abnormal gene to his or her offspring. The chance that their children will inherit the changed/deleted gene and actually develop retinoblastoma is approximately 45%.

Some people with retinoblastoma have inherited a non-functioning or missing RB1 gene from either their mother or father even though their parents have never developed retinoblastoma. It is possible that one parent has a changed or missing RB1 gene in every somatic cell but has not developed retinoblastoma because their remaining RB1 gene has remained functional. It is also possible that the parent had developed a retinal tumor that was destroyed by the body. In other cases, one parent has two normal RB1 genes in every somatic cell, but some of their egg or sperm cells contain a changed or missing RB1 gene. This is called gonadal mosaicism.

Retinoblastoma can also result when both RB1 genes become spontaneously changed or deleted in a retinal cell but the RB1 genes are normal in all the other cells of the body. Approximately 60% of people with retinoblastoma have this type of disease, called sporadic retinoblastoma. A person with sporadic retinoblastoma does not have a higher chance of having children with the disease. Their relatives do not have a higher risk of developing retinoblastoma themselves or having children who develop retinoblastoma. Sporadic retinoblastoma is usually unifocal and has an average age of onset of approximately two years.

Symptoms

The most common symptom of retinoblastoma is leukocoria. Leukocoria results when the pupil reflects a white color rather than the normal black or red color that is seen on a flash photograph. It is often most obvious in flash photographs since the pupil is exposed to a lot of light, and the duration of the exposure is so short that the pupil does not have time to constrict. Children with retinoblastoma can also have problems seeing and this can cause them to appear cross-eyed (strabismus). People with retinoblastoma may also experience red, painful, and irritated eyes, inflamed tissue around the eye, enlarged pupils, and possibly different-colored eyes.

Diagnosis

Children who have symptoms of retinoblastoma are usually first evaluated by their pediatrician. The pediatrician will often perform a red reflex test to diagnose or confirm leukocoria. Prior to this test the doctor inserts medicated eye drops into the child's eyes so that the pupils will remain dilated and not contract when exposed to bright light. The doctor then examines the eyes with an ophthalmoscope, which shines a bright light into the eyes and allows the doctor to check for leukocoria. Leukocoria can also be diagnosed by taking a flash Polaroid photograph of a patient who has been in a dark room for three to five minutes.

If the pediatrician suspects retinoblastoma on the basis of these evaluations, he or she will most likely refer the patient to an ophthalmologist (eye doctor) who has experience with retinoblastoma. The ophthalmologist will examine the eye using an indirect ophthalmoscope. The opthalmoscope shines a bright light into the eye, which helps the doctor to visualize the retina. This evaluation is usually done under general anesthetic, although some very young or older patients may not require it. Prior to the examination, medicated drops are put into the eyes to dilate the pupils, and anesthetic drops may also be used. A metal clip is used to keep the eyes open during the evaluation. During the examination, a cotton swab or a metal instrument with a flattened tip is used to press on the outer lens of the eye so that a better view of the front areas of the retina can be obtained. Sketches or photographs of the tumor as seen through the ophthalmoscope are taken during the procedure.

An ultrasound evaluation is used to confirm the presence of the tumor and to evaluate its size. **Computed tomography** (CT, or CAT, scan) is used to determine whether the tumor has spread outside of the eye and to the brain. Sometimes **magnetic resonance imaging** (MRI) is also used to look at the eyes, eye sockets, and the brain to see if the cancer has spread.

In most cases the cancer has not spread beyond the eye, and other evaluations are unnecessary. If the cancer appears to have spread beyond the eye, then other assessments such as a blood test, spinal tap (**lumbar puncture**), and/or **bone marrow biopsy** may be recommended. During a spinal tap, a needle is inserted between the vertebrae of the spinal column and a small sample of the fluid surrounding the spinal cord is obtained. In a bone marrow **biopsy**, a small amount of tissue (bone marrow) is taken from inside the hip or breast bone for examination.

Genetic testing

Establishing whether someone is affected with an inherited or non-inherited form of retinoblastoma can help to ascertain whether other family members such as siblings, cousins, and offspring are at increased risk for developing retinoblastoma. It can also sometimes help guide treatment choices, since patients with an inherited form of retinoblastoma may be at increased risk for developing recurrent tumors or other types of cancers, particularly when treated with radiation. It is helpful for the families of a child diagnosed with retinoblastoma to meet with a genetic specialist such as a genetic counselor and/or geneticist. These specialists can help to ascertain the chances that the retinoblastoma is inherited and facilitate **genetic testing** if desired.

If a patient with unilateral or bilateral retinoblastoma has a relative or relatives with retinoblastoma, it can be assumed that they have an inherited form of retinoblastoma. However, it cannot be assumed that a patient without a family history of the disease has a sporadic form.

Even when there is no family history, most cases of bilateral and trilateral retinoblastoma are inherited, as are most cases of unilateral, multifocal retinoblastoma. However, only 15% of unilateral, unifocal retinoblastoma cases are inherited.

The only way to establish whether someone has an inherited form of retinoblastoma is to see if the retinoblastoma gene is changed or deleted in the blood cells obtained from a blood sample. Approximately 5% to 8% of individuals with retinoblastoma possess a chromosomal abnormality involving the RB1 gene that can be detected by looking at their chromosomes under the microscope. The chromosomes can be seen by obtaining a blood sample. If this type of chromosomal abnormality is detected in a child, then analysis of the parents' chromosomes should be performed. If one of the parents possesses a chromosomal abnormality, then they are at higher risk for having other offspring with retinoblastoma. Chromosome testing would be recommended for the blood relatives of the parent with the abnormality.

Usually, however, a chromosomal abnormality is not detected in a child with retinoblastoma. In this case, specialized DNA tests that look for small RB1 gene changes need to be performed on the blood cells. DNA testing can be difficult, time consuming, and expensive, since there are many possible RB1 gene changes that can cause the gene to become nonfunctional.

If a sample of tumor is available, then it is recommended that DNA testing be performed on the tumor cells prior to DNA testing of the blood cells. This testing can usually identify the gene changes/deletions in the RB1 genes that caused the tumor to develop. In some cases, RB1 gene changes/deletions are not found in the tumor cells (as of 2001, approximately 20% of RB1 gene changes or deletions are not detectable). In these cases, DNA testing of the blood cells will not be able to ascertain whether someone is affected with an inherited or non-inherited form of retinoblastoma.

If the changes in both RB1 genes are detected in the tumor cell, then these same changes can be looked for in the blood cells. If an RB1 gene is deleted or changed in all of the blood cells tested, the patient can be assumed to have been born with a changed/deleted RB1 gene in all of their cells. This person has a 50% chance of passing the RB1 gene change/deletion on to his or her children. Most of the time, this change/deletion has been inherited from a parent. Occasionally the gene change/deletion occurred spontaneously in the original cell that was formed when the egg and sperm came together at conception (de novo).

If an RB1 gene change/deletion is found in all of the blood cells tested, both parents should undergo blood testing to check for the same RB1 gene change/deletion. If the RB1 gene change/deletion is identified in one of the parents, it can be assumed that the retinoblastoma was inherited and that siblings have a 50% chance of inheriting the altered gene. More distant blood relatives of the parent with the identified RB1 gene change/deletion may also be at risk for developing retinoblastoma. Siblings and other relatives could undergo DNA testing to see if they have inherited the RB1 gene change/deletion.

If the RB1 gene change/deletion is not identified in either parent, then the results can be more difficult to interpret. In this case, there is a 90-94% chance that the retinoblastoma was not inherited.

In some cases, a person with retinoblastoma will have an RB1 gene change/deletion detected in some of their blood cells and not others. It can be assumed that this person did not inherit the retinoblastoma from either parent. Siblings and other relatives would therefore not be at increased risk for developing retinoblastoma. Offspring would be at increased risk since some of the egg or sperm cells could have the changed/deleted RB1 gene. The risks to offspring would probably be less than 50%.

In families where there are multiple family members affected with retinoblastoma, blood samples from multiple family members are often analyzed and compared through DNA testing. Ninety-five percent of the time, this type of analysis is able to detect patterns in the DNA that are associated with a changed RB1 gene in that particular family. When a pattern is detected, at-risk relatives can be tested to establish whether they have inherited an RB1 gene change/deletion.

PRENATAL TESTING. If chromosome or DNA testing identifies an RB1 gene/deletion in someone's blood cells, then prenatal testing can be performed on this person's offspring. An amniocentesis or chorionic villus sampling can be used to obtain fetal cells which can be analyzed for the RB1 gene change/deletion or chromosomal abnormality.

Treatment team

If possible, a person with retinoblastoma should be referred to a medical center with a team of cancer specialists. It is important that this team include specialists such as a primary care pediatrician, an ophthalmologist with extensive experience in treating retinoblastoma, pediatric surgeons, radiation oncologists, pediatric medical oncologists, rehabilitation specialists, pediatric nurse specialists, genetic specialists, and social workers.

Clinical staging, treatments, and prognosis

A number of different classification (staging) systems are used to establish the severity of retinoblastoma and aid in choosing an appropriate treatment plan. The most widely used staging system is the Reese-Ellsworth system. This system is used to classify intraocular tumors and predict which tumors are favorable enough that sight can be maintained. The Reese-Ellsworth classification system is divided into:

- Group I (very favorable for maintenance of sight): small solitary or multiple tumors, less than 6.4 mm in size (1 inch = 25.4 mm), located at or below the equator of the eye
- Group II (favorable for maintenance of sight): solitary or multiple tumors, 6.4mm-16mm in size, located at or behind the equator of the eye
- Group III (possible for maintenance of sight): any tumor located in front of the equator of the eye, or a solitary tumor larger than 16 mm in size and located behind the equator of the eye
- Group IV (unfavorable for maintenance of sight): multiple tumors, some larger than 16 mm in size, or any tumor extending in front of the outer rim of the retina (ora serrata)
- Group V (very unfavorable for maintenance of sight): large tumors involving more than half of the retina, or vitreous seeding, in which small pieces of tumor are broken off and floating around the inside of the eye

When choosing a treatment plan, the first important criteria to ascertain is whether the cancer is localized within the eye (intraocular) or has spread to other parts of the body (extraocular). An intraocular retinoblastoma may only involve the retina or could involve other parts of the eye. An extraocular retinoblastoma could involve only the tissues around the eye or could result from the spread of cancer to the brain or other parts of the body.

It is also important to establish whether the cancer is unilateral (one eye) or bilateral (both eyes), multifocal or unifocal. In order for the tumors to be considered multifocal, they must have arisen independently and not as the result of the spread of cancer cells. It is also important to check for trilateral retinoblastoma.

Treatments

The treatment chosen depends on the size and number of tumors, whether the cancer is unilateral or bilateral, and whether the cancer has spread to other parts of the body. The goal of treatment is to cure the cancer and prevent as much loss of vision as possible. Since the late 1990s, doctors treating patients with retinoblastoma have tended to avoid enucleation and external beam **radiation therapy** whenever possible, in favor of **chemotherapy** to reduce the tumor in addition to focal therapies. Improved methods of chemoreduction have led to increasing success in saving patients' eyes, often with some visual function.

TREATMENT OF INTRAOCULAR TUMORS. Surgical removal of the affected eye (enucleation) is used when the tumor(s) are so large and extensive that preservation of sight is not possible. This surgery is performed under general anesthetic and usually takes less than an hour. Most children who have undergone this surgery can leave the hospital on the same day. A temporary ball is placed in the eye socket after the surgery. Approximately three weeks after the operation, a plastic artificial eye (prosthesis) that looks like the normal eye is inserted into the eye socket.

Radiation therapy is often used for treatment of large tumors when preservation of sight is possible. External beam radiation therapy involves focusing a beam of radiation on the eye. If the tumor has not spread extensively, the radiation beam can be focused on the cancerous retinal cells. If the cancer is extensive, radiation treatment of the entire eye may be necessary. External beam radiation is performed on an outpatient basis and usually occurs over a period of three to four weeks. Some children may need sedatives prior to the treatment. This type of therapy can result in a temporary loss of a patch of hair on the back of the head and a small area of "sun-burned" skin. Long-term side effects of radiation treatment can include cataracts, vision problems, bleeding from the retina, and decreased growth of the bones on the side of the head. People with an inherited form of retinoblastoma have an increased risk of developing other cancers as a result of this therapy. Some consideration should therefore be given to alternative treatment therapies for those with an inherited form of retinoblastoma.

Photocoagulation therapy is often used in conjunction with radiation therapy but may be used alone to treat small tumors that are located on the back of the eye. Photocoagulation involves using a laser to destroy the cancer cells. This type of treatment is done under local or general anesthesia and is usually not associated with post-procedural pain.

Thermotherapy is also often used in conjunction with radiation therapy or drug therapy (chemotherapy). Thermotherapy involves the use of heat to help shrink tumor cells. The heat is either used on the whole eye or localized to the tumor area. It is done under local or general anesthesia and is usually not painful.

Cryotherapy is a treatment often used in conjunction with radiation therapy but can also be used alone on small tumors located on the front part of the retina. Cryotherapy involves the use of intense cold to destroy cancer cells and can result in harmless, temporary swelling of the external eye and eyelids that can last for up to five days. Eye drops or ointment are sometimes provided to reduce the swelling.

Brachytherapy involves the application of radioactive material to the outer surface of the eye at the base of the tumor. It is generally used for tumors of medium size. A patient undergoing this type of procedure is usually hospitalized for three to seven days. During that time, he or she undergoes one surgery to attach the radioactive material and one surgery to remove it. Eye drops are often administered for three to four weeks following the operation to prevent inflammation and **infection**. The long-term side effects of this treatment can include cataracts and damage to the retina, which can lead to impaired vision.

Intravenous treatment with one or more drugs (chemotherapy) is often used for treatment of both large and small tumors. Chemotherapy is sometimes used to shrink tumors prior to other treatments such as radiation therapy or brachytherapy. Occasionally, it is also used alone to treat very small tumors.

TREATMENT OF INTRAOCULAR AND UNILATERAL RETINOBLASTOMA. Often, by the time that unilateral retinoblastoma is diagnosed, the tumor is so large that useful vision cannot be preserved. In these cases removal of the eye (enucleation) is the treatment of choice. Other therapies are unnecessary if enucleation is used to treat intraocular unilateral retinoblastoma. If the tumor is small enough, other therapies such as external beam radiation therapy, photocoagulation, cryotherapy, thermotherapy, chemotherapy, and brachytherapy may be considered.

TREATMENT OF INTRAOCULAR AND BILATERAL RETINOBLASTOMA. If vision can be preserved in both eyes, radiation therapy of both eyes may be recommended. Smaller, more localized tumors can sometimes be treated by local therapies such as cryotherapy, photocoagulation therapy, thermotherapy, or brachytherapy. Some centers may use chemotherapy in place of radiation therapy when the tumors are too large to be treated by local therapies or are found over the optic nerve of the eye. Many centers are moving away from radiation treatment and toward chemotherapy because it is less likely to induce future tumors. Enucleation is performed on the more severely affected eye if sight cannot be preserved in both.

EXTRAOCULAR RETINOBLASTOMA. There is no proven effective therapy for the treatment of extraocular retinoblastomas. Commonly, radiation treatment of the eyes and chemotherapy is provided.

Prognosis

Individuals with intraocular retinoblastoma who do not have trilateral retinoblastoma usually have a good survival rate with a 90% chance of disease-free survival for five years. Those with extraocular retinoblastoma have less than a 10% chance of disease-free survival for the same amount of time. Trilateral retinoblastoma generally has a very poor prognosis. Patients with trilateral retinoblastoma who receive treatment have an average survival rate of approximately eight months, while those who remain untreated have an average survival rate of approximately one month. Patients with trilateral retinoblastoma who are asymptomatic at the time of diagnosis may have a better prognosis than those who experience symptoms.

Patients with an inherited form of unilateral retinoblastoma have a 70% chance of developing retinoblastoma in the other eye. Retinoblastoma recurs in the other eye in approximately 5% of people with a non-inherited form of retinoblastoma, so it is advisable for even these patients to be closely monitored. People with an inherited form of retinoblastoma who have not undergone radiation treatment have approximately a 26% chance of developing cancer in another part of the body within 50 years of the initial diagnosis. Those with an inherited form who have undergone radiation treatment have a 58% chance of developing a secondary cancer by 50 years after the initial diagnosis. Most of the secondary cancers are skin cancers, bone tumors (osteosarcomas), and soft-tissue sarcomas. Soft-tissue sarcomas are malignant tumors of the muscle, nerves, joints, blood vessels, deep skin tissues, or fat. The prognosis for retinoblastoma patients who develop secondary cancers, however, is very poor as of the early 2000s.

Survivors of retinoblastoma are likely to have visual field defects after their cancer treatment is completed, most commonly scotomas, which are areas of lost or depressed vision within an area of normal vision. The size and type of these visual defects are determined by the size and type of the original tumor and the form of therapy used to treat it.

Alternative and complementary therapies

There are no alternative or complementary therapies specific to the treatment of retinoblastoma. Since most people diagnosed with retinoblastoma are small children, most drug-based alternative therapies designed to treat general cancer would not be recommended. Many specialists would, however, stress the importance of establishing a well-balanced diet, including certain fruits, vegetables, and vitamin supplements, to ensure that the body is strengthened in its fight against cancer. Some advocate the use of visualization strategies, in which patients would visualize the immune cells of their body attacking and destroying the cancer cells.

The most common side effects of chemotherapy include **nausea**, **vomiting**, and temporary hair loss (**alopecia**). This treatment can result in a temporary decrease in blood cells, including white blood cells, red blood cells, and platelets.

Coping with cancer treatment

Both retinoblastoma itself and treatments such as enucleation and radiation can result in vision impairment and cause some mild disfigurement around the eye. Children with resulting vision impairment can often be helped by centers and programs for the visually impaired. It is recommended that children who have undergone enucleation should wear protective glasses to protect the remaining eye. Special glasses may be recommended for those who are involved in contact sports. **Reconstructive surgery** following enucleation or radiation treatment may be recommended to improve the cosmetic appearance of the area around the eye. Eye drops and ointments may also be used to counteract side effects such as swelling and inflammation that can be associated with cancer treatments such as brachytherapy and cryotherapy.

If chemotherapy is used, the child may experience side effects such as nausea, vomiting, and hair loss. The patient may also experience a decreased level of: white blood cells, which can cause an increased susceptibility to infection; red blood cells, which can result in **fatigue** or shortness of breath; and platelets, which can cause an increased risk of bruising or prolonged bleeding after an injury. These symptoms are generally temporary and can often be treated. There are a number of drugs on the market that can decrease or even eliminate **nausea and vomiting**. Early recognition of infections and treatments with **antibiotics** are very important. All high fevers should be reported to a physician immediately and may require hospitalization. Platelet transfusions are sometimes necessary for the replacement of platelets. Loss of hair can be very traumatic to an older child, but the use of a wig, until the hair grows back, may be helpful.

Clinical trials

As of 2004, the National Cancer Institute is conducting four **clinical trials** for the treatment of retinoblastoma and one intensive study of individuals and families at high risk for cancer. The treatment trials include two forms of combination chemotherapy; the use of **arsenic trioxide**; and combination chemotherapy followed by **bone marrow transplantation**.

Prevention

Although retinoblastoma cannot be prevented, appropriate screening and surveillance should be applied to all at-risk individuals to ensure that the tumor(s) are diagnosed at an early stage. The earlier the diagnosis, the more likely that an eye can be salvaged and vision maintained.

Screening of people diagnosed with retinoblastoma

Children who have been diagnosed with retinoblastoma should receive periodic dilated retinal examinations until the age of five. Young children will need to undergo these evaluations under anesthetic. After five years of age, periodic eye examinations are recommended. It may be advisable for patients with bilateral retinoblastoma or an inherited form of retinoblastoma to undergo periodic screening for the **brain tumors** found in trilateral retinoblastoma. There are no specific screening protocols designed to detect non-ocular tumors. All lumps and complaints of **bone pain**, however, should be thoroughly evaluated.

Screening of relatives

When a child is diagnosed with retinoblastoma, it is recommended that parents and siblings receive a dilated retinal examination by an ophthalmologist who is experienced in the diagnosis and treatment of the disease. It is also recommended that siblings continue to undergo periodic retinal examinations under anesthetic until they are three years of age. From three to seven years of age, periodic eye examinations are recommended. The retinal examinations can be avoided if DNA testing indicates that the patient has a non-inherited form of retinoblastoma or if the sibling has not inherited the RB1 gene change/deletion. Any relatives who are found through DNA testing to have inherited an RB1 gene change/deletion should undergo the same surveillance procedures as siblings.

The children of someone diagnosed with retinoblastoma should also undergo periodic retinal examinations under anesthetic. Retinal surveillance should be performed unless DNA testing proves that their child does not possess the RB1 gene change/deletion. If desired, prenatal detection of tumors using ultrasound may also be performed. During the ultrasound procedure, a hand-held instrument is placed on the maternal abdomen or inserted vaginally. The ultrasound produces sound waves that are reflected back from the body structures of the fetus, producing a picture that can be seen on a video screen. If a tumor is detected through this evaluation, the affected baby may be delivered a couple of weeks earlier. This can allow for earlier intervention and treatment.

Special concerns

Since retinoblastoma most often affects children, parents have the difficult task of helping the doctor explain the condition and prognosis to their child. It is very important for parents to be open and honest about the disease, and some have found it helpful to read their child a story about another child who has faced the same condition.

Dealing with a diagnosis of retinoblastoma can be very stressful and frightening for children. Talking to other children with the same diagnosis can be helpful. Talking to a counselor or using relaxation therapies may also help a child deal with the emotions and fear associated with retinoblastoma.

Children with retinoblastoma may experience difficulties with their **self image** because of the temporary loss of hair or the loss of one or both eyes. It is important to remind these children of their many positive qualities. It is also important to teach children strategies for coping with others who may tease them or ask them questions about their condition.

The diagnosis of retinoblastoma can greatly impact the whole family. For some, therapy may be necessary to ensure that the family can cope with the stresses associated with this diagnosis. Talking with other families who have children with retinoblastoma can also be of help.

In general, most children and families cope very well with the diagnosis of retinoblastoma. Since the prognosis is usually very good, it is important that parents strive to maintain a positive outlook.

Resources

BOOKS

Beers, Mark H., MD, and Robert Berkow, MD, editors. "Retinoblastoma." Section 19, Chapter 266 In*The Merck Manual of Diagnosis and Therapy*. Whitehouse Station, NJ: Merck Research Laboratories, 2002.

PERIODICALS

Abramson, D. H., M. R. Melson, and C. Servodidio. "Visual Fields in Retinoblastoma Survivors." *Archives of Ophthalmology* 122 (September 2004): 1324–1330.

Aerts, I., H. Pacquement, F. Doz, et al. "Outcome of Second Malignancies after Retinoblastoma: A Retrospective Analysis of 25 Patients Treated at the Institut Curie." *European Journal of Cancer* 40 (July 2004): 1522–1529.

Lohmann, D. R., and B. L. Gallie. "Retinoblastoma: Revisiting the Model Prototype of Inherited Cancer." *American Journal of Medical Genetics, Part C: Seminars in Medical Genetics* 129 (August 15, 2004): 23–28.

Provenzale, J. M., S. Gururangan, and G. Klintworth. "Trilateral Retinoblastoma: Clinical and Radiologic Progression." *AJR: American Journal of Roentgenology* 183 (August 2004): 505–511.

Shields, C. L., A. Mashayeki, J. Cater, et al. "Chemoreduction for Retinoblastoma. Analysis of Tumor Control and Risks for Recurrence in 457 Tumors." *American Journal of Ophthalmology* 138 (September 2004): 329–337.

Shields, C. L., and J. A. Shields. "Diagnosis and Management of Retinoblastoma." *Cancer Control* 11 (September-October 2004): 317–327.

OTHER

Abramson, David, and Camille Servodidio. "A Parent's Guide to Understanding Retinoblastoma.". [cited June 20, 2001]. http://www.retinoblastoma.com/guide/guide.html.

Kid's Eye Cancer. [cited June 20, 2001]. http://www.kidseyecancer.org.

Lohmann, Dietmar, N. Bornfeld, B. Horsthemke, and E. Passarge. "Retinoblastoma." *Gene Clinics*. July 17, 2000. [cited June 20, 2001]. http://www.geneclinics.org/profiles/retinoblastoma.

McCusick, Victor. "Retinoblastoma; RB1." *Online Mendelian Inheritance in Man*. February 14, 2001. [cited June 20, 2001]. http://www.ncbi.nlm.nih.gov/Omim.

"Retinoblastoma" *CancerNet*. <http://cancernet.nci.nih.gov/Cancer_Types/Retinoblastoma.shtml>.

Solutions by Sequence. [cited June 20, 2001]. http://www.solutionsbysequence.com.

ORGANIZATIONS

American Academy of Ophthalmology (AAO). P. O. Box 7424, San Francisco, CA 94120-7424. (415) 561-8500. Fax: (415) 561-8533. http://www.aao.org.

Institute for Families with Blind Children. PO Box 54700, Mail Stop 111, Los Angeles, CA 90054-0700. (213) 669-4649.

National Retinoblastoma Parents Group. PO Box 317, Watertown, MA 02471 (800) 562-6265. Fax: (617) 972-7444. napvi@perkins.pvt.k12.ma.us.

Retinoblastoma International. 4650 Sunset Blvd., Mail Stop #88, Los Angeles, CA 90027. (323) 669-2299. info@retinoblastoma.net. http://www.retinoblastoma.net/rbi/index_rbi.htm.

The Retinoblastoma Society. Saint Bartholomew's Hospital, London, UK EC1A 7BE. Phone: 020 7600 3309 Fax: 020 7600 8579. <http://ds.dial.pipex.com/rbinfo>.

Lisa Andres, M.S., C.G.C.
Rebecca J. Frey, PhD

Rhabdomyosarcoma

Definition

Rhabdomyosarcoma is a childhood **cancer**. It begins in cells that will become skeletal muscle cells. Skeletal muscle is attached to bones and is different from the smooth muscle that lines the intestinal tract (esophagus, stomach, small and large intestines). With rhabdomyosarcoma, these muscle cells grow uncontrollably and form masses or lumps called tumors. They can start almost anywhere in the body where there is skeletal muscle.

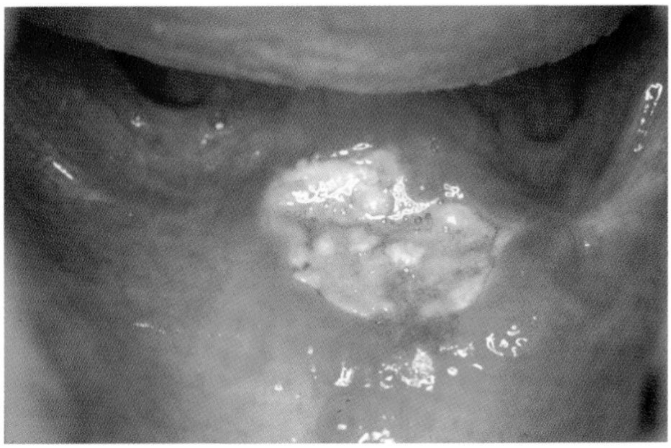

Rhabdomyosarcoma, a malignant tumor affecting the inside of the mouth. *((c) Eamonn McNulty, SPL/Photo Researchers. Reproduced by permission.)*

Description

Rhabdomyosarcomas can start in any organ that contains skeletal muscle cells, but most commonly tumors are found in the head and neck and in the prostate, bladder, and vagina. From 5–8% of all cancers diagnosed in children are rhabdomyosarcomas.

Demographics

Rhabdomyosarcoma occurs most frequently in children ages 2 to 6 and 15 to 19 years old. More males than females develop rhabdomyosarcomas. Among younger children, the tumor is usually in the head and neck and may involve the area surrounding the eye. Less often, young children develop rhabdomyosarcomas of the genitourinary tract (bladder, prostate, vagina).

In the older age group, the most likely site is the male genitourinary tract, especially the testes and surrounding area. Other body parts where rhabdomyosarcoma may begin are on the arms, legs, trunk, or deep inside the abdomen (retroperitoneum).

Some cases of rhabdomyosarcoma run in families and are linked to genetic syndromes. Immediate family members of children with rhabdomyosarcoma are at increased risk of developing certain cancers that are not rhabdomyosarcomas, such as breast and **brain tumors**.

KEY TERMS

Biopsy—The surgical removal and microscopic examination of living tissue for diagnostic purposes.

Chemotherapy—Treatment of cancer with synthetic drugs that destroy the tumor either by inhibiting the growth of cancerous cells or by killing them.

Metastasize—The spread of cancer cells from a primary site to distant parts of the body.

Oncologist—A doctor who specializes in cancer medicine.

Pathologist—A doctor who specializes in the diagnosis of disease by studying cells and tissues under a microscope.

Radiation therapy—Treatment using high energy radiation from X-ray machines, cobalt, radium, or other sources.

Stage—A term used to describe the size and extent of spread of cancer.

Causes and symptoms

The causes of rhabdomyosarcoma are not known. Certain inherited conditions that run in families increase the risk of developing this cancer. Rhabdomyosarcoma has been linked to medical conditions such as fetal alcohol syndrome, neurofibromatosis, Gorlin's syndrome, and **Li-Fraumeni syndrome**.

The symptoms of rhabdomyosarcoma depend on the site of the tumor and whether it has spread. When rhabdomyosarcoma begins in the head, it may involve the area surrounding the eye, the nasal passages or the ear and throat. Tumors in these areas may cause swelling, especially around the eye; blocked nasal passages or sinuses; ear pain and bleeding; and difficulties swallowing. Rhabdomyosarcomas in the head and neck may also put pressure on the brain or nerves.

When rhabdomyosarcoma affects an arm, leg or other body part, the swelling may be mistaken for a bruise or other injury. When the genitals or urinary tract are involved, there may be symptoms such as recurring urinary tract infections, blood in the urine, **incontinence**, or blockage of the urinary tract or rectum.

Rhabdomyosarcoma affecting the testes may cause swelling of the scrotum. When the uterus or vagina is affected, there may be a mass or small tumor pushing into the vaginal canal.

QUESTIONS TO ASK THE DOCTOR

- What stage is the rhabdomyosarcoma?
- What are the recommended treatments?
- What are the side effects of the recommended treatment?
- Is treatment expected to cure the disease or only to prolong life?

Diagnosis

Some patients who have rhabdomyosarcomas go to the doctor because they have discovered a lump or mass or swelling on a body part. Others have symptoms related to the part of the body that is affected by the tumor. The patient's doctor will take a detailed medical history to find out about the symptoms. The history is followed by a complete physical examination with special attention to the suspicious symptom or body part.

Depending on the location of the tumor (mass or lump), the doctor will order **imaging studies** such as x ray, ultrasound, **computed tomography** (CT) scans and **magnetic resonance imaging** (MRI) to help determine the size, shape and exact location of the tumor. The doctor may also order bone scans to determine if the tumor has spread to bones. Blood tests will be done and an examination of the bone marrow also may be performed.

A **biopsy** of the tumor is necessary to make the diagnosis of rhabdomyosarcoma. During a biopsy, some tissue from the tumor is removed. The tissue sample is examined by a pathologist, a doctor who specializes in the study of diseased tissue.

Types of biopsy

The type of biopsy done depends on the location of the tumor. For some small tumors, such as those on the arm or leg, the doctor may perform an excisional biopsy, removing the entire tumor and a margin of surrounding normal tissue. Most often, the doctor will perform an incisional biopsy, a procedure that involves cutting out only a piece of the tumor. This biopsy provides a core of tissue from the tumor that is used to determine its type and grade.

Treatment team

Patients with rhabdomyosarcoma are usually cared for by a multidisciplinary team of health professionals.

The patient's pediatrician, or primary care doctor may refer the patient to other physician specialists, such as surgeons and oncologists (doctors who specialize in cancer medicine). Radiologic technicians perform x ray, CT and MRI scans, and nurses and laboratory technicians may obtain samples of blood, urine, and other laboratory tests.

Before and after any surgical procedures, specially trained nurses may explain the procedures and help to prepare patients and families. Depending on the tumor location and treatment plan, patients may also benefit from rehabilitation therapy with physical therapists and nutritional counseling from dieticians.

Clinical staging, treatments, and prognosis

Staging

The purpose of staging a tumor is to determine how far it has advanced. This is important because treatment varies depending on the stage. Stage is determined by the size of the tumor, whether the tumor has spread to nearby lymph nodes, and whether the tumor has spread elsewhere in the body.

Tumors are staged using numbers to designate Stages I through IV. The higher the number, the more the tumor has advanced. Stage I rhabdomyosarcomas have not extended beyond the site where they began; they are limited to a single muscle or organ. Stage II tumors show signs of spread beyond the muscle or organ where they began. Stage III rhabdomyosarcomas are tumors that could not be removed in their entirety by surgery. As a result, some tumor remains at the site where it began. Stage IV rhabdomyosarcomas have involved either lymph nodes or have spread to distant parts of the body.

Treatment

Treatment for rhabdomyosarcoma varies depending on the location of the tumor, its size and grade, and the extent of its spread. By the time most cases of rhabdomyosarcoma are diagnosed, there has already been some spread of the disease. For these patients, the goals of treatment are to remove or control the tumor and combat the spread of the cancer.

Generally, when completely removing the tumor will not sharply reduce function, rhabdomyosarcoma tumors are surgically removed. The site, size, and extent of the tumor determine the type of surgery performed. The goal of removing as much tumor as possible is to reduce the amount of radiation needed after surgery. The part of the body where the tumor was removed is treated with radiation to destroy remaining tumor cells. Many patients also receive **chemotherapy**.

When the disease has spread throughout the body, there may be no benefit from surgical removal of the tumor. These cases, usually patients with Group IV tumors, are treated with chemotherapy.

Side effects

The surgical treatment of rhabdomyosarcoma carries risks related to the surgical site, such as loss of function resulting from head and neck surgeries. Head and neck surgeries may also result in deformities that may be cosmetically unsatisfactory. There are also the medical risks associated with any surgical procedure, such as reactions to general anesthesia or **infection** after surgery.

The side effects of **radiation therapy** depend on the site being radiated. Radiation therapy can produce side effects such as **fatigue**, skin rashes, **nausea**, **diarrhea**, and secondary cancers. Most of the side effects lessen or disappear completely after the radiation therapy has been completed.

The side effects of chemotherapy vary depending on the medication, or combination of **anticancer drugs**, used. Nausea, **vomiting**, **anemia**, lower resistance to infection, and hair loss are common side effects. Medication may be given to reduce the unpleasant side effects of chemotherapy.

Alternative and complementary therapies

Many patients explore alternative and complementary therapies to help to reduce the stress associated with illness, improve immune function and feel better. While there is no evidence that these therapies specifically combat disease, activities such as biofeedback, relaxation, therapeutic touch, massage therapy and guided imagery have been reported to enhance well-being.

Prognosis

The outlook for patients with rhabdomyosarcoma varies. It depends on the site of the tumor, how the cancer cells look under the microscope, and extent of spread. For example, patients with tumors affecting the area around the eye and the bladder are more likely to do well than patients with tumors that begin deep within the chest or abdomen.

Rhabdomyosarcoma may spread to areas near the tumor and it can spread to nearby lymph glands. To spread to distant parts of the body, the cells travel in the blood or through the lymph glands. The most common sites for **metastasis** (spread) are the lymph glands near the tumor, the lung, liver, bone marrow, and brain. In general, tumors that have spread widely throughout the body are not associated with favorable survival rates.

Patients with Stage I tumors that are completely removed surgically have excellent prognoses; eight-year survival is nearly 75%. Sixty five percent of patients with Stage II tumors are disease free after 8 years. Stage I and II rhabdomyosarcomas account for about 40% of all cases.

About 40% of patients with Stage III and 15% of those with Stage IV rhabdomyosarcomas are disease free after 8 years. Patients with tumors that do not respond to treatment and those who suffer recurrences have poor outlooks for long-term survival.

Coping with cancer treatment

Toddlers, children, and teens undergoing cancer treatment have special needs. The diagnosis of a life-threatening illness, surgery, and radiation or chemotherapy may cause fear, anxiety, **depression**, and loss of self-esteem. Toddlers may be especially fearful when they are separated from their parents for medical tests and hospital stays. Disruption of their normal routines and discomfort from diagnostic tests and treatment may also cause anxiety. Older children face additional social problems including making up missed school work, explaining the illness and treatment to friends, and coping with physical limitations or disability.

Teens with serious illnesses and disabilities face special conflicts and challenges. One conflict is between the teen's growing desire for independence and the reality of dependence on others for the activities of daily living. It is important for teens to be fully informed about their disease and treatment plan and involved in treatment decision making. Many teens benefit from continuing contact with friends, classmates, teachers, and family during hospital stays and recovery at home.

Depression, emotional distress, and anxiety associated with the disease and its treatment may respond to counseling from a mental health professional. Play therapy often helps toddlers and young children to reveal and express their feelings about illness and treatment. Many cancer patients and their families find participation in mutual aid and group support programs help to relieve feelings of isolation and loneliness. By sharing problems with others who have lived through similar difficulties patients and families can exchange ideas and coping strategies.

Clinical trials

About 102 clinical studies were underway during 2009. For example, in one clinical trial at John Hopkins Oncology Center, patients with recurring or widespread rhabdomyosarcoma were being treated with chemotherapy to stop tumor cells from dividing and simultaneously being given stem cells (**bone marrow transplantation**) to replace the immune cells killed by chemotherapy.

Other **clinical trials** compare different combinations of chemotherapy drugs to find out which combination is most effective. For example, in one study, patients with previously untreated rhabdomyosarcoma were randomly assigned to two different combinations of chemotherapy drugs. Along with radiation therapy, patients in one group received three drugs, **vincristine**, **dactinomycin**, and **cyclophosphamide** once a week. Patients in the other group were given vincristine, cyclophosphamide, and **topotecan**, instead of dactinomycin.

Other types of clinical research study individuals and families at high risk of cancer to help identify cancer genes. To learn more about clinical trials visit the National Cancer Institute (NCI) CancerNet web site at <http://cancernet.nci.nih.gov/> or the Pediatric Oncology Branch of the National Cancer Institute web site at http://www.dcs.nci.nih.gov/pedonc.

Prevention

Since the causes of rhabdomyosarcoma are not known, there are no recommendations about how to prevent its development. Among families with an inherited tendency to develop soft tissue sarcomas, careful monitoring may help to ensure early diagnosis and treatment of the disease.

Special concerns

Rhabdomyosarcoma, like other cancer diagnoses, may produce a range of emotional reactions in patients and families. Education, counseling, and participation in group support programs can help to reduce feelings of guilt, fear, anxiety, and hopelessness. For many parents suffering from spiritual distress, visits with clergy members and participation in organized prayer may offer comfort.

Resources

BOOKS

Pelletier, Kenneth R. *The Best of Alternative Medicine*. New York: Simon & Schuster, 2000.

PERIODICALS

Arndt, Carola A. R., and William M. Crist. "Medical Progress: Common Musculoskeletal Tumors of Childhood and Adolescence." *New England Journal of Medicine* 341, no. 5 (July 29, 1999): 342–352.

ORGANIZATIONS

American Cancer Society. 1599 Clifton Road, N.E., Atlanta, GA 30329. (800)227–2345.

Cancer Research Institute. 681 Fifth Avenue, New York, NY 10022. (800)992–2623.

National Cancer Institute Clinical Cancer Trials. <http://cancertrials.nci.nih.gov.>.

National Cancer Institute (National Institutes of Health). 9000 Rockville Pike, Bethesda, MD 20892. (800)422–6237.

The Pediatric Oncology Branch of the National Cancer Institute. (877) 624–4878 or (301)496–4256. http://www.dcs.nci.nih.gov/pedonc/Index.html.

Barbara Wexler, M.P.H.

Richter's syndrome

Definition

Richter's syndrome is a rare and aggressive type of acute adult leukemia that results from a transformation of **chronic lymphocytic leukemia** into diffuse large cell **lymphoma**.

Description

Leukemia is a group of cancers of the white blood cells. In adults, white blood cells are made in the bone marrow of the flat bones (skull, shoulder blades, ribs, hip bones). There are three main types of white blood cells: granulocytes, monocytes, and lymphocytes. Richter's syndrome concerns only the lymphocytes.

Lymphocytic leukemia develops from lymphocytes in the bone marrow. Unlike many other cancers in which a tumor starts growing in one particular location, lymphocytic leukemia is a disease of blood cells that travel throughout the body. In chronic (long-term) lymphocytic leukemia (CLL), lymphocytes do not follow a normal life cycle, and eventually, too many will exist in the blood. They are abnormal and do not fight infections well.

In a small percentage of people, CLL, even when it is treated, transforms into a new kind of aggressive blood **cancer** called diffuse large cell lymphoma. When this transformation occurs, it is called Richter's syndrome. The disease is named for the American pathologist Maurice Nathaniel Richter, who practiced medicine early in the twentieth century.

KEY TERMS

Lymph nodes—Small, bean-shaped collections of tissue found in lymph vessels. They produce cells and proteins that fight infection and filter lymph. Nodes are sometimes called lymph glands.

Lymph system—Primary defense against infection in the body. The tissues, organs, and channels (similar to veins) that produce, store, and transport lymph and white blood cells to fight infection.

Lymphoma—A cancer of the lymph system.

Demographics

Richter's syndrome is a disease of older adults. It is an extremely rare disease. The American Cancer Society estimates that in 2000, there were 8,100 new cases of chronic lymphocytic leukemia, and that 98% of these were in adults. Of these 8,100 new cases, only a handful will develop into Richter's syndrome. In general, people who are more likely to get CLL are those who smoke, have been exposed to high doses of radiation, or who have had long-term exposure to herbicides and pesticides. People who have close relatives (parent, siblings or children) with CLL are also more likely to develop the disease. However, none of these risk factors predict whether CLL will develop into Richter's syndrome.

Causes and symptoms

Scientists have yet to understand why some people develop Richter's syndrome and others do not. So far, no firm genetic or environmental links have been found.

When the transformation from CLL to Richter's syndrome occurs, a change occurs in the way the lymphocytes look under the microscope. In addition, lymph nodes swell, tumors grow rapidly in the lymph system, and the patient may experience **fever**, **night sweats**, and **weight loss**. The patient's health deteriorates rapidly and severely.

Diagnosis

Diagnosis is made by examining blood cells under microscope and by a **bone marrow biopsy**. This is the same test used to diagnose CLL. A small amount of bone marrow from one of the flat bones is drawn out

QUESTIONS TO ASK THE DOCTOR

- What kind of changes in my body can I expect to see from this cancer?
- What is the treatment plan?
- What are the likely side effects of the treatment plan?
- How long am I likely to survive?
- Since Richter's syndrome is rare, how much experience do you have with this disease?
- Are there hospitals that specialize in the treatment of Richter's syndrome where I might receive treatment unavailable here?

with a needle for laboratory examination. In some cases, lymph nodes are also removed and examined in the laboratory.

Treatment team

Since a person who develops Richter's syndrome is already a cancer patient, a treatment team is already in place. This team usually includes an oncologist (cancer specialist), a hematologist (blood specialist) and possibly a radiation oncologist (specialist in **radiation therapy**), radiation or **chemotherapy** technicians, and nurses with special training in cancer care. With the development of Richter's syndrome, a social worker or counselor may be added to the team.

Clinical staging, treatments, and prognosis

Richter's syndrome is not staged. Chemotherapy is used to treat Richter's syndrome, although treatments are often unsuccessful. In addition, allogenic **bone marrow transplantation** is currently being tried in some patients. This treatment is not common and is not done at many cancer centers. For Richter's syndrome, the median survival rate (the time to which half the patients survive) is less than one year.

Alternative and complementary therapies

Alternative and complementary therapies range from herbal remedies, vitamin supplements, and special diets to spiritual practices, acupuncture, massage, and similar treatments. When these therapies are used in addition to conventional medicine, they are called complementary therapies. When they are used instead of conventional medicine, they are called alternative therapies.

There are no specific alternative therapies directed toward Richter's syndrome. However, good nutrition and activities that reduce stress and promote a positive view of life have no unwanted side effects and may help improve the quality of life.

Unlike traditional pharmaceuticals, complementary and alternative therapies are not evaluated by the United States Food and Drug Administration (FDA) for either safety or effectiveness. Patients should be wary of "miracle cures." In order to avoid any harmful side effects or interference with regular cancer treatment, patients should notify their doctors if they are using any herbal remedies, vitamin supplements, or other unprescribed treatments. Alternative and experimental treatments normally are not covered by insurance.

Coping with cancer treatment

Richter's syndrome is usually fatal within a short time. Coming to grips with this is tremendously stressful for both the patient and family members. In addition, chemotherapy treatments can cause **fatigue**, **nausea**, **vomiting**, and other uncomfortable side effects. Some patients decide to end treatment rather than undergo this discomfort when their chance of recovery is almost non-existent. Others wish to continue full treatment.

This and many other personal decisions are issues to discuss with loved ones. It is often helpful for loved ones to have the support of a therapist, religious leader, or other counselor at this time when emotions are intense and often conflicting. Hospice staff members or hospital social workers or chaplains can direct patients and family members to resources that address their individual needs.

Clinical trials

Many ongoing **clinical trials** related to chronic lymphocytic lymphoma may be appropriate for people with Richter's syndrome. Participation is always voluntary. The selection of clinical trials underway changes frequently. Current information on what clinical trials are available and where they are being held is available by entering the search term "chronic lymphocytic lymphoma" at the following web sites:

- National Cancer Institute: <http://cancertrials.nci.nih.gov> or (800) 4-CANCER
- National Institutes of Health Clinical Trials: <http://clinicaltrials.gov>
- Center Watch: A Clinical Trials Listing: <http://www.centerwatch.com>

Prevention

There is no known way to prevent the transformation of CLL into Richter's syndrome.

Resources

PERIODICALS

Rodriguez, J., et al. "Allogenic Haematopoietic Transplantation for Richter's Syndrome." *British Journal of Haematology*. 110 (April 2000): 897–9.

ORGANIZATIONS

American Cancer Society. National Headquarters, 1599 Clifton Rd. NE, Atlanta, GA 30329. 800(ACS)-2345). http://www.cancer.org.

Cancer Information Service, National Cancer Institute. Building 31, Room 10A19, 9000 Rockville Pike, Bethesda, MD 20892. (800) 4-CANCER. http://www.nci.nih.gov/cancerinfo/index.html.

Leukemia & Lymphoma Society. 1311 Mamaroneck Ave., 3rd floor, White Plains, NY 10605. (800) 955-4572. http://www.leukemia-lymphoma.org.

National Leukemia Research Association, Inc. 585 Stewart Ave., Suite 536, Garden City, NY 11530. (516) 222-1944.

Tish Davidson, A.M.

Rituximab

Definition

Rituximab is a humanized monoclonal antibody that selectively binds to CD20, a protein found on the surface of normal and malignant B cells and is used to reduce the numbers of circulating B cells in patients who have B-cell **non-Hodgkin's lymphoma** (NHL). Rituximab is sold as Rituxan in the United States.

Purpose

Rituximab is a monoclonal antibody used to treat NHL characterized by overgrowth of B cells, the cell involved in about 85% of NHL malignancies. Of all the B-cell cancers more than 90% express the CD20 protein on the cell surface, a requirement for the proper function of rituximab. By binding the CD20 protein on the B cell, the antibody targets it for removal from the circulation. Based on data gathered in the laboratory developers believe that rituximab triggers both cell-mediated and complement-mediated means to kill the B cells, two different methods that the immune system uses to eliminate foreign cells. Binding of the antibody may also trigger apoptosis, or programmed cell death, of the B cells.

KEY TERMS

Antibody—A protective protein made by the immune system in response to an antigen, also called an immunoglobulin.

Apoptosis—Internal system for cell death, also called programmed cell death.

CD20—A protein found on the surface of normal and malignant B cells.

Humanization—Fusing the constant and variable framework region of one or more human immunoglobulins with the binding region of an animal immunoglobulin, done to reduce human reaction against the fusion antibody.

Monoclonal—Genetically engineered antibodies specific for one antigen.

Rituximab has been most effective against low-grade (indolent) or follicular B-cell NHL. Low-grade (slow progression) NHL often responds well to initial treatment, but frequently relapses, making rituximab a welcome addition to the treatment options. Additionally, rituximab has been used for a second course of treatments after relapse with some success. As most patients with NHL are in stage III or IV by the time of diagnosis and treatment, experience with rituximab treatment are primarily with those stages of the disease.

As of spring 2001 **clinical trials** were being held testing the ability of this drug to work against several other types of cancers, including newly diagnosed NHL, intermediate- or high-grade (aggressive) NHL, AIDS-associated NHL, **Waldenström's macroglobulinemia**, **Hodgkin's disease**, **hairy cell leukemia** (HCL), **chronic lymphocytic leukemia** (CLL), **multiple myeloma**, **mantle cell lymphoma**, and large cell **lymphoma**.

Description

Rituximab is produced in the laboratory using genetically engineered single clones of B cells. Like all antibodies it is a Y-shaped molecule that can bind to one particular substance, the antigen for that monoclonal antibody. For rituximab that antigen is CD20, a protein found on the surface of B cells. Rituximab is a humanized antibody, meaning that the regions that bind CD20, located on the tips of the Y branches, are derived from mouse antibodies but the rest of the antibody is human sequence. The presence of the human sequences helps to reduce the **immune response** by the patient against the antibody itself—a problem seen when complete mouse antibodies were used for **cancer** therapies. The human sequences also help to ensure that the various cell-destroying mechanisms of the human immune system are properly triggered with binding of the antibody.

In 1997 Rituximab was the first unconjugated (not linked to a radioactive isotope or toxin) antibody approved for use by the FDA to treat cancer. It is specifically approved for treatment of low-grade or follicular B-cell NHL. Administration of the antibody resulted in either complete or partial responses in a little less than half of those patients.

Rituximab can be used alone or in combination with other chemotherapeutic drugs. Specifically, very good results have been seen when used in combination with the CHOP **chemotherapy** regimen (**cyclophosphamide**, **doxorubicin**, **vincristine**, and prednisone). When used in combination, dosages of the antibody given before beginning chemotherapy, alternating with the other drugs, then after the chemotherapy as a "mop-up" have proven effective.

There are a number of clinical trials in progress testing the ability of rituximab to work in combination with other chemotherapy drugs, treatments, and cytokines. Some substances and treatments being tested include interleukins 2 and 11, stem cell transplantation, radioimmunotherapy, vaccination, and a wide variety of other chemotherapy combinations.

Recommended dosage

The recommended dosage for patients with low-grade or follicular NHL is 375 mg/m2 infused intravenously. The infusion is given at weekly intervals for four total dosages. Acetominophen and diphenhydramine hydrochoride are given 30-60 minutes before the infusion to help reduce side effects. If given as a retreatment the dosage is the same. Clinical trials were ongoing in 2001 to help clarify the ideal dosage and treatment schedule for this drug. Generally, decrease in symptoms occurs at an average of 55 days after the last administration of the antibody.

Precautions

Serious (even fatal) infusion reactions, especially with the first infusion, have been known with this drug. There are a number of patient conditions that can make taking this drug more dangerous. Specifically, heart problems such as arrhythmias and high blood pressure, and the medications taken to treat those conditions, can be a problem with this treatment.

Side effects

The majority of side effects occur after or during the first infusion of the drug. Some common side effects include dizziness, feeling of swelling of tongue or throat, **fever** and chills, flushing of face, headache, **itching**, **nausea and vomiting**, runny nose, shortness of breath, skin rash, and unusual **fatigue**.

Less common side effects include black, tarry stools; blood in urine or stools; fever or chills with cough or hoarseness; lower back or side pain, or painful or difficult urination; pain at place of injection; pinpoint red spots on skin; red, itchy lining of eye; swelling of feet or lower legs; unusual bleeding or bruising; and unusual weakness.

Although they are very rare this drug does have serious side effects such as chest pain and irregular heartbeat, particularly in patients already having heart conditions. It can also cause serious effects on the blood cells such as low red blood cell count (**anemia**) and low white blood cell count (**neutropenia**). Additionally, this drug has caused low blood pressure (hypotension).

In patients with high tumor burden (a large number of circulating malignant B cells) this drug can cause a side effect called **tumor lysis syndrome**. Thought to be due to the release of the lysed cells' contents into the blood stream, it can cause a misbalance of urea, uric acid, phosphate, and calcium in the urine and blood. Patients at risk for this side effect must keep hydrated and can be given **allopurinol** (an anitgout medication) before infusion.

Interactions

There have been no formal drug interaction studies done with rituximab.

See also Monoclonal antibodies.

Michelle Johnson, M.S., J.D.

Rofecoxib *see* **Cyclooxygenase 2 inhibitors**

S

Salivary gland tumors

Definition

A salivary gland tumor is an uncontrolled growth of cells that originates in one of the many saliva-producing glands in the mouth.

Description

The tongue, cheeks, and palate (the hard and soft areas at the roof of the mouth) contain many glands that produce saliva. In saliva there are enzymes, or catalysts, that begin the breakdown (digestion) of food while it is still in the mouth. The glands are called salivary glands because of their function.

There are three big pairs of salivary glands in addition to many smaller ones. The parotid glands, submandibular glands and sublingual glands are the large, paired salivary glands. The parotids are located inside the cheeks, one below each ear. The submandibular glands are located on the floor of the mouth, with one on the inner side of each part of the lower jaw, or mandible. The sublingual glands are also in the floor of the mouth, but they are under the tongue.

The parotids are the salivary glands most often affected by tumors. Yet most of the tumors that grow in the parotid glands are benign, or not cancerous. Approximately 8 out of 10 salivary tumors diagnosed are in a parotid gland. One in 10 diagnosed is in a submandibular gland. The remaining 10% are diagnosed in other salivary glands.

In general, glands more likely to show tumor growth are also glands least likely to show malignant tumor growth. Thus, although tumors of the sublingual glands are rare, almost all of them are malignant. In contrast, about one in four tumors of the parotid glands is malignant.

Cancers of the salivary glands begin to grow in epithelial cells, or the flat cells that cover body surfaces. Thus, they are called carcinomas.

Demographics

Cancers in the mouth account for fewer than 2% of all cases of **cancer** and about 1.5% of cancer deaths. About 7% of all cancers diagnosed in the head and neck region are diagnosed in a salivary gland. Men and women are at equal risk.

Mortality from salivary gland tumors in the United States is higher among male African Americans below the age of 50 than among older workers of any race or either sex. The reasons for these findings are not clear as of early 2004.

Causes and symptoms

When survivors of the 1945 atomic bombings of Nagasaki and Hiroshima began to develop salivary gland tumors at a high rate, radiation was suspected as a cause. Ionizing radiation, particularly gamma radiation, is a factor that contributes to tumor development. So is **radiation therapy**. Adults who received radiation therapy for enlarged adenoids or tonsils when they were children are at greater risk for salivary gland tumors.

Another reported risk factor is an association between wood dust inhalation and **adenocarcinoma** of the minor salivary glands of the nose and paranasal sinuses. There is also evidence that people infected with herpes viruses may be at greater risk for salivary gland tumors. And individuals infected with human immunodeficiency virus (HIV) have more salivary gland disease in general, and may be at greater risk for salivary gland tumors.

Although there has been speculation that the electromagnetic fields generated by cell phones increase the risk of salivary gland tumors, a recent study done

KEY TERMS

Adenoids—Common name for the pharyngeal tonsils, which are lymph masses in the wall of the air passageway (pharynx) just behind the nose.

Biopsy—Tissue sample is taken from the body for examination.

Computed tomography (CT)—X rays are aimed at slices of the body (by rotating equipment) and results are assembled with a computer to give a three-dimensional picture of a structure.

Lymph—Tissue that is part of the lymphatic system, the system that collects and returns fluid to the blood vessels and produces substances that fight infection.

Magnetic resonance imaging (MRI)—Magnetic fields and radio frequency waves are used to take pictures of the inside of the body.

Tonsils—Common name for the palatine tonsils, which are lymph masses in the back of the mouth, on either side of the tongue.

in Denmark has concluded that the use of cell phones, pagers, and similar devices is not a risk factor.

Symptoms are often absent until the tumor is large or has metastasized (spread to other sites). In many cases, the tumor is first discovered by the patient's dentist. During regular dental examinations, the dentist looks for masses on the palate or under the tongue or in the cheeks, and such checkups are a good way to detect tumors early. Some symptoms are:

- lump or mass in the mouth
- swelling in the face
- pain in the jaw or the side of the face
- difficulty swallowing
- difficulty breathing
- difficulty speaking

Diagnosis

A tissue sample will be taken for study via a **biopsy**. Usually an incision is necessary to take the tissue sample. Sometimes it is possible to take a tissue sample with a needle.

Magnetic resonance imaging (MRI) and **computed tomography** (CT) scans are also used to evaluate the tumor. They help determine whether the cancer has spread to sites adjacent to the salivary gland where it is found. MRI offers a good way to examine the tonsils and the back of the tongue, which are soft tissues. CT is used as a way of studying the jaw, which is bone.

QUESTIONS TO ASK THE DOCTOR

- Which type of salivary gland tumor do I have?
- Is this the best place to have the salivary gland tumor treated?

Treatment team

Generally, physicians with special training in the organs of the nose and throat take responsibility for the care of a patient with a salivary gland cancer. They are called otolaryngologists or occasionally by a longer name, otorhinolaryngologists.

For short, otolaryngologists are usually labeled ENT (for Ear, Nose and Throat) specialists. An ENT specializing in cancer will probably lead the team. An oncologist or radiation therapist may be involved, and nurses, as well as a nutritionist, speech therapist and social worker, will also be part of the team. Depending on the extent of the cancer when diagnosed, some surgery and treatments result in extensive changes in the throat, neck and jaw. The social worker, speech therapist and nutritionist are important in helping the patient cope with the changes caused by surgery and radiation treatment. If there is great alteration to the neck because of surgery, rehabilitation will also be part of the recovery process and a rehabilitation therapist will become a member of the team.

Clinical staging, treatments, and prognosis

To assess the stage of growth of a salivary gland tumor, many features are examined, including how big it is and the type of abnormal cell growth. Analysis of the types of abnormal cell growth in tissue is so specific that many salivary gland tumors are given unique names.

In stage I cancer the tumor is less than one inch in size and it has not spread. Stage II salivary gland cancers are larger than one inch and smaller than two and one-half inches, but they have not spread. Stage III cancers are smaller than one inch, but they have spread to a lymph node. Stage IV cancers have spread to adjacent sites in the head, which may include the base of the skull and nearby nerves, or they are larger than two and one-half inches and have invaded a lymph node.

Surgical removal (excision) of the tumor is the most common treatment. **Chemotherapy** and radiation therapy may be part of the treatment, particularly if the cancer has metastasized, or spread to other sites; chemotherapy of salivary gland cancers, however, does not appear to extend survival or improve the patient's quality of life. Because there are many nerves and blood vessels near the three major pairs of salivary glands, particularly the parotids, the surgery can be quite complicated. A complex surgery is especially true if the tumor has spread.

A promising form of treatment for patients at high risk of tumor recurrence in the salivary glands near the base of the skull is gamma knife surgery. Used as a booster treatment following standard neutron radiotherapy, gamma knife surgery appears to be well tolerated by the patients and to have minimal side effects.

Tumors in small salivary glands that are localized and can usually be removed without much difficulty. The outlook for survival once the tumor is removed is very good if it has not metastasized.

For parotid cancers, the five-year survival rate is more than 85% whether or not a lymph node is involved at diagnosis. The ten-year survival rate is just under 50%.

Most early stage salivary gland tumors are removed, and they do not return. Those that do return, or recur, are the most troublesome and reduce the chance an individual will remain cancer-free.

Alternative and complementary therapies

Such techniques as yoga, meditation, or biofeedback can help a patient cope with anxiety over the condition and discomfort from treatment and should be explored as an option.

Coping with cancer treatment

A support group helps during the course of treatment and follow-up. Patients are encouraged to join one. They should also be encouraged to take an active role in following the recommendations and decisions made by the treatment team.

Clinical trials

There are a number of **clinical trials** in progress. For example, the more researchers understand the nature of cancer cells, the better they are able to design drugs that attack only cancer cells. Or, in some cases, drugs that make it easier to kill cancer cells have also been designed.

The Cancer Information Service at the National Institutes of Health offers information about clinical trials that are looking for participants. The service can be contacted at (800) 422-6237.

Prevention

Minimizing intake of alcoholic beverages may be important. Avoiding unnecessary exposure of the head to radiation may also be considered preventative. Anything that reduces the risk of contracting a sexually transmitted disease, such as the use of condoms, also may lower the risk of salivary gland cancer.

Special concerns

Salivary gland tumors are considered rare. Because there are so many salivary glands, and so many types of salivary tumors, most physicians (even those who specialize in diseases of the ears, nose and throat) are challenged when they must interpret results of study of tumor tissue. For treatment of a salivary gland tumor, it is best to find a medical facility that specializes in diseases of the head and neck. Such a facility will be better able to match treatment to the specific characteristics of the tumor.

See also Oral cancer; Oropharyngeal cancer.

Resources

BOOKS

Beers, Mark H., MD, and Robert Berkow, MD, editors. "Disorders of the Oral Region: Neoplasms." Section 9, Chapter 105 In *The Merck Manual of Diagnosis and Therapy*. Whitehouse Station, NJ: Merck Research Laboratories, 2002.

PERIODICALS

Day, T. A., J. Deveikis, M. B. Gillespie, et al. "Salivary Gland Neoplasms." *Current Treatment Options in Oncology* 5 (February 2004): 11–26.

Douglas, J. G., D. L. Silbergeld, and G. E. Laramore. "Gamma Knife Stereotactic Radiosurgical Boost for Patients Treated Primarily with Neutron Radiotherapy for Salivary Gland Neoplasms." *Stereotactic and Functional Neurosurgery* 82 (March 2004): 84–89.

Johansen, C. "Electromagnetic Fields and Health Effects—Epidemiologic Studies of Cancer, Diseases of the Central Nervous System and Arrhythmia-Related Heart Disease." *Scandinavian Journal of Work and Environmental Health* 30, Supplement 1 (2004): 1–30.

Lawler, B., A. Pierce, P. J. Sambrook, et al. "The Diagnosis and Surgical Management of Major Salivary Gland Pathology." *Australian Dental Journal* 49 (March 2004): 9–15.

Wilson, R. T., L. E. Moore, and M. Dosemeci. "Occupational Exposures and Salivary Gland Cancer Mortality among African American and White Workers in the United States." *Journal of Occupational and Environmental Medicine* 46 (March 2004): 287–297.

Zheng, R., L. E. Wang, M. L. Bondy, et al. "Gamma Radiation Sensitivity and Risk of Malignant and Benign Salivary Gland Tumors: A Pilot Case-Control Analysis." *Cancer* 100 (February 1, 2004): 561–567.

OTHER

Oral Cavity and Pharyngeal Cancer Online text. American Cancer Society. Revised 05/22/2000. [cited July 18, 2001]. <http://www3.cancer.org/cancerinfo>.

ORGANIZATIONS

SPOHNC, Support for People with Oral and Head and Neck Cancer. P.O. Box 53, Locust Valley, NY 11560-0053. (800) 377-0928. http://www.spohnc.org.

Diane M. Calabrese
Rebecca J. Frey, PhD

Samarium SM 153 Lexidronam *see* **Radiopharmaceuticals**

Sarcoma

Definition

A general term for any **cancer** of the bone, cartilage, fat, muscle, blood vessels, or other connective or supportive tissues. Sarcomas can be divided into soft tissue and bone (osteogenic) sarcomas. Liposarcomas (cancerous tumors of fat tissue) are an example of soft tissue sarcomas, while **Ewing's sarcoma** is considered an osteogenic sarcoma.

Kate Kretschmann

Sargramostim

Definition

Sargramostim is a medicine used to increase the blood cell counts after bone marrow transplants and **chemotherapy**. Sargramostim may be referred to as GM-CSF or granulocyte-macrophage colony stimulating factor.

KEY TERMS

Antibiotics—Specific drugs used to treat infections.

Apheresis—The process of removing and collecting specific cells from the blood through a machine.

Bone marrow transplant—A procedure that destroys all of a patient's diseased bone marrow and replaces it with healthy bone marrow.

Chemotherapy—Specific drugs used to treat cancer.

Food and Drug Administration (FDA)—A government agency that oversees public safety in relation to drugs and medical devices. The FDA gives the approval to pharmaceutical companies for commercial marketing of their products.

Intravenous—Entering the body directly through a vein.

Neutropenia—A condition involving low levels of the white blood cells responsible for fighting infections.

Peripheral blood stem cell transplant—A procedure that collects and stores healthy young and non-developed blood stem cells. These are then given back to a patient to help them recover from high doses of chemotherapy.

Reinfusion—The transfer through a vein of healthy stem cells or bone marrow to a patient that has received large doses of chemotherapy.

Subcutaneous—Underneath the initial layer of skin.

Purpose

Sargramostim is a drug approved by the Food and Drug Administration (FDA) to decrease the time it takes for the bone marrow blood counts to recover after a bone marrow transplant. This decreases the risk of **infection**, the amount of time patients are treated with **antibiotics**, and the amount of time patients are in the hospital

Sargramostim is approved for use after chemotherapy to increase the recovery of the white cell counts and decrease the length of time a patient may have a **fever** and infection due to a low white count.

Sargramostim can be used after **bone marrow transplantation**. Once the new healthy bone marrow has been given back to a patient, sargramostim can be administered to help increase the blood cell counts and decrease the risk of fever and infection. Sargramostim can be used in patients when bone marrow is not recovering after a bone marrow transplant.

Sargramostim can be used for patients who will undergo a peripheral blood stem cell transplant. Patients will receive the sargramostim before the transplant. The sargramostim in these patients causes young, non-developed blood cells, known as stem or progenitor cells, to move from the bone marrow to the blood where they will then be removed from a patient by the process of apheresis. These blood cells are stored until after the patient receives larges doses of chemotherapy that destroy the bone marrow and the **cancer**. The patient then receives these stored cells back by an intravenous infusion. The stored cells repopulate the bone marrow and develop into the many types of functioning blood cells.

Description

Sargramostim is known as the brand name Leukine or Prokine. It has been available for use in bone marrow transplant patients for almost a decade. In cancer patients, chemotherapy destroys white blood cells temporarily. These white blood cells will grow again, but during the time that the levels are low patients are at an increased risk of developing fevers and infection. Sargramostim acts to stimulate the bone marrow to make more white blood cells which can either prevent the white count from dropping below normal or decrease the time that the level is low. This helps the patient avoid fevers and infections and allows them to receive their next doses of chemotherapy without delay.

Recommended dosage

Sargramostim is a clear colorless liquid that is dosed based on a mathematical calculation that measures a person's body surface area (BSA). This number is dependent on a patient's height and weight. The larger the person the greater the body surface area. Body surface area is measured in the units known as square meter (m^2). The body surface area is calculated and then multiplied by the drug dosage in milligrams per square meter (mg/m^2). This calculates the actual dose a patient is to receive.

It is kept refrigerated until ready to use and it is administered to patients as an injection directly underneath the skin, subcutaneously. Subcutaneous is the preferred way to give the drug; it can be given in the back of the arms, upper legs, or stomach area. Sargramostim can also be administered to patients as a short intravenous infusion into a vein over 15 to 30 minutes.

To treat chemotherapy caused neutropenia in AML patients

The starting dose for AML patients who have just finished induction chemotherapy is 250 micrograms per square meter per day. This is given beginning four days after the chemotherapy has ended or approximately day number eleven of therapy. The dose is administered as intravenous infusion over a period of four hours. The doctor will inform the patient when it is time to stop the sargramostim based on blood count monitoring.

For patients receiving bone marrow transplant

The recommended dose is 250 micrograms per square meter per day administered as a two-hour infusion intravenously. This medication should begin within 2 to 4 hours of the patient receiving the bone marrow infusion.

If the patient's counts are not returning after the bone marrow has been received, sargramostim can be administered at a dose of 250 micrograms per square meter per day intravenously over a two hour time period for 14 consecutive days. This can be repeated after a seven-day rest for two more cycles. The doctor may increase the dose to 500 micrograms per square meter per day if the white count does not rise.

For patients prior to receiving a peripheral blood stem cell transplant

The recommended dose is 250 micrograms per square meter per day. This can be given either as a once daily dose administered under the skin, or intravenously administered as a continuous infusion over 24 hours. This dosing should continue until the last day of collection.

For patients after receiving a peripheral blood stem cell transplant

The recommended dose is 250 micrograms per square meter per day. This can be given either as a once daily dose administered under the skin, or intravenously administered as a continuous infusion over 24 hours. This dosing should begin right after the patient receives the stem cell infusion and continue until the white count rises to acceptable levels.

Precautions

Sargramostim should not be received by a patient in the 24-hour time frame before or after receiving chemotherapy.

Blood counts will be monitored frequently while on sargramostim. This allows the doctor to determine if the drug is working and when to stop treatment.

Sargramostim can affect patients who have kidney or liver problems before beginning treatment. These patients will be monitored by the doctor for any changes in kidney or liver function.

It is not recommended to give sargramostim to patients who have certain types of leukemias.

Sargramostim should be used with caution in patients who have fluid problems, including heart and lung problems.

Patients with a known previous allergic reaction to sargramostim or yeast-derived substances should tell their doctor before receiving this drug.

Patients who may be pregnant or trying to become pregnant should tell their doctor before receiving sargramostim.

Side effects

One of the most common side effects of sargramostim is **bone pain**. The sargramostim causes bone marrow to produce more white blood cells, and the process causes the patient to experience pain in their bones.

Other common side effects due to sargramostim administration are fever, muscle aches, chills, and weakness.

An uncommon, but serious side effect of sargramostim is increased fluid in patients. This swelling with fluid can occur in the body as a whole, legs, arms, around the heart, and in the lungs.

Patients who have received sargramostim treatment have reported: **nausea and vomiting**, muscle pain, abdominal pain, rash, **diarrhea**, hair loss (**alopecia**), mouth sores, **fatigue**, allergic reactions and **itching**, shortness of breath, weakness, dizziness, heart problems, pain at the injection site, blood clots, headache, cough, rash, constipation, and change in kidney and/or liver function. These side effects may be due to the chemotherapy administration patients have received prior to the sargramostim.

Interactions

Sargramostim should not be given at the same time as chemotherapy or **radiation therapy**. Dosing should begin at least 24 hours after the last dose of treatment.

Patients on lithium or steroids should tell their doctor before starting sargramostim therapy, as these drugs can affect the white blood cell count.

Nancy J. Beaulieu, RPh.,BCOP

Saw palmetto

Definition

Saw palmetto is a natural plant remedy used to treat men who are experiencing difficulty when urinating. According to the American Dietetic Association, saw palmetto is one of the most commonly used dietary supplements among Americans between the ages of 50 and 76.

Purpose

Saw palmetto is not used to treat **cancer**. It is used to treat non-malignant enlargement of the prostate gland, also called benign prostatic hyperplasia (BPH).

Although saw palmetto has also been used to treat prostatitis and chronic pelvic pain syndrome (CPPS) in men, it does not appear to be useful for these conditions. A group of researchers at Columbia University reported in early 2004 that men given saw palmetto for CP/CPPS showed no appreciable improvement at the end of a year-long trial.

Description

The prostate gland is found only in men. It is located where the bladder drains into the urethra. The urethra is the tube that takes urine out of the body. The prostate gland contributes to the fluid in which sperm are ejaculated (semen).

It is common for the prostate to enlarge in men over age 50. This enlargement often is not malignant. It is thought to occur because of the action of **testosterone**, a male hormone, on the cells of the prostate. As the prostate grows, it can press on the urethra and narrow it. This causes men to have problems with urination that include the frequent urge to urinate (especially at night) and a week, dribbling, interrupted urine stream.

Saw palmetto is the bushy palm, *Serenoa repens* that grows to a height of about 18 feet (6 m) along the coast of the United States from South Carolina to Florida, and in Southern California. It is also found in Europe along the Mediterranean. Other names for

KEY TERMS

Malignant—Cancerous. Cells tend to reproduce without normal controls on growth and form tumors or invade other tissues.

Testosterone—The main male hormone. It is produced in the testes and is responsible for the development of primary and secondary male sexual traits.

this plant are American dwarf palm, cabbage palm, serenoa, or sable. The medicinal part of the saw palmetto is an extract from the dark, olive-sized berries.

Saw palmetto has a long history of use by Native Americans in treating bladder inflammation, urinary difficulties, sexual difficulties, and respiratory tract infections. Of these uses, the only scientifically substantiated claim is that saw palmetto eases urinary difficulties and increases urine output. Although the exact mechanism of action of saw palmetto has not been determined, it is believed to interfere with the action of testosterone on the prostate gland. Finasteride (Proscar, also known as Permixon) is a prescription drug used to treat BPH that works in the same way. It is important to remember that BPH is not cancer, and saw palmetto is not a treatment for cancer.

Recommended dosage

Extract of saw palmetto is available in health food stores in capsules, liquid concentrate, tablets, and as dried, ground berries. An average daily dose of the drug is 1–2 grams of which 320 mg are the active ingredients. Dosage may vary from manufacturer to manufacturer.

Saw palmetto is classified as a dietary supplement. The United States Food and Drug Administration does not test or certify it. Unlike traditional pharmaceuticals, its manufacture is largely unregulated. Dietary supplements such as saw palmetto are not required to meet standards of purity or effectiveness in controlled **clinical trials**. Men interested in using saw palmetto should look for a reputable manufacturer of supplements who provides adequate testing and label information. The cost of dietary supplements is not covered by insurance.

Precautions

Men who are having trouble urinating should see a doctor before taking any remedies on their own. **Prostate cancer** is a serious, sometimes life-threatening disease, and its symptoms can be similar to BPH. A blood test and physical examination are used to diagnose prostate cancer. It is believed that saw palmetto may interfere with this blood test (called a prostate specific antigen or PSA test). Men should have this blood test done before they begin taking saw palmetto to make sure they get correct results.

Side effects

Saw palmetto has few side effects, and is generally regarded as safe. Medical authorities in Germany, France, and Italy all officially recognize it as a safe and generally effective treatment for symptoms of BPH. Side effects that have been reported are uncommon but include headache, upset stomach, and **diarrhea**.

Interactions

Since saw palmetto is a natural remedy, few controlled studies have been done on how it interacts with other herbal remedies or traditional pharmaceuticals. In general, however, persons taking birth control pills, estrogen replacement therapy, or testosterone replacement therapy should consult their doctor before taking saw palmetto.Patients taking any supplements such as **vitamins** or herbs should tell their doctor.

Resources

BOOKS

Foster, Steven W. *Guide to Herbal Dosages*. Loveland, CO: Interweave Press, 2000.

PERIODICALS

D'Epiro, Nancy Walsh. "Saw Palmetto and the Prostate." *Patient Care* April 15, 1999: 29.

Gong, E. M., and G. S. Gerber. "Saw Palmetto and Benign Prostatic Hyperplasia." *American Journal of Chinese Medicine* 32 (March 2004): 331–338.

Gunther, S., R. E. Patterson, A. R. Kristal, et al. "Demographic and Health-Related Correlates of Herbal and Specialty Supplement Use." *Journal of the American Dietetic Association* 104 (January 2004): 27–34.

Kaplan, S. A., M. A. Volpe, and A. E. Te. "A Prospective, 1-Year Trial Using Saw Palmetto Versus Finasteride in the Treatment of Category III Prostatitis/Chronic Pelvic Pain Syndrome." *Journal of Urology* 171 (January 2004): 284–288.

Peng, C. C., P. A. Glassman, L. E. Trilli, et al. "Incidence and Severity of Potential Drug-Dietary Supplement Interactions in Primary Care Patients: An Exploratory Study of 2 Outpatient Practices." *Archives of Internal Medicine* 164 (March 22, 2004): 630–636.

ORGANIZATIONS

National Institute on Aging (NIA) Information Center. P. O. Box 8057, Gaithersburg, MD 20892-8057. (800) 222-2225. http://www.nih.gov/nia.

Tish Davidson, AM
Rebecca J. Frey, PhD

Scintigraphy *see* **Nuclear medicine scans**

Scopolamine

Definition

Scopolamine, also called hyoscine hydrobromide, is used in **cancer** treatment to prevent **nausea and vomiting** that results from movement of the head.

Purpose

Chemotherapy causes **nausea** and **vomiting** in many people. These conditions can occur for several different reasons. Scopolamine is used to treat nausea and vomiting that result from movement of the head. In many ways, this type of nausea is similar to motion sickness.

Other uses of scopolamine include pre-anesthesia sedation. In combination with morphine, scopolamine may be given to women in childbirth to induce "twilight sleep." Lastly, scopolamine is used in an ophthalmic solution to dilate the pupil of the eye before an eye examination.

Description

Scopolamine is a natural product and is familiar to many people as a motion sickness medicine. In its most common form, it comes as a patch that a person with motion sickness wears behind the ear. It is also known by the brand names Transderm-Scop and Transderm-V.

As a motion sickness drug, scopolamine has been used for many years with few side effects. It is approved by the United States Food and Drug Administration (FDA), and its cost is usually covered by insurance. In cancer treatment, scopolamine is used to treat a particular type of nausea and vomiting that occur as a result of chemotherapy.

Scopolamine is classified as an anticholinergic drug. This means it works by blocking the nerve impulses that send information from the part of the inner ear that controls the sense of balance. In motion sickness, a person vomits because conflicting information arrives in the brain from the inner ear and the eye. Some chemotherapy drugs also cause the brain to receive conflicting information, so that when patients move their head, they feel nauseated. People vary in their sensitivity to this condition. This drug is effective in helping most people control nausea and vomiting that arises from this source.

KEY TERMS

Narrow-angle glaucoma—Glaucoma is a disease where increased pressure in the eye causes damage and changes to the field of vision. Narrow-angle refers to a specific type of damage.

Recommended dosage

Scopolamine comes in a patch that the patient applies behind the ear. The patch stays in place for three days and releases a continuous supply of the drug. To be effective, the patch must be applied at least four hours before chemotherapy is begun. After three days, the patch is removed. Unused patches should be stored at room temperature.

Precautions

People applying or removing a scopolamine patch should wash their hands well immediately after handling the patch so that they do not accidentally transfer any of the drug to other parts of their body (for example, by rubbing their eyes). Scopolamine should not be used in children, should be kept away from pets, and should be used with caution in the elderly.

The patch should be used with caution in patients with a history of either seizures or psychosis, because scopolamine may make either of these disorders worse.

Side effects

About 65% of the people who use scopolamine get a dry mouth. About 17% of people report feeling drowsy from the drug. Other less common side effects include blurred vision, disorientation, restlessness, confusion, dizziness, difficulty urinating, constipation, skin rash, dry red itchy eyes, extreme sensitivity to light, and narrow-angle glaucoma.

Interactions

Many drugs interact with nonprescription (over-the-counter) drugs and herbal remedies. Patients should always tell their health care providers about these remedies, as well as prescription drugs they are taking. Patients should also mention if they are on a special diet such as low salt or high protein.

Scopolamine interferes with the absorption of ketoconazole (Nizoral), an antifungal drug, sometimes used to treat **prostate cancer**. It may also interact with other anticholinergic drugs (drugs that block nerve impulses), antidepressants, and antihistamines. Scopolamine decreases the absorption of phenothiazines (antipsychotic drugs), and interfers with the effectiveness of levodopa, a drug given to treat Parkinson's disease.

Resources

BOOKS

Beers, Mark H., MD, and Robert Berkow, MD, editors. "Drugs in Pregnancy." Section 18, Chapter 249 In*The Merck Manual of Diagnosis and Therapy*. Whitehouse Station, NJ: Merck Research Laboratories, 2002.

Beers, Mark H., MD, and Robert Berkow, MD, editors. "Motion Sickness." Section 20, Chapter 282 In*The Merck Manual of Diagnosis and Therapy*. Whitehouse Station, NJ: Merck Research Laboratories, 2002.

Beers, Mark H., MD, and Robert Berkow, MD, editors. "Ophthalmologic Disorders." Section 8, Chapter 96 In*The Merck Manual of Diagnosis and Therapy*. Whitehouse Station, NJ: Merck Research Laboratories, 2002.

Karch, A. M. *Lippincott's Nursing Drug Guide*. Springhouse, PA: Lippincott Williams & Wilkins, 2003.

PERIODICALS

Spinks, A. B., J. Wasiak, E. V. Villanueva, and V. Bernath. "Scopolamine for Preventing and Treating Motion Sickness." *Cochrane Database Systems Review* 3 (2004): CD002851.

ORGANIZATIONS

United States Food and Drug Administration (FDA). 5600 Fishers Lane, Rockville, MD 20857-0001. (888) INFO-FDA. www.fda.gov.

Tish Davidson, A.M.
Rebecca J. Frey, PhD

Screening test

Definition

A screening test is a procedure that is performed to detect the presence of a specific disease. The individual or group of individuals (as in mass screenings) does not present any symptoms of the disease.

KEY TERMS

BRCA-1 and BRCA-2—These are tumor suppressor genes whose inherited mutations have been associated with hereditary forms of breast cancer.

Digital rectal exam—The physician will feel the prostate for irregular symmetry by going into the rectum.

Genetic test—This tests for the presence of specific genes or the presence of mutations on specific genes.

Prostate-specific antigen test—This test measures the level of prostate antigen in the blood to identify presence of prostate cancer.

Transrectal ultrasonography—This test uses a small rectal probe to create an image of the prostate gland.

Purpose

The purpose of a **cancer** screening test is to identify the presence of a specific cancer in an individual that does not demonstrate any symptoms. Screening allows for early detection of cancer and can save the life of the person who might have died if the cancer was not detected by screening. If cancers are detected early, the treatment can be more effective and often less costly than if the cancer had progressed and needed drastic treatment.

Precautions

Most screening tests have been developed to be non-invasive or mildly invasive. For example breast self-exams, mammograms, and pelvic exams may be uncomfortable but are non-invasive. Therefore, most screening tests will not be affected by medications that a patient may be taking or other unrelated conditions a patient may be experiencing.

Description

Before developing or administering a screening test, the effectiveness of the test needs to be evaluated. There are several criteria to consider when deciding whether or not to screen. First, is the cancer highly fatal and common? If yes, then it is suitable for screening. Second, in order to screen a cancer, there must be detectable pre-symptomatic indicators. Finally, the reliability of results needs to be evaluated. A test can have one of the four following outcomes: true positive, false positive, true negative, and false negative.

QUESTIONS TO ASK THE DOCTOR

- What medications interfere with the results of this test?
- What tests can be performed to confirm that the results of this screening test are accurate?
- What is the most accurate and cost-effective screening test for the type of cancer in question?
- Can this test be performed anonymously?
- Will my insurance company pay for this test?

Randomized controlled trials also help to identify effective screening.

Screening tests exist for many of the more common cancers such as **prostate cancer**, **breast cancer**, **colon cancer**, lung cancer, and **cervical cancer**. Each screening test has an advisable age to begin screening and a recommended frequency at which the test should be performed. As people age, cancer becomes more prevalent; therefore, more screening tests are recommended.

Prostate cancer screening

Prostate cancer affects many men each year. Screening includes a digital rectal exam, tests for prostate-specific antigen (PSA), and transrectal **ultrasonography** (TRUS). Each of these tests takes less than half an hour to perform. The PSA test is an excellent tool as it is highly sensitive, reasonably priced, and well-tolerated by patients. Men should be counseled about the benefits and risks of detecting and treating an indolent tumor (this cancer may not have caused symptoms). The treatment may cause urinary and sexual problems.

Breast cancer screening

After **skin cancer**, breast cancer is the most common malignancy that is diagnosed in women. There are several screening methods that can be performed, including **breast self-exam** (performed by the patient), clinical breast exam, **mammography**, and BRCA-1 and BRCA-2 **genetic testing**. Genetic testing is offered to patients who have a familial history of breast cancer. All of these tests can be performed in the doctor's office and take less than half an hour. Genetic testing requires a blood sample, and it takes a few days to receive the results. Counseling is strongly advised prior to genetic testing.

Colon cancer

Colon cancer (colorectal cancer) is the third leading cause of cancer death in the United States and is the third most diagnosed cancer among both men and women. Screening tests include **fecal occult blood test**, flexible **sigmoidoscopy**, **barium enema**, and **colonoscopy**. High-risk patients (significant familial history) should begin screening at puberty or 10 years prior to occurrence of family member's tumor. Sigmoidoscopy and colonoscopy are slightly invasive, completed under mild sedative in the hospital on an outpatient basis, and take about 15 and 30 minutes respectively. Screening with colonoscopy is unique and reliable, because it allows visualization of the entire colon.

Preparation

Most screening procedures are non-invasive in order to make them convenient for patients and cost effective. Screening such as breast exams, mammography, pelvic exams, digital rectal exams, and tests that require blood samples require no preparation by the patient. However, barium enema, sigmoidoscopy, and colonoscopy all require prior preparation of the bowel. Patients will be asked to consume a clear liquid diet 24 hours prior to the exams, followed by liquid laxative about 2 hours prior to the exam. An enema or two may be required until the stool is clear.

Aftercare

Since most of the exams are non-invasive, there is no required aftercare. However, patients are encouraged to monitor themselves for any related symptoms of the cancer in question.

Risks

Since no medical tests are perfect, there are several negative consequences associated with screening. First, if a patient's prognosis would be the same with or without the screening, then the patient experiences a longer time of being sick. Second, if the results of the tests are a false negative, then the patient may be negligent in identifying symptoms and warning signals. Conversely if the results of the test are a false positive, then the patient may be subjected to unnecessary diagnostic procedures and psychological trauma. Finally, insurance companies or employers that possess results of a positive genetic test could use that information unethically, impacting coverage and employment advances.

Normal results

Normal results vary for each test and need to be analyzed for false negative results.

Abnormal results

Doctors schedule more diagnostic testing if abnormal results arise. Normally, a **biopsy** is administered on the tissue in question in order to view the cells for typical cancer traits.

See also Pap smear; Tumor grading; Tumor staging.

Resources

BOOKS

Bast, Robert C. *Cancer Medicine*. Hamilton, Ontario: B.C. Decker Inc., 2000.

PERIODICALS

Ruffin, Mack T., M.D., et al. "Predictors of Screening for Breast, Cervical, Colorectal, and Prostatic Cancer Among Community-Based Primary Care Practices." *The Journal of the American Board of Family Practice* January/February 2000: 1–10.

Sally C. McFarlane-Parrott

Second cancers

Definition

A second **cancer** is a malignancy that develops in someone who has survived an earlier cancer.

Description

Formally referred to as second primary neoplasms, second cancers are also described as late effects of the original disease or of the treatment used to cure it.

Blood-based malignancies usually occur within a few years of treatment. Solid tumors may not become evident until 20 years later. Most second cancers affect parts of the body that have been exposed to radiation and are near the site of the original tumor.

Demographics

Having once had cancer almost doubles an individual's risk of having cancer a second time. A child who develops cancer before the age of 15 is eight times more susceptible to a new cancer than a boy or girl the same age who has not had the disease. Age does not seem to decrease the likelihood that any cancer survivor will develop a second malignancy.

KEY TERMS

Late effect—A consequence of illness or therapy that becomes evident only after long-term patient monitoring.

Neoplasm—A new, abnormal growth of tissue. A neoplasm may be benign or malignant.

Solid tumor—A cancer that originates in an organ or tissue rather than in bone marrow or the lymph system.

Each year, almost 100,000 new malignancies are diagnosed among the more than 8,000,000 children, teenagers, and adults who have previously been treated for cancer. Although still rare, the incidence of new cancers in patients cured of one or more malignancies more than doubled (from approximately 6.4% to 15.3%) between 1973 and 1997. The rate of second cancers will continue to rise as the number of long-term cancer survivors continues to grow.

Children who have been treated for **Hodgkin's disease** are most at risk for developing a second cancer within 20 years. The likelihood is lowest for individuals who survive five years or longer after being treated for **non-Hodgkin's lymphoma**.

Causes

Some second cancers result from the risk factors responsible for the original disease. Some are caused by radiation or **chemotherapy** treatments that damage normal cells or suppress the patient's immune system.

Chemotherapy generally increases the likelihood of leukemia. Radiation raises the risk of developing **breast cancer** or other solid tumors.

Scientists do not fully understand why chemotherapy causes some cancer survivors to develop new malignancies. They believe radiation's role in second cancers is influenced by:

- the kind of radiation exposure the patient receives
- how much radiation the patient receives
- how old the patient is at the time of treatment
- the patient's personal and family medical history

Research

Although second cancers can occur following treatment for any type of cancer, researchers are

QUESTIONS TO ASK THE DOCTOR

- Am I likely to develop a second cancer?
- How can I reduce my risk of developing a second cancer?
- What symptoms might mean that I have developed a new cancer?
- What should I do if any of these symptoms occur?

concentrating on **lymphoma**, leukemia, and **testicular cancer** because these are the diseases that most often affect children and young adults.

Researchers are also trying to determine which types of cell damage can be characterized as precancerous and how:

- the patient's gender
- the patient's age at the time of diagnosis
- the stage of the original cancer at the time of diagnosis
- the length of the patient's survival affect the risk of developing a second cancer.

Other studies focus on whether administering both radiation and chemotherapy raises or lowers a patient's risk of developing a second cancer and how specific chemotherapy drugs, the number of times a patient is exposed to radiation, and the total amount of radiation a patient receives during a course of treatment affect the chances of developing a new malignancy.

In 1993, the National Cancer Institute (NCI) initiated the Childhood Cancer Survivor Study (CCSS). The most extensive study of its kind ever undertaken, the ongoing investigation involves more than 20,000 patients diagnosed with cancer before the age of 21. It is designed to:

- provide new information about long-term effects of cancer and cancer treatments
- enable doctors to design treatments that increase survival rates and reduce the incidence and severity of unpleasant or harmful side effects
- help survivors understand how diagnosis and treatment can continue to affect their health
- implement programs for the prevention and early detection of second cancers and other late effects

In 1996, NCI established an Office of Cancer Survivorship (OCS) to identify and provide education and support for the special physical and emotional needs of cancer survivors.

OCS's mission is improving cancer survivors' quality of life. Priority research focuses on increasing awareness of the challenges associated with cancer survivorship and developing programs to lessen the burdens of cancer survivors.

NCI's Pediatric Oncology Branch conducts **clinical trials** for children whose cancer has recurred or has not responded to treatment.

Prevention

Researchers are:

- investigating the process that transforms cancer treatments into sources of new tumors
- studying ways to maintain or improve survival rates while treating patients with gentler types of chemotherapy or doses of radiation too low to inflict the cell damage that causes second cancers
- confident that further research into causes of second cancers will enable them to develop strategies to prevent the development of new malignancies

Even though only a small percentage of cancer survivors develop second malignancies, everyone who has had cancer must:

- follow a healthy lifestyle
- avoid known causes of cancer, like smoking or prolonged exposure to the sun
- diligently follow their doctor's recommendations regarding cancer screenings and other forms of medical surveillance
- see a doctor as soon as they develop new symptoms or notice any changes in the way they look or feel

Special concerns

Improved long-term cancer survival rates have increased concern about the physical and psychological effects of the disease and the treatments used to cure it.

Doctors must monitor cancer patients carefully to make sure radiation and chemotherapy dosages low enough to eliminate unwanted side effects are strong enough to eradicate all a patient's cancer cells.

A patient who has had cancer should be aware of the risk of developing a second cancer. However, patients should not refuse or discontinue treatment for fear of developing a second malignancy. The benefits of cancer treatment far outweigh the risk of developing a new cancer.

Resources

OTHER

Key cancer statistics. National Cancer Institute. [cited 29 April 2001]. <http://search.nci.nih.gov/search97cgi/s97_cgi>.

Long-term follow-up study.University of Minnesota. [cited April 10, 2001 and April 27, 2001]. http://www.cancer.umn.edu/ltfu.

Platz, Elizabeth A., et al. *Second cancers. Cancer medicine.*http://www.cancernetwork.com/canmed/ch188/188-0.htm.

ORGANIZATIONS

Division of Cancer Control and Population Sciences, National Cancer Institute. 6130 Executive Blvd., Executive Plaza North, Rockeville, MD 20852. (301) 594-6776. <http://dccps.nci.nih.gov/ocs>.

National Childhood Cancer Foundation.440 E. Huntington Dr., PO Box 60012, Arcadia, CA 91066-6012. (800) 458-NCCF. http://www.nccf.org/NCCF/Advocacy/program.asp.

Maureen Haggerty

KEY TERMS

Adhesion—A band of internal scar tissue that develops after injury or surgery.

Anastomosis (plural, anastomoses)—The surgical connection of two structures, such as blood vessels or sections of the intestine.

Cholesteatoma—A destructive and expanding sac that develops in the middle ear or mastoid process.

Debulking—The removal of part of a malignant tumor in order to make the remainder more sensitive to radiation or chemotherapy.

Endometriosis—The growth of tissue like the lining of a woman's uterus (endometrium) outside the uterus in other parts of the body.

Endoscopy—A surgical technique that uses an endoscope (a thin, lighted, telescope-like instrument) to visualize structures inside the human body.

Infertility—The inability to become pregnant or carry a pregnancy to term.

Ischemia—Inadequate blood supply to an organ or area of tissue due to obstruction of a blood vessel.

Kidney stones—Small solid masses that form in the kidney.

Second-look surgery

Definition

Second-look surgery is performed after a procedure or course of treatment to determine if the patient is free of disease. If disease is found, additional procedures may or may not be performed at the time of second-look surgery.

Purpose

Second-look surgery may be performed under numerous circumstances on patients with various medical conditions.

Cancer

A second-look procedure is sometimes performed to determine if a **cancer** patient has responded successfully to a particular treatment. Examples of cancers that are assessed during second-look surgery are **ovarian cancer** and colorectal cancer. In many cases, before a round of **chemotherapy** and/or **radiation therapy** is started, a patient will undergo a surgical procedure called cytoreduction to reduce the size of a tumor. This debulking increases the sensitivity of the tumor and decreases the number of necessary treatment cycles. Following cytoreduction and chemotherapy, a second-look procedure may be necessary to determine if the area is cancer-free.

An advantage to second-look surgery following cancer treatment is that if cancer is found, it may be removed during the procedure in some patients. In other cases, if a tumor cannot be entirely removed, the surgeon can debulk the tumor and improve the patient's chances of responding to another cycle of chemotherapy. However, second-look surgery cannot definitively prove that a patient is free of cancer; some microscopic cancer cells can persist and begin to grow in other areas of the body. Even if no cancer is found during second-look surgery, the rate of cancer relapse is approximately 25%.

Pelvic disease

Second-look surgery may benefit patients suffering from a number of different conditions that affect the pelvic organs. Endometriosis is a condition in which the tissue that lines the uterus grows elsewhere in the body, usually in the abdominal cavity, leading to pain and scarring. Endometrial growths may be surgically removed or treated with medications. A second-look procedure may be performed following the initial surgery or course of medication to determine if treatment was successful in reducing the number of growths. Additional growths may be removed at this time.

Second-look surgery may also be performed following the surgical removal of adhesions (bands of scar tissue that form in the abdomen following surgery or injury) or uterine fibroids (noncancerous growths of the uterus). If the results are positive, an additional procedure may be performed to remove the adhesions or growths. Patients undergoing treatment for infertility may benefit from a second-look procedure to determine if the cause of infertility has been cured before ceasing therapy.

Abdominal disease

In patients suffering from bleeding from the gastrointestinal (GI) tract, recurrence of bleeding after attempted treatment remains a significant risk; approximately 10–25% of cases do not respond to initial treatment. Second-look surgery following treatment for GI bleeding may be beneficial in determining if bleeding has recurred and treating the cause of the bleeding before it becomes more extensive.

Patients suffering from a partial or complete blockage of the intestine are at risk of developing bowel ischemia (death of intestinal tissue due to a lack of oxygen). Initial surgery is most often necessary to remove the diseased segment of bowel; a second-look procedure is commonly performed to ensure that only healthy tissue remains and that the new intestinal connection (called an anastomosis) is healing properly.

Other conditions

A variety of other conditions can be assessed with second-look surgery. Patients who have undergone surgical repair of torn muscles in the knee might undergo a procedure called second-look arthroscopy to assess whether the repair is healing. A physician may use second-look mastoidoscopy to visualize the middle ear after removal of a cholesteatoma (a benign but destructive growth in the middle ear). A second endoscopic procedure may be performed on a patient who underwent endoscopic treatment for sinusitis (chronic **infection** of the sinuses) to evaluate the surgical site and remove debris.

Description

Second-look surgery may be performed within hours, days, weeks, or months of the initial procedure or treatment. This time interval depends on the patient's condition and the type of procedure.

Laparotomy

A laparotomy is a large incision through the abdominal wall to visualize the structures inside the abdominal cavity. After placing the patient under general anesthesia, the surgeon first makes a large incision through the skin, then through each layer under the skin in the region that the surgeon wishes to explore. The area will be assessed for evidence of remaining disease. For example, in the case of second-look laparotomy following treatment for endometriosis, the abdominal organs will be examined for evidence of endometrial growths. In the case of cancer, a "washing" of the abdominal cavity may be performed; sterile fluid is instilled into the abdominal cavity and washed around the organs, then extracted with a syringe. The fluid is then analyzed for the presence of cancerous cells. Biopsies may also be taken of various abdominal tissues and analyzed.

If the surgeon discovers evidence of disease or a failed surgical repair, additional procedures may be performed to remove the disease or repair the dysfunction. For example, if adhesions are encountered during a second-look procedure on an infertile female patient, the surgeon may remove the adhesions at that time. Upon completion of the procedure, the incision is closed.

Laparoscopy

Laparoscopy is a surgical technique that permits a view of the internal abdominal organs without an extensive surgical incision. During laparoscopy, a thin lighted tube called a laparoscope is inserted into the abdominal cavity through a tiny incision. Images taken by the laparoscope are seen on a video monitor connected to the scope. The surgeon may then examine the abdominal cavity, albeit with a more limited operative view than with laparotomy. Procedures such as the removal of growths or repair of deformities can be performed by instruments inserted through other small incisions in the abdominal wall. After the procedure is completed, any incisions are closed with stitches.

Other procedures

Depending on the area of the body in question, other procedures may be used to perform second-look surgery. These include:

- Arthroscopy. Arthroscopy uses a thin endoscope to visualize the inner space of a joint such as the knee or elbow. Second-look arthroscopy may be used to determine if previous surgery on the joint is healing properly.

- Percutaneous nephrolithotomy (PNL). This minimally invasive procedure is used to remove kidney stones. Second-look PNL may be used to remove fragments of stones that could not be removed during the initial procedure.
- Hysteroscopy. A hysteroscope is an instrument used to visualize and perform procedures on the inner cavity of the uterus. Second-look hysteroscopy may be used after surgery or medical treatment to treat adhesions or benign growths in the uterus to determine if they have been effectively removed.
- Mastoidectomy. This surgical procedure is used to treat cholesteatoma; a second-look procedure is generally performed to ensure that the entire cholesteatoma was removed during the initial procedure.

Resources

BOOKS

Cushner, Fred D., W. Norman Scott, and Giles R. Scuderi, eds. *Surgical Techniques for the Knee* . New York: Thieme, 2005.

Hatch, Kenneth D. *Laparoscopy for Gynecology and Oncology*. Philadelphia: Wolters Kluwer/Lippincott Williams and Wilkins Health, 2008.

Sabel, Michael S., Vernon K. Sondak, and Jeffrey J. Sussman, eds. *Surgical Foundations: Essentials of Surgical Oncology* . Philadelphia: Mosby Elsevier, 2007.

PERIODICALS

Ahn, J. H., J. C. Yoo, H. S. Yang, et al. "Second-Look Arthroscopic Findings of 208 Patients after ACL Reconstruction." *Knee Surgery, Sports Traumatology, Arthroscopy* 15 (March 2007): 242–248.

Barakate, M., and I. Bottrill. "Combined Approach Tympanoplasty for Cholesteatoma: Impact of Middle-Ear Endoscopy." *Journal of Laryngology and Otology*, June 7, 2007, 1–5.

Gershenson, D. M. "Management of Ovarian Germ Cell Tumors." *Journal of Clinical Oncology* 25 (July 10, 2007): 2938–2943.

Marmo, Riccardo, Gianluca Rotandano, Maria Antonia Bianca, Roberto Piscopo, Antonio Prisco, and Livio Cipolletta. "Outcome of Endoscopic Treatment for Peptic Ulcer Bleeding: Is a Second Look Necessary?" *Gastrointestinal Endoscopy* 57, no. 1 (January 2003): 62–7.

Sood, A. K. "Second-Look Laparotomy for Ovarian Germ Cell Tumors: To Do or Not to Do?" *Journal of Postgraduate Medicine* 52 (October-December 2006): 246–247.

Yanar, H., K. Taviloglu, C. Ertekin, et al. "Planned Second-Look Laparoscopy in the Management of Acute Mesenteric Ischemia." *World Journal of Gastroenterology* 13 (June 28, 2007): 3350–3353.

ORGANIZATIONS

American College of Surgeons. 633 N. Saint Clair St., Chicago, IL 60611-3211. (312) 202-5000. http://www.facs.org.

Society of Surgical Oncology. 85 W. Algonquin Rd., Suite 550, Arlington Heights, IL 60005. (847) 427-1400. http://www.surgonc.org.

OTHER

Horlbeck, Drew, and Matthew Ng. "Middle Ear Endoscopy." *eMedicine*. June 12, 2006. [cited January 12, 2008] http://www.emedicine.com/ENT/topic483.htm.

Johnson, Darren L., and Jeffrey B. Selby. "Meniscal Transplantation: Indications and Results." *Medscape General Medicine,* August 3, 2001. [cited May 20, 2003] http://www.medscape.com/viewarticle/408541_1.

Stephanie Dionne Sherk
Rebecca Frey, Ph.D.

Segmentectomy

Definition

Segmentectomy is the excision (removal) of a portion of any organ or gland. The procedure has several variations and many names, including wide excision, **lumpectomy**, tumorectomy, **quadrantectomy**, and partial **mastectomy**.

Purpose

The purpose of this procedure is to surgically remove a portion (in this case, with a cancerous tumor) of an organ or gland as a treatment.

Precautions

Because of the need for radiotherapy after segmentectomy, some patients, such as pregnant women and those with syndromes not compatible with radiation treatment, may not be candidates for this procedure. As with any surgery, patients should alert their physician about all allergies and any medications they are taking.

Description

Common organs that have segments are the breasts, lungs, and liver. When **cancer** is confined to a segment, removal of that portion may offer cancer-control results equivalent to larger operations. This is especially true for breast and liver cancers. In cases of lung cancer, **lobectomy** (surgical removal of all or part of the lung) is preferable, but if the patient does not have sufficient pulmonary function to tolerate this larger operation,

KEY TERMS

Conservation surgery—Surgery that preserves the aesthetics of the area to be worked on.

Excision—To surgically remove.

Lymph nodes—Small, bean-shaped organs located throughout the lymphatic system. Lymph nodes store special cells that can trap cancer cells and bacteria that are traveling through the body.

Radiotherapy—The treatment of disease with high-energy radiation, such as x or gamma rays.

then a segmentectomy may be necessary. For breast and lung cancers, this procedure is often combined with removal of some or all regional lymph nodes.

Preparation

Routine preoperative preparations, such as having nothing to eat or drink the night before surgery, are typically ordered for a segmentectomy. Information about expected outcomes and potential complications is also part of the preparation for this surgery.

Aftercare

After a segmentectomy, patients are usually cautioned against any moderate lifting for several days. Other activities may be restricted (especially if lymph nodes were removed) according to individual needs. Pain is often enough to limit inappropriate motion. Women who undergo segmentectomy of the breast are often instructed to wear a well-fitting support bra both day and night for approximately one week after surgery. Pain is usually well-controlled with prescribed medication. If it is not, the patient should contact the surgeon, as severe pain may be a sign of a complication, which needs medical attention.

Radiation therapy is usually started four to six weeks after surgery and will continue for four to five weeks. The timing of additional therapy is specific to each individual patient.

Risks

Risk of **infection** in the area affecting a segmentectomy only occurs in 3% to 4% of patients.

Normal results

Successful removal of the tumor.

QUESTIONS TO ASK THE DOCTOR

- Is segmentectomy an option for treatment?
- How will I know that all the cancer has been removed?
- What is the risk of tumor recurrence if I undergo this procedure?
- What should I do to prepare for surgery?
- What future care will I need?

Abnormal results

Major bleeding and/or infection at the wound after surgery.

Clinical Trials

Using a segmentectomy to remove breast cancers (as a technique that conserves the aesthetics of a breast) is being investigated for large tumors after several cycles of preoperative **chemotherapy**. Segmentectomy is also being investigated for treating small-cell lung cancers. Information about clinical trial options is available from the National Cancer Institute at http://www.nci.nih.gov.

Resources

BOOKS

Zurrida, S., and Giovanna Gatti."Breast Conservation: Quandrantectomy: Its Current Role and Technical Aspects." In *Breast Cancer Diagnosis and Management*. Elsevier Science, 2000.

PERIODICALS

Korst, R.J., et al."Appropriate Surgical Treatment of Resectable Non-small-cell Lung Cancer." *World Journal of Surgery* February 2001: 184–8.

Okada, M., et al."Is Segmentectomy With Lymph Node Assessment an Alternative to Lobectomy for Non-Small Cell Lung Cancer of 2 cm or Smaller?" *Annual Thoracic Surgery* March 2001: 956–61.

Sagawa, M., et al."Segmentectomy for Roentgenographically Occult Bronchogenic Squamous Cell Carcinoma." *Annual Thoracic Surgery* April 2001: 1100–4

Veronesi, U., and S. Zurrida. ldquo;Treatment of Breast Cancer." *Annales Chirurgiae et Gynaecologiae* 2000: 187–90.

Veronesi, U., and S. Zurrida. "Quandrantectomy for Malignant Disease." *Operative Techniques in General Surgery* June 2000: 132–6.

Zurrida, S., et al."The Veronesi Quadrantectomy: An Established Procedure for the Conservative Treatment of Early Breast Cancer." *International Journal of Surgical Investigation* 2000:1–9.

Laura Ruth, Ph.D.

Self image *see* **Body image**

Semustine

Definition

Semustine, also known as methyl-CCNU, is one of a group of antineoplastic (antitumor) drugs known as alkylating agents. As of mid-2001, it was an investigational drug.

Purpose

Semustine has been used in the treatment of **brain tumors**, lymphomas, colorectal **cancer**, and **stomach cancer**. It is not clearly superior to other treatments for these diseases. It has also been associated with an increased risk of secondary (that is, treatment-related) leukemia. Thus, semustine is not widely used in the U.S.

Description

Like many antineoplastic (antitumor) therapies, semustine acts by killing quickly growing cells. Since cancerous cells are generally growing faster than normal cells, drugs that kill quickly growing cells generally affect tumors more than normal cells. However, some normal cells, such as white blood cells and platelets, also grow quickly, and can be severely affected by antineoplastic drugs. Antitumor therapies create a situation where the drug is racing to kill the tumor before it causes irreparable damage to normal tissues. The ideal situation is one in which the growth of the tumor is severely affected, but the growth of normal cells is unaffected. However, not every situation is ideal. Some patients taking antitumor drugs may have to discontinue treatment or decrease the dose because of side effects.

Semustine is included in the group of **anticancer drugs** known as alkylating agents.

Semustine is an investigational drug in the United States. This means that the FDA has not approved this drug for marketing in the U.S. as of mid-2001. Generally, **investigational drugs** are made available through participation in research studies.

Many drugs have toxic side effects, some of which are difficult to detect. **Clinical trials** are used to determine the side effects, drug interactions, and precautions for medicines, as well as their efficacy. Successful completion of multi-step clinical trials results in FDA approval of a drug. Many drugs that are used in clinical trials never gain FDA approval, however, possibly because of severe side effects that outweigh the benefits of the medication, or because the medication does not perform the function for which it was tested. Final approval of a drug is also expensive. Some drugs may not receive the financial support necessary to achieve final approval.

KEY TERMS

Investigational drug—A drug that has not been approved for marketing by the FDA. These drugs are generally available to patients through participation in research studies.

Recommended dosage

Since semustine is investigational, there is no recommended dosage. Different dosing schedules have been reported in the literature for different cancers.

Precautions and side effects

In the published reports of semustine use, a common side effect is **myelosuppression**, the damage to white blood cells and platelets. Such damage may result in **infection** and bleeding, respectively. The myelosuppression from semustine is prolonged, meaning that it takes longer for blood cells to recover than is seen with many other anticancer drugs. Therefore, the interval between courses of semustine is longer than with other agents. Semustine also causes **nausea and vomiting**. Sometimes **anorexia**, or loss of appetite, persists after **nausea** and **vomiting**. As noted above, semustine has also been associated with the development of secondary leukemia.

Interactions

Semustine has been linked with other alkylating agents that can cause leukemia.

Michael Zuck, Ph.D.

Senna *see* **Laxatives**

Senokot *see* **Laxatives**

Sentinel lymph node biopsy

Definition

Sentinel **lymph node biopsy** (SLNB) is a minimally invasive procedure in which a lymph node near the site of a cancerous tumor is first identified as a sentinel node and then removed for microscopic analysis. SLNB was developed by researchers in several different **cancer** centers following the discovery that the human lymphatic system can be mapped with radioactive dyes, and that the lymph node(s) closest to a tumor serve to filter and trap cancer cells. These nodes are known as sentinel nodes because they act like sentries to warn doctors that a patient's cancer is spreading.

The first descriptions of sentinel nodes come from studies of penile and testicular cancers done in the 1970s. A technique that uses blue dye to map the lymphatic system was developed in the 1980s and applied to the treatment of **melanoma** in 1989. The extension of sentinel lymph node **biopsy** to the treatment of **breast cancer** began at the John Wayne Cancer Institute in Santa Monica, California, in 1991. As of 2003, SLNB is used in the diagnosis and treatment of many other cancers, including cancers of the head and neck, anus, bladder, lung, and male breast.

Purpose

Sentinel lymph node biopsy has several purposes:

- Improving the accuracy of cancer staging. Cancer staging is a system that classifies malignant tumors according to the extent of their spread in the body. It is used to guide decisions about treatment.
- Catching the spread of cancer to nearby lymph nodes as early as possible.
- Defining homogeneous patient populations for clinical trials of new cancer treatments.

Description

A sentinel lymph node biopsy is done in two stages. In the first part of the procedure, which takes one to two hours, the patient goes to the nuclear medicine department of the hospital for an injection of a radioactive tracer known as technetium 99. A doctor who specializes in nuclear medicine first numbs the area around the tumor with a local anesthetic and then injects the radioactive technetium. He or she usually injects a blue dye as well. The doctor will then use a gamma camera to take pictures of the lymph nodes before surgery. This type of imaging study is called lymphoscintigraphy.

After the lymphoscintigraphy, the patient must wait several hours for the dye and the radioactive material to travel from the tissues around the tumor to the sentinel lymph node. He or she is then taken to the operating room and put under general anesthesia. Next, the surgeon injects more blue dye into the area around the tumor. The surgeon then uses a hand-held probe connected to a gamma ray counter to scan the area for the radioactive technetium. The sentinel lymph node can be pinpointed by the sound made by the gamma ray counter. The surgeon makes an incision about 0.5 in long to remove the sentinel node. The blue dye that has been injected helps to verify that the surgeon is removing the right node. The incision is then closed and the tissue is sent to the hospital laboratory for examination.

Preparation

Some cancer patients should not be given an SLNB. They include women with cancer in more than one part of the breast; women who have had previous breast surgery, including plastic surgery; women with breast cancer in advanced stages; and women who have had **radiation therapy**. Melanoma patients who have undergone wide excision (removal of surrounding skin as well as the tumor) of the original **skin cancer** are also not candidates for an SLNB.

Apart from evaluating the patient's fitness for an SLNB, no additional preparation is necessary.

Aftercare

A sentinel lymph node biopsy does not require extensive aftercare. In most cases, the patient goes home after the procedure or after an overnight stay in the hospital.

The surgeon will discuss the laboratory findings with the patient. If the sentinel node was found to contain cancer cells, the surgeon will usually recommend a full axillary **lymph node dissection** (ALND). This is a more invasive procedure in which a larger number of lymph nodes—usually 12–15—is surgically removed. A drainage tube is placed for two to three weeks, and the patient must undergo physical therapy at home.

Risks

Risks associated with an SLNB include the following:

- Mild discomfort after the procedure.
- Lymphedema (swelling of the arm due to disruption of the lymphatic system after surgery).

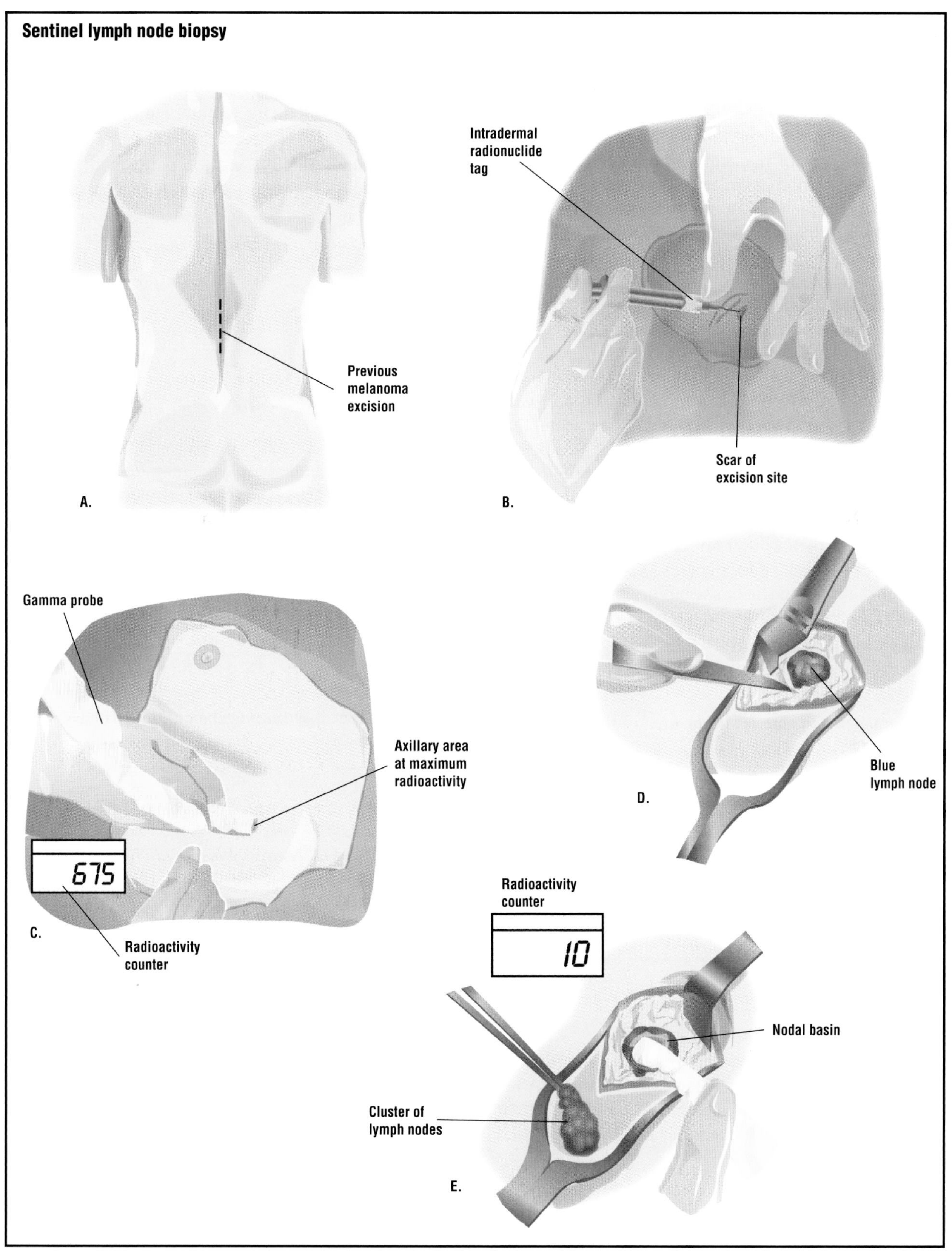

(Illustration by Argosy Publishing. Reproduced by permission of The Gale Group.)

WHO PERFORMS THE PROCEDURE AND WHERE IS IT PERFORMED?

An SLNB is usually performed in a hospital that has a department of nuclear medicine, although it is sometimes done as an outpatient procedure. The radioactive material or dye is injected by a physician who specializes in nuclear medicine. The sentinel lymph node is removed by a surgeon with experience in the technique. It is then analyzed in the hospital laboratory by a pathologist, who is a doctor with special training in studying the effects of disease on body organs and tissues.

The accuracy of a sentinel lymph node biopsy depends greatly on the skill of the surgeon who removes the node. Recent studies indicate that most doctors need to perform 20–30 SLNBs before they achieve an 85% success rate in identifying the sentinel node(s) and 5% or fewer false negatives. They can gain the necessary experience through special residency programs, fellowships, or training protocols. It is vital for patients to ask their surgeon how many SLNBs he or she has performed, as those who do these biopsies on a regular basis generally have a higher degree of accuracy.

- Damage to the nerves in the area of the biopsy.
- Temporary discoloration of the skin in the area of the dye injection.
- False negative laboratory report. A false negative means that there is cancer in other lymph nodes in spite of the absence of cancer in the sentinel node. False negatives usually result from either poor timing of the dye injection, the way in which the pathologist prepared the tissue for examination, or the existence of previously undiscovered sentinel nodes.

Normal results

Sentinel lymph node biopsies have a high degree of accuracy, with relatively few false negatives. A negative laboratory report means that there is a greater than 95% chance that the other nearby lymph nodes are also free of cancer.

Morbidity and mortality rates

Compared to axillary lymph node dissection, sentinel lymph node biopsy has a significantly lower rate of complications, including a lower rate of post-operative pain and **infection**, as well as a lower long-term risk of lymphedema.

QUESTIONS TO ASK THE DOCTOR

- Am I a candidate for sentinel lymph node biopsy?
- How many SLNBs have you performed?
- Do you perform this procedure on a regular basis?
- What is your false negative rate?

Alternatives

Breast cancer patients who should not have a sentinel lymph node biopsy usually undergo an axillary lymph node dissection to determine whether their cancer has spread. Melanoma patients who have already had a wide excision of the original melanoma may have nearby lymph nodes removed to prevent the cancer from spreading. This procedure is called a prophylactic lymph node dissection.

Resources

BOOKS

Abeloff, MD et al. *Clinical Oncology*. 3rd ed. Philadelphia: Elsevier, 2004.

Habif, TP. *Clinical Dermatology*. 4th ed. St. Louis: Mosby, 2004.

Katz, VL et al. *Comprehensive Gynecology*. 5th ed. St. Louis: Mosby, 2007.

Khatri, VP and JA Asensio. *Operative Surgery Manual*. 1st ed. Philadelphia: Saunders, 2003.

Townsend, CM et al. *Sabiston Textbook of Surgery*. 17th ed. Philadelphia: Saunders, 2004.

PERIODICALS

Burak, W. E., S. T. Hollenbeck, E. E. Zervos, et al. "Sentinel Lymph Node Biopsy Results in Less Postoperative Morbidity Compared with Axillary Lymph Node Dissection for Breast Cancer." *American Journal of Surgery* 183 (January 2002): 23-27.

Burrall, Barbara, and Vijay Khatri. "Still Debating Sentinel Lymph Node Biopsy?" *Dermatology Online Journal* 7 (2):1 [April 22, 2003].

Golshan, M., W. J. Martin, and K. Dowlatshahi. "Sentinel Lymph Node Biopsy Lowers the Rate of Lymphedema When Compared with Standard Axillary Lymph Node Dissection." *American Surgeon* 69 (March 2003): 209-211.

Peley, C., E. Farkas, I. Sinkovics, et al. "Inguinal Sentinel Lymph Node Biopsy for Staging Anal Cancer." *Scandinavian Journal of Surgery* 91 (2002): 336-338.

Pow-Sang, Julio, MD. "The Spectrum of Genitourinary Malignancies." *Cancer Control* 9 (July-August 2002): 275-276.

Schmalbach, C. E., B. Nussenbaum, R. S. Rees, et al. "Reliability of Sentinel Lymph Node Mapping with Biopsy for Head and Neck Cutaneous Melanoma." *Archives of Otolaryngology—Head and Neck Surgery* 129 (January 2003): 61-65.

Uren, R. F., R. Howman-Giles, and J. F. Thompson. "Patterns of Lymphatic Drainage from the Skin in Patients with Melanoma." *Journal of Nuclear Medicine* 44 (April 2003): 570-582.

ORGANIZATIONS

American Cancer Society (ACS). (800) ACS-2345. www.cancer.org.

National Cancer Institute (NCI). NCI Public Inquiries Office, Suite 3036A, 6116 Executive Boulevard, MSC8332, Bethesda, MD 20892-8322. (800) 4-CANCER or (800) 332-8615 (TTY). www.nci.nih.gov.

Society of Nuclear Medicine (SNM). 1850 Samuel Morse Drive, Reston, VA 20190. (703) 708-9000. www.snm.org.

Rebecca Frey, Ph. D.

Sentinel lymph node mapping

Definition

Sentinel lymph node mapping is a method of determining whether **cancer** has metastasized (spread) beyond the primary tumor and into the lymph system. The mapping procedure is used in conjunction with **sentinel lymph node biopsy** or dissection.

Purpose

The lymph system is the body's primary defense against **infection**. Lymph vessels carry clear, slightly yellow fluid called lymph that contains proteins to help rid the body of infection. Lymph nodes are small, bean-shaped collections of tissue found along the lymph vessels. Cancer cells can break off from the original tumor and spread through the lymph system to distant parts of the body where secondary tumors are formed. One job of the lymph nodes is to clean the lymph by trapping foreign cells, such as bacteria or cancer cells, and identifying foreign proteins for antibody response.

The sentinel lymph node is the first lymph node that filters the fluid draining away from the primary tumor. If cancer cells are breaking off and entering the lymph system, the first filtering node (not necessarily the closest to the tumor) will be most likely to contain the breakaway cancer cells.

QUESTIONS TO ASK THE DOCTOR

- Am I a good candidate for sentinel lymph node mapping and biopsy?
- How much experience do you have with this procedure?
- If you have limited experience, can you refer me to a center where this operation is frequently performed?
- Where can I find out about clinical trials involving sentinel node mapping and biopsy?
- If I am not a good candidate for sentinel lymph node biopsy, why not, and what are my options?

There are about 600 lymph nodes in the body. About 200 are in the head and neck and another 30–50 are in the armpit. Others are located in the groin. The sentinel node, or first filtering lymph node, will be different for each tumor and for each individual. Sentinel lymph node mapping is a technique for pinpointing which node is the most likely to receive the primary drainage from the tumor and therefore the most likely to contain cancer, so that it can be surgically removed and examined under the microscope for cancer.

If the sentinel node is cancer-free, there is a very high probability that cancer has not spread to any other node. If cancer cells are present in the sentinel node, it is likely that other nodes in the lymph system also contain cancer cells. This information is important in staging the cancer and individualizing cancer treatment for maximum benefit.

Sentinel lymph node mapping is a relatively new technique. It was first used in 1977 by researchers studying cancer of the penis. Later it was used successfully in staging **melanoma** (a type of **skin cancer**). In 1993, researchers first used the technique in **breast cancer** patients. Since then, **clinical trials** in breast cancer patients have demonstrated the accuracy and effectiveness of sentinel lymph node mapping and dissection in the staging of breast cancer. Researchers hope to be able to apply the sentinel node technique to other cancers in the future.

Advantages of sentinel lymph node mapping

Before sentinel node mapping was developed, there was no way of knowing whether and how far cancer had spread without removing and examining samples from many lymph nodes under the microscope. For example, in breast cancer patients, after a **lumpectomy** or **mastectomy** it was conventional treatment to remove most of the axillary nodes. These are the lymph nodes in the armpit. Removing axillary nodes causes frequent complications in as many as 80% of women. These complications include swelling (lymphedema), numbness, burning sensation in the armpit, reduction in arm and shoulder movement, and increased risk of infection.

Sentinel **lymph node dissection** limits the extent of surgery. It provides the following advantages:

- Less surgical trauma because only one lymph node or a small cluster of nodes is removed. For example, in breast cancers, two or three nodes are generally removed.
- Fewer side effects from surgery.
- The lymph system is left intact and is better able to transport fluid and fight infection.
- Fewer risks of impairment of arm and shoulder movements.
- With only a small amount of tissue being removed, it can be studied much more exhaustively in the laboratory for the presence of cancer.
- Significant reduction in post-mastectomy pain.

How accurate are sentinel lymph node mapping and dissection?

Sentinel lymph node mapping is being used primarily in cases of melanoma and breast cancer. The technique is relatively new, and several breast cancer clinical trials are underway. One purpose is to determine the most accurate methods of finding the sentinel node. Another is to compare the control of cancer and survival rates of sentinel node **biopsy** with conventional axillary lymph node dissection in women whose sentinel nodes are both positive and negative for cancer. Up-to-date information about these clinical trials can be obtained from the National Cancer Institute at http://www.cancertrials.nci.nih.gov or (800) 4-CANCER.

Since sentinel lymph node mapping and dissection are relatively new, they are not done at every hospital. Doctors need special training in order to perform these procedures. Studies consistently have shown that the ability to locate the sentinel node increases the more experience doctors have with the procedure. Experienced physicians can pinpoint the sentinel node with about 95% to 98% accuracy. Similarly, studies have shown that there is a learning curve for surgeons and pathologists (doctors who examine the nodes in the laboratory) in sentinel lymph node dissection. The more experience they have, the more accurate they are.

Overall, accurate diagnoses from sentinel lymph node dissection are very high (92% or more). However, it is important that the patient find out how much training and experience the treatment team has with this procedure, and if necessary ask for a referral to another facility with more experienced staff. Some insurers may also consider the procedure experimental. Patients should check with their insurers about coverage, as the acceptance of this procedure is evolving.

KEY TERMS

Lumpectomy—Surgical removal of a tumor in the breast.

Lymph—Clear, slightly yellow fluid carried by a network of thin tubes to every part of the body. Cells that fight infection are carried in the lymph.

Lymph nodes—Small, bean-shaped collections of tissue found in lymph vessels. They produce cells and proteins that fight infection and filter lymph. Nodes are sometimes called lymph glands.

Lymph system—Primary defense against infection in the body. The tissues, organs, and channels (similar to veins) that produce, store, and transport lymph and white blood cells to fight infection.

Mastectomy—Surgical removal of the entire breast.

Metastasize—Spread of cells from the original site of the cancer to other parts of the body where secondary tumors are formed.

Precautions

Women with breast cancer who are the best candidates for sentinel node dissection are those with early stage breast cancer with low to moderate risk of lymph node involvement. Women who are not good candidates for sentinel node dissection are those who:

- Are believed to have cancer in the lymph nodes.
- Have had prior surgery (such as breast reduction surgery) that would change the normal pattern of lymph flow near the primary tumor.
- Have already received chemotherapy, because chemotherapy can create tissue changes that alter normal lymph flow.

- Are older, because lymph flow alters with age and the sentinel node may not be accurately detected.

To get valid results, people with melanoma must have sentinel **lymph node biopsy** performed before wide excision of the original melanoma.

Description

Sentinel lymph node mapping and dissection is done in a hospital under general anesthesia. There are two methods of detecting the sentinel node. In the dye method, a vital blue tracer dye is injected near the tumor. The dye enters the lymph system and then collects in the sentinel or first filtering node. The surgeon looks for the accumulation of dye and removes the blue node.

In the radioactive technique, a low-level radioactive tracer is injected near the tumor. It is absorbed into the lymph system and travels to the sentinel node. A hand-held Geiger counter (a device that measures radioactivity) is passed over the area near the tumor until the spot with the most radioactivity is located. The radioactive ("hot") node is then removed. Because accuracy in locating the sentinel node is increased by 10% to 15% if both radioactive and dye tracers are used together, this is generally done.

Once the sentinel nodes are removed, they are sent to the laboratory to be examined for cancer. If no cancer cells are present, there is rarely a need to remove more lymph nodes. If cancer cells are present, it is likely that more lymph nodes will be removed. In any event, information from the sentinel node biopsy will be used to determine the best way to treat the cancer.

Preparation

Standard pre-operative blood and liver function tests are performed before sentinel node mapping and dissection. The patient will also meet with an anesthesiologist before the operation and should tell the anesthesiologist about all medication (prescription, non-prescription, or herbal) that he or she is taking and all drug allergies.

Aftercare

Since only a small amount of tissue is removed, patients generally recover quickly from sentinel node mapping and dissection. They may feel tired from the anesthesia and may experience minor burning, pain, and slight swelling at the site of the incision. If tracer dye is used, the dye stays in the body for up to nine months and may be visible under the skin.

Risks

The greatest risk associated with sentinel lymph node mapping is that the sentinel node cannot be identified and conventional removal of many lymph nodes will be necessary. Failure to locate the sentinel node happens in less than 5% of patients.

The second greatest risk is of a false-negative reading (approximately 5% to 8% for breast cancer), finding no cancer in the tissue sample when it is actually present. As discussed above, this test is extremely accurate when performed by an experienced treatment team.

Other risks associated with sentinel lymph node mapping are allergic reaction to the dye, infection at the incision site, and allergic reaction to anesthesia.

Normal results

If no cancer cells are found in the sentinel node, other lymph nodes do not need to be removed.

Abnormal results

If cancer cells are found in the sentinel lymph node the treatment team may recommend an operation to remove more lymph nodes and/or radiation or **chemotherapy** to control the cancer.

Resources

PERIODICALS

Hsueh, Eddy C., Nora Hansen, and Armando Giuliano, "Intraoperative Lymphatic Mapping and Sentinel Lymph Node Dissection in Breast Cancer." *CA: A Cancer Journal for Clinicians* 50 (2000): 279–91.

ORGANIZATIONS

American Cancer Society. National Headquarters, 1599 Clifton Rd. NE, Atlanta, GA 30329. 800 (ACS)-2345. http://www.cancer.org.

Cancer Information Service. National Cancer Institute, Building 31, Room 10A19, 9000 Rockville Pike, Bethesda, MD 20892. (800) 4-CANCER. http://www.nci.nih.gov/cancerinfo/index.html.

Tish Davidson, A.M.

Sexual dysfunction in cancer patients

Definition

Sexual dysfunction is a common side effect of **cancer** and cancer treatments, effecting all aspects of a cancer patient‘s **sexuality**, including sexual desire and physical and psychological problems. Sexual dysfunction includes infertility, erectile dysfunction, pain during sex, negative **body image**, early menopause, **depression**, anxiety, feelings of guilt about the origin of the cancer, and a general lack of interest in sex.

Demographics

Sexual dysfunction in cancer patients occur in men and women of all ages and ethnicities, including heterosexuals, bisexuals, and homosexuals. More than half of all survivors of breast, prostate, colorectal, and **gynecologic cancers** experience post-treatment sexual problems, according to the Dana-Farber Cancer Institute in Boston. About half of all women treated for breast and gynecologic cancers experience long term sexual dysfunction, according to the National Cancer Institute (NCI). Gynecologic cancers include those of the ovaries, uterus, and vagina. The NCI estimates that the rates of sexual dysfunction following various cancer treatments range from 40% to 100%. Erectile dysfunction (ED) in men following treatment for **prostate cancer** is 60% to 90% following radical **prostatectomy** and 67% to 85% following external-beam **radiation therapy**, according to NCI estimates. The NCI also reports the rates of sexual dysfunction in people with Hodgkin‘s **lymphoma** and **testicular cancer** is 25%.

Men who are under the age of 50 and those who were able to get and maintain erections before prostate cancer treatment are more likely to be capable of healthy erections after treatment. Men with prostate cancer that has spread beyond the prostate gland are more likely to experience erection problems, according to the American Cancer Society.

Description

Sexual dysfunction in cancer patients is a common problem that occurs in about half of all people with cancer of the breast or reproductive organs. Many people experience problems having sex following their cancer treatment. Depending on the type of cancer, the problems may be of short duration or long-term. Many of these people were unprepared for changes in their sex lives, reports the NCI. The main problems reported are worrying about intimacy after treatment, not being able to have satisfactory sex, having symptoms of menopause, and not being able to have children. Some people have a negative image of their body after cancer treatment; even the thought of being seen naked can be stressful. Other concerns are that sex will be painful, that they will not be able to perform sexually, and feelings of being unattractive.

For some cancer patients and survivors, changes in their body cause them to fear being rejected by a sexual partner and thus become less involved in social situations, including dating. The NCI offers the following recommendations to help people regain their social life:

- Focus on activities that are enjoyable but don‘t take up a lot of time, such as taking a class or joining a club.
- Don‘t let having or surviving cancer be an excuse for not dating or meeting people.
- Don‘t tell a new date or friend about any sexual problems until there is a sense of trust and friendship.
- Think of dating as a learning process with the goal of having an enjoyable social life. Not all dates or budding friendships work regardless of whether a person has cancer or not.

Risk factors

There are no specific risk factors for sexual dysfunction in cancer patients. People with certain types of cancer have a greater chance of experiencing sexual problems. These cancer types include breast, cervical, ovarian, uterine, vaginal, anal, penile, testicular, and prostate.

Causes and symptoms

Physical and psychological factors lead to the development of sexual problems in people with cancer and cancer survivors. Physical causes include losing the ability to have sex due to the side effects of cancer treatments, general **fatigue**, and pain. Treatments that can lead to physical factors include surgery, radiation treatment, and chemical therapy, commonly called **chemotherapy**. Other factors include pain medications, depression, feelings of guilt regarding the patient‘s belief about what caused the cancer, changes in body image following surgery, and stresses relating to personal and sexual relationships. For example, aging is often associated with a decrease or loss of sexual desire and performance so people who are middle-aged or older may feel more stressful than a younger person with cancer.

Diagnosis

The diagnosis of sexual dysfunction in cancer patients is generally determined by each patient since “normal” sexual functioning has a wide range, defined by the patient and their sexual partner based on age, gender, personal attitudes, and religious and cultural values. Physicians treating cancer patients should bring up the topic of sexual problems associated with the specific type of cancer. If they do not, the patient should question the doctor on potential sexual problems from the time the cancer is diagnosed, through treatment, and post-treatment.

Examination

A physical examination in women during or following cancer treatment may reveal potential problems with normal sexual function, such as dryness in the vagina. A physical examination is generally not useful and rarely used in men.

Tests

There are no tests that measure sexual function and dysfunction in women other than their own belief that here is a problem. In men, the primary test is the ability or inability to get and maintain an erection sufficient enough to have sex.

Procedures

The primary procedure used to diagnose sexual dysfunction in cancer patients is a series of questions asked by the patient's primary care doctor or more commonly, by a specialist, such as oncologist, gynecologist, or urologist. In some cases, the questioner may be a sex therapist or counselor. Commonly asked questions include:

- Do you enjoy sex?
- Do you have sufficient energy for sex?
- Do you reach orgasm during sex?
- Do you have any pain during sex?
- When did the sexual problems start?
- Did you have any sexual problems before being diagnosed with cancer?

Treatment

There are a variety of medical treatments available to cancer patients with sexual dysfunction, including counseling with a psychologist or sex therapist. Many hospitals and cancer treatment centers have programs that can help people with cancer and cancer survivors reclaim their ability and desire to have sex. Often, the goal of a particular treatment is to help cancer patients, survivors, and their sexual partners to discover or rediscover their sense of sexual pleasure and sensuality. Sometimes this means approaching sex from a perspective that may be different that what the person experienced before developing cancer.

Traditional

Traditional, non-drug treatments are available to men and women. In men, these include surgery and medical devices such as penile implants that can treat erectile dysfunction in men who do not respond to medications. Treatments for women include vaginal lubricants and vaginal dilators that can ease pain during sex.

Drugs

In women, hormone replacement therapy involving estrogen and progesterone, either alone or together, if often used. In men, erectile dysfunction (ED) drugs are commonly prescribed. These drugs include Viagra (sildenafil), Levitra (vardenafil), and Cialis (tadalafil).

Alternative

Alternative and complementary treatments include over-the-counter medications such as yohimbe, meditation, biofeedback, acupuncture, and hypnosis. In states where the use of marijuana for medical purposes is legal, the otherwise illegal drug may be recommended, usually by a physician that specializes in medical marijuana use.

Home remedies

There are few home remedies that are considered useful by medical professionals. Several that are used to varying degrees of success include yoga, creative imagery, **vitamins** and minerals such as zinc and **saw palmetto**, herbs, and special diets.

Prognosis

As in most medical conditions, there are some people who do not respond at all to treatment. Others will respond in varying degrees. In many cases, a cancer patient can resume the same type and degree of sexual activity that they had before their cancer. So the prognosis is very patient-specific and often depends of the type of cancer and its severity. Many cancer patients can learn to adapt to changes in their sexual function. More testing and research is needed to evaluate and compare the effectiveness of various treatments, including medical and psychological approaches, according to the National Cancer Institute, a branch of the U.S. government's National Institutes of Health.

Sexual problems may not be resolved within the first two years following treatment, reports the NCI.

QUESTIONS TO ASK YOUR DOCTOR

- What can be done prior to cancer treatment to help minimize my chances of having sexual problems after treatment?
- What can my sexual partner do to help with my sexual dysfunction?
- Would a sex counselor or therapist be helpful?
- Is it okay to have sex during treatment?
- Will treatment or lack of treatment effect my ability to have children?

Sexual problems can increase over time and can interfere with returning to the cancer survivor's return to their pre-cancer sexual behavior.

Prevention

There are no sure ways to prevent sexual dysfunction in cancer patients or survivors. However, there are treatment alternatives that can reduce the risk of having sexual problems related to cancer and cancer treatments. Radiation therapy is a big culprit in causing sexual problems in cancer patients since it can destroy tissue, especially when used against ovarian and prostate cancers. In men with prostate cancer, those that have nerve-sparing radical prostatectomy surgery are less likely to develop sexual problems than men who have radiation therapy.

Resources

BOOKS

Carr, Kris. *Crazy Sexy Cancer Survivor: More Rebellion and Fire For Your Healing Journey*Charleston, SC: Skirt Publishing, 2008.

Frank, Richard C. *Fighting Cancer with Knowledge and Hope: A Guide for Patients, Families, and Health Care Providers* New Haven, CT: Yale University Press, 2009.

Goldstein, Andrew, et al. *Female Sexual Pain Disorders: Evaluation and Management*Hoboken, NJ: Wiley-Blackwell, 2009.

Mulhall, John P. *Sexual Function in the Prostate Cancer Patient*New York: Humana Press, 2009.

PERIODICALS

Amsterdam, Alison, and Michael Krychman. "Sexual Function in Gynecologic Cancer Survivors." *Expert Review of Obstetrics &Gynecology*(May 30, 2008): 331–337.

Derzko, C., et al. "Management of Sexual Dysfunction in Postmenopausal Breast Cancer Patients Taking Aromatase Inhibitor Therapy." *Current Oncology*(Dec. 14, 2007): S20–S40.

Hordem, Amanda, and Annette F. Street. "Communicating About Patient Sexuality and Intimacy After Cancer: Mismatched Expectations and Unmet Needs." *Medical Journal of Australia*(March 5, 2007): 224–227.

Kendirci, M, et al. "Update on Erectile Dysfunction in Prostate Cancer Patients." *Current Opinions in Urology*(May 2006): 186–195.

Pietrangeli, Alberto, et al. "Sexual Dysfunction Following Surgery for Rectal Cancer—A Clinical and Neurophysiological Study." *Journal of Experimental & Clinical Cancer Research*(Sept. 17, 2009): N/A.

ORGANIZATIONS

American Cancer Society, 250 Williams St., Atlanta, GA, 30303, (800) 227-2345, http://www.cancer.org.

American Psychosocial Oncology Society, 154 Hansen Rd., Ste. 201, Charlottesville, VA, 22911, (434) 293-5350, (866) 276-7443, (434) 977-1856, info@apos-society.org, http://www.apos-society.org.

National Cancer Institute, 6116 Executive Blvd., Room 3036A, Bethesda, MD, 20892-8322, (800) 422-6237, cancergovstaff@mail.nih.gov, http://www.cancer.gov.

National Center for Complementary and Alternative Medicine, P.O. Box 7923, Gaithersburg, MD, 20898, (888) 644-6226, (866) 464-2616, Email form on Website, http://www.nccam.nih.gov.

Breast Cancer Society of Canada, 420 East St. N., SarniaON, Canada, N7T 6Y5, (519) 336-0748, (800) 567-8767, (519) 336-5725, bcsc@bcsc.ca, http://www.bcsc.ca.

Canadian Cancer Society, 10 Alcorn Ave., Ste. 200, TorontoON, Canada, M4V 3B1, (416) 961-7223, (416) 961-4189, ccs@cancer.ca, http://www.cancer.ca.

Cancer Council Australia, GPO Box 4708, SydneyNSW, Australia, 2001, 61 2 8063 4100, 61 2 8063 4101, info@cancer.org.au, http://www.cancer.org.au.

European Society of Gynaecologocal Oncology, 1-3 Rue Chantepoulet, P.O. Box 1726, Geneva 1, Switzerland, CH-1211, 41 22 906 9150, info@esgo.org, http://www.esgo.org.

Irish Cancer Society, 43/45 Northumberland Road, Dublin 4, Ireland, (800) 200 700, helpline@irishcancer.ie, http://www.cancer.ie.

Ken R. Wells

Sexuality

Definition

Sexuality can be defined as the quality or state of being sexual. Quite often it is an aspect of one's need for closeness, caring, and touch.

Cancer and sexuality

Faced with a disease such as **cancer** most people initially lose interest in sex. Sexual desire is overshadowed by concern for one's health. Certain cancers directly affect sexual organs making sexual activity impossible or painful. **Chemotherapy**, radiation and surgical treatments of cancer can affect sexual activity making it difficult or undesirable. The side effects of cancer treatments such as **nausea** and pain can lessen sexual desire. Cancer treatments that disturb the normal hormone balance can also lessen desire. Many cancer patients are also worried that their partner may feel negatively about them because of the changes in their body and the fact that they have cancer.

Sexuality can be expressed in many different ways. It is possible to continue a healthy and satisfying relationship and maintain a healthy sexual image even after any changes brought about by cancer. Sexual intimacy can be a source of comfort during treatment and recovery from cancer. This may require some adaptation and change of the patient's current sexual patterns but with the right support groups and encouragement from the partner it should be possible to maintain healthy sexual activity.

Cancer and female sexuality

Women undergoing chemotherapy, **radiation therapy**, or pelvic surgery may experience pain during intercouse. This could be caused by changes in the size and moistness of the vagina, or **infection** of the bladder or vagina. Sometimes the pain is so severe that it sets off an involuntary contraction of the vagina called vaginismus. This contraction makes intercourse impossible. Extra lubrication is necessary to make intercourse comfortable. Vaginisimus can be treated by counseling and special relaxation training.

Radical surgery that will drastically change the physical aspects of the vagina and vulva pose an additional challenge for the affected woman and her partner. The woman may be affected psychologically by the change in appearance and also by the fear of pain or bleeding. The genitals may be physically altered so that sexual intercourse is difficult or impossible. Sex therapy, **reconstructive surgery**, or altering habits so that sexual needs are met without intercourse all may be options after surgery that radically affects the genitals.

Another common effect of cancer treatment is premature menopause. This may follow removal of ovaries by surgery, suppression of ovaries by chemotherapy or radiation therapy of the pelvis. The symptoms are much more severe than normal menopause causing vaginal dryness and tightness, hot flashes and sometimes low androgen levels which can also reduce sexual desire. Women who do not have hormone-sensitive tumors may want to consider hormone replacement therapy, after consultation with their doctor. Radiation treatment of the pelvis, cervix or vagina may cause scarring of the vagina. This makes it tighter and difficult to penetrate. Series of vaginal dilators of different sizes can help to relieve this problem. It is important to use these early to prevent vaginal shrinkage. Counseling may also be beneficial for the affected woman and her partner.

Cancer and male sexuality

Radiation therapy of the pelvis can impair sexual function. Circulating **testosterone** levels may come down temporarily and during this time men may have a loss of sexual desire. But this does not seem to be a permanent effect in all cases. It may be possible to get aroused by taking more time and experimenting with different kinds of caressing and love making. If erection does not occur after a significant period of time the doctor may suggest tests to check for sleep erections. Some are take-home tests and if they suggest that erection occurs normally during sleep, it is clear the physiological mechanism is intact and sexual counseling may relieve the problem. Sexual counseling may also be helpful to allow enjoyment with sexual caressing in the absence of erections. Men with medical impotence may also be helped by the use of Viagra. Men need replacement with hormones in only very rare cases. In fact, extra testosterone can cause undetected **prostate cancer** to grow.

Surgery for various cancers can cause sexual problems. Surgery for **bladder cancer** can lead to decreased sexual desire, lowered ability to obtain an erection, and less frequent or less intense orgasms. Surgery for **penile cancer** and **testicular cancer** can result in decreased fertility and desire, difficulties with erections and orgasms, and decreased volume of semen. In treating prostate cancer, the **biopsy** obtained to confirm diagnosis may decrease semen levels, and, after a man has had his prostate gland removed (**prostatectomy**), he may be unable to obtain an erection. However, new surgical advances and new chemotherapy options may help reduce these effects.

If, during surgery, the blood supply to the penis is affected, the surgeon may take an abdominal artery and try to connect it the penis. This operation is only successful in a quarter of the patients. Penile injection therapy and vacuum devices have been used to produce erections in the absence of sufficient blood flow. Medications that produce erections are risky and may lead to the formation of scar tissue. Vacuum erection devices are safer but intrude in the lovemaking. Medical erection problems may also be treated by penile prosthesis. This is one of the best ways to treat a permanent erection problem.

Sexual problems of specific cancer treatments

Urostomy or colostomy

Before sexual activity one must ensure that the **urostomy** fits correctly. The appliance should be emptied to reduce the chance of a leak. A patterned pouch can be worn over it to cover it. Sexual activity with a **colostomy** can be performed with the same precautions. One can plan sexual activity at a time when the colostomy is not active and avoid gas-producing foods that day. Direct communication and reassurances from a loving partner can be extremely helpful.

Mastectomy

The breast symbolizes sexuality and when the treatment of **breast cancer** involves **mastectomy**, psychological counseling is helpful to regain desire and sexual enjoyment. There may be fewer problems when a **lumpectomy** is done. Women who feel awkward about the change after surgery may consider using a prosthesis covered with a nightgown or bra, or they may consider reconstruction either with or without implantation.

Limb amputation

Treatment mainly of primary tumors of bone often includes amputating a limb. If the partners can openly communicate they can decide whether the prosthesis needs to be worn during lovemaking. Prosthesis can help with movement and balance but the straps that attach it can get in the way. If the prosthesis is not used, pillows could be used instead for balance.

Treatment of facial cancer

Some cancers of the head and neck may be treated by partial removal of the facial bony structure. This can be psychologically very damaging as the scar is so public and affects the face, a vital part of the human personality. Following such surgery, speech may also be affected. Recent advances in facial prosthesis and plastic surgery may help regain a more natural appearance and speech.

Professional help for sexual problems

The first step is to discuss sexual problems with one's doctor. Sometimes doctors themselves may not be at ease discussing sexual issues. Cancer centers may have sexual rehabilitation centers with experts on staff comfortable dealing with these issues. Medical schools and some private practice groups run sexual dysfunction clinics that provide comprehensive care to treat sexual problems. Sex therapists can provide sexual counseling. It is important that the sex therapist be a psychiatrist, social worker, or psychologist with special training in treating sexual problems. Professional societies such as American Association for Marriage and Family Therapy can give information about these specialists. It is important to avoid untrained people who provide useless and sometimes harmful therapy.

See also Body image; Fertility issues.

Resources

OTHER

The American Cancer Society. *Sexuality and Cancer: For the Man Who Has Cancer and His Partner.Sexuality and Cancer: For the Woman Who Has Cancer and Her Partner*. Other publications also available free from the American Cancer Society. Telephone: 1-800-ACS-2345. Also available through the web site: http://www.cancer.org.

"For Women:Body Image Issues." *Gillette Women's Cancer Connection*.http://www.gillettecancerconnect.org.

ORGANIZATIONS

The American Association for Marriage and Family Therapy. 1133 15th Street NW, Suite 300, Washington D.C. 20005. Telephone: (202) 452-0109 Web site: http://www.aamft.org.

American Cancer Society. Telephone: 1-800-ACS-2345. Web site: http://www.cancer.org.

Malini Vashishtha, Ph.D.

Sézary syndrome

Definition

Sézary syndrome is a type of **cutaneous T-cell lymphoma**, characterized by skin abnormalities, extreme **itching**, enlarged lymph glands, and abnormal blood cells.

Description

Sézary syndrome is a type of **lymphoma**, which is a disease where lymphocytes (a type of white blood cell) increase to very large numbers in a person's blood. Sézary syndrome is a type of lymphoma known as a cutaneous T-cell lymphoma, meaning

KEY TERMS

Eczema—A superficial inflammation of the skin, generally with itching and a red rash.

Interferon —A substance produced by cells that can enhance the immune system.

Monoclonal antibodies —Antibodies made in the lab that can identify and target specific infectious agents and cancers.

Psoriasis—A chronic skin condition, causing red, scaling patches to appear to the skin.

that it is a disease where the white blood cells known as T-lymphocytes increase to large numbers.

Sézary syndrome can affect many organs. In early stage disease, the skin is the only organ affected; however, later stage disease can affect other organ systems.

Demographics

Sézary syndrome is relatively rare, affecting about one in one million people. The incidence of the syndrome increases with age, with most cases appearing in people in their 50s or 60s. Men appear to be affected more often than women, and black males appear to be at higher risk of developing the syndrome than white males.

Causes and symptoms

There are no known causes of Sézary syndrome. Early in the course of study of the syndrome, it was thought that exposure to certain chemicals could trigger the disease. However, later studies have not shown any relation between industrial chemical exposure and Sézary syndrome

The symptoms of Sézary syndrome can be very subtle; because of this, it is often not diagnosed for many years. Early symptoms include skin lesions that can look like eczema and psoriasis. Later symptoms can include skin tumors, especially in body folds. Enlarged lymph glands in the neck, armpits, and groin can accompany the skin tumors. Later in the course of Sézary syndrome symptoms may relate to other areas of disease involvement.

Diagnosis

The diagnosis of Sézary syndrome is made by careful clinical evaluation. Generally, a patient with Sézary syndrome seeks treatment for skin lesions that are not responsive to ordinary medications. If the doctor suspects a cutaneous T-cell lymphoma, a blood test is ordered to see if there are any abnormalities, such as an increase or decrease in lymphocytes and the presence or absence of Sézary cells, which are certain white blood cells with a distinctive shape when viewed under a microscope. Finally, a sample (**biopsy**) of one the skin lesions is done to see if the lesion is part of Sézary syndrome or caused by some other disease.

Clinical staging, treatment, prognosis

Staging for cutaneous T-cell lymphoma, including Sézary syndrome, is based on the extent of skin involvement and the presence or absence of other manifestations of the syndrome. Stage I is characterized by mild skin involvement. In stage II there is extensive skin involvement, including skin tumors. Patients in stage III and IV have extensive skin involvement, blood abnormalities including Sézary cells, and swollen lymph nodes.

There are multiple therapies for Sézary syndrome. However, unless the disease is in an early stage, the chances for a complete cure are small. Nonspecific treatment includes skin lubricants and moisturizers to help treat the skin irritation and dryness that is common with the syndrome. Low potency steroid creams or ointments may be used to help treat itching and skin inflammation.

The first therapy used with some success against Sézary syndrome is **mechlorethamine**, or nitrogen mustard. It is applied daily to the entire skin surface (except for sensitive areas such as eyelids and genitalia) for six to twelve months, then three times a week for one to two years more. Several studies have investiagted the effectiveness of nitrogen mustard therapy, and have found that in stage I or II disease, the therapy causes complete remission in 60–80% of patients. Side effects are minimal, but dry skin, irritation, and change in skin pigmentation can occur.

Another treatment that has been used for many years, especially for stage II and III disease, is electron beam **radiation therapy**. Treatment with electron beam radiation therapy has been used since 1953, with good response rates seen in 50–70% of patients. Side effects can include excessive skin dryness, skin blistering, loss of hair on treated areas, and increased risk of **skin cancer**.

ECP, or photophoresis, has been approved by the FDA as a treatment for Sézary syndrome. In this mode of treatment, phototherapy with ultraviolet light is combined with leukapheresis. In leukapheresis, a person's blood is taken out and passed through special filters that remove circulating Sézary cells; the cells are treated with ultraviolet radiation, then reinfused into the patient. Response rates range from 55% to 75%, with some reports showing a 15–25% cure rate. Side effects can include **nausea** and **fever**.

Systemic **chemotherapy** is often used in patients who are in later stages of the disease. Using standard **cancer** chemotherapeutic agents such as **cyclophosphamide**, **vincristine**, and **doxorubicin**, response rates up to 19 months have been seen. No studies have shown an increased survival rate in patients getting aggressive, high-dose chemotherapy versus those getting more standard doses.

The prognosis for patients with Sézary syndrome is based on placing the patient in one of three categories: good, intermediate, or poor. Patients with good prognosis have the condition limited to their skin. Their general survival time is more than 10 years. Patients in the intermediate category have skin lesions including tumors and plaques, but no blood involvement. Their survival time is five years. Patients in the poor risk category have extensive skin lesions along with blood abnormalities, including high levels of Sézary cells. Patients in this category, even with extensive treatment, generally have survival rates of only one year or less.

Coping with cancer treatment

There are multiple ways to help patients cope with side effects brought about by the treatment of Sézary syndrome. Lubricants can be used to help dryness, scaling, and itching of the skin caused by the use of topical treatments such as nitrogen mustard and electron beam therapy. Symptoms such as **nausea and vomiting**, caused by ECP and systemic chemotherapy, can be treated with standard anti-nausea and **vomiting** medication.

Clinical trials

In 2009, many **clinical trials** are underway to investigate several forms of innovative treatment for cutaneous T-cell lymphoma and Sézary syndrome. Interferon has been used with some success in both early and late stage disease. Common side effects include a decrease in white blood cells and chronic **fatigue**. The use of **monoclonal antibodies** in treating late stage disease (III and IV) has been recently studied. Early studies have shown response rates of around 30%. Side effects include allergies to the monoclonal antibodies, fever, and fatigue.

Prevention

As of 2001, there are no known ways to prevent Sézary syndrome.

Resources

BOOKS

Abeloff, D. Martin, et al. *Clinical Oncology*. New York: Churchill Livingstone, 2000.

PERIODICALS

Macey, William H. "A Primary Care Approach to Cutaneous T-Cell Lymphoma." *The Nurse Practioner* 25, no.4 (April 2000): 82-98.

Edward R Rosick, D.O., M.P.H., M.S.

Shingles *see* **Herpes zoster**

Shunt *see* **Peritoneovenous shunt**

Sigmoidoscopy

Definition

Sigmoidoscopy is a procedure by which a doctor inserts either a short and rigid or slightly longer and flexible fiber-optic tube into the rectum to examine the lower portion of the large intestine (or bowel).

Purpose

Sigmoidoscopy is used most often in screening for colorectal **cancer** or to determine the cause of rectal bleeding. It is also used for the diagnosis of inflammatory bowel disease and other benign diseases of the lower intestine.

Cancer of the rectum and colon is the second most common cancer in the United States, claiming the lives of about 56,000 people annually. As a result, The American Cancer Society recommends that people age 50 and over be screened for colorectal cancer every five years. The screening includes a flexible sigmoidoscopy. Screening at an earlier age should be done on patients who have a family history of colon or **rectal cancer**, or small growths in the colon (polyps).

Individuals with inflammatory bowel disease (Crohn's colitis or ulcerative colitis) are at increased risk for colorectal cancer and should begin their screenings at a younger age, and be screened more frequently. Many doctors screen such patients more often than every three to five years. Those with ulcerative colitis should be screened beginning 10 years after the onset of disease; those with Crohn's colitis beginning 15 years after the onset of disease.

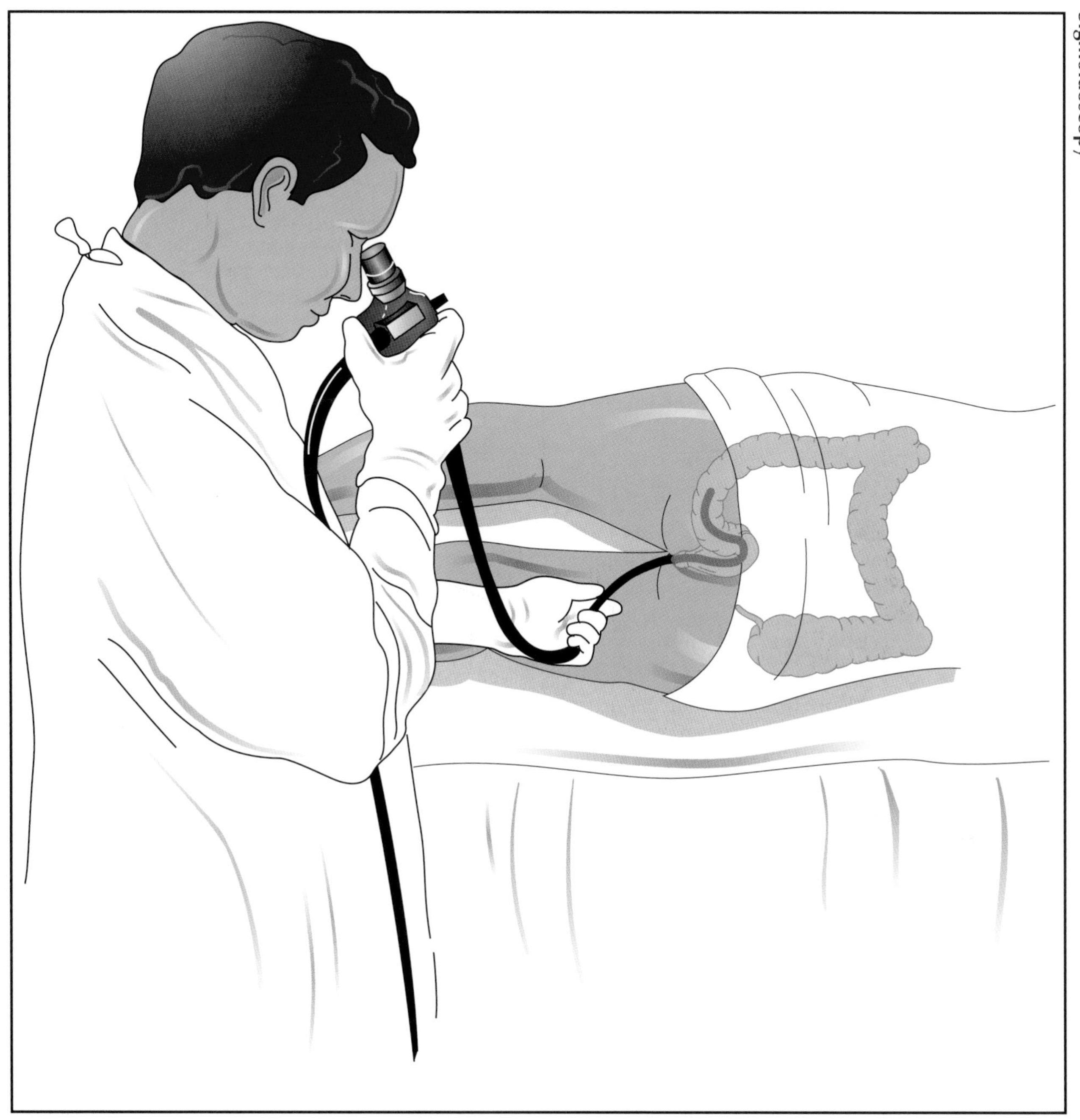

Sigmoidoscopy is a procedure most often used in screening for colorectal cancer and as a test in diagnosis of possible inflammatory bowel disease. As illustrated above, the physician can view the rectum and colon through a sigmoidoscope, a flexible fiber-optic tube which contains a light source and a lens. *(Illustration by Electronic Illustrators Group, Cengage Learning, Gale.)*

Some doctors prefer to do this screening with a colonoscope, which allows them to see the entire colon (certain patients, such as those with Crohn's colitis or ulcerative colitis, must be screened with a colonoscope). However, compared with sigmoidoscopy, **colonoscopy** is a longer process, causes more discomfort, and is more costly.

Studies have indicated that about one-fourth of all precancerous or small cancerous growths in the colorectal region can be seen with a rigid sigmoidoscope. The longer, flexible version, which is the primary type of sigmoidoscope used in the screening process, can detect more than one-half of all growths in this region. This examination is usually performed in combination

QUESTIONS TO ASK THE DOCTOR

- Why do I need a sigmoidoscopy?
- Should I undergo a colonoscopy instead?
- If a biopsy is done, how long before I get the results?
- Will I need to have this test again in the future? When?

KEY TERMS

Biopsy—A procedure where a piece of tissue is removed from a patient for diagnostic testing.

Colorectal cancer—Cancer of the large intestine, or colon and rectum (the last 16 inches of the large intestine before the anus).

Inflammatory bowel disease—Ulcerative colitis or Crohn's colitis; chronic conditions characterized by periods of diarrhea, bloating, abdominal cramps, and pain, sometimes accompanied by weight loss and malnutrition because of the inability to absorb nutrients.

Polyp—A small growth that can be precancerous when it appears in the colon.

with a **fecal occult blood test**, in an effort to increase detection of polyps and cancers that lie beyond the scope's reach.

Precautions

The exam is not always adequate. A 2004 study reported that among older patients and women, sigmoidoscopy is not always effective, particularly because insertion depth is not adequate. For unknown reasons, this is almost twice as true for women as for men.

Sigmoidoscopy can usually be conducted in a doctor's office or a health clinic. However, some individuals should have the procedure done in a hospital day surgery facility. These include patients with rectal bleeding, and patients whose blood does not clot well (possibly as a result of blood-thinning medications).

Description

Most sigmoidoscopy is done with a flexible fiberoptic tube. The tube contains a light source and a camera lens. The doctor moves the sigmoidoscope up beyond the rectum (the first 1 ft/30 cm of the colon), examining the interior walls of the rectum. If a 2 ft/60 cm scope is used, the next portion of the colon can also be examined for any irregularities.

The procedure takes 20 to 30 minutes, during which time the patient will remain awake. Light sedation may be given to some patients. There is some discomfort (usually bloating and cramping) because air is injected into the bowel to widen the passage for the sigmoidoscope. Pain is rare except in individuals with active inflammatory bowel disease.

In a colorectal cancer screening, the doctor is looking for polyps or tumors. Studies have shown that over time, many polyps develop into cancerous lesions and tumors. Using instruments threaded through the fiberoptic tube, cancerous or precancerous polyps can either be removed or biopsied during the sigmoidoscopy. People who have cancerous polyps removed can be referred for full colonoscopy, or more frequent sigmoidoscopy, as necessary.

The doctor may also look for signs of ulcerative colitis, which include a loss of blood flow to the lining of the bowel, a thickening of the lining, and sometimes a discharge of blood and pus mixed with stool. The doctor can also look for Crohn's disease, which often appears as shallow or deep ulcerations, or erosions and fissures in the lining of the colon. In many cases, these signs appear in the first few centimeters of the colon above the rectum, and it is not necessary to do a full colonoscopic exam.

Private insurance plans often cover the cost of sigmoidoscopy for screening in healthy individuals over 50, or for diagnostic purposes. Medicare covers the cost for diagnostic exams, and may cover the costs for screening exams.

Preparation

The purpose of preparation for sigmoidoscopy is to clean the lower bowel of stool so that the doctor can see the lining. Many patients are required to consume only clear liquids on the day before the test, and to take two enemas on the morning of the procedure. The bowel is cleaner, however, if patients also take an oral laxative preparation of 1.5 oz phospho-soda the evening before the sigmoidoscopy.

Certain medications should be avoided for a week before having a sigmoidoscopy. These include:

- apirin, or products containing aspirin
- ibuprofen products (Nuprin, Advil, or Motrin)

- iron or vitamins containing iron

Although most prescription medication can be taken as usual, patients should check with their doctor in advance.

Aftercare

Patients may feel mild cramping after the procedure that will improve after passing gas. Patients can resume their normal activities almost immediately.

Risks

There is a slight risk of bleeding from the procedure. This risk is heightened in individuals whose blood does not clot well, either due to disease or medication, and in those with active inflammatory bowel disease. The most serious complication of sigmoidoscopy is bowel perforation (tear). This complication is very rare, however, occurring only about once in every 7,500 procedures.

Normal results

A normal exam shows a smooth bowel wall with no evidence of inflammation, polyps or tumors.

Abnormal results

For a cancer screening sigmoidoscopy, an abnormal result involves one or more noncancerous or precancerous polyps or tumors. Patients showing polyps have an increased risk of developing colorectal cancer in the future.

Small polyps can be completely removed. Larger polyps or tumors usually require the doctor to remove a portion of the growth for diagnostic testing. Depending on the test results, the patient is then scheduled to have the growth removed surgically, either as an urgent matter if it is cancerous, or as an elective surgery within a few months if it is noncancerous.

In a diagnostic sigmoidoscopy, an abnormal result shows signs of active inflammatory bowel disease, either a thickening of the intestinal lining consistent with ulcerative colitis, or ulcerations or fissures consistent with Crohn's disease.

Resources

PERIODICALS

Manoucheri, Manoucher, et al. "Bowel Preparations for Flexible Sigmoidoscopy: Which Method Yields the Best Results?" *The Journal of Family Practice* 48, no. 4 (April 1999): 272–4.

"Office Procedures—Flexible Sigmoidoscopy." *American Family Physician* 63, no. 7 (2001).

"Women are Twice as Likely as Men to Have an Inadequate Signoidoscopy Examination." *Doctor* February 5, 2004: 13.

OTHER

"Diagnostic Tests." *The National Digestive Diseases Information Clearinghouse (National Institutes of Health).* [cited July 5, 2001]. http://www.niddk.nih.gov/health/digest/pubs/diagtest/index.htm.

Jon H. Zonderman
Teresa G. Odle

Simple mastectomy

Definition

Simple **mastectomy** is the surgical removal of one or both breasts. The adjacent lymph nodes and chest muscles are left intact. If a few lymph nodes are removed, the procedure is called an extended simple mastectomy. Breast-sparing techniques may be used to preserve the patient's breast skin and nipple, which is helpful in cosmetic **breast reconstruction**.

Purpose

Removal of a patient's breast is usually recommended when **cancer** is present in the breast or as a prophylactic when the patient has severe fibrocystic disease and a family history of **breast cancer**. The choice of a simple mastectomy may be determined by evaluating the size of the breast, the size of the cancerous mass, where the cancer is located, and whether any cancer cells have spread to adjacent lymph nodes or other parts of the body. If the cancer has not been contained within the breast, it calls for a **modified radical mastectomy**, which removes the entire breast and all of the adjacent lymph nodes. Only in extreme circumstances is a radical mastectomy, which also removes part of the chest wall, indicated.

A larger tumor usually is an indication of more advanced disease and will require more extensive surgery such as a simple mastectomy. In addition, if a woman has small breasts, the tumor may occupy more area within the contours of the breast, necessitating a simple mastectomy in order to remove all of the cancer.

Very rapidly growing tumors usually require the removal of all breast tissue. Cancers that have spread to adjacent tissues such as the chest wall or skin make simple mastectomy a good choice. Similarly, multiple sites of cancer within a breast require that the entire breast be removed. In addition, simple mastectomy is also recommended when cancer recurs in a breast that has already undergone a **lumpectomy**, which is a less invasive procedure that just removes the tumor and some surrounding tissue without removing the entire breast.

Sometimes, surgeons recommend simple mastectomy for women who are unable to undergo the adjuvant **radiation therapy** required after a lumpectomy. Radiation treatment is not indicated for pregnant women, those who have had previous therapeutic radiation in the chest area, and patients with collagen vascular diseases such as scleroderma or lupus. In these cases, simple mastectomy is the treatment of choice.

Some women with family histories of breast cancer and who test positive for a cancer-causing gene choose to have one or both of their breasts removed as a preventative for future breast cancer. This procedure is highly controversial. Though prophylactic mastectomy reduces the occurrence of breast cancer by 90% in high-risk patients, it is not a foolproof method. There has been some incidence of cancer occurring after both breasts were removed.

Demographics

According to the American Cancer Society in 2003, it was estimated that more than 260,000 new cases of breast cancer in women would occur that year. New cases of breast cancer in men were expected to reach 1,300. Rates of incidence have increased since 1980, due in part to the aging of the population. During the 1990s, breast cancer incidence increased only in women age 50 and over.

For approximately 80% of women, the first indication of cancer is the discovery of a lump in the breast, found either by themselves in a monthly self-exam or by a partner or by a mammogram, a special X-ray of the breast that looks for anomalies. Early detection of breast cancer means that smaller tumors are found, which require less intensive surgery and have better treatment outcomes. Simple mastectomy has been the standard treatment of choice for breast cancer for the past 60 years. Newer breast-conserving surgery techniques have gained acceptance since the mid-1980s. For larger hospitals, facilities in urban areas, and health care institutions with a cancer center or high cancer patient volume, these newer techniques are being utilized at a more rapid rate, especially on the East Coast.

KEY TERMS

Lumpectomy—A less-invasive procedure that just removes the tumor and some surrounding tissue, without removing the entire breast.

Lymphedema—Swelling, usually of the arm after a mastectomy, caused by the accumulation of fluid from faulty drainage in the lymph system.

Mammogram—A special X-ray of the breast that looks for anomalies in the breast.

In 2003, the National Cancer Institute found that American women were 21% more likely to have a mastectomy than their counterparts in the United Kingdom. Though breast-conserving procedures are available and have proven to be viable options, some physicians and women still think breast removal will also remove all of their risk of cancer recurrence. It is clear that treatment options for cancer are highly individual and often emotionally charged.

Description

Simple mastectomy is one of several types of surgical treatments for breast cancer. Some techniques are rarely used; others are quite common. These common surgical procedures include:

- Radical mastectomy. Radical mastectomy is rarely used, and then only in cases where cancer cells have invaded the chest wall and the tumor is very large. The breast, muscles under the breast, and all of the lymph nodes are removed. This produces a large scar and severe disability to the arm nearest the removed breast.
- Modified radical mastectomy. Modified radical mastectomy was the most common form of mastectomy until the 1980s. The breast is removed along with the lining over the chest muscle and all of the lymph nodes.
- Simple mastectomy. Simple, sometimes called total, mastectomy has been the treatment of choice in the late 1980s and 1990s. Generally, only the breast is removed; though, sometimes, one or two lymph nodes may be removed as well.
- Partial mastectomy. Partial mastectomy is used to remove the tumor, the lining over the chest muscle underneath the tumor, and a good portion of breast tissue, but not the entire breast. This is a good treatment choice for early stage cancers.

- Lumpectomy. Lumpectomy or breast-conserving surgery just removes the tumor and a small amount of tissue surrounding it. Some lymph nodes may be removed as well. This is the most commonly used surgical procedure for the treatment of breast cancer in the early twenty-first century.

Two other surgical procedures are variations on the simple mastectomy. The skin-sparing mastectomy is a new surgical procedure in which the surgeon makes an incision, sometimes called a keyhole incision, around the areola. The tumor and all breast tissue are removed, but the incision is smaller and scarring is minimal. About 90% of the skin is preserved and allows a cosmetic surgeon to perform breast reconstruction at the same time as the mastectomy. The subcutaneous mastectomy, or nipple-sparing mastectomy, preserves the skin and the nipple over the breast.

During a simple mastectomy, the surgeon makes a curved incision along one side of the breast and removes the tumor and all of the breast tissue. A few lymph nodes may be removed. The tumor, breast tissue, and any lymph nodes will be sent to the pathology lab for analysis. If the skin is cancer-free, it is sutured in place or used immediately for breast reconstruction. One or two drains will be put in place to remove fluid from the surgical area. Surgery takes from two to five hours; it is longer with breast reconstruction.

Breast reconstruction

Breast reconstruction, especially if it is begun at the same time as the simple mastectomy, can minimize the sense of loss that women feel when having a breast removed. Although there may be other smaller surgeries later to complete the breast reconstruction, there will not be a second major operation nor an additional scar.

If there is not enough skin left after the mastectomy, a balloon-type expander is put in place. In subsequent weeks, the expander is filled with larger amounts of saline (salt water) solution. When it has reached the appropriate size, the expander is removed and a permanent breast implant is installed.

If there is enough skin, an implant is installed immediately. In other instances, skin, fat, and muscle are removed from the patient's back or abdomen and repositioned on the chest wall to form a breast.

None of these reconstructions have nipples at first. Nipples are later reconstructed in a separate surgery. Finally, the areola is tattooed in to make the reconstructed breast look natural.

Breast reconstruction does not prevent a potential recurrence of breast cancer.

Diagnosis/Preparation

If a mammogram has not been performed, it is usually ordered to verify the size of the lump the patient has reported. A **biopsy** of the suspicious lump and/or lymph nodes is usually ordered and sent to the pathology lab before surgery is discussed.

When a simple mastectomy has been determined, preoperative tests such as blood work, a chest X-ray, and an electrocardiogram may be ordered. Blood-thinning medications such as aspirin should be stopped several days before the surgery date. The patient is also asked to refrain from eating or drinking the night before the operation.

At the hospital, the patient will sign a consent form, verifying that the surgeon has explained what the surgery is and what it is for. The patient will also meet with the anesthesiologist to discuss the patient's medical history and determine the choice of anesthesia.

Aftercare

If the procedure is performed as an outpatient surgery, the patient may go home the same day of the surgery. The length of the hospital stay for inpatient mastectomies ranges from one to two days. If breast reconstruction has taken place, the hospital stay may be longer.

The surgical drains will remain in place for five to seven days. Sponge baths will be necessary until the stitches are removed, usually in a week to 10 days. It is important to avoid overhead lifting, strenuous sports, and sexual intercourse for three to six weeks. After the surgical drains are removed, stretching exercises may be begun, though some physical therapists may start a patient on shoulder and arm mobility exercises while in the hospital.

Since breast removal is often emotionally traumatic for women, seeking out a support group is often helpful. Women in these groups offer practical advice about matters such as finding well-fitting bras and swimwear, and emotional support because they have been through the same experience.

For women who chose not to have breast reconstruction, it may be necessary to find the proper fitting breast prosthesis. Some are made of cloth, and others are made of silicone, which are created from a mold from the patient's other breast.

In some case, the patient may be required to undergo additional treatments such as radiation, chemotheraphy, or hormone therapy.

WHO PERFORMS THE PROCEDURE AND WHERE IS IT PERFORMED?

Simple mastectomy is performed by a general surgeon or a gynecological surgeon. If reconstructive breast surgery is to be done, a cosmetic surgeon performs it. Patients undergo simple mastectomies under general anesthesia as an inpatient in a hospital. There is a growing trend, due to reductions in insurance coverage and patient preference, to perform simple mastectomies without reconstructive breast surgery as outpatient procedures.

Risks

The risks involved with simple mastectomy are the same for any major surgery; however, there may be a need for more extensive surgery once the surgeon examines the tumor, the tissues surrounding it, and the lymph nodes nearby. A biopsy of the lymph nodes is usually performed during surgery and a determination is made whether to remove them. Simple mastectomy usually has limited impact on range of motion of the arm nearest the breast that is removed, but physical therapy may still be necessary to restore complete movement.

There is also the risk of **infection** around the incision. When the lymph nodes are removed, lymphedema may also occur. This condition is a result of damage to the lymph system. The arm on the side nearest the affected breast may become swollen. It can either resolve itself or worsen.

As in any surgery, the risk of developing a blood clot after a mastectomy is a serious matter. All hospitals use a variety of techniques to prevent blood clots from forming. It is important for the patient to walk daily when at home.

Finally, there is the risk that not all cancer cells were removed. Further treatment may be necessary.

Normal results

The breast area will fully heal in three to four weeks. If the patient had breast reconstruction, it may take up to six weeks to recover fully. The patient should be able to participate in all of the activities she has engaged in before surgery. If breast reconstruction is done, the patient should realize that the new breast will not have the sensitivity of a normal breast. In addition, dealing with cancer emotionally may take time, especially if additional treatment is necessary.

QUESTIONS TO ASK THE DOCTOR

- Why is this procedure necessary?
- How big is my tumor?
- Are there other breast-saving or less-invasive procedures for which I might be a candidate?
- What can I expect after surgery?
- Do you work with a cosmetic surgeon?
- Will I have to undergo radiation or chemotherapy after surgery?

Morbidity and mortality rates

Deaths due to breast cancer have declined by 1.4% each year between 1989 and 1995, and by 3.2% each year thereafter. The largest decreases have been among younger women, as a result of cancer education campaigns and early screening, which encourages more women to go to their physicians to be checked.

Research performed between 2000 and 2004 demonstrated that the five-year survival rate for cancers confined to the breast is 98%. For cancers that had spread to areas within the chest region, the rate was 83.5%, and it is only 26.7% for cancers occurring in other parts of the body after breast cancer treatment. The best survival rates were for early-stage tumors.

Two 20-year longitudinal studies concluded in 2002 indicated that the survival rate for patients with modified radical mastectomy (the removal of the entire breast and all lymph nodes) was no different from that of breast-conserving lumpectomy (the removal of the tumor alone). These studies suggest that the removal of the entire breast may not afford greater protection against future cancer than breast-conserving techniques; however, the majority of cancer recurrences happen within the first five years for both those with mastectomies and those with lumpectomies.

Alternatives

Skin-sparing mastectomy, also called nipple-sparing mastectomy, is becoming a treatment of choice for women undergoing simple mastectomy. In this procedure, the skin of the breast, the areola, and the nipple are peeled back to remove the breast and its inherent tumor. Biopsies of the skin and nipple areas are performed immediately to assure that they do not have cancer cells in them. Then, a cosmetic surgeon performs a breast reconstruction at the same time as the mastectomy. The breast regains its normal contours once prostheses are inserted. Unfortunately, the nipple will lose its sensitivity and, of course, its function, since all underlying tissue has been removed. If cancer is found near the nipple, this procedure cannot be done.

Resources

BOOKS

Abeloff, M. D., J. Armitage, J. Niederhuber, M. Kastan, and W. G. McKenna. *Clinical Oncology*, 3rd ed. Philadelphia: Elsevier, 2004.

Katz V. L., G. Lentz, R. A. Lobo, and D. Gershenson. *Comprehensive Gynecology*, 5th ed. St. Louis: Mosby, 2007.

Khatri, V. P., and J. A. Asensio. *Operative Surgery Manual*, 1st ed. Philadelphia: Saunders, 2002.

Townsend, C.M., R. D. Beauchamp, B. M. Evers, and K. Mattox. *Sabiston Textbook of Surgery*, 17th ed. Philadelphia: Saunders, 2004.

PERIODICALS

"American Women Still Having Too Many Mastectomies." *Women's Health Weekly* (February 6, 2003): 20.

Jancin, Bruce. "High U.S. Mastectomy Rate Is Cause for Concern." *Family Practice News* 33, no.2 (January 15, 2003): 31.

"Procedure Preserves Natural Appearance after Mastectomy." *AORN Journal* 77, no.1 (January 2003): 213.

Zepf, Bill. "Mastectomy vs. Less Invasive Surgery for Breast Cancer." *American Family Physician* 67, no.3 (February 1, 2003): 587.

ORGANIZATIONS

American Cancer Society, 1875 Connecticut Avenue, NW, Suite 730, Washington, DC, 20009, (800) ACS-2345, http://www.cancer.org.

American Society of Plastic Surgeons, 444 E. Algonquin Rd., Arlington Heights, IL, 60005, (847) 228-9900, http://www.plasticsurgery.org.

National Cancer Institute, 6116 Executive Boulevard, MSC8322, Suite 3036A, Bethesda, MD, 20892-8322, (800) 422-6237, http://www.cancer.gov.

Janie Franz

Sirolimus

Definition

Sirolimus is indicated by the Food and Drug Administration (FDA) to be used after a kidney transplant to prevent the body from rejecting the new kidney. Sirolimus may also have a role in prevention of organ rejection in heart or lung transplantation, and prevention of graft-versus-host disease in patients undergoing **bone marrow transplantation**. Sirolimus (formerly known as rapamycin) became available at the end of 1999 and is marketed under the brand name Rapamune by Wyeth-Ayerst Laboratories.

KEY TERMS

Immune system—The body's mechanism to fight infections, toxic substances, and to recognize and neutralize or eliminate foreign material (for example, a body organ transplanted from another person).

Immunosuppressant—An agent that decreases activity of immune system (for example, radiation or drugs).

Lymphocele—A mass surrounded by an abnormal sac that contains lymph (fluid that is collected from tissues throughout the body) from diseased or injured lymphatic channels.

Lymphoma—Any malignant (cancerous) disorder of lymphoid tissue.

Steroids—Drugs such as prednisone or dexamethasone, which resemble body's natural hormones and are often used to decrease inflammation or to suppress activity of immune system.

Transplant—Tissue transferred from one part of the body to another or from one person to another.

Description

Sirolimus belongs to a class of macrolide **antibiotics** and is isolated from an organism named *streptomyces hygriscopicus*.

Sirolimus prevents the immune system from attacking the transplanted organ by decreasing the growth of certain chemicals in the body responsible for the immune function (B and T lymphocytes). Sirolimus works differently from other immunosuppressants used to prevent organ rejection after transplantation (**azathioprine**, **mycophenolate mofetil**, **tacrolimus**, **cyclosporine**, and steroids). It should be given in combination with cyclosporine and steroids to prevent acute rejection of a transplanted kidney. This drug is available as a tablet and a liquid and can be used in children and adults.

Recommended dosage

Adults

KIDNEY TRANSPLANTATION. The first dose of 3 tablets (2 mg each) or 6 milliliters of oral solution should be given as soon as possible after a kidney is transplanted. Then, a maintenance dose of 2 mg should be given once a day.

Children over 13 years of age and Adults less than 40 kg (88 lbs)

KIDNEY TRANSPLANTATION. 3 mg of sirolimus per square meter of body surface area on day 1 after transplantation, followed by a maintenance dose of 1 mg per square meter per day.

Children less than 13 years of age

Check with a physician.

Administration

Sirolimus should be administered in combination with cyclosporine and steroids. To decrease the risk of side effects, sirolimus should be given four hours after cyclosporine. To avoid variations in blood levels, sirolimus should be taken consistently— either always with food or always without food. Sirolimus oral solution should only be mixed with water or orange juice and consumed immediately. Juices or liquids other than water or orange juice should not be used to mix sirolimus. Bottled sirolimus solution should be stored in the refrigerator, but not frozen. Refrigerated sirolimus solution may develop a slight haze. If haze is noticed, the drug should be left at room temperature and gently shaken until haze disappears. If a dose is missed, it should taken as soon as possible unless it is almost time for the next dose. Two doses at the same time should not be taken.

Precautions

Sirolimus may increase the risk of the following conditions:

- infections caused by viruses and bacteria
- lymphoma or skin cancer
- elevated blood lipids (cholesterol and triglycerides)
- decreased kidney function
- lymphocele formation after a kidney transplantation

Patients with the following conditions should use sirolimus with caution:

- an allergic reaction to tacrolimus (has a similar structure to sirolimus)
- liver disease (dose of sirolimus may need to be decreased)
- treatment with medications that are broken down in the liver and that may interact with sirolimus
- Pregnancy. These patients should use an effective method of birth control started before therapy with sirolimus and continued for 12 weeks after stopping this medication.

Patients should immediately alert their doctor if any of these symptoms develop:

- fever, chills, sore throat
- fast heartbeat
- trouble breathing
- unusual bleeding or bruising

Sirolimus should be taken consistently with regard to meals (either always taken with food or always taken on an empty stomach) and at least four hours after cyclosporine to decrease variability of blood sirolimus levels. Patients should avoid grapefruit or grapefruit juice because it may increase sirolimus levels in the blood. Those taking sirolimus will need to see a physician regularly to check blood and urine.

Side effects

The most common side effects include mild dose-related risk of bleeding, elevated blood cholesterol and triglyceride values, decreased kidney function, high blood pressure, **diarrhea** or constipation, rash, acne, joint pain, **nausea**, **vomiting**, stomachache, and decreased blood potassium and phosphate values. Sirolimus can decrease the number of red blood cells, which can cause a patient to look pale, feel tired, short of breath, and drowsy, and experience heart palpitations. People who are allergic to tacrolimus may develop an allergy when taking sirolimus.

Interactions

Sirolimus is broken down in the liver by the same enzyme system that also breaks down cyclosporine and tacrolimus. Because cyclosporine can increase sirolimus blood levels, sirolimus should be given four hours after the morning cyclosporine dose to decrease the risk of side effects. Diltiazem (Cardizem, Tiazac, Dilacor) and ketoconazole (Nizoral) can increase sirolimus blood levels. The use of ketoconazole should be avoided in patients taking sirolimus. Other drugs that are likely to increase sirolimus blood levels and increase its side effects include calcium channel blockers (used to treat high blood pressure), drugs that treat fungal infections (ketoconazole, itraconazole, fluconazole), macrolide antibiotics (erythromycin, clarithromycin), and anti-HIV drugs (ritonavir, nelfinavir, indinavir). Rifampin can greatly decrease sirolimus blood levels, potentially making it less effective. Other drugs that may decrease effectiveness of sirolimus include phenobarbital, **carbamazepine**, rifabutin, and **phenytoin**. Anyone who is taking these drugs should ask their physician if they could safely take sirolimus.

Olga Bessmertny, Pharm.D.

Sjögren's syndrome

Description

Sjögren's syndrome (SS) is an autoimmune disease, which means that the immune system has mounted an attack against specific tissues of the body. For example, most patients with Sjögren's syndrome carry antibodies to molecules found in the nucleus of cells (antinuclear antibodies). Although Sjögren's syndrome can affect practically any organ in the body, it is characterized by dry mouth (**xerostomia**) and dry eyes (xerophthalmia). These hallmark symptoms are known as "sicca symptoms." Sjögren's syndrome goes by many names which include Sjögren's disease, dry-mouth and dry-eyes disease, sicca complex, and sicca syndrome. The disorder is named for Henrik Sjögren, a Swedish ophthalmologist.

Symptoms of Sjögren's syndrome include dry mouth, difficulty or inability to swallow (dysphagia), tooth decay (dental caries), impaired taste and smell, dry eyes, eye pain, eye redness, muscle pain (myalgia), and **fatigue**. Many patients develop a variety of skin problems that include dry patches, vasculitis, and cutaneous B-cell **lymphoma**. Other less common symptoms include **diarrhea**, headaches, joint pain (arthralgia), muscle weakness, hair loss (**alopecia**), and dry cough. About 33% of patients develop arthritis. Patients with **cancer** of lymphoid tissue (lymphoma) and Sjögren's syndrome have **fever**, nerve involvement, low numbers of red blood cells (**anemia**) and white blood cells (lymphopenia), inflammation of blood vessels of the skin (skin vasculitis), and disease of the lymph nodes (lymphadenopathy) much more frequently than patients with Sjögren's syndrome alone.

The symptoms of Sjögren's syndrome can have a pronounced effect on quality of life. Besides causing discomfort, the symptoms also disrupt sleep, which can have side effects such as fatigue, difficulty concentrating, and **depression**. Patients with Sjögren's syndrome are at risk for tooth decay and yeast infections in the mouth (erythematous candidiasis). Approximately 5% of the patients with Sjögren's syndrome develop malignant lymphoma.

SS is found in all races and ethnic groups. It is thought to affect between 0.1% and 3% of the population in the United States; this range reflects the lack of a uniform set of diagnostic criteria. According to the American College of Rheumatology, between 1 million and 4 million Americans have Sjögren's syndrome.

Causes

The cause of Sjögren's syndrome is unknown, although several viruses are suspected triggers of the autoimmune reaction. In 2004 a team of researchers in Greece presented evidence that a coxsackievirus may be the cause of SS. The sicca symptoms of Sjögren's syndrome are caused by the invasion and multiplication of white blood cells (lymphocytes) into the salivary glands and tear glands. The lymphocytes destroy the gland tissue and cause the glands to malfunction, reducing the production of tears and saliva. This invasion by lymphocytes, however, does not fully account for the sicca symptoms. Other, as yet unidentified, factors play a role in the development of the sicca symptoms.

Sjögren's syndrome can occur in combination with certain cancers. For more than half of the patients with non-Hodgkin lymphoma, the lymphoma is located in the salivary glands, causing them to malfunction. **Graft-vs.-host disease** in patients who have undergone **bone marrow transplantation** can cause eye problems similar to those seen in Sjögren's syndrome. Both **chemotherapy** and **radiation therapy** to the head and neck can cause xerostomia.

Treatments

There is no cure for Sjögren's syndrome. Therefore, treatment is aimed at relieving symptoms. Dry eyes may be treated with eye drops and avoidance of drying conditions such as wind, hair dryers, and medications that cause dry eyes (e.g. tricyclic antidepressants). Eyeglasses may protect the eyes from wind. The lower tear ducts may be blocked with silicone plugs (punctal occlusion) to conserve natural tears. Use of humidifiers, both at home and at work, can significantly reduce sicca symptoms. Saliva substitutes and sugar-free hard candies or chewing gum, which stimulate salivation, can reduce sicca symptoms. The drugs **pilocarpine** (Salagen) and cevimeline (Evoxac) can increase salivation. Cevimeline also has been found effective in relieving the symptom of dry eye in SS as well. Pain may be relieved by nonsteroidal anti- inflammatory drugs (e.g. Aleve) or other pain medications.

The patient with Sjögren's syndrome should faithfully conduct routine daily oral hygiene consisting of tooth brushing two to three times, flossing once, and utilizing medicated rinses as prescribed by the physician. Fluoride varnishes applied by a dentist and nightly fluoride treatments can help to prevent dental caries. Brushing and flossing should be performed carefully to prevent damage to the weakened oral mucosa.

Alternative and complementary therapies

In a controlled clinical study, the herbal vitamin supplement LongoVital was shown to increase the rate of salivation. Sicca symptoms may be reduced by acupuncture. Papayas contain papain, which is an enzyme that breaks up proteins. Eating papayas, drinking papaya juice, or drinking a solution of crushed papain tablets in water can liquefy thick saliva. Drinking a solution of meat tenderizer (which contains papain) in water is another alternative.

Resources

BOOKS

Beers, Mark H., MD, and Robert Berkow, MD, editors. "Diffuse Connective Tissue Disease." Section 5, Chapter 50 In*The Merck Manual of Diagnosis and Therapy*. Whitehouse Station, NJ: Merck Research Laboratories, 2002.

Iwamoto, Ryan R. "Xerostomia." In *Cancer Symptom Management*, edited by Connie H. Yarbro, Margaret H. Frogge, and Michelle Goodman, 2nd ed. Sudbury, MA: Jones and Bartlett Publishers, 1999.

PERIODICALS

Bell, Mary, et al. "Sjögren's Syndrome: A Critical Review of Clinical Management." *The Journal of Rheumatology* 26, no. 9 (2001): 2051–2059.

Daniels, Troy E. "Evaluation, Differential Diagnosis, and Treatment of Xerostomia." *Current Opinion in Rheumatology* 27 (2001): 6–9.

Fox, Robert I., and Paul Michelson. "Approaches to the Treatment of Sjögren's Syndrome." *Current Opinion in Rheumatology* 27 (2000): 15–20.

Fox, Robert I. "Update in Sjögren Syndrome." *Current Opinion in Rheumatology* 12 (2000): 391–398.

Francis, Mark L., MD. "Sjogren Syndrome." *eMedicine* July 1, 2004. <http://emedicine.com/med/topic2136.htm>.

Ono, M., E. Takamura, K. Shinozaki, et al. "Therapeutic Effect of Cevimeline on Dry Eye in Patients with Sjögren's Syndrome: A Randomized, Double-Blind Clinical Study." *American Journal of Ophthalmology* 138 (July 2004): 6–17.

Roguedas, A. M., L. Misery, B. Sassolas, et al. "Cutaneous Manifestations of Primary Sjögren's Syndrome Are Underestimated." *Clinical and Experimental Rheumatology* 22 (September-October 2004): 632–636.

Stevenson, H. A., M. E. Jones, J. L. Rostron, et al. "UK Patients with Primary Sjögren's Syndrome Are at Increased Risk from Clinical Depression." *Gerodontology* 21 (September 2004): 141–145.

Triantafyllopoulou, A., N. Tapinos, and H. M. Moutsopoulos. "Evidence for Coxsackievirus Infection in Primary Sjögren's Syndrome." *Arthritis and Rheumatism* 50 (September 2004): 2897–2902.

OTHER

American College of Rheumatology Fact Sheet. "Sjögren's Syndrome." http://www.rheumatology.org/public/factsheets/sjogrens_new.asp?aud = pat.

MGH Virtual Brain Tumor Center. [cited June 22, 2001]. <http://brain.mgh.harvard.edu>.

ORGANIZATIONS

American College of Rheumatology. 1800 Century Place, Suite 250, Atlanta, GA 30345-4300. (404) 633-3777. Fax: (404) 633-1870. http://www.rheumatology.org.

Sjögren's Syndrome Foundation, Inc. 8120 Woodmont Avenue, Bethesda, MD 20814. (800) 475-6473. Fax: (301) 718-0322.http://www.sjogrens.org.

Belinda Rowland, Ph.D.
Rebecca J. Frey, PhD

Skin cancer

Definition

Skin **cancer** refers to abnormal cells of the skin that grow uncontrollably. If untreated these cells can grow deeper into the skin and invade other tissues. There are three main types of skin cancer: **basal cell carcinoma**, squamous cell **carcinoma** and **melanoma**. All three types are related to excessive sun exposure.

Demographics

Cancer of the skin is the most common type of cancer among all of the cancer types. Skin cancers account for as much as 50% of all cases of cancer. The estimated incidence of basal skin cancer is between 800,000 to 900,000 new cases per year while between 200,000 and 300,000 new cases of squamous cell skin cancers are diagnosed each year.

It is estimated that there will be 68,720 new melanomas cases will be diagnosed and 8,650 deaths will occur in the U.S. due to melanoma in 2009.

The incidence of skin cancers continues to rise. This increase is attributed to better detection practices, increased exposure to the ultraviolet radiation in sunlight, and to the increasing age of the general population.

Deaths from skin cancers are relatively uncommon with about 2,000 deaths occurring from non-melanoma type skin cancers each year. Despite increasing incidence rates of skin cancer, deaths from skin cancers have continued to decline over the last three decades.

Description

Cancer which is also called a neoplasm, carcinoma or malignancy is a group of diseases where abnormal cells continuously grow out of control. These cells can spread to other organs and if not controlled can result in death. Skin cancer is the most common type of cancer but certainly not the most fatal. Although skin cancer most often occurs on areas of the skin that are exposed to sunlight, this is not always the case.

There are three main types of skin cancer; melanoma, basal cell cancer and squamous cell cancer. Each develops from a different cell type of the skin's epidermal layer. Basal cell carcinoma and squamous cell carcinoma are the most common and most treatable if they are found early. Melanoma is a more serious form of skin cancer affecting deeper layers of the skin and has a higher potential to spread to other parts of the body.

Basal cell cancer is the most common type of skin cancer, accounting for about 80% of all skin cancers. It develops from cells of the lowest layer of the epidermis, the basal cells. These are the cells which produce new skin cells. It occurs primarily on the parts of the skin exposed to the sun and is most common in people living in equatorial regions or areas of high ozone depletion. Light-skinned people are at greater risk of developing basal cell cancer than dark-skinned people. Basal cell cancer grows very slowly; however if it is not treated it can invade deeper skin layers causing extensive damage and can be fatal. This type of cancer can appear as a shiny, translucent nodule on the skin or as a red, wrinkled and scaly area.

Squamous cell cancer is the second most frequent type of skin cancer. It arises from the outer keratinizing layer of skin just below the surface. Squamous cell cancer grows faster than basal cell cancer and is more likely to metastasize to the lymph nodes as well as to distant sites. Squamous cell cancer most often appears on the arms, head, and neck. Fair-skinned people of Celtic descent are at high risk for developing squamous cell cancer. This type of cancer is rarely life-threatening but can cause serious problems if it spreads and can also cause disfigurement. Squamous cell cancer usually appears as a scaly, slightly elevated area of damaged skin. Squamous cell cancer can spear in an area of chronic inflammation on the skin.

Malignant melanoma is the most serious type of skin cancer. It develops from the melanocytes or pigment producing cells of the skin. These cells are found in the lower part of the epidermis. Melanocytes are stimulated by the sun to produce more melanin or pigment. It is this pigment that protects skin cells from sun damage and explains why darker skinned persons have a lower risk of melanoma. Although melanoma is the least common skin cancer, it is the most aggressive. It spreads (metastasizes) to other parts of the body– especially the lungs and liver– as well as invading surrounding tissues. Melanomas in their early stages resemble moles. In Caucasians, melanomas appear most often on the trunk, head, and neck in men and on the arms and legs in women. Melanomas in African Americans, however, occur primarily on the palms of the hand, soles of the feet, and under the nails. Melanomas appear only rarely in the eyes, mouth, vagina, or digestive tract. Although melanomas are associated with exposure to the sun, the greatest risk factor for developing melanoma might be genetic. People who have a first-degree relative with melanoma have an increased risk up to eight times greater of developing the disease.

Besides the three major types of skin cancer, there are a few other less common forms of skin cancer as well as some precancerous skin lesions.

- Kaposi's sarcoma (KS) occurs primarily in people whose immune system is depressed, such as AIDS patients, or those who have had organ transplants. When KS occurs with AIDS it is usually more aggressive.
- Merkel cell carcinoma is a rare skin cancer usually found on sun-exposed areas. Merkel cell carcinoma grows more rapidly than basal and squamous cell carcinomas and can spread.
- Sebaceous gland carcinoma is an aggressive cancer that begins in the oil glands of the skin. They are hard, painless nodules that can develop anywhere, but most often on the eyelid.

Precancerous skin lesions include:

- Actinic keratosis or AK is also known as solar keratosis. It appears as rough, scaly patches that are red, pink or brown. They appear most often on the face, ears, lower arms and hands. This condition is not cancer but may develop into squamous cell carcinoma.
- Leukoplakia occurs inside the mouth as white patches. It is related to constant irritation as might

be caused by smoking, rough edges on teeth, dentures or fillings.

- Actinic chelitis is a type of actinic keratosis or leukoplakia that occurs on the lips.
- Bowen disease. This is a type of skin inflammation (dermatitis) that sometimes looks like squamous cell cancer. This may be a superficial type of squamous cell carcinoma that appears as a persistent, scaly patch. It can resemble eczema or psoriasis.
- Keratoacanthoma is a dome-shaped tumor that can grow quickly and appear like squamous cell cancer. Although it is usually benign, it should be removed.

Risk factors for skin cancer include the following

- Excessive exposure to ultraviolet light or a history of sunburns. Severe sunburns as a child increases the risk for skin cancer later in life.
- Having fair skin or less pigmentation in the skin.
- A family history of skin cancer or a personal history of previously having skin cancer.
- Exposure to certain environmental chemicals including arsenic, pitch, creosote, radium or coal tar.
- Age—skin cancer takes years to develop and is more common with age. The sunburn you get as a teen can increase your risk of skin cancer when you are 40.
- A weakened immune system due to HIV/AIDS, leukemia, or drugs that suppress the immune system.
- Having a high number of moles on the body; more than 100.

The biggest risk for skin cancer is excessive exposure to the sun and getting sunburned. The risk of skin cancer is also hereditary, with the risk increasing with a first degree relative having the disease. Those who are fair skinned are more at risk. Age is also a risk factor as skin cancers tend to take years to develop they rarely appear before age 30 or 40. Melanoma is 10 times more likely to occur in whites than in African Americans. People having a high number of moles on their body are also at higher risk.

Frequent use of tanning beds and tanning booths has been linked to the development of skin cancer. Women who use tanning beds or booths more frequently than once per month are at greatest risk and are 55% more likely to develop malignant melanoma. Risk is greatest for individuals who are fair-skinned, who have blonde or red hair, and who have blue, green or gray-colored eyes. People who burn easily after sun exposure, those who have previously been treated for skin cancer and individuals with a family member diagnosed with skin cancer are at greater risk for the development of skin cancer after using tanning beds or booths.

Exposure to toxic chemicals such as arsenic, tar, coal, paraffin and certain types of oil can increase the risk of **non-melanoma skin cancer**. **Radiation therapy** used for cancer as well as drugs used to treat psoriasis can also increase the risk of non-melanoma skin cancer. Skin cancer most often develops on areas of the skin that are exposed to the sun. The most common locations are the scalp, face, lips, ears, neck, chest, arms and hands. It can however also occur on areas that do not see much light such as the palms, between the toes and the genital area.

Causes and symptoms

All three main types of skin cancer are related to excessive sun exposure. Ultraviolet light from the sun damages the DNA found in the cells. This damage to the DNA causes changes in the cell that can lead to increased and out of control growth. Although it was once thought that only UVB rays were responsible for the DNA damage that leads to cancer we now know it is both UVA and UVB rays. Since tanning beds deliver high levels of UVA, they can put people at significant risk for the development of skin cancer.

Basal cell carcinoma appears as a pearly or waxy bump or a flat, flesh colored or brown mark. It is difficult to distinguish this type of mark from a normal mole without performing a **biopsy**. A basal cell carcinoma can take months or years before it becomes sizable. Squamous cell carcinoma can appear as a firm, red nodule or a flat mark with scaly, crusted surface.

Melanoma, the most serious of the skin cancers, appears as a large brownish spot. This spot can change in color or size or have an irregular border. It can also appear as a shiny, firm, dome-shaped bump. Melanomas can vary greatly in their appearance, but often the first sign is a change in a mole. Early detection of melanoma is important for successful treatment.

Kaposi **sarcoma** appears as red or purple patches on the skin or mucous membranes. This type of cancer tends to be more common in people with immune suppression such as those with AIDS or who have undergone organ transplants.

It used to be the ABCD rule was used as a guide for examining moles. Recently, the American Cancer Society added E to their visual grading system. This ABCDE system provides an easy way to remember the important characteristics of moles when one is examining the skin:

- Asymmetry. A normal mole is round, whereas a suspicious mole is unevenly shaped.
- Border. A normal mole has a clear-cut border with the surrounding skin, whereas the edges of a suspect mole are often irregular or scalloped.
- Color. Normal moles are uniformly tan or brown, but cancerous moles may appear as mixtures of red, white, blue, brown, purple, or black.
- Diameter. Normal moles are usually less than 5 millimeters in diameter. A skin lesion greater than 1/4 inch across may be suspected as cancerous.
- Evolving. A mole that changes over time in color or shape or develops itchiness or bleeding can be suspect.

Diagnosis

Examination

A person who finds a suspicious-looking mole, a change in the appearance or texture of a mole, new areas of skin growth or a bothersome area of skin should consult a physician. As with many cancers, early detection and treatment is important in increasing the chances of treating the cancer successfully. A physician can do a thorough inspection of the skin, noting any suspicious looking areas. If any suspect areas are found, the patient's primary care physician will most likely refer him or her to a physician who specializes in skin diseases (a dermatologist).

Procedures

A proper diagnosis of skin cancer requires that a biopsy or a small sample of skin be taken and analyzed by a lab. The skin sample is often done in the physician's office under local anesthesia.

If cancer is present, the stage of the cancer is then determined. This is a rating of how advanced the cancer is and will help determine the appropriate treatment for the cancer. Stages include stage 0, stage I, stage II, stage III, and stage IV, often with substages as well. Each stage represents a progressively larger sized tumor. Stage 0 refers to a precancerous lesion of suspicious cells and stage IV refers to a more severe tumor that has spread to other parts of the body.

Treatment

Treatment depends upon the type of cancer and the severity. Basal cell carcinoma is fairly easy to treat when detected early as is squamous cell. There are four main types of treatment for skin cancer. They include surgery, radiation therapy, **chemotherapy** and **photodynamic therapy**. There are always new types of treatment being tested in **clinical trials**. One new type is biologic therapy which stimulates the patient's immune system to remove the cancer.

Surgery is often the best choice if the tumor is localized and easily removable. There are several different surgical procedures used. Excision surgery involves using a scalpel cutting around the tumor to remove it from the skin. This can also be done by shaving the tumor off the surface of the skin. Mohs micrographic surgery involves taking the skin lesion off in small sections and immediately examining it in the microscope to see when the surgery has gone deep enough to remove the cancerous cells. Mohs micrographic surgery has the highest cure rates of all surgical treatments for basal skin cancers with a 96% cure rate. It is a more time consuming surgery though and not always available. Cryosurgery freezes and destroys the tumor cells. Laser surgery uses a laser beam to cut the skin to remove the tumor. Dermabrasion removes the upper layer of skin and can be used for very small superficial tumors.

Radiation therapy uses high energy **x rays** directed towards the tumor to kill cancer cells. It is often used for cancers that occur on the face or ears where **reconstructive surgery** would be difficult.

Chemotherapy refers to drugs taken internally either by injection or orally that travel through the bloodstream. Chemotherapy is intended to either stop the growth of cancer cells or to kill the cancer cells. Chemotherapy often has rather serious side effects as it affects other cells in the body besides the cancer cells. Occasionally, for non-melanoma skin cancers, the chemotherapy drug 5-FU can be delivered in a cream form to use topically.

Photodynamic therapy uses both a drug and a laser to kill cancer cells. The drug is a photosensitizer which becomes active only after light of a specific wavelength from the laser contacts it. This allows more control over preventing damage to healthy tissue. Photodynamic therapy is relatively new and not always available.

Prognosis

Prognosis depends upon the type of cancer and its severity. Skin cancer is the most common type of cancer in the United States but accounts for less than 1% of cancer deaths. Basal cell carcinoma is fairly easy to treat when caught early. Squamous cell carcinoma also is not usually serious and can be 100% treatable if caught early. If not detected and diagnosed in early stages, skin cancer can be more difficult to treat and treatment for the cancer can result in some disfigurement.

QUESTIONS TO ASK YOUR DOCTOR

- What type of skin cancer do I have?
- What are my various treatment options?
- Are there any clinical trials that would be relevant for my type of cancer?
- What is your experience in treating this type of cancer?
- What stage or how advanced is my cancer?
- What is the goal of treatment, to eradicate the cancer or to alleviate symptoms?
- Should I go to a specialized cancer center?

A small number of squamous cell carcinomas can spread to other organs.

Melanoma is a more serious type of skin cancer, however, if it is caught early is still curable. Melanoma is the most likely skin cancer to spread to other parts of the body which worsens the prognosis. According to the American Cancer Society, for stage I melanoma, the 5-year survival rates range from 92 to 99%. The 5-year survival rate for stage II melanomas is from 56-78%. The 5-year survival rate for stage III melanoma decreases to 50-68% and for stage IV melanoma, 5-year survival drops to 18%. Patients over the age of 70 typically have 5-year survival rates on the lower side.

Prevention

There are many interventions to decrease risk for skin cancer such as avoid prolonged exposure to the sun and minimizing risk for sunburn. Recently, there has been some controversy in the area of sun exposure and cancer. Although there is a definite relationship to excessive sun exposure and skin cancer, the risk of sensible exposure to the sun may have been over exaggerated. Exposure to sunlight is necessary for our bodies to make vitamin D and vitamin D deficiencies have been increasing recently, putting people at risk of vitamin D deficiency diseases. Vitamin D has also been found to decrease the rate of several types of cancer. There is also some evidence that certain sunscreen ingredients may actually contribute to cancer risks. However, recommendations are still to prevent overexposure to the sun.

- Wear protective clothing (long sleeves and hat) while in the sun.
- Use sunscreen of at least 15 SPF when outside.
- Avoid being outside when the sun is brightest, between 10 a.m. and 4 p.m.
- Avoid tanning beds and booths.
- Check your skin periodically for abnormal moles. The American Academy of Dermatologists recommends doing this on your birthday: "Check your birthday suit on your birthday." Although this will not prevent skin cancer, early detection improves prognosis.

See also Basal cell Carcinoma; Bowen's disease; Melanoma; Meckel cell carcinoma

Resources

PERIODICALS

Holick, M.F., Sunlight and vitamin D for bone health and prevention of autoimmune diseases, cancers, and cardiovascular disease. Am. Journ. Clin. Nutr. 2004; 80:1678S-1688S. http://www.ajcn.org/cgi/content/full/80/6/1678S

Moan, J., Porojnicu, A.C., Dahlback, A., Setlow, R.B., Addressing the health benefits and risks, involving vitamin D or skin cancer, or increased sun exposure. PNAS 2008; 105: http://www.pnas.org/cgi/reprint/0710615105v1

van der Pols, J.C., Williams, G.M., & Pandeya, N., etal. "Prolonged Exposure of Squamous Cell Carcinoma of the Skin by Regular Sunscreen Use."*Cancer Epidemiol Biomarkers Prev*.2006, 15(2):2546–8.

OTHER

National Cancer Institute http://www.cancer.gov/cancertopics/pdq/treatment/skin/Patient/page3. 1/04/2008 [cited September 20, 2009].

National Cancer Institute http://www.cancer.gov/cancertopics/pdq/prevention/skin/healthprofessionals.

ORGANIZATIONS

American Cancer Society, 1-800-ACS-2345, http://www.cancer.org.

Skin Cancer Foundation, 149 Madison Avenue, Suite 901, New York, NY, 10016, 1-212-725-5176, http://www.skincancer.org.

Cindy L. Jones, Ph.D.
Melinda Granger Oberleitner, R.N., D.N.S., A.P.R.N., C.N.S.

Skin cancer, non-melanoma

Definition

Non-melanoma **skin cancer** is a malignant growth of the external surface or epithelial layer of the skin. The main types of non-melanoma skin **cancer** are basal cell and squamous cell carcinomas of the skin.

Demographics

Cancer of the skin is the most common type of cancer among all of the cancer types. Skin cancers account for as much as 50% of all cases of cancer. The estimated incidence of basal skin cancer is between 800,000 to 900,000 new cases per year while between 200,000 and 300,000 new cases of squamous cell skin cancers are diagnosed in the United States each year.

The incidence of skin cancers continues to rise. This increase is attributed to better detection practices, increased exposure to the ultraviolet radiation in sunlight, and to the increasing age of the general population.

Deaths from skin cancers are relatively uncommon with about 2,000 deaths occurring from non-melanoma type skin cancers each year. Despite increasing incidence rates of skin cancer, deaths from skin cancers have continued to decline over the last three decades.

Description

Skin cancer is the growth of abnormal cells capable of invading and destroying other associated skin cells. Skin cancer is often subdivided into either **melanoma** or non-melanoma. Melanoma is a dark-pigmented, usually malignant tumor arising from a skin cell capable of making the pigment melanin (a melanocyte). Non-melanoma skin cancer most often originates from the external skin surface as a squamous cell **carcinoma** or a **basal cell carcinoma**.

The cells of a cancerous growth originate from a single cell that reproduces uncontrollably, resulting in the formation of a tumor. Exposure to sunlight is documented as the main cause of more than 1 million cases of non-melanoma skin cancer diagnosed each year in the United States. The incidence increases for those living where direct sunshine is plentiful, such as near the equator.

Basal cell carcinoma affects the skin's basal layer and has the potential to grow progressively larger in size, although it rarely spreads to distant areas (metastasizes). Basal cell carcinoma accounts for 80% of skin cancers (excluding melanoma), whereas squamous cell cancer makes up about 20%. Squamous cell carcinoma is a malignant growth of the external surface of the skin. Squamous cell cancers metastasize at a rate of 2–6%, with up to 10% of lesions affecting the ear and lip.

Risk factors

Risk factors for skin cancer include the following:

- Excessive exposure to ultraviolet light or a history of sunburns. Severe sunburns as a child increases the risk for skin cancer later in life.
- Having fair skin or less pigmentation in the skin.
- A family history of skin cancer or a personal history of previously having skin cancer.
- Exposure to certain environmental chemicals including arsenic, pitch, creosote, radium or coal tar.
- Age—skin cancer often takes years to develop and is more common with age. The sunburn you get as a teen can increase your risk of skin cancer when you are 40.
- A weakened immune system due to HIV/AIDS, leukemia, or drugs that suppress the immune system.
- Having a high number of moles on the body; more than 100.

The biggest risk for skin cancer is excessive exposure to the sun and getting sunburned. The risk of skin cancer is also hereditary, with the risk increasing with a first degree relative having the disease. Those who are fair skinned are more at risk. Age is also a risk factor as skin cancers tend to take years to develop; they rarely appear before age 30 or 40.

Exposure to toxic chemicals such as arsenic, tar, coal, paraffin and certain types of oil can increase the risk of non-melanoma skin cancer. **Radiation therapy** used for cancer as well as drugs used to treat psoriasis can also increase the risk of non-melanoma skin cancer. Skin cancer most often develops on areas of the skin that are exposed to the sun. The most common locations are the scalp, face, lips, ears, neck, chest, arms and hands. It can however also occur on areas that do not see much light such as the palms, between the toes and the genital area.

Causes and symptoms

Cumulative sun exposure is considered a significant risk factor for non-melanoma skin cancer. There is evidence suggesting that early, intense exposure causing blistering sunburn in childhood may also play an important role in the cause of non-melanoma skin cancer. Basal cell carcinoma most frequently affects the skin of the face, with the next most common sites being the ears, the backs of the hands, the shoulders, and the arms. It is prevalent in both sexes and most commonly occurs in people over 40.

About 1–2% of all skin cancers develop within burn scars; squamous cell carcinomas account for about 95% of these cancers, with 3% being basal cell carcinomas and the remainder malignant melanomas.

Basal cell carcinomas usually appear as small skin lesions that persist for at least three weeks. This form of non-melanomatous skin cancer looks flat and waxy, with the edges of the lesion translucent and rounded. The edges also contain small fresh blood vessels. An ulcer in the center of the lesion gives it a dimpled appearance. Basal cell carcinoma lesions vary from 4–6mm in size, but can slowly grow larger if untreated.

Squamous cell carcinoma also involves skin exposed to the sun, such as the face, ears, hands, or arms. This form of non-melanoma is also most common among people over 40. Squamous cell carcinoma presents itself as a small, scaling, raised bump on the skin with a crusting ulcer in the center, but without pain and **itching**.

Basal cell and squamous cell carcinomas can grow more easily when people have a suppressed immune system because they are taking immunosuppressive drugs or are exposed to radiation. Some people must take immunosuppressive drugs to prevent the rejection of a transplanted organ or because they have a disease in which the immune system attacks the body's own tissues (autoimmune illnesses); others may need radiation therapy to treat another form of cancer. Because of this, everyone taking these immunosuppressive drugs or receiving radiation treatments should undergo complete skin examination at regular intervals. If proper treatment is delayed and the tumor continues to grow, the tumor cells can spread (metastasize) to muscle, bone, nerves, and possibly the brain.

Diagnosis

Examination

To diagnose skin cancer, doctors must carefully examine the lesion and ask the patient about how long it has been there, whether it itches or bleeds, and other questions about the patient's medical history.

Procedures

If skin cancer cannot be ruled out, a sample of the tissue is removed and examined under a microscope (a **biopsy**). A definitive diagnosis of squamous or basal cell cancer can only be made with microscopic examination of the tumor cells. Once skin cancer has been diagnosed, the stage of the disease's development is determined. The information from the biopsy and staging allows the physician and patient to plan for treatment and possible surgical intervention.

Treatment

A variety of treatment options are available for those diagnosed with non-melanoma skin cancer. Some carcinomas can be removed by cryosurgery, the process of freezing with liquid nitrogen. Uncomplicated and previously untreated basal cell carcinoma of the trunk and arms is often treated with curettage and electrodesiccation, which is the scraping of the lesion and the destruction of any remaining malignant cells with an electrical current. Removal of a lesion layer-by-layer down to normal margins (Mohs' surgery) is an effective treatment for both basal and squamous cell carcinoma. Radiation therapy is best reserved for older, debilitated patients or when the tumor is considered inoperable. Laser therapy in combination with a photosensitizing drug, a treatment known as **photodynamic therapy**, can be used to treat some non-melanoma skin cancers. The topical application of the **chemotherapy** drug, 5-FU, may be used as treatment option for non-melanoma skin cancers.

Alternative treatment

Alternative medicine aims to prevent rather than treat skin cancer. **Vitamins** have been shown to prevent sunburn and, possibly, skin cancer. Some dermatologists have suggested that taking vitamins E and C may help prevent sunburn. In one particular study, men and women took these vitamins for eight days prior to being exposed to ultraviolet light. The researchers found that those who consumed vitamins required about 20% more ultraviolet light to induce sunburn than did people who didn't take vitamins. This is the first study that indicates the oral use of vitamins E and C increases resistance to sunburn. These **antioxidants** are thought to reduce the risk of skin cancer, and are expected to provide protection from the sun even in lower doses. Other anitoxidant nutrients, including beta carotene, selenium, zinc, and the bioflavonoid quercetin have been suggested as possibly preventing skin cancer. However, a 2003 study reported that selenium was not effective in preventing basal cell carcinoma and may even increase risk of squamous cell carcinoma and total non-melanoma skin cancer. Antioxidant herbs such as bilberry (*Vaccinium myrtillus*), hawthorn (*Crataegus laevigata*), tumeric (*Curcuma longa*), and ginkgo (*Ginkgo biloba*) also have been presented as helpful in preventing skin cancers.

Researchers are also looking at botanical compounds that could be added to skin care products applied externally to lower the risk of skin cancer. Several botanical compounds had been tested on animals and found to be effective in preventing skin cancer, but further research needs to be done on human subjects.

QUESTIONS TO ASK YOUR DOCTOR

- What type of skin cancer do I have?
- What are the recommended treatment options for my type of skin cancer
- How long will treatment last?
- Are the recommended treatments available in my community?
- How long will I need follow-up after treatment?
- What can I do to prevent a recurrence of my skin cancer after treatment?

Prognosis

Both squamous and basal cell carcinoma are curable with appropriate treatment, although basal cell carcinomas have about a 5% rate of recurrence. Early detection remains critical for a positive prognosis. Although it is rare for basal cell carcinomas to metastasize, their metastases can rapidly lead to death if they invade the eyes, ears, mouth, or the membranes covering the brain.

Prevention

Avoiding exposure to the sun reduces the incidence of non-melanoma skin cancer. Sunscreen with a sun-protective factor of 15 or higher is helpful in prevention, along with a hat and clothing to shield the skin from sun damage. People should examine their skin monthly for unusual lesions, especially if previous skin cancers have been experienced.

Advances in photographic technique have now made it easier to track the development of moles with the help of whole-body photographs. A growing number of hospitals are offering these photographs as part of outpatient mole-monitoring services.

Resources

BOOKS

Po-lin, So.*Skin Cancer*New York: Chelsea House Publications, 2007.

Ringborg, Ulrik, et al.*Skin Cancer Prevention*New York: Informa Healthcare, 2006.

White, Danielle M.*Only Skin Deep? An Essential Guide to Effective Skin Cancer Programs and Resources*Lincoln, NE: iUniverse, 2007.

PERIODICALS

Babbington, Gabrielle. "Safe Sun Level Policy Released."*Australian Doctor* (June 29, 2007): 12.

Bedevian, Rima. "Skin Cancer—The Burning Truth."*Plastic Surgery Products* (June 2007): 10–11.

Burfeind, Daniel B. "Women Nearly Three Times More Likely to Die of Genital Non-Melanoma Skin Cancer Than Men."*Dermatology Nursing* (June 2007): 309–310.

Chira, Sandy. "Skin Cancer: Tips on Prevention, Clues to Detection."*Consultant* (May 1, 2007): 589.

Lens, M. & Medenica, L."Systemic Retinoids in Chemoprevention of Non-melanoma Skin Cancer." *Expert Opin Pharmacother* (June 2008):1363–74.

ORGANIZATIONS

American Academy of Dermatology. P.O. Box 4014, Schaumburg, IL 60168-4014. Telephone: (866) 503-7546. Website: http://www.aad.org.

American Cancer Society. 250 Williams St., Atlanta, GA 30303. Telephone: (800)227-2345. Website: http://www.cancer.org.

Canadian Cancer Society. 10 Alcorn Ave., Suite 200, Toronto, ON M4V 3B1 Canada. Telephone: (416) 961-7223. Website: http://www.cancer.ca.

National Cancer Institute. 6116 Executive Blvd., Room 3036A, Bethesda, MD 20892. Telephone: (800) 422-6237. Website: http://www.cancer.gov.

Skin Cancer Foundation. 149 Madison Ave., Suite 901, New York, NY 10016. Telephone: (800) 754-6490. Website: http://www.skincancer.org.

Jeffrey P. Larson, RPT
Melinda Granger Oberleitner, R.N., D.N.S., A.P.R.N., C.N.S.

Small intestine cancer

Definition

Cancer of the small intestine is a rare disease that results when abnormal, malignant cells divide out of control. Cancers in this location consist primarily of **adenocarcinoma**, **lymphoma**, **sarcoma**, and carcinoid tumors.

Description

The small intestine is a long tube inside the abdomen divided into three sections: the duodenum, jejunum, and ileum. The function of the small intestine is to break down food and to remove proteins, carbohydrates, fats, **vitamins**, and minerals. Obstruction of the small intestine by cancer may impair normal passage and digestion of food and nutrients.

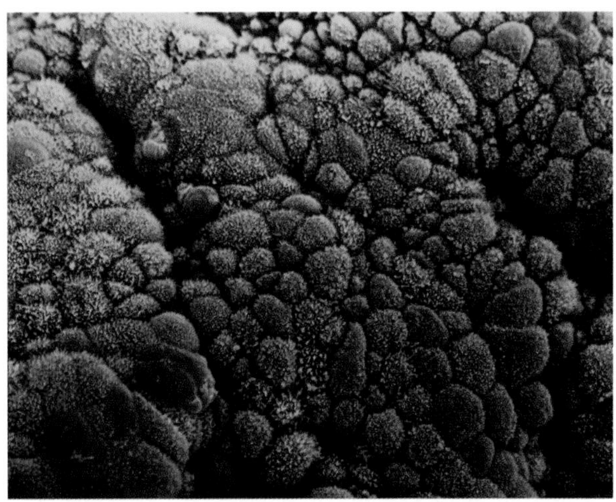

Colored scanning electron micrograph (SEM) of cancer cells in the intestine. *(© Quest, Science Source/Photo Researchers, Inc. Reproduced by permission.)*

Adenocarcinoma

These malignancies most often start in the lining of the small intestine, most frequently occurring in the duodenum and jejunum, the sections closest to the stomach. These tumors may obstruct the bowel, causing digestive problems. Adenocarcinoma is the most common cancer of the small intestine, but only accounts for 2% of all tumors in the gastrointestinal tract and 1% of all deaths related to cancer of the gastrointestinal tract. Carcinomas of the small intestine may appear at multiple sites.

Lymphoma

This fairly uncommon cancer is typically a non-Hodgkin's type that starts in the lymph tissue of the small intestine. (The body's immune system is comprised of lymph tissue, which assists in fighting infections.) Malignant lymphoma is not often found as a solitary lesion.

Sarcoma

Sarcoma malignancies of the small intestine are usually **leiomyosarcoma**. They most often occur in the smooth muscle lining of the ileum, the last section of the small intestine. Liposarcoma and angiosarcoma occur more rarely in the small intestine.

Carcinoid tumors

Carcinoid tumors are most often found in the ileum. In approximately 50% of cases, they appear in multiples.

KEY TERMS

Adenocarcinoma—A cancer that starts in glandular tissue.

Angiosarcoma—A malignant tumor that develops either from blood vessels or from lymphatic vessels.

Carcinogen—A substance that causes cancer.

Carcinoid—A tumor that develops from neuroendocrine cells.

Leiomyosarcoma—A cancerous tumor of smooth (involuntary) muscle tissue.

Liposarcoma—A cancerous tumor of fat tissue.

Lymphoma—A cancer of the lymphatic tissue.

Malignant—Cancerous; a tumor or growth that often destroys surrounding tissue and spreads to other parts of the body.

Metastasis—The spread of cancer from the original site to other body parts.

Radiation therapy—Also called radiotherapy, it uses high-energy rays to kill cancer cells.

Sarcoma—A malignant tumor of the soft tissue including fat, muscle, nerve, joint, blood vessel, and deep skin tissues.

Staging—Performing exams and tests to learn the extent of the cancer within the body, especially whether the disease has spread from the original site to other parts of the body.

Demographics

Approximately 50% of small intestine cancers are adneocarcinomas; 20% are lymphomas; 20% are carcinoid; and about 10% are sarcomas.

Causes and symptoms

The causes of this cancer are not known, but factors that contribute to its development include exposure to carcinogens such as chemicals, radiation, and viruses. In addition, smoking and a poor diet may contribute to the incidence of small intestine cancer. The incidence of cancer is higher in obese individuals.

Often cancer of the small intestine does not initially produce any symptoms. Gastrointestinal bleeding is perhaps the most common symptom. A doctor should be consulted if any of these symptoms are present:

QUESTIONS TO ASK THE DOCTOR

- What is my diagnosis?
- Is there any evidence the cancer has spread?
- What is the stage of the disease?
- What are my treatment choices?
- What new treatments are being studied?
- Would a clinical trial be appropriate for me?
- What are the expected benefits of each kind of treatment?
- What are the risks and possible side effects of each treatment?
- How often will I have treatments?
- How long will treatment last?
- Will I have to change my normal activities?
- What is the treatment likely to cost?
- Is infertility a side effect of cancer treatment? Can anything be done about it?
- What is my prognosis?

- involuntary weight loss
- a lump in the abdominal region
- blood in the stool
- pain or cramping in the abdominal region

Diagnosis

Evaluation begins by taking a patient's medical history and conducting a physical examination. If a patient experiences symptoms, a doctor may suggest the following tests:

- Upper gastrointestinal x ray/upper GI series: To allow the stomach to be seen easier on an x ray, the patient drinks a liquid called barium. This test can be conducted in either a doctor's office or a radiology department at a hospital.
- CT scan (computed tomography): A computerized x ray that takes a picture of the abdomen.
- MRI scan (magnetic resonance imaging): A imaging technique that uses magnetic waves to take a picture of the abdomen.
- Ultrasound: An imaging technique that uses sound waves to locate tumors.
- Endoscopy: An endoscope is a thin, lighted tube which is placed down the throat to reach the first section of the small intestine (duodenum). During this procedure, the doctor may take a biopsy, in which a small piece of tissue is removed for examination of cancereous cells under a microscope.

If small intestine cancer is evident, more tests will be conducted to determine if cancer has spread to other parts of the body.

Treatment team

Cancer treatment often requires a team of specialists and may include a surgeon, medical oncologist, radiation oncologist, nurse, physical therapist, occupational therapist, dietitian, and or a social worker.

Clinical staging, treatments, and prognosis

As with many other types of cancer, malignancies of the small intestine can be classified as localized, regional spread, or distant spread.

- Localized: The cancer has not spread beyond the wall of the organ it developed in.
- Regional spread: The cancer has spread from the organ it started in to other tissues such as muscle, fat, ligaments, or lymph nodes.
- Distant spread: The cancer has spread to tissues or organs outside of where it originated such as the liver, bones, or lungs.

Treatment options for small intestine cancer most often include surgery, and possibly **radiation therapy**, **chemotherapy**, and/or biological therapy. Cancer of the small intestine is treatable and sometimes curable depending on the histology. Removing the cancer through surgery is the most common treatment. If the tumor is large, a small portion may be removed if resection of the small intestine is possible. For larger tumors, surgery requires removing a greater amount of the surrounding normal intestinal tissue, in addition to some surrounding blood vessels and lymph nodes.

Radiation therapy kills cancer cells and reduces the size of tumors through the use of high-energy **x rays**. Radiation therapy may come from an external source using a machine or an internal source. Internal-based therapy involves the use of radioisotopes to administer radiation through thin plastic tubes to the area of the body where cancer cells are found. Side effects of radiation therapy include:

- fatigue
- loss of appetite
- nausea and vomiting
- diarrhea
- gas
- bloating
- mild temporary, sunburn-like skin changes

- difficulty tolerating milk products

Chemotherapy kills cancer cells with drugs taken orally or by injection in a vein or muscle. It is referred to as a systemic treatment due to fact that it travels through the bloodstream and kills cancer cells outside the small intestine. **Adjuvant chemotherapy** may be given following surgery to ensure all cancer cells are killed. Some side effects of chemotherapy are:

- nausea and vomiting
- loss of appetite (anorexia)
- temporary hair loss (alopecia)
- mouth sores
- fatigue, as a result of a low red blood cell count
- higher likelihood of infection or bleeding due to low white blood cell counts and low blood platelets, respectively

Radiation and chemotherapy are seldom beneficial in small intestinal cancers.

Utilizing the body's immune system, biological therapy stimulates the body to combat cancer. Natural materials from the body or other laboratory-produced agents are designed to boost, guide, or restore the body's ability to fight disease.

Treatment options for small interstine cancers are based on the type of cells found—adenocarcinoma, lymphoma, sarcoma, or carcinoid tumor—rather than the clinical staging system.

Treatment of adenocarcinoma of the small intestine may consist of:

- surgical removal of the tumor
- If the cancer cannot be removed by resection of the small intestine, surgery may be performed to bypass the cancer to allow food to travel through the intestine.
- symptom relief with radiation therapy
- chemotherapy or biological therapy in a clinical trial setting
- a clinical trial involving radiation and drug therapy (with or without chemotherapy) to elicit greater sensitivity to radiation using radiosensitizers

Treatment of lymphoma of the small intestine may consist of:

- surgical removal of the cancer and lymph nodes in close proximity to it
- Surgery accompanied by radiation therapy or adjuvant chemotherapy. If the disease is localized to the bowel wall, then surgical resection alone or combined chemotherapy should be considered. If the disease has extended to the regional lymph nodes, then surgical resection and combination chemotherapy is suggested at the time of diagnosis.
- For extensive lymphoma or lymphoma that cannot be removed surgically, chemotherapy with or without additional radiation therapy is frequently used to reduce the risk of recurrence.

Treatment of leiomyosarcoma of the small intestine may consist of:

- surgical removal of the cancer
- When cancer cannot be removed by resection, surgical bypass of the tumor is recommended to allow food to pass.
- radiation therapy
- For unresectable metastatic disease, surgery, radiation therapy, or chemotherapy is suggested in order to alleviate symptoms.
- For unresectable primary or metastatic disease, a clinical trial evaluating the benefits of new anticancer drugs (chemotherapy) and biological therapy.

For recurrent small intestine cancer, treatment may consist of the following measures, if the cancer has returned to one area of the body only:

- surgical removal of the cancer
- symptom relief using chemotherapy or radiation therapy
- a clinical trial using radiation and drug therapy (with or without chemotherapy) to elicit greater sensitivity to radiation using radiosensitizers

For recurrent metastatic adenocarcinoma or leiomyosarcoma, there is no standard effective chemotherapy treatment. Patients should be regarded as candidates for clinical studies assessing new **anticancer drugs** or biological agents.

For carcinoid tumors less than 1 cm in size, surgical removal of the tumor and surrounding tissue is possible. Carcinoid tumors often grow and spread slowly, therefore, approximately half are found at an early or localized stage. By the time of sugery, 80% of the tumors over 2 cm in diameter have metastasized locally or to the liver.

The prognosis or likelihood of recovery depends on the type of cancer, the overall health of the patient, and whether the cancer has spread to other regions or is only localized in the small intestine. A cure depends on the ability to remove the cancer completely with surgery. Adenocarcinoma is most common in the duodenum, however, patient survival is less likely for individuals with cancer is in this area compared with those patients with tumors in the jejunum or ileum due to reduced rates of surgery to remove cancer. In 2009, there will be 2,000 cases of adenocarcinoma of the small intestine. Of these malignancies, 55% occurred in the duodenum, 13% in the ileum, 18% in the jejunum, and 14% were in unspecified areas. The National Cancer Database reported a median survival of 19.7 months for these patients with an overall 5-year disease survival rate of 30.5%. For resectable adenocarcinoma, the National Cancer Institute reports an overall five-year survival rate of only 20%, whereas resectable leiomyosarcoma's survival rate is reported at approximately 50%. One study found the overall rate of metastatic spread of leiomyosarcoma ranged from 24–50%; this cancer most often spread to the liver. Five-year survival in 705 patients with leiomyosarcoma was reported at 28%. Surgery is the preferred treatment for smooth muscle tumors. Little benefit was found for irradiation or chemotherapy, or for these therapies combined. Patients over 75 years of age have a significantly poorer survival rate than younger people. In addition, patients with poorly differentiated tumors have a poorer prognosis than those with moderately or well-differentiated tumors. Survival rate decreases with progression of disease by stage: localized 47.6%; regional 31%; distant 5.2%.

Alternative and complementary therapies

Bovine and shark cartilage is currently being explored in **clinical trials** for antitumor properties, but there is not enough evidence to warrant its use. Some popular herbs that are purported to have therapeutic effects in cancer treatment include echinacea, garlic, ginseng, and ginger. Laboratory studies have shown that echinacea has the potential to control the growth of cancerous cells, but more studies are needed to confirm efficacy in humans. In addition, dosage and toxicity levels still need to be established. Some studies suggest that diets high in garlic reduce the risk of stomach, esophageal, and colon cancers. There is still debate regarding the best form of garlic to take—whole raw garlic or garlic in tablet form; aged or fresh garlic; garlic with odor or "deodorized" garlic. Ginger is often recommended for its beneficial effects on the digestive system, but evidence has not confirmed efficacy in cancer treatment. Ginseng in excessive amounts can be very toxic, causing **vomiting**, bleeding, and death. Patients should not take herbal remedies without consulting their physicians, particularly if they intend to combine the herbs with prescription drugs. Herb and drug combinations can sometimes result in toxic interactions.

Coping with cancer treatment

Pain is a common problem for people with some types of cancer, especially when the cancer grows and presses against other organs and nerves. Pain may also be a side effect of treatment. However, pain can generally be relieved or reduced with prescription medicines or over-the-counter drugs as recommended by the doctor. Other ways to reduce pain, such as relaxation exercises, may also be useful. It is important for patients to report pain to their doctors, so that steps can be taken to help relieve it.

Depression may affect approximately 15–25% of cancer patients, particularly if the prognosis for recovery is poor. A number of antidepressant medications are available from physicians to alleviate feelings of depression. Counseling with a psychologist or psychiatrist also may help patients deal with depression.

Clinical trials

Glivec (STI-571, or **imatinib mesylate**) is in clinical trials for treatment of gastrointestinal stromal tumors, as well as for leukemia and glioblastoma, a type of brain tumor. An open trial (GIST trial SWOG-S0033) led by Southwest Oncology Group will test those individuals with metastatic or recurrent disease using two doses of the drug.

Clinical trials may be suitable for patients suffering from small intestine cancer. The principal investigator should be contacted regarding participation in appropriate trials. For information about cancer trials, patients can visit the National Cancer Institute web site at http://cancertrials.nci.nih.gov.

Prevention

Most people who develop cancer do not have inherited genetic abnormalities. Their genes have been damaged after birth by substances in their environment. A substance that damages deoxyribonucleic acid (DNA) in a way that can lead to cancer is called a carcinogen. Carcinogens include certain chemicals, certain types of radiation, and viruses. Asbestos is one substance that is suspected of contributing to the development of small intestinal cancer. Although the precise causes of cancer are not known, a variety of factors are known to contribute to the development of cancer including tobacco smoke, and poor dietary habits such as high-fat diet. Eating a diet rich in fruits and vegetables and low in fat may reduce the likelihood of cancer. Studies have demonstrated that individuals who were protected from cancer ate a greater variety of foods and nutrients compared to those with cancer.

Several fruits, vitamins, and minerals were found particularly protective against intestinal cancer including vitamin B_6, folate, niacin, and iron. Some studies have linked eating large amounts of salt-cured, salt-pickled, and smoked foods to cancers of the digestive system. Other studies have linked stomach cancers, specifically intestinal cancer, to a lack of fruits, vegetables, and fiber in the diet. For prevention of cancer, it is important to avoid carcinogens (smoking, chemicals) and known risk factors, and to pursue a healthy lifestyle which includes moderate alcohol intake, regular exercise, a low-fat diet, and a diet rich in fruits and vegetables. Modifying genetic predispositions through risk factor reduction can also assist in prevention.

Special concerns

Due to the side effects of radiation and chemotherapy, individuals must make a deliberate effort to eat as nutritiously as possible. Those who experience pain, **nausea**, or **diarrhea** may want to discuss treatments options with their doctor to ease these side effects.

Eating well during cancer treatment means getting enough calories and protein to help prevent **weight loss** and maintain strength. Eating nutritiously may also help an individual feel better.

Resources

BOOKS

Kelsen, David, Bernard Levin, and Joel Tepper. *Principles and Practice of Gastrointestinal Oncology* . Philadelphia: Lippincott Williams & Wilkins Publishers, 2001.

PERIODICALS

Howe, J.R., et al. "The American College of Surgeons Commission on Cancer and the American Cancer Society. Adenocarcinoma of the Small Bowel: Review of the National Cancer Data Base, 1985-1995." *Cancer* 86 (1999): 2693-2706.

ORGANIZATIONS

The National Cancer Institute (NCI). For information contact the Public Inquiries Office: Building 31, Room 10A31, 31 Center Drive, MSC 2580, Betheseda, MD 20892-2580 USA. (301) 435-3848 or 1-800-4-CANCER. <http://cancer.gov/publications/> or <http://cancer trials.nci.nih.gov> or <http://cancernet.nci.nih.gov>.

National Center for Complementary and Alternative Medicine (NCCAM). 31 Center Dr., Room #5B-58, Bethesda, MD 20892-2182. (800) NIH-NCAM. Fax: (301) 495-4957. <http://nccam.nih.gov>.

Crystal Heather Kaczkowski, MSc.

Smoking cessation

Definition

Smoking cessation is the medical term for quitting smoking. It is a vital part of **cancer prevention** because smoking is the single most preventable cause of death from **cancer**. As early as 1982, the Surgeon General reported that tobacco causes more cancer deaths in the United States than any other factor–30% of all cancer deaths, including 87% of deaths from lung cancer. Although people think of smoking most often in connection with lung cancer, smoking is also associated with cancers of the mouth, throat, voice box (larynx), esophagus, pancreas, kidney, and bladder. Women who smoke increase their risk of cancer of the cervix. Quitting smoking, however, significantly reduces the risk of cancer; 15 years after quitting, a former smoker's risk is almost as low as that of someone who has never smoked.

Description

Smoking cessation covers several different approaches, ranging from medications and psychotherapy to special classes and programs. Smoking is a habit difficult to break because it involves many different aspects of a person's emotions and social life as well as physical addiction to nicotine. Most people who quit smoking successfully use a combination of treatments or techniques for quitting.

Special concerns

People who are trying to quit smoking are often concerned about:

- Withdrawal symptoms. Nicotine, the substance in tobacco that gives smokers a pleasurable feeling, is as addictive as heroin or cocaine. Withdrawal from nicotine may produce depression, anger, fatigue, headaches, problems with sleep or concentration, or increased appetite for food. These symptoms usually start several hours after the last cigarette. They may last for several days or several weeks.
- Weight gain. Many people, particularly women, gain between two and 10 pounds after giving up smoking. This mild weight gain, however, is not nearly as great a danger to health as continuing to smoke. Getting more exercise can help.
- Stress. Many smokers started to smoke as a way to cope with stress and tension. Finding other methods—exercise, meditation, biofeedback, massage, and others, can reduce the temptation to smoke when stress arises.

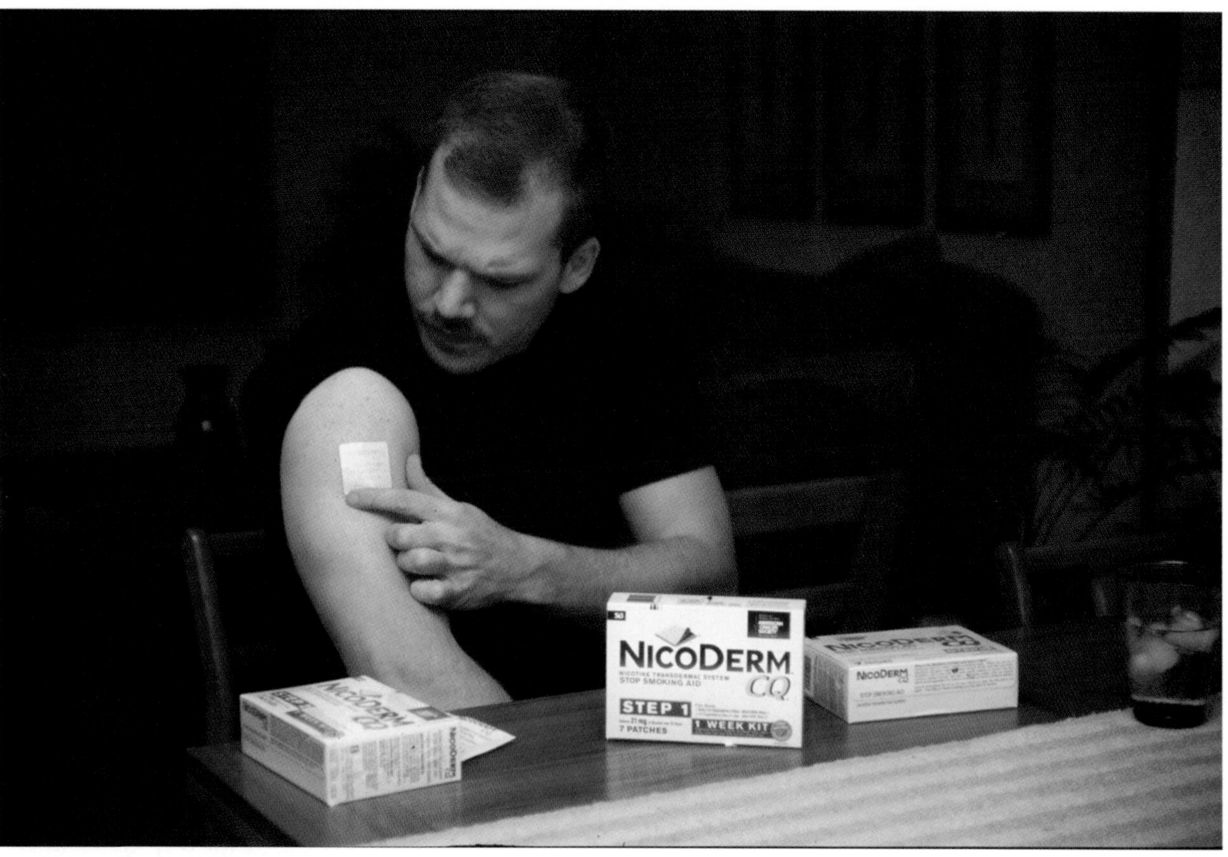

A man with a nicotine patch. *(Photo Researchers, Inc. Reproduced by permission.)*

- Side effects of nicotine replacement products. Smokers who are using these products to help them quit may experience headaches, nausea, sore throat, or long-term dependence. Side effects can often be reduced or eliminated by using a lower dosage of the product or switching to another form of nicotine replacement.

Treatments

Nicotine replacement therapy

Nicotine replacement therapy gives the smoker a measured supply of nicotine without the other harmful chemicals in tobacco. It reduces the physical craving for **cigarettes** so that the smoker can handle the psychological aspects of quitting more effectively.

As of 2001, the Food and Drug Administration (FDA) had approved four forms of nicotine replacement therapy:

- Transdermal patches. Patches, which are nonprescription items, supply measured doses of nicotine through the skin. The doses are lowered over a period of weeks, thus helping the smoker to reduce the need for nicotine gradually.
- Nicotine gum. Nicotine gum provides a fast-acting nicotine replacement that is absorbed through the mouth tissues. The smoker chews the gum slowly and then keeps it against the inside of the cheek for 20 to 30 minutes. The gum is also available without prescription.
- Nasal spray. Nicotine nasal spray provides nicotine through the tissues that line the nose. It acts much more rapidly than the patches or gum, but requires a doctor's prescription.
- Inhalers. Nicotine inhalers are plastic tubes containing nicotine plugs. The plug gives off nicotine vapor when the smoker puffs on the tube. Some smokers prefer inhalers because they look more like cigarettes than other types of nicotine replacement. They also require a doctor's prescription.

Other medications

Bupropion, which is sold under the trade name Zyban, is an antidepressant medication given to lower

KEY TERMS

Bupropion—An antidepressant medication given to smokers for nicotine withdrawal symptoms. It is sold under the trade name Zyban.

Buspirone—An anti-anxiety medication that is also given for withdrawal symptoms. It is sold under the trade name BuSpar.

Nicotine—A colorless, oily chemical found in tobacco that makes people physically dependent on smoking. It is poisonous in large doses.

QUESTIONS TO ASK THE DOCTOR

- What methods would you recommend to help me quit smoking?
- How can I cope with withdrawal symptoms and other side effects of quitting?
- Are there any stop-smoking programs in this area that you would recommend?

the symptoms of withdrawal from nicotine. Bupropion by itself can help people quit smoking, but its success rate is even higher when it is used together with nicotine replacement therapy. Another drug that is sometimes given for nicotine withdrawal is buspirone (BuSpar), which is an antianxiety medication.

Stop-smoking programs and groups

Stop-smoking programs help by reinforcing a smoker's decision to give up tobacco. They teach people to recognize common problems that occur during quitting and they offer emotional support and encouragement. While stop-smoking programs do not have as high a success rate by themselves as medications or nicotine replacement therapy, they are very helpful as part of an overall quitting plan. The most effective programs include either individual or group psychological counseling. Many state Medicaid plans now cover the costs of smoking cessation programs; further information is available from the American Association of Respiratory Care at http://www.aarc.org/advocacy/state/smoking_treatment.html.

The Great American Smokeout has been held annually since 1977 on the third Thursday in November to call attention to the high human costs of smoking. Smokers are asked to quit for the day and donate the money saved on cigarettes to high school scholarship funds.

Nicotine Anonymous is an organization that applies the Twelve Steps of Alcoholics Anonymous (AA) to tobacco addiction. Its group meetings are free of charge.

Alternative and complementary therapies

Some people find that hypnosis helps them to quit. Acupuncture has also been used, but there are no large-scale studies comparing it to other stop-smoking treatments. A list of physicians who are also licensed acupuncturists is available from the American Academy of Medical Acupuncture at (800) 521-2262.

Other complementary approaches that have been shown to be useful in quitting smoking include movement therapies like yoga, t'ai chi, and dance. Prayer and meditation have also helped many smokers learn to handle stress without using tobacco.

See also Cigarettes.

Resources

BOOKS

American Cancer Society. *Quitting Smoking*. New York: American Cancer Society, 2000. [cited June 29, 2001].http://www.cancer.org/tobacco/quitting.

Beers, Mark H., MD, and Robert Berkow, MD, editors. "Smoking Cessation.". In *The Merck Manual of Diagnosis and Therapy*. Whitehouse Station, NJ: Merck Research Laboratories, 1999.

United States Public Health Service. *You Can Quit Smoking*. Consumer Guide, June 2000. [cited June 29, 2001]. Government Publications Clearinghouse, P.O. Box 8547, Silver Spring, MD 20907. <http:www.surgeongeneral.gov/tobacco/consquits.htm./>

OTHER

United States Public Health Service Fact Sheet. *Treating Tobacco Use and Dependence*. June, 2000. [cited June 29, 2001]. http://www.surgeongeneral.gov/tobacco/smokfact.htm..

ORGANIZATIONS

American Association for Respiratory Care. 11030 Ables Lane, Dallas, TX 75229. [cited June 29, 2001]. http://www.aarc.org.

American Cancer Society (ACS). 1599 Clifton Road, NE, Atlanta, GA 30329. (404) 320-3333 or (800) ACS-2345. Fax: (404) 329-7530. [cited June 29, 2001]. http://www.cancer.org/.

American Lung Association. 1740 Broadway, 14th Floor, New York, NY 10019. (212) 315-8700 or (800) 586-4872 (LUNG USA).

National Cancer Institute, Office of Cancer Communications. 31 Center Drive, MSC 2580, Bethesda, MD 20892-2580. (800) 4-CANCER (1-800-422-6237). TTY: (800) 332-8615.[cited June 29, 2001]. http://www.nci.nih.gov./.

National Heart, Lung, and Blood Institute. Information Center, P. O. Box 30105, Bethesda, MD 20824. (301) 251-1222.

Nicotine Anonymous. (415) 750-0328.[cited June 29, 2001]. http://www.nicotine-anonymous.org/.

Rebecca J. Frey, Ph.D.

Sodium iodide I 131 *see* **Radiopharmaceuticals**

Sodium phosphate P 32 *see* **Radiopharmaceuticals**

Soft tissue sarcoma

Definition

Soft tissue sarcomas are cancerous (malignant) tumors that develop in mesodermal tissues that surround, support, and connect the structures and organs of the body.

Description

Soft tissues include muscles, fibrous (connective) tissues, fat, blood and lymph vessels, synovial tissues surrounding the joints, peripheral nerve tissues, and deep skin tissues. As soft tissue sarcomas grow, they may invade surrounding tissue, or spread (metastasize) to distant sites in the body. Together they account for less than 1% of all newly diagnosed cancers.

About one-half of all soft tissue sarcomas develop in the arms, legs, hands, or feet. About 40% occur in the trunk, internal organs, or the retroperitoneum—the back of the abdominal cavity. The remaining 10% occur in the head and neck.

Muscle tissue sarcomas

Rhabdomyosarcoma (RMS)—a skeletal muscle tumor—is the most common soft tissue **sarcoma** in children. Embryonal rhabdomyosarcoma (ERMS) is more common than alveolar rhabdomyosarcoma (ARMS). ERMS commonly develops in the head, neck, or reproductive or urinary tract organs. ARMS develops in the large muscles of the arms, legs, or trunk. All other soft tissue sarcomas in children are classified as non-rhabdomyosarcoma or non-RMS.

Leiomyosarcomas are smooth muscle tumors that occur most often in the retroperitoneum or internal organs but also may occur in the deep soft tissues of the arms or legs.

Fibrous tissue sarcomas

Soft tissue sarcomas often occur in connective tissue:

- Fibrosarcoma is a cancer of the tendons and ligaments.
- Malignant fibrous histiocytoma (MFH) is the most common soft tissue tumor of the limbs, although it also occurs in the retroperitoneum. MFH accounts for 40% of all soft tissue sarcomas.
- Dermatofibrosarcoma protuberans (DFSP) is a low-grade cancer of fibrous tissue under the skin, usually in the limbs or trunk.
- Desmoid tumors may be low-grade fibrosarcomas or a unique type of fibrous tissue tumor.

Fat tissue sarcomas

Liposarcomas develop in fat tissue anywhere in the body but occur most often in the thigh or the retroperitoneum. They range from very slow to very fast growing and account for 25% of all soft tissue sarcomas.

Blood and lymph vessel sarcomas

- Angiosarcoma is called hemangiosarcoma if it occurs in a blood vessel and lymphangiosarcoma if it occurs in a lymph vessel.
- Hemangioendothelioma—usually called epithelioid hemangioendothelioma (EHE) in adults—is a low-grade cancer in the blood vessels of soft tissue or internal organs such as the lungs or liver.
- Hemangiopericytoma is a sarcoma of the perivascular tissue around blood vessels that help control blood flow. It most often develops in the legs, pelvis, or retroperitoneum.
- Kaposi's sarcoma is a tumor formed by cells similar to those that line blood and lymph vessels.

Synovial sarcoma

Synovial sarcomas are tumors of the synovium—the tough tissue that surrounds the joints. They occur most often in leg and arm joints, especially the knee. They are the most common non-RMS in children. Approximately 30% of synovial sarcomas occur in those under age 20.

KEY TERMS

Alveolar rhabdomyosarcoma, ARMS—A type of soft tissue sarcoma in the large muscles of the arms, legs, or trunk that primarily affects older children.

Brachytherapy—Irradiation in direct contact with a sarcoma.

Cytogenetics—The combined study of heredity and the structure and function of cells.

Dermatofibrosarcoma protuberans, DFSP—A low-grade cancer of fibrous tissue under the skin, usually in the limbs or trunk.

Embryonal rhabdomyosarcoma, ERMS—The most common type of RMS in children, occurring in the head, neck, or genitourinary tract and resembling fetal skeletal muscle tissue.

Epithelioid hemangioendothelioma, EHE—Hemangioendothelioma in adults.

Extraosseous Ewing's tumor, EOE—A type of Ewing's tumor in soft tissue outside of the bone tissue with some characteristics of embryonic nerve tissue.

Fine needle aspiration, FNA—A type of biopsy that uses a very thin needle to remove small pieces of a superficial suspected sarcoma.

Hemangioendothelioma—A low-grade sarcoma of the blood vessels of soft tissues or internal organs such as the lungs or liver.

Lymph nodes—The filtering system for the lymph that carries white blood cells of the immune system throughout the body via lymph vessels.

Mesoderm—The middle layer of embryonic cells that gives rise to skin, connective tissue, blood and lymph vessels, the urogenital system, and most muscles.

Malignant fibrous histiocytoma, MFH—The most common soft tissue tumor of the limbs, occurring primarily in older adults and accounting for 40% of all soft tissue sarcomas.

Non-RMS—All soft tissue sarcomas in children that are not RMS.

Primitive neuroectodermal tumor, PNET—A type of Ewing's tumor in soft tissue with some characteristics of embryonic nerve tissue.

Retroperitoneum—The space between the lining of the abdominal and pelvic walls and the back wall of the body.

Rhabdomyosarcoma, RMS—A cancerous tumor of the skeletal muscle and the most common soft tissue sarcoma in children.

TNM—A cancer staging system in which T is the primary tumor size and location, N is lymph node involvement, and M is metastasis to distant parts of the body.

Peripheral nerve sarcomas

Malignant peripheral nerve sheath tumors—also called malignant schwannomas, neurofibrosarcomas, or neurogenic sarcomas—are tumors in cells surrounding the peripheral nerves that run throughout the body. Ewing's tumors are a group of related cancers that share characteristics with nerve tissue in a developing embryo. Ewing's tumors that occur in soft tissue are extraosseous (outside of the bone) Ewing's (EOE) and primitive neuroectodermal tumors (PNET).

Other soft tissue sarcomas

Some soft tissue sarcomas are of uncertain origin:

- Mesenchymonia is a combination of tissue types that resemble fibrosarcoma and others.
- Alveolar soft-part sarcoma most commonly develops in the legs.
- Epithelioid sarcoma usually develops under the skin of the hands, forearms, lower legs, or feet.
- Clear cell sarcoma—also called malignant melanoma of the soft parts (MMSP), clear cell sarcoma of tendons, aponeuroses—is a rare sarcoma of the tendons and related tissues. It has some characteristics of malignant melanoma or skin cancer.
- Desmoplastic small cell tumors usually occur in the abdomen, pelvis, or tissues around the testes, primarily in males.

Demographics

It is estimated that 1,270 new cases of soft tissue sarcomas will be diagnosed in the United States during 2008. Every year in the United States 850–900 children under age 20 are diagnosed with soft tissue sarcoma, accounting for 7.4% of cancers in that age group. During 2008 an estimated 5,150 American males and females will die of soft tissue sarcoma.

Childhood soft tissue sarcomas occur most frequently during infancy or after age 10. Male children have a slightly higher incidence than females and black

QUESTIONS TO ASK YOUR DOCTOR

- What type of sarcoma do I have?
- Has the cancer spread?
- What stage is the cancer and what does that mean for me?
- What are the treatment options?
- What treatment do you recommend and why?
- What are the risks and side effects of each treatment?
- What are the risks of recurrence after each treatment?
- How should I prepare for the treatment?
- How much work or school will be missed?
- What is the recovery time after treatment?
- What is my estimated survival time?

children have a slightly higher incidence than white children, particularly among 15–19-year-olds.

More than 85% of RMS occur in infants, children, and teenagers. Almost 60% of soft tissue sarcomas in children up to age four are RMS. The prevalence of RMS declines steadily with increasing age, accounting for only 23% of soft tissue sarcomas in 16–19-year-olds. ERMS accounts for 75% of RMS in children aged 1–14. ARMS can affect children in all age groups but is more prevalent among older children.

Other soft tissue sarcomas also affect different age groups:

- Adolescents are more likely to develop leiomyosarcoma in the trunk, whereas in adults it is more common in the uterus or digestive tract.
- Infantile fibrosarcoma affects children up to age four.
- Adolescents are more likely to develop fibrosarcoma in the arms or legs and MFH in the legs.
- Adults are more likely to develop fibrosarcoma in the arms, legs, or trunk, or DFSP in the trunk; MFH is most common in older adults.
- Liposcarcoma can occur in the arms and legs of older teenagers and in the arms, legs, or trunk of adults; however it is most common in people aged 60–65.
- Adults are more likely to develop hemangiosarcoma in the arms, legs, or trunk, lymphangiosarcoma in the arms, or Kaposi's sarcoma in the legs or trunk.
- Hemangiopericytoma is more common in adults, although infantile hemangiopericytoma occurs in children up to age four.
- Synovial sarcomas usually occur in young adults.
- Teenagers and adults can develop malignant peripheral nerve sheath tumors in the arms, legs, or trunk.
- Soft tissue Ewing's tumors are relatively common in children and very rare in adults.
- Mesenchymonia is a rare sarcoma of children.
- Aveolar soft-part sarcoma is rare, usually affecting young adults.
- Alveolar soft-part sarcoma of the muscular nerves of the arms or legs can affect children in all age groups but is more prevalent in older children.
- Epithelioid sarcoma usually affects adolescents and young adults.
- Desmoplastic small cell tumors are rare and affect primarily male teenagers and young adults.

Causes & symptoms

Causes

Although most soft tissue sarcomas have no known cause, those in children generally are associated with chromosomal changes. Other soft tissue sarcomas are caused by changes in the DNA carried on the chromosomes. Some of these changes or mutations are inherited but most are acquired during a person's lifetime, possibly from exposure to radiation or cancer-causing chemicals.

In addition:

- Leiomyosarcoma and some other soft tissue sarcomas have been linked to the Epstein-Barr virus in people with AIDS.
- Some hormones, particularly estrogen, cause desmoid tumors to grow.
- Angiosarcomas sometimes develop in an area that has been exposed to radiation.
- Kaposi's sarcoma appears to be related to infection by human herpesvirus-8.

Symptoms

During their early stages most soft tissue sarcomas do not cause symptoms. However as they grow larger the tumors begin to press against normal tissue causing soreness or pain. Synovial sarcoma causes tenderness, pain, or swelling in a joint.

Symptoms of soft tissue sarcoma can include:

- a new or growing lump anywhere in the body
- a usually painless swelling or lump in an arm or leg that grows over weeks or months.

About one-third of abdominal sarcomas cause increasing pain. Although symptoms may be nonspecific, abdominal tumors can grow large enough to be felt or to cause blockage or bleeding in the stomach or bowels. This leads to blood in vomit or stools and may cause stools to be very black and tarry.

RMS often develops in easily detectable regions such as a lump just under the skin or around the testes:

- RMS in an eye muscle can cause bulging eye
- RMS in the nasal cavity may cause nosebleeds
- RMS often occurs in the bladder or genitourinary tract causing difficult urination or blood in the urine
- RMS in the abdomen or pelvis may cause vomiting, abdominal pain, or constipation

Diagnosis

Only about 50% of soft tissue sarcomas are diagnosed at early stages before the **cancer** has spread. Soft tissue sarcomas in children may be particularly difficult to diagnose.

Diagnosis may include:

- a medical history to uncover any risk factors
- a physical examination
- ultrasound imaging for visualizing internal organs and masses
- a computed tomography (CT) scan—sometimes in conjunction with a radiocontrast dye—to help determine whether a sarcoma has spread to the liver or other organs
- magnetic resonance imaging (MRI)—sometimes with radiocontrast dyes—to obtain detailed images of organs or masses
- chest x rays to determine whether a sarcoma has spread to the lungs
- positron emission tomography (PET) to scan the entire body for metastasized cancer

Biopsies

Unlike most cancers, the size of a soft tissue sarcoma may be less important than the appearance of the cancer cell. Cells that appear similar to normal cells of the same tissue are called well-differentiated or moderately differentiated. Sarcoma cells that appear very different from normal tissue are referred to as poorly differentiated or undifferentiated. For example, ERMS cells resemble developing skeletal muscle cells in a 6–8-week-old fetus and ARMS cells resemble the normal muscle cells of a 10-week-old fetus. Therefore microscopic examination of sarcoma cells obtained by a biopsy—the removal of sarcoma tissue—is very important for determining the clinical stage, the probable growth rate of the cancer, the likelihood of **metastasis**, and the prognosis.

A fine needle aspiration (FNA) **biopsy** uses a very thin needle and syringe to remove small fragments of a superficial (near the surface), easily accessed sarcoma. The needle may be guided by feeling a mass near the surface or using a CT scanner. Although much less invasive than other types of biopsies, FNA may not provide enough tissue to identify a sarcoma, determine its type, and grade it. However it is useful for determining whether a suspected sarcoma is a benign tumor, another type of cancer, an **infection**, or some other disease. FNA also is used to determine whether tumors in other organs are metastases of the sarcoma.

If FNA indicates a sarcoma, another type of biopsy is used to confirm the diagnosis:

- A core needle biopsy removes a cylindrical piece of tissue of about one-sixteenth in. (0.15 cm) diameter and 0.5 in. (1.3 cm) long. A CT scanner may be used to guide the needle into tumors located in internal organs. Although a core biopsy avoids an incision and may not require general anesthesia, the small sample size may cause a cancer to be missed or misdiagnosed.
- If the sarcoma is small, near the surface, and away from vital tissues, an excisional biopsy may be used to remove the entire mass and surrounding normal tissue. This combines a diagnostic biopsy with surgical treatment.
- An incisional biopsy removes a small portion of a large sarcoma.
- An open surgical biopsy under general anesthesia is used to diagnose RMS in children. In addition to the tumor sample, nearby lymph nodes may be removed for testing.

Testing

In addition to histological examination under a microscope, biopsy samples may require special testing to identify a sarcoma and its type and grade:

- An immunohistochemical test treats the sample with antibodies that recognize cell proteins that are typical of some types of sarcomas. When an antibody binds such a cell protein, a color change is detected microscopically.
- For cytogenetic techniques biopsied cells are grown in the laboratory for about a week and examined microscopically to determine whether chromosomal changes have occurred.

- Fluorescent *in situ* hybridization (FISH) may be used to detect chromosome abnormalities without first growing the cells.

Treatment team

Soft tissue sarcomas are treated by a multidisciplinary team of cancer specialists including:

- pathologists
- hematologists
- oncologists
- surgeons
- radiation oncologists

Children and adolescents with soft tissue sarcomas are treated at medical centers specializing in **childhood cancers** with treatment teams that include:

- a primary care physician
- pediatric hematologists/oncologists
- pediatric surgeons
- radiation oncologists
- pediatric oncology nurses
- nurse practitioners
- rehabilitation and physical therapists
- psychologists
- child-life specialists
- nutritionists
- social workers
- educators

Clinical staging, treatments, and prognosis

Staging systems

TNM. Soft tissue sarcomas often are staged according to the TNM system of the American Joint Committee on Cancer, in which T is the primary tumor size and location:

- TX—cannot be assessed
- T0—no evidence of a primary tumor
- T1—the sarcoma is 2 in. (5 cm) or less
- T2—the sarcoma is more than 2 in. (5 cm)
- a—the tumor is superficial
- b—the tumor is deep in a limb or the abdomen.

N represents lymph node involvement in the region of the sarcoma:

- NX—cannot be assessed
- NO—lymph nodes free of sarcoma cells
- N1—regional lymph nodes have sarcoma cells.

Although RMS and synovial and epithelioid sarcomas commonly spread to lymph nodes, overall lymph node involvement occurs with less than 3% of adult soft tissue sarcomas.

M represents metastasis to distant organs:

- MX—cannot be assessed
- MO—sarcoma has not spread
- M1—distant metastases

GRADING. In addition to a standard staging system, soft tissue sarcomas are graded according to the microscopic appearance of the cells, where G is the histological grade:

- GX—cannot be assessed
- G1 or low grade—cells appear normal, well-differentiated, slow-growing; these rarely metastasize
- G2 or intermediate—cells are moderately differentiated and fast growing
- G3 or high grade—cells are poorly differentiated and faster growing
- G4—cells are abnormal, poorly or undifferentiated, and very fast growing.

Clinical staging

Stage I sarcomas are low-grade cancers:

- Stage IA—G1–2, T1a or b, N0, M0
- Stage IB—G1–2, T2a, N0, M0

Stage II, III, and IV sarcomas are high-grade cancers:

- Stage IIA—G1–2, T2b, N0, M0
- Stage IIB—G3–4, T1a–b, N0, M0
- Stage IIC—G3—4, T2a, N0, M0
- Stage III—G3–4, T2b, N0, M0
- Stage IVA—any G, any T, N1, M0
- Stage IVB—any G, any T, any N, M1.

Treatments

In addition to the stage, treatment depends on other factors including the location of the sarcoma. Treatment of children with non-RMS usually follows the standard treatment for adults. However potential long-term effects of treatment are a greater concern in children, who are much more susceptible to radiation and are expected to live much longer than adults.

SURGERY. Most stage I, II, and III soft tissue sarcomas are surgically removed, with the goal of completely removing (resectioning) the tumor, as well as at least 0.8–1.2 in. (2–3 cm) of surrounding tissue. Many soft tissue sarcomas in infants and young children can be treated successfully by surgery alone. Only about 5% of arm or leg sarcomas require **amputation** of the limb. Most patients have limb-sparing surgery followed by **radiation therapy**, although these procedures are more difficult in children than in adults. Amputation may be necessary when invading sarcoma cells surround essential nerves, arteries, or muscles, or when limb-sparing surgery would result in a dysfunctional limb or chronic pain. Amputation is not recommended if the sarcoma has metastasized to the lungs or other organs. Abdominal sarcomas are difficult to remove because they can be quite large and adjacent to vital organs.

Stage IVA sarcomas and nearby lymph nodes are surgically removed. Sometimes the removal of stage IVB sarcomas and all of their metastases is attempted. Surgery may be preceded by high-dose radiation and/or **chemotherapy** to shrink the tumor or for high-grade sarcomas that are at risk of metastasizing. If the only metastasis is in the lungs, sometimes the lung tumor can be removed.

RADIATION THERAPY. Radiation therapy uses high-energy rays such as **x rays** to kill cancer cells:

- External beam radiation—delivered from outside the body—is aimed directly into the sarcoma and is the most common radiation treatment for soft tissue sarcomas.
- Internal radiation therapy (brachytherapy) delivers small pellets of radioactive material directly into the sarcoma through thin plastic tubes. It may be used alone or in combination with external beam radiation.

Radiation may be used:

- before and/or after surgery for all sarcoma stages
- for inoperable stage I and II sarcomas
- as the primary treatment for patients with health conditions that preclude surgery
- to kill small clusters of cancer cells
- to relieve symptoms of stage IVB sarcoma
- as an adjunct treatment 6–9 weeks after chemotherapy
- for recurrent sarcomas that were not treated previously with radiation
- to treat pain accompanying recurrences

Tumors of the retroperitoneum, trunk, head, or neck may be treated with fast neutron therapy.

Short-term side effects of radiation therapy may include:

- fatigue
- mild skin conditions
- infections
- nausea, vomiting, and diarrhea after irradiation of the abdomen
- mouth sores and loss of appetite after head or neck irradiation
- swelling, weakness, or pain following irradiation of large portions of a limb

Longer-term radiation effects can include:

- worsening of chemotherapy side effects
- breathing difficulties and lung damage from chest irradiation
- bone fractures, sometimes occurring years later
- headaches and mental problems one to two years after radiation therapy for metastatic sarcoma in the brain

CHEMOTHERAPY. Chemotherapy may be used:

- as primary therapy for some sarcomas
- to shrink a stage II tumor prior to surgery
- as postoperative treatment for stage II sarcomas
- before or after surgery for stage III sarcomas to reduce the risk of recurrence
- to treat metastasized sarcomas
- to reduce pain with stage IV sarcomas
- for recurrence at a distant site

Synovial sarcomas respond more readily to chemotherapy than other soft tissue sarcomas. Chemotherapy usually does not prevent metastasis and the benefits of postoperative chemotherapy in children have been questioned.

Ifosfamide and **doxorubicin** (Adriamycin) are the most common drugs for treating soft tissue sarcoma. They may be used alone, together, or in combination with other drugs including:

- dacarbazine
- methotrexate
- vincristine
- cisplatin
- paclitaxel
- mesna for protecting the bladder from severe irritation caused by ifosfamide

When used alone only doxorubicin and ifosfamide have response rates above 20%. Doxorubicin alone or in combination with **dacarbazine** is the most frequently used chemotherapy for advanced sarcomas. High-dose ifosfamide is used to relieve symptoms of inoperable sarcomas.

Postoperative chemotherapy for ERMS is usually **vincristine** and **dactinomycin** (actinomycin-D). For group II and III RMS, **cyclophosphamide** is added for a three-drug combination called VAC. **Topotecan** also may be included.

Temporary side effects of chemotherapy may include:

- nausea and vomiting
- loss of appetite
- hair loss
- mouth sores

Chemotherpy can damage blood-producing bone marrow cells, increasing the risk of:

- fatigue
- bruising or bleeding
- infection

Most side effects disappear when chemotherapy ends, although it sometimes causes infertility. Doxorubicin can weaken the heart and ifosfamide and cyclophosphamide can cause permanent kidney or bladder damage.

RECURRENCES. Treatment of recurrent soft tissue sarcomas depends on the initial type and treatment. If the initial treatment was minimal, a local recurrence may be treated with surgery and radiation. If the original treatment was aggressive, limb amputation may be necessary. The lungs are the most common distant site of sarcoma recurrences, usually within two to three years after the initial diagnosis. These are treated as stage IV disease. In older patients symptoms of recurrence may be treated by the sequential use of single chemotherapy drugs. Synovial sarcomas tend to recur locally and involve regional lymph nodes; however distant metastasis occurs in about 50% of cases, sometimes many years later.

Prognosis

Stage I and II soft tissue sarcomas rarely metastasize although they may recur locally if inadequately treated:

- Stage I sarcomas have a five-year-survival rate of 99% and only a 20% chance of recurrence within five years.
- Stage II sarcomas have an 82%-five-year-survival rate and a five-year-recurrence risk of 35%.
- Stage III sarcomas have a five-year-survival rate of 50% and a five-year-recurrence risk of about 65%.
- Stage IV sarcomas are usually incurable with a five-year-survival rate of 10–15%.
- Surgery to remove metastatic lung sarcomas has a five-year-survival rate of 20–30% and occasionally a complete cure.
- Patients over age 60 have a poorer prognosis than younger adults.

In children:

- stage I: 90% never have a recurrence
- stage II: about 89% survive long term and about 50% of recurrences are cured in the second round of treatment
- stage III: about 70% survive long term
- stage IV: a five-year-survival rate of less than 30%, although children under age 10 with metastatic embryonal tumors have a 50% chance of survival.

Younger children with RMS have higher survival rates than older children and adolescents and ERMS has a more favorable prognosis than ARMS. More than 70% of children survive ERMS and second malignancies arise in less than 25% of survivors, usually in children with more advanced disease.

Children with non-RMS generally have a better prognosis than adults, although if the sarcoma is not removed completely, metastasizes, or recurs, the prognosis is poor:

- Leiomyosarcoma has a good prognosis unless it is within the gastrointestinal tract.
- Infantile fibrosarcoma—which occurs in children under five—has an excellent prognosis when treated with surgery alone.
- Adult-type fibrosarcomas have a survival rate of about 60% in both children and adults.
- MFH has a survival rate of about 50%.
- Desmoid tumors rarely metastasize and have an excellent prognosis.
- Liposarcomas have a good prognosis if completely removed.
- The prognosis for angiosarcomas and hemangioendotheliomas depends on their removal, the extent of the disease, and the grade of the malignancy.
- Hemangiopericytoma has an excellent prognosis in young children and an overall survival rate of 30–70%.
- Synovial sarcoma has a survival rate of 80%.
- Neurofibrosarcoma has a very good prognosis with complete removal; otherwise the prognosis is poor.
- Alveolar and clear cell soft-part sarcomas have a 50% survival rate and late relapses are common.

High-grade retroperitoneal sarcoma has a less favorable prognosis because of the difficulty of completely removing the tumor and the limitations on high-dose radiation therapy. Local recurrence is the most common cause of death in these patients.

Clinical trials

As of 2005 numerous **clinical trials** for treating soft tissue sarcomas in children and adults were underway, including trials to evaluate:

- chemotherapy prior to surgery
- regional chemotherapy in which drugs are injected directly into the artery that supplies an affected limb
- new drugs for reducing heart damage from doxorubicin, so that higher doses can be used
- the use of radiation therapy during surgery for abdominal and retroperitoneal sarcomas
- drugs such as interleukin-2 to boost the immune system
- vaccines that may cause the immune system to recognize abnormal chemicals in sarcomas and destroy the cells
- stem-cell transplantations that allow higher levels of chemotherapy for treating RMS.

Prevention

Most soft tissue sarcomas develop in people with no known risk factors. Since early detection is very important, a healthcare professional should be consulted about unexplained lumps, growths, or other symptoms. Less than 5% of soft tissue sarcomas are caused by radiation exposure. Lymphangiosarcomas can develop where lymph nodes have been damaged by radiation or surgically removed.

A high percentage of patients with angiosarcoma of the liver have been exposed to vinyl chloride. Although exposures to other chemicals—including dioxin, herbicides containing phenoxyacetic acid, and chlorophenols in wood preservations—have been suggested as risk factors for soft tissue sarcoma, there are no proven connections.

The only known risk factors in children are congenital (present at birth) abnormalities and genetic (inherited) conditions:

- Li-Fraumeni syndrome increases the risk of soft tissue sarcomas as well as other types of cancer and there is a high risk of developing soft tissue sarcoma in an area that was irradiated to treat another cancer.
- Children with inherited retinoblastoma—an eye cancer—are at increased risk for soft tissue sarcoma.
- Children with Beckwith-Wiedemann syndrome are at risk for developing RMS.
- Gardner's syndrome increases the risk of desmoid tumors in the abdomen.
- Neurofibromatosis or von Recklinghausen's disease is characterized by benign neurofibromas; in about 5% of cases these develop into malignant peripheral nerve sheath tumors.

Those with a family history of sarcomas or other cancers occurring at a young age may have **genetic testing** to assess their risk.

Special concerns

Since advanced soft tissue sarcoma has a high risk of metastasis and recurrence, following treatment a patient may have:

- frequent physical examinations
- chest x rays, ultrasound, or CT or MRI scans

See also AIDS-related cancers; Osteosarcoma.

Resources

BOOKS

Meyer, W. H. 'Soft Tissue Sarcomas.' In *Cancer Medicine*. 6th ed., edited by D. W. Kufe, et al. Hamilton, Ontario: BC Decker, 2003: 2377–82.

Pizzo, P. A., and D. G. Poplack, editors. *Prinicples and Practice of Pediatric Oncology*. 4th ed. Philadelphia: Lippincott, Williams and Wilkins, 2002.

Pollack, Raphael E. *Soft Tissue Sarcomas*. Atlanta: American Cancer Society, 2002.

Weiss, S. W., and J. R. Goldblum. *Enzinger and Weiss's Soft Tissue Tumors*. 4th ed. St. Louis: Mosby, 2001.

Yasko, A., et al. 'Sarcomas of Soft Tissue and Bone.' In *Clinical Oncology*, edited by R. E. Lenhard Jr, et al. Atlanta: American Cancer Society, 2001: 611-32.

PERIODICALS

O'Sullivan, B., et al. 'Preoperative Versus Postoperative Radiotherapy in Soft-Tissue Sarcoma of the Limbs: A Randomized Trial.' *The Lancet* 359, no. 9325 (2002): 2235–41.

OTHER

Adult Soft Tissue Sarcoma (PDQ): Treatment, Health Professional Version. February 1, 2005. National Cancer Institute. March 30, 2005. <http://cancernet.nci.nih.gov/cancertopics/pdq/treatment/adult-soft-tissue-sarcoma/healthprofessional>.

Adult Soft Tissue Sarcoma (PDQ): Treatment, Patient Version. April 22, 2004. National Cancer Institute. March 30, 2005. <http://cancernet.nci.nih.gov/cancertopics/pdq/treatment/adult-soft-tissue-sarcoma/patient>.

Childhood Soft Tissue Sarcoma (PDQ): Treatment, Health Professional Version. February 17, 2005. National Cancer Institute. March 30, 2005. <http://cancernet.nci.nih.gov/cancertopics/pdq/treatment/child-soft-tissue-sarcoma/healthprofessional>.

Childhood Soft Tissue Sarcoma (PDQ): Treatment, Patient Version. February 16, 2005. National Cancer Institute. March 30, 2005. <http://cancernet.nci.nih.gov/cancertopics/pdq/treatment/child-soft-tissue-sarcoma/patient>.

Gurney, James G., et al. 'Soft Tissue Sarcomas.' *SEER Pediatric Monograph*. National Cancer Institute. March 30, 2005. <http://seer.cancer.gov/publications/childhood/softtissue.pdf>.

Rhabdomyosarcoma. September 11, 2003. American Cancer Society. March 30, 2005. <http://documents.cancer.org/5020.00/5020.00.pdf>.

Sarcoma—Adult Soft Tissue Cancer. January 5, 2005. American Cancer Society. March 30, 2005. <http://documents.cancer.org/188.00/188.00.pdf>.

'Soft Tissue Sarcomas: Questions and Answers.' *Cancer Facts*. May 6, 2002. National Cancer Institute. March 30, 2005. <http://cis.nci.nih.gov/fact/6_12.htm>.

ORGANIZATIONS

American Cancer Society. PO Box 102454, Atlanta, GA 30368-2454. 800-ACS-2345. http://www.cancer.org. Information, research, and patient support.

CureSearch. 4600 East West Highway, #600, Bethesda, MD 20814-3457. 800-458-6223. 240-235-2200. http://www.curesearch.org. Children's Oncology Group and the National Childhood Cancer Foundation. Information, research, and advocacy.

National Cancer Institute. Public Inquiries Office, Suite 30361, 6116 Executive Blvd., MSC-8322, Bethesda, MD 20892-8322. 800-4-CANCER (800-422-6237). http://www.nci.nih.gov. Information, research, and clinical trials.

National Children's Cancer Society. 1015 Locust, Suite 600, St. Louis, MO 63101. 800-5-FAMILY (800-532-6459). 314-241-1600. <http://nationalchildrenscancersociety.com<. Financial assistance, support services, advocacy, and education.

Margaret Alic, Ph.D.

Sorafenib

Definition

Sorafenib is a anti-cancer drug used to treat some types of **kidney cancer** and **liver cancer**.

Purpose

Sorafenib is used to treat a type of kidney **cancer** known as renal cell **carcinoma**. Sorafenib is used for renal cell carcinoma specifically when it is not amenable to surgery and methods other than surgery need to be used to remove the cancer, when the carcinoma has reached an advanced stage resistant to other treatments, and when the cancer is metastatic (has traveled from other sites in the body). Sorafenib is also used for a type of liver cancer known as hepatocellular carcinoma. Sorafenib is used for hepatocellular carcinoma specifically when it is not amenable to surgery and methods other than surgery need to be used to remove the cancer.

KEY TERMS

Angiogenesis—Physiological process involving the growth of new blood vessels from pre-existing blood vessels, process used by some cancers to create their own blood supply

Blood electrolytes—Ions present in the blood that are necessary for health such as sodium and potassium

Blood platelets—Blood component responsible for normal blood clotting to seal wounds

Cytochrome P450— Enzymes present in the liver that metabolize drugs

Erectile dysfunction—Sexual disorder involving the inability to develop or maintain a penile erection

Hemorrhage—Extensive bleeding that may be life threatening

Hepatocellular carcinoma—Malignant cancer of the liver that may arise in the liver or metastasize from elsewhere in the body

Metastasize—The process by which cancer spreads from its original site to other parts of the body

Receptor tyrosine kinase—Cell surface receptors that interact with growth factors and hormones to affect the normal life cycle of a cell

Renal cell carcinoma—Cancer of the kidney that originates in the very small tubes in the kidney that filter the blood and remove waste products

Serine/threonine kinases— Cell surface receptors that interact with growth factors and hormones to affect the normal life cycle of a cell

Description

Sorafenib is manufactured by Bayer HealthCare Pharmaceuticals and Onyx Pharmaceuticals under the trade name Nexavar. It is manufactured in pill form taken by the oral route of administration. Sorafenib is an anti-cancer drug that acts on receptor tyrosine kinases to inhibit the growth of tumors. Receptor tyrosine kinases are receptors for growth factors that are a natural part of cell development and necessary for normal cell growth. When tyrosine kinase receptors are activated, they initiate chemical signals that

QUESTIONS TO ASK YOUR DOCTOR OR PHARMACIST

- How long will I need to take this drug before you can tell if it helps for me?
- Do I have to have blood work and other laboratory tests done to check the effect the drug is having?
- Is this drug safe to take with the other drugs that I am currently taking?
- What side effects should I watch for? When should I call the doctor about them?
- Are there any clinical trials of this drug combined with other therapies that might benefit me?

tell the cell how to grow and develop. Normal tyrosine kinase receptors turn on and off as needed for usual amounts of growth. However, when cells have constantly activated tyrosine kinase receptors, it can lead to abnormal growth and cancer. Drugs in the class of sorafenib inhibit these overly active tyrosine kinase receptors, thereby inhibiting the proliferation of tumor cells. Sorafenib acts on other drug targets that affect tumor growth called serine/threonine kinases. By acting at these additional kinases, sorafenib increases the range of tumor cell surface targets and the effectiveness of **chemotherapy**.

Once they reach a certain size, solid tumor cells need to form their own blood supply in order to grow and remain alive. New blood vessels need to be formed for the tumor to survive. This process is known as angiogenesis. Angiogenesis is a part of tumor progression, one of the processes critical to tumor growth and survival. Sorafenib is thought to act on many different tumor cell surface receptors, which in addition to inhibiting individual tumor cell growth, inhibit the angiogenesis process as well.

Studies have shown that use of sorafenib increases progression-free survival compared to placebo. The term progression-free survival describes the length of time during and after treatment in which a patient is living with a disease that does not get worse. In a clinical trial designed to test out a cancer drug in humans, progression-free survival is a way to measure how effective a treatment is.

Recommended Dosage

Sorafenib is taken orally in pill form. The usual adult dose for either renal cell carcinoma or hepatocellular carcinoma is 400 mg taken twice a day. The presence of fat in food decreases the amount of sorafenib available to fight cancer in the body. Sorafenib needs to be taken either 1 hour before or 2 hours after meals, and should be swallowed with water. Therapy with sorafenib is continued for as long as there is clinical benefit, or until the development of intolerable side effects or toxicity. In patients that develop severe side effects the dose may be adjusted to 400 mg taken once daily or discontinued altogether if toxicity occurs.

Studies done in Japanese patients suggest that less drug may be present in the body after the usual dose when compared with white patients. The clinical significance of this finding and its implications for dosing are unknown. Patients should never take higher doses of sorafenib than those set by their physician. If a dose of sorafenib is missed and remembered near the time of the next dose, that dose is skipped. Patients should never double dose to catch up on missed doses.

Precautions

Sorafenib is a pregnancy category D drug. Pregnancy category D drugs are drugs for which there is evidence of human fetal risk based on data from marketing experience or studies in done in humans, but for which the potential medical benefit is great enough that it may warrant use of the drug in pregnant women despite the risks. Sorafenib use during pregnancy may result in death to the fetus. Sorafenib is only used in pregnancy if medically necessary for survival of the mother, and is not recommended for use in breastfeeding. Both male and female patients undergoing sorafenib treatment should avoid the conception of a pregnancy. At least two forms of reliable birth control methods need to be used during treatment and for 2 weeks after the last dose.

Sorafenib has not been approved for use in individuals less than 18 years of age. Patients should not have any vaccinations while taking sorafenib without the consent of their treating physician, and live **vaccines** should not be given. Patients taking sorafenib should also avoid being around people who have recently had the oral polio vaccine or the inhaled flu vaccine, as these are both live vaccines.

Sorafenib may not be appropriate for use in patients with pre-existing heart disease or disorders, recent heart attack, excessive bleeding or bleeding disorders, inflammation of the pancreas, depressed immune system, decreased blood platelets, impaired kidneys or kidney disease, impaired liver or liver disease, or damage to the gastrointestinal tract. Sorafenib may not be appropriate for use in patients who have recently had surgical procedures. Sorafenib increases risk of causing high blood pressure or exacerbation of existing high blood pressure, especially within the first 6 weeks of treatment. Blood pressure is monitored regularly while in treatment with sorafenib.

Side Effects

Sorafenib is used when the medical benefit is judged to be greater than the risk of side effects. Many patients undergoing sorafenib treatment do not develop medically serious side effects. The most commonly seen side effects associated with sorafenib treatment are abdominal pain and cramping, **nausea**, **vomiting**, **diarrhea**, constipation, bone and joint pain, muscle pain, weakness, **fatigue**, flu-like symptoms, **fever**, flushed skin, rash, peeling inflamed skin, hair loss, acne, headache, loss of appetite, **weight loss**, difficulty breathing, cough, hoarseness, **anemia**, high blood pressure, inflammation of the inner lining of the mouth, **depression**, erectile dysfunction, hemorrhage (severe bleeding) of the gastrointestinal and respiratory tracts, blood electrolyte imbalances, depressed immune system, nervous system damage in the arms and legs, and blood disorders such as decreased blood platelets.

Sorafenib also commonly causes severe hand foot syndrome, caused by leakage of sorafenib out of small blood vessels in the hands and feet. During some types of chemotherapy, small amounts of medication in the blood stream leak out of capillaries in the palms of the hands and the soles of the feet. Drug leakage is increased by heat exposure or friction. The result is redness, tenderness, and sometimes peeling of the skin of the palms and soles. The appearance of sunburn, numbness, and tingling may develop, and may interfere with the activity level of the patient.

Rarely, sorafenib treatment is associated with chronic heart failure, heart attacks, and other cardiac disorders, severe inflammation of the pancreas, inflammation of the gastrointestinal tract, heartburn, abnormal breast development in males, extreme high blood pressure, ringing in the ears, and short periods of decreased oxygen flow to the brain.

Interactions

Patients should make their doctor aware of any and all medications or supplements they are taking before using sorafenib. Sorafenib interacts with many other drugs. Some drug interactions may make sorafenib unsuitable for use, while others may be monitored and attempted. Use of sorafenib with the agent **docetaxel** may cause docetaxel toxicity, caution is advised. Multiple agents may have toxic effects when used in the same time period as sorafenib. Sorafenib may have dangerous additive effects with other drugs that also cause bleeding disorders. Drugs that interact with sorafenib in this way include **warfarin** and **heparin**.

Sorafenib is metabolized by a set of liver enzymes known as cytochrome P450 (CYP-450) subtype 3A4. Drugs that induce, or activate these enzymes increase the metabolism of sorafenib. This results in lower levels of therapeutic sorafenib, thereby negatively affecting treatment of cancer. For this reason drugs that induce CYP-450 subtype 3A4 may not be used with sorafenib. This includes some anti-epileptic drugs such as **carbamazepine**, some anti-inflammatory drugs such as **dexamethasone**, anti-tuberculosis drugs such as rifampin, and the herb St. John's Wort.

Drugs that act to inhibit the action of CYP-450 subtype 3A4 may cause undesired increased levels of sorafenib in the body. This could lead to toxic doses. Some examples are **antibiotics** such as clarithromycin, antifungal drugs such as ketoconazole, antiviral drugs such as indinavir, antidepressants such as fluoxetine, and some cardiac agents such as verapamil. Grapefruit juice may also increase the amount of sorafenib in the body. Patients should avoid drinking grapefruit juice or eating grapefruit while taking sorafenib.

Resources

BOOKS

*Goodman and Gilman's The Pharmacological Basis of Therapeutics, Eleventh Edition*McGraw Hill Medical Publishing Division, 2006.

*Tarascon Pharmacopoeia Library Edition*Jones and Bartlett Publishers, 2009.

OTHER

Medscape*Sorafenib*.<http://www.medscape.com.>

RxList*Nexavar*.<http://www.rxlist.com.>

Epocrates*Sorafenib*.<http://www.epocrates.com.>

ORGANIZATIONS

National Cancer Institute. 6116 Executive Boulevard, Room 3036A, Bethesda, MD 20892-8322. (800)4-CANCER <http://www.cancer.gov.>

FDA U.S. Food and Drug Administration. 10903 New Hampshire Ave, Silver Spring, MD 20993. (888)INFO-FDA <http://www.fda.gov.>

Maria Basile, Ph.D.

Sperm banking *see* **Fertility issues**

Spinal axis tumors

Definition

Spinal axis tumors are tumors that affect the spinal cord—the bundle of nerves that lies inside the backbone. Another term for spinal axis tumors is spinal cord tumors.

Description

Spinal axis tumors form on or near the spinal cord and produce pressure on the associated nerves and blood vessels. There are three types of spinal axis tumors: extradural, extramedullary intradural, and intramedullary.

Extradural spinal axis tumors

Extradural tumors are found outside the dura mater, the membrane that encases the spinal cord. Extradural tumors are wedged between the dura mater and the bone of the spine. Types of extradural tumors include chordomas, osteoblastomas, osteomas, and hemangiomas.

Extramedullary intradural spinal axis tumors

Extramedullary intradural tumors are found inside the dura mater but outside the nerves of the spinal cord itself. Types of extramedullary tumors include meningiomas and neurofibromas.

Intramedullary spinal axis tumors

Intramedullary tumors are found inside the nerves of the spinal cord. Types of intramedullary tumors include astrocytomas, ependymomas, and hemangioblastomas.

Benign vs. malignant

Spinal axis tumors are classified as either benign or malignant. The cells of malignant tumors are very different from normal cells, grow quickly, and usually spread easily to other parts of the body. Benign tumors have cells that are similar to normal cells, grow slowly, and tend to be localized. However, even benign tumors can cause significant problems when they grow within the confined space inside the backbone.

Demographics

Primary spinal axis tumors, or tumors that originate in the spinal axis itself, are extremely rare and represent only 0.5% of all diagnosed tumors. Malignant primary spinal axis tumors comprise about 65% of all spinal axis tumors. However, most spinal axis tumors result from **metastasis**, or spreading, of other types of **cancer** to the spinal axis. Other cancers that can spread to the spinal axis include head and neck cancer, **thyroid cancer**, **skin cancer**, **prostate cancer**, lung cancer, **breast cancer**, and others. The American Cancer Society estimates that brain and spinal cord cancers (primary only) represent approximately 1.4% of all cancers and 2.4% of all cancer-related deaths, but separate statistics for spinal cord cancers only are unavailable.

Half of all spinal axis tumors occur in the thoracic, or chest, region as opposed to the neck (cervical) or lower back (lumbar) region.

Spinal axis tumors occur with equal frequency in members of all races and ethnic groups. There does not appear to be any relationship between spinal axis

KEY TERMS

Astrocytoma—A tomor that begins in the brain or spinal cord in cells called astrocytes.

Chordoma—A type of bone cancer.

Dura mater—The tough membrane that encases the nerves of the spinal cord.

Ependymoma—A tumor that begins in the tissue that lines the central canal of the spinal cord and the ventricles of the brain. About 85% of these tumors are benign.

Hemangioblastoma—A tumor composed of capillaries and disorganized clumps of capillary cells or angioblasts.

Hemangioma—A benign tumor consisting of a mass of blood vessels.

Meningioma—A tumor that occurs in the meninges, the membranes that cover the brain and spinal cord. Meningiomas usually grow slowly and primarily affect adults.

Metastasic tumor—A tumor that results from the spreading of one type of cancer to other parts of the body.

Neurofibroma—A fibrous tumor of nerve tissue.

Osteoblastoma—A benign tumor that most frequently occurs in the vertebrae, leg bones, or arm bones of children and young adults.

Osteoma—A usually benign tumor of bone tissue.

Spinal cord—The bundle of nerves that runs inside the backbone.

QUESTIONS TO ASK THE DOCTOR

- Which type of spinal axis tumor do I have?
- Is my tumor operable?

tumors and any geographic region. Males and females are affected in equal numbers by spinal axis tumors.

Causes and symptoms

The cause, or causes, of primary spinal axis tumors are not known. The cause of metastatic spinal axis tumors is the originating cancer in another part of the body.

The symptoms of spinal axis tumors are the result of increased pressure on the nerves of the spine. These symptoms include:

- constant, severe, burning or aching pain
- numbness of the skin or decreased temperature sensation
- muscle weakness, wasting, or even paralysis
- problems with bladder and bowel control
- muscle spasticity or problems in walking normally

The location of the tumor determines where the symptoms are most noticeable. A tumor in the cervical region can cause symptoms in the neck or arms, while a tumor in the thoracic region may cause chest pain. A tumor in the lumbar region can result in observable symptoms in the back, bladder and bowel, and legs.

Diagnosis

The diagnosis of spinal axis tumors begins with a medical history and physical examination when the patient brings his or her symptoms to the doctor's attention. The diagnosis may be difficult to make due to the similarity of tumor symptoms to those caused by disc herniation or other spinal cord injuries.

If the doctor suspects a spinal axis tumor may be present, further diagnostic tests are ordered. These tests are performed by a neurological specialist. Imaging tests that may be ordered include:

- magnetic resonance imaging (MRI)
- computed tomography (CT)
- bone scan
- spinal tap and myelogram, a specialized x-ray technique

Treatment team

Treatment of any primary central nervous system tumor, including spinal axis tumors, is different from treating tumors in other parts of the body. Spinal cord surgery requires much more precision than most other surgeries. Also, the thoracic area, where the majority of spinal axis tumors are located, is highly sensitive to radiation. The most up-to-date treatment opportunities are available from experienced, multi-disciplinary medical professional teams made up of doctors, nurses, and technologists who specialize in cancer (oncology), neurosurgery, medical imaging, drug or **radiation therapy**, and anesthesiology.

Clinical staging, treatments, and prognosis

Malignant tumors of the spinal axis may spread (metastasize) to other parts of the central nervous system, but almost never spread to other parts of the body. As of mid-2001, there is no staging system for spinal axis tumors. The most important factors in determining prognosis for individuals with these tumors are the type of cell involved (eg. astrocyte, ependyma, etc.) and the grade of the tumor (an indicator of the aggressiveness of the tumor cells). Grade I tumors have cells that are not malignant and are nearly normal in appearance. Grade II tumors have cells that appear to be slightly abnormal. Grade III tumors have cells that are malignant and clearly abnormal. Grade IV tumors contain fast-spreading and abnormal cells. In general, the survival rate for some types of spinal cord tumors, such as extradural tumors and low-grade astrocytomas, is better than for other types, such as ependymomas.

The treatment of spinal axis tumors depends on the location of the tumor and the severity of the symptoms. Many spinal axis tumors can be treated by surgical removal of the tumor. Medical advances in surgical techniques, such as microsurgery and laser surgery, have greatly improved the success rate of spinal cord surgeries.

In some instances of spinal axis tumors, the tumor is inoperable. Patients with inoperable spinal axis tumors are generally treated with radiation therapies.

Other treatments may include the use of steroids to reduce swelling and pressure on the spinal cord, surgical decompression and fusion of the spine, and **chemotherapy** in selected cases. These may be the only treatments used if the spinal axis tumor is due to the metastasis of another primary cancer.

Prevention

Because the causes of spinal axis tumors are not known, there are no known preventative measures.

Special concerns

If left untreated, spinal axis tumors can cause loss of muscle function up to and including paralysis. This makes the proper diagnosis of spinal axis tumors important.

See also Astrocytoma; Brain and central nervous system tumors; Chordoma; Ependymoma.

Resources

OTHER

Brain and Spinal Cord Tumors—Hope Through Research. National Institute of Neurological Disorders and Stroke. [cited April 15, 2001]. http://www.ninds.nih.gov/health_and_medical/pubs/brain_tumor_hope_through_research.htm.

Spinal Cord Tumor Support. [cited April 15, 2001]. http://www.spinalcordtumor.homestead.com.

ORGANIZATIONS

The Brain Tumor Society. 124 Watertown Street, Suite 3-H, Watertown, MA 02472. (617) 924-9997. Fax: (617) 924-9998. http://www.tbts.org/.

National Brain Tumor Foundation. 785 Market Street, Suite 1600, San Francisco, CA 94103. (415) 284-0208. http://www.braintumor.org/.

Paul A. Johnson, Ed.M.

Spinal cord compression

Description

In order to understand spinal cord compression, it is useful to understand the structure of the spinal cord and to understand the difference between the spinal cord and the vertebral column. The vertebral column includes the bony structure surrounding the spinal cord and the spinal cord itself. Also an important part of the vertebral column, the intervertebral disks, are found between vertebrae. They act as shock absorbers. The spinal cord, however, is the series of nerves that runs down the hollow part of the vertebrae. Thus, the bony vertebrae and shock-absorbing disks protect the spinal cord from physical damage and compression.

Spinal cord compression occurs when something presses down with sufficient force on the nerves within the spinal cord so that they lose their ability to function properly. Although trauma, degenerative back disease, and genetic disorders can cause pressure on the spinal cord, the term spinal cord compression is usually reserved for cases in which the presence of a tumor results in pressure on the spinal cord. The tumor may originate in a number of areas and either directly or indirectly put pressure on the cord.

The spinal cord is a series of nerves bundled together that are responsible for most functions of the body, including, but not limited to, the "fight or flight" response, the movement of arms and legs, and feeling below the neck. Each nerve is responsible for different functions, such as movement, and each has a different position within the structure of the spinal cord. Thus, depending on which angle the spinal cord is compressed from, a person could experience numbness versus a loss of the ability to control muscles (often seen as an odd limp), depending on which area is compressed.

Not only do the different nerve clusters of the spinal cord have different functions, but each has nerves branching off from the spinal cord at many levels. Each of these branches controls different parts of the body. For example, nerves branching off the spinal cord in the low back control movement of the legs, and nerves branching off the spinal cord at the level of the neck are responsible for most of the movements of the arm. Thus, compression of the spinal cord at different levels can result in very different symptoms.

Vertebrae are, in order, divided into cervical, thoracic, lumbar, and sacral sections. The cervical vertebrae correspond to the neck, the thoracic vertebrae correspond to most of the torso, the lumbar vertebrae are found in the low back, and the sacral vertebrae correspond to the area of the buttocks. There are seven cervical, twelve thoracic, five lumbar, and five sacral vertebrae (although the sacrum is one bony structure and contains no intervertebral disks). The level of compression is indicated by using the first letter of the type of vertebra and then the number of the vertebra within the group. The topmost vertebrae are numbered lowest, so the first cervical vertebra is the vertebra closest to the head, and is known as C1. C7 is the cervical vertebra furthest down the spine. Compression of the spinal cord in this region would be known as compression at C7. The closer the compression is to the head, the more symptoms the patient is likely to have, since compression of the spinal cord affects all the levels of nerves below the area of compression that are part of the same nerve branch. For example, if movement were affected at C2 and below, a person would have difficulty using both arms and legs, whereas compression at T12 might result in just difficulty using the legs.

Importantly, the first symptom patients usually display prior to actual spinal cord compression is pain, especially pain that is not relieved by lying down, and which has lasted one month or more. This kind of pain should be sufficient to suspect imminent spinal cord compression due to cancerous causes. Also, there may be damage to nerve roots at the level of compression that can lead to symptoms in other parts of the body. For example, if the cord compression is in the lower part of the spine, then parts of the legs may be affected with numbness, tingling and loss of power and movement. Similarly, if the problem lies in the upper part of the spinal column, there may be a loss of power and sensation in parts of the arms or hands. If the cord compression becomes more severe, it can affect lower muscle functions such as bowel and bladder.

Causes

The most common cause of cancerous spinal cord compression is a vertebral **metastasis**. A metastasis is a cancerous lesion that arises from another tumor somewhere else in the body. Vertebral metastases account for 85% of cases of spinal cord compression, and 70% of those metastases occur in the thoracic vertebrae. About 5% to 10% of patients with **cancer** will develop metastases to the spinal cord. Tumors may also grow from the nerves themselves, from the connective tissue surrounding the nerves, or, rarely, from the bony vertebrae themselves. Tumors that grow from outside the vertebral column may cause pressure by either growing into the hollow space in the vertebral column or by pressuring the vertebrae into an abnormal conformation. More rarely, tumors in the vertebrae may cause compression indirectly by causing the vertebrae to collapse. Tumors that originate in the spinal cord or in the connective tissue overlying the spinal cord cause direct pressure because there is a limited area in which they can grow before impinging on the cord directly.

Treatments

If symptoms develop, prompt diagnosis and rapid treatment are crucial in order to avoid any permanent damage to the sensitive nerve tissue of the spinal cord. Usually, **magnetic resonance imaging** (MRI) or **computed tomography** (CT) scans will be performed to confirm cord compression and fully define the level and extent of the lesion. High-dose **corticosteroids** (oral or IV **dexamethasone**) may be promptly administered in order to reduce inflammation and pressure.

The goal of therapy for spinal cord compression includes pain control, avoidance of complications, preserving or improving neurologic functions, or reversing impaired neurologic functions. Treatment usually involves treatment of the underlying tumor. For most patients with cancer-induced compression, **radiation therapy** is the treatment of choice. However, if radiation therapy is unavailable or if neurologic signs worsen despite medical therapy, surgical decompression should be performed. Surgery is also indicated when a **biopsy** is needed, when the spine is unstable, when tumors have recurred after radiation therapy, or when any abscess is present. Finally, in some tumors known to be highly chemoresponsive, **chemotherapy** alone or in combination with other modalities may be used.

Resources

BOOKS

Beers, Mark H., and Robert Berkow, editors. *The Merck Manual of Diagnosis and Therapy*. 17th ed. Whitehouse Station, NJ, 1999.

PERIODICALS

Abrahm, Janet L. "Management of Pain and Spinal Cord Compression in Patients with Advanced Cancer." *Annals of Internal Medicine* 131 (July 6, 1999): 37.

Garner, C.M. "Cancer-related Spinal Cord Compression." *American Journal of Nursing* 99, no. 7 (July 1999): 34.

Michael Zuck, Ph.D.

Splenectomy

Definition

Splenectomy is the surgical removal of the spleen, which is an organ that is part of the lymphatic system. The spleen is a dark purple, bean-shaped organ located in the upper left side of the abdomen, just behind the bottom of the rib cage. In adults, the spleen is about 4.8 × 2.8 × 1.6 in in size, and weighs about 4 or 5 oz. (It measures 12 × 7 × 4 cm, and weighs between 113 and 141 grams.) Its functions include: playing a role in the immune system, filtering foreign substances from the blood, removing worn-out blood cells from the blood, regulating blood flow to the liver, and sometimes storing blood cells. The storage of blood cells is called sequestration. In healthy adults, about 30% of blood platelets are sequestered in the spleen.

Purpose

Splenectomies are performed for a variety of different reasons and with different degrees of urgency. Most splenectomies are done after the patient has been diagnosed with hypersplenism. Hypersplenism is not a specific disease but a group of symptoms, or a

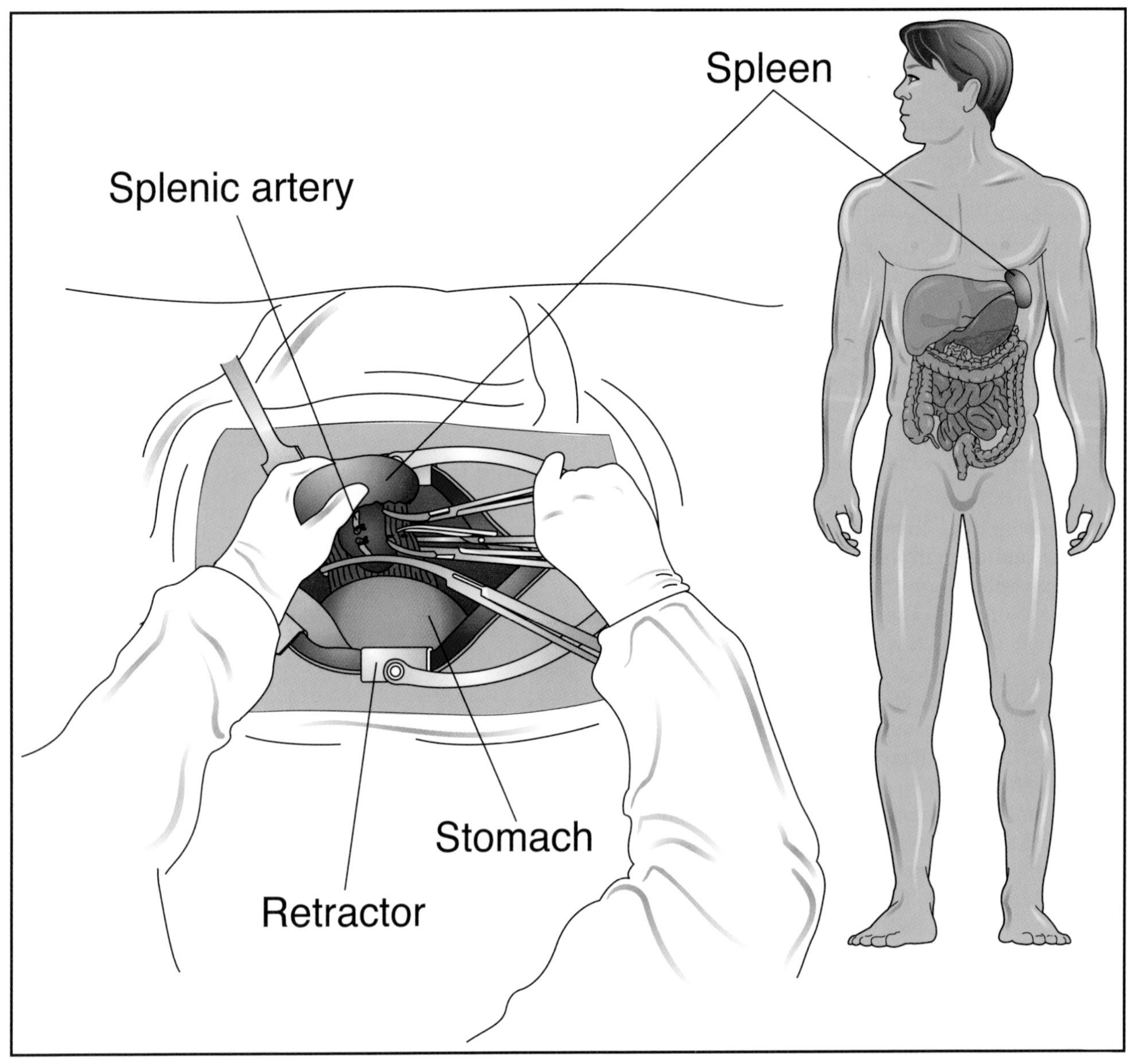

Splenectomy is the surgical removal of the spleen. This procedure is performed as a last resort in most diseases involving the spleen. In some cases, such as in many types of cancer, splenectomy does not cure the condition causing the splenomegaly—it only relieves the symptoms from the enlarged spleen. *(Illustration by Electronic Illustrators Group. Cengage Learning, Gale.)*

syndrome, that can be produced by a number of different disorders. Hypersplenism is characterized by enlargement of the spleen (splenomegaly), defects in the blood cells, and an abnormally high turnover of blood cells. It is almost always associated with splenomegaly caused by specific disorders such as cirrhosis of the liver or certain cancers, such as leukemia or lymphomas (both Hodgkin's and non-Hodgkin's). Because serious consequences may result from removal of immune system organs such as the spleen, the decision to perform a splenectomy depends on the severity and prognosis of the disease or condition causing the hypersplenism.

Splenectomy always necessary

There are two diseases for which splenectomy is the only treatment—primary cancers of the spleen and a blood disorder called hereditary spherocytosis (HS). In HS, the absence of a specific protein in the red blood cell membrane leads to the formation of relatively fragile cells that are easily damaged when they pass through the spleen. The cell destruction does not occur elsewhere in the body and ends when the spleen is removed. HS can appear at any age, even in newborns, although doctors prefer to put off removing the spleen until the child is five or six years old.

KEY TERMS

Embolization—An alternative to splenectomy that involves injecting silicone or similar substances into the splenic artery to shrink the size of the spleen.

Hereditary spherocytosis (HS)—A blood disorder in which the red blood cells are relatively fragile and are damaged or destroyed when they pass through the spleen. Splenectomy is the only treatment for HS.

Hypersplenism—A syndrome marked by enlargement of the spleen, defects in one or more types of blood cells, and a high turnover of blood cells.

Immune or idiopathic thrombocytopenic purpura (ITP)—A blood disease that results in destruction of platelets, which are blood cells involved in clotting.

Laparoscope—An instrument used to view the abdominal cavity through a small incision and perform surgery on a small area, such as the spleen.

Pneumovax—A vaccine that is given to splenectomy patients to protect them against bacterial infections. Other vaccines include Pnu-Imune and Menomune.

Sepsis—A generalized infection of the body, most often caused by bacteria.

Sequestration—A process in which the spleen withdraws some normal blood cells from circulation and holds them in case the body needs extra blood in an emergency. In hypersplenism, the spleen sequesters too many blood cells.

Splenomegaly—Abnormal enlargement of the spleen.

Thromboembolism—A clot in the blood that forms and blocks a blood vessel. It can lead to infarction, or death of the surrounding tissue due to lack of blood supply.

Splenectomy usually necessary

There are some disorders in which splenectomy is usually recommended. They include:

- Immune (idiopathic) thrombocytopenic purpura (ITP). ITP is a disease involving platelet destruction. Splenectomy has been regarded as the definitive treatment for this disease and is effective in about 70% of chronic ITP cases. More recently, however, the introduction of new drugs in the treatment of ITP has reopened the question as to whether splenectomy is always the best treatment option.
- Trauma. The spleen can be ruptured by blunt as well as penetrating injuries to the chest or abdomen. Car accidents are the most common cause of blunt traumatic injury to the spleen. Occasionally, the spleen is injured during an operation within the abdomen. Sometimes, the spleen can be repaired (splenorrhaphy) rather than removed.
- Abscesses in the spleen. These are relatively uncommon but have a high mortality rate.
- Rupture of the splenic artery. Rupture sometimes occurs as a complication of pregnancy.
- Hereditary elliptocytosis. This is a relatively rare disorder. It is similar to HS in that it is characterized by red blood cells with defective membranes that are destroyed by the spleen.

Due to more sophisticated imaging techniques, nonoperative splenic preservation is becoming more common for injuries due to splenic trauma. Splenectomy should be avoided whenever possible as the advantages of splenic preservation have been well established. Specifically, splenectomy increases the risks of postoperative and long-term **infection**, and the procedure is associated with excessive transfusion requirements.

Splenectomy sometimes necessary

In other disorders, the spleen may or may not be removed.

- Hodgkin's disease, a serious form of cancer that causes lymph nodes to enlarge and causes the immune system to malfunction. Treatments such as radiation, chemotherapy, and surgical removal of the spleen can exacerbate this malfunction, increasing the likelihood of infection. Splenectomy is sometimes performed in order to find out how far the disease has progressed. However, splenectomy has been shown to increase the risk of secondary acute leukemia in patients with Hodgkin's disease.
- Hairy cell leukemia. Patients may suffer discomfort due to a very enlarged spleen caused by leukemia cells growing in the spleen. Splenectomy was once the only treatment for this disease; but due to the complications associated with splenectomy (low blood cell counts, fatigue, frequent infections, and easy bleeding or bruising), physicians are now more often recommending chemotherapy.
- Chronic myeloid disorders. These disorders include chronic myelocytic leukemia, polycythemia vera, essential thrombocythemia, and agnogenic myeloid metaplasia (myelofibrosis); they enlarge the spleen to

various degrees. In early stages of chronic myelocytic leukemia, splenectomy does not provide much benefit.

- Myelofibrosis. Myelofibrosis is a disorder in which bone marrow is replaced by fibrous tissue. It produces severe and painful splenomegaly. Splenectomy does not cure myelofibrosis but may be performed to relieve pain caused by the swollen spleen.
- Thrombotic thrombocytopenic purpura (TTP). TTP is a rare disorder marked by fever, kidney failure, and an abnormal decrease in the number of platelets. Splenectomy is one part of treatment for TTP.
- Autoimmune hemolytic disorders. These disorders may appear in patients of any age but are most common in patients over 50. The red blood cells are destroyed by antibodies produced by the patient's own body (autoantibodies).
- Thalassemia. Thalassemia is a hereditary form of anemia that is most common in people of Mediterranean origin. Splenectomy is sometimes performed if the patient's spleen has become painfully enlarged.

Precautions

Patients should be carefully assessed regarding the need for a splenectomy. Because of the spleen's role in protecting against infection, it should not be removed unless necessary. The operation is relatively safe for young and middle-aged adults. Older adults, especially those with cardiac or pulmonary disease, are more vulnerable to post-surgical infections. Thromboembolism following splenectomy is another complication for this patient group, which has about 10% mortality following the surgery. Splenectomies are performed in children only when the benefits outweigh the risks.

The most important part of the assessment is the measurement of splenomegaly. The normal spleen cannot be felt when the doctor examines the patient's abdomen. A spleen that is large enough to be felt indicates splenomegaly. In some cases the doctor will hear a dull sound when he or she thumps (percusses) the patient's abdomen near the ribs on the left side. **Imaging studies** that can be used to demonstrate splenomegaly include ultrasound tests, technetium-99m sulfur colloid imaging, and **computed tomography** (CT) scans. The rate of platelet or red blood cell destruction by the spleen can be measured by tagging blood cells with radioactive chromium or platelets with radioactive indium.

Description

Complete splenectomy

REMOVAL OF ENLARGED SPLEEN. Splenectomy is performed under general anesthesia. The most common technique is used to remove greatly enlarged spleens. After the surgeon makes a cut (incision) in the abdomen, the artery to the spleen is tied to prevent blood loss and reduce the spleen's size. It also helps prevent further sequestration of blood cells. The surgeon detaches the ligaments holding the spleen in place and removes it. In many cases, tissue samples will be sent to a laboratory for analysis.

REMOVAL OF RUPTURED SPLEEN. When the spleen has been ruptured by trauma, the surgeon approaches the organ from its underside and fastens the splenic artery.

In some cases, the doctor may prefer conservative (nonsurgical) management of a ruptured spleen, most often when the patient's blood pressure is stable and there are no signs of other abdominal injuries. In the case of multiple abdominal trauma, however, the spleen is usually removed.

Partial splenectomy

In some cases the surgeon removes only part of the spleen. This procedure is considered by some to be a useful compromise that reduces pain from an enlarged spleen while leaving the patient less vulnerable to infection.

Laparoscopic splenectomy

Laparoscopic splenectomy, or removal of the spleen through several small incisions, has been more frequently used in recent years. Laparoscopic surgery involves the use of surgical instruments, with the assistance of a tiny camera and video monitor. Laparoscopic procedures reduce the length of hospital stay, the level of post-operative pain, and the risk of infection. They also leave smaller scars. Laparoscopic splenectomy is not, however, the best option for many patients.

A laparoscopic splenectomy using a hanger wall-lifting procedure may provide a better technique and can avoid the usual complications associated with pneumoperitoneum. The patient's left lower chest and left abdominal wall are lifted by three wires in two directions, left laterally and vertical to the abdominal wall.

Laparoscopic splenectomy is gaining increased acceptance in the early 2000s as an alternative to open splenectomy for a wide variety of disorders, although splenomegaly still presents an obstacle to laparoscopic splenectomy; massive splenomegaly has been considered a contraindication. In patients with enlarged spleens, however, laparoscopic splenectomy is associated with less morbidity, decreased transfusion rates, and shorter hospital stays than when the open approach is used. Patients with enlarged spleens usually have more severe hematologic diseases related to greater morbidity; therefore, laparoscopic splenectomy has potential advantages.

The most frequent serious complication following laparoscopic splenectomy is damage to the pancreas. Application of a hydrogel sealant to the pancreas during surgery, however, appears to significantly reduce the risk of leakage from the pancreas.

Splenic embolization

Splenic embolization is an alternative to splenectomy that is used in some patients who are poor surgical risks. Embolization involves plugging or blocking the splenic artery to shrink the size of the spleen. The substances that are injected during this procedure include polyvinyl alcohol foam, polystyrene, and silicone. Embolization is a technique that needs further study and refinement.

Preparation

Preoperative preparation for nonemergency splenectomy includes:

- correction of abnormalities of blood clotting and the number of red blood cells and/or platelets
- treatment of any infections
- Control of immune reactions. Patients are usually given protective vaccinations about a month before surgery. The most common vaccines used are Pneumovax or Pnu-Imune 23 (against Pneumococcal infections) and Menomune-A/C/Y/W-135 (against meningococcal infections).

Aftercare

Immediately following surgery, patients should follow instructions and take all medications intended to prevent infection. Blood transfusions may be indicated for some patients to replace defective blood cells. The most important part of aftercare, however, is long-term caution regarding vulnerability to infection. Patients should see their doctor at once if they have a **fever** or any other sign of infection, and avoid travel to areas where exposure to malaria or similar diseases is likely. Children with splenectomies may be kept on antibiotic therapy until they are 16 years old. All patients can be given a booster dose of pneumococcal vaccine five to ten years after splenectomy.

Risks

The chief risk following splenectomy is overwhelmingly bacterial infection, or postsplenectomy **sepsis**. This vulnerability results from the body's decreased ability to clear bacteria from the blood, and lowered levels of a protein in blood plasma that helps to fight viruses (immunoglobulin M). The risk of dying from infection after splenectomy is highest in children, especially in the first two years after surgery. The risk of postsplenectomy sepsis can be reduced by vaccinations before the operation. Some doctors also recommend a two-year course of penicillin following splenectomy or long-term treatment with ampicillin.

Other risks following splenectomy include inflammation of the pancreas and collapse of the lungs. In some cases, splenectomy does not address the underlying causes of splenomegaly or other conditions. Excessive bleeding after the operation is an additional possible complication, particularly for ITP patients. Infection immediately following surgery may also occur.

Normal results

Results depend on the reason for the operation. In blood disorders, the splenectomy will remove the cause of the blood cell destruction. Normal results for patients with an enlarged spleen are relief of pain and of the complications of splenomegaly. It is not always possible, however, to predict which patients will respond well or to what degree.

See also Infection and sepsis.

Resources

BOOKS

Beers, Mark H., MD, and Robert Berkow, MD, editors. "Disorders of the Spleen." Section 11, Chapter 141 In*The Merck Manual of Diagnosis and Therapy*. Whitehouse Station, NJ: Merck Research Laboratories, 2002.

Wilkins, Bridget S., and Dennis H. Wright. *Illustrated Pathology of the Spleen*. Cambridge, UK:Cambridge University Press, 2000.

PERIODICALS

Balague, C., E. M. Targarona, G. Cerdan, et al. "Long-Term Outcome after Laparoscopic Splenectomy Related to Hematologic Diagnosis." *Surgical Endoscopy* 18 (August 2004): 1283–1287.

Bemelman, W. A., et al. "Hand-assisted Laparoscopic Splenectomy." *Surgical Endoscopy* 14, no. 11 (November 2000): 997–8.

Bjerke, H. Scott, MD, and Janet S. Bjerke, MSN. "Splenic Rupture." *eMedicine* 19 (June 2002). http://www.emedicine.com/med/topic2792.htm.

Bolton-Maggs, P. H., R. F. Stevens, N. J. Dodd, et al. "Guidelines for the Diagnosis and Management of Hereditary Spherocytosis." *British Journal of Haematology* 126 (August 2004): 455–474.

Brigden, M.L. "Detection, Education and Management of the Asplenic or Hyposplenic Patient." *American Family Physician* 63, no. 3: 499–506, 508.

Kahn, M. J., and K. R. McCrae. "Splenectomy in Immune Thrombocytopenic Purpura: Recent Controversies and Long-term Outcomes." *Current Hematology Reports* 3 (September 2004): 317–323.

Lo, A., A. M. Matheson, and D. Adams. "Impact of Concomitant Trauma in the Management of Blunt Splenic Injuries." *New Zealand Medical Journal* 117 (September 10, 2004): U1052.

Rosen, M., R. M. Walsh, and J. R. Goldblum. "Application of a New Collagen-Based Sealant for the Treatment of Pancreatic Injury." *Surgical Laparoscopy, Endoscopy and Percutaneous Techniques* 14 (August 2004): 181–185.

ORGANIZATIONS

Leukaemia Research Fund. 43 Great Ormond St., London WCIN 3JJ. <http://dspace.dial.pipex.com/lrf-//>.

National Heart, Lung and Blood Institute. Building 31, Room 4A21, Bethesda, MD 20892. (301)496-4236. http://www.nhlbi.nih.gov.

Teresa G. Norris
Crystal Heather Kaczkowski, MSc.
Rebecca J. Frey, PhD

Squamous cell carcinoma of the skin

Definition

A squamous cell **carcinoma** is a **skin cancer** that originates from squamous keratinocytes in the epidermis, the top layer of the skin. *Squamous* is a term that indicates a surface with a scaly nature.

Description

Squamous keratinocytes are flattened unpigmented skin cells in the middle of the epidermis. When they become cancerous, these cells invade the dermis (the layer of skin just below the epidermis) and spread out into the normal skin. They become visible as a small growth or area of change in the skin's appearance.

Most squamous cell carcinomas appear on areas that have been exposed to the sun: the head and neck, forearms, backs of the hands, upper part of the torso, and lower legs. Many develop in precancerous patches called actinic keratoses. Actinic keratoses are rough, scaly patches on the skin that usually start to show up in middle age. They are associated with a lifetime's exposure to the sun. Estimates of the chance that an actinic keratosis will turn into a squamous cell carcinoma vary from 0.24% to 20%.

Squamous cell carcinomas can also originate in old scars and burns, long-standing sores, and other areas of chronic skin irritation. These tumors tend to be more dangerous than those that arise in actinic keratoses.

The least dangerous type of squamous cell carcinoma is called **Bowen's disease**, intraepithelial squamous cell carcinoma, or squamous cell carcinoma *in situ*. Bowen's disease can show up anywhere on the skin, but it is especially common on the head and neck. This **cancer** usually grows slowly; but may evolve into a more serious, spreading form if it is not removed.

Other types of squamous cell carcinomas grow fairly quickly and can develop within a few months. These tumors may spread in the skin along the blood vessels, nerves, and muscles. They can also metastasize, or spread to other areas. On the average, 2–6% of squamous cell carcinomas metastasize, but the rate varies with the tumor site. At least 95% of the tumors that originate in actinic keratoses remain in the skin; but up to 38% of the cancers from scars are metastatic. **Metastasis** is also more likely when the cancer originates on the ear, lip, or genitalia, is large or deep, or develops in someone with a severely suppressed immune system. Cancers that regrow after treatment, and tumors that spread along the nerves are particularly dangerous.

Demographics

Squamous cell carcinoma is the second most common type of skin cancer in North America. There are between 80,000 and 100,000 cases diagnosed each year in the United States.

Squamous cell carcinomas are more common in the older adult population rather than the young. Overall, the chance of developing one is about 7%–11%. The likelihood increases with exposure to the sun, and is greatest for fair-skinned individuals who tan poorly. Living near the equator, where ultraviolet light is more intense, also increases the risk. A weakened immune system— for instance, from an organ transplant, or AIDS—can also increase the risk of developing a squamous cell carcinoma by a factor of 5 to 250.

Squamous cell carcinomas tend to be most dangerous in individuals with dark skin. The mortality rate for African-Americans with squamous cell carcinomas is 17–24%, much higher than the 2% death rate for white males with nonmelanoma skin cancer. One

KEY TERMS

Actinic keratosis (plural actinic keratoses)—A rough, dry, scaly patch on the skin associated with sun exposure.

Albinism—A genetic disease characterized by the absence of the normal skin pigment, melanin.

Antioxidant—A substance that can neutralize free radicals. Free radicals are damaging molecules formed from oxygen. Antioxidant vitamins include vitamin E, C, and beta-carotene, a form of vitamin A.

Biopsy—A sample of an organ taken to look for abnormalities. Also, the technique used to take such samples.

Chronic—Long-standing.

Dermis—A layer of skin sandwiched between the epidermis and the fat under the skin. It contains the blood vessels, nerves, sweat glands, and hair follicles.

Epidermis—The thin layer of skin cells at the surface of the skin.

Fluorouracil—A cancer drug.

Interferon alpha—A chemical made naturally by the immune system and also manufactured as a drug.

Local anesthetic—A liquid used to numb a small area of the skin.

Lymph node—A small organ full of immune cells, found in clusters throughout the body. Lymph nodes are where reactions to infections usually begin.

Nonmelanoma skin cancer—A squamous cell carcinoma or basal cell carcinoma.

Nonsteroidal anti-inflammatory drugs (NSAIDS)—A class of drugs that suppresses inflammation. Includes a wide variety of drugs, including aspirin.

Papillomavirus—A member of a group of viruses associated with warts and cervical cancer.

Pathologist—A doctor who specializes in examining cells and other parts of the body for abnormalities.

Precancerous—Abnormal and with a high probability of turning into cancer, but not yet a cancer.

Oncologist—A doctor who specializes in the treatment of cancer.

Retinoids—A class of drugs related to vitamin A.

Selenium—A mineral needed in extremely small quantities by the body. Large amounts can be very toxic.

Xeroderma pigmentosum—A genetic disease characterized by the inability to repair damaged DNA. Individuals with this disease develop an excessive number of skin cancers.

reason for this disparity is that the cancers that develop in dark skin are more likely to come from old scars and burns than from actinic keratoses.

Causes and symptoms

Squamous cell carcinoma is caused by genetic damage to a skin cell. A number of factors can increase the risk that this will happen, but the exact cause is rarely known.

Any of the following changes may be a warning sign that an actinic keratosis is developing into a squamous cell carcinoma:

- pain
- increased redness
- sores or bleeding
- hardening or thickening
- increased size

Most squamous cell carcinomas begin as a small red bump on the skin. More advanced squamous cell carcinomas have the following characteristics:

- a few millimeters to a few centimeters in diameter
- reddish-brown, flesh-colored, pink, or red
- bumpy or flat
- sharp, irregular edges in Bowen's disease; others may have no definite edge
- may be crusted or scaly
- may contain bleeding sores

Diagnosis

Squamous cell carcinomas are usually diagnosed with a skin **biopsy** taken in the doctor's office. This is generally a brief, simple procedure. After numbing the skin with an injection of local anesthetic, the doctor snips out the tumor or a piece of it. This skin sample is sent to a pathologist to be read. It can take up to a week for the biopsy results to come back. Squamous cell carcinomas are graded into categories of one through four. The grading is based on how deeply the tumor penetrates in the skin and how abnormal its cells are. Higher grades are more serious.

QUESTIONS TO ASK THE DOCTOR

- What treatment(s) would you recommend for my tumor?
- How effective would you expect each of them to be, for a tumor of this size and in this location?
- How much cosmetic damage am I likely to see with each?
- Are there any alternatives?
- How should I prepare for the procedure?
- What is the risk that my tumor in particular will grow again?

Treatment team

Primary care physicians remove some squamous cell carcinomas; other cancers, including larger or more complicated tumors, may be referred to a dermatologist. The services of a plastic surgeon are occasionally necessary. Metastatic tumors are often treated by an oncologist, surgeons, specially trained nurses, and specialists in radiation treatment.

Clinical staging, treatments, and prognosis

Staging

In stage 0 (Bowen's disease), the cancer is very small and has not yet spread from the epidermis to the dermis.

In stage I, the cancer is less than 2 cm (0.8 inches) in diameter. No cancer cells can be found in lymph nodes or other internal organs.

In stage II, the cancer is more than 2 cm (0.8 inches) in diameter. No cancer cells can be found in lymph nodes or other internal organs.

In stage III, cancer cells have been found in nearby lymph nodes or in the bone, muscle, or cartilage beneath the skin.

A stage IV cancer can be any size. In this stage, cancer cells have been discovered in internal organs that are distant from the skin. Squamous cell carcinomas tend to spread to nearby lymph nodes, the liver, and the lungs.

Treatment

The treatment options for a squamous cell carcinoma depend on the size of the tumor, its location, and the likelihood that it will spread aggressively or metastasize. All of the treatments described below generally have cure rates of approximately 90% to 99% for small, localized cancers. The five-year cure rates are highest with Moh's surgery, also called Mohs micrographic surgery.

One option is conventional surgery. The doctor numbs the area with an injection of local anesthetic, then cuts out the tumor and a small margin of normal skin around it. The wound is closed with a few stitches. One advantage of conventional surgery is that the wound usually heals quickly. Another benefit is that the complete cancer can be sent to a pathologist for evaluation. If cancer cells are found in the skin around the tumor, additional treatments can be done.

Laser surgery may be an alternative. A disadvantage to laser surgery is that the wounds from some lasers heal more slowly than cuts from a scalpel. The advantage is that bleeding is minimal.

Another option is Moh's micrographic surgery. This technique is a variation of conventional surgery. In this procedure, the surgeon examines each piece of skin under the microscope as it is removed. If any cancer cells remain, another slice is taken from that area and checked. These steps are repeated until the edges of the wound are clear of tumor cells, then the wound is closed. The advantage to this technique is that all of the visible cancer cells are removed but as much normal skin as possible is spared. Mohs surgery is often used for larger or higher risk tumors and when cosmetic considerations are important. The main disadvantage is that it takes much longer than conventional surgery and requires a specially trained surgeon.

In cryosurgery, liquid nitrogen is used to freeze the tumor and destroy it. This treatment is another type of blind destruction; there is no skin sample to make sure the cancer cells have all been killed. Patients report swelling and pain after cryosurgery, and a wound appears a few days later where the cells were destroyed. Healing takes about four to six weeks. When the site heals, it has usually lost its normal pigment. There is a risk of nerve damage with this technique. Cryosurgery is generally used only for small cancers in stage 0 and stage I.

In electro dessication and curettage, the physician scoops out the cancer cells with a spoon-shaped instrument called a curette. After most of the tumor is gone, the rest is destroyed with heat from an electrical current. The wound is left open to heal like an abrasion. It leaks fluid, crusts over, and heals during the next two to six weeks. This method is generally used only for the smallest squamous cell carcinomas (stage 0 and stage I). One disadvantage is that there is no skin sample to confirm that the tumor is completely gone. The electrical current used during this surgery can interfere with some pacemakers.

Some cases of Bowen's disease can be treated by applying a lotion containing 5-fluorouracil (**fluorouracil** or 5-FU) for several weeks. This treatment usually gives good cosmetic results. The side effects from 5-fluorouracil include allergies to the ingredients, infections, redness, peeling, and crusting, sensitivity to the sun, and changes in skin color. The main disadvantage to this treatment is that the drug cannot penetrate very far and cancer cells in the deeper parts of the tumor may not be destroyed.

Radiation therapy is sometimes used for squamous cell carcinomas, especially when the tumor is at a site where surgery would be difficult or remove a sizeable amount of tissue. This treatment is sometimes combined with surgery for cancers that have metastasized or are likely to. One disadvantage is that tumors returning after radiation tend to grow more quickly than the original cancer. In addition, **x rays** may promote new skin cancers. The cosmetic results are usually good. In some cases the skin may lose a little pigment, or develop spider veins. Some doctors reserve radiation treatment for those over 60. One drawback of radiation therapy for squamous cell carcinomas in or near the mouth is that the radiation may cause the tissues inside the mouth to break down.

Chemotherapy is often added to surgery or radiation for stage IV cancers. Retinoids and interferon are experimental treatments that may be helpful.

Prognosis

Because many squamous cell carcinomas are not staged, precise five-year survival rates for each stage are not available. In general, the prognosis is very good for small squamous cell carcinomas that originate in actinic keratoses. However, cancers that were not completely destroyed may regrow. Tumors can redevelop in the scar from the surgery, on the edges of the surgery site, or deep in the skin. Larger or higher-risk tumors, cancers that regrow after treatment, and tumors that have invaded local tissues or metastasized are more difficult to cure. Most metastases show up within the first two years after a skin tumor has been removed. The five-year survival rate for metastatic cancers is 34%.

Alternative and complementary therapies

Alternative treatments for squamous cell carcinoma usually attempt to prevent rather than treat this cancer. Options being tested include antioxidant **vitamins**, minerals, and green tea extracts.

Coping with cancer treatment

Most squamous cell carcinomas are removed with techniques that cause few, if any, lasting side effects. Patients who have cosmetic concerns may wish to discuss them with their doctors.

Clinical trials

The medical community considers the following treatments to be experimental.

Clinical trials are testing whether interferon alpha, injected into the tumor, can destroy some squamous cell carcinomas. An early report from a combination of interferon alpha and retinoids is promising.

Ongoing trials are also evaluating whether small squamous cell carcinomas can be cured with photodynamic laser therapy. In this technique, a dye activated by laser light destroys the cancer. This dye is spread onto the skin, injected, or drunk. During a waiting period, normal cells clear the dye, then a laser activates the remainder. As of 2001, this technique was only useful for cancers very near the surface of the skin. One side effect after treatment is a period of excessive sun-sensitivity.

Other clinical trials are testing whether retinoids spread onto the skin can prevent or treat squamous cell carcinoma.

Another new experimental approach to squamous cell carcinoma is gene therapy. Researchers in Texas reported in 2003 on a Phase III investigation that uses an adenovirus as a vector to carry an altered p53 gene into the cancerous squamous cells. The function of the p53 gene is to maintain the structure of the cell's DNA and to induce the cell to die if its DNA is damaged beyond repair. Phase I and phase II trials have indicated that this approach to treatment has lengthened the survival time in patients with recurrent squamous cell carcinoma.

Prevention

The most important risk factor for squamous cell carcinoma is exposure to the sun (or other source of ultraviolet light) combined with a lighter complexion and inability to tan. Other risk factors include:

- increasing age
- actinic keratoses
- a previous skin cancer
- exposure to arsenic or the chemicals in coal tars

- radiation treatments
- treatment with psoralen and ultraviolet light for psoriasis
- chronic skin damage such as burn scars and ulcers
- infection with some varieties of human papillomavirus
- genetic disorders such as xeroderma pigmentosum and albinism
- a weakened immune system

Most people will receive 80% of their lifetime exposure to the sun before they reach the age of 20. For this reason, prevention should start during childhood and adolescence. Some important steps to prevent squamous cell carcinoma, as well as other skin cancers include:

- Wear protective clothing and a wide-brimmed hat in the sun.
- Stay out of the sun from 10 A.M. to 4 P.M..
- Use a sunscreen that has a sun protection factor (SPF) of at least 15.
- Avoid suntanning booths.

Drugs related to vitamin A (including beta-carotene and retinoids), vitamin E, **nonsteroidal anti-inflammatory drugs** (NSAIDS), and selenium might be able to prevent some skin cancers. In 2001, their effectiveness was still in question.

Special concerns

Because many squamous cell carcinomas are found on the face and neck, cosmetic concerns are a priority for many patients. If there is a risk of noticeable scarring or damage, a patient may wish to ask about alternative types of removal or inquire about the services of a plastic surgeon.

After treatment, it is important to return to the doctor periodically to check for regrowth or new skin cancers. Approximately a third to a half of all patients with nonmelanoma skin cancers find a new skin cancer within the next five years. Having a squamous cell carcinoma before the age of 60 may also increase the chance of developing other cancers in internal organs; however, this idea is still very controversial.

See also Basal cell carcinoma; Chemoprevention; Reconstructive surgery.

Resources

BOOKS

Beers, Mark H., MD, and Robert Berkow, MD, editors. "Squamous Cell Carcinoma." Section 10, Chapter 126 In*The Merck Manual of Diagnosis and Therapy.* Whitehouse Station, NJ: Merck Research Laboratories, 2002.

Keefe, Kristin A., and Frank L. Meyskens, Jr. "Cancer Prevention." In *Clinical Oncology*, edited by Martin D. Abeloff, James O. Armitage, Allen S. Lichter, and John E. Niederhuber, 2nd ed. Philadelphia: Churchhill Livingstone, 2000, pp.339–42.

Rohrer, Thomas E. "Cancer of the Skin." In *Conn's Current Therapy; Latest Approved Methods of Treatment for the Practicing Physician*, edited by Robert E. Rakel, et al., 52nd ed. Philadelphia: W. B. Saunders, 2000, pp.763–5.

Waldorf, Heidi A. "Premalignant Lesions." In *Conn's Current Therapy; Latest Approved Methods of Treatment for the Practicing Physician*, edited by Robert E. Rakel, et al., 52nd ed. Philadelphia: W. B. Saunders, 2000, pp.792–4.

Wolfe, Jonathan. "Nonmelanoma Skin Cancers: Basal Cell and Squamous Cell Carcinoma." In *Clinical Oncology*, edited by Martin D. Abeloff, James O. Armitage, Allen S. Lichter, and John E. Niederhuber, 2nd ed. Philadelphia: Churchhill Livingstone, 2000, pp.1351–8.

PERIODICALS

Edelman, J., J. Edelman, and J. Nemunaitis. "Adenoviral p53 Gene Therapy in Squamous Cell Cancer of the Head and Neck Region." *Current Opinion in Molecular Therapeutics* 5 (December 2003): 611–617.

Elmets C.A., D. Singh, K. Tubesing, M. Matsui. S. Katiyar, and H. Mukhtar. "Cutaneous photoprotection from ultraviolet injury by green tea polyphenols." *Journal of the American Academy of Dermatology* 44, no. 3 (March 2001): 425–32.

Garner, Kyle L., and Wm. Macmillian Rodney. "Basal and Squamous Cell Carcinoma." *Primary Care; Clinics in Office Practice* 27, no. 2 (June 2000): 477–8.

Huber, M. A., and G. T. Terezhalmy. "The Head and Neck Radiation Oncology Patient." *Quintessence International* 34 (October 2003): 693–717.

Jerant, Anthony F., Jennifer T. Johnson, Catherine Demastes Sheridan, and Timothy J. Caffrey. "Early Detection and Treatment of Skin Cancer." *American Family Physician* 62 (July 15, 2000): 357–68, 375–6, 381–2.

Shamsadini, S., A. Taheri, S. Dabiri, et al. "Grouped Skin Metastases from Laryngeal Squamous Cell Carcinoma and Overview of Similar Cases." *Dermatology Online Journal* 9 (December 2003): 27.

OTHER

"Non-melanoma Staging." *Oncology Channel.* Mar. 2001. [cited June 26, 2001]. <http://oncologychannel.com/nonmelanoma/staging.shtml>.

"Nonmelanoma Skin Cancer Treatment—Health Professionals." *CancerNet.* Aug. 2000 National Cancer Institute. [cited Mar. 15, 2001]. <http://cancernet.nci.nih.gov/pdq.html>.

"Prevention of Skin Cancer. Prevention—Health Professionals." *CancerNet.* Mar. 2001 National Cancer Institute.

[cited June 26, 2001]. <http://cancernet.nci.nih.gov/pdq.html>.

Skin Cancer. CancerLinksUSA. 1999. [cited June 26, 2001]. http://www.cancerlinksusa.com/skin/index.htm.

ORGANIZATIONS

American Skin Association. 150 East 58th Street, 32nd Floor, New York, NY, 10155-0002. (212) 753-8260.

NIH/National Arthritis and Musculoskeletal and Skin Diseases Information Clearinghouse One AMS Circle, Bethesda, MD, 20892-3675.(301)495-4484. [cited July 2, 2001]. http://www.nih.gov/niams. The NIAMS conducts and supports basic, clinical, and epidemiologic research and research training and disseminates information on diseases that include many forms of arthritis and diseases of the musculoskeletal system and the skin.

Skin Cancer Foundation. 245 Fifth Avenue, Suite 2402, New York, NY 10016. (212) 725-5176.

Anna Rovid Spickler, D.V.M., Ph.D.
Rebecca J. Frey, PhD

Staging *see* **Tumor staging**

Stem cell transplant *see* **Bone marrow transplantation**

Stenting

Definition

Stenting is a procedure in which a cylindrical structure (stent) is placed into a hollow tubular organ to provide artificial support and maintain the patency of the opening. Although it is most often used for cardiovascular functioning, it is also utilized to manage obstructions in **cancer** patients.

Purpose

Stents are used in cancer patients to relieve obstructions due to:

- direct blockages within the tube (or lumen) due to cancer growth
- narrowing of the lumen from tumor growth outside pressing on the tube and narrowing the lumen
- occasionally from the build up of scar tissue (fibrosis) from radiation therapy

Tumors most likely to cause obstruction requiring stent placement include **esophageal cancer**, bronchogenic **carcinoma**, **pancreatic cancer**, cancers of the bile duct, and occasionally colorectal carcinomas.

QUESTIONS TO ASK THE DOCTOR

- Am I a good candidate for this procedure?
- Do I have any contraindications that should be considered before having the procedure?
- Will I experience any improvement in my quality of life?
- What are the advantages and disadvantages of the procedure?
- Does the physician performing the procedure do this often or only occasionally?

Precautions

Every patient should be viewed individually with special consideration given to the patient's present status. Generally, surgical procedures are for the correction of a problem; but in many cancer cases, relief of symptoms is the only therapeutic option. Since it is extremely difficult to remove or reposition these stents after they are placed, the degree of relief to be offered by its insertion should be significant. The physician and the patient should discuss all alternatives and come to a mutual decision.

Description

Endoscopic retrograde cholangiopancreatography (ERCP) is the name of the procedure utilized to place most stents for pancreatic and biliary tumors. The ERCP is a flexible endoscope, which can be directed and moved around the many bends in the upper gastrointestinal tract. The newer video endoscopes have a tiny, optically sensitive computer chip at the end which transmits electronic signals up the scope to a computer that displays an image on a large video screen. The scope has an open channel that permits other instruments to be passed through it to perform biopsies, inject solutions, or place stents. Since ERCP uses x-ray films, the procedure takes place in an x-ray area. Initially the throat is anesthetized with a spray solution and the patient is also usually mildly sedated. The endoscope is inserted into the upper esophagus and a thin tube is inserted through it to the main bile duct entering the intestinal area. Dye is injected into the bile duct and/or the pancreatic duct and x-ray films are taken. The patient usually lies on the left side and then turns onto the stomach to allow complete visualization of the ducts. The patient is able to breathe easily throughout the

KEY TERMS

Endoscope—An instrument used for direct visual inspection of hollow organs or body cavities.

Esophagus—The muscular, membranous structure that extends from the throat to the stomach.

Lumen—The cavity or channel within a tube or tubular organ, such as a blood vessel or the intestine.

exam and rarely gags. Any gallstones found may be removed or if the duct has become narrowed, an incision can be made using electrocautery (electrical heat) to relieve the blockage. It is also possible to widen narrowed ducts by placing stents in these areas to keep them open. The patient is taken to recovery following the procedure, which takes 20–40 minutes.

Other endoscopes are used to place stents elsewhere in the body. For example, an esophagoscope is used to place stents in cases of esophageal cancer, a bronchoscope is used for procedures involving endobronchial obstructions, and a colonoscope is used in cases of colorectal obstructions.

Preparation

The patient is instructed not to eat or drink anything for eight hours prior to the procedure. Some physicians may request that no asprin be taken for a certain time period prior to the procedure to prevent excessive bleeding.

Aftercare

The patient may go home after the procedure or may spend one or two nights in the hospital. **Antibiotics** may be given especially if there has been longstanding biliary obstruction. Dietary restrictions are common after esophageal and colorectal stenting.

Risks

The most serious risk associated with the placement of a stent is the risk of perforation. If a tear is made, leakage with life-threatening **infection** may occur. Migration or recurrent obstruction may necessitate repeat stenting if possible. Occasionally bleeding may occur.

Normal results

Relief of the obstruction with resumption of the ability to eat, breathe, normally clear fluids from the liver or pancreas, or allow normal passage of stool is the desired result of this procedure.

Abnormal results

A sudden change in the degree of pain and/or **fever** that persists as well as any unusual changes should be communicated immediately to a physician.

Resources

BOOKS

Dolmath, Bart L., and Ulrich Blum, editors. *Stent-Grafts: Current Clinical Practice*. New York: Thieme, 2000.

OTHER

American Cancer Society, P.O. Box 102454, Atlanta, GA 30368-2454. http://www.ca.cancer.org.

American Society of Clinical Oncology. 1900 Duke Street, Suite 200, Alexandria, VA 22314. Phone: 703-299-0150. http://www.asco.org.

Jackson Gastroenterology. http://www.gicare.com.

National Digestive Diseases Information Clearinghouse. *ERCP (Endoscopic Retrograde Cholangiopancreatography)*. http://www.niddk.nih.gov/health/digest/pubs/diagtest/ercp.htm.

Linda K. Bennington, C.N.S., M.S.N.

Stereotactic needle biopsy

Definition

Stereotactic needle **biopsy** (SNB) is an ultrasound-guided and mammogram-directed needle aspiration biopsy of breast tissue. It is a diagnostic procedure used to determine the cause of radiographic abnormalities in breast tissue.

Purpose

Stereotactic needle biopsy is performed when nonpalpable (unable to be felt) abnormalities are identified by mammogram. The abnormality is generally located on a routine screening mammogram. This biopsy procedure uses a large (core) or small (fine) needle that withdraws samples of the abnormal breast tissue. The doctor uses either the mammogram or an ultrasound image of the abnormal tissue to guide the needle to the biopsy site. The needle is used to remove tissue samples of the site for laboratory analysis.

QUESTIONS TO ASK THE DOCTOR

- What type of physician performs a stereotactic needle biopsy?
- How long will it take to interpret the biopsy results?
- What type of pain management will be used during the procedure?
- Can the biopsy give false negative results?
- Will I have a fine needle biopsy or core biopsy? Why?

Description

The patient is made comfortable with a local anesthesia injection prior to the start of the procedure. Special imaging techniques are used to localize (easily see) the abnormal spot. First, the patient lies face down on a table with breasts suspended through an opening. Then mammograms are taken of the suspicious site from several different angles. This technique creates a virtual three-dimensional (stereotactic) picture of the abnormal area. A computer is used to guide the needle to the site for sample removal. If the abnormality can be seen easily on ultrasound, the biopsy may be performed with the patient lying on her back while ultrasound imaging localizes the abnormality. The samples are examined in the laboratory by a pathologist (a physician trained in identification of pathological or abnormal findings) to determine if **cancer** cells are present.

There are two different types of needles used for stereotactic needle biopsy. The procedures are similar, but the size of the needle varies. A fine-needle biopsy is most often used, in conjunction with ultrasound imaging, when a cyst is suspected. The doctor is able to suction a sample of fluid or tissue through the needle and send it for analysis. The needle is smaller and so is the sample of fluid or tissue extracted. In a core needle biopsy, the needle is larger, has a cutting edge, and enables the physician to extract a larger tissue sample from the suspicious area. A larger tissue sample can enhance laboratory accuracy in identifying the presence of cancer cells.

Preparation

Prior to ordering a breast biopsy, the physician gathers as much information from the patient as possible by asking questions that provide a medical history. The physician will perform a clinical breast examination through palpation to determine any changes from previous exams or to determine a baseline exam. The physician orders a routine screening mammogram (x ray) and interprets the results. If something abnormal is revealed on mammogram, further radiologic exams are requested. After confirming the presence of a radiographic abnormality, the physician will order a biopsy. A patient's written informed consent is necessary before any invasive procedure. The document should explain, in understandable language, the patient's treatment options, risks and benefits of the procedure, and potential complications.

General anesthesia is not used for the stereotactic needle biopsy procedure. Usually the physician will use a local injectable anesthetic agent at the needle insertion site to numb the area. When the anesthetic is injected at the biopsy site, the patient will feel a stinging sensation. The physician will wait until the numbing agent takes effect, then proceed with the biopsy. At this point, the patient should only feel a pressure sensation as the needle is guided to the biopsy site.

Precautions

Patients should discuss the indications (reasons for) and contraindications (reasons why not) of having a stereotactic needle biopsy performed with their doctor. While the procedure has been studied extensively with positive outcomes for accuracy of results, it is most indicated in cases where there is a non-palpable area of abnormal tissue identified by mammogram. However, vaguely palpable abnormalities can also be managed in this way. Physicians divide "abnormal findings" into several categories. A probable benign finding is a category 3, a suspicious abnormal finding is a category 4, and a highly suggestive of malignancy finding is a category 5.

When there is a probable benign finding (category 3), frequently there is no previous mammogram for comparison study. A stereotactic needle biopsy is done on a category 3 finding when there is a strong family history of **breast cancer**. Usually, a category 3 finding requires only a six month follow-up with **mammography**.

When there is a suspicious abnormality (category 4), a sterotactic needle biopsy is most useful, as well as indicated. In this category, stereotactic needle biopsy is used to differentiate those patients requiring surgical intervention from those needing clinical and mammographic (x-ray) follow-up.

In a category 5 finding, highly suggestive of malignancy, the physician can use information from a stereotactic needle biopsy to confirm a diagnosis and expedite surgical intervention in this category.

Stereotactic needle biopsy is not indicated in all cases where there is nonpalpable breast tissue abnormality. The size of the patient and size of the breast must be considered because a certain breast thickness is necessary for mammogram-guided biopsy. There is no such requirement for ultrasound-guided procedures. Abnormalities just under the skin are technically difficult for the placement of the biopsy needle and are best excised (removed) in an open surgical procedure. Also, areas of breast tissue micro-calcification (tiny areas of thickened breast tissue) that are not closely clustered together can be difficult to visualize in a stereotactic system and therefore difficult to retrieve during biopsy. Finally, the patient must be able to remain still and lie face down for the duration of the biopsy procedure (20 to 40 minutes). Any movement by the patient can render the localization of the abnormal site invalid.

Aftercare

After the procedure, the patient may experience pain or discomfort at the biopsy site. Mild bruising can also occur at the site. For these reasons, the physician may suggest that activities be limited for 24 to 48 hours post-procedure. The physician will suggest or prescribe a medication for discomfort relief. Often, a sport bra or other firm support garment will minimize breast movement and increase post-procedure comfort. Icing the area may also be reccommended. The physician will inform the patient of further follow-up care needed to monitor the patient's ongoing breast health and the subsequent intervals for follow-up imaging.

Risks

It is very important for the patient who is facing a stereotactic needle biopsy procedure to know that there is the possibility of needing a repeat biopsy procedure. A repeat biopsy is necessary if there is a discrepancy between the radiology reports and the pathologist's findings from laboratory analysis of the sample (concordance). As with any procedure, there is a slight risk of allergic reaction to anesthesia. To be well informed, patients should consult with their physician about the risks prior to undergoing SNB.

Results

Stereotactic needle biopsy is a diagnostic tool used to determine the presence of cancer cells. It is not a therapy used to obliterate an area of abnormal tissue. The results of the biopsy help the physician to determine the best medical or surgical options available to the patient. The biopsy results are reviewed by the physician performing the SNB and by the pathologist who analizes the sample. Results are reviewed and discussed with the patient and options for further treatment or follow up are presented. The patient, with the guidance and expertise of the physician, selects a course of therapy.

Resources

BOOKS

DeVita, Vincent T., Jr., Samuel Hellman, and Steven A. Rosenberg, editors. *Cancer: Principles and Practice of Oncology*. Philadelphia: Lippincott Williams & Wilkins, 2001.

PERIODICALS

Norris, T. "Stereotactic Breast Biopsy." *Radiologic Technology* 72, no. 1 (May 2001): 431.

OTHER

Bassett l., D. P. Winchester, R. B. Caplan, D. D. Dershaw, et al. "Stereotactic Core-Needle Biopsy Of The Breast: A Report of the Joint Task Force of the American College of Radiology, American College of Surgeons, and College of American Pathologists."

Molly Metzler, R.N., B.S.N.

Stereotactic surgery

Definition

Stereotactic surgery is an approach to **cancer** diagnosis and treatment that makes use of a system of three-dimensional coordinates to locate a site (most commonly within the brain) as precisely as possible for **biopsy** or surgery. The English word *stereotactic* is a combination of a Greek root, *stereo-*, which means "solid" or "having three dimensions," and the Latin word *tactus*, which means "touch." Stereotactic neurosurgery may make use of a conventional incision and drill to enter the patient's skull or precisely focused beams of radiation to destroy cancerous tissue. This second method, which is called stereotactic radiosurgery, is not surgery in the usual sense of the word because no incision is involved.

Purpose

Stereotactic surgery may be performed either to obtain a tissue sample for biopsy or to remove or destroy the tumor itself. Stereotactic biopsies are the

QUESTIONS TO ASK YOUR DOCTOR

- Is stereotactic radiosurgery an option for treatment of my tumor?
- How much experience have you had with this form of treatment?
- What do you consider the advantages and drawbacks of gamma knife and linear accelerator radiosurgery?
- What are the risks of this treatment in my particular case?

preferred method of confirming a diagnosis of a brain tumor, because of their precision and because they may offer the only method of obtaining a tissue sample if the tumor is located deep within the brain or close to structures that control vital functions. Stereotactic surgery may also be used in the diagnosis of epilepsy; since the areas of abnormal brain activity in epilepsy cannot always be identified by **imaging studies**, a neurosurgeon can use a stereotactic system to place electrodes for recording brain waves in the areas suspected of being the focus of seizures.

Stereotactic surgery can be used to treat movement disorders as well as **brain tumors**. In fact, the first clinical application of stereotactic systems in human medicine was in the treatment of schizophrenia in the late 1940s, followed by the use of stereotactic surgery to treat Parkinson's disease and chronic pain in the 1950s. As of the early 2000s, stereotactic surgery is used to treat such other movement disorders as Huntington's chorea and essential tremor, and to insert catheters into the brain to drain abnormal collections of fluid resulting from head injuries, hydrocephalus, or cysts.

Stereotactic radiosurgery can be used to treat movement disorders, malformations of blood vessels, and benign tumors (acoustic neuromas, pituitary adenomas, and meningiomas) as well as malignant tumors of the brain and spinal cord. It may also be used to treat cancers in the nose or other small and well-defined parts of the body, or as a follow-up "booster" treatment for patients with recurrent tumors who have already received the maximum safe dose of conventional **radiation therapy**.

Precautions

Stereotactic surgery or radiosurgery should be done only by qualified specialists who are experienced in these techniques, and performed only in treatment centers with the necessary high-level equipment.

Stereotactic radiosurgery with a gamma knife is most effective in treating relatively small tumors (an inch or less in diameter) with well-defined borders that have not invaded the brain; in addition, it is usually reserved for patients with a life expectancy of six months or longer. Large brain tumors may require partial removal by conventional open surgery prior to treatment with radiosurgery.

Description

Stereotactic surgery

The earliest forms of stereotactic surgery in humans developed out of an apparatus that was designed by Victor Horsley and Henry Clarke in 1906 to study brain functions in monkeys. It was not until 1946, however, that two American researchers designed a stereotactic frame to guide brain surgery in humans. There were two difficulties in transferring a stereotactic system from other mammals to humans, however; one problem was the much greater degree of variation among humans in the location of various bony landmarks on the skull that were used to identify the approximate location of various parts of the brain. The other problem was the lack of a reliable imaging method for visualizing internal brain structures.

By the 1940s, a method known as positive contrast ventriculography, in which some of the cerebral fluid in the ventricles of the brain was withdrawn and replaced with air or another contrast medium that would show up on an x-ray, allowed surgeons to identify structures within the brain in relation to one another. Ventriculography made it possible to use such internal structures as the posterior commissure or pineal gland rather than various points on the outside of the skull as landmarks for brain surgery. Researchers compiled stereotactic atlases, or collections of photographs of cross-sections of brain tissue, with reference grids around the borders of each photograph. A surgeon could consult one of these atlases in order to calculate the exact location of a targeted brain structure with reference to the posterior commissure. Present-day stereotactic surgery still makes use of atlases, although they are now compiled from computer images rather than photographs.

The first frame that was used in stereotactic surgery in the 1940s consisted of a plaster cap fitted to the individual patient with a head ring and electrode carrier mounted to it. In the early 2000s, however, stereotactic surgery made use of a base ring attached to the patient's skull, a CT or MRI scan, and an arc ring to

KEY TERMS

Atlas—In anatomy, a collection of medical illustrations of one specific subject, such as the brain or heart. Detailed atlases of the brain are important guides for surgeons performing stereotactic neurosurgery.

Collimator—A metal tube designed to control the size and direction of a beam of radiation.

Cyclotron—A machine that accelerates charged atomic particles within a constant magnetic field.

Fractionated—In radiotherapy, treatment that is divided into several sessions of smaller doses of radiation rather than one large dose delivered in a single session.

Gamma knife—The name for a specific type of radiosurgery that uses highly focused cobalt-60 radiation to destroy cancerous tissue in the brain. It is not a knife in the conventional sense.

Hydrocephalus—A condition marked by the buildup of cerebrospinal fluid within the skull, causing increased pressure on the brain and a variety of neurologic symptoms. Stereotactic surgery may be used to place a catheter within the brain in order to drain the excess fluid.

Landmark—An anatomical structure that is easy to recognize and suitable as a reference point in locating other structures or making measurements.

Photon—A quantum of electromagnetic radiation with no mass and no charge.

Posterior commissure—A bundle of fibers that connects the two cerebral hemispheres near the third ventricle of the brain.

Radiosurgery—A form of cancer treatment in which tissue is destroyed by radiation from an external source or an implant rather than by manual removal. In spite of its name, radiosurgery is not surgery in the usual sense of making an incision, removing tissue, and then closing the incision.

Ventricles—Small cavities within the brain filled with cerebrospinal fluid.

guide the surgeon in drilling a hole through the skull. After the base ring is attached to the patient's scalp, he or she is taken to the operating room, where the base ring is attached to the operating table in order to hold the patient's head steady. The entry site for the surgeon's drill is selected, and the entry site and area of the tumor are located on a phantom image that relates these points to the patient's head. Coordinates derived from the phantom image are entered into a computer that determines the final path of the surgeon's instruments. An arc ring is then attached to the base ring to guide the surgeon's movements. This stereotactic system allows the surgeon to make only a very small incision (less than one-quarter in. long) in the scalp, and drill a hole smaller in diameter than a pencil in order to insert a biopsy needle or electrode.

Some medical centers use a frameless method for stereotactic brain surgery. In this method, images of the patient's head from CT or MRI scans are uploaded into a computer for display on a monitor. Markers on the patient's skin are registered by a probe linked to the computer by a camera, which joins the position of the patient's head on the operating table to the images on the computer monitor. In addition, the surgeon's instruments contain light-emitting diodes (LEDs) that are tracked by the computer during the operation.

Stereotactic radiosurgery and radiotherapy

Stereotactic radiosurgery (SRS) can be performed with three different types of machines to provide the radiation used to kill the tumor cells. The gamma knife is a stationary unit that contains 201 sources of gamma rays derived from cobalt-60 that can be focused by a computer on a single small area of the brain. The radiation can be directed very precisely to the tumor without destroying nearby healthy tissue. The patient lies on a couch with a large helmet attached to his or her headframe. The helmet contains holes that allow beams of radiation to enter. The couch is then slid into a gantry containing the cobalt-60. Treatment time varies from several minutes to over an hour, depending on the size, shape, and location of the tumor. Gamma knife radiosurgery is usually a single-dose treatment.

Radiosurgery can also be performed with a linear accelerator (also called a LINAC), which is a device that produces high-energy photons that can be used to treat larger tumors, metastatic tumors, or arteriovenous malformations. Linear accelerators are preferred for multisession treatments using smaller doses of radiation. Radiosurgery performed with divided doses is known as fractionated radiosurgery; some doctors prefer to call it fractionated stereotactic radiotherapy, or FSR. The advantage of fractionated treatment is that it allows a higher total dose of radiation to be delivered to the tumor without harming nearby normal tissues. The beams of radiation from a LINAC are shaped to a very high degree of accuracy by metal tubes known as collimators. Unlike the gamma knife unit, the LINAC moves around the patient during treatment, delivering arcs of radiation matched by computer to the shape of the tumor.

The third type of machine that can be used for radiosurgery is a cyclotron, which is a nuclear reactor used to accelerate charged particles (usually protons or ions) to high levels of energy that can be used for radiosurgery. Cyclotrons are available in very few locations, however, and there have been few **clinical trials** comparing radiosurgery performed with a cyclotron to radiosurgery using a gamma knife or LINAC.

Preparation

Some cancer centers use an invasive form of preparation for stereotactic surgery or radiosurgery. In this method, the patient is not allowed food or drink after midnight the night before the procedure. He or she is given an intravenous sedative in the morning; local anesthetic is then applied at four points on the scalp. It is not necessary to shave the head. After the skin has been numbed, the surgeon fastens the base ring to the patient's skull with four pins, the insertion points of the pins determined by the location of the brain tumor. The patient is then given a CT or MRI scan. The resultant image allows the surgeon to calculate the exact area of the tumor in three dimensions. The planning and procedure may take anywhere from three to 12 hours.

Other cancer centers use a less invasive form of patient preparation that consists of an individualized mouthpiece used to attach a headframe (or "halo" to the patient's head. The headframe is used to prevent the head from moving during treatment as well as to position the head precisely.

Stereotactic radiosurgery is always preceded by a careful review of the patient's records to make sure that this type of treatment is appropriate for the tumor. The patient may be given steroid medications to control swelling of brain tissue or antiepileptic drugs to prevent seizures prior to radiosurgery.

If the patient is to receive fractionated radiosurgery or FSR, he or she will be given a simulation scan prior to treatment. The simulation scan allows the neurosurgeon to plan the treatment by making a set of images that show the exact location of the tumor in relation to normal brain tissue. The first step is the creation of a thermoplastic mask that will allow the doctor to position the patient's head precisely each time the patient receives a treatment. Next, the patient is positioned in a scanner while wearing the mask. The simulation scan takes about two and a half hours. When the patient returns for a treatment session about a week later, the molded thermoplastic mask is used to reposition the patient's head in the exact location that was used for the simulation scan. Fractionated treatments usually take between 30 and 90 minutes to complete.

A preparatory scan is not needed with some newer lightweight linear accelerators, which make use of a robot to position the dose of radiation rather than a frame to hold the patient's head in place. If the patient moves during treatment, the robot detects the movement and repositions the linear accelerator before delivering the radiation beam.

Aftercare

Stereotactic surgery

After the surgeon has completed the procedure, he or she closes the scalp incision—usually with only one stitch—and removes the base ring from its attachment points on the scalp by unscrewing the pins. These holes are small and do not require stitches, although an antibiotic medication is applied to prevent **infection**. The patient is taken to a recovery room, remains in the hospital overnight for observation, and goes home the next day. Patients must arrange for a friend or relative to drive them home. A follow-up visit with the neurosurgeon is scheduled for six to 12 weeks after treatment.

Stereotactic radiosurgery and radiotherapy

Patients receiving gamma knife treatment can be treated as outpatients, returning home after the procedure. If pins were used to attach a headframe to the patient's scalp, the head will be wrapped with gauze for about two hours before the patient is discharged.

Risks

Stereotactic surgery

The risks of stereotactic surgery are similar to those of other surgical procedures involving open incisions in the head or neck:

- infection
- scarring
- pain
- incomplete removal of the tumor

- swelling of brain tissue
- worsening of neurologic symptoms
- anesthesia reaction

Stereotactic radiosurgery

The risks of stereotactic radiosurgery are similar to those for other forms of radiation treatment of the brain or spinal cord:

- nausea and vomiting
- headaches
- dizziness
- fatigue
- hair loss
- radiation necrosis (a group or collection of dead brain cells)
- leukoencephalopathy (damage to the white matter of the brain)
- swelling of brain tissue

Normal results

Normal results of stereotactic surgery include the obtaining of an appropriate tissue sample for biopsy or the removal of cancerous tissue. Normal results of stereotactic radiosurgery include the shrinkage or death of cancer cells in the brain or spinal cord, the drainage of excess cerebrospinal fluid, or improvement in tremor and other symptoms of Parkinson's disease or Huntington's chorea.

Abnormal results

Abnormal results for stereotactic radiosurgery would include the failure of the tumor to respond to treatment.

See also Brain tumors; Radiation therapy.

Resources

BOOKS

"Intracranial Neoplasms (Brain Tumors)." Section 14, Chapter 177 in *The Merck Manual of Diagnosis and Therapy*, edited by Mark H. Beers, MD, and Robert Berkow, MD. Whitehouse Station, NJ: Merck Research Laboratories, 2004.

PERIODICALS

Jagannathan, J., J. H. Petit, K. Balsara, et al. "Long-Term Survival after Gamma Knife Radiosurgery for Primary and Metastatic Brain Tumors." *American Journal of Clinical Oncology* 27 (October 2004): 441–444.

Mindermann, T. "Tumor Recurrence and Survival Following Gamma Knife Surgery for Brain Metastases." *Journal of Neurosurgery* 102 (January 2005) (Supplement): 287–288.

Solberg, T. D., S. J. Goetsch, M. T. Selch, et al. "Functional Stereotactic Radiosurgery Involving a Dedicated Linear Accelerator and Gamma Unit: A Comparison Study." *Journal of Neurosurgery* 101 (November 2004) (Supplement 3): 373–380.

OTHER

American Brain Tumor Association (ABTA). *Focusing on Treatment: Stereotactic Radiosurgery*. Des Plaines, IL: ABTA, 2004.

Levy, Robert, MD. "A Short History of Stereotactic Neurosurgery." *Cyber Museum of Neurosurgery*, 2005. http://www.neurosurgery.org/cubermuseum/stereotactichall/stereoarticle.html.

National Institute of Neurological Disorders and Stroke (NINDS). *Brain and Spinal Tumors: Hope Through Research*. NIH Publication No. 93-504. Bethesda, MD: NINDS, 2005.

National Institute of Neurological Disorders and Stroke (NINDS) Report. *Brain Tumors: Detection and Diagnosis*. Bethesda, MD: NINDS, 2005. http://www.ninds.nih.gov/find_people/groups/brain_tumor_prg/detection_pr.htm.

Rebecca Frey, PhD

STI-571 *see* **Imatinib mesylate**

Stomach cancer

Definition

Stomach **cancer** (also known as gastric cancer) is a disease in which the cells forming the inner lining of the stomach become abnormal and start to divide uncontrollably, forming a mass called a tumor.

Demographics

In 2009, the American Cancer Society estimated that 21,130 Americans would be diagnosed with stomach cancer and approximately 10,620 deaths would result from the disease. The risk for developing stomach cancer in the United States is about 1 in 100. The risk is higher for men than for women. The average age at time of diagnosis of stomach cancer is 71 years. Two-thirds of stomach cancer cases are diagnosed in people older than age 65, but in families with a hereditary risk for stomach cancer, cases in younger individuals are more frequently seen.

Although stomach cancer incidence has been decreasing, it is the fourth most commonly diagnosed

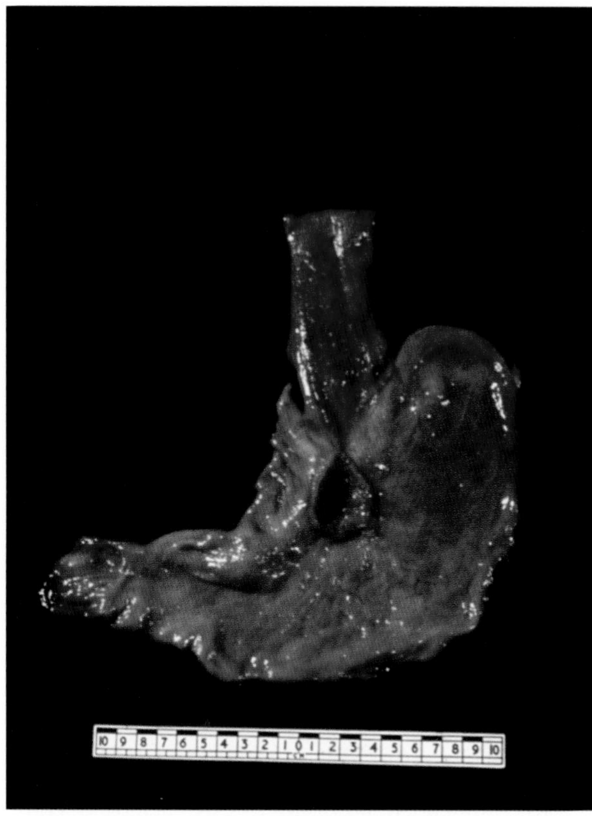

An excised section of a human stomach showing a cancerous tumor (center, triangular shape). *(Custom Medical Stock Photo. Reproduced by permission.)*

cancer and the second leading cause of cancer deaths worldwide. Stomach cancer is one of the leading causes of cancer deaths in several areas of the world, most notably in Japan and China and in countries in Eastern Europe and Latin America.

In Japan, gastric cancer is diagnosed almost ten times as frequently as in the United States. The number of new stomach cancer cases is decreasing in some areas, however, especially in developed countries. In the United States, incidence rates of stomach cancer have declined. The use of refrigerated foods and increased consumption of fresh fruits and vegetables, instead of preserved foods with high salt content, may be a reason for the decline. Another reason for the decrease may be that **antibiotics**, which are given to treat childhood illnesses, can kill the bacterium *Helicobacter pylori,* which is a major cause of stomach cancer.

Description

The stomach is a J-shaped organ that lies in the left and central portion of the abdomen. The stomach produces many digestive juices and acids that mix with the food and aid in the process of digestion. There are five regions of the stomach that doctors refer to when determining the origin of stomach cancer. These are:

- the cardia, area surrounding the cardiac sphincter which controls movement of food from the esophagus into the stomach
- the fundus, upper expanded area adjacent to the cardiac region
- the antrum, lower region of the stomach where it begins to narrow
- the prepyloric region, just before or nearest the pylorus
- the pylorus, the terminal region where the stomach joins the small intestine.

Cancer can develop in any of the five sections of the stomach. Symptoms and outcomes of the disease will vary depending on the location of the cancer.

In the last twenty years a trend of decreasing incidence of gastric tumors diagnosed in the gastric body and distal stomach has been noted while the incidence of cancers in the gastroesophageal junction and cardia areas has increased dramatically. The reason for this change in incidence patterns is not yet fully understood.

Most gastric cancers are adenocarcinomas. Adenocarcinomas comprise 90 to 95% of stomach tumors. Other less common types of stomach cancers are lymphomas, carcinoid tumors and gastrointestinal stromal tumors (GIST).

Risk factors

Factors associated with the development of stomach cancer include:

- infection with the bacterium helicobacter pylori
- history of smoking
- increased consumption of foods containing nitrates which are commonly found in foods such as cured meats
- increased consumption of smoked foods and foods high in salt
- consumption of a diet low in fresh fruits and vegetables
- personal history of prior gastric surgery
- history of pernicious anemia
- history of atrophic gastritis, a precancerous condition
- blood type A
- mutations in the E-cadherin (CDH1) gene which are associated with a hereditary form of gastric cancer

Causes and symptoms

The exact cause for stomach cancer has not yet been identified. However, several factors have been identified which appear to play a significant role in the development of stomach cancer.

Studies have shown that eating foods with high quantities of salt and nitrites increases the risk of stomach cancer. The diet in a specific region can have a great impact on its residents. Making changes to the types of foods consumed has been shown to decrease likelihood of disease, even for individuals from countries with higher risk. For example, Japanese people who move to the United States or Europe and change the types of foods they eat have a far lower chance of developing the disease than do Japanese people who remain in Japan and do not change their dietary habits. Eating recommended amounts of fruit and vegetables may lower a person's chances of developing this cancer.

Several studies have identified a bacterium (*Helicobacter pylori*) that causes stomach ulcers (inflammation in the inner lining of the stomach). Chronic (long-term) **infection** of the stomach with these bacteria may lead to a particular type of cancer (lymphomas or mucosa-associated lymphoid tissue [MALT]) in the stomach.

A hereditary form of gastric cancer, which is more likely to develop in younger individuals, has been linked to people with blood group A, a history of pernicious **anemia** and with a genetic mutation in the E-cadherin gene. Prophylactic **gastrectomy** may be recommended for younger patients known to have this specific genetic mutation.

A history of smoking also increases the risk for developing stomach cancer. Smoking doubles the risk for the development of stomach cancer.

Stomach cancer is a slow-growing cancer. It may be years before the tumor grows very large and produces distinct symptoms. In the early stages of the disease, the patient may only have mild discomfort, indigestion, heartburn, a bloated feeling after eating (also known as early satiety), and mild **nausea**. In the advanced stages, a patient has loss of appetite and resultant **weight loss**, stomach pains, **vomiting**, difficulty in swallowing, and blood in the stool. Stomach cancer often spreads (metastasizes) to adjoining organs such as the esophagus, adjacent lymph nodes, liver, or colon.

Diagnosis

Unfortunately, many patients diagnosed with stomach cancer experience pain for two or three years before informing a doctor of their symptoms. When a doctor suspects stomach cancer from the symptoms described by the patient, a complete medical history is conducted to check for any related risk factors.

Examination

A thorough physical examination is conducted to assess all the symptoms. Advanced gastric cancer may be diagnosed by noting palpable nodes in the left supraclavicular area and in the left axillary region which are typically nodes where **metastasis** from stomach cancer may occur. Other areas which may harbor metastatic disease include ovarian or pelvic masses which may be palpable.

The physician may also note changes to the skin including acanthosis nigricans (areas of dark, thick, velvety skin in the body folds such as the armpits, groin, under the breasts or behind the neck) or the appearance of new areas of seborrheic keratoses (itchy, crusty, wart-like skin lesions).

Tests

Recommended laboratory tests include a complete blood count (CBC) and blood chemistry profile. Laboratory tests may be ordered to check for blood in the stool (**fecal occult blood test**) and anemia (low red blood cell count), which often accompany gastric cancer.

The H. pylori test will also be ordered to determine if the patient is infected with the bacterium. If the H. pylori test is positive, treatment will be initiated.

In some countries, such as Japan, it is appropriate for patients to undergo routine screening examinations for stomach cancer, as the risk of developing cancer in that society is very high. Such screening might be useful for all high-risk populations. Due to the low prevalence of stomach cancer in the United States, routine screening is usually not recommended unless a family history of the disease exists.

Imaging tests which may be ordered if a diagnosis of gastric cancer is suspected include X-rays of the chest, abdominal **computed tomography** (CT) scan with contrast, CT and ultrasound of the pelvis in females, and PET/CT or PET (**positron emission tomography**) scans.

During another test, known as **upper gastrointestinal endoscopy**, a thin, flexible, lighted tube (endoscope) is passed down the patient's throat and into the stomach. The doctor can view the lining of the esophagus and the stomach through the tube. Sometimes, a small ultrasound probe is attached at the end of the endoscope. This probe sends high frequency sound waves that bounce off the stomach wall. A computer creates an image of the stomach wall by translating the pattern of echoes generated by the reflected sound waves. This procedure is known as an endoscopic ultrasound, or EUS.

Endoscopy has several advantages because the physician is able to see any abnormalities directly. In addition, if any suspicious-looking patches are seen, **biopsy** forceps can be passed painlessly through the tube to collect some tissue for microscopic examination. This is known as a biopsy. Endoscopic ultrasound (EUS) is beneficial because it can provide valuable information on depth of tumor invasion.

After stomach cancer has been diagnosed and before treatment starts, another type of x-ray scan is taken. Computed tomography (CT) is an imaging procedure that produces a three-dimensional picture of organs or structures inside the body. CT scans are used to obtain additional information in regard to how large the tumor is and what parts of the stomach it borders; whether the cancer has spread to the lymph nodes; and whether it has spread to distant parts of the body (metastasized), such as the liver, lung, or bone. A CT scan of the chest, abdomen, and pelvis is taken. If the tumor has gone through the wall of the stomach and extends to the liver, pancreas, or spleen, the CT will often show it. Although a CT scan is an effective way of evaluating whether cancer has spread to some of the lymph nodes, it is less effective than EUS in evaluating whether the nodes closest to the stomach are free of cancer.

Clinical staging

More than 95% of stomach cancers are caused by adenocarcinomas, malignant cancers that originate in glandular tissues. The remaining 5% of stomach cancers include lymphomas and other types of cancers.

It is important that gastric lymphomas be accurately diagnosed because these cancers have a much better prognosis than stomach adenocarcinomas. Approximately half of the people with gastric lymphomas survive five years after diagnosis.

Treatment for gastric **lymphoma** involves surgery combined with **chemotherapy** and **radiation therapy**.

Staging of stomach cancer is based on how deep the growth has penetrated the stomach lining; to what extent (if any) it has invaded surrounding lymph nodes; and to what extent (if any) it has spread to distant parts of the body (metastasized). The more confined the cancer, the better the chance for a cure.

One important factor in the staging of **adenocarcinoma** of the stomach is whether the tumor has invaded the surrounding tissue and, if it has, how deep it has penetrated. If invasion is limited, prognosis is favorable. Diseased tissue that is more localized improves the outcome of surgical procedures performed to remove the diseased area of the stomach. This is called a resection of the stomach.

Stomach cancer is staged using the Tumor(T), Node(N), Metastasis(M), classification system. After stage 0, where the cancer has not grown beyond the layers of the tissue lining the stomach, the tumor is labeled stage I through IV. Stage 1 indicates less tumor involvement; stage IV indicates the tumor has spread outside of the stomach and has invaded other tissues or organs in the body.

Treatment

Because symptoms of stomach cancer are so mild, treatment often does not commence until the disease is well advanced. The three standard modes of treatment for stomach cancer are surgery, radiation therapy, and chemotherapy. While deciding on the patient's treatment plan, the doctor takes into account many factors. The location of the cancer and its stage are important considerations. In addition, the patient's age, general health status, and personal preferences are also taken into account.

Surgery

In the early stages of stomach cancer, surgery may be used to remove the cancer. Surgical removal of adenocarcinoma is the only treatment capable of eliminating the cancer. Prior to surgery, CT scans and endoscopic ultrasound are performed to determine the extent of tumor involvement. If the cancer is widespread and cannot be removed with surgery, an attempt is made to remove blockage and control symptoms such as pain or bleeding. This is known as palliative surgery.

Depending on the location of the cancer, a portion of the stomach may be removed, a procedure called a partial or subtotal gastrectomy. In a surgical procedure known as total gastrectomy, the entire stomach may be removed. However, doctors prefer to leave at least part of the stomach if possible.

Partial or total gastrectomy is often accompanied by other surgical procedures. Lymph nodes are frequently removed during gastric cancer surgery. The current recommendation in the United States is that a gastrectomy done to remove a gastric tumor include removal of at least 15 lymph nodes in the areas near the cancer to offer the best hope of survival for the patient. Because stomach cancer is a relatively rare cancer in the U.S., it is recommended that surgery for stomach cancer be done by a surgeon experienced in this type of procedure and in a center with experience in treating large numbers of gastric cancer cases. In addition to total or partial removal of the stomach along with adjacent lymph nodes, nearby organs, or parts of these organs, may be removed if cancer has spread to them. Such organs may include the pancreas, colon, or spleen.

Preliminary studies suggest that patients who have tumors that cannot be removed by surgery at the start of therapy may become candidates for surgery later. Combinations of chemotherapy and radiation therapy are sometimes able to reduce disease for which surgery is not initially appropriate. Preliminary studies were being performed as of 2008 to determine if some of these patients can become candidates for surgical procedures after such therapies are applied.

Chemotherapy

Chemotherapy involves administering anti-cancer drugs either intravenously (through a vein in the arm) or orally (in the form of pills). This method can either be used as the primary mode of treatment or after surgery to destroy any cancerous cells that may have migrated to distant sites.

Although chemotherapy using a single medicine (the chemotherapy drug 5-FU) is sometimes used, the best response rates are often achieved with combinations of medicines. Therefore, in addition to studies exploring the effectiveness of new medicines, as of 2008 there were many **clinical trials** in progress attempting to evaluate how to best combine existing forms of chemotherapy to bring the greatest degree of help to patients.

Some of the more commonly used chemotherapy drugs used to treat stomach cancer include 5-FU, **doxorubicin**, **methotrexate**, **epirubicin**, **etoposide**, and **cisplatin**.

Radiation therapy

Radiation therapy is often used after surgery to destroy the cancer cells that may not have been completely removed during surgery. To treat stomach cancer, external beam radiation therapy is generally used. In this procedure, high-energy rays from a machine that is outside of the body are concentrated on the area of the tumor. In the advanced stages of stomach cancer, radiation therapy is used to ease the symptoms such as pain and bleeding. However, studies of radiation treatment for stomach cancer have shown that the way it has been used it has been ineffective for many patients.

As of 2009 researchers were actively assessing the role of chemotherapy and radiation therapy used before a surgical procedure is conducted. They were searching for ways to use both chemotherapy and radiation therapy so that they increase the length of survival of patients more effectively than existing methods were able to do.

QUESTIONS TO ASK YOUR DOCTOR

- Has the cancer spread to the lymph nodes?
- Has the cancer spread to the lungs, liver, or spleen?
- (If surgery is recommended) Do recent studies show that it might be a good idea to also use chemotherapy or radiation therapy?
- (If gastrectomy or partial gastrectomy was performed) How should I alter my diet and eating patterns?
- (Following surgery) What foods should I eat? Is there a registered dietitian I can speak with on a regular basis about what I should eat?

Prognosis

In 2009, the American Cancer Society reported approximately only 10–15% of patients with stomach cancer live at least five years following diagnosis. Patients diagnosed with stomach cancer in the earliest stages have a far better prognosis than those diagnosed in the later stages. In the early stages, the tumor is small, lymph nodes are unaffected, and the cancer has not migrated to the lungs or the liver. Unfortunately, only about 10–20% of patients with stomach cancer are diagnosed before the cancer has spread to the lymph nodes or formed a distant metastasis. Over 50% of patients diagnosed in the very early stages of stomach cancer are able to achieve a cure for their cancer.

Prevention

Avoiding many of the risk factors associated with stomach cancer may prevent its development. Excessive amounts of salted, smoked, and pickled foods should be avoided, as should foods high in nitrates. A diet that includes recommended amounts of fruits and vegetables is believed to lower the risk of several cancers, including stomach cancer. The American Cancer Society recommends eating at least five servings of fruits and vegetables daily and choosing six servings of food from other plant sources, such as grains, pasta, beans, cereals, and whole grain bread. Following a healthy diet and balancing caloric intake with recommended amounts of physical activity may reduce obesity, which may itself be a risk for developing stomach cancer.

Abstaining from tobacco and excessive amounts of alcohol reduces the risk for many cancers. In countries where stomach cancer is common, such as Japan, early detection is important for successful treatment.

Treatment for H. pylori infection, especially for those individuals with chronic infections, may reduce the risk for developing stomach cancer.

Resources

PERIODICALS

Khushalani, N."Cancer of the Esophagus and Stomach." *Mayo Clinic Proceedings* 83(June 2008):712–22.

Quiros, R.M. & Bui, C.L."Multidisciplinary Approach to Esophageal and Gastric Cancer."*Surgical Clinics of North American* 89(February 2009):79–96.

OTHER

"Gastric Cancer Treatment(PDQ)." National Cancer Institute (NCI). July 2, 2009 [cited September 12, 2009]. http://www.cancer.gov/cancertopics/pdq/treatment/gastric/HealthProfessional.

"Gastric Cancer v.1.2009." National Comprehensive Cancer Network (NCCN) Practice Guidelines in Oncology [cited September 12, 2009]http://www.nccn.org/professionals/physician_gls/PDF/gastric.pdf.

"Overview: Stomach Cancer." American Cancer Society (ACS). May 14, 2009 [cited September 12, 2009] http://www.cancer.org/docroot/CRI/content/CRI_2_4_1X_What_is_stomach_cancer_40.asp?sitearea = .

ORGANIZATIONS

American Cancer Society, (800) ACS-2345, https://www.cancer.org/.

National Cancer Institute, 6116 Executive Blvd., Room 3036A, Bethesda, MD, 20892-8322, (800)-4-CANCER, http://www.cancer.gov/.

National Coalition for Cancer Survivorship, 1010 Wayne Avenue, 5th Floor, Suite 300, Silver Spring, MD, 20910, (888) 650-9127, http://www.canceradvocacy.org/.

Lata Cherath, Ph.D.
Bob Kirsch
Melinda Oberleitner, R.N., D.N.S.

Stomatitis

Description

Stomatitis describes an inflammation of the mucous membranes of the mouth. This condition, frequently referred to as **mucositis**, can result from **cancer** treatments such as **chemotherapy** and **radiation therapy**. It is characterized by mouth ulcers or sores, and pain in the mouth. The first symptoms may be sensitivity to spicy foods and reddened mucous membranes. The patient with stomatitis may also experience a dry or swollen tongue, difficulty swallowing, and an inability to eat or drink. It is usually a short-term condition, lasting from just a few days to a few weeks. Reddened areas in the mouth may appear as early as three days after receiving chemotherapy, but normally it is within five to seven days. As time goes on, ulceration occurs. The inflammation can range from mild to severe. If such complications as **infection** do not occur, stomatitis usually heals completely within two to four weeks.

Although stomatitis is often a short-term problem, it is of concern to cancer patients and health care professionals because it can interfere with the patient's receiving adequate nutrition as well as cause pain and discomfort.

Causes

Stomatitis is most often caused by such cancer treatments as chemotherapy and radiation therapy. Chemotherapy medications work because they are attracted to rapidly growing cells like cancer cells. However, many of the body's normal cells also grow

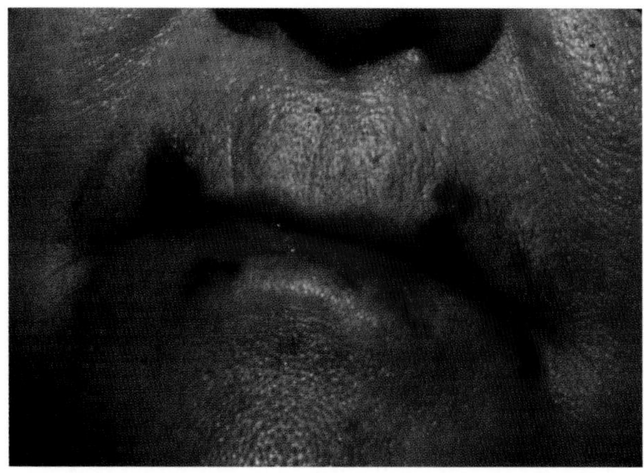

A close-up view of patient's mouth with gingivostomatitis cold sores. *(Custom Medical Stock Photo. Reproduced by permission.)*

rapidly, and chemotherapy kills them as well. The mouth includes several structures that together are referred to as the oral cavity: the lips, teeth, gums, tongue, pharynx, and the salivary glands. Most of these structures are covered by mucous membranes, the shiny, pink moist lining of the mouth. The outer layer of mucous membranes grows very rapidly, and because of this characteristic they can easily be damaged by chemotherapy and radiation therapy. When these cells are damaged, they slough off, and the lining of the mouth is left vulnerable and without protection. This exposed lining may become inflamed, swollen, and dry, and will often develop ulcers or sores.

Stomatitis caused by radiation therapy normally develops in the area where the radiation is given. It generally begins seven to fourteen days after starting radiation. It will usually exhibit improvement about two to three weeks after the treatment stops.

Stomatitis may also develop as an indirect result of cancer treatment or the cancer itself. Chemotherapy can frequently cause the patient's infection-fighting white blood cells to drop down below normal levels. When this happens, the body may be unable to keep the normal organisms in the oral cavity in balance and stomatitis, as well as such infections as **thrush** (oral candidiasis), may result. The severity of the stomatitis is dependent on various factors, including the diagnosis, the patient's age, the patient's oral condition before cancer treatment, and the level of oral care during therapy. The duration and severity of the low white blood count is another factor.

Stomatitis may also be caused or worsened by wearing dentures, braces, or other dental appliances that irritate the tissues of the mouth. According to the American Dental Association, about 8.4% of all Americans over the age of 17 have denture stomatitis.

Treatments

Various measures can be taken by the cancer patient to help prevent the occurrence or severity of stomatitis. A carefully followed program of good oral care started before cancer treatment can reduce the severity of stomatitis. The primary preventative measures include good nutritional intake, good oral hygiene practices, and early detection of any oral lesions by either the patient or a health care professional.

Once cancer treatment has started, the patient should carefully observe the mouth daily. The patient should inform their health care professional if any symptoms such as reddened areas, swelling, blisters, sores, white patches, or bleeding are noted. Meticulous oral hygiene and comfort measures are the focus of care. Sometimes, no matter what the patient does, stomatitis occurs. However, if good oral care is performed, the severity of symptoms is usually lessened. The following measures may be recommended to treat stomatitis:

- Rinsing the oral cavity after meals and before bedtime with a mild salt-water or baking soda and water solution will help keep the mouth clean and free of debris.
- A soft-bristled toothbrush or soft foam tooth-cleaning device should be used to keep the mouth and teeth very clean.
- Maintaining a good nutritional intake and drinking adequate amounts of fluids helps the body heal the stomatitis.
- The use of any tobacco products and alcohol should be avoided, as they can irritate the lining of the mouth.
- Avoid spicy or acidic foods, or very hot foods.
- Patients who wear dentures should remove them at night rather than leaving them in the mouth overnight, and should clean them carefully with an antiseptic solution.

Sometimes stomatitis develops in spite of the patient's best efforts. If the mouth sores are painful enough to prohibit eating and drinking, pain medications, including numbing medicines and both non-narcotic and narcotic pain medicines, may be prescribed.

Alternative and complementary therapies

Some preliminary studies have shown **glutamine**, an amino acid, to be effective in shortening the duration of stomatitis. Topical Vitamin E has also been studied and it shows some suggestions of being an effective therapy in patients with stomatitis. Other small studies suggest that using ice chips or a chamomile mouthwash will decrease the severity of symptoms. However, most of these studies have been small in scope, and cannot definitively claim the effectiveness of the varying treatments. As with anyone undergoing cancer treatment, the patient with stomatitis should consult with their physician or other health care professional regarding the usage of these alternative approaches.

More recently, a group of researchers in Brazil have reported that an extract made from the leaves of *Trichilia glabra*, a plant found in South America, is effective in killing several viruses that cause stomatitis.

Resources

BOOKS

Beers, Mark H., MD, and Robert Berkow, MD, editors. "Disorders of the Oral Region." In *The Merck Manual of Diagnosis and Therapy*. Whitehouse Station, NJ: Merck Research Laboratories, 2007.

Sonis, Stephen T. "Oral Complications of Cancer Chemotherapy." In *Cancer Medicine*. 5th ed. Hamilton: B.C. Decker, 2000.

PERIODICALS

Cella, M., D. A. Riva, F. C. Coulombie, and S. E. Mersich. "Virucidal Activity Presence in *Trichilia glabra* Leaves." *Revista Argentina de microbiologia* 36 (July-September 2004): 136–138.

Sciubba, James J., DMD, PhD. "Denture Stomatitis." *eMedicine* June 11, 2002. http://www.emedicine.com/derm/topic642.htm.

Shulman, J. D., M. M. Beach, and F. Rivera-Hidalgo. "The Prevalence of Oral Mucosal Lesions in U.S. Adults: Data from the Third National Health and Nutrition Examination Survey, 1988–1994." *Journal of the American Dental Association* 135 (September 2004): 1279–1286.

Wohlschlaeger, A. "Prevention and Treatment of Mucositis: A Guide for Nurses." *Journal of Pediatric Oncology Nursing* 21 (September-October 2004): 281–287.

Wojtaszek, Cynthia. "Management of Chemotherapy-induced Stomatitis." *Clinical Journal of Oncology Nursing* 4 (November-December 2000).

OTHER

"Oral Complications of Chemotherapy and Head/Neck Radiation: Supportive Care." National Cancer Institute. [cited July 3, 2001]. <http://cancernet.nci.nih.gov>.

Deanna Swartout-Corbeil, R.N.
Rebecca J. Frey, PhD

Streptozocin

Definition

Streptozocin is one of the anticancer (antineoplastic) drugs called alkylating agents. It is available in the United States under the brand name Zanosar.

Purpose

Streptozocin is primarily used to treat **cancer** of the pancreas, specifically advanced islet-cell **carcinoma**.

Description

Streptozocin chemically interferes with the synthesis of the genetic material (DNA) of cancer cells, which prevents these cells from being able to reproduce.

KEY TERMS

Antineoplastic—A drug that prevents the growth of a neoplasm by interfering with the maturation or proliferation of the cells of the neoplasm.

Neoplasm—New abnormal growth of tissue.

Recommended dosage

Streptozocin is given by injection. The dosage prescribed varies widely depending on the patient, the cancer being treated, and whether or not other medications are also being taken.

Precautions

Streptozocin carries a risk of renal (kidney) toxicity. While receiving streptozocin, patients are encouraged to drink extra fluids, since this can increase the amount of urine passed and help prevent kidney problems.

Streptozocin may cause an allergic reaction in some people. Patients with a prior allergic reaction to streptozocin should not take this medication.

Streptozocin also may cause serious birth defects if either the man or the woman is taking this drug at the time of conception or if the woman takes this drug during pregnancy. Streptozocin also may cause miscarriage.

It is not known whether streptozocin is passed from mother to child through breast milk. However, since many drugs are excreted in breast milk and since streptozocin has the potential to adversely affect an infant, breast feeding is not recommended while this medication is being taken.

Streptozocin suppresses the immune system (by damaging white blood cells) and interferes with the normal functioning of certain organs and tissues. For these reasons, it is important that the prescribing physician is aware of any of the following pre-existing medical conditions:

- a current case of, or recent exposure to, chicken pox
- diabetes mellitus
- herpes zoster (shingles)
- a current case, or history of, gout or kidney stones
- all current infections
- kidney disease
- liver disease

Also, because streptozocin damages white blood cells and platelets, patients taking this drug must exercise extreme caution to avoid contracting any new infections or sustaining any injuries that result in bruising or bleeding.

Side effects

The common side effects of streptozocin include:

- fatigue
- loss of appetite (anorexia)
- nausea and vomiting
- increased susceptibility to infection and bleeding
- swelling of the feet or lower legs
- unusual decrease in urination
- temporary hair loss (alopecia)

Diarrhea is a less common side effect that may also occur.

Because streptozocin can damage the kidneys, liver, white blood cells, and platelets, patients taking this medication should be closely monitored for evidence of these adverse side effects. Laboratory tests, including renal function, urinalysis, complete blood count, and liver function, should be done at frequent intervals (approximately weekly) during drug therapy. If evidence of these adverse side effects is found, treatment with streptozocin may be discontinued or the dose may be decreased.

Interactions

Streptozocin should not be taken in combination with any prescription drug, over-the-counter drug, or herbal remedy without prior consultation with a physician. It is particularly important that the prescribing physician be aware of the use of any of the following drugs:

- anti-infection drugs
- carmustine (an anticancer drug)
- cisplatin (an anticancer drug)
- cyclosporine (an immunosuppressive drug)
- deferoxamine (used to remove excess iron from the body)
- gold salts (used for arthritis)
- inflammation or pain medication other than narcotics
- narcotic pain medication containing acetaminophen (Tylenol) or aspirin
- lithium (used to treat bipolar disorder)
- methotrexate (an anticancer drug also used for rheumatoid arthritis and psoriasis)
- penicillamine (used to treat Wilson's disease and rheumatoid arthritis)
- phenytoin (an anticonvulsant)
- plicamycin (an anticancer drug)
- tiopronin (used to prevent kidney stones)

See also Pancreatic cancer, endocrine.

Paul A. Johnson, Ed.M.

Strontium-89 *see* **Radiopharmaceuticals**

Substance abuse

The therapeutic use of drugs for symptom control in the **cancer** population requires careful management. In general, substance abuse among cancer patients is quite uncommon. Cancer patients who haven't had previous substance abuse problems do not tend to develop them as the result of a cancer diagnosis or treatment. However, cancer patients with a history of substance abuse are a high risk of developing problems while being treated for cancer. For example, the use of illegal drugs may interfere with the effectiveness of the drugs prescribed to treat cancer. Cancer patients that are actively using illegal substances may become even more ill or develop serious complications. To make matters worse, patients who abuse drugs, or have done so in the past, are likely to be reluctant to disclose the truth to their treatment team and family members. Physicians that know about the problem can adjust a patient's treatment accordingly; therefore, every effort should be made by both the treatment team and the patient to deal with each other openly and honestly. In doing so, it will be easier for the treatment team to accurately assess and manage the patient's cancer therapy.

Recovering addicts may fear that they cannot handle the use of any potentially addictive substance. That is why it is so important for the treatment goals to be realistic and individualized for each patient. Recovering addicts may have reservations using **opioids** for their pain, fearing a relapse. Indeed, it is true that they are at a higher risk of relapse due to the stress associated with cancer and the availability of the drugs. Therefore, knowing that a relapse is possible, the patient and treatment team can create a therapy plan that embraces plenty of social and emotional support. Limits can be set to reduce the occurrence of relapse and control the damage when, and if, they occur.

On the other hand, patients who have never had drug problems may fear the use of opioids, too, but for different reasons. They may be concerned that the therapeutic use of opioids will turn them into addicts. Usually this concern stems from a misunderstanding of what constitutes an addict. Being physically dependent on a drug and being an addict are two different things. The National Cancer Institute explains addiction as "the use of a substance in a manner that is out of control, compulsive, used in increasing amounts, and is continued despite the risk of harm." Therefore, cancer patients that uses opioids to relieve their pain may become physically dependent on their medication, but that is not the same as being addicted to it. Furthermore, cancer patients taking opioids for pain don't tend to become physically dependent on them anyway, especially if the doses are correct and the medication is properly. However, if physical dependence does occur, the patient can be gently weaned off the drug and other methods of pain control can be utilized. All cancer patients can develop drug tolerances, but developing a drug tolerance has not been shown to lead to drug addiction or substance abuse problems.

Understanding the cause of substance abuse in the cancer population is difficult, because so many factors are involved. Emotional and psychological issues could play a part in it, as well as the progression of the disease itself. As the disease progresses, the pain could worsen. Under-treatment could cause patients to self-medicate in an effort to relieve the intense pain. When the treatment plan is adjusted correctly and the pain is eliminated or at least manageable, the patient no longer needs to use the medications improperly. Unfortunately, patients with addictive personalities are more likely to develop an addiction to the prescription drugs if they cannot obtain adequate pain relief. If this should occur, every effort should be made not to judge them, but instead to show compassion and render the appropriate treatment necessary to help them deal with their pain.

However, it is very important to note, once again, that patients without a history of drug abuse are highly unlikely to develop addiction problems from using opioids to control their pain. In fact, it is actually the under-treatment of pain that is more likely to lead to problems that the proper use of opioids, which is why health care professionals should talk openly with their patients about any concerns they have regarding their treatment regime. In fact, the National Cancer Institute points out that "the feeling of euphoria that a drug addict experiences does not happen in patients taking drugs to control pain. A patient taking opioids therapeutically more typically experiences a sense of **depression** rather than euphoria, thereby reducing the risk that the patient will become addicted to the drug."

In their article published in *Oncology*, Dr. Passik and colleagues noted that a comprehensive approach is needed when treating cancer patients who are either actively abusing substances or have a history of substance abuse. This approach, they explain, "goes beyond simply avoiding certain drugs or routes of administration and provides practical means to manage risk during cancer treatment."

Clinical experts in **pain management** and palliative care suggest considering the following guidelines when developing a treatment plan for patients with current or past drug or alcohol abuse problems:

- Create a multidisciplinary team
- Consider the whole patient: mind, body, and spirit
- Recognize specific drug abuse behaviors
- Utilize nondrug approaches when possible

Creating a multidisciplinary team is an especially good idea for cancer patients in general and is critically important for patients with special needs, such as those who have substance abuse problems. The team should be comprised of health care practitioners best suited to meet the needs of the patient. Patients with substance abuse issues are likely to benefit from a physician who specializes in pain medicine and palliative care, as well as a social worker and psychologist that specializes in addiction. Physicians specializing in the treatment of pain, for example, come from a variety of medical backgrounds, such as anesthesiology, oncology, psychiatry, and surgery. Ideally, a pain management team should be formed that works with the patient's primary care physician, oncologist, and radiologist to provide comprehensive care to the patient.

This concept is referred to as holistic medicine. It is one that embraces a variety of therapy options designed to see the patient as a whole person (mind, body, and spirit). Numerous studies, such as the one by Reuben and colleagues published in 1998 in the *Archives of Internal Medicine*, have validated that a patient with advanced cancer is likely to have a number of symptoms in addition to pain, such as insomnia, depression, and **fatigue**. Helping a patient cope emotionally with cancer can be just as important as helping the patient physically, especially when a person has a history of substance abuse. Some patients really benefit from group therapy, whereas others find individual therapy more helpful. As Dr. Passik and colleagues state in the second part of their two-part article on substance abuse in cancer patients, "to optimize long-term opioid therapy, well-established guidelines for cancer pain management must be applied." In doing so, the patient is less likely to be under-treated for pain, which may help to prevent relapses. In addition, the spiritual needs of a patient should also be addressed. For example, this kind of spiritual healing is one of the principles embraced by many hospices around the country.

All patients should be monitored for the development of signs that might indicate they are developing substance abuse problems. This is especially important when a patient has a history of substance abuse problems. The environment of the patient needs to be assessed to be sure that the patient's caretakers are not contributing to the problem by enabling him or her to abuse substances. A cooperative effort needs to be established that encourages honesty and disclosure.

Educational interventions that help patients communicate better with their doctors can enhance the quality of their treatment. Music and art therapy can be helpful, especially for patients who enjoy expressing themselves creatively. Some patients find it easier to deal with their pain by utilizing alternative medicine techniques, such as yoga, acupuncture, and massage therapy.

Given the complex nature of pain management in cancer patients, much more research is needed regarding the best treatment options for patients with substance abuse problems coupled with cancer-related pain.

Resources

BOOKS

Raj, P. P., Paradise, L. A., editors. 10th ed. New York, NY: Bantam Books, 2002.

PERIODICALS

Passik, S. D., Portenoy, R. K., Ricketts, P. L."Substance abuse issues in cancer patients. Part 2: Evaluation and Treatment. 12 (1998): 729–741.

Passik, S. D., Portenoy, R. K., Ricketts, P. L."Substance abuse issues in cancer patients. Part 1: Prevalence and diagnosis. 12 (1998): 517–524.

Reuben, D. B., Mor, V., Hiris, J. "Clinical symptoms and length of survival in patients with terminal cancer." 148 (1998): 1586.

OTHER

American Medical Association "Pain Management: Assessing and Treating Pain in Patients with Substance Abuse Concerns." December 2003. American Medical Association. 1 April 2009 http://www.ama-cmeonline.com/pain_mgmt/module04/05man/03_01.htm#.

National Cancer Institute "Substance Abuse Issues in Cancer. 23 Jan 2003 National Cancer Institute. [24 Feb. 2009] http://www.cancer.gov/.

Lee Ann Paradise

Sunitinib

Definition

Sunitinib is marketed by Pfizer under the trade name Sutent. It is a type of anti-cancer drug in a class called receptor tyrosine kinase inhibitors. It has been approved for use in a type of **kidney cancer** called renal cell **carcinoma** and gastrointestinal (GI) tumors called GISTs (gastrointestinal stromal tumors).

Purpose

Sunitinib is used to treat patients with renal cell carcinoma. Renal cell carcinoma occurs in small tubules in the kidney that help filter blood. It is a very common type of kidney **cancer** in adults. Sunitinib is also used for GISTs that are resistant to other agents or in patients who cannot tolerate the first regimen (imatinib) usually used to treat GISTs. GISTs are tumors that derive from connective tissue in the GI tract, and are generally benign when small to medium in size. When large enough they may metastasize. Sunitinib was the first anti-cancer agent that was approved for use in treating two different types of cancer at the same time, and is part of the standard of care for these diseases.

Description

Sunitinib is an anti-cancer drug that acts on receptor tyrosine kinases to inhibit the growth of tumors. Receptor tyrosine kinases are receptors for growth factors that are a natural part of cell development and necessary for normal cell growth. When tyrosine kinase receptors are activated, they initiate chemical signals that tell the cell how to grow and develop. Normal tyrosine kinase receptors turn on and off as needed for usual amounts of growth. However, when cells have constantly activated tyrosine kinase receptors, it can lead to abnormal growth and cancer. Drugs in the class of sunitinib inhibit these overly active tyrosine kinase receptors.

Once they reach a certain size, solid tumor cells need to form their own blood supply in order to grow and remain alive. New blood vessels need to be formed

KEY TERMS

Angiogenesis—Physiological process involving the growth of new blood vessels from pre-existing blood vessels, process used by some cancers to create their own blood supply

Catheter—Tube inserted into a body cavity or blood vessel to allow drainage of fluids (as in a urinary catheter), injection of drugs, or insertion of a surgical instrument

Cytochrome P450— Enzymes present in the liver that metabolize drugs

Epilepsy—Neurological disorder characterized by recurrent seizures

Gastrointestinal stromal tumor—Tumor of the gastrointestinal tract derived from connective tissue

Hemolytic anemia—Type of anemia involving destruction of red blood cells

Metastasize—The process by which cancer spreads from its original site to other parts of the body

QT prolongation—Potentially dangerous heart condition that affects the rhythm of the heart beat and alters the ECG reading of the heart

Receptor tyrosine kinase—Cell surface receptors that interact with growth factors and hormones to affect the normal life cycle of a cell

Renal cell carcinoma—Cancer of the kidney that originates in the very small tubes in the kidney that filter the blood and remove waste products

Teratogen—Drug or chemical agent that has the potential to cause birth defects in a developing fetus

Tuberculosis—Potentially fatal infectious disease that commonly affects the lungs, is highly contagious, and is caused by an organism known as mycobacterium

for the tumor to survive. This process is known as angiogenesis. Angiogenesis is a part of tumor progression, one of the processes critical to tumor growth and survival. Sunitinib is thought to act on many different receptor tyrosine kinases, which in addition to inhibiting individual tumor cell growth, inhibit the angiogenesis process as well.

Studies have shown that sunitinib is an effective drug, affecting both time to tumor progression and progression-free survival. The term time to tumor progression describes a period of time from when disease is diagnosed (or treated) until the disease starts to get worse. Progression-free survival describes the length of time during and after treatment in which a patient is living with a disease that does not get worse. Both time to tumor progression and progression-free survival may be used in a clinical study or trial to help find out how well a new treatment works. In studies done on sunitinib, patients receiving sunitinib had a longer median time to tumor progression and a longer median progression-free survival than those receiving placebo and other drugs tested.

Recommended Dosage

Sunitinib is taken orally in capsule form. The drug is made in dosages of 12.5, 25, and 50 mg. The dose used to treat both kidney cancer and GISTs are often 50 to 100 mg per day, but may vary according to the patient's medical condition. A regimen of 100 mg a day would involve taking two 50 mg capsules once a day. Sunitinib is usually taken in 4 week time periods with 2 weeks off in between.

For the treatment of GIST in adults sunitinib may be given in 6 week cycles at a dosage of 50 mg once daily for 4 consecutive weeks, followed by a 2 week period without taking any drug. For the treatment of advanced renal cell carcinoma in adults, sunitinib is administered in 6 week cycles at a recommended dosage of 50 mg once daily for 4 consecutive weeks, followed by a 2 week period without the drug. In clinical studies done with sunitinib, these regimens were maintained for as long as the patient derived clinical benefit from sunitinib or until unacceptable toxicity occurred.

Dosage of sunitinib is adjusted in increasing or decreasing doses of 12.5 mg daily (considered 1 dose level). Adjustments are made depending on the individual patient health and ability to tolerate the treatment. Studies have shown that sunitinib does not act significantly differently in the body based on the adult age, ethnicity, or gender of a patient. However, sunitinib has not been evaluated in pediatric patients. Following an oral dose, peak blood concentrations of sunitinib are reached within 6 to 12 hours. It is administered without regard to meals. Taking food with sunitinib has no effect on the dose absorbed or the dose available to the body.

Precautions

Sunitinib is not recommended for use in pregnant women. Birth control is recommended while using this drug. Sunitinib is a pregnancy Category D drug. Category D describes drugs in which there is evidence of potential human fetal risk based on adverse reaction data from investigational or marketing experience or studies in humans, but potential benefits may warrant use of the drug in pregnant women despite potential risks. For Category D drugs, medical necessity must be great enough to warrant risking harm to the fetus. Sunitinib is both a teratogen and lethal to fetuses in animal studies. Sunitinib is not recommended for use in breast feeding women. Sunitinib is only used in adults as the safety for use in patients less than 18 years of age has not been established. Caution must be used in patients greater than 65 years of age, as sunitinib may cause increased toxic side effects in this age group. All patients taking sunitinib must remain well hydrated. Patients should not have any vaccinations while taking sunitinib without the consent of their treating physician. Patients taking sunitinib should avoid being around people who have recently had the oral polio vaccine or inhaled flu vaccine.

Sunitinib may not be suitable for patients with a history of liver failure, inflammation of the pancreas, bleeding disorders, heart failure, imbalances in body potassium or magnesium, very high blood pressure, seizure disorders, some heart rhythm abnormalities, or other heart conditions. Sunitinib may cause a heart condition that affects the rhythm of the heartbeat known as QT prolongation. Sometimes QT prolongation can cause a serious cardiac condition that includes a fast and irregular heartbeat, with severe dizziness and fainting. The risk of developing QT prolongation syndrome may be increased if the patient is taking other drugs that also affect the rhythm of the heart, or if the patient has cardiac problems. Low blood levels of potassium or magnesium may also increase risk of QT prolongation. Sunitinib toxicity may cause other adverse side effects affecting heart function, and multiple other medical heart conditions may result from use of sunitinib.

Sunitinib may also negatively affect function of the thyroid gland. A set of baseline thyroid function tests are done before patients receive sunitinib therapy. Patients are also monitored closely for evidence of thyroid dysfunction. Other precautionary tests such as blood pressure checks, heart function tests, pancreatic inflammation, and blood chemistry need to be monitored during sunitinib therapy.

Side Effects

Sunitinib is used when the medical benefit is judged to be greater than the risk of side effects. Many patients who are prescribed sunitinib do not develop serious side effects. The most frequent side effects of sunitinib are abdominal pain and cramping, dizziness, changes in liver enzymes, loss of appetite, altered taste in the mouth, **nausea and vomiting**, joint pain, constipation or **diarrhea**, cough, dry skin, **fatigue**, **fever**, increased blood pressure, difficulty breathing, increased bleeding, hair loss, and rash. Less frequently seen side effects include eye tearing, muscle pain, thyroid dysfunction, increased infections such as **pneumonia** or catheter infections, nerve damage, black stool, vomit that looks like coffee grounds, changes in hair or skin color, and sore tongue. Sunitinib may decrease the ability of the body to fight off an **infection**, as it suppresses the immune system.

QUESTIONS TO ASK YOUR DOCTOR OR PHARMACIST

- How long will I need to take this drug before you can tell if it helps for me?
- Is this drug safe to take with the other drugs that I am currently taking?
- What side effects should I watch for? When should I call the doctor about them?
- Are there any clinical trials of this drug combined with other therapies that might benefit me?

Interactions

Patients should make their doctor aware of any and all medications or supplements they are taking before using sunitinib. Sunitinib interacts with many other drugs. Some drug interactions may make sunitinib unsuitable for use, while others may be monitored and attempted.

Sunitinib may have dangerous additive effects with other drugs that also cause QT prolongation. Drugs that interact with sunitinib in this way include amiodarone, dofetilide, pimozide, procainamide, quinidine, sotalol, and macrolide **antibiotics** such as erythromycin. Sunitinib has been combined with multiple other agents in **clinical trials** with no clinical problems. However, sunitinib is known to interact with one other **chemotherapy** agent called **bevacizumab**, causing a severe form of **anemia** known as **hemolytic anemia**.

Sunitinib is metabolized by a set of liver enzymes known as cytochrome P450 (CYP-450) subtype 3A4. Drugs that induce, or activate these enzymes increase the metabolism of Sunitinib. This results in lower levels of therapeutic sunitinib, thereby negatively affecting treatment of cancer. For this reason drugs that induce CYP-450 subtype 3A4 may not be used with sunitinib. This includes some anti-epileptic drugs such as **carbamazepine**, some anti-inflammatory drugs such as **dexamethasone**, anti-tuberculosis drugs such as rifampin, and the herb St. John's Wort.

Drugs that act to inhibit the action of CYP-450 subtype 3A4 may cause undesired increased levels of sunitinib in the body. This could lead to toxic doses. Some examples are antibiotics such as clarithromycin, antifungal drugs such as ketoconazole, antiviral drugs such as indinavir, antidepressants such as fluoxetine, and some cardiac agents such as verapamil. Grapefruit juice may also increase the amount of sunitinib in the body. Patients should avoid drinking grapefruit juice or eating grapefruit while taking sunitinib.

Resources

BOOKS

Goodman and Gilman's The Pharmacological Basis of Therapeutics, Eleventh Edition McGraw Hill Medical Publishing Division, 2006.

Tarascon Pharmacopoeia Library Edition Jones and Bartlett Publishers, 2009.

OTHER

Medscape*Sunitinib*<http://www.medscape.com.>

RxList*Sunitinib*<http://www.rxlist.com.>

ORGANIZATIONS

National Cancer Institute. 6116 Executive Boulevard, Room 3036A, Bethesda, MD 20892-8322. (800)4-CANCER http://www.cancer.gov.

FDA U.S. Food and Drug Administration. 10903 New Hampshire Ave, Silver Spring, MD 20993. (888)INFO-FDA. http://www.fda.gov.

Maria Basile, Ph.D.

Sun's soup

Definition

A combination of vegetables and herbs, Sun's soup is a complementary therapy and dietary supplement used for its apparent anticancer properties and as a stimulant for the immune system.

Selected Vegetables and *Sun's Soup* are names of various mixtures of vegetables and herbs. These mixtures were developed by Alexander Sun, a Taiwanese biochemist. Two formulations of these products are marketed in the United States as dietary supplements.

Purpose

As a complementary therapy, these products are believed to lengthened the survival of patients with advanced **non-small cell lung cancer** or other types of malignant tumors. In general, Sun's soup is used in conjunction with traditional cancer-fighting therapies, such as surgery, radiation, and **chemotherapy**.

Description

Also known as Selected vegetables, Sun's soup was developed by Alexander Sun, a biochemist, in the mid-1980s. Initially, the mixture contained shitake mushroom, mung bean, Hedyotis diffusa, and Scutellaria barbata, all of which are thought to fight **cancer** and stimulate the immune system. A 1999 study published in *Hepatogastroenterology* by Nakano and colleagues, lentinan, a beta-glucan found in shitake mushrooms, was used as adjunctive therapy with positive results. The authors reported that not only was the survival of the patients with gastric cancer prolonged, but their quality of life was improved. However, the National Cancer Institute asserted that lentinan may not be active when consumed as an ingredient in the soup. But the National Cancer Institute did other substances in shitake mushrooms may offer health benefits.

Sun began to treat other patients with a variant of the original mixture that excluded Hedyotis diffusa and Scutellaria barbata. This second formulation, a freeze-dried powder, was named Selected Vegetables (SV) or Dried Selected Vegetables (DSV). In 1992, Sun began a phase I/II clinical trial to evaluate DSV as a treatment for patients diagnosed with non-small cell lung cancer. By 1999, Sun and colleagues reported their results in an article published in *Nutrition and Cancer*. Knowing that DSV contained anti-tumor components, Sun and colleagues designed their study to measure how well patients tolerated using it on a long-term basis and its influence on the survival of patients with advanced non-small cell lung cancer. Therefore, there were two parts to the study: the toxicity arm and the survival arm. The toxicity arm was comprised of five patients with stage I non-small cell lung cancer, all of whom were asked to add DSV to their daily diet. Sun and colleagues refer to this group as the "toxicity study group (TG)." The survival arm was comprised of 19 patients with stage III or IV non-small cell lung cancer. Six of the 19 patients added DSV to their daily diet; Sun and colleagues referred to these patients as the "treatment group (SVG)." The remaining 13 patients who did not add DSV to their daily diet served as the "control group (CG)."

KEY TERMS

Adjunctive therapy—Sometimes referred to as "secondary therapy," adjunctive therapy is used in conjunction with the primary therapy.

Beta-glucan—Found in a variety of mushrooms, beta-glucan is a type of polysaccharide believed by some researchers to contain anti-tumor properties and the ability to boost the immune system.

Bioavailability—The ability of a drug to be absorbed and used by the body.

Hedyotis diffusa—In ancient Chinese medicine, this herb has been used to boost the immune system.

Median survival time—The National Cancer Institute defines median survival time as "the time from either diagnosis or treatment at which half the patients with a disease are found to be, or expected to be, still alive." With regard to a clinical trial, median survival time is a common measurement used to determine the effectiveness of a treatment.

Non-small cell cancer—The National Cancer Institute defines non-small cell cancer as "a group of lung cancers, which includes squamous cell carcinoma, adenocarcinoma, and large cell carcinoma."

Scutellaria barbata—Commonly used in traditional Chinese medicine to treat lung cancer, Scutellaria barbata is an herb that belongs to the skullcap family.

Stage I non-small cell cancer—The National Cancer Institute defines this stage as "cancer [that] is present in the lung only. Stage I is also divided into stages IA and IB based on the size and location of the tumor."

Stage III non-small cell cancer—The National Cancer Institute defines this stage "as cancer that has spread to structures near the lung; to the lymph nodes in the area that separates the two lungs (mediastinum); or to the lymph nodes on the other side of the chest or in the lower neck." Stage III is also divided into stage IIIA (resection likely) and stage IIIB (resection unlikely).

It is important to note that all the patients were treated with conventional therapies as deemed appropriate for them. TG patients had surgery plus **radiation therapy** or radiation therapy alone. SVG patients had radiation therapy alone or chemotherapy alone. CG patients had radiation therapy alone, chemotherapy alone, surgery plus radiation therapy, or chemotherapy plus radiation therapy with the exception of one patient who received palliative care, which is care that focuses on symptom management and quality of life issues.

With regard to the toxicity arm of the study, Sun and colleagues reported that "no clinical signs of toxicity were found in the TG patients in the 24-month study period." In fact, all five patients had either gained weight or maintained their weight. Another way the researchers measured how well the patients were tolerating the use of DSV was by recording changes in Karnofsky Performance Status (KPS), which is a common way of assessing a cancer patient's ability to perform routine tasks. A scoring system of 0 to 100 is used with a greater ability to handle everyday tasks associated with higher scores. Four out of the five TG patients had improved scores, which were measured at the time they entered the study and three months later. One TG patient's score remained the same. Two years after diagnosis, all five TG patients had survived and no recurrent tumors were found during follow-up. Furthermore, Sun and colleagues reported that the TG patients used DSV from 17 months to longer than 24 months. This led Sun and his team to conclude that DSV was "safe, nontoxic, and well tolerated."

With regard to the survival arm of the study, Sun and his team stated that "age, KPS, and body mass index of the SVG and CG patients were comparable" when the study began. Almost five months later a second weight measurement was taken that included 9 of the 13 CG patients and all six of the SVG patients. The average **weight loss** for the SVG group was 2.1%, whereas the average weight loss for the CG group was 11.6%. Reported as statistically significant, the group that added DSV to their daily diet clearly retained more body weight than the group that did not. A statistically significant difference was also noted with regard to the KPS scores between the CG group and the SVG group. One to three months after entering the trial, the KPS scores were improved for the SVG group, whereas the scores for the CG group declined. In other words, adding DSV to the daily diet of the patients in the SVG group not only appeared to help them avoid a decline in condition, but it was also associated with an actual improvement in condition. Furthermore, the median survival time of the CG patients was four months, whereas the median survival time of the SVG patients was 15.5 months. This statistically significant difference reported by Sun and his team supports the notion that adding DSV to the daily diet of a stage III or IV non-small cell lung cancer patient helps to prolong his or her life.

Encouraged by these results, Sun and his team reformulated the mixture and embarked on a pilot study to investigate its anticancer components, which was published in 2001 in *Nutrition and Cancer*. This third formulation was referred to as frozen selected vegetables (FSV). Through the use of a lung tumor model, tumor growth was assessed in mice. According to Sun and his team, a daily portion of FSV was "found to contain 63 mg of inositol hexaphosphate [found in legumes], 4.4 mg of daidzein [found in soy products], 2.6 mg of genistein [found in soy products], and 16 mg of coumestrol [estrogen-like substance found in plants]." Sun et al reported that mouse food containing 5% of FSV "was associated with a 53–74% inhibition of tumor growth rate." Fourteen patients with stage IIIB and stage IV non-small cell lung cancer who added FSV to their daily diet for 2 to 46 months were also evaluated. According to Sun et al, "the lead case remained tumor free for more than 133 months; the second case showed complete regression of multiple brain lesions after using FSV and radiotherapy. The median survival time of the remaining 12 patients was 33.5 months and one-year survival was greater than 70%." Ultimately, Sun et al concluded that not only was ingesting FSV nontoxic, but its ingestion was also "associated with objective responses, prolonged survival, and attenuation of the normal pattern of the progression of stage IIIB and stage IV of non-small cell lung cancer."

Though these results appear promising (as do the results of the previous 1999 clinical trial by Sun et al), the results should be viewed with some degree of caution, because more research is needed. For example, in order to confirm the results of the 2001 study, a large randomized controlled clinical trial should be conducted. Furthermore, as the National Cancer Institute points out, "all of the patients [in the 2001 study] were aware of the reported benefits of Sun's soup and had actively sought treatment." Therefore, the National Cancer Institute states cautions that "the results obtained with such highly motivated, self-selected patients might not be typical of those obtained with most patients diagnosed with advanced non-small cell lung cancer." In addition, both the 1999 and 2001 Sun studies share a weakness: the small number of patients involved. Another problem is that the formulations in both studies differ, making a comparison between the two difficult. Therefore, more studies testing both formulations on larger samples sizes are needed to confirm the results.

Recommended dosage

Patients should consult their physicians for dosage clarification, including how much and how often any dietary supplement should be taken, as well as the best formulation to use. For example, in the study conducted by Sun et al that was published in *Nutrition and Cancer* in 1999, the mixture tested was in the freeze-dried powder form and the participants orally consumed 30 grams of it a day, which they mixed with water or soup. In the subsequent study conducted by Sun that was published in *Nutrition and Cancer* in 2001, the participants orally consumed 10 ounces a day, which is approximately 283 grams, of the reformulated, frozen mixture. Both forms are available in the United States, but consumers should be aware that dietary supplements are not regulated by the United States Food and Drug Administration. Therefore, Sun's soup should be purchased only from a reputable supplier, preferably one who is recommended by a physician.

Precautions

Patients should consult with their physician regarding all food or over-the-counter medications before they are consumed.

The National Cancer Institute indicates that there is no information on the safety or the efficacy of this treatment.

Side effects

No toxic side effects are known to be associated with the use of Sun's soup. A bloated sensation was reported by participants in the 1999 study conducted by Sun and colleagues. Participants in the 2001 study did not experience any negative side effects. However, an important distinction between the two studies should be noted. In the 1999 study, the mixture of Sun's soup was in a freeze-dried powder form and was mixed with water or soup. In the 2001 study, a reformulated, frozen mixture of Sun's soup was used. This difference could explain why the participants reported different responses.

Interactions

Although Sun's soup is not known to interact with other medications, it is best for patients to consult a pharmacist and/or physician regarding the safety of its use.

Resources

PERIODICALS

Borchers, A. T., et al. "Mushrooms, tumors, and immunity." *Proceedings of the Society for Experimental Biology and Medicine* 221 (1999): 281–293.

Nakano, H., K. Namatame, H. Nemoto, et al. "A multi-institutional prospective study of lentinan in advanced gastric cancer patients with unresectable and recurrent diseases: effect on prolongation of survival and improvement of quality of life. Kanagawa Lentinan Research Group." *Hepatogastroenterology* 46 (1999): 2662–2668.

Sun, A. S., O. Ostadal, V. Ryznar, et al. "Phase I/II of stage III and IV non-small cell lung cancer patients taking a specific dietary supplement." *Nutrition and Cancer* 34 (1999): 62–69.

Sun, A. S., H. C. Yeh, L. H. Wang, et al. "Pilot study of a specific dietary supplement in tumor-bearing mice and in stage IIIB and IV non-small cell lung cancer patients." *Nutrition and Cancer* 39 (2001): 85–95.

OTHER

"Selected Vegetables/Sun's Soup (PDQ[R]) Health Professional Version." *National Cancer Institute*. June 2004. [cited February 17, 2005]. http://www.nci.nih.gov/cancertopics/pdq/cam/vegetables-sun-soup/Health/Professional.

Lee Ann Paradise

Superior vena cava syndrome

Definition

The superior vena cava is a large vein in the chest that drains the blood from the upper body back to the heart. Compression or occlusion (blocking off) of this vein creates superior vena cava syndrome.

Description

When the superior vena cava (SVC) becomes compressed or occluded, the blood from the upper body cannot drain back to the heart properly. This creates suffusion (the spreading of bodily fluids into surrounding tissue) which causes varying degrees of airway obstruction, swelling and cyanosis (purple discoloration due to lack of oxygenation) of the face, neck, arms and chest area.

Causes

Cancer is the most common cause of superior vena cava Syndrome. Lung cancer, **lymphoma**, **breast cancer**, and **germ cell tumors** of the chest are commonly associated with SVC syndrome. Any cancer that invades or constricts the blood vessels in the chest can cause SVC syndrome. Other non-cancer causes of SVC Syndrome are thyroid goiter, fungal infections, pericardial constriction, aortic aneurysm, and any other disease that creates swelling in the mediastinum (organs and vessels of the chest). Occasionally, SVC syndrome can be caused by a central vein catheter (an IV catheter that is placed into central circulation with its tip in the superior vena cava), which may cause a thrombosis (blockage) of the SVC.

QUESTIONS TO ASK THE DOCTOR

- What is the most likely cause of my SVC syndrome?
- What tests will be done to determine the cause of my SVC syndrome?
- What are my treatment options for SVC syndrome?
- Am I a candidate for a stent?
- If I am a candidate for thrombolytic therapy, will ongoing anticoagulation be used? Will it interfere with my cancer therapy?
- If I choose to do nothing (opt for no therapy), what may be the consequence?
- Is my SVC syndrome presenting an oncologic medical emergency?

Symptoms

Patients with superior vena cava syndrome (SVC syndrome) might experience facial swelling causing the shirt collar to feel tight, shortness of breath, coughing, a change of voice, or confusion. A patient might also notice distention or enlargement of veins near the surface of the skin. The development of these signs and symptoms is usually a gradual process taking up to four weeks from onset of symptoms to diagnosis.

Diagnosis

The physician diagnoses SVC syndrome by starting with a complete patient history and physical examination. The physician will ask about onset of symptoms and timeframes of symptom development. The physician will recommend a chest x ray and a **computed tomography** scan to visualize the chest area in order to confirm the presence of SVC syndrome. The physician may also order venous patency (flow of blood through the vein) studies using contrast dye and scanning techniques. The physician may order a scan done in a **Magnetic resonance imaging** (MRI) lab, ultrasound lab, or in nuclear medicine to help assess the cause of the superior vena cava syndrome. These tests help the physician identify the site and nature of the obstruction. If cancer of the bronchi is suspected, the patient should also anticipate other testing such as sputum collection, **bronchoscopy**, and **biopsy** of the suspected cancer site. These tests are very important to the oncologist (a physician who specializes in the treatment of cancer), because they will help to identify the disease, determine the stage, and hence the appropriate course of treatment.

Risks

Many patients have the symptoms of superior vena cava syndrome for more than a week before seeing their doctor. Sometimes the diagnosis of SVC syndrome is the first sign that there is cancer present in the body (only 3–5% of patients with SVC syndrome do not have cancer). Most patients with SVC syndrome do not die from the syndrome itself, but from the underlying disease, and the extent of the cancer invasion causing the syndrome. Physicians consider the presence of superior vena cava syndrome a life-threatening oncologic medical emergency when there is tracheal (airway) obstruction present. Further, if there is extensive suffusion causing swelling in the vessels in the brain, the patient's condition can rapidly deteriorate. Once the diagnosis of SVC syndrome is made, the physician will immediately commence determining the cause of the syndrome to avoid or minimize these risks.

Treatment

There are several treatment options to alleviate the symptoms of SVC syndrome. The feasibility of these options depends on the primary cause of the obstruction, the severity of the symptoms, the prognosis of the patient, and the patient's preferences and ultimate goals for therapy. The physician will need to determine the histology (cellular origin) of the obstructing cancer before proceeding with SVC syndrome treatment. Unless there is airway obstruction or swelling in the brain, treatment of SVC syndrome can be delayed to determine the stage of the underlying disease.

Medical management of SVC syndrome includes elevating the head, using steroids to minimize swelling, and diuretics to remove fluid from circulation. Some patient may develop collateral circulation (development of smaller vessel branches to assist with the excess fluid load on the SVC) and not need further treatment.

Chemotherapy is used on lymphomas or small cell lung cancers because they are sensitive to the drugs. Rapid initiation of chemotherapy in these situations can dramatically reduce the unpleasant symptoms of SVC syndrome in most patients. When chemotherapy is not the best choice for the cancer type, **radiation therapy** can provide some relief from symptoms.

Other treatment options include thrombolysis where a fibrolytic agent (agent that breaks down a thrombus or clot) is injected into the obstructed SVC. This option is used when it is determined that the obstruction is inside the vein. Stent placement (placing a sterile mesh tube inside the SVC to keep the vessel open) has been used successfully in some patients, but may require ongoing anticoagulation therapy after placement. Finally, surgical bypass of the obstructed SVC is a possible option for some patients, however the procedure is extensive and the patient must have appropriate healthy veins to graft to the affected area.

Resources

PERIODICALS

Abner, A. "Approach to the Patient who Presents with Superior Vena Cava Obstruction." *Chest* 103, suppl. 4 (1993): 394–7s.

Baker, G. L., and H. J. Barnes. "Superior Vena Cava Syndrome: Etiology, Diagnosis, and Treatment." *American Journal of Critical Care* 1 (1992): 54–64.

Chan, R. H., A. R. Dar, E. Yu, et al. "Superior Vena Cava Obstruction in Small-Cell Lung Cancer." *International Journal of Radiation Oncology, Biology, Physics* 38, no.3 (1997): 513–20.

Dyet, J. F.; A. A. Nicholson, and A. M. Cook. "The Use of the Wallstent Endovascular prosthesis in the Treatment of Malignant Obstruction of the Superior Vena Cava." *Clinical Radiology* 48, no. 6 (1993): 381–5.

Schraufnagel, D.E.; R. Hill, J.A. Leech, et al. "Superior Vena Caval Obstruction: Is it a Medical Emergency?" *American Journal of Medicine* 70, no. 6 (1981): 1169–74.

Molly Metzler, R.N., B.S.N.

Supratentorial primitive neuroectodermal tumors

Definition

Supratentorial primitive neuroectodermal tumors, or SPNETs, are primary **brain tumors** found mostly in children. The word *supratentorial* refers to the location of these tumors in the part of the brain called the cerebrum, above the tentorium (the tentlike membrane that covers the cerebellum). This term is used to differentiate these tumors from medulloblastomas, which are

KEY TERMS

Blastoma—An abnormal growth of embryonic cells. Supratentorial primitive neuroectodermal tumors are sometimes called cerebral neuroblastomas.

Calcification—A deposit of calcium within cells or tissues. Calcifications in the brain are often visible on imaging studies of SPNETs.

Cerebellum—The part of the brain that lies within the lower back portion of the skull behind the brain stem. The cerebellum helps to coordinate voluntary movements.

Cerebrum—The largest part of the brain in humans, occupying the upper part of the skull cavity. Supratentorial primitive neuroectodermal tumors are located in the cerebrum.

Medulloblastoma—A malignant tumor of the cerebellum that occurs mostly in children and is considered a type of primitive neuroectodermal tumor. Medulloblastomas are sometimes classified as infratentorial primitive neuroectodermal tumors because they develop underneath the tentorium.

Primary brain tumor—A tumor that starts in the brain, as distinct from a metastatic tumor that begins elsewhere in the body and spreads to the brain.

Primitive—Simple or undifferentiated. SPNETs are classified as primitive tumors because they arise from cells that have not yet separated into groups of more specialized cells.

Shunt—A tube inserted by a surgeon to relieve pressure on the brain from blocked cerebrospinal fluid. The tube allows the fluid to bypass the tumor that is blocking its flow.

Supratentorial—Located above the tentorium, which is the tentlike membrane that covers the cerebellum.

Ventricle—One of the small cavities located within the brain.

sometimes called infratentorial primitive neuroectodermal tumors (IPNETs) because they are located beneath the tentorium. *Primitive* refers to the fact that SPNETs arise from cells that have not yet separated into more specialized types of cells. The word *neuroectodermal* means that these tumors develop out of a layer of cells in the embryo that eventually gives rise to the baby's nervous system. Supratentorial primitive neuroectodermal tumors are also called cerebral neuroblastomas.

QUESTIONS TO ASK YOUR DOCTOR

- Which risk group has my child been assigned to?
- What treatments would you recommend for a child in that group, and why would you recommend them?
- Is my child eligible for any current clinical trials for children with SPNETs?
- Would you recommend any of the treatments currently considered experimental?
- If the tumor recurs, what is my child's life expectancy? What can I do to make the remaining time as pain-free and enjoyable as possible?

Description

SPNETs are rapidly growing tumors that are considered highly malignant. While they resemble medulloblastomas in terms of the type of cells that give rise to them, they are far less common; the ratio of medulloblastomas to SPNETs is thought to be about 25: 1.

The location of SPNETs in the cerebrum means that they occur in the largest part of the brain—the portion that governs speech, emotions, voluntary muscular movements, and the ability to think, reason, and solve problems. These tumors may metastasize, or spread, to other parts of the central nervous system (CNS) via the cerebrospinal fluid. A doctor looking at a CT scan of one of these tumors will usually see a large mass with clear margins that contains cysts, calcifications (deposits of calcium within the brain cells), and patches of dead tumor cells. In some cases the doctor will also see evidence of bleeding into nearby tissue.

Demographics

These tumors are extremely rare, accounting for only 0.5–2 percent of childhood tumors of the central nervous system (CNS). About 2,200 children below the age of 15 are diagnosed with malignant tumors of the brain and spinal cord each year in the United States; between 10 and 40 of these children will be diagnosed with SPNETs.

It is difficult to evaluate the statistical significance of racial or gender differences in such a small group; however, the available evidence from American **cancer** registries suggests that these cancers occur more frequently in Caucasian children than in African Americans, and more frequently in males than in females. The male: female ratio is thought to be about 1.8: 1.

SPNETs occur almost exclusively in younger children, with very few cases reported in adolescents or adults. About 75% of these tumors occur in children below the age of 15, with 50% diagnosed in children below the age of 10. Most SPNETs diagnosed in adults occur in young adults between the ages of 21 and 40.

Causes and symptoms

The causes of SPNETs are not well understood. They do not run in families and are not known to be associated with carcinogens in the environment. It is thought that they result from sporadic (random) gene mutations, possibly associated with abnormalities in the short arm of chromosome 17.

The symptoms of a supratentorial primitive neuroectodermal tumor are often insidious, which means that they are gradual in onset. They are caused by the increased pressure of cerebrospinal fluid inside the skull. Depending on the size of the tumor and the child's age, symptoms may include the following:

- headache, usually worse in the morning, sometimes relieved by vomiting
- blurred vision
- nausea and intermittent vomiting
- weakness or loss of sensation on one side of the body
- difficulty with balance
- frequent crying (in children below the age of three)
- decreased interaction with other people
- lowered energy level or unusual need for sleep
- irritability and other personality changes
- unexplained changes in weight or appetite

Parents should note, however, that none of these symptoms are unique to SPNETs; they may be produced by other types of brain tumors, head trauma, meningitis, migraine headaches, or several other medical conditions. In any event, a child with these symptoms should be seen by a doctor at once.

Diagnosis

The diagnosis of a supratentorial primitive neuroectodermal tumor begins with a review of the child's medical history and a thorough physical examination. The child may be given several vision tests if he or she is seeing double or having other visual disturbances. The doctor may notice one or more of the following signs, although none of them are distinctive features of SPNETs:

- Papilledema. Papilledema refers to swelling of the optic disk, usually caused by increased fluid pressure behind the eye.
- Ataxia. This term refers to loss of muscular coordination.
- Nystagmus. This refers to rapid involuntary movement of the eyeball. The doctor may be able to detect it by having the child look to the right or the left.
- Palsy of the lower cranial nerve.
- Dysmetria. This term refers to the loss of ability to estimate distance when using the muscles; an example would be overreaching when trying to pick up a small object.

The child's doctor will then order both laboratory tests and **imaging studies**. The laboratory tests are done to rule out such diseases as meningitis and to see whether the child's liver and other organs are functioning normally. The imaging studies are performed to determine the extent of the cancer and to assign the child to a risk group.

The diagnosis of SPNET cannot be confirmed, however, on the basis of a clinical examination. Instead, a neurosurgeon will perform what is known as an open **biopsy**. He or she will drill a small hole in the child's skull and remove a small piece of the tumor for examination by a pathologist.

Imaging tests

Imaging tests for SPNETs include the following:

- Magnetic resonance imaging (MRIs)
- Computed tomography (CT) scan
- Chest x ray
- Bone scan (This test is necessary to determine whether the tumor has spread beyond the central nervous system.)

Laboratory tests

Standard laboratory tests for children with brain tumors include a complete blood count (CBC), electrolyte analysis, tests of kidney, liver, and thyroid function, and tests that determine whether the child has been recently exposed to certain viruses. In addition, a **lumbar puncture** will usually be performed to look for cancer cells in the child's spinal fluid.

Treatment team

Since the 1960s, most children diagnosed with brain tumors have been treated in specialized children's cancer centers. A child with a SPNET will usually have a pediatric oncologist as his or her primary doctor, along with one or more specialists. These specialists may include a neurosurgeon, pathologist, neuroradiologist, radiation oncologist, medical oncologist, endocrinologist, nutritionist, physical therapist or rehabilitation specialist, and psychologist or psychiatrist. The team will also include social workers, clergy, and other professionals to help the parents cope with the stresses of their child's illness and treatments.

Clinical staging, treatments, and prognosis

Staging

Supratentorial primitive neuroectodermal tumors are not staged in the same way as cancers elsewhere in the body. Instead, children with these tumors are divided into two risk groups, average risk and poor risk. Assignment to these groups is based on the following factors:

- child's age
- size and location of the tumor
- whether the tumor has spread to other parts of the central nervous system
- whether the tumor has spread beyond the CNS to other parts of the body

Average-risk children are those older than three years, with most or all of the tumor removed by surgery and no evidence that the cancer has spread beyond the cerebrum. Poor-risk children are those who are younger than three years, whose cancer was located near the center of the brain or could not be removed completely by surgery, and whose cancer has spread to or beyond other parts of the CNS. The risk of recurrence is higher for children in the poor risk group.

Treatments

Treatments for SPNETs depend on the child's age and his or her risk group. Children younger than three years are not usually given **radiation therapy** because it can affect growth and normal brain development. They are usually treated with surgery first to remove as much of the tumor as possible, followed by **chemotherapy** if they are considered poor-risk patients. The drugs most commonly used to treat SPNETs include **lomustine**, **cisplatin**, **carboplatin**, and **vincristine**.

In addition to removing the tumor, the surgeon may also place a shunt to reduce pressure on the child's brain if the tumor is blocking the flow of cerebrospinal fluid. A shunt is a plastic tube with one end placed within the third ventricle of the brain. The rest of the shunt is routed under the skin of the head, neck, and chest with the other end placed in the abdomen or near the heart. About 30% of children treated for SPNETs require shunt placement.

Children three years and older are treated with surgery first, followed by radiation treatment of the entire brain and spinal cord. Those considered poor risks may also be given chemotherapy. Recurrent SPNETs are treated with further surgery and an additional course of chemotherapy.

Treatments for supratentorial primitive neuroectodermal tumors that are considered experimental as of 2005 include the following:

- Gamma knife surgery (GKS).
- Gene therapy.
- High-dose chemotherapy. Chemotherapy with topotecan has been reported to give promising results in treating SPNETs, as does high-dose chemotherapy combined with stem cell transplantation.
- Photodynamic therapy.
- Bone marrow transplantation.
- Newer drugs: Irinotecan, tipifarnib, lapatinib, ixabepilone, cilengitide, and tariquidar.

Prognosis

The prognosis for children with SPNETs depends largely on their risk group. In general, however, these tumors have a poorer prognosis than other types of brain tumors in children, in part because of the difficulty of removing the complete tumor due to its large size, its extensive blood supply, and its location within the cerebrum. The overall five-year survival rate of children with supratentorial primitive neuroectodermal tumors is reported to be 50–60 percent, but is much lower in children younger than three years and in older children who do not respond to radiation therapy.

Recurrent tumors of this type are almost always fatal; there are no effective therapies for recurrent SPNETs as of the early 2000s.

Alternative and complementary therapies

Some complementary therapies that are reported to help children with SPNETs include pet therapy, humor therapy, art therapy, and music therapy. All of these can be pleasurable for the child as well as relaxing. Ginger or peppermint may help to relieve the **nausea and vomiting** associated with chemotherapy.

Coping with cancer treatment

Children being treated for SPNETs can be given additional medications to treat **nausea** and other side effects of chemotherapy. With regard to homesickness and other emotional reactions to being away from home, children's cancer centers have social workers and child psychologists who can educate the child's family about the cancer as well as help the child deal with separation issues.

The side effects of radiation therapy in children with brain tumors may include the formation of dead tissue at the site of the tumor. This formation is known as radiation necrosis. It occurs in about 5% of children who receive radiation therapy and may require surgical removal. Radiation necrosis, however, is not as serious as recurrence of the tumor.

Children who have difficulty speaking after brain surgery, or who experience physical weakness, difficulty walking, visual impairment, or other sensory problems, are given physical therapy and/or speech therapy on either an inpatient or outpatient basis.

Clinical trials

Because SPNETs are so rare, the American Cancer Society recommends that children diagnosed with these tumors be enrolled in an appropriate clinical trial. As of the mid 2000s, there we are about 30 **clinical trials** in the United States for children with various types of PNETs. Some of these trials involve gene testing to improve diagnosis of children with brain tumors, while others are exploring various combinations of chemotherapy (including new agents), **photodynamic therapy**, stem cell transplantation, and **bone marrow transplantation** as treatments for primitive neuroectodermal tumors.

Prevention

There is no way to prevent SPNETs because their cause is still unknown.

Special concerns

Children with SPNETs are like children with other long-term illnesses in that they may develop emotional problems in reaction to restrictions on their activities, uncomfortable treatments, or being treated in a cancer center away from home. These children may withdraw from others, become angry or bitter, or feel inappropriately guilty about their illness. It is important for parents to reassure the child that he or she did not cause the cancer or deserve it as a punishment for being "bad." Parents may benefit from consulting a child psychiatrist about these and other emotional problems.

Another special concern is the task of explaining the child's illness and treatments to other family members and friends in ways that they can understand. Members of the child's treatment team can be helpful in providing simplified descriptions for siblings or schoolmates.

A third area of concern with **childhood cancers** is the parents' relationships with their other children and with each other. Siblings may resent the amount of time and attention given to the child with cancer, or they may fear that they too will develop a brain tumor. Support groups for families of children with cancer can help by sharing strategies for coping with these problems as well as allowing members to express anxiety and other painful feelings in a safe setting.

See also Medulloblastoma; Pineoblastoma.

Resources

BOOKS

American Brain Tumor Association (ABTA). *A Primer of Brain Tumors*. Des Plaines, IL: ABTA, 2004. The entire book can be downloaded free of charge as one large PDF file from the ABTA website.

"Intracranial Neoplasms (Brain Tumors)." Section 14, Chapter 177 in *The Merck Manual of Diagnosis and Therapy*, edited by Mark H. Beers, MD, and Robert Berkow, MD. Whitehouse Station, NJ: Merck Research Laboratories, 2007.

Pelletier, Kenneth R., MD. *The Best Alternative Medicine*. New York: Simon & Schuster, 2002.

PERIODICALS

Dai, A. I., J. W. Backstrom, P. C. Burger, and P. K. Duffner. "Supratentorial Primitive Neuroectodermal Tumors of Infancy: Clinical and Radiologic Findings." *Pediatric Neurology* 29 (November 2003): 430–434.

Gardner, Sharon L., MD. "Application of Stem Cell Transplant for Brain Tumors." *Pediatric Transplantation* 8 (June 2004) (Supplement 5): 28–32.

Ghosh, Subrata, MD, and Draga Jichici, MD. "Primitive Neuroectodermal Tumors of the Central Nervous System." *eMedicine*, 14 December 2001. http://www.emedicine.com/neuro/topic326.htm.

MacDonald, Tobey, MD. "Medulloblastoma." *eMedicine*, 29 July 2004. http://www.emedicine.com/ped/topic1396.htm.

Perez-Martinez, A., A. Lassaletta, M. Gonzalez-Vincent, et al. "High-Dose Chemotherapy with Autologous Stem Cell Rescue for Children with High-Risk and Recurrent Medulloblastoma and Supratentorial Primitive Neuroectodermal Tumors." *Journal of Neurooncology* 71 (January 2005): 33–38.

Young, Guy, MD, Jeffrey A. Toretsky, MD, Andrew B. Campbell, MD, and Allen E. Eskenazi, MD.

"Recognition of Common Childhood Malignancies." *American Family Physician* 61 (April 1, 2000): 2144–2154.

OTHER

American Academy of Child and Adolescent Psychiatry (AACAP). *The Child with a Long-Term Illness.* AACAP Facts for Families #19. Washington, DC: AACAP, 1999.

American Cancer Society (ACS), Cancer Reference Information. *Brain and Spinal Cord Tumors in Children.*. <http://documents.cancer.org/144.00/144.00.pdf>.

ORGANIZATIONS

American Academy of Child and Adolescent Psychiatry. 3615 Wisconsin Avenue, NW, Washington, DC 20016-3007. (202) 966-7300. Fax: (202) 966-2891. http://www.aacap.org..

American Brain Tumor Association (ABTA). 2720 River Road, Des Plaines, IL 60018. (800) 886-2282 or (847) 827-9910. http://www.abta.org. This independent non-profit association supports research as well as providing patient and family education materials.

CureSearch Children's Oncology Group (COG) Research Operations Center. 440 East Huntington Drive, P. O. Box 60012, Arcadia, CA 91066-6012. CureSearch is a joint effort of two organizations, the Children's Oncology Group (COG) and the National Childhood Cancer Foundation (NCCF). The COG conducts research and clinical trials while the NCCF conducts fundraising and advocacy initiatives.

Rebecca Frey, PhD

Suramin

Definition

Suramin (suramin hexasodium; CI-1003) is a polysulfonated naphthylurea. It is a growth factor antagonist for palliative treatment in hormone-refractory **prostate cancer** and hormone-responsive metastatic prostate **cancer**.

KEY TERMS

Antagonist—A drug that binds to a cellular receptor for a hormone, neurotransmitter, or another drug. Antagonists block the action of the substance without producing any physiologic effect itself.

Antineoplastic—Antineoplastic therapy is a regimen of chemotherapy aimed at destroying malignant cells using a variety of agents that directly affect cellular growth and development.

Anthelmintic—An agent destructive to worms. Many anthelmintic drugs are toxic and should be given with care; the patient should be observed carefully for toxic effects after the drug is given.

Antiprotozoal—An agent destructive to protozoa.

Clinical trials—Highly regulated and carefully controlled patient studies, where either new drugs to treat cancer or novel methods of treatment are investigated.

DNA—Deoxyribonucleic acid. Genetic information carried in chromosomes.

Growth factors—Growth factors or human growth factors are compounds made by the body that function to regulate cell division and cell survival. Some growth factors are also produced in the laboratory by genetic engineering and are used in biological therapy. Growth factors are significant because they can induce angiogenesis, the formation of blood vessels around a tumor. These growth factors also encourage cell proliferation, differentiation, and migration on the surfaces of the endothelial cells.

Metastatic—The term used to describe a secondary cancer, or one that has spread from one area of the body to another.

Palliative—To alleviate disease without curing it.

Tumor—An abnormal mass of tissue that serves no purpose. Tumors may be either benign (noncancerous) or malignant (cancerous).

Purpose

Suramin has been used for years to combat African sleeping sickness and river blindness but it has also been found beneficial in slowing the progression of prostate cancer. This drug is classified as an antiprotozoal or anthelminitic. In addition to combating prostate cancer, suramin has demonstrated antitumor activity against many types of tumors including endometrial, breast, ovarian, and lung cancer. It has a number of important biological functions for cancer treatment; it inhibits a number of growth factors and receptors needed for tumor growth including epidermal growth factor (EGF), platelet-derived growth factor (PDGF), fibroblast growth factor, and vascular endothelial growth factor. Suramin decreases blood plasma levels of insulin-like growth factors 1 and 2. Suramin also inhibits tumor antigen, DNA synthesis, cell motility, and urokinase activity. It has also demonstrated significant improvements in pain response.

In one of the most recent clinical studies, published in 2001, suramin delayed disease progression, by inhibition of prostate-specific antigen levels, thus prolonging survival in prostate cancer patients. This study also demonstrated suramin delayed two other clinical study endpoints: progression-free survival (i.e. delaying disease progression) and time to pain progression.

Description

While conducting research into suramin as a potential anti-HIV agent, it was found that tumors regressed in HIV-associated cancers. This discovery led investigators to evaluate the antineoplastic effects of suramin. Unfortunately, suramin did not prove effective as an anti-HIV agent.

Suramin, under the brand name Metaret, was submitted for Food and Drug Administration (FDA) approval for treatment of hormone-refractory prostate cancer in 1997 by Warner-Lambert. However, a review by the Oncologic Drugs Advisory Committee in 1998 did not support FDA approval. It was given approval for the "List of Orphan Designations and Approvals." It has been reported to be under development by the Cooperative Research and Development Agreement (CRADA) with the National Cancer Institute (NCI) and the National Institute of Health (NIH). This drug was withdrawn in 2000 and will not be pursued for FDA approval by Pfizer, who merged with Warner-Lambert.

Recommended dosage

Since this drug is not FDA approved for cancer treatment, dosing information is not readily obtainable. Original research on suramin with continuous infusions was associated with severe toxicities. Due to these toxicities, a long half-life, and a narrow therapeutic range, there was a desire to avoid prolonged continuous infusions. During **clinical trials**, outpatient doses of suramin were aimed at maintaining plasma concentrations at 150 to 250 mcg/mL for three months' duration to minimize treatment exposure.

Precautions

The majority of the precautions listed below are based on suramin's use as an antiprotozoal agent.

The following precautions should be considered:

- Allergies. Alert the doctor if any unusual or allergic reaction to suramin occurs or to any other substances, such as foods, preservatives, or dyes.
- Pregnancy. Suramin has not been studied in pregnant women, but animal studies in animals have shown that suramin may cause birth defects or death of the fetus. Before receiving this medicine, alert the doctor if you are pregnant or if you may become pregnant.
- Breast-feeding. It is not known whether suramin passes into breast milk. This issue should be discussed with a doctor for a mother who wishes to breast-feed.
- Children. Suramin can cause serious side effects in any patient, so prior to adminstration to children, discuss the risks with a doctor.
- Older adults. Elderly people are especially sensitive to the effects of suramin. This may increase the chance of side effects during treatment.
- Other medical problems. The presence of other medical problems may affect the use of suramin. Make sure to tell the doctor about any other medical problems, especially kidney or liver disease. Patients with kidney or liver disease may have an increased chance of side effects

Due to a risk of adrenal insufficiency (which results from the inadequate production of adrenal hormones) and coagulopathy (a defect that interferes with the blood clotting mechanism), patients receiving suramin should be administered hydrocortisone and vitamin K.

Significant toxicities are associated the use of suramin. However, with careful monitoring of serum concentrations, these toxicities are manageable.

Side effects

Rash, edema, and asthenia are commonly reported, but generally mild to moderate. Malaise and **fatigue** are the most common dose-limiting toxicities, affecting 41% of patients in clinical trials for prostate cancer. The majority of the side effects listed below are based on suramin's use as an antiprotozoal agent. Different doses used for cancer treatment may effect the side effect profile. Abdominal pain, **fever**, metallic taste, and a general feeling of discomfort may be bothersome but do not usually require medical attention. These effects may disappear during treatment as the body adjusts to the medicine. Other common side effects are: cloudy urine; crawling or tingling sensation of the skin; **diarrhea**; faintness (particularly after missing meals); headache; increased skin color; irritability; **itching**; joint pain; loss of appetite (**anorexia**); **nausea and vomiting**; numbness or weakness in arms, hands, legs, or feet; stinging sensation on skin;

swelling on skin; tenderness of the palms and the soles; and becoming easily tired.

Less common side effects may include: extreme fatigue or weakness; increased sensitivity of eyes to light; changes in or loss of vision; watery eyes; swelling around eyes; ulcers or sores in mouth; as well as painful and tender glands in the neck, armpits, or groin.

Side effects that may occur rarely include:

- cold and clammy skin
- convulsions
- decreased blood pressure
- difficulty breathing
- fever and sore throat
- fever with or without chills
- increased heartbeat
- loss of consciousness
- pale skin
- pinpoint red spots on skin
- red, thickened, or scaly skin
- swelling and/or tenderness in upper abdominal or stomach area
- swollen and/or painful glands
- unusual bleeding or bruising
- unusual fatigue or weakness
- yellow discoloration of the eyes or skin

Some patients may experience other side effects not listed above. Patients experiencing any other side effects should check with the attending physician.

Interactions

Drug interaction information is not readily available for suramin. However, as with any treatment, patients should alert their doctor to any prescription, over-the-counter, or herbal remedies they are taking in order to avoid possible drug interactions.

Crystal Heather Kaczkowski, MSc.

Surgical oncology

Definition

Surgical oncology is a specialized area of oncology that engages surgeons in the cure and management of **cancer**.

Purpose

Cancer has become a medical specialty warranting its own surgical area because of advances in the biology, pathophysiology, diagnostics, and staging of malignant tumors. Surgeons have traditionally treated cancer patients with resection and radical surgeries of tumors, and left the management of the cancer and the patient to other specialists. Advances in the early diagnosis of cancer, the staging of tumors, microscopic analyses of cells, and increased understanding of **cancer biology** have broadened the range of nonsurgical cancer treatments. These treatments include systematic **chemotherapy**, hormonal therapy, and radiotherapy as alternatives or adjunctive therapy for patients with cancer.

Not all cancer tumors are manageable by surgery, nor does the removal of some tumors or metastases necessarily lead to a cure or longer life. The oncological surgeon looks for the relationship between tumor excision and the risk presented by the primary tumor. He or she is knowledgeable about patient management with more conservative procedures than the traditional excision or resection.

Demographics

According to the American Cancer Society and the National Cancer Institute, about 559,650 people were projected to die of cancer in the year 2007. 66% of those diagnosed with cancer within the year 2007 are expected to survive for at least five years after diagnosis. The most common newly diagnosed cancers for males in the United States during 2007, with total of over 766,860 cases for all races, were:

- prostate—29%;
- lung—15%;
- colon and rectum—10%;
- bladder—7%; and
- non-Hodgkin's lymphoma—4%.

The most common newly diagnosed cancers for females in the United States during 2007, with total of over 678,060 cases for all races, were:

- breast—26%;
- lung—15%;
- colon and rectum—11%;
- uterine corpus—6%; and
- non-Hodgkin's lymphoma—4%.

Description

Surgical oncology is guided by principles that govern the routine procedures related to the cancer

KEY TERMS

Biopsy—The surgical excision of tissue to diagnose the size, type, and extent of a cancerous growth.

Cancer surgery—Surgery in which the goal is to excise a tumor and its surrounding tissue found to be malignant.

Resection—Cutting out tissue to eliminate a cancerous tumor; usually refers to a section of the organ, (e.g., colon, intestine, lung, stomach) that must be cut to remove the tumor and its surrounding tissue.

Tumor staging—The method used by oncologists to determine the risk from a cancerous tumor. A number—ranging from 1A–4B— is assigned to predict the level of invasion by a tumor, and offer a prognosis for morbidity and mortality.

patient's cure, palliative care, and quality of life. Surgical oncology performs its most efficacious work by local tumor excision, regional lymph node removal, the handling of cancer recurrence (local or widespread), and in rare cases, with surgical resection of metastases from the primary tumor. Each of these areas plays a different role in cancer management.

Excision

Local excision has been the hallmark of surgical oncology. Excision refers to the removal of the cancer and its effects. Resection of a tumor in the colon can end the effects of obstruction, for instance, or removal of a breast **carcinoma** can stop the cancer. Resection of a primary tumor also stops the tumor from spreading throughout the body. The cancer's spread into other body systems, however, usually occurs before a local removal, giving resection little bearing upon cells that have already escaped the primary tumor. Advances in oncology through pathophysiology, staging, and **biopsy** offer a new diagnostic role to the surgeon using excision. These advances provide simple diagnostic information about size, grade, and extent of the tumor, as well as more sophisticated evaluations of the cancer's biochemical and hormonal features.

Regional lymph node removal

Lymph node involvement provides surgical oncologists with major diagnostic information. The sentinel node biopsy is superior to any biological test in terms of prediction of cancer mortality rates. Nodal biopsy offers very precise information about the extent and type of invasive effects of the primary tumor. The removal of nodes, however, may present pain and other morbid conditions for the patient.

Local and regional recurrence

Radical procedures in surgical oncology for local and regional occurrences of a primary tumor provide crucial information on the spread of cancer and prognostic outcomes; however, they do not contribute substantially to the outcome of the cancer. According to most surgical oncology literature, the ability to remove a local recurrence must be balanced by the patient's goals related to aesthetic and pain control concerns. Historically, more radical procedures have not improved the chances for survival.

Surgery for distant metastases

In general, a cancer tumor that spreads further from its **primary site** is less likely to be controlled by surgery. According to research, except for a few instances where **metastasis** is confined, surgical removal of a distant metastasis is not warranted. Since the rapidity of discovering a distant metastasis has little bearing upon cancer survival, the usefulness of surgery is not time dependent. In the case of liver metastasis, for example, a cure is related to the pathophysiology of the original cancer and level of cancer antigen in the liver rather than the size or time of discovery. While surgery of metastatic cancer may not increase life, there may be indications for it such as pain relief, obstruction removal, control of bleeding, and resolution of **infection**.

Diagnosis/Preparation

Surgery removes cancer cells and surrounding tissues. It is often combined with **radiation therapy** and chemotherapy. It is important for the patient to meet with the surgical oncologist to talk about the procedure and begin preparations for surgery. Oncological surgery may be performed to biopsy a suspicious site for malignant cells or tumor. It is also used for tumor removal from organs such as the tongue, throat, lung, stomach, intestines, colon, bladder, ovary, and prostate. Tumors of limbs, ligaments, and tendons may also be treated with surgery. In many cases, the biopsy and surgery to remove the cancer cells or tissues are done at the same time.

The impact of a surgical procedure depends upon the diagnosis and the area of the body that is to be treated by surgery. Many cancer surgeries involve major organs and require open abdominal surgery, which is the most extensive type of surgical procedure. This surgery requires medical tests and work-ups to judge the health of the patient prior to surgery, and to make decisions about adjunctive procedures like radiation or chemotherapy. Preparation for cancer surgery requires psychological readiness for a hospital stay, postoperative pain, sometimes slow recovery, and anticipation of complications from tumor excision or resection. It also may require consultation with stomal therapists if a section of the urinary tract or bowel is to be removed and replaced with an outside reservoir or conduit called an ostomy.

Aftercare

After surgery, the type and duration of side effects and the elements of recovery depend on where in the body the surgery was performed and the patient's general health. Some surgeries may alter basic functions in the urinary or gastrointestinal systems. Recovering full use of function takes time and patience. Surgeries that remove conduits such as the colon, intestines, or urinary tract require appliances for urine and fecal waste and the help of a stomal therapist. Breast or prostate surgeries yield concerns about cosmetic appearance and intimate activities. For most cancer surgeries, basic functions like tasting, eating, drinking, breathing, moving, urinating, defecating, or neurological ability may be changed in the short-term. Resources to attend to deficits in daily activities need to be set up before surgery.

Risks

The type of risks that cancer surgery presents depends almost entirely upon the part of the body being biopsied or excised. Risks of surgery can be great when major organs are involved, such as the gastrointestinal system or the brain. These risks are usually discussed explicitly when surgerical decisions are made.

Normal results

Most cancers are staged; that is, they are described by their likelihood of being contained, spreading at the original site, or recurring or invading other bodily systems. The prognosis after surgery depends upon the stage of the disease, and the pathology results on the type of cancer cell involved. General results of cancer surgery depend in large part on norms of success based upon the study of groups of patients with the same diagnosis. The results are often stated in percentages of the chance of cancer recurrence or its spread after surgery. After five disease-free years, patients are usually considered cured. This is because the recurrence rates decline drastically after five years. The benchmark is based upon the percentage of people known to reach the fifth year after surgery with no recurrence or spread of the primary tumor.

WHO PERFORMS THE PROCEDURE AND WHERE IS IT PERFORMED?

A surgeon who specializes in cancer surgery or oncology performs oncology surgery in a general hospital or cancer research center.

QUESTIONS TO ASK THE DOCTOR

Who is recommended for a second opinion?

What are the alternatives to surgery for this cancer?

What is the likelihood that this surgery will entirely eliminate the cancer?

Is this a surgical procedure that is often performed in this hospital or surgical center?

Morbidity and mortality rates

Morbidity and mortality of oncological surgery are high if there is organ involvement or extensive excision of major parts of the body. Because there is an ongoing disease process and many patients may be very ill at the time of surgery, the complications of surgery may be quite complex. Each procedure is understood by the surgeon for its likely complications or risks, and these are discussed during the initial surgical consultations.

There are comprehensive surgical procedures for many cancers, and complications may be extensive due to the use of general anesthetic and the opening of body cavities. Open surgery has general risks associated with it that are not related to the type of procedure. These risks include possibility of blood clots and cardiac events.

There is an extensive body of literature about the complication and morbidity rates of surgery performed by high-volume treatment centers. Data show that in general, large volumes of surgery affect the quality outcomes of surgery, with smaller hospitals having lower rates of procedural success and higher operative and postoperative complications than larger facilities. It is not known whether the surgeon's experience or the advantages of institutional resources in operative or postoperative care contributes to these statistics.

Alternatives

Alternatives to cancer surgery exist for almost every cancer treated in the United States. Research into alternatives has been very successful for some—but not all—cancers. There are many alternatives to surgery, and chemotherapy and radiation after surgery. Most organizations dealing with cancer patients suggest alternative treatments. Physicians and surgeons expect to be asked about alternatives to surgery, and are usually quite knowledgeable about their use as cancer treatments or as adjuncts to surgery.

Resources

BOOKS

Abeloff, M. D., J. Armitage, J. Niederhuber, M. Kastan, and W. G. McKenna. *Clinical Oncology,* 3rd ed. Philadelphia: Elsevier, 2004.

Cummings, C. W., et al.*Otolaryngology: Head and Neck Surgery,* 4th ed. St. Louis: Mosby, 2004.

Katz V. L., G. Lentz, R. A. Lobo, and D. Gershenson. *Comprehensive Gynecology,* 5th ed. St. Louis: Mosby, 2007.

Khatri, V. P., and J. A. Asensio. *Operative Surgery Manual,* 1st ed. Philadelphia: Saunders, 2002.

Townsend, C.M., R. D. Beauchamp, B. M. Evers, and K. Mattox. *Sabiston Textbook of Surgery,* 17th ed. Philadelphia: Saunders, 2004.

Wein, A. J., L. R. Kavoussi, A. C. Novick, A. W. Partin, and C. A. Peters. *Campbell-Walsh Urology,* 9th ed. Philadelphia: Saunders, 2006.

OTHER

Cancer Trends Progress Report—2007 Update. National Cancer Institute. December 2007. http://progressreport.cancer.gov/ (April 7, 2008).

ORGANIZATIONS

American Cancer Society, 1875 Connecticut Avenue, NW, Suite 730, Washington, DC, 20009, (800) ACS-2345, http://www.cancer.org.

National Breast Cancer Coalition, 1101 17th Street, NW, Suite 1300, Washington, DC, 20036, (800) 622-2838, (202) 265-6854, http://www.stopbreastcancer.org/.

Office of Cancer Complementary and Alternative Medicine, National Cancer Institute, 6116 Executive Boulevard, Suite 609, MSC 8339, Bethesda, MD, 20892, (800) 422-6237, http://www.cancer.gov/cam/.

Nancy McKenzie, Ph.D.
Rosalyn Carson-DeWitt, M.D.

Syndrome of inappropriate antidiuretic hormone

Description

The syndrome of inappropriate antidiuretic hormone production (SIADH) is a condition in which the body develops an excess of water and a decrease in sodium (salt) concentration, as a result of improper chemical signals. Patients with SIADH may become severely ill, or may have no symptoms at all.

A syndrome is a collection of symptoms and physical signs that together follow a pattern. SIADH is one of the **paraneoplastic syndromes**, in which a **cancer** leads to widespread ill effects due to more than just the direct presence of tumor.

Normal physiology

The body normally maintains very tight control over its total amount of water and its concentration of sodium. Many organs including the kidneys, heart, and the adrenal, thyroid, and pituitary glands participate in this regulation. One important contribution is the release of a chemical substance, or hormone, by the pituitary gland into the bloodstream. This chemical substance, called antidiuretic hormone (ADH), is also known as arginine vasopressin, or AVP.

The pituitary releases ADH into the bloodstream when receptors in various organs detect that the body has too little water or too high a concentration of salt. ADH then affects the way the kidneys control water and salt balance. ADH causes the kidneys to decrease their output of urine. The body thus saves water by undergoing antidiuresis, that is, not excreting urine.

Simultaneously, the concentration of sodium in the body serum decreases. This decrease results from a second effect of ADH on the kidneys. When the kidneys retain extra water, the existing concentration of sodium in the body decreases slightly as a result of dilution. These functions are all part of the body's extremely precise control over water and salt balance in health.

Abnormal physiology in SIADH

Certain disease states can upset the delicate balance of water and salt in the body. If there is too much ADH in the body, or if the kidneys overreact to the ADH they receive, the body retains excess water and the serum sodium concentration becomes diluted and falls to abnormal levels. The patient with SIADH develops symptoms based on the degree of abnormality in the serum sodium concentration and the speed with which this concentration falls.

Normal serum sodium concentration is 135-145 mEq/L (milliEquivalents of sodium per liter of body fluid). When the sodium concentration is 125–135 mEq/L the patient may have mild **nausea**, loss of appetite, **fatigue**, headache, or still remain free of symptoms. As the sodium level drops below 120 mEq/L, the patient experiences greater weakness, confusion, sleepiness, **vomiting**, and weight gain. As the sodium concentration approaches 110 mEq/L, the patient may suffer seizures, coma, and death.

Causes

SIADH has many known causes, some of which particularly relate to cancer or its treatment. These causes include specific types of cancer, drugs used to treat cancer itself, drugs used to treat the effects of cancer, and conditions that arise as a consequence of cancer or its treatment.

Specific types of cancer

SIADH results from numerous different types of cancer. The malignancies known to cause SIADH include:

- Lung cancer, small cell type
- Gastrointestinal cancers (pancreatic cancer, exocrine; duodenal or stomach cancer)
- Genitourinary cancer (bladder cancer, prostate cancer, ovarian cancer)
- Lymphoma, including Hodgkin's disease
- Head and neck cancers (oral cancers, laryngeal cancer, nasopharyngeal cancer)
- Thymoma
- Brain and central nervous system tumors
- Breast cancer
- Melanoma

Certain cancers produce and secrete ADH themselves. This production occurs without regard for the needs of the body. Thus, the kidneys receive repeated signals to save water, even when the body already has a marked excess of fluid. Of all the types of cancer that produce ADH themselves, small-cell lung cancer is by far the most common. Small-cell cancer of the lung is the cause in 75% of cases of SIADH caused directly by a tumor. In some cases, the appearance of SIADH may be the first indication that a cancer exists.

Also, primary or metastatic tumors in the brain may lead to SIADH. SIADH here results from an increase in intracranial pressure (pressure within the head), or from other effects of intracranial disease on the brain. Increased intracranial pressure commonly causes various parts of the brain to work improperly.

Drugs used to treat cancer itself

A variety of drugs used in cancer treatment may lead to SIADH. The mechanism of this effect may be that the drug causes the abnormal release of ADH, or that the drug makes existing ADH work in a stronger fashion than usual. **Chemotherapy** drugs that cause SIADH include:

- Vincristine, vinblastine, vinorelbine and other vinca alkaloids (Oncovin, Velban, Navelbine)
- Cyclophosphamide, ifosfamide, melphalan and other nitrogen mustards (Cytoxan, Ifex, Alkeran)
- Cisplatin (Platinol-AQ)
- Levamisole (Ergamisol)

Drugs used to treat the effects of cancer

SIADH may occur as a reaction to drugs used to treat effects of cancer such as pain, **depression**, or seizures. SIADH also may result from general anesthesia.

- Narcotic pain medications (morphine, Oramorph SR, fentanyl, Duragesic)
- Tricyclic antidepressants (amitriptyline, Elavil)
- Carbamazepine (Tegretol)
- General anesthetics

Conditions that arise as a consequence of cancer

SIADH may result from some of the debilitating consequences of cancer. For example, a person with cancer who is weak or unsteady will have a tendency to fall and hit the head. Skull fracture and other types of head injury may damage the brain or increase the intracranial pressure, and thus lead to SIADH.

Also, cancer patients who are weak, malnourished, receiving chemotherapy, or spending excessive time in bed have an increased risk of **pneumonia** and other infections. Infections including pneumonia, meningitis, and tuberculosis can cause SIADH.

Treatments

The treatment of SIADH involves relief of the urgent symptoms and correction of the underlying problem. For immediate improvement, all patients with SIADH require sharp restriction of their daily water intake. As little as two cups of liquid, about 500 ml, may be the daily limit for some patients. In cases where the sodium concentration is already dangerously low, doctors may cautiously give an intravenous infusion of fluid with a high concentration of sodium (hypertonic saline solution). However, this treatment carries some risk of damaging the brain. Physicians may also use a medicine such as furosemide (Lasix) that promotes water excretion (diuresis). Another drug, **demeclocycline**, blocks the action of ADH in the kidney.

The most definitive way to relieve SIADH is to address the underlying problem itself. Thus, if a tumor produces abnormal ADH, then surgery, **radiation therapy**, or chemotherapy may help by reducing tumor size. If SIADH results from use of a drug, then the patient must discontinue the medicine. Finally, doctors try to identify and treat any other correctable cause, such as an **infection**.

Prognosis

The prognosis of SIADH depends largely on its cause. Until recently, many physicians believed that the appearance of SIADH indicated a poor prognosis for cancer. However, more recent reports contradict this idea. The patient's ability to observe severe restriction of fluid intake may determine the degree of ongoing symptoms. SIADH usually improves after stopping a drug or curing an infection when that is the cause. When cancer is the direct cause of SIADH, one hopes for similar improvement of SIADH from treatments that reduce the amount of cancer in the body.

Resources

BOOKS

DeVita, Vincent T. Jr., Samuel Hellman, and Steven A. Rosenberg, editors. *Cancer: Principles and Practice of Oncology*. Philadelphia: Lippincott Williams & Wilkins, 2001.

Kenneth J. Berniker, M.D.

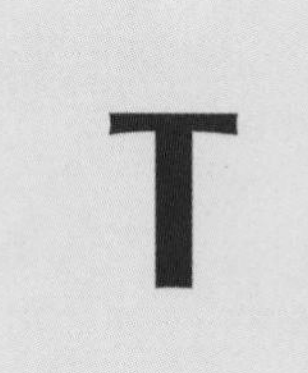

Tacrolimus

Definition

Tacrolimus belongs to a group of medicines known as immunosuppressive agents. It is used primarily to lower the body's natural immunity in order to prevent the rejection of organ transplants and to prevent graft-versus-host disease. Tacrolimus is also known as Prograf and FK506.

Purpose

Tacrolimus first saw use in transplant patients. By suppressing the activity of the immune system, tacrolimus makes it more likely that the recipient of a transplanted organ will accept that organ. It is especially used for kidney transplants.

In the fight against leukemia, grafts of stem cells from donors are sometimes given to the patient to encourage the blood of a recipient to begin production of normal cells. Tacrolimus may be given during the graft process because it seems to make the patient more receptive to the donated stem cells.

Description

Tacrolimus somehow suppresses, or prevents activity of, the cells in the lymphatic system, which are known as T cells. Under normal circumstances T cells mount an **immune response** to foreign materials in the body. However, during a transplant, T cells can cause the reaction that can lead to the rejection of a donor organ. The exact reason for the activity of tacrolimus is not understood.

Recommended dosage

Given by mouth, in a capsule, or by intravenous line, tacrolimus doses range from about 0.03 milligrams to 0.05 milligrams per kilogram (1 kilogram equals approximately 2.2 pounds) of body weight per day. Individuals with liver or kidney problems must be given a lower dose.

KEY TERMS

Intravenous line—A tube that is inserted directly into a vein to carry medicine directly to the blood stream bypassing the stomach and other digestive organs that might alter the medicine.

Lymphatic system—The system that collects and returns fluid in tissues to the blood vessels and produces defensive agents for fighting infection and invasion by foreign bodies.

Stem cell—Cell that gives rise to a lineage of cells. Particularly used to describe the most primitive cells in the bone marrow from which all the various types of blood cell are derived.

Precautions

Tacrolimus should be taken without food and long after a meal. If there is food in the stomach it will interfere with the way the drug makes its way into the body. Grapefruit juice can increase the activity of tacrolimus and should be avoided.

Side effects

Many serious side effects are associated with tacrolimus. Conditions affecting the brain brought on by the use of tacrolimus include coma (unconscious state) and delirium (uncontrolled and erratic conscious state). Most times the brain conditions are reversible. Headache, skin rashes, hair loss (**alopecia**), pain, sensitivity to light, and shock (anaphylaxis) are all side effects. Kidney damage, which cannot be reversed, is also a danger.

Use of tacrolimus greatly increases the likelihood a person will get **skin cancer** and **lymphoma**. Anyone using the drug should be monitored closely for changes in the skin, and all normal precautions for avoiding skin **cancer**, such as avoiding direct exposure to ultraviolet light, should be taken.

Interactions

This drug interacts with a long list of other drugs. It is important to tell the physician in charge of the care plan, each and every drug being taken, so that interactions can be avoided. Tacrolimus prevents effective vaccination, and vaccinations should not be given while the drug is in use.

Diane M. Calabrese

Tamoxifen

Definition

Tamoxifen (also known as Nolvadex) is a synthetic compound similar to estrogen. It mimics the action of estrogen on the bones and uterus, but blocks the effects of estrogen on breast tissue.

Purpose

Tamoxifen is used as adjuvant hormonal therapy immediately after surgery in early stages of **breast cancer** and in advanced metastatic breast **cancer** (stages III and above) in women and men. Adjuvant therapy is treatment added to curative procedures (such as surgery) to prevent the recurrence of cancer. Although tamoxifen is also used to treat malignant **melanoma**, **brain tumors**, and uterine cancer, these uses are not indicated on the product label. According to U.S. Food and Drug Administration (FDA) guidelines, women who are at high risk of developing breast cancer may take tamoxifen to reduce their risk; however, prolonged use may increase the risk of developing **endometrial cancer** (also called uterine cancer).

In 2003, researchers described the use of high-dose tamoxifen along with follicle-stimulating hormone (FSH) in stimulating ovary production for women who have had breast cancer who want to undergo in vitro fertilization. Standard in vitro therapies can increase estrogen and risk of breast cancer recurrence. The combination of tamoxifene and FSH may offer some breast cancer protection and hope for pregnancy.

KEY TERMS

Anticoagulant—An agent preventing the coagulation (clotting) of blood.

Apoptosis—A type of cell death where cells are induced to commit suicide.

Double-blind study—A study where neither the participant nor the physician know who has received the drug in question.

Oncogene—A gene whose presence can cause cancer; usually arising through mutation of a normal gene.

Thromboembolism—A blood clot that blocks a blood vessel in the cardiovascular system.

Description

First synthesized in 1966 in Great Britain as an antifertility drug, tamoxifen was evaluated to treat cancer in 1970. In 1998, the FDA approved tamoxifen to reduce the risk of breast cancer. While tamoxifen can be given to patients alone, it is often given in combination with other chemotherapeutic drugs such as 5-fluorouracil (5-FU, or **fluorouracil**).

Tamoxifen belongs to a family of compounds called **antiestrogens**. Antiestrogens are used in cancer therapy to inhibit the effects of estrogen on target tissues. Estrogen is a steroid hormone secreted by the female ovary. Depending on the target tissue, estrogen can stimulate the growth of female reproductive organs and breast tissue, play a role in the female menstrual cycle, and protect against bone loss by binding to estrogen receptors on the outside of cells within the target tissue. Antiestrogens act selectively against the effects of estrogen on target cells in a variety of ways, thus they are called selective estrogen receptor modulators (SERMs).

Tamoxifen selectively inhibits the effects of estrogen on breast tissue, while selectively mimicking the effects of estrogen on bone (by increasing bone mineral density) and uterine tissues. These qualities make tamoxifen an excellent therapeutic agent against breast cancer. Although researchers are unclear about precisely how tamoxifen kills breast cancer cells, it is known to compete with estrogen by binding to estrogen receptors on the membrane of target cells. This limits the effects of estrogen on breast tissue. Tamoxifen also may be involved in other anti-tumor activities affecting oncogene expression, promotion of apoptosis (cancer cell death), and growth factor secretion. (Growth factors are hormones that influence cell division and proliferation, and these hormones can encourage cancers to grow.)

In 2000, the STAR (Study of Tamoxifen and **Raloxifene**) study began. The purpose of this double-blind study was to evaluate the use of tamoxifen and raloxifene (another type of SERM) over a five-year period in 19,747 postmenopausal women 35 years or older and at high risk for developing breast cancer. The study found both drugs to be equally effective in reducing the risk for breast cancer in high-risk, postmenopausal women.

Another National Cancer Institute study that is relevant to the discussion of tamoxifen is the Breast **Cancer Prevention** Trial. This trial began in 1992 and was designed to see if tamoxifen was effective as a preventive against breast cancer. The study also was a double-blind study, and participants were receiving either tamoxifen or a placebo (an inactive pill that looks like tamoxifen). About four years into the study, in 1998, researchers reported that the women receiving tamoxifen:

- had 49% fewer diagnoses of invasive breast cancer
- had 50% fewer diagnoses of noninvasive breast cancer (such as ductal carcinoma in situ)
- had fewer fractures of the hip, wrist, and spine
- had more than twice the chance of developing endometrial cancer
- had increased chance of developing blood clots, both in the lung and in major veins when compared to the women receiving the placebo

Because of these findings, in 1998, the FDA approved the use of tamoxifen as a breast cancer preventive for high-risk women, as mentioned above. A final report released in 2005 supported the 1998 findings.

Recommended dosage

Tamoxifen is taken orally and is available in 10- and 20-milligram (mg) tablets. Although it can be given within the range of 10 mg to 80 mg, the typical dosage is 20 to 40 mg daily for both adult females and males using tamoxifen for treatment of advanced breast cancer. At this dosage, there is an observed 30% response rate with complete remission in 10% of patients. It appears that patients 60 years and older have higher response rates. For patients using tamoxifen for adjuvant therapy after surgery, the typical dosage is 20 mg once daily for two to five years following surgery. Women at high risk for developing breast cancer usually take 20 mg daily for five years. If a dosage is missed, patients should not double the next dosage. Instead, they should go back to their regular schedule and contact their doctor.

Tamoxifen doesn't work for everyone. In 2003, scientists announced development of a new test that may predict whether patients' tumors are responding to tamoxifen treatment and warn clinicians if the tumor becomes resistant to the drugs.

Precautions

Tamoxifen is not recommended for use in children. Women who are pregnant or nursing should not use this drug since it has several side effects that, although rare, can be severe. It is known to cause miscarriages and birth defects. Women are encouraged to use birth control while taking tamoxifen. However, oral contraceptives can negatively alter the effects of tamoxifen. Therefore, patients should explore other, nonhormonal birth control options.

Great care should be exercised when tamoxifen is used with **warfarin**, an anticoagulant, because tamoxifen can interfere with the effects of warfarin, and dose adjustments may be necessary. Patients who are predisposed to the formation of thromboembolisms, or blood clots, should use tamoxifen with caution. It should be noted that smokers are at a higher risk for thromboembolism than nonsmokers.

In late 2003, cancer experts were beginning to recommend a new group of drugs called **aromatase inhibitors** (Arimidex, common name anastrozole or Femara and Novartis, common name letrozole) as an alternative to tamoxifen or following tamoxifen therapy. These drugs fight breast cancer differently, but early research shows they fight it as effectively and with fewer side effects. However, these drugs also may be added after a course of tamoxifen to improve overall treatment results.

Side effects

Although tamoxifen is usually well tolerated by patients, there are some side effects. About 25% of patients experience side effects such as mild **nausea**, **vomiting**, hot flashes, weight gain, **bone pain**, and hair thinning. These side effects are usually not severe enough to stop therapy. Patients using tamoxifen for long periods of adjuvant therapy may face unwanted effects years into therapy, which warrant discontinued use of the drug. Some of these effects include possible increased risk of developing liver **adenoma** as well as increased risk of uterine (endometrial) cancer; eye problems such as retinal lesions, macular edema, and corneal changes (most resolve after use is discontinued); neurological problems such as **depression**, dizziness, confusion, and **fatigue**; and genital problems such as vaginal bleeding, vaginal discharge, and endometriosis.

Interactions

Tamoxifen can interfere with the anticoagulant drug warfarin, and if these two drugs are used together, patients will need to be monitored very closely. Oral contraceptives can also interfere with the action of tamoxifen. In 2003, researchers discovered that paroxetine, an antidepressant used to ease hot flashes that accompany treatment with tamoxifene, was interfering with tamoxifene's effectiveness.

See also Alopecia; Nausea and vomiting; Toremifene.

Resources

PERIODICALS

"Breast Cancer Guidelines Suggest Alternative to Standard Therapy." *Drug Topics* August 18, 2003: 22.

"Drug that Eases Tamoxifen Side Effect May also Hinder its Effectiveness." *Drug Week* December 26, 2003: 54.

Johnson, Kate. "High-dose Tamoxifen for IVF in Breast Cancer Survivors: Combine with FSH." *OB GYN News* December 15, 2003: 8–11.

MacReady, Nora. "Post-tamoxifen Letrozole May Cut Breast Ca Risk: More than 5,000 Women Studied." *Internal Medicine News* November 15, 2003: 18–19.

"New Test Could Predict Response to Tamoxifen and Anastrozole." *Drug Week* November 28, 2003: 64.

Sally C. McFarlane-Parrott
Teresa G. Odle

Taste alteration

Description

Taste alteration refers to a decrease in the ability to taste foods (hypogeusia), changes in how food tastes (dysgeusia), or the complete loss of the ability to taste foods (ageusia). It also refers to the presence of a metallic or medicine-like taste in the mouth. Taste alterations may occur as a result of **cancer** treatment, **infection** within the mouth, or the cancer itself.

Taste alteration can have a significant effect on the nutritional status of a cancer patient. Patients with taste alteration may avoid certain foods, lose their appetite (**anorexia**), and lose weight. Eating can be a chore when the patient also has a dry mouth (**xerostomia**) or a mouth infection, such as **thrush**.

Causes

Humans have the ability to taste bitter, salty, sour, and sweet flavors with the taste buds. Taste buds are on the tongue, back portion of the roof of the mouth (soft palate), and the back of the throat. The taste buds are composed of taste cells. Taste cells have tiny hairs (microvilli) the take up microscopic particles of food in the mouth. Taste alteration occurs when the taste buds are damaged by cancer therapy or as a symptom of xerostomia or infection.

Taste alteration may be caused by the cancer itself. Invasion of the mouth by the tumor can alter taste. Between 88% and 93% of the patients with head and neck tumors have taste alterations. Cancer can cause the patient to become deficient in nutrients such as copper, niacin, nickel, vitamin A, and zinc, which can lead to taste alterations. In addition, it is believed that cancer-related chemicals in the bloodstream may affect taste.

Taste alteration can occur in patients who are receiving **radiation therapy** to the head, neck, or chest. The taste buds are very sensitive to radiation and taste alteration can occur within the first two weeks of radiation therapy. Also, radiation therapy can cause decreases in the production of saliva, which can alter taste. Reduced amounts of saliva can change the taste of salty and bitter foods.

Patients undergoing **chemotherapy** may experience taste alterations. Chemotherapy drugs damage the taste cells. The resulting alterations in taste are varied but the most common complaints include: a metallic taste, enhanced taste of bitter flavors (such as beef, pork, coffee, chocolate), and reduced taste of sweet flavors. Between 36% and 71% of the patients undergoing chemotherapy experience taste changes. **Antibiotics**, pain relievers (analgesics), antidepressants, and many other drugs can also affect taste. Chemotherapy drugs that are frequently associated with taste changes include:

- carboplatin
- cisplatin
- cyclophosphamide
- dacarbazine
- doxorubicin
- 5-fluorouracil (5-FU, or fluorouracil)
- levamisole
- methotrexate
- nitrogen mustard
- vincristine

Surgery to the head or neck can also cause taste alteration. Metallic or medicine-like tastes can be caused by a zinc deficiency or by increased levels of calcium or lactate.

Taste alteration is usually a temporary condition, although it may take a few months for taste to return to normal. However, surgery of the roof of the mouth (hard palate), tongue, or throat or high-dose radiation therapy can cause permanent taste alteration.

Treatments

There is no cure or treatment for taste alteration. Patients with this condition are counseled on methods to overcome the affect of taste alteration on eating. However, some studies have shown that zinc supplements, given at the first sign of taste alteration, can reduce radiation-induced taste changes.

The patient's teeth should be brushed and flossed before eating to remove old tastes and refresh the mouth. Rinsing the mouth with salted water, water containing baking soda, tea, or ginger ale before eating may be helpful. Brushing and flossing should be performed carefully to prevent damage to the weakened mouth tissues.

There are a variety of measures that can be taken to make food more tasteful and less offensive. Dietary recommendations include:

- eating foods that are cool or at room temperature
- adding tart flavors to foods such as lemon, citrus, and vinegar, unless mouth sores are present
- using mints, gum, or lemon drops to remove bad tastes after eating
- adding more sugar to foods to reduce salty, acid, or bitter tastes
- using barbecue sauce, basil, catsup, chili powder, garlic, mint, mustard, onion, oregano, rosemary, or tarragon to add flavor to foods
- eating frozen fruits such as grapes, melons, or oranges
- eating fresh vegetables, which may taste better than frozen or canned ones

Alternative and complementary therapies

Taste alteration related to a zinc deficiency can be treated by the addition of zinc to the diet. Zinc deficiency can be relieved by taking zinc picolinate supplements. Foods that are rich sources of zinc include oysters, crab, beef, pork, eggs, nuts, yogurt, and whole grains.

See also Sjögren's syndrome.

Belinda Rowland, Ph.D.

Temozolomide

Definition

A **chemotherapy** medicine used to reduce the size of a cancerous tumor and prevent the growth of new **cancer** cells. In the United States, temozolomide is known by the brand name Temodar and in the European Union as Temodal.

Purpose

Temozolomide is used as a treatment for a type of brain tumor called an anaplastic **astrocytoma**. Specifically, it is a treatment for patients who have experienced a relapse (or recurrence) of this disease while being treated with the drug **procarbazine**, one of a group of **anticancer drugs** known as nitrosoureas, which include **carmustine** and **lomustine**. As of the early 2000, it is being investigated as a treatment of newly diagnosed and advanced stages of other brain/central nervous system tumors, such as oligodendrogliomas and ependymomas, and for an advanced malignant **melanoma** that has spread to the central nervous system.

Description

Temozolomide was first made in a British laboratory in the early 1980s and was approved for use in the United States in 1999.

It is included in the cancer drug category termed **antineoplastic agents**. These drugs slow or prevent the growth of cancerous tumors. Temozolomide is among a subset of antineoplastic agents that were designed to target rapidly dividing cells in the body, such as the cancerous cells that form tumors. These drugs work by altering the structure of the DNA in fast-growing cells, causing a cell to die or to fail to replicate itself.

The use of temozolomide as a treatment for cancers other than brain cancer and in combination with different cancer therapies is still experimental. Many ongoing **clinical trials** focus on the use of temozolomide as a cancer treatment not only for newly diagnosed and recurrent brain/central nervous system tumors, but also for advanced stages of **germ cell tumors**, lung cancer (non-small cell), **mycosis fungoides**, **Sézary syndrome**, and **gastrointestinal cancers**. Some clinical trials also involve experimental treatment of advanced brain cancer or malignant melanomas using a combination of temozolomide and other cancer drugs or therapies, such as **radiation therapy** and the drugs interleukin-12, **aldesleukin**, **thalidomide**, carmustine, **interferons**, and lomustine.

KEY TERMS

Anaplasia—Characteristics of a cell, such as shape and orientation, that make it identifiable as a cancer cell.

Anaplastic astrocytoma—The advanced stage of a rapidly growing brain tumor. This type of tumor originates in the brain, unlike other brain tumors that may occur due to the spreading of cancer from another part of the body.

DNA (Deoxyribonucleic acid)—The genetic material found in each cell in the body that plays an important role in controlling many cell functions. When a cell divides to create two new cells, an identical copy of its DNA is found in each. If there is an error in a cell's DNA, division may not occur.

Drug clearance—The amount of a drug that is removed from the body through urination.

It is not yet known if temozolomide is more effective than other treatments, but it has been shown to stop or slow disease progression in patients with recurrent **brain tumors** who have not responded to other treatments, including other chemotherapy drugs, radiation therapy, or surgery. However, the duration of the response varies.

For the treatment of a malignant melanoma, temozolomide is as equally effective as **dacarbazine**, the drug most frequently used for this cancer. If the cancer spreads to the central nervous system, temozolomide may be more effective than dacarbazine, because it, unlike dacarbazine, is able to move from the blood into the central nervous system.

A possible advantage to the use of temozolomide over other therapy options is that a patient may be able to continue the treatment over a longer period of time. Decreased bone marrow activity (**myelosuppression**) is a common reaction to many chemotherapy drugs, including temozolomide. But unlike other drugs, this condition is temporary in temozolomide patients; therefore, patients can physically tolerate a more extended treatment. Also, the side effects experienced with temozolomide are usually less severe compared to other drug treatment options, resulting in patients with a better quality of life.

Recommended dosage

Temozolomide is available in capsules and is taken orally. Dosage is determined based on a patient's body height and weight. The typical dose for the first treatment cycle is 150 mg per day taken for five consecutive days, with each treatment cycle lasting 28 days. The number of treatment cycles depends on how well a patient tolerates the treatment and its effectiveness in treating the cancer. The optimal number of treatment cycles is not known.

Because myelosuppression is a common reaction to this drug treatment, white blood cell and platelet counts are carefully monitored, particularly in the first few treatment cycles. A complete blood count is made on day 22 and day 29 of a treatment cycle. If blood counts are below a certain level, treatment is either postponed or the dosage is decreased in the next treatment cycle. The minimum recommended dosage is 100 mg. Blood counts within an acceptable range can result in an increased dosage for the next cycle.

Precautions

Food decreases the rate at which temozolomide is absorbed into the bloodstream. Although there are no foods that should be avoided while taking this drug, it should be taken on an empty stomach and swallowed whole with a glass of water.

Side effects

The most common side effects for patients treated with temozolomide are **nausea and vomiting**, headache, **fatigue**, and constipation. In a study of 158 brain tumor patients, 53% experienced **nausea** and 42% experienced **vomiting**, and most of these cases were moderate, with only about 10% of the patients experiencing severe forms of either condition. Avoiding food prior to taking temozolomide can decrease the occurrence of these effects, or they can be controlled with medication. In the same study, 41% of the patients reported headaches, 34% reported feeling fatigued, and 33% experienced constipation.

Between 10% and 20% of the patients in the study experienced convulsions, partial paralysis, **diarrhea**, **fever**, feeling weak, a **infection**, dizziness, coordination problems, a **memory change**, or insomnia. Less than 10% of the 158 patients experienced **anorexia**, rash or **itching**, inflammation in the throat region, **incontinence**, back pain, an overactive adrenal gland, anxiety, comprehension problems, coughing, muscle pain, weight gain, **depression**, sinus problems, or abnormal vision.

Myelosuppression is experienced by 4% to 19% of patients. **Neutropenia** and **thrombocytopenia** are the most common forms, and the more severe cases of both are higher in women and in the elderly (patients older than age 70) than in men. When myelosuppression occurs, it usually appears late in the first few treatment cycles and does not worsen over time. On average, blood count levels return to normal 14 days after the lowest blood count is recorded.

Coping with side effects may require making some lifestyle changes or, in some cases, taking medication. For example, to treat constipation, patients may be told to increase the amount of fluid they drink, perform regular exercise, and eat more dietary fiber, while any infection will require medication. Treatment options for side effects should be discussed with a doctor.

Interactions

Valproic acid, a drug used to treat seizures, decreases the clearance of temozolomide from the body by about 5%. No other negative drug interaction has been reported, although its interaction with many conventional and alternative drugs has yet to be studied.

See also Cancer genetics; Chemoprevention; DNA cytometry; Drug resistance; Vaccines.

Monica McGee, M.S.

KEY TERMS

Angiogenesis—Physiological process involving the growth of new blood vessels from pre-existing blood vessels; used by some cancers to create their own blood supply.

Cytochrome P450— Enzymes present in the liver that metabolize drugs.

Hemolytic anemia—Type of anemia involving destruction of red blood cells.

Humanized monoclonal antibody—Human-like antibodies usually genetically engineered in mice and used in a therapeutic manner.

Metastasize—The process by which cancer spreads from its original site to other parts of the body.

Renal cell carcinoma—Cancer of the kidney that originates in the very small tubes in the kidney that filter the blood and remove waste products.

Thrombophlebitis—Vein inflammation related to a blood clot.

Triglycerides—Blood component measured with cholesterol to make up the lipid profile, which helps determine the likelihood of an individual to develop heart disease.

VEGF—Vascular endothelial growth factor, chemical compound in the body that contributes to the growth of new blood vessels.

Temsirolimus

Definition

Temsirolimus is an anti-cancer drug designed to inhibit the synthesis of proteins that regulate proliferation, growth, and survival of tumor cells.

Purpose

Temsirolimus is used to treat renal cell **carcinoma**, a type of **kidney cancer**. Renal cell carcinoma originates in the very small tubes in the kidney that filter the blood and remove waste products.

Description

Temsirolimus was developed for the treatment of renal cell carcinoma by Wyeth Pharmaceuticals and approved for use by the U.S. Food and Drug Administration (FDA) in 2007. It is a derivative of the anti-cancer drug **sirolimus**. Temsirolimus is sold under the brand name Torisel. It is designed to inhibit an enzyme called mTOR in tumor cells that regulate their proliferation, growth, and survival. The enzyme mTOR is activated in the tumor cells of renal cell carcinoma. Activation of this enzyme leads to a series of chemical events called a signaling cascade. Renal cell carcinoma mTOR signaling causes an increase in two cellular signaling molecules called hypoxia-inducible factor 1a (HIF-1a) and vascular endothelial growth factor (VEGF). Both HIF-1a and VEGF are needed for tumor growth and survival. Hypoxia-inducible factor 1a affects cellular processes for tumor growth and survival and increases the amount of VEGF. Vascular endothelial growth factor is responsible for the formation of tumor blood vessels in the process of angiogenesis. Angiogenesis is the process of a tumor growing a new blood vessel system for tumor use. Once a solid tumor reaches a certain size, it needs blood vessels in order for its cells to remain alive, and to continue to grow. Blood vessels that grow in tumors also contribute to its **metastasis** to other parts of the body.

By inhibiting mTOR, temsirolimus inhibits tumor cell replication and growth, as well as inhibiting the process of angiogenesis. Studies done on renal cell carcinoma have shown that use of temsirolimus increases median survival time and progression-free survival compared to placebo or other agents tested. Median survival time is a term used to describe the time from either diagnosis or treatment at which half of the patients with a given disease are expected to still be alive. The term progression-free survival describes the length of time during and after treatment in which a patient is living with a disease that does not get worse. In a clinical trial designed to test out a **cancer** drug in humans, both median survival time and progression-free survival are ways to measure how effective a treatment is.

QUESTIONS TO ASK YOUR DOCTOR OR PHARMACIST

- How long will I need to take this drug before you can tell if it helps for me?
- Is this drug safe to take with the other drugs that I am currently taking?
- What side effects should I watch for? When should I call the doctor about them?
- Are there any clinical trials of this drug combined with other therapies that might benefit me?

Recommended dosage

Temsirolimus is administered intravenously over 30 to 60 minute intervals. For adults with renal cell carcinoma, it is given at a dose of 25 mg once weekly. Therapy with temsirolimus is continued as long as clinical benefit to the patient is seen or until unacceptable levels of toxicity occur. The goal of temsirolimus administration is to use the dose that will be effective in the treatment of cancer while still avoiding toxicity. Once toxicity occurs either treatment is discontinued or the dose is adjusted. A dose of 20 mg per week may be attempted instead. In patients with diabetes, doses of anti-diabetes medication may need to be increased as temsirolimus may increase blood sugar levels. To minimize risk of hypersensitivity reactions, patients are intravenously pre-medicated with the antihistamine drug diphenhydramine hydrochloride at a dose of 25 to 50 mg about 30 minutes before beginning a temsirolimus infusion.

Precautions

Temsirolimus is a category D pregnancy drug. Category D pregnancy drugs are drugs in which there is evidence of risk to a human fetus based on clinical studies done in humans or marketing experience but that may be used during pregnancy if potential benefits to the patient are determined to outweigh potential risks to the fetus. Temsirolimus is contraindicated for use during pregnancy unless medically necessary, and may cause serious harm to a fetus. Birth control must be started prior to beginning treatment with temsirolimus and continued for at least 12 weeks after treatment. Both women and men receiving temsirolimus therapy need to use at least two reliable forms of contraception for this time period. Studies have shown fetal harm in animals. Temsirolimus should not be used during breast feeding. Temsirolimus has not been approved for use in individuals less than 18 years of age.

Patients should not have any vaccinations while taking temsirolimus without the consent of their treating physician. Patients taking temsirolimus should avoid being around people who have recently had the oral polio vaccine or the inhaled form of the flu vaccine, as these are live **vaccines**. If a physician determines that a patient taking temsirolimus requires a non-live vaccine during therapy, it should be administered during a treatment free period in the **chemotherapy** cycle of at least 14 days.

Treatment with temsirolimus increases risk for gastrointestinal perforations in susceptible individuals. There is also a possible increase in risk of adverse or toxic side effects in patients with history of stroke, diabetes mellitus, liver disease, high blood lipid levels, brain metastases, lung disease, kidney disease and those undergoing surgery. Fatal lung disease, bowel perforations, and kidney failure have occurred in treatment with temsirolimus.

Side Effects

Temsirolimus is used when the medical benefit is judged to be greater than the risk of side effects. Potential side effects include abdominal pain and cramping, loss of appetite, **nausea**, **vomiting**, **anemia**, joint pain, muscle pain, back pain, chest pain, chills, **fever**, flushed skin, **diarrhea**, constipation, altered taste perception, headache, high blood sugar, difficulty breathing, **fatigue**, weakness, acne, high blood pressure, nose bleeds, increased blood lipids and triglycerides, insomnia, mouth and throat sores, inflamed throat, itchy skin, rash, **weight loss**, **depression**, impaired wound healing, compromised immune system, thrombophlebitis, and abnormal liver function tests. Temsirolimus also causes an increased risk of infections including urinary tract infections, **pneumonia**, and other upper respiratory tract infections.

Interactions

Patients should make their doctor aware of any and all medications or supplements they are taking before using temsirolimus. Temsirolimus interacts with many other drugs. Some drug interactions may make temsirolimus unsuitable for use, while others may be monitored and attempted. Medications such as ACE inhibitors have shown negative effects when used with temsirolimus. Use of anticoagulants with temsirolimus has resulted in bleeding reactions in the brain. Temsirolimus causes toxicity when used with another cancer drug called sirolimus. Oral contraceptive pills may cause toxic levels of temsirolimus during treatment. Use of the herb Echinacea may decrease the efficacy of temsirolimus if taken in the same time period.

Temsirolimus is metabolized by a set of liver enzymes known as CYP-450 subtype 3A4. Drugs that induce, or activate, these enzymes increase the metabolism of temsirolimus. This results in lower levels of therapeutic temsirolimus, thereby negatively affecting treatment of cancer. For this reason drugs that induce CYP-450 subtype 3A4 may not be used with temsirolimus. This includes some anti-epileptic drugs such as **carbamazepine**, some anti-inflammatory drugs such as **dexamethasone**, anti-tuberculosis drugs such as rifampin, and the herb St. John's Wort.

Drugs that act to inhibit the action of CYP-450 subtype 3A4 may cause undesired increased levels of temsirolimus in the body. This could lead to toxic doses and be very dangerous. Some examples are **antibiotics** such as clarithromycin or erythromycin, antifungal drugs such as ketoconazole, antiviral drugs such as indinavir, antidepressants such as fluoxetine, and some cardiac agents such as amiodarone or verapamil. Grapefruit juice may also increase the amount of temsirolimus in the body. Eating grapefruit or drinking grapefruit juice is not advised while taking temsirolimus. If drugs that induce or inhibit CYP450 3A4 are medically necessary during treatment with temsirolimus, the dose of temsirolimus given may need to be adjusted.

Resources

BOOKS

Brunton, Laurence L., et al. *Goodman and Gilman's The Pharmacological Basis of Therapeutics, Eleventh Edition* McGraw Hill Medical Publishing Division, 2006.

Hamilton, Richard J., editor. *Tarascon Pharmacopoeia Library Edition*Jones and Bartlett Publishers, 2009.

OTHER

Medscape. *Temsirolimus.* http://www.medscape.com.

RxList. *Temsirolimus.* http://www.rxlist.com.

ORGANIZATIONS

National Cancer Institute. 6116 Executive Boulevard, Room 3036A, Bethesda, MD 20892-8322. (800)4-CANCER. http://www.cancer.gov.

U.S. Food and Drug Administration. 10903 New Hampshire Ave, Silver Spring, MD 20993. (888)INFO-FDA. http://www.fda.gov.

Maria Basile, Ph.D.

Teniposide

Definition

Teniposide is a **chemotherapy** medicine used to treat **cancer** by destroying cancerous cells. Teniposide is also known as the brand name Vumon and may also be referred to as VM-26.

Purpose

Teniposide is approved by the Food and Drug Administration (FDA) as induction therapy (an initial, intensive course of chemotherapy) for refractory childhood acute lymphoblastic leukemia. Teniposide is used in combination with other chemotherapy drugs. It has also been used in some adult leukemias and lung cancers.

Description

Teniposide is a clear liquid for infusion into a vein. Teniposide is a semisynthetic derivative of podophyllotoxin found in extracts of the mandrake plant. It is a member of the group of chemotherapy drugs known as topoisomerase II inhibitors. Topoisomerase II is one of the enzymes involved in rearrangement of DNA structures, such as temporarily breaking DNA strands and resealing them. This process is necessary for cell replication, and topoisomerase II inhibitors interfere with this important process as it prevents the cells from further dividing and multiplying and the cells subsequently die.

Recommended dosage

A teniposide dose can be determined using a mathematical calculation that measures a person's body surface area (BSA). This number is dependent upon a patient's height and weight. The larger the

KEY TERMS

Anemia—Red blood cell count that is lower than normal.

Chemotherapy—Specific drugs used to treat cancer.

DNA—Deoxyribonucleic acid, the genetic material inside cells that allows cells to function, separate, into two cells, and make more cells.

Food and Drug Administration—A government agency that oversees public safety in relation to drugs and medical devices. The FDA gives the approval to pharmaceutical companies for commercial marketing of their products.

Induction therapy—Initial intensive course of chemotherapy designed to wipe out abnormal cells and allow regrowth of normal cells.

Intravenous—Administered into the body through a vein.

Neutropenia—White blood cell count that is lower than normal.

Refractory cancer—Cancer that is not responding to treatment.

person the greater the body surface area. Body surface area is measured in the units known as square meter (m^2). The body surface area is calculated and then multiplied by the drug dosage in milligrams per square meter (mg/m^2). This calculates the actual dose a patient is to receive.

To treat refractory childhood leukemia

Teniposide is dosed at 165 mg per square meter as an infusion into a vein over 30-60 minutes and is given with the chemotherapy drug **cytarabine** at a dose of 300 mg per square meter. This combination is given twice a week for eight to nine doses.

Other leukemia dosing includes teniposide 100 mg per square meter once or twice weekly, and teniposide 250 mg per square meter with the chemotherapy drug **vincristine** 1.5 mg per square meter given into a vein each week for four to eight weeks.

Patients with significant kidney and liver problems may need to receive a smaller dose of teniposide than patients with normal kidney and liver function.

Patiets with Down syndrome should receive a smaller dose with the initial treatment.

Precautions

Blood counts will be monitored regularly while on teniposide therapy. During a certain time period after receiving this drug, there is an increased risk of getting infections. Caution should be taken to avoid unnecessary exposure to germs. Patients with a known previous allergic reaction to chemotherapy drugs should tell their doctor before treatment. Patients who may be pregnant or trying to become pregnant should tell their doctor before receiving teniposide. Chemotherapy can cause men and women to be sterile (unable to have children). Patients should check with their doctors before receiving live virus **vaccines** while on chemotherapy.

Side effects

The most common side effect of teniposide is low blood counts, referred to as **myelosuppression**. When the white blood cell count is lower than normal, known as **neutropenia**, patients are at an increased risk of developing a **fever** and infections. Teniposide also causes the platelet count to fall. Platelets are blood cells in the body that allow for the formation of clots. When the platelet count is low patients are at an increased risk for bruising and bleeding. If the platelet count remains too low, a platelet blood transfusion is an option. Low red blood cell counts, referred to as **anemia**, may make patients feel tired, dizzy, and lacking energy. A drug known as **erythropoietin** may be given to increase a patient's red blood cell count.

Teniposide infusions given too quickly into the vein can cause a significant drop in blood pressure. This can usually be avoided by administering the drug over a time period of at least 30-60 minutes. Teniposide can also cause mild to moderate **nausea and vomiting**. Patients will be given medicines known as **antiemetics** before receiving teniposide to help prevent or decrease this side effect. **Diarrhea**, loss of appetite (**anorexia**), and mouth sores and inflammation are also common. Rarely, allergic or anaphylactic-type reactions that include fever, sweating, tongue swelling, chest tightness, **itching**, shortness of breath, low blood pressure, and increased heart rate have occurred.

Other less common side effects caused by teniposide include rash, itching, hair loss (**alopecia**), liver and kidney problems, **fatigue**, seizures, tingling, fever, development of another type of cancer or leukemia due to taking the drug, and redness and pain at the site of injection into the vein. All side effects a patient experiences should be reported to their doctor.

Interactions

There is an increase risk of worsening some of the side effects of teniposide when it is administered with the medicines sodium salicylate, tolbutamide (a drug to lower blood sugar levels), or sulfamethizole (an antibiotic).

Nancy J. Beaulieu, R.Ph., B.C.O.P.

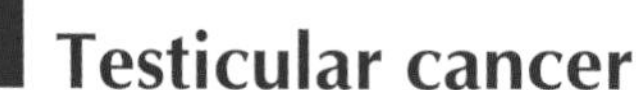

Testicular cancer

Definition

Testicular **cancer** is a disease in which cancer cells are discovered in one or both testicles. The testicles, also known as testes or gonads, are located in a pouch beneath the penis called the scrotum.

Demographics

The American Cancer Society estimates that approximately 8,400 new cases of testicular cancer will be diagnosed in American men in 2009. In addition, about 380 men will die of the disease in 2009. There is a 1 in 300 probability of developing testicular cancer. The disease is highly curable and the risk of dying from testicular cancer is very low. Only 1 in every 5,000 men diagnosed with testicular cancer die from their cancer. Although the incidence of testicular cancer is rising, having doubled since the 1970s, it is still rare. Scandinavian countries have the highest rate in the world. Germany and New Zealand also have high rates. The lowest incidences of testicular cancer are in Asia and Africa.

Description

The testicles make up one portion of the male reproductive system. Normally, they are each somewhat smaller than a golf ball in size and are contained within the scrotum. The testicles are a man's primary source of male hormones, particularly **testosterone**. They also produce sperm.

There are several types of cells contained in the testicles, and any of these may develop into one or more types of cancer. Over 95% of all testicular cancers begin in cells called germ cells. There are two main types of **germ cell tumors** in men: seminomas and nonseminomas. Seminomas make up about 40% of all testicular germ cell tumors. Nonseminomas make up a group of cancers, which include choriocarcinoma, yolk sac tumors, embryonal **carcinoma**, and teratoma. Clinically, nonseminomatous tumors are the more aggressive tumor type.

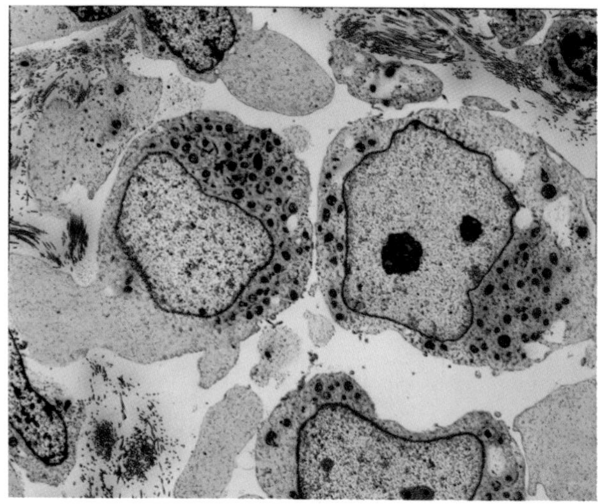

Colored transmission electron micrograph (TEM) of a section through teratoma cancer cells in a testis. Three rapidly dividing cells are seen at center left, center right, and lower right. They have large, irregular nuclei (pale brown) and green cytoplasm. *(Copyright Quest, Science Source/Photo Researchers, Inc. Reproduced by permission.)*

Although testicular cancer accounts for less than 2% of all cancers in men, it is the most commonly seen cancer in young men aged 15 to 35. It is also one of the most curable.

Risk factors

There is research showing that some men are more likely to develop testicular cancer than others. The risk

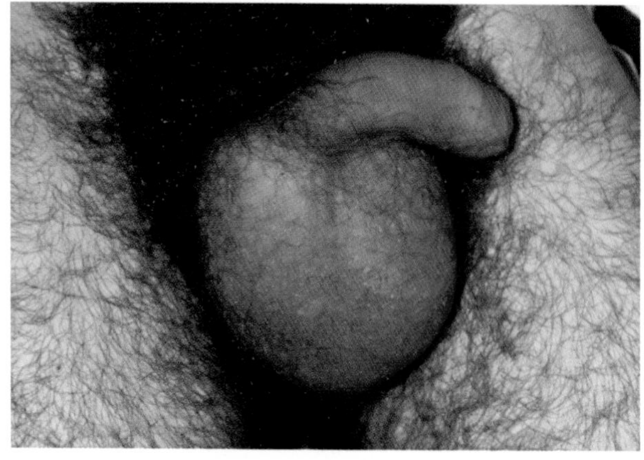

The swollen scrotum of a man suffering from cancer of the testis. *(Copyright Dr. P. Marazzi, Science Source/Photo Researchers, Inc. Reproduced by permission.)*

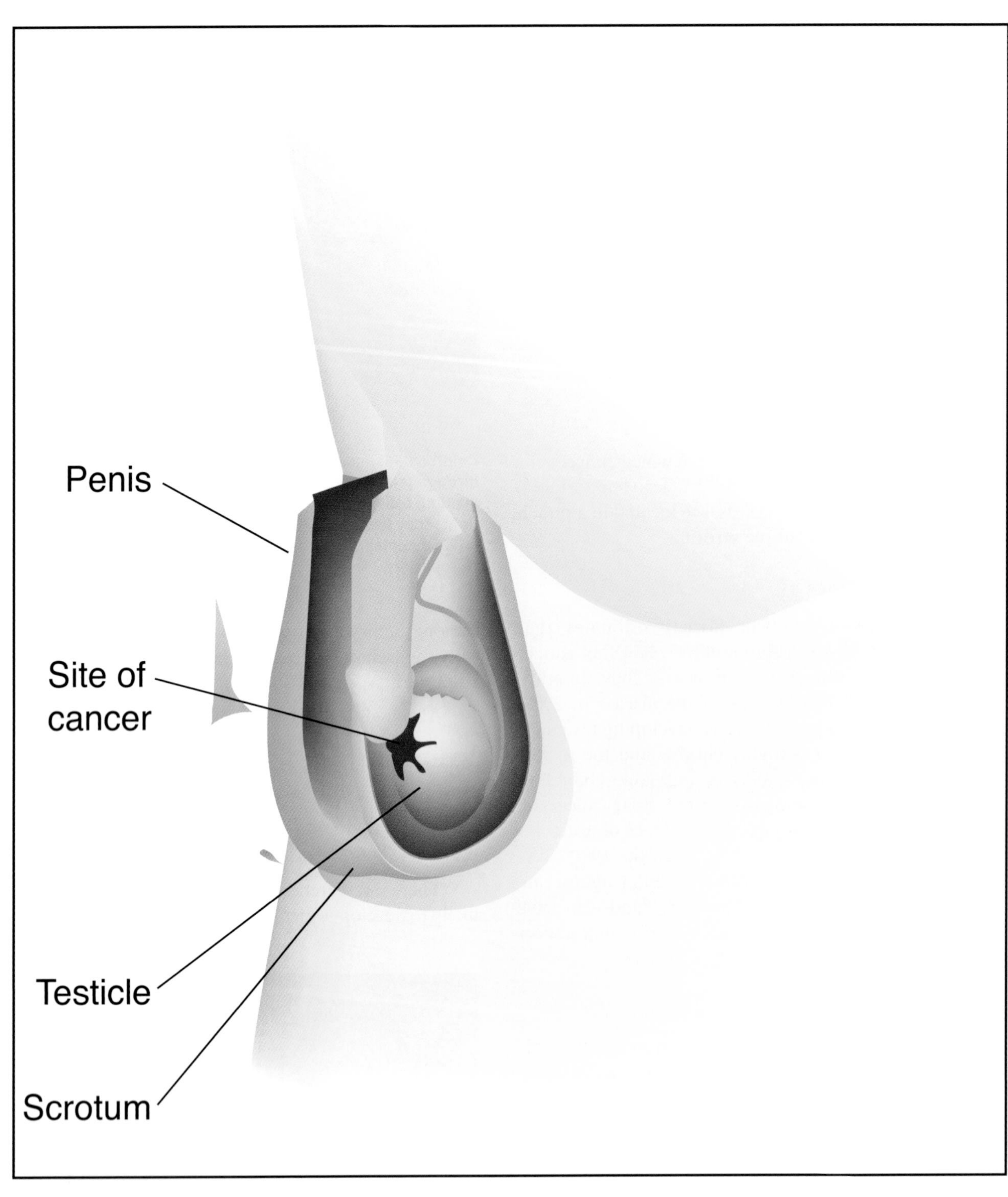

Mesothelioma occurs when malignant cells are found in the mesothelium—tissue that lines the chest and abdominal cavities, the pericardial sac, and also surrounds the outer surface of most internal organs, like the lungs. Here, mesothelioma affects the lining surrounding the patient's left lung (right side of image). *(Illustration by Argosy Publishing. Cengage Learning, Gale.)*

for testicular cancer is much higher for boys born with one or both of their testicles located in the lower abdomen rather than in the scrotum. This condition is called cryptorchidism or undescended testicles. The lifetime risk of being diagnosed with testicular cancer is four times higher for boys with cryptorchidism than the risk in the general population. This risk factor remains even if surgery is done to place the testicle back into the scrotum.

Boys born with Down syndrome are also at higher risk of developing testicular cancer, although the reasons for this increased risk are not yet fully understood.

There are other risk factors as well. Men who have had abnormal development of their testicles are at increased risk, as are men with Klinefelter's syndrome (a disorder of the sex chromosomes). A family history of testicular cancer increases the possibility of getting the disease. Men infected with the human immunodeficiency virus (HIV), especially those with AIDS, have a higher incidence, as do infertile men. Certain testicular tumors appear more frequently among men who work in certain occupations, like miners, oil workers, and utility workers. There is no conclusive evidence that injuries to the testicles, or environmental exposure to various chemicals causes the disease.

Causes and symptoms

The exact causes of testicular cancer are unknown although a number of risk factors have been identified which, when present, seem to place some men at higher risk for the development of this type of cancer.

Testicular cancer usually shows no early symptoms with only 25% of men experiencing symptoms. It is suspected when a mass or lump is felt in the testes, although a testicular mass does not always indicate cancer and is usually painless.

Symptoms of testicular cancer include:

- a lump in either testicle (usually pea-sized, but may be as large as a marble or an egg)
- any enlargement or significant shrinking of a testicle
- a sensation of heaviness in the scrotum
- a dull ache in the groin or lower abdomen
- any sudden collection of fluid in the scrotum
- tenderness or enlargement of the breasts
- pain or discomfort in a testicle or in the scrotum

Other symptoms, such as pain in the lower back, shortness of breath, chest pain, cough, abdominal pain, and headaches, may be present if the cancer is advanced and has spread to the lymph nodes in the abdomen, the lungs and/or the brain.

Diagnosis

When a man exhibits symptoms that suggest a possibility of testicular cancer, several diagnostic steps will occur before a definitive diagnosis is made.

Examination

The physician conducts a personal and family medical history and a complete physical examination is performed. The doctor will examine the scrotum as well as the abdomen and other areas to check for additional masses.

Tests

If a mass is found, an ultrasound of the testicles is performed. Through the use of sound waves, ultrasounds can help visualize internal organs and may be useful in telling the difference between fluid-filled cysts and solid masses.

Computed tomography (CT scan) as well as ultrasound may be used to diagnose malignant germ cell tumors in undescended testes. CT scans are also used to determine if the cancer has spread to other areas of the body outside of the testes.

A chest x ray may be done to see if the cancer has spread to the lungs and/or to the lymph nodes in the thoracic area. Other imaging tests that may be ordered include a **magnetic resonance imaging** (MRI) scan and/or a **positron emission tomography** (PET) scan.

Certain blood tests can be helpful in diagnosing some testicular tumors. **Tumor markers** are substances often found in higher-than-normal amounts in cancer patients. Some testicular cancers secrete high levels of certain proteins such as alpha-fetoprotein (AFP), human chorionic gonadotropin (HCG), and enzymes like lactate dehydrogenase (LDH). These markers may help find a tumor that is too small to be felt during a physical examination. In addition, these tests are also helpful in determining how much cancer is actually present, and in evaluating the response to treatment to make sure the tumor has not returned.

AFP is a tumor marker produced by nonseminomatous testicular tumors. Elevated HCG levels may be secreted by seminomas and nonseminoma tumors. Pure seminomas are not associated with elevated AFP levels. Some testicular tumors contain elements of both seminoma and nonseminoma tumors. In that case, the tumor is clinically managed as a nonseminoma.

Procedures

If a suspicious growth is found, a surgeon will need to remove the tumor and send it to the laboratory for testing. A pathologist examines the testicular tissue microscopically to determine whether cancer cells are present. If cancer cells are found, the pathologist sends back a report describing the type and extent of the cancer. In almost all cases, the surgeon removes the entire affected testicle through an incision in the groin, though not through the scrotum. This procedure is called radical inguinal **orchiectomy**.

Once testicular cancer is determined, further tests are necessary to find out if the cancer has metastasized (spread) to other parts of the body, and to ascertain the stage or extent of the disease. This information helps the doctor plan appropriate treatment. These tests may include abdominopelvic computed tomography (CT scan), bone scans, and chest **x rays**.

Treatment

Staging

One method the cancer treatment team uses to describe the scope of a patient's cancer is the use of a staging system. Testicular cancer is classified using the TNM system. However, in order to simplify and summarize this information, the TNM description can be grouped according to stages.

Stages of testicular cancer:

- Stage I. This stage refers to a cancer found only in the testicle, with no spread to the lymph nodes or to distant organs.
- Stage II. This indicates that the cancer has spread to the lymph nodes in the abdomen, but not to lymph nodes in other parts of the body.
- Stage III. In this stage, the cancer has spread beyond the lymph nodes in the abdomen, and/or the cancer is in parts of the body far away from the testicles, such as the lungs or the liver.
- Recurrent. Recurrent disease indicates that the cancer has come back after it has already been treated. Testicular cancer can come back in the same testicle (if it was not surgically removed) or in some other body part.

Treatment

The treatment decisions for testicular cancer are dependent on the stage and cell type of the disease, as well as the patient's age and overall health. The four kinds of treatment most commonly used are surgery, **radiation therapy**, **chemotherapy**, and bone marrow or stem cell transplantation.

Patients diagnosed with testicular cancer should be provided with information regarding fertility preservation options, including sperm banking, prior to the start of treatment.

Surgery is normally the first line of treatment for testicular cancer and involves the removal of the affected testicle. This procedure is known as a radical inguinal orchiectomy. Depending on the type and stage of the cancer, some lymph nodes may also be removed at the same time, or possibly in a second operation. This procedure is called a retroperitoneal **lymph node dissection**, and can be a major operation. Some patients will experience temporary complications after surgery, including infections and bowel obstruction. If both of the testicles are taken out, a man will have no ability to produce sperm cells and will become infertile (unable to father a child). Surgery removing the lymph nodes may cause some damage to nearby nerves, which may interfere with the ability to ejaculate. Men undergoing surgery for testicular cancer may wish to discuss nerve-sparing surgery with their doctor, as well as sperm banking.

Radiation therapy for testicular cancer is delivered from a machine and is known as external beam radiation. One potential problem with this type of radiation is that it can also destroy nearby healthy tissue as well as cancer cells. Other potential side effects include **nausea**, **diarrhea**, and **fatigue**. A special device can be used to protect the unaffected testicle to preserve fertility. Seminomas are very sensitive to the effects of radiation therapy.

Chemotherapy refers to the use of drugs in treating cancer. Since the drugs enter the bloodstream and circulate throughout the body, chemotherapy is considered a systemic treatment. The drugs primarily used in the treatment of testicular cancer are **cisplatin**, **vinblastine**, **bleomycin**, **carboplatin**, **cyclophosphamide**, **etoposide**, **ifosfamide**, paclitaxel, **mesna**, **gemcitabine**, and oxaliplatin. These drugs are given in various combinations, since the use of two or more drugs is considered more effective than using only one drug.

Since chemotherapy agents can affect normal as well as cancerous cells, several side effects are possible. These side effects include:

- **nausea and vomiting**
- changes in appetite (**anorexia**)
- temporary hair loss (**alopecia**)
- mouth sores
- increased risk of infections
- bleeding or bruising
- fatigue
- diarrhea or constipation

Several drugs are available to assist in treating these side effects, most of which will disappear after the treatment is completed. However, some of the

QUESTIONS TO ASK THE DOCTOR

- How do I perform a testicular self-examination?
- What kind of testicular cancer do I have?
- What treatment choices do I have?
- How long will my treatments last?
- What side effects can I expect from my treatment?
- How long will it take me to recover?
- What are the chances that the cancer will come back?
- Is there a chance I will become infertile?

chemotherapy agents used during treatment of testicular cancer may cause long-term side effects. These include hearing loss, nerve damage, and possible kidney or lung damage. Another potentially serious long-term complication is an increased risk of leukemia. This is a rare side effect, however, as it occurs in less than 1% of testicular cancer patients who receive chemotherapy. Chemotherapy may also interfere with sperm production. This may be permanent for some, but many will regain their fertility within a few years.

Studies are ongoing to determine whether high doses of chemotherapy combined with stem-cell transplantation will prove effective in treating some patients with advanced testicular cancer. In this treatment, blood-forming cells called stem cells are taken from the patient (either from the bone marrow or filtered out of the patient's blood). These cells are kept frozen while high-dose chemotherapy is administered. After receiving the chemotherapy, the patient is given the stem cells through an infusion. This treatment enables the use of extra large doses of chemotherapy that might increase the cure rate for some testicular cancers.

Preferred treatment plans by stage of disease

Stage I: Stage I seminomas are normally treated with a radical inguinal orchiectomy followed by radiation treatment aimed at the lymph nodes. More than 95% of Stage I seminomas are cured through this method. Another treatment approach is treatment with a single dose of the chemotherapy drug carboplatin as an alternative to radiation therapy. Patients in this stage can experience relapse of the disease, however, as long five years or more after orchiectomy. Therefore, follow-up surveillance is strongly recommended. Current recommendations in 2009 regarding follow-up include a history and physical examination with measurement of tumor markers every three to four months in the first year, every six months in the second year, and then annually after the second year. For those patients not undergoing radiation therapy, more intense follow-up is currently recommended. Stage I non-seminomas are also highly curable with surgery, followed by one of three options. These options include the performance of a retroperitoneal lymph node dissection, two cycles of chemotherapy, or careful observation for several years.

Stage II: Stage II seminomas and non-seminomas are cured in 90% to 95% of the cases. For the purposes of treatment, stage II testicular cancers are classified as either bulky or nonbulky. Nonbulky seminomas (no lymph nodes can be felt in the abdomen) are treated with an orchiectomy followed by radiation to the lymph nodes. Men with bulky seminomas have surgery, which is followed by a course of chemotherapy. Nonbulky Stage II non-seminomas are treated with surgery and lymph node removal, with possible chemotherapy. Men with bulky disease have surgery followed by chemotherapy.

Stage III: Stage III seminomas and non-seminomas are treated with surgery followed by chemotherapy. Those who are not cured may be eligible to participate in **clinical trials** of other chemotherapy agents. Virtually all patients with advanced seminoma, approximately 80% of patients, are cured after receiving chemotherapy receiving the drug cisplatin.

Recurrent: Treatment of recurrent testicular cancer is dependent upon the initial stage and the treatment given. This might include further surgery and chemotherapy. Many men whose disease comes back after chemotherapy are treated with high-dose chemotherapy followed by autologous stem cell transplantation.

Prognosis

The overall five-year survival rate for testicular cancer is 95%, making testicular cancer one of the most curable forms of cancer. According to the American Cancer Society, almost 200,000 American men have survived testicular cancer. When the cancer is detected before it has had the time to spread outside of the testicle the five-year survival rate is 99%. The survival rates for testicular cancers that have spread to the local lymph nodes and for those cancers that have spread beyond the lymph nodes in the immediate area are 96% and 71% respectively. The key is early diagnosis. Delay in diagnosis results in the patient's presentation in a more advanced stage of the disease at the time of diagnosis.

Prevention

The main risk factors associated with testicular cancer—cryptorchidism, family history of the disease, and being Caucasian—are unavoidable since they are present at birth. In addition, many men diagnosed with the disease have no known risk factors. Because of these reasons, it is not possible to prevent most incidences of testicular cancer.

Special concerns

For many men, testicles are symbolic of manhood, and the removal of one can lead to embarrassment, or fear about a partner's reaction. Indeed, after surgical removal, the affected side of the scrotum does look and feel empty. To correct this, a patient can have a testicular prosthesis implanted in his scrotum. This prosthesis looks and feels like a real testicle, and the surgical procedure usually leaves only a small scar.

See also Fertility issues; Sexuality.

Resources

PERIODICALS

Carver, B.S., Shienfield, J. "The Current Status of Laparoscopic Retroperitoneal Lymph Node Dissection for Non-Seminomatous Germ Cell Tumors." *Nature Clinical Practice Urology* 2(2005):330-335.

Dahm, P., Rosser, C.J., & McKiernan, J.M. "Quality of Care for Testicular Cancer." *Urologic Oncology* 27(Jul-Aug 2009):448–53.

Fossa, S.D., Chen, J., Schonfeld, S.J., et al. "Risk of Contralateral Testicular Cancer: A Population Based Study of 29,515 US Men. "*Journal of the National Cancer Institute* 97(2005):1056-1066.

Mercer, E. S., B. Broecker, E. A. Smith, et al. "Urological Manifestations of Down Syndrome." *Journal of Urology* 171 (March 2004): 1250–1253.

Oliver, R.T., Mason, M.D., Fogarty, P.J, et al. "Radiotherapy versus Carboplatin in Stage I Seminoma: Updated Analysis of the MRC/EROTC Randomized Trial." *Journal of Clinical Oncology* 26(2008):1 (abstract).

OTHER

American Cancer Society. *Testicular Cancer*. http://www.cancer.org/docroot/CRI/content/CRI_2_4_1X_What_is_testicular_cancer? August 3, 2009 [cited September 20, 2009].

National Comprehensive Cancer Network. *NCCN Practice Guidelines in Oncology Testicular Cancer v.1.2010*.www.nccn.org [cited September 20, 2009].

ORGANIZATIONS

American Cancer Society. (800) ACS-2345.

National Cancer Institute. Cancer Information Service. (800) 4-CANCER.

Deanna Swartout-Corbeil, R.N.
Rebecca J. Frey, PhD
Melinda Oberleitner, R.N., D.N.S., A.P.R.N., C.N.S.

Testicular self-exam

Definition

A testicular self-examination (TSE) is the procedure by which a man checks the appearance and consistency of his testes.

Purpose

Most testicular cancers are first noticed by the man himself, many times after a blow or other injury to the scrotum. Men should perform a TSE every month to find out if the testes contain any suspicious lumps or other irregularities, which could be signs of **cancer** or **infection**.

It is particularly important for adult male survivors of **childhood cancers** to perform TSE on a regular basis. A group of researchers at the University of Minnesota reported in 2004 that only 17% of male survivors of childhood cancer examine their own testes as a form of cancer screening. The researchers urged primary care physicians to teach cancer survivors about the importance of regular self-examination in adult life.

Precautions

None.

Description

A TSE should take place during a warm shower or bath, when the skin is warm, wet, and soapy. The man needs to step out of the tub so that he is in front of a mirror. The heat from the tub or shower will relax the scrotum (sac containing the testes) and the skin will be softer and thinner, making it easier to feel a lump. It is important that the exam be done very gently.

The man should stand facing his mirror and look for swelling on the scrotum. Using both hands, the scrotum should be gently lifted so that the area underneath can be checked.

The next step is the exam by hand. The index and middle fingers should be placed under each testicle,

QUESTIONS TO ASK THE DOCTOR

- How long should a testicular self-examination take?
- What should be done if the presence of a lump is uncertain during a TSE?
- What action should be taken if a lump or abnormality is definitely found during TSE?
- What medical tests are done to confirm testicular cancer?
- How often is a testicular examination performed as part of a physical examination?
- What are the other signs of testicular cancer?

with the thumbs on top. The testes should be examined one at a time. The man should roll each testicle between his fingers and thumbs. He should feel for lumps of any size (even as small as a pea) particularly on the front or side of each testicle. He should also look for soreness or irregularities. Next, the epididymis and vas deferens, located on the top and back of the testes, should be felt. This area feels like a cord, and should not be tender.

Normal results

It is normal for one testicle to be larger than the other, and for them to hang at different levels, but the size should stay the same from one month to the next. The testes should be free from lumps, pain, irregularities, and swelling.

Abnormal results

A TSE is considered abnormal if any swelling, tenderness, lumps, or irregularities are found. Hard, unmoving lumps are abnormal, even if they are painless. A lump could be a sign of an infection or a cancerous tumor. A change in testicle size from one month to the next is also abnormal. A feeling of heaviness in the scrotum is another abnormal sign. If any abnormality is found, a man is encouraged to check with his doctor as soon as possible because **testicular cancer** is highly curable if found early.

KEY TERMS

Epididymis—A tube in the back of the testes that transports sperm.

Scrotum—The pouch containing the testes.

Testes (singular, testis)—Egg-shaped male gonads located in the scrotum. Testes is the plural form of testis, which is a testicle.

Vas deferens (plural, vasa deferentia)—A tube that is a continuation of the epididymis. This tube transports sperm from the testis to the prostatic urethra.

Resources

BOOKS

Beers, Mark H., MD, and Robert Berkow, MD, editors. "Overview of Cancer." Section 11, Chapter 142 In*The Merck Manual of Diagnosis and Therapy*. Whitehouse Station, NJ: Merck Research Laboratories, 2002.

Hainsworth, John D., and F. Anthony Greco. "Testis." In *Cancer Treatment*, edited by Charles M. Haskell, 5th ed. Philadelphia: W.B. Saunders, 2001.

Seidel, Henry M., et al. *Mosby's Guide to Physical Examination*. 4th ed. St. Louis: Mosby, Inc., 1999.

PERIODICALS

Yeazel, M. W., K. C. Oeffinger, J. G. Gurney, et al. "The Cancer Screening Practices of Adult Survivors of Childhood Cancer: A Report from the Childhood Cancer Survivor Study." *Cancer* 100 (February 1, 2004): 631–640.

OTHER

"Questions and Answers About Testicular Cancer." Feb. 2000. *National Cancer Institute*. http://cis.nci.nih.gov/fact/6_34.htm.

Rhonda Cloos,, RN
Rebecca J. Frey, PhD

Testolactone

Definition

Testolactone is a synthetic drug related to the male hormone **testosterone**. It is used to reduce the size of tumors in some women with advanced **breast cancer**. Testolactone is available in the U.S. under the brand name Teslac.

Purpose

Testolactone is used in treating advanced breast **cancer** in postmenopausal women and in women who have had their ovaries removed. It is never used in treating breast cancer in men.

KEY TERMS

Malignant—Cancerous. Malignant cells tend to reproduce without normal controls on growth and form tumors or invade other tissues.

Ovaries—A pair of female reproductive organs that release eggs. They are the main source of the female hormone estrogen.

Postmenopausal—Older women who no longer menstruate because of their age.

Testosterone—The main male hormone. It is produced in the testes and is responsible for the development of primary and secondary male sexual traits.

Description

Testolactone is approved by the United States Food and Drug Administration (FDA), and its cost usually is covered by insurance. It is classified as an antineoplastic agent, which means that it stops or slows the growth of malignant cells. One advantage of testolactone is that, although it is related to testosterone, it does not cause women to develop male characteristics such as a deep voice or facial hair.

As noted above, testolactone is related to the male hormone testosterone. The way in which it inhibits the growth of breast cancer cells is not clear. However, it is known that the hormone estrogen stimulates the growth of some breast cancer cells, and testolactone seems to interfere with estrogen production. The resulting reduction in estrogen levels may slow the growth of breast cancers sensitive to this hormone.

In breast cancer, testolactone is a palliative treatment. This means that it helps relieve symptoms, but does not cure the cancer. It is effective only in about 15% of the women who take it. In these women, however, it helps reduce the size of half or more tumors. Normally testolactone is used along with other **chemotherapy** drugs for fighting advanced breast cancer.

Recommended dosage

Testolactone comes as a 50 mg tablet. The dose will depend on the patient's body weight and her general health, as well as other drugs she may be taking. However, a standard dose is 250 mg (5 tablets) four times a day for three months. It takes at least several weeks before the drug begins to be effective. Tablets should be stored at room temperature.

Precautions

People with a history of heart or kidney disease should be sure to tell their doctor, as this may affect their use of testolactone.

Side effects

Testolactone often causes **nausea**, **vomiting**, and loss of appetite (**anorexia**). Because testolactone must be taken over many months to be effective, people who experience these symptoms should talk to their doctor about medications to relieve the **nausea and vomiting** so that they can continue to take testolactone.

Other side effects reported with testolactone include numbness or tingling in the toes, fingers, and face; **diarrhea**; swelling and water retention in the feet and legs, and swelling of the tongue; hair loss (**alopecia**), and abnormal nail growth. However, since women who take this drug are receiving other chemotherapy drugs and are in an advanced stage of cancer, it is difficult to pinpoint whether testolactone is exclusively responsible for some of these side effects.

Interactions

Many drugs interact with nonprescription (over-the-counter) drugs and herbal remedies. Patients should always tell their health care providers about these remedies, as well as any prescription drugs they are taking. Patients should also mention if they are on a special diet such as low salt or high protein. They should not take calcium supplements, since testosterone already has the potential to increase circulating calcium to dangerous levels.

Testolactone may increase the effect of anticoagulants (blood thinning medication). In women where cancer has spread to the bones, testolactone may increase the circulating level of calcium in the body. Calcium levels need to be tested regularly.

Tish Davidson, A.M.

Testosterone

Definition

Synthetic derivatives of the natural hormone testosterone are used to reduce the size of hormone-responsive tumors.

KEY TERMS

Hormone—A chemical produced by a gland in one part of the body that travels through the circulatory system and affects only specific receptive tissues at another location in the body.

Postmenopausal—Women have stopped menstruating, usually because of their age.

Testes—Egg-shaped male sexual organs contained in the scrotum that produce testosterone and sperm.

Purpose

Testosterone-related drugs are used to treat advanced disseminated **breast cancer** in women.

Description

Testosterone belongs to a class of hormones called androgens. These are male hormones responsible for the development of the male reproductive system and secondary male sexual characteristics such as voice depth and facial hair. Testosterone is normally produced by the testes in large quantities in men. It also occurs normally in smaller quantities in women.

Several man-made derivatives of testosterone are used to treat advanced disseminated breast **cancer** in women, especially when cancer has spread to the bones. The most common of these testosterone-like drugs are **fluoxymesterone** (Halotestin) and methyltestosterone (Testred). These androgens are used only in women who have late-stage breast cancer and who meet specific criteria. These criteria include:

- The patient is postmenopausal.
- The tumors have been shown to be hormone-dependent.
- The tumors have spread, often to the bone, or recurred after other hormonal cancer treatments.

Using testosterone derivatives to treat breast cancer is a palliative treatment. This means that the treatment helps relieve symptoms but does not cure the cancer. These drugs are approved by the United States Food and Drug Administration (FDA), and their cost is usually covered by insurance.

Clinical trials are currently underway that involve the use of testosterone-related androgens in varying combinations with other drugs to treat advanced cancers. The selection of clinical trials changes constantly. Current information on the availability and location of clinical trials can be found at the following web sites:

- National Cancer Institute: (800) 4-CANCER or http://cancertrials.nci.nih.gov.
- National Institutes of Health Clinical Trials: http://clinicaltrials.gov.
- Center Watch: A Clinical Trials Listing: http://www.centerwatch.com.

Recommended dosage

Dosage is individualized and depends on the patient's body weight and general health, as well as the other drugs she is taking and the way her cancer responds to hormones. Halotestin comes in tablets of 2 mg, 5 mg, or 10 mg. A standard dose of Halotestin for inoperable breast cancer is 10 to 40 mg in divided doses daily for several months. Tablets should be stored at room temperature. Testred comes in 10 mg capsules. A standard dose for women with advanced breast cancer is 50 to 200 mg daily.

Precautions

Women who take testosterone derivatives for advanced breast cancer are postmenopausal, so the usual precautions about avoiding pregnancy when receiving androgen therapy do not apply.

Side effects

The most serious side effect of these drugs is **hypercalcemia**, a condition in which too much calcium circulates in the blood. This occurs because these drugs liberate calcium from bones. Calcium levels are monitored regularly, and the drug is discontinued if hypercalcemia occurs. Another serious (but less common) side effect is the development of tumors in the liver. Other side effects include deepening of the voice, development of facial hair and acne, fluid retention, and **nausea**.

Interactions

As with any course of treatment, patients should alert their physician to any prescription, over-the-counter, or herbal remedies they are taking in order to avoid harmful drug interactions. Patients should also mention if they are on a special diet, such as low salt or high protein. They should not take calcium supplements, since testosterone already has the potential to increase circulating calcium to dangerous levels.

Testosterone derivatives may interact with anticoagulant drugs (blood thinners) such as Coumadin.

Tish Davidson, A.M.

Tetrahydrocannabinol

Definition

Tetrahydrocannabinol (THC) is the main psychoactive substance found in the hemp plant *Cannabis sativa*, or marijuana.

Purpose

A number of studies indicate medical benefits of THC for **cancer** and AIDS patients by increasing appetite and decreasing **nausea**, blocking the spread of some cancer-causing **herpes simplex** viruses. It has been shown to assist some glaucoma patients by reducing pressure within the eye, and is used, in the form of cannabis, by a number of multiple sclerosis patients for relieving spasms. Effects include relaxation; euphoria; altered space-time perception; enhancement of visual, auditory, and olfactory senses; disorientation; and appetite stimulation. Synthetic THC, also known under the substance name *dronabinol*, is available as a prescription drug under the trade name Marinol in several countries including the United States, Netherlands, and Germany.

Description

The issue of medical uses of THC is politicized in the United States because of its status as a Schedule I drug under the U.S. Controlled Substances Act of 1970. Schedule I drugs are defined as those considered to have high potential for abuse, with no recognized medical use in treatment in the United States. In this drug's case, its recreational use is distinguished from its medical use. Marijuana is Schedule I, but tetrahydrocannabinol (THC, Marinol) is Schedule II.

There have been major advances in THC pharmacology and in the understanding of the cancer disease process. In particular, research has demonstrated the presence of numerous cannabinoid (chemical constituents of marijuana) receptors in the nucleus of the solitary tract, a brain center that is important in the control of **vomiting**. While other anti-vomiting drugs are equally or more effective than oral THC, Marinol, or smoked cannabis for certain individuals unresponsive to conventional anti-emetic drugs, the use of smoked cannabis can provide relief more effectively than oral preparations, which may be difficult to swallow or be expelled in vomit before having a chance to take effect. The euphoria effect of THC or smoked cannabis improves mood, whereas several conventional tranquilizers, also used in the treatment of psychoses such as schizophrenia, may produce unwanted side effects such as excessive sedation, flattening of mood, and distressing physical symptoms such as uncontrolled or compulsive movements.

There would appear to be growing evidence of direct anti-tumor activity of cannabinoids, specifically CB1 and CB2 agonists, in a range of cancer types, including brain (gliomas), skin, pituitary, prostate, and bowel. The anti-tumor activity has led in laboratory animals and in-vitro human tissues to regression of tumors, reductions in vascularisation (blood supply) and metastases (secondary tumors), as well as direct inducement of death among cancer cells. Indeed, the complex interactions of cannabinoids and receptors contribute to scientific understanding of the mechanisms by which cancers develop. However, smoking of cannabis releases a number of non-cannabinoid carcinogens into the lungs and upper respiratory tract, and a number of researchers have identified pre-cancerous changes in lung cells. The failure of these researchers to discover significant evidence of actual cancer cells in the lung may be attributed to these anti-cancer activities of cannabinoids, including THC, counteracting the effects of other carcinogens in smoked cannabis. Some researchers have investigated the link between mental and spiritual state and cancer remission, associating the cannabinoid system with the expression of pleasure on the one hand and stress on the other.

Recommended dosage

The average dose of Marinol is 5–20 mg daily. Most patients respond to 5 mg three or four times daily. Dosage may be escalated during a **chemotherapy**

KEY TERMS

Cannabinoid—Chemical constituents of marijuana, such as THC.

Carcinogens—Cancer-causing agents.

Chemotherapy—The use of chemical agents to treat diseases, especially cancer.

Glaucoma—An eye disorder marked by abnormally high pressure within the eyeball.

Herpes simplex—Either of two viral diseases marked by clusters of small watery blisters, one affecting the area of the mouth and lips and the other the genitals.

Multiple sclerosis—A serious progressive disease of the central nervous system.

cycle or at subsequent cycles, based upon initial results. Therapy should be initiated at the lowest recommended dosage and increased based on clinical response. Marinol is a small soft gel and is available in three strengths: 2.5, 5, and 10 mg. The pediatric dosage for the treatment of chemotherapy-induced emesis is the same as in adults. Caution is recommended in prescribing Marinol for children because of the psychoactive effects.

Precautions

THC and Marinol should be carefully evaluated in patients with the following medical conditions because of individual variation in response and tolerance to the effects of the drugs: patients with cardiac disorders; patients with a history of **substance abuse**, including alcohol abuse or dependence; mania (a psychiatric disorder characterized by excessive physical activity, rapidly changing ideas, and impulsive behavior); **depression**; or schizophrenia. Marinol and THC should be used with caution in patients receiving sedatives, hypnotics, or other psychoactive drugs because of the potential for additive or synergistic effects on the central nervous system. Marinol should be used with caution in pregnant patients, nursing mothers, or pediatric patients because it has not been studied in these populations.

Side effects

Some negative effects are associated with constant, long-term use, including memory loss, depression, and loss of motivation. The long-term effects of THC on humans is highly disputed.

Interactions

No clinically significant drug-to-drug interactions were discovered in Marinol **clinical trials**.

Ken R. Wells,

Thalidomide

Definition

Thalidomide, which is also known as Thalomid, is a drug used to fight aggressive cancers, particularly those that have metastasized, or spread. It became infamous as a teratogen in the 1960s for the severe birth defects that it caused in 46 countries around the world. Thalidomide was never approved for use in the United States but it was widely available elsewhere from 1957 to 1961 as a sedative and treatment for **nausea** during pregnancy. It was withdrawn from the market in 1961 after what has been called the largest medical tragedy of modern times. The number of children with birth defects caused by thalidomide is estimated to be between 10,000 and 20,000.

Purpose

Thalidomide is presently classed as an immunomodulatory agent, which means that it is a drug that affects the immune system. It appears to change the levels of certain proteins that the body normally uses to control the activity of cells.

There are many studies, either in progress or recently completed, that suggest thalidomide can slow or stop the spread of **cancer** of the brain, breast, colon, and prostate, as well as **multiple myeloma** (MM: a cancer of the bone marrow). Thalidomide appears to be useful in treating patients with MM who have not benefited from other therapies. Research studies that consider the benefit of thalidomide in treating other cancers are multiplying rapidly. The use of the drug in cancer therapy is likely to increase.

The same action of thalidomide that harms babies makes it useful as a powerful cancer fighter. Thalidomide interferes with the formation of blood vessels, a process known as angiogenesis. It is therefore called an antiangiogenic drug as well as an immunomodulator.

Cancers that spread have a lot of blood vessels (are highly vascularized). Thus, when cancer cells are not nourished by a blood supply, they die. One way to stop the spread of cancer is to stop the formation of the blood vessels that carry nourishment to the cancer cells, and that is what thalidomide is thought to do. Researchers also are interested in other activities of thalidomide, particularly the ones that make it capable of eliminating such skin eruptions as sores or ulcers in the mouths of patients with AIDS and leprosy.

Other diseases for which thalidomide is being tested as a therapy as of 2009 include:

- Crohn's disease
- Behçet's disease, a rare autoimmune disorder
- Amyotrophic lateral sclerosis (Lou Gehrig's disease)
- Congestive heart failure
- Diarrhea
- HIV infection
- Chronic pain
- Rheumatoid arthritis

- Tuberculosis
- Thyroid cancer
- Systemic lupus erythematosus
- Malignant melanoma
- Macular degeneration
- Graft-versus-host disease

Demographics

Thalidomide is given primarily to adult patients to treat either multiple **myeloma** or erythema nodosum, but can be prescribed for children as young as 11 years of age.

Precautions

In 1998 the Food and Drug Administration (FDA) required the company that sells thalidomide to establish a System for Thalidomide Education and Prescribing Safety (S.T.E.P.S) oversight program. The program includes: limiting prescription and dispensing rights to authorized prescribers and pharmacies; keeping a registry of all patients who are prescribed thalidomide; providing extensive patient education about the risks associated with the drug; and providing periodic pregnancy tests for women who take it.

Thalidomide can also be detected in male sperm; therefore four men who are taking the drug and having sexual relations with women of childbearing age must use latex condoms during and at least four weeks after completing treatment with thalidomide.

Because thalidomide can make people drowsy, patients who take it should avoid driving a car, operating heavy machinery, or performing other tasks that could be made dangerous by sleepiness.

Pediatric

Thalidomide has been used to treat children as young as 11; however, the S.T.E.P.S. program requires that a child or adolescent under 18 years of age must understand the nature of the drug, have received warnings about its risks and possible side effects, show sufficient maturity to comply with contraceptive measures (if applicable), and have a parent or guardian sign a statement guaranteeing the young person's compliance with the program.

Pregnant or breastfeeding

The serious threat thalidomide poses to fetuses cannot be overstated. No pregnant woman and no woman who has any chance of becoming pregnant should take thalidomide. (Only women who have had a hysterectomy or who are at the age of menopause and have been in a menopausal state, which is no menses, or periods, for 24 consecutive months, can be considered as having no chance of becoming pregnant.)

Interactions

Barbiturates, salts, esters used to encourage sleep, and alcohol increase the effect of thalidomide's power of sedation. They should not be taken with the drug. Thalidomide also intensifies the action of chlorpromazine (Thorazine) and reserpine, which are antipsychotic drugs.

Patients taking griseofulvin, rifampin, **carbamazepine**, **phenytoin**, or certain herbal supplements (particularly St. John's wort) must use at least two other effective methods of contraception or abstain from sexual relations while taking thalidomide, as these other drugs interfere with the effectiveness of oral contraceptives.

Food interferes with the absorption of thalidomide; the drug should therefore be taken only when the stomach is empty.

Description

Origins

There is some debate about the origin of the research that led to thalidomide. Although the drug was patented in 1954 by a German company named Grünenthal, some evidence indicates that thalidomide was first developed by a Nazi scientist in 1944 as a possible antidote for nerve gas. Other historians claim that the drug was first synthesized by British scientists working at the University of Nottingham in 1949.

Thalidomide was first introduced under the name of Contergan on the European market in 1957 as a tranquilizer, a medication prescribed particularly for imparting drowsiness and sleep. The drug was sold over the counter; it was not a prescription medication. Ironically, Contergan was considered a safe sedative because unlike barbiturates, it could not be used in high doses to commit suicide. It was then given to pregnant women to provide them with relief from morning sickness. Soon after being given to pregnant women, thalidomide was linked to death or severe disabilities in newborns. Some children who had been exposed to thalidomide while in the womb (in utero) failed to develop limbs or had very short limbs, a condition called phocomelia. Other children were born blind or deaf or with other physical problems.

The connection between thalidomide and birth defects was suspected in 1960 by two doctors, an

Australian obstetrician named William McBride (1927–) and a German pediatrician named Widukind Lenz (1919–95). Dr. Lenz was able to prove that the drug was the cause of the birth defects in 1961. Dr. Frances Kelsey (1914–), a Canadian physician who became an American citizen in the 1930s, became a heroine in 1962 for her work in preventing the licensing of Contergan (under the trade name Kevadon) in the United States. Dr. Kelsey began working for the FDA in 1960 and withheld approval of thalidomide because she was not satisfied that it had been tested adequately. Her concern was vindicated by the following year by Dr. Lenz's publications.

Interest in thalidomide as a treatment for leprosy and a skin disease called erythema nodosum (EN) began in Israel in 1964 and was continued by researchers at Rockefeller University in New York in the 1990s. In 1998 the FDA approved the use of thalidomide for leprosy and EN; it approved the use of thalidomide for newly diagnosed multiple myeloma patients in 2006.

Preparation

Recommended dosage

Thalidomide is given as a capsule taken by mouth. There are four sizes: 50 mg, 100 mg, 150 mg, and 200 mg. Dosages used are highly individualized and depend on the type of cancer or other disease being attacked. For example, in one study of multiple myeloma therapy, a starting dose of 200 mg per day was increased to 800 mg per day over a two-week period. As of 2009 there is no standard dosage for thalidomide; some patients benefit from low doses of the drug alone, while others need to use it in combination with steroid medications like **dexamethasone**. Selection of an appropriate treatment regimen is made on a case-by-case basis.

In a **colon cancer** study, 400 mg per day of thalidomide were given in combination with the anticancer drug **irinotecan**. The dose of irinotecan was between 300 and 350 mg per day. Used in combination with irinotecan, thalidomide contributed its own cancer-fighting properties and it also seemed to reduce the side effects of irinotecan.

In a trial using thalidomide to treat **prostate cancer**, both low doses (as low as 200 mg per day) and high doses (as high as 1200 mg per day) were tried. The patients taking high doses fared somewhat better.

Aftercare

Patients should contact their doctor about any side effects with thalidomide, particularly if they experience peripheral **neuropathy**. The doctor may lower the dosage or take the patient off the drug. Patients should not, however, change their dosage or discontinue the drug on their own but should consult their doctor.

QUESTIONS TO ASK YOUR DOCTOR

- Would you recommend thalidomide for my disease?
- Do you consider the drug safe to take provided that the S.T.E.P.S. procedure is followed?
- How many patients have you treated with thalidomide? What were their outcomes?
- Should I consider participating in a clinical trial of thalidomide therapy?
- What is the risk of a severe side effect from thalidomide?

Risks

Side effects

Besides the extreme risk thalidomide poses to fetuses, it also produces side effects in the person taking the drug. The side effects of thalidomide are milder than those of many other **anticancer drugs**, and because the drug poses less discomfort than other cancer-fighting drugs, it is particularly attractive to oncologists, or physicians who treat cancer patients.

Among the side effects are erratic heartbeat, swelling (edema), digestive upsets of all sorts, including both constipation and **diarrhea**, pain in back and neck muscles, low blood pressure, and skin rashes.

More serious side effects include:

- Drowsiness
- Dizziness
- Peripheral neuropathy (tingling sensations or numbness in the arms, legs, hands, or feet)
- Leukopenia (low level of white blood cells)
- Stevens-Johnson syndrome and toxic epidermal necrolysis (TEN), life-threatening skin disorders that require immediate medical care; TEN in particular has a death rate of 30–40%
- Increased risk of blood clot formation in the venous circulation, which increases the risk of heart attack or stroke
- Seizures

Results

Thalidomide appears to be most effective in treating newly diagnosed patients with multiple **melanoma**, with a response rate of 60–70%. It is also highly effective in treating patients with erythema nodosum, having a higher response rate than prednisolone and other steroid medications.

Health care team roles

Patients taking thalidomide will have to be under the care of an oncologist or other specialist authorized to prescribe the drug and experienced in interpreting the results of treatment as well as monitoring the patient for side effects. The patient's pharmacist may be helpful in providing additional information about drug interactions and precautions.

Alternatives

Other prescription drugs that are being used as alternatives to thalidomide include lenalidomide (Revlimid), a derivative of thalidomide made by the same company that manufactures Thalomid; and **bortezomib** (Velcade), a proteasome inhibitor approved by the FDA in 2003. Revlimid was approved by the FDA in 2006 for use with dexamethasone in treating patients with multiple myseloma. Velcade is also used to treat multiple myeloma. Both drugs have the advantage of having fewer side effects than thalidomide itself, particularly a lower risk of blood clot formation.

Another derivative of thalidomide, pomalidomide (Actimid), is in phase 2 **clinical trials** for treatment of multiple myeloma as of late 2009. It is reported to show promising results.

Caregiver concerns

Caregiver concerns include monitoring the patient for side effects, particularly such potentially life-threatening conditions as TEN; and checking to see that the patient is complying with the S.T.E.P.S. requirements.

Resources

BOOKS

Brynner, Rock, and Trent Stephens. *Dark Remedy: The Impact of Thalidomide and Its Revival as a Vital Medicine*. New York: Basic Books, 2001.

Chabner, Bruce A., and Dan L. Longo, eds. *Cancer Chemotherapy and Biotherapy: Principles and Practice*, 4th ed. Philadelphia : Lippincott Williams and Wilkins, 2006.

Schlich, Thomas, and Ulrich Trohler. *The Risks of Medical Innovation: Risk Perception and Assessment in Historical Context*. New York: Routledge, 2006.

PERIODICALS

Holaday, J.W., and B.A. Berkowitz. "Antiangiogenic Drugs: Insights into Drug Development from Endostatin, Avastin and Thalidomide." *Molecular Interventions* 9 (August 2009): 157–66.

Kaur, I., et al. "Comparative Efficacy of Thalidomide and Prednisolone in the Treatment of Moderate to Severe Erythema nodosum leprosum: A Randomized Study." *Australasian Journal of Dermatology* 50 (August 2009): 181–85.

Laubach, J.P., et al. "Hematology: Thalidomide Maintenance in Multiple Myeloma." *Nature Reviews: Clinical Oncology* 6 (October 2009): 565–66.

Layzer, R., and J. Wolf. "Myeloma-associated Polyneuropathy Responding to Lenalidomide." *Neurology* 73 (September 8, 2009): 812–13.

Lee, S.M., et al. "Anti-angiogenic Therapy Using Thalidomide Combined with Chemotherapy in Small Cell Lung Cancer: A Randomized, Double-blind, Placebo-controlled Trial." *Journal of the National Cancer Institute* 101 (August 5, 2009): 1049–57.

Martin, M.G., and R. Vij. "Arterial Thrombosis with Immunomodulatory Derivatives in the Treatment of Multiple Myeloma: A Single-center Case Series and Review of the Literature." *Clinical Lymphoma and Myeloma* 9 (August 2009): 320–23.

Pretz, J., and B.C. Medeiros. "Thalidomide-induced Pneumonitis in a Patient with Plasma Cell Leukemia: No Recurrence with Subsequent Lenalidomide Therapy." *American Journal of Hematology* 84 (July 16, 2009): 698–99.

Zangari, M., et al. "Thrombotic Events in Patients with Cancer Receiving Antiangiogenesis Agents." *Journal of Clinical Oncology* 27 (October 10, 2009): 4865–4873.

OTHER

AIDS Treatment Data Network. *Fact Sheet: Thalidomide*. http://www.aegis.com/factshts/network/simple/thalid.html.

Grünenthal GmbH. *Thalidomide: The Facts*. http://www.contergan.grunenthal.info/ctg/en_EN/html/ctg_en_en_history.jhtml?CatId=ctg_en_en_history_a_01.

International Myeloma Foundation (MF). *Understanding Thalidomide Therapy*. http://myeloma.org/pdfs/Understanding_Thalidomide.pdf.

ORGANIZATIONS

American Society of Health-System Pharmacists (ASHP), 7272 Wisconsin Avenue, Bethesda, MD, 20814, 301-657-3000, http://www.ashp.org/.

Celgene Corporation [manufacturer of Thalomid], 86 Morris Avenue, Summit, NJ, 07901, 908-673-9000, 888-423-5436, http://www.thalomid.com/.

European Medicines Agency (EMEA), 7 Westferry Circus, Canary Wharf, London, United Kingdom, E14 4HB, +44 2074188400, +44 2074188416, http://www.emea.europa.eu/.

International Myeloma Foundation (IMF), 12650 Riverside Drive, Suite 206, North Hollywood, CA, United States, 91607-3421, 818-487-7455 , 800-452-2873 (U.S. and Canada), 818-487-7454, TheIMF@myeloma.org, http://myeloma.org/.

Multiple Myeloma Research Foundation (MMRF), 383 Main Avenue, Fifth Floor, Norwalk, CT, 06851, 203-229-0464, 203-229-0572, info@themmrf.org, http://www.multiplemyeloma.org/.

U.S. Food and Drug Administration (FDA), 10903 New Hampshire Ave., Silver Spring, MD, 20993, 888-463-6332, http://www.fda.gov/.

Diane M. Calabrese
Rebecca J. Frey, PhD

Thioguanine

Definition

Thioguanine is an anticancer (antineoplastic) agent belonging to the class of drugs called antimetabolites. It also acts as a suppressor of the immune system. It is available only in the generic form in the United States, or under the brand name Lanvis in Canada. Other common designations for thioguanine include 6-thioguanine (6-TG) and TG.

Purpose

Thioguanine is used to treat various forms of acute and nonlymphocytic leukemias. It is usually used in combination with other **chemotherapy** drugs, such as **cyclophosphamide**, **cytarabine**, prednisone, and/or **vincristine**.

Description

Thioguanine chemically interferes with the synthesis of genetic material of **cancer** cells. It acts as a false building block for DNA and RNA, which, when used to copy DNA and RNA, leads to cell death.

Recommended dosage

Thioguanine is administered orally. It is generally given once per day in a dosage of 2 mg per kg (2.2 pounds) of body weight. This dosage may be increased to 3 mg per kg if the patient does not respond to the medication within three weeks.

KEY TERMS

Antineoplastic—A drug that prevents the growth of a neoplasm by interfering with the maturation or proliferation of the cells of the neoplasm.

Neoplasm—New abnormal growth of tissue.

Precautions

Thioguanine can cause an allergic reaction in some people. Patients with a prior allergic reaction to thioguanine or **mercaptopurine** should not take thioguanine.

Thioguanine can cause serious birth defects if either the man or the woman is taking this drug at the time of conception or if the woman is taking this drug during pregnancy. Because thioguanine is easily passed from mother to child through breast milk, breast feeding is not recommended while thioguanine is being taken.

This drug suppresses the immune system and interferes with the normal functioning of certain organs and tissues. For these reasons, it is important that the prescribing physician is aware of any of the following pre-existing medical conditions:

- a current case of, or recent exposure to, chicken pox
- herpes zoster (shingles)
- a current case, or history of, gout or kidney stones
- all current infections
- kidney disease
- liver disease

Also, because thioguanine is such a potent immunosuppressant, patients receiving this drug must exercise extreme caution to avoid contracting any new infections, and should make an effort to:

- avoid any individual with any type of infection
- avoid bleeding injuries, including those caused by brushing or flossing the teeth
- avoid contact of the hands with the eyes or nasal passages
- avoid contact sports or any other activity that could cause a bruising or bleeding injury

Side effects

A common side effect of thioguanine use is **myelosuppression** with decreases in white blood cell and platelet counts. Other possible side effects include:

- increased susceptibility to infection

- **nausea and vomiting**
- **diarrhea**
- mouth sores
- skin rash, itching, or hives
- swelling in the feet or lower legs

A doctor should be consulted immediately if the patient experiences:

- black, tarry or bloody stools
- blood in the urine
- persistent cough
- fever and chills
- pain in the lower back or sides
- painful or difficult urination
- unusual bleeding or bruising

Interactions

Thioguanine should not be taken in combination with any prescription drug, over-the-counter drug, or herbal remedy without prior consultation with a physician. It is particularly important that the prescribing physician be aware of the use of any of the following drugs:

- antithyroid agents
- azathioprine
- chloramphenicol
- colchicine
- flucytosine
- interferon
- plicamycin
- probenecid
- sulfinpyrazone
- zidovudine
- any radiation therapy or chemotherapy medicines

See also Cancer genetics; Chemoprevention; DNA flow cytometry; Drug resistance.

Paul A. Johnson, Ed.M.

Thiotepa

Definition

Thiotepa is a **chemotherapy** drug used to reduce the size of a cancerous tumor and prevent the growth of new **cancer** cells. This drug is sometimes referred by the brand name Thioplex.

KEY TERMS

DNA (Deoxyribonucleic acid)—The genetic material found in each cell in the body that plays an important role in controlling many of the cell's functions. When a cell divides to create two new cells, an identical copy of its DNA is found in each. If there is an error in a cell's DNA, division may not occur.

Effusion—The collection of fluid in a body cavity or tissue due to the rupture of a blood or other body vessel, resulting from a type of trauma, cancer, or other condition.

Lymph system—This system is involved in preventing bacteria and other infection-causing particles from entering into the bloodstream. It is made up of small organs called lymph nodes, which make and store infection-fighting cells, and thin tubes, or vessels, that branch into all parts of the body.

Myelosuppression— The suppression of bone marrow activity, resulting in reduction in the number of platelets, red cells, and white cells found in the circulation.

Purpose

Thiotepa has been used in the treatment of many types of tumors, but it is most often used as a treatment for the advanced stages of **breast cancer**, **ovarian cancer**, the middle and late stages of **bladder cancer**, and to control body cavity effusions, such as **pleural effusion** and **pericardial effusion**, that occur with some cancers. It is also sometimes used for the treatment of **Hodgkin's disease** and other lymph system cancers.

Description

Thiotepa was developed in the 1950s. It has been an approved cancer drug in the United States for over 20 years.

This drug is included in the cancer drug category termed **antineoplastic agents**, which slow or prevent the growth of cancerous tumors. Specifically, thiotepa is among a group of antineoplastic agents that were designed to alter the structure of the DNA in cells, causing a cell to die or to fail to replicate itself. These drugs do not distinguish between normal and cancerous cells and thus affect both equally.

Thiotepa is among several chemotherapy drugs being investigated for use in experimental high-dose chemotherapy, where a cancer patient is given a combination of several chemotherapy drugs at higher than normal dose levels. This treatment approach has been the focus of numerous **clinical trials**, most commonly for advanced breast cancer. One high-dose breast cancer chemotherapy treatment uses a combination of thiotepa, **cyclophosphamide**, and **carboplatin**. However, based on results from studies dating from 1999 to 2000, the effect of high-dose chemotherapy treatments, including those using thiotepa, have not conclusively improved the outcome or quality of life for breast cancer patients.

One approved chemotherapy treatment for advanced stages of breast cancer, where patients have not responded to other chemotherapy treatments or have experienced a relapse after a chemotherapy treatment, is a combination drug therapy of thiotepa, **doxorubicin**, and **vinblastine**. However, the results of this and other treatment options for late-stage breast cancer are not good. Treatment with a combination of chemotherapy drugs results in approximately 10% to 20% of patients showing no signs of cancer, and the duration of this response is usually less than 12 months.

Thiopeta is about as equally effective as the other chemotherapy drugs recommended for treating bladder cancer, including **mitomycin-C**, doxorubicin, ethoglucid, or **epirubicin**. Research results suggest that these drugs may reduce the chance for cancer recurrence but has little effect on reducing the **metastasis** of the disease. After surgical removal of a tumor, thiotepa has been shown to reduce the size of the remaining tumor in 29% of bladder cancer patients.

Body cavity effusions are a known complication for the advanced stages of many cancers, including lung cancer and breast cancer. Fluid in the heart cavity, or pericardial effusion, can be managed with the use of a procedure called a **pericardiocentesis** and the injection of thiotepa into the cavity. This treatment has been shown to result in the absence of pericardial effusion in approximately 70% to 90% of all cancer patients for at least 30 days. In a 1998 study of 23 cancer patients with pericardial effusion, 83% responded to this treatment, and the condition did not worsen for about nine months.

Recommended dosage

Patients are usually given thiotepa intravenously (directly into the vein) either as a rapid injection or through an intravenous (IV) infusion (drip). It can also be administered as an injection into a muscle or into the fluid that surrounds the spinal cord. For the treatment of body cavity effusions, it is injected through a tube into the site where this condition occurs. In bladder cancer patients, it is instilled directly into the bladder.

Each dosage is calculated based on a patient's weight at the start of each treatment. The correct dosage is carefully matched and adjusted to an individual's overall condition and response to the treatment. There is a range of doses for each method used to administer the drug, and the initial dose is usually the higher value in the range. How well the patient tolerates the treatment and the effectiveness of the dosage in treating the cancer will determine the final dosage on which the patient is maintained for the duration of the therapy.

When given intravenously, such as for breast or ovarian cancer, the initial dose is 0.4 milligram per kilogram (mg/kg) of body weight. Once the best dose for an individual patient is determined, it is given every one to four weeks.

For bladder cancer patients, an initial treatment of 60 mg of thiotepa that has been dissolved in 60 milliliters (ml) of sodium chloride is instilled directly into the bladder. If a patient has difficulty retaining this volume for two hours, the dose is reduced to 30 ml. The typical treatment cycle is once a week over a four-week period.

The dosage of thiotepa for the treatment of effusion ranges from 0.6 to 0.8 mg/kg. The dosage and duration of treatment varies with the specific site of the condition, and can be as frequent as one to two times per week.

Because **myelosuppression** is a common reaction to this drug treatment, white blood cell and platelet counts are carefully monitored, usually weekly during the treatment and for three weeks after. This condition may limit the dose level that a patient can tolerate. If blood counts are below a certain level, treatment is either postponed or the dosage is decreased in the next treatment cycle.

Precautions

As with many chemotherapy drugs, **vaccines** should not be given to patients taking thiotepa, and patients should avoid contact with people who have recently taken the oral polio vaccine. Myelosuppression can increase the chance for **infection** and bleeding. Contact with people who have an infection should be avoided. To decrease the chance for bleeding, aspirin or aspirin-containing medicines should not be taken. High doses of thiotepa can lead to severe cases of myelosuppression and may increase a patient's chance for a later occurrence of leukemia.

Side effects

Myelosuppression, usually **neutropenia** (decrease of the infection-fighting white cells) or **thrombocytopenia** (decrease of the platelets responsible for blood clotting), is common and usually occurs one to three weeks after each treatment, but may last throughout the therapy. **Nausea and vomiting** are uncommon and are most likely to occur six to twelve hours after the drug is given. Dizziness or a mild headache can occur within the first few hours after a treatment. **Anorexia**, **stomatitis**, **diarrhea**, infertility, **fever**, and **alopecia** are uncommon. Severe myelosuppression, stomatitis, **memory change**, and problems with thinking or speaking may result from high dose treatments. Side effects for bladder cancer treatment can include pain when urinating, blood in the urine, or inflammation of the bladder.

Coping with side effects may require making some life-style changes or in some cases, such as **nausea**, taking medication. Treatment options for side effects should be discussed with a doctor.

According to reports, Thiotepa conditioning regimen in patients with advanced hematologic neoplasms is associated with renal and hepatic toxicity. Relapse of hematologic malignancies after allogeneic stem cell transplantation remains a common problem, in particular for patients who have advanced disease at the time of transplantation. Researchers concluded that this regimen requires modification to reduce toxicity.

Interactions

Thiotepa combined with nitrogen mustard chemotherapy drugs such as cyclophosphamide or combined with **radiation therapy** does not improve the response to this treatment and can intensify some side effects, such as myelosuppression and infertility.

See also Cancer genetics; Chemoprevention; DNA cytometry; Drug resistance.

Monica McGee, M.S.

Thoracentesis

Definition

Also known as pleural fluid analysis, thoracentesis is a procedure that removes an abnormal accumulation of fluid or air from the chest through a needle or tube.

QUESTIONS TO ASK THE DOCTOR

- How will thoracentesis benefit me?
- Will I have to have this procedure more than once?
- How soon after this procedure can I resume my normal activities?
- Will this procedure cure my problem?
- Will I require hospitalization?

Purpose

Thoracentesis can be performed as a diagnostic or treatment procedure. For diagnosis, only a small amount of fluid is removed for analysis. For treatment, larger amounts of air or fluid are removed to relieve symptoms.

The lungs are lined on the outside with two thin layers of tissue called pleura. The space between these two layers is called the pleural space. Normally, there is only a small amount of lubricating fluid in this space. Liquid and/or air accumulates in this space between the lungs and the ribs from many conditions. The liquid is called a **pleural effusion**; the air is called a pneumothorax. Most pleural effusions are complications emanating from metastatic malignancy, or the movement of **cancer** cells from one part of the body to another; these are known as malignant pleural effusions. Other causes include trauma, **infection**, congestive heart failure, liver disease, and renal disease. Most malignant pleural effusions are detected and controlled by thoracentesis.

Symptoms of a pleural effusion include shortness of breath, chest pain, **fever**, **weight loss**, cough, and edema. Removal of air is often an emergency procedure to prevent suffocation from pressure on the lungs. Negative air pressure within the chest cavity allows normal respiration. The accumulation of air or fluid within the pleural space can eliminate these normal conditions and disrupt breathing and the movement of air within the chest cavity. Fluid removal is performed to reduce the pressure in the pleural space and to analyze the liquid.

Thoracentesis often provides immediate abatement of symptoms. However, fluid often begins to re-accumulate. A majority of patients will ultimately

KEY TERMS

Axilla—Armpit.

Catheter—A tube that is moved through the body for removing or injecting fluids into body cavities.

Hypovolemic shock—Shock caused by a lack of circulating blood.

Osmotic pressure—The pressure in a liquid exerted by chemicals dissolved in it. It forces a balancing of water in proportion to the amount of dissolved chemicals in two compartments separated by a semi-permeable membrane.

Pleura—Two thin layers lining the lungs on the outside.

require additional therapy beyond a simple thoracentesis procedure.

Precautions

Thoracentesis should never be performed by inserting the needle through an area with an infection. An alternative site needs to be found in these cases. Before undergoing this procedure, a patient must make their doctor aware of any allergies, bleeding problems or use of anticoagulants, pregnancy, or possibility of pregnancy.

Description

Prior to thoracentesis, the location of the fluid is pinpointed through x ray, **computed tomography** (CT) scan, or ultrasound. Ultrasound and CT are more accurate methods when the effusion is small or walled off in a pocket (loculated). A sedative may be administered in some cases but is generally not recommended. Oxygen may be given to the patient.

The usual place to tap the chest is below the armpit (axilla) or in the back. Under sterile conditions and local anesthesia, a needle, a through-the-needle-catheter, or an over-the-needle catheter may be used to perform the procedure. Overall, the catheter techniques may be safer. Once fluid is withdrawn, it is sent to the laboratory for analysis. If the air or fluid continue to accumulate, a tube is left in place and attached to a one-way system so that it can drain without sucking air into the chest.

Preparation

Patients should check with their doctor about continuing or discontinuing the use of any medications (including over-the-counter drugs and herbal remedies). Unless otherwise instructed, patients should not eat or drink milk or alcohol for at least four hours before the procedure, but may drink clear fluids like water, pulp-free fruit juice, or tea until one hour before. Patients should not smoke for at least 24 hours prior to thoracentesis. To avoid injury to the lung, patients should not cough, breathe deeply, or move during this procedure.

Aftercare

After the tube is removed, **x rays** will determine if the effusion or air is reaccumulating, though some researchers and clinicians believe chest x rays do not need to be performed after routine thoracentesis.

Risks

Reaccumulation of fluid or air are possible complications, as are hypovolemic shock (shock caused by a lack of circulating blood) and infection. Patients are at increased risk for poor outcomes if they have a recent history of anticoagulant use, have very small effusions, have significant amounts of fluid, have poor health leading into this condition, have positive airway pressure, or have adhesions in the pleural space. A pneumothorax can sometimes be caused by the thoracentesis procedure. The use of ultrasound to guide the procedure can reduce the risk of pneumothorax.

Thoracentesis can also result in hemothorax, or bleeding within the thorax. In addition, internal structures, such as the lung, diaphragm, spleen, or liver, can be damaged by needle insertion. Repeat thoracenteses can increase the risk of developing hypoproteinemia (a decrease in the amount of protein in the blood).

Resources

BOOKS

Abeloff, Martin D., et al., editors. *Clinical Oncology*. New York: Churchill Livingstone, 2000.

Celli, R. Bartolome. "Diseases of the Diaphragm, Chest Wall, Pleura and Mediastinum." In *Cecil Textbook of Medicine*, edited by Claude J. Bennett. Philadelphia: W. B. Saunders, 2000.

PERIODICALS

Colt, Henri G. "Factors Contributing to Pneumothorax After Thoracentesis." *Chest* 117 (February 2000).

Petersen, W.G. "Limited Utility of Chest Radiograph After Thoracentesis." *Chest* 117 (April 2000): 1038–42.

J. Ricker Polsdorfer, M.D.
Mark A. Mitchell, M.D.

Thoracic surgery

Definition

Thoracic surgery is any surgery performed in the chest (thorax).

Purpose

The purpose of thoracic surgery is to treat diseased or injured organs in the thorax, including the esophagus (muscular tube that passes food to the stomach), trachea (windpipe that branches to form the right bronchus and the left bronchus), pleura (membranes that cover and protect the lung), mediastinum (area separating the left and right lungs), chest wall, diaphragm, heart, and lungs.

General thoracic surgery is a field that specializes in diseases of the lungs and esophagus. The field also encompasses accidents and injuries to the chest, esophageal disorders (**esophageal cancer** or esophagitis), lung **cancer**, lung transplantation, and surgery for emphysema.

Description

The most common diseases requiring thoracic surgery include lung cancer, chest trauma, esophageal cancer, emphysema, and lung transplantation.

Lung cancer

Lung cancer is one of the most significant public health problems in the world. Approximately 213,380 new cases of lung and bronchial cancer occurred in 2007. It is the leading cause of cancer deaths among both men and women, killing more than 160,390 people annually. The overall five-year survival rate for all types of lung cancer is about 15.5%, as compared to 64.8% for **colon cancer**, 89% for **breast cancer**, and 99.9% for **prostate cancer**.

Lung cancer develops primarily by exposure to toxic chemicals. Cigarette smoking is the most important risk factor responsible for the disease. Other environmental factors that may predispose a person to lung cancer include industrial substances such as arsenic, nickel, chromium, asbestos, radon, organic chemicals, air pollution, and radiation.

Most cases of lung cancer develop in the right lung because it contains the majority (55%) of lung tissue. Additionally, lung cancer occurs more frequently in the upper lobes of the lung than in the lower lobes. The tumor receives blood from the bronchial artery (a major artery in the pulmonary system).

Adenocarcinoma of the lung is the most frequent type of lung cancer, accounting for 45% of all cases. This type of cancer can spread (metastasize) earlier than another type of lung cancer called squamous cell **carcinoma** (which occurs in approximately 30% of lung cancer patients). Approximately 66% of squamous cell carcinoma cases are centrally located. They expand against the bronchus, causing compression. Small-cell carcinoma accounts for 20% of all lung cancers; the majority (80%) are centrally located. Small-cell carcinoma is a highly aggressive lung cancer, with early **metastasis** to distant sites such as the brain and bone marrow (the central portion of certain bones, which produce formed elements that are part of blood).

Most lung tumors are not treated with thoracic surgery since patients seek medical care later in the disease process. **Chemotherapy** increases the rate of survival in patients with limited (not advanced) disease. Surgery may be useful for staging or diagnosis. Pulmonary resection (removal of the tumor and neighboring lymph nodes) can be curative if the tumor is less than or equal to 1.8 in (3 cm), and presents as a solitary nodule. Lung tumors spread to other areas through neighboring lymphatic channels. Even if thoracic surgery is performed, postoperative chemotherapy may also be indicated to provide comprehensive treatment (i.e., to kill any tumor cells that may have spread via the lymphatic system).

Genetic engineering has provided insights related to the growth of tumors. A genetic mutation called a k-ras mutation frequently occurs, and is implicated in 90% of genetic mutations for adenocarcinoma of the lung. Mutations in the cancer cells make them resistant to chemotherapy, necessitating the use of multiple chemotherapeutic agents.

Chest trauma

Chest trauma is a medical/surgical emergency. Initially, the chest should be examined after an airway is maintained. The mortality (death) rate for trauma patients with respiratory distress is approximately 50%. This figure rises to 75% if symptoms include both respiratory distress and shock. Patients with respiratory distress require endotracheal intubation (passing a plastic tube from the mouth to the windpipe) and mechanically assisted ventilator support. Invasive thoracic procedures are necessary in emergency situations.

Trauma requiring urgent thoracic surgery may include any of the following problems: a large clotted hemothorax, massive air leak, esophageal injury, valvular cardiac (heart) injury, proven damage to blood vessels in the heart, or chest wall defect.

Esophageal cancer

The number of new cases of esophageal cancer is slowly rising, with about 14,500 people diagnosed annually. While the cause of esophageal cancer is not precisely known, the greatly increased rate of esophageal cancer seems to be tied to the epidemic of obesity in the United States. Obesity results in acid reflux into the esophagus, chronic esophageal irritation, and progression to abnormal cell types that result in esophageal cancer, specifically of adenocarinoma of the esophagus. Smoking and alcohol seem to also result in chronic esophageal irritation, leading to an association with squamous cell carcinoma of the esophagus.

Difficulty swallowing (dysphagia) is the cardinal symptom of esophageal cancer. Radiography, endoscopy, computerized axial tomography (CT scan), and **ultrasonography** are part of a comprehensive diagnostic evaluation. The standard operation for patients with resectable esophageal carcinoma includes removal of the tumor from the esophagus, a portion of the stomach, and the lymph nodes (within the cancerous region).

Emphysema

Lung volume reduction surgery (LVRS) is the term used to describe surgery for patients with emphysema. LVRS is intended to help persons whose disabling dyspnea (difficulty breathing) is related to emphysema and does not respond to medical management. Breathlessness is a result of the structural and functional pulmonary and thoracic abnormalities associated with emphysema. Surgery will assist the patient, but the primary pathogenic process that caused the emphysema is permanent because lung tissues lose the capability of elastic recoil during normal breathing (inspiration and expiration).

Patients are usually transferred out of the intensive care unit (ICU) within one day of surgery. Physical therapy and rehabilitation (coughing and breathing exercises) begin soon after surgery, and the patient is discharged when deemed clinically stable.

Lung transplantation

There are various types of lung transplantations: unilateral (one lung, the most common type); bilateral (both lungs); heart-lung; and living donor lobe transplantation.

The survival rate for persons receiving a single lung transplant is more than 82% at one year, almost 60% at three years, and more than 43% at five years. Double-lung transplants have similar success rates: 82% at one year, 64% at three years, and 48% at five years. A successful outcome is highly dependent on the patient's general medical condition. Those who have symptomatic osteoporosis (severe disease of the musculoskeletal system) or are users of **corticosteroids** may not have favorable outcomes.

The death rate occurs due to infections (pulmonary infections) or chronic rejection (bronchiolitis obliterans) if the donor lung was not a perfect genetic match. Patients are given postoperative **antibiotics** to prevent bacterial infections during the early period following surgery.

Bacterial **pneumonia** is usually severe. A bacterial genus known as *Pseudomonas* accounts for 75% of post-transplant pneumonia cases. Patients can also acquire viral and fungal infections, and an **infection** caused by a cell parasite known as *Pneumocystis carinii.* Infections are treated with specific medications intended to destroy the invading microorganism. Viral infections require treatment of symptoms.

Acute (quick onset) rejection is common within the first weeks after lung transplantation. Acute rejection is treated with steroids (bolus given intravenously), and is effective in 80% of cases. Chronic rejection is the most common problem, and typically begins with symptoms of **fatigue** and a vague feeling of illness. Treatment is difficult, and the results are unrewarding. There are several immunosuppressive protocols currently utilized for cases of chronic rejection. The goal of immunosuppressive therapy is to prevent the host's immune reaction from destroying the genetically foreign organ.

Diagnosis/Preparation

The surgeon may use two common incisional approaches: sternotomy (incision through and down the breastbone) or via the side of the chest (**thoracotomy**).

An operative procedure known as video-assisted thoracoscopic surgery (VATS) is minimally invasive. During VATS, a lung is collapsed and the thoracoscope and surgical instruments are inserted into the thorax through any of three or four small incisions in the chest wall.

Another approach involves the use of a mediastinoscope or bronchoscope to visualize the internal anatomical structures during thoracic surgery or diagnostic procedures.

WHO PERFORMS THE PROCEDURE AND WHERE IS IT PERFORMED?

Thoracic surgery is performed in a hospital by a specialist in general surgery who has received advanced training in thoracic surgery.

Preoperative evaluation for most patients (except emergency cases) must include cardiac tests, blood chemistry analysis, and physical examination. Like most operative procedures, the patient should not eat or drink food 10–12 hours prior to surgery. Patients who undergo thoracic surgery with the video-assisted approach tend to have shorter inpatient hospital stays.

Aftercare

Patients typically experience severe pain after surgery, and are given appropriate pain medications. In uncomplicated cases, chest and urine (Foley catheter) tubes are usually removed within 24–48 hours. A highly trained and comprehensive team of respiratory therapists and nurses is vital for postoperative care that results in improved lung function via deep breathing and coughing exercises.

Risks

Precautions for thoracic surgery include coagulation blood disorders (disorders that prevent normal blood clotting) and previous thoracic surgery. Risks include hemorrhage, myocardial infarction (heart attack), stroke, nerve injury, embolism (blood clot or air bubble that obstructs an artery), and infection. Total lung collapse can occur from fluid or air accumulation, as a result of chest tubes that are routinely placed after surgery for drainage.

Resources

BOOKS

Abeloff, M. D., et al. *Clinical Oncology*, 3rd ed. Philadelphia: Elsevier, 2004.

Khatri, V. P., and J. A. Asensio. *Operative Surgery Manual*, 1st ed. Philadelphia: Saunders, 2003.

Libby, P., et al. *Braunwald's Heart Disease*, 8th ed. Philadelphia: Saunders, 2007.

Marx, John A., et al. *Rosen's Emergency Medicine*, 6th ed. St. Louis, MO: Mosby, Inc., 2006.

Mason, R. J., et al. *Murray & Nadel's Textbook of Respiratory Medicine*, 4th ed. Philadelphia: Saunders, 2007.

Townsend, C. M., et al. *Sabiston Textbook of Surgery*, 17th ed. Philadelphia: Saunders, 2004.

PERIODICALS

Krupnick, A. S. "Operative Thoracic Surgery," 5th ed. *Journal of the American College of Surgery* 204, no. 5 (May 2007).

Ng, T. "Evolution to video-assisted thoracic surgery lobectomy after training: Initial results of the first 30 patients." *Journal of the American College of Surgery* 203, no. 4 (October 2006).

ORGANIZATIONS

American Association for Thoracic Surgery. 900 Cummings Center, Suite 221-U, Beverly, MA 01915. (978) 927-8330. Fax: (978) 524-8890. E-mail: aats@prri.com.

Laith Farid Gulli, MD, MS
Abraham F. Ettaher, MD
Nicole Mallory, MS, PA-C

Thoracoscopy

Definition

Thoracoscopy is the insertion of an endoscope, a narrow diameter tube with a viewing mirror or camera attachment, through a very small incision (cut) in the chest wall.

Purpose

Thoracoscopy makes it possible for a physician to examine the lungs or other structures in the chest cavity, without making a large incision. It is an alternative to **thoracotomy** (opening the chest cavity with a large incision). Many surgical procedures, especially taking tissue samples (biopsies), can also be accomplished with thoracoscopy. The procedure is done to:

- assess lung cancer
- take a biopsy for study
- determine the cause of fluid in the chest cavity
- introduce medications or other treatments directly into the lungs
- treat accumulated fluid, pus (empyema), or blood in the space around the lungs

For many patients, thoracoscopy replaces thoracotomy. It avoids many of the complications of open chest surgery and reduces pain, hospital stay, and recovery time.

Precautions

Because one lung is partially deflated during thoracoscopy, the procedure cannot be done on patients whose lung function is so poor that they do not receive

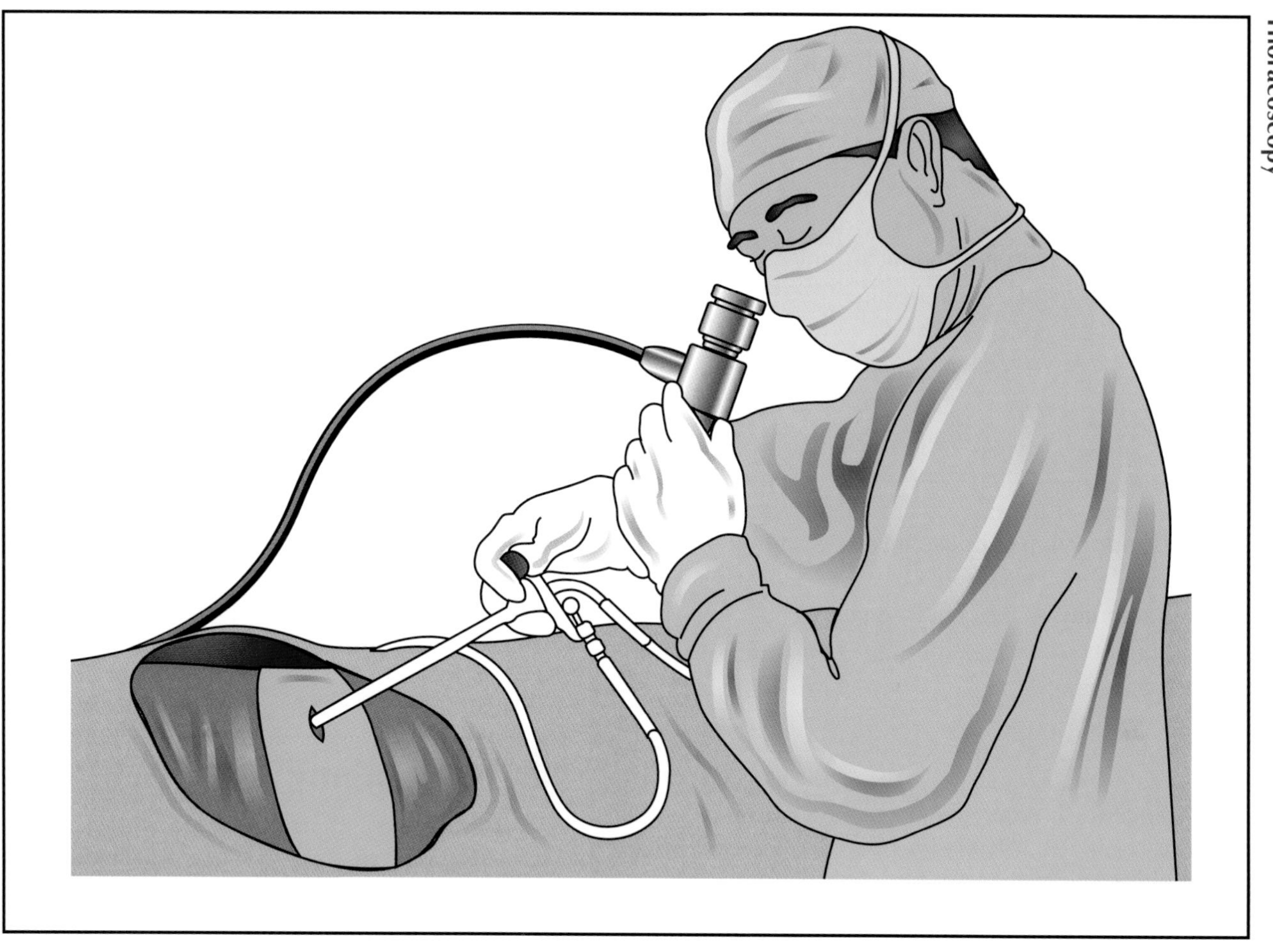

Thoracoscopy is a procedure in which a physician can view the chest cavity and the lungs by inserting an endoscope through the chest wall. Thoracoscopy is less invasive than surgical lung biopsy. *(Illustration by Electronic Illustrators Group. Cengage Learning, Gale).*

enough oxygen with only one lung. Patients who have had previous surgery that involved the chest cavity, or who have blood-clotting problems, are not good candidates for this procedure.

Thoracoscopy gives physicians a good but limited view of the organs, such as lungs, in the chest cavity. Endoscope technology is being refined every day, as is what physicians can accomplish by inserting scopes and instruments through several small incisions instead of making one large cut.

Description

Thoracoscopy is most commonly performed in a hospital, and general anesthesia is used. Some of the procedures are moving toward outpatient services and local anesthesia. More specific names are sometimes applied to the procedure, depending on what the target site of the effort is. For example, if a physician intends to examine the lungs, the procedure is often called pleuroscopy. The procedure takes two–four hours.

The surgeon makes two or three small incisions in the chest wall, often between the ribs. By making the incisions between the ribs, the surgeon minimizes damage to muscle and nerves and the ribs themselves. A tube is inserted in the trachea and connected to a ventilator, which is a mechanical device that assists the patient with inhaling and exhaling.

The most common reason for a thoracoscopy is to examine a lung that has a tumor or a metastatic growth of **cancer**. The lung to be examined is deflated to create a space between the chest wall and the lung. The patient breathes with the other lung with the assistance of the ventilator.

A specialized endoscope, or narrow diameter tube, with a video camera or mirrored attachment, is inserted through the chest wall. Instruments for taking necessary tissue samples are inserted through other

QUESTIONS TO ASK THE DOCTOR

- How soon will you know the results?
- When can I resume any medications that were stopped?
- When can I resume normal activities?
- What future care will I need?

KEY TERMS

Endoscope—Instrument designed to allow direct visual inspection of body cavities, a sort of microscope in a long access tube.

Thoracotomy—Open chest surgery.

Trachea—Tube of cartilage that carries air into and out of the lungs.

small incisions. After tissue samples are taken, the lung is re-inflated. All incisions, except one, are closed. The remaining open incision is used to insert a drainage tube. The tissue samples are sent to a laboratory for evaluation.

Preparation

Prior to thoracoscopy, the patient will have several routine tests, such as blood, urine, and chest x ray. Older patients must have an electrocardiogram (a trace of the heart activity) because the anesthesia and the lung deflation put a big load on the heart muscle. The patient should not eat or drink from midnight the night before the thoracoscopy. The anesthesia used can cause **vomiting**, and, because anesthesia also causes the loss of the gag reflex, a person who vomits is in danger of moving food into the lungs, which can cause serious complications and death.

Aftercare

After the procedure, a chest tube will remain in one of the incisions for several days to drain fluid and release residual air from the chest cavity. Hospital stays range from two to five days. Medications for pain are given as needed. After returning home, patients should do only light lifting for several weeks.

Risks

The main risks of thoracoscopy are those associated with the administration of general anesthesia. Sometimes excessive bleeding, or hemorrhage, occurs, necessitating a thoracotomy to stop it. Another risk comes when the drainage tube is removed, and the patient is vulnerable to lung collapse (pneumothorax).

Resources

PERIODICALS

Dardes, N., E.P. Graziani, I. Fleishman, and M. Papale. "Medical Thoracoscopy in Management of Pleural Effusions." *Chest* 118, no. 4 (October 2000): 129s.

Shawgo, T., T.M. Boley, and S. Hazelrigg."The Utility of Thoracoscopic Lung Biopsy for Diagnosis and Treatment." *Chest* 118, no. 4 (October 2000): 114s.

Tish Davidson, A.M.

Thoracotomy

Definition

Thoracotomy is the process of making of an incision (cut) into the chest wall.

Purpose

A physician gains access to the chest cavity (called the thorax) by cutting through the chest wall. Reasons for the entry are varied. Thoracotomy allows for study of the condition of the lungs; removal of a lung or part of a lung; removal of a rib; and examination, treatment, or removal of any organs in the chest cavity. Thoracotomy also provides access to the heart, esophagus, diaphragm, and the portion of the aorta that passes through the chest cavity.

Lung **cancer** is the most common cancer requiring a thoracotomy. Tumors and metastatic growths can be removed through the incision (a procedure called resection). A **biopsy**, or tissue sample, can also be taken through the incision, and examined under a microscope for evidence of abnormal cells.

A resuscitative or emergency thoracotomy may be performed to resuscitate a patient who is near death as a result of a chest injury. An emergency thoracotomy provides access to the chest cavity to control injury-related bleeding from the heart, cardiac compressions to restore a normal heart rhythm, or to relieve pressure on the heart caused by cardiac tamponade

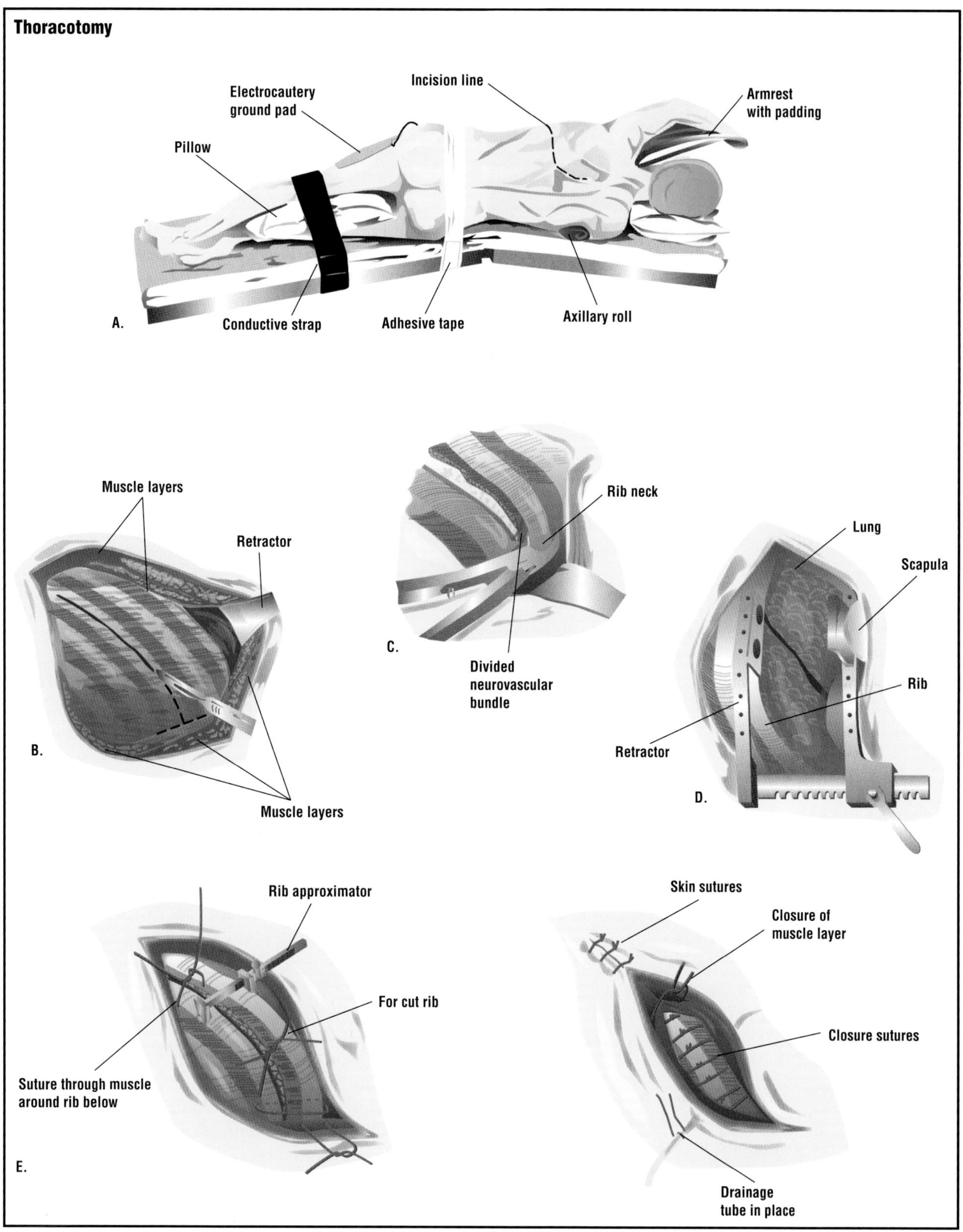

For a thoracotomy, the patient lies on his or her side with one arm raised (A). An incision is cut into the skin of the ribcage (B). Muscle layers are cut, and a rib may be removed to gain access to the cavity. (C). Retractors hold the ribs apart, exposing the lung (D). After any repairs are made, the cut rib is replaced and held in place with special materials (E). Layers of muscle and skin are stitched. *(Illustration by GGS Information Services. Cengage Learning, Gale.)*

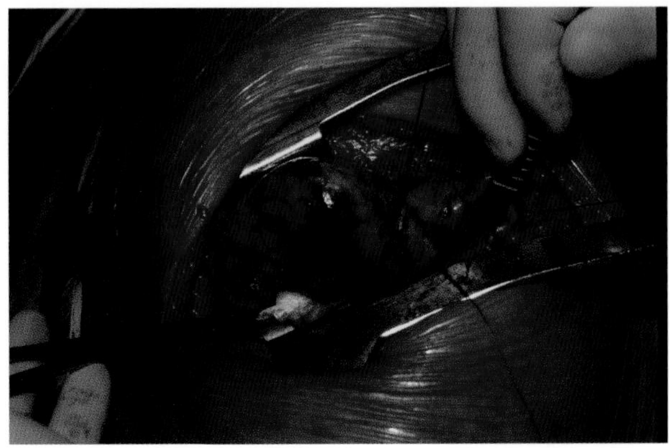

Thoracotomy for left upper lobectomy. The cancer is visible just above the sponge stick. *(Custom Medical Stock Photo. Reproduced by permission.)*

KEY TERMS

Aorta—The major artery carrying blood away from the heart.

Catheter—A tube inserted into a body cavity to drain fluid. An example would be a urinary catheter used to drain urine from the urethra.

Diaphragm—The large flat muscle that runs horizontally across the bottom of the chest cavity.

Esophagus—The muscular tube that connects the mouth and the stomach.

Trachea—The tube made of cartilage that carries air from the nose and mouth to the lungs.

Urethra—The tube that carries urine from the bladder to the outside of the body.

(accumulation of fluid in the space between the heart's muscle and outer lining).

Demographics

Thoracotomy may be performed to diagnose or treat a variety of conditions; therefore, no data exist as to the overall incidence of the procedure. Lung cancer, a common reason for thoracotomy, is diagnosed in approximately over 196,000 people each year and affects more men than women (108,355 diagnoses in men compared to 87,897 in women).

Description

The thoracotomy incision may be made on the side, under the arm (axillary thoracotomy); on the front, through the breastbone (median sternotomy); slanting from the back to the side (posterolateral thoracotomy); or under the breast (anterolateral thoracotomy). The exact location of the cut depends on the reason for the surgery. In some cases, the physician is able to make the incision between ribs (called an intercostal approach) to minimize cuts through bone, nerves, and muscle. The incision may range from just under 5–10 in (12.7–25 cm).

During the surgery, a tube is passed through the trachea. It usually has a branch to each lung. One lung is deflated for examination and surgery, while the other one is inflated with the assistance of a mechanical device (a ventilator).

A number of different procedures may be commenced at this point. A **lobectomy** removes an entire lobe or section of a lung (the right lung has three lobes and the left lung has two). It may be done to remove cancer that is contained by a lobe. A **segmentectomy**, or wedge resection, removes a wedge-shaped piece of lung smaller than a lobe. Alternatively, the entire lung may be removed during a **pneumonectomy**.

In the case of an emergency thoracotomy, the procedure performed depends on the type and extent of injury. The heart may be exposed so that direct cardiac compressions can be performed; the physician may use one hand or both hands to manually pump blood through the heart. Internal paddles of a defibrillating machine may be applied directly to the heart to restore normal cardiac rhythms. Injuries to the heart causing excessive bleeding (hemorrhaging) may be closed with staples or stitches.

Once the procedure that required the incision is completed, the chest wall is closed. The layers of skin, muscle, and other tissues are closed with stitches or staples. If the breastbone was cut (as in the case of a median sternotomy), it is stitched back together with wire.

Diagnosis/Preparation

Patients are told not to eat after midnight the night before surgery. They must tell their physicians about all known allergies so that the safest anesthetics can be selected. Older patients must be evaluated for heart ailments before surgery because of the additional strain on the heart.

Aftercare

Opening the chest cavity means cutting through skin, muscle, nerves, and sometimes bone. It is a major procedure that often involves a hospital stay of five to

WHO PERFORMS THE PROCEDURE AND WHERE IS IT PERFORMED?

Thoracotomy may be performed by a thoracic surgeon, a medical doctor who has completed surgical training in the areas of general surgery and surgery of the chest area, or an emergency room physician (in the case of emergency thoracotomy). The procedure is generally performed in a hospital operating room, although emergency thoracotomies may be performed in an emergency department or trauma center.

seven days. The skin around the drainage tube to the thoracic cavity must be kept clean, and the tube must be kept unblocked.

The pressure differences that are set up in the thoracic cavity by the movement of the diaphragm (the large muscle at the base of the thorax) make it possible for the lungs to expand and contract. If the pressure in the chest cavity changes abruptly, the lungs can collapse. Any fluid that collects in the cavity puts a patient at risk for **infection** and reduced lung function, or even collapse (called a pneumothorax). Thus, any entry to the chest usually requires that a chest tube remain in place for several days after the incision is closed.

The first two days after surgery may be spent in the intensive care unit (ICU) of the hospital. A variety of tubes, catheters, and monitors may be required after surgery.

Risks

The rich supply of blood vessels to the lungs makes hemorrhage a risk; a blood transfusion may become necessary during surgery. General anesthesia carries risks such as **nausea**, **vomiting**, headache, blood pressure issues, or allergic reaction. After a thoracotomy, there may be drainage from the incision. There is also the risk of infection; the patient must learn how to keep the incision clean and dry as it heals.

After the chest tube is removed, the patient is vulnerable to pneumothorax. Physicians strive to reduce the risk of collapse by timing the removal of the tube. Doing so at the end of inspiration (breathing in) or the end of expiration (breathing out) poses less risk. Deep breathing exercises and coughing should be emphasized as an important way that patients can improve healing and prevent **pneumonia**.

QUESTIONS TO ASK THE DOCTOR

Why is thoracotomy being recommended?

What diagnostic tests will be performed to determine if thoracotomy is necessary?

What type of incision will be used and where will it be located?

What type of procedure will be performed?

How long is the recovery time and what is expected during this period?

If a biopsy is the only reason for the procedure, is a thoracoscopy or a guided needle biopsy an option (instead of thoracotomy)?

Normal results

The results following thoracotomy depend on the reasons why it was performed. If a biopsy was taken during the surgery, a normal result would indicate that no cancerous cells are present in the tissue sample. The procedure may indicate that further treatment is necessary; for example, if cancer was detected, **chemotherapy**, **radiation therapy**, or more surgery may be recommended.

Morbidity and mortality

One study following lung cancer patients undergoing thoracotomy found that 10–15% of patients experienced heartbeat irregularities, readmittance to the ICU, or partial or full lung collapse; 5–10% experienced pneumonia or extended use of the ventilator (greater than 48 hours); and up to 5% experienced wound infection, accumulation of pus in the chest cavity, or blood clots in the lung. The mortality rate in the study was 5.8%, with patients dying as a result of the cancer itself or of postoperative complications.

Alternatives

Video-assisted **thoracic surgery** (VATS) is a less invasive alternative to thoracotomy. Also called **thoracoscopy**, VATS involves the insertion of a thoracoscope (a thin, lighted tube) into a small incision through the chest wall. The surgeon can visualize the structures inside the chest cavity on a video screen. Instruments such as a stapler or grasper may be inserted through other small incisions. Although initially used as a diagnostic tool (to visualize the lungs or to remove a sample of lung tissue for further examination), VATS is being increasingly used to remove some lung tumors, and is usually appropriate for those under 2.4 in (6 cm). In some practices, as many as 8% of all lobectomies are now performed using VATS technique.

An alternative to emergency thoracotomy is a tube thoracostomy, a tube placed through the chest wall to drain excess fluid. Over 80% of patients with a penetrating chest wound can be successfully managed with a thoracostomy.

Resources

BOOKS

Khatri, V. P., and J. A. Asensio. *Operative Surgery Manual*, 1st ed. Philadelphia: Saunders, 2003.

Mason, R. J., et al. *Murray & Nadel's Textbook of Respiratory Medicine*, 4th ed. Philadelphia: Saunders, 2007.

Townsend, C. M., et al. *Sabiston Textbook of Surgery*, 17th ed. Philadelphia: Saunders, 2004.

PERIODICALS

Blewett, C. J., et al. "Open Lung Biopsy as an Outpatient Procedure." *Annals of Thoracic Surgery* (April 2001): 1113–1115.

Handy, John R., et al. "What Happens to Patients Undergoing Lung Cancer Surgery? Outcomes and Quality of Life Before and After Surgery." *Chest* 122, no.1 (August 14, 2002): 21–30.

Swanson, Scott J. and Hasan F. Batirel. "Video-Assisted Thoracic Surgery (VATS) Resection for Lung Cancer." *Surgical Clinics of North America* 82, no.3 (June 1, 2002): 541–9.

ORGANIZATIONS

American Cancer Society. 1599 Clifton Rd. NE, Atlanta, GA 30329-4251. (800) 227-2345. http://www.cancer.org (accessed April 10, 2008).

Society of Thoracic Surgeons. 663 N. Saint Clair St., Suite 2320, Chicago, IL 60611-3658. (312) 202-5800. http://www.sts.org (accessed April 10, 2008).

OTHER

"Detailed Guide: Lung Cancer." *American Cancer Society* [cited April 28, 2003]. http://www.cancer.org/docroot/CRI/CRI_2_3x.asp?dt=15 (accessed April 10, 2008).

Diane M. Calabrese
Stephanie Dionne Sherk

Thrombocytopenia

Description

Thrombocytopenia (thrombocythemia) is a blood disorder characterized by an abnormally low number of circulating platelets (thrombocytes) in the bloodstream. Because platelets play an important role in the process of coagulation (blood clotting) and in the plugging of damaged blood vessels, persons with decreased platelets bruise easily and can have episodes of excessive bleeding (hemorrhage). Thrombocytopenia is usually an acquired disorder, but it can also be congenital, as in neonatal rubella (German measles).

Platelets are irregular, disc-shaped fragments of large cells called megakaryocytes, which are found in the spongy center of long bones (bone marrow). They are the smallest cell-like structures in the blood. When a blood vessel is punctured or damaged, normal mature platelets have a tendency to aggregate (group) together at the site, forming a plug that stops the bleeding. The lifespan of platelets in the blood is relatively short (five to ten days), so the bone marrow of healthy individuals is continually producing new platelets to replace the old ones.

Doctors usually use a combination of the physical examination, the medical history, and laboratory testing to diagnose this disorder. The platelet count, which is part of a complete blood count (CBC), is a key diagnostic tool. It measures the number of platelets in a volume of blood. The blood normally contains between 150,000 and 400,000 platelets per microliter (cubic millimeter or mm^3) of blood. (A million microliters is equal to one liter, or about 1.1 quarts.) In adults, a platelet count of less than 100,000/microliter is considered low, but might occur without symptoms. Abnormal bleeding often occurs when the platelet count is below 30,000/microliter. If the count falls below 10,000/microliter, abnormal external bleeding is usually evident, and serious internal bleeding can be life threatening.

Causes

Thrombocytopenia occurs when any of the following abnormal conditions exist:

- decreased production of platelets by the bone marrow
- increased destruction of circulating platelets
- increased trapping of platelets by the spleen
- platelet loss from hemorrhage

The most common cause of thrombocytopenia is a decrease in the production of platelets by the bone marrow. When abnormalities develop in the bone marrow, the megakaryocytes (platelet precursors) can lose their ability to produce platelets in sufficient amounts. This is a common side effect of blood cancers such as leukemia, which causes an abnormal growth of white blood cells in the bone marrow. These abnormal cells crowd out the normal bone marrow cells, including the platelets. Other diseases that cause this condition are tumors that spread (metastasize) to the bone, aplastic **anemia**, and viral infections such as rubella. Radiation and drugs used in **cancerchemotherapy** and in the treatment of other serious diseases can also cause the bone marrow to malfunction in this way, especially if they are used together. Some drugs, such as aspirin or **heparin**, do not actually cause a decrease in the number of platelets, but they destroy the functional ability of the platelets to aggregate.

Platelets can break down in unusually high amounts in persons with abnormalities in their blood vessel walls, with blood clots, or with man-made replacement heart valves. Devices (stents) placed inside blood vessels to keep them from closing (because of weakened walls or fat build-up) can also cause an increased destruction of platelets. In addition, severe microbial infections, **infection** with the human immunodeficiency virus (HIV)—the virus that causes AIDS—and other changes in the immune system can speed up the removal of platelets from the circulation.

Normally, the spleen holds about one-third of the body's platelets as part of this organ's function to recycle certain aging or damaged blood cells. When liver disease or cancer of the spleen is present, the spleen can become enlarged (a condition called splenomegaly) and trap many more platelets than normal. Because a greater number of platelets remain in the enlarged organ, fewer platelets are circulating in the bloodstream.

Treatments

Sometimes this disorder is asymptomatic and does not require any treatment. This is often the case when thrombocytopenia occurs in children following a viral infection. Even when the disorder is a side effect of both **radiation therapy** and chemotherapy, if the thrombocytopenia is not severe, it is often reversible on its own once the therapies end.

Treatments, when necessary, vary with the severity of the disorder, the abnormal condition that caused the disorder, and any underlying or secondary cause. When possible, the best form of treatment is to eliminate whatever is causing the condition. For example, if a drug is causing the thrombocytopenia, eliminating that drug would be the ideal solution. However, when the disorder is a side effect of chemotherapy, the patient might need to continue the drug therapy. In such cases, the doctor must decide whether it is in the best interest of the patient to continue with the same dosage, to lower the dosage, to try an alternative drug, or to give the patient a platelet transfusion. For diseases other than blood cancers, doctors can sometimes continue the chemotherapy at full dosage by also giving the patient a platelet growth factor called **Oprelvekin** (marketed as Neumega) to boost the production of normal platelets in the bone marrow.

If a dysfunctional immune system is destroying the patient's platelets, the doctor might use a corticosteroid (such as prednisone) or gamma globulin to suppress the patient's **immune response** and to help maintain adequate platelet levels. **Corticosteroids** can also have unwanted side effects, so doctors usually do not use this treatment for very long.

If an enlarged spleen is the underlying cause of the thrombocytopenia, the doctor might want to try corticosteroids or epinephrine to release platelets from the spleen. If these methods fail, surgical removal of the spleen (**splenectomy**) can help to raise the platelet level since the spleen is no longer there to capture the platelets. However, the disease that caused the enlarged spleen, such as **lymphoma** or cancer that spread to the spleen from another area of the body, should be treated as well.

If the patient is having severe external or internal bleeding as the result of injury or disease, a platelet transfusion might be necessary for immediate results. This is especially true if laboratory tests show a decreased production of platelets in the bone marrow.

Alternative and complementary therapies

A natural substance called **thrombopoietin** shows promise as a regulator of platelet production.

Many over-the-counter medicines, herbal supplements (such as garlic, ginger, feverfew, and ginko biloba) and **vitamins** can affect the ability of platelets to function properly. To determine the best treatment for a patient and to avoid drug interactions, the doctor needs to know every drug and remedy a patient is taking.

Resources

BOOKS

Altman, Roberta, and Michael J. Sarg. *The Cancer Dictionary*, rev. ed. New York: Checkmark Books, 2000.

Komaroff, Anthony L. *Harvard Medical School Family Health Guide*. New York: Simon & Schuster, 1999.

PERIODICALS

Henderson, C.W. "Study Results Suggest Hope for Previously Untreatable Patients." *Blood Weekly* 16 November 2000: 20.

OTHER

"Side Effect Management Series: Low Blood Platelets (Thrombocytopenia)." *Oncology.com*. 2001. [cited June 28, 2001]. http://www.oncology.com.

Beverly Miller, MT(ASCP)
Dominic De Bellis

Thrombopoietin

Definition

Thrombopoietin is an investigational or experimental drug that may increase the number of platelets in the bloodstream.

Purpose

Thrombopoietin is an experimental drug that may be used to treat **thrombocytopenia** (a reduced number of platelets in the blood).

Description

Thrombocytopenia, or a low number of platelets in the blood, can be a life-threatening condition. Platelets are necessary for the normal process of blood clotting. When someone experiences thrombocytopenia, a cut or bruise might not heal quickly, or at all, without medical intervention. Therefore, patients with a low platelet cell count must take special precautions, and suffer significant risk.

Thrombocytopenia is a common side effect from many common **chemotherapy** agents. These agents temporarily decrease the production of platelets, as well as white blood cells that fight **infection** and red blood cells that carry oxygen. **Carboplatin** is an example of an agent that has a tendency to lower platelet counts. Like other cells of the blood (white blood cells and red blood cells), the number of platelets will generally increase and return to normal over days and weeks following the administration of chemotherapy.

By reducing the severity of platelet-related side effects, thrombopoietin could allow the antitumor medication to be used at higher doses and/or for longer periods of time. Thrombopoietin may also be used in other situations in which patients have low platelet cell counts.

Thrombopoietin is derived from the gene of the same name. A laboratory-synthesized version of the human gene product encourages the development of platelet cells from precursor cells in the blood.

KEY TERMS

Investigational drug—A drug that has not been approved for marketing by the FDA. These drugs are generally available to patients through participation in clinical trials/research studies.

Thrombocytopenia—A condition characterized by a reduced number of platelets in the blood.

Thrombopoietin is an investigational, or an experimental, drug in the U.S. Generally, **investigational drugs** are made available through participation in **clinical trials**.

Recommended dosage, precautions, side effects, and interactions

As noted above, investigational drugs generally are prescribed as part of a clinical trial. Clinical trials seek to determine how effective a drug is at treating the targeted condition, the effective dose of the drug, any precautions patients should take before the drug is administered, any side effects the drug may have, and any interactions the investigational drug may have with other drugs. Since thrombopoietin is investigational, it is premature to discuss dosage, precautions, side effects, and interactions.

Michael Zuck, Ph.D.

Thrush

Description

Thrush (Candidiasis) is a superficial yeast **infection** of the mouth and throat. Other names for this common condition include oral candidiasis, oropharyngeal candidiasis, pseudomembranous candidiasis, and mycotic **stomatitis**. Thrush is characterized by the presence of thick, curd-like white patches on the tongue and inside of the cheeks. The underlying tissue is red and inflamed. The roof and floor of the mouth and the gums may also be affected. Thrush may be easily diagnosed by the appearance of the lesion. To confirm the diagnosis, a sample for microscopic analysis may be taken by scraping the lesion with a tongue depressor.

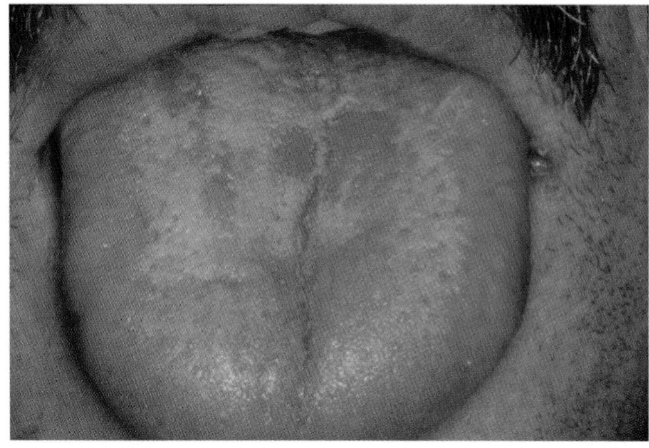

This patient's tongue is infected with oral candidiasis, or thrush. *(Photograph by Edward H. Gill. Custom Medical Stock Photo. Reproduced by permission.)*

Thrush itself is a harmless infection; however, *Candida* may spread throughout the body (systemic infection) to the kidneys, lungs, joints, bones, and brain and spinal cord (central nervous system). A systemic infection can be very serious, especially in a **cancer** patient with a weakened immune system.

Causes

Thrush may be caused by several different species of *Candida*. Thrush rarely occurs in healthy persons. Three factors contribute to infection *Candida*: impairment of the immune system (immunosuppression), injury to the tissues (mucosa, mucous membranes) of the mouth, and decrease in saliva flow. In addition, thrush can occur following treatment with **antibiotics**, when normal mouth (oral) bacteria have been eliminated allowing for overgrowth of *Candida*. In addition to standard intravenous chemotherapeutic agents, **corticosteroids**, **cyclosporine** A, and interleukin-2 (**aldesleukin**) suppress the immune system, placing the patient at a higher risk of infection. Patients who have been treated with myeloablative therapy, as in preparation for **bone marrow transplantation**, are at a very high risk of infection. In addition, certain cancers predispose the patient to developing candidiasis, including **multiple myeloma**, **chronic lymphocytic leukemia**, **hairy cell leukemia**, **Hodgkin's disease**, and **adrenal tumors**. Malnutrition, which is not uncommon among cancer patients, also suppresses the immune system.

Patients undergoing **chemotherapy** and/or head and neck radiation are at an increased risk of developing thrush. These therapies target the rapidly dividing cancer cells.The mucosal cells which line the mouth are also rapidly dividing. The skin and mucous membranes make up the first line of defense against invading organisms and, when damaged by cancer treatments, these tissues become susceptible to infection. Chemotherapy can decrease the number of neutrophils, a type of white blood cell, causing a condition called **neutropenia**. Neutropenia significantly increases the patient's risk of infection. **Radiation therapy** reduces the number of white blood cells which impairs the immune system.

Thrush is a temporary side effect of cancer treatment. It can take up to a year for the immune system to recover from intensive radiation therapy. Thrush that is related to the cancer may be persistent or recurrent.

Treatments

Thrush is usually treated with the antifungal drugs clotrimazole, nystatin, or amphotericin. Clotrimazole is taken as a lozenge which is allowed to dissolve slowly in the mouth. The commonly used nystatin is taken as a solution that is swished through the mouth, although recent studies have shown that nystatin may not be as effective as the newer antifungals. Amphotericin is taken as a tablet or solution. The duration of treatment may range from five to 14 days. Often, thrush resolves with local treatment alone, however, systemic medication (such as fluconazole) may be used in some cases.

The patient with thrush should faithfully conduct a daily oral hygiene routine consisting of tooth brushing two to three times, flossing once, utilizing medicated rinses as prescribed by the physician. Brushing and flossing should be performed carefully to prevent damage to the weakened oral mucosa. Dentures and other mouth appliances, which can harbor the yeast and be a source for possible reinfection, need to be disinfected.

Alternative and complementary therapies

Because there is the risk that *Candida* may spread and cause a serious systemic infection, thrush should be treated with antifungal drugs. The patient with thrush can help fight the infection by eating a well-balanced diet to counteract immunosuppression caused by malnutrition. Nutritional supplements may also be useful. Some practitioners claim that herbs (such as goldenseal or garlic) can be used to kill yeasts and boost the immune system. However, these complementary therapies should be discussed with the patient's physician because of thrush's potentially serious threat to the cancer patient.

See also Chemoprevention.

Resources

OTHER

The Cancer Center at the University of Virginia. "What to do when you have taste changes." [cited July 5, 2001]. http:www.med.virginia.edu/medcntr/cancer/taste changes.html.

On-line Medical Dictionary. "Candidiasis" [cited July 5, 2001]. http://www.graylab.ac.uk/cgi-bin/omd?query=thrush.

ORGANIZATIONS

National Cancer Institute. *CancerNet*. [cited July 5, 2001]. http://www.nci.nih.gov.

Belinda Rowland, Ph.D.

Thymic cancer

Definition

Thymic **cancer** refers to any one of several different types of tumors that have originated within the thymus gland.

Description

The thymus is located in the upper chest just below the neck. It is a small organ that produces certain white blood cells before birth and during childhood. These white blood cells are called lymphocytes and are an important part of the body's immune system. Once released from the thymus, lymphocytes travel to lymph nodes where they help to fight infections. The thymus gland becomes smaller in adulthood and is gradually taken over by fat tissue.

Three cell types of the thymus can give rise to cancer. The epithelial cells that make up the outer covering of the thymus can become cancerous resulting in thymic **carcinoma** and **thymoma**. When the lymphocytes in the thymus or lymph nodes become cancerous, the resulting cancers are called **Hodgkin's disease** or non-Hodgkin's lymphomas. A third, less common, cell type in the thymus is called Kulchitsky cells (neuroendocrine cells). These cells release chemical messengers called hormones. Cancer that originates from Kulchitsky cells is called thymic carcinoid tumors. Another type of thymic cancer, thymolipoma, is composed of thymic tissue and fatty tissue.

Although rare, thymomas are the most common type of thymic cancer. With fewer than 200 cases reported each, thymic cancer and thymic carcinoid tumors are very rare. Thymic carcinomas tend to spread more rapidly and are more aggressive than thymomas. Taken together, thymic cancers represent only about 1.5% of all malignancies.

KEY TERMS

Adjuvant therapy—A treatment that is intended to aid the primary treatment. Adjuvant treatments for thymic cancer are radiation therapy and chemotherapy.

Lymphocyte—A type of white blood cell that is found in the thymus.

Neoadjuvant therapy—Radiation therapy or chemotherapy used to shrink a tumor before surgical removal of the tumor.

Paraneoplastic syndrome—A set of symptoms that is associated with cancer but is not directly caused by the cancer.

Pleura—The outer covering of the lungs.

Resection—Surgical removal of all or part of an organ or tissue.

Demographics

Thymic cancer is more common in the middle-aged and elderly; according to the National Cancer Institute (NCI), most patients diagnosed with these cancers are between 40 and 60 years of age. Thymoma and thymic carcinoma affect men and women equally. Thymic carcinoid tumors most frequently afflict men.

Causes and symptoms

The cause of thymic cancer is unknown. Cancer is caused when the normal mechanisms that control cell growth become disturbed, causing the cells to grow continually without stopping. This is caused by damage to the DNA in the cell.

Although some researchers think that previous exposure to radiation of the upper chest may be a risk factor for thymic cancer, the association has not been proved as of 2004.

Thymic tumors are not usually evident until the enlarged thymus presses on the windpipe (trachea) or blood vessels, which cause symptoms. The symptoms of thymic cancer will vary depending on what type of cancer is present. Symptoms of any thymic tumor may include shortness of breath, swelling of the face, coughing, and chest pain.

QUESTIONS TO ASK THE DOCTOR

- What type of thymic cancer do I have?
- What stage of cancer do I have?
- Has the cancer spread?
- What is the five-year survival rate for patients with this type of cancer?
- Will you perform a biopsy?
- What type of biopsy will you perform?
- What is the risk of seeding cancerous cells during a biopsy?
- What are my treatment options?
- What are the risks and side effects of these treatments?
- What medications can I take to relieve treatment side effects?
- Are there any clinical studies underway that would be appropriate for me?
- What effective alternative or complementary treatments are available for thymic cancer?
- How debilitating is the treatment? Will I be able to continue working?
- What is the chance that the cancer will recur?
- What are the signs and symptoms of recurrence?
- What can be done to prevent recurrence?
- How often will I have follow-up examinations?

Thymic carcinoid tumors can release hormones that may cause symptoms. Symptoms of thymic carcinoid tumors may also include red and warm skin, (flushing), **diarrhea**, and asthma.

Approximately 40% of the patients diagnosed with thymoma have no symptoms. The signs and symptoms of thymoma are vast and are related to the many disorders caused by thymoma. The most common conditions related to thymoma (**paraneoplastic syndromes**) are red cell aplasia, **myasthenia gravis**, and hypogammaglobulinemia. These conditions are autoimmune diseases, those in which the body mounts an attack against certain normal cells of the body. About 47% of thymomas are associated with myasthenia gravis. Symptoms of thymoma may also include:

- muscle weakness (especially in the eyes, neck, and chest, causing problems with vision, swallowing, and breathing)
- weakness
- dizziness
- shortness of breath
- fatigue

Diagnosis

The physician will conduct a complete physical examination. He or she may be able to feel a fullness in the lower neck region. Routine blood tests may be performed. **Imaging studies** are necessary because the symptoms of thymic cancer can be caused by many other diseases. Thymic tumors can be identified by chest x ray, **magnetic resonance imaging** (MRI), and **computed tomography** (CT). About half of these tumors can be detected by a plain-film chest x-ray.

A **biopsy** may be performed, in which a small sample of the tumor is removed and examined under the microscope. However, because of the risk of "seeding" cancerous cells, biopsies are not routinely performed. Because other tumors can lie in the region of the thymus, thymic cancer can be diagnosed only by identification of the cells that make up the tumor. There are a few different methods for biopsy of a thymic tumor. For a **mediastinoscopy**, a wand-like lighted camera (endoscope) and special instruments are passed through a small cut in the lower neck. The surgeon can see the tumor on a monitor and can cut off small samples for microscopic analysis. Mediastinoscopy is performed under general anesthesia. Alternatively, a needle biopsy will be taken in which a long needle is passed through the skin and into the tumor. Fine needle biopsy uses a thin needle and larger-core needle biopsy uses a wider needle. Needle biopsies may be performed in conjunction with computed tomography imaging.

Patients who are having difficulty breathing may have a **bronchoscopy** performed to examine the wind pipe. An endoscope, in this case a bronchoscope, is inserted through the mouth and into the windpipe. The physician will look for tumors and may perform biopsies.

Treatment team

The treatment team for thymic cancer may include a hematologist, pulmonologist, immunologist, oncologist, thoracic surgeon, cardiologist, radiation oncologist, nurse oncologist, psychiatrist, psychological counselor, and social worker.

Clinical staging, treatments, and prognosis

Clinical staging

There is more than one type of staging system for thymic cancer but the Masaoka system is used most often. This staging system was developed for thymoma; however, it is sometimes used to stage the other thymic cancers as well. Thymic carcinoma is graded (low or high) based on the cell type present in the tumor. Thymoma is categorized into four stages (I, II, III, and IV) which may be further subdivided (A and B) based on the spread of cancerous tissue. The Masaoka staging system is as follows:

- Stage I. The thymoma lies completely within the thymus.
- Stage II. The thymoma has spread out of the thymus and invaded the outer layer of the lung (pleura) or nearby fatty tissue.
- Stage III. The thymoma has spread to other neighboring tissues of the upper chest including the outer layer of the heart (pericardium), the lungs, or the heart's main blood vessels.
- Stage IVA. The thymoma has spread throughout the pericardium and/or the pleura.
- Stage IVB. The thymoma has spread to organs in other parts of the body.

Treatments

The treatment for thymic cancer depends on the type and stage of cancer and the patient's overall health. Because thymic cancers are so rare, there are no defined treatment plans. Treatment options include surgery, **radiation therapy**, and/or **chemotherapy**. Surgical removal of the tumor is the preferred treatment. Surgery is often the only treatment required for stage I thymic cancers. A treatment that is intended to aid the primary treatment is called adjuvant therapy. For instance, chemotherapy may be used along with surgery to treat thymic cancer. Stages II, III, and IV thymic cancers are often treated with surgery and some form of adjuvant therapy.

As of 2004, the preferred approach to thymic carcinoma is a combination of aggressive surgical treatment, chemotherapy using platinum-based compounds, and radiation treatments.

SURGERY. Thymic cancer may be treated by resection (surgical removal) of the tumor and some of the nearby healthy tissue. Removal of the entire thymus is called a thymectomy. Surgery on the thymus is usually performed through the chest wall by splitting open the breast bone (sternum), a procedure called a median sternotomy. When complete removal of the tumor is impossible, the surgeon will remove as much of the tumor as possible (debulking surgery, subtotal resection). In these cases, if the tumor has spread, surgery may include removal of other tissues such as the pleura, pericardium, blood vessels of the heart, lung, and nerves.

RADIATION THERAPY. Radiation therapy uses high-energy radiation from **x rays** and gamma rays to kill the cancer cells. Radiation given from a machine that is outside the body is called external radiation therapy. Radiation therapy is often used as adjuvant therapy following surgery to reduce the chance of cancer recurrence. Radiation may be used to kill cancer cells in cases in which the tumor was only partially removed. It may be used before surgery to shrink a large tumor. Radiation therapy is not very effective when used alone, although it may be used alone when the patient is too sick to withstand surgery.

The skin in the treated area may become red and dry and may take as long as a year to return to normal. Radiation to the chest may damage the lung causing shortness of breath and other breathing problems. Also, the tube that goes between the mouth and stomach (esophagus) may be irritated by radiation causing swallowing difficulties. **Fatigue**, upset stomach, diarrhea, and **nausea** are also common complaints of patients having radiation therapy. Most side effects go away about two to three weeks after radiation therapy has ended.

CHEMOTHERAPY. Chemotherapy uses **anticancer drugs** to kill the cancer cells. The drugs are given by mouth (orally) or intravenously. They enter the bloodstream and can travel to all parts of the body. Chemotherapy may be given before surgery to shrink a tumor, which is called neoadjuvant therapy. Thymic tumor cells are very sensitive to anticancer drugs, especially **cisplatin**, **doxorubicin**, and **ifosfamide**. Generally, a combination of drugs is given because it is more effective than a single drug in treating cancer.

The side effects of chemotherapy are significant and include stomach upset, **nausea and vomiting**, appetite loss (**anorexia**), hair loss (**alopecia**), mouth sores, and fatigue. Women may experience vaginal sores, menstrual cycle changes, and premature menopause. There is also an increased chance of infections.

Prognosis

The approximate five-year survival rates are 35% for thymic carcinomas and 60% for thymic carcinoids. The five-year survival rates for thymomas are 96% for stage I, 86% for stage II, 69% for stage III, and 50% for stage IV.

Thymomas rarely spread (metastasize) but thymic carcinomas frequently spread to distant organs. Thymic carcinomas spread most often to the pleura, lung, local lymph nodes (bean-sized structures that contain lymphocytes), bone, and liver. Thymic carcinoid tumors commonly spread to local lymph nodes.

Thymomas are prone to recurrence, even 10–15 years following surgery. For thymomas, recurrence rates are drastically reduced and the five-year survival rates are drastically increased in patients who receive adjuvant radiation therapy. Recurrence of thymic carcinoid tumors is common.

Thymomas are also associated with an increased risk of second malignancies.

Alternative and complementary therapies

Although alternative and complementary therapies are used by many cancer patients, very few controlled studies on the effectiveness of such therapies exist. Mind-body techniques such as prayer, biofeedback, visualization, meditation, and yoga have not shown any effect in reducing cancer but they can reduce stress and lessen some of the side effects of cancer treatments. Gerson, macrobiotic, orthomolecular, and Cancell therapies are ineffective treatments for cancer.

Clinical studies of hydrazine sulfate found that it had no effect on cancer and even worsened the health and well-being of the study subjects. One clinical study of the drug amygdalin (Laetrile) found that it had no effect on cancer. Laetrile can be toxic and has caused deaths. Shark cartilage, although highly touted as an effective cancer treatment, is an improbable therapy that has not been the subject of clinical study. Although the results are mixed, clinical studies suggest that melatonin may increase the survival time and quality of life for cancer patients.

Selenium in safe doses may delay the progression of thymic cancer. Laboratory and animal studies suggest that curcumin, the active ingredient of turmeric, has anticancer activity. Maitake mushrooms may boost the immune system, according to laboratory and animal studies. The results of laboratory studies suggest that **mistletoe** has anticancer properties; however, clinical studies have not been conducted.

For more comprehensive information, the reader may wish to consult the book on complementary and alternative medicine published by the American Cancer Society listed in the Resources section.

Coping with cancer treatment

The patient should consult his or her treatment team regarding any side effects or complications of treatment. Many of the side effects of chemotherapy can be relieved by medications. Patients should consult a psychotherapist and/or join a support group to deal with the emotional consequences of cancer and its treatment.

Clinical trials

As of late 2009, there was one active **clinical trial** studying thymic cancer, sponsored by the National Cancer Institute. The trial was studying the effectiveness and toxicity of AZ00530 on thymic cancers. This study was open to patients with invasive, relapsed, or metastatic thymoma or thymic carcinoma. The National Cancer Institute website has information on this and other studies. Patients should consult with their treatment team to determine if they are candidates for any ongoing studies.

Prevention

Because there are no risk factors for the development of thymic cancer known with certainty, there are no preventive measures. However, there may be an association between thymic cancer and exposure of the chest to radiation.

Special concerns

Damage to the lungs and/or esophagus caused by radiation therapy to the upper chest is a concern. Biopsy runs the risk of seeding tumor cells to other parts of the body.

Because of the increased risk of second malignancies, patients diagnosed with thymomas should have lifelong surveillance.

See also Thoracotomy.

Resources

BOOKS

Beers, Mark H., MD, and Robert Berkow, MD, editors. "Disorders of the Peripheral Nervous System." In *The Merck Manual of Diagnosis and Therapy*. Whitehouse Station, NJ: Merck Research Laboratories, 2007.

Bruss, Katherine, Christina Salter, and Esmeralda Galan, editors. *American Cancer Society's Guide to Complementary and Alternative Cancer Methods*. Atlanta: American Cancer Society, 2000.

Cameron, Robert, Patrick Loehrer, and Charles Thomas. "Neoplasms of the Mediastinum." In *Cancer: Principles & Practice of Oncology*, edited by Vincent T. DeVita, Samuel Hellman, and Steven Rosenberg. Philadelphia: Lippincott Williams & Wilkins, 2001, pp. 1019–36.

PERIODICALS

Chetty, G. K., O. A. Khan, C. V. Onyeaka, et al. "Experience with Video-Assisted Surgery for Suspected Mediastinal Tumours." *European Journal of Surgical Oncology* 30 (September 2004): 776–780.

Eng, T. Y., C. D. Fuller, J. Jagirdar, et al. "Thymic Carcinoma: State of the Art Review." *International Journal of Radiation Oncology, Biology, Physics* 59 (July 1, 2004): 654–664.

Giaccone, Giuseppe. "Treatment of Thymoma and Thymic Carcinoma." *Annals of Oncology* 11, Supplement 3 (2000): 245–6.

OTHER

American Cancer Society. "Thymus Cancer." November 1999. [cited April 29, 2001 and July 6, 2001]. http://www3.cancer.org/cancerinfo.

National Cancer Institute. *Thymoma and Thymic Carcinoma (PDQ): Treatment*, Health Professional Version. http://www.cancer.gov/cancertopics/pdq/treatment/malignant-thymoma/HealthProfessional.

ORGANIZATIONS

American Cancer Society. 1599 Clifton Rd. NE, Atlanta, GA 30329. (800) ACS-2345. http://www.cancer.org.

Cancer Research Institute, National Headquarters. 681 Fifth Ave., New York, NY 10022. (800) 992-2623. http://www.cancerresearch.org.

National Institutes of Health. National Cancer Institute. 9000 Rockville Pike, Bethesda, MD 20982. Cancer Information Service: (800) 4-CANCER. http://cancernet.nci.nih.gov.

Belinda Rowland, Ph.D.
Rebecca J. Frey, PhD

Thymoma

Definition

Thymomas are the most common tumor of the thymus.

Description

The thymus is located in the upper chest just below the neck. It is a small organ that produces certain white blood cells before birth and during childhood. These white blood cells are called lymphocytes and are an important part of the body's immune system. Once released from the thymus, lymphocytes travel to lymph nodes where they help to fight infections. The thymus gland becomes smaller in adulthood and is gradually taken over by fat tissue.

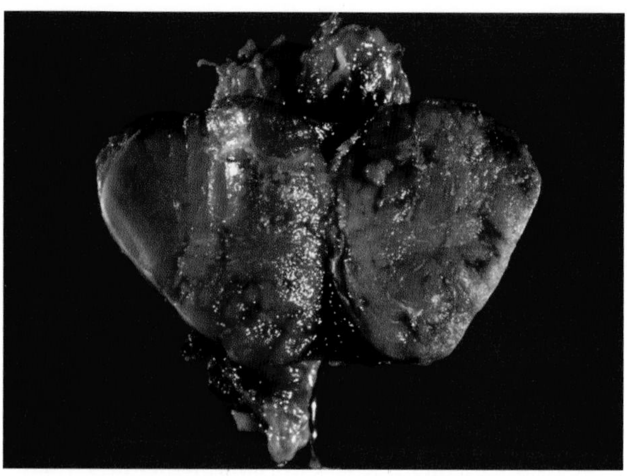

Gross specimen of the human thymus gland cut through showing a tumor (thymoma). *(Copyright Science Source/Photo Researchers, Inc. Reproduced by permission.)*

Although rare, thymomas are the most common type of thymic tumor. The term thymoma traditionally refers to a non-invasive, localized (only in the thymus) type of thymic tumor. Thymomas arise from thymic epithelial cells, which make up the covering of the thymus. Thymomas frequently contain lymphocytes, which are noncancerous. Thymomas are classified as either noninvasive (previously called benign) or invasive (previously called malignant). Noninvasive thymomas are those in which the tumor is encapsulated and easy to remove. Invasive thymomas have spread to nearby structures (such as the lungs) and are difficult to remove. Approximately 30% to 40% of thymomas are of the invasive type.

Demographics

Thymoma affects men and women equally. It is usually diagnosed between the ages of 40 and 60 years. Thymomas are uncommon in children.

Causes and symptoms

The cause of thymoma is unknown. **Cancer** is caused when the normal mechanisms that control cell growth become disturbed, causing the cells to grow continually without stopping. This is caused by damage to the DNA in the cell.

Approximately 40% of the patients diagnosed with thymoma have no symptoms. The symptoms in the remaining 60% of patients are caused by pressure from the enlarged thymus on the windpipe (trachea) or blood vessels or by **paraneoplastic syndromes**. Paraneoplastic syndromes are collections of symptoms in cancer patients that cannot be explained by the tumor.

KEY TERMS

Adjuvant therapy—A treatment that is intended to aid the primary treatment. Adjuvant treatments for thymic cancer are radiation therapy and chemotherapy.

Invasive—A descriptive term for thymoma that has spread beyond the outer wall of the thymus.

Lymphocyte—A type of white blood cell that is found in the thymus.

Neoadjuvant therapy—Radiation therapy or chemotherapy used to shrink a tumor before surgical removal of the tumor.

Paraneoplastic syndrome—A set of symptoms that is associated with cancer but is not directly caused by the cancer.

Pleura—The outer covering of the lungs.

Seventy-one percent of thymomas are associated with paraneoplastic syndromes. The most common syndromes related to thymoma are pure red cell aplasia (having abnormally low levels of red blood cells), **myasthenia gravis** (a muscular disorder), and hypogammaglobulinemia (having abnormally low levels of antibodies). These conditions are autoimmune diseases, those in which the body mounts an attack against certain normal cells of the body. Regarding myasthenia gravis, 15% of patients with this syndrome have thymomas. Alternately, 50% of patients with thymomas have myasthenia gravis. The relationship between the two entities is not clearly understood, though it is believed that the thymus may give incorrect instructions about the production of acetypcholine receptor antibodies, thus setting the state for faulty neuromuscular transmission. The confirmed presence of either thymomas or myasthenia gravis should prompt investigation for the other condition.

Symptoms of thymoma may include:

- shortness of breath
- swelling of the face
- coughing
- chest pain
- muscle weakness (especially in the eyes, neck, and chest, causing problems with vision, swallowing, and breathing)
- weakness
- dizziness
- shortness of breath
- fatigue

QUESTIONS TO ASK THE DOCTOR

- What histologic class of thymoma do I have?
- What stage of cancer do I have?
- Has the cancer spread?
- What is the five-year survival rate for patients with this stage of thymoma?
- Will you perform a biopsy?
- What type of biopsy will you perform?
- What is the risk of seeding during a biopsy?
- What are my treatment options?
- What are the risks and side effects of these treatments?
- What medications can I take to relieve treatment side effects?
- Are there any clinical studies underway that would be appropriate for me?
- What effective alternative or complementary treatments are available for thymoma?
- How debilitating is the treatment? Will I be able to continue working?
- What is the chance that the cancer will recur?
- What are the signs and symptoms of recurrence?
- What can be done to prevent recurrence?
- How often will I have follow-up examinations?

Diagnosis

The physician will conduct a complete physical exam. He or she may be able to feel a fullness in the lower neck region. Routine blood tests may be performed. **Imaging studies** are necessary because the symptoms of thymoma can be caused by many other diseases. Thymomas can be identified by chest x ray, **magnetic resonance imaging** (MRI), and **computed tomography** (CT).

A **biopsy** may be performed, in which a small sample of the tumor is removed and examined under the microscope. However, because of the risk of "seeding" cancerous cells, biopsies are not routinely performed. There are a few different methods to biopsy a thymoma. For a **mediastinoscopy**, a wand-like lighted camera (endoscope) and special instruments are passed through a small cut in the lower neck. The surgeon can see the tumor on a monitor and can cut off small samples for microscopic analysis. Mediastinoscopy is performed under general anesthesia. Alternatively, a needle biopsy will be taken in which a long needle is passed through the skin and into the tumor. Fine needle biopsy uses a thin needle and larger-core needle biopsy uses a wider needle. Needle biopsies may be performed in conjunction with computed tomography imaging.

Patients who are having difficulty breathing may have a **bronchoscopy** performed to examine the wind pipe. An endoscope, in this case a bronchoscope, is inserted through the mouth and into the windpipe. The physician will look for tumors and may perform biopsies.

Treatment team

The treatment team for thymoma may include a hematologist, pulmonologist, immunologist, oncologist, thoracic surgeon, cardiologist, radiation oncologist, nurse oncologist, psychiatrist, psychological counselor, and social worker.

Clinical staging, treatments, and prognosis

Clinical staging

There is more than one type of staging system for thymoma but the Masaoka system, a surgical staging system developed in 1981, is used most often. Thymoma is categorized into four stages (I, II, III, and IV) which may be further subdivided (A and B) based on the spread of cancerous tissue. The Masaoka staging system is as follows:

- Stage I. The thymoma lies completely within the thymus.
- Stage II. The thymoma has spread out of the thymus and invaded the outer layer of the lung (pleura) or nearby fatty tissue.
- Stage III. The thymoma has spread to other neighboring tissues of the upper chest including the outer layer of the heart (pericardium), the lungs, or the heart's main blood vessels.
- Stage IVA. The thymoma has spread throughout the pericardium and/or the pleura.
- Stage IVB. The thymoma has spread to organs in other parts of the body.

In 1999, the World Health Organization (WHO) adopted a new classification system for thymic tumors. This system is a histologic classification, which means that it is based on the microscopic features of the cells that make up the tumor. The WHO classification system ranks thymomas into types A, AB, B1, B2, B3, and C, by increasing severity.

Treatments

The treatment for thymoma cancer depends on the stage of cancer and the patient's overall health. Because thymomas are so rare, there are no defined treatment plans. Treatment options include surgery, **radiation therapy**, and/or **chemotherapy**. Surgical removal of the tumor is the preferred treatment. Surgery is often the only treatment required for stage I tumors. Treatment of thymoma often relieves the symptoms caused by paraneoplastic syndromes.

A treatment that is intended to aid the primary treatment is called adjuvant therapy. For instance, chemotherapy may be used along with surgery to treat thymoma. Stages II, III, and IV thymomas are often treated with surgery and some form of adjuvant therapy.

SURGERY. Thymoma may be treated by surgically removing (resecting) the tumor and some of the nearby healthy tissue. Removal of the entire thymus gland is called a thymectomy. Surgery on the thymus is usually performed through the chest wall by splitting open the breast bone (sternum), a procedure called a median sternotomy. When complete removal of the tumor is impossible, the surgeon will remove as much of the tumor as possible (debulking surgery, sub-total resection). In these cases, if the tumor has spread, surgery may include removal of other tissues such as the pleura, pericardium, blood vessels of the heart, lung, and nerves.

RADIATION THERAPY. Radiation therapy uses high-energy radiation from **x rays** and gamma rays to kill the cancer cells. Radiation given from a machine that is outside the body is called external radiation therapy. Radiation therapy is often used as adjuvant therapy following surgery to reduce the chance of cancer recurrence. Radiation may be used to kill cancer cells in cases in which the tumor was only partially removed. It may be used before surgery to shrink a large tumor. Radiation therapy is not very effective when used alone, although it may be used alone when the patient is too sick to withstand surgery.

The skin in the treated area may become red and dry and may take as long as a year to return to normal. Radiation to the chest may damage the lung causing shortness of breath and other breathing problems. Also, the tube that goes between the mouth and stomach (esophagus) may be irritated by radiation causing swallowing difficulties. **Fatigue**, upset stomach, **diarrhea**, and **nausea** are also common complaints of patients having radiation therapy. Most side effects go away about two to three weeks after radiation therapy has ended.

CHEMOTHERAPY. Chemotherapy uses **anticancer drugs** to kill the cancer cells. The drugs are given by mouth (orally) or intravenously. They enter the bloodstream and can travel to all parts of the body. Chemotherapy may be given before surgery to shrink a tumor, which is called neoadjuvant therapy. Thymoma cells are very sensitive to anticancer drugs, especially **cisplatin**, **doxorubicin**, and **ifosfamide**. Generally, a combination of drugs is given because it is more effective than a single drug in treating cancer. **Corticosteroids** are also used to treat thymoma.

The side effects of chemotherapy are significant and include stomach upset, **nausea and vomiting**, appetite loss (**anorexia**), hair loss (**alopecia**), mouth sores, and fatigue. Women may experience vaginal sores, menstrual cycle changes, and premature menopause. There is also an increased chance of infections.

Prognosis

The five-year survival rates for thymomas are 96% for stage I, 86% for stage II, 69% for stage III, and 50% for stage IV. Thorough (radical) surgery is associated with a longer survival rate. Almost 15% of thymoma patients develop a second cancer.

Thymomas rarely spread (metastasize) outside of the chest cavity. **Metastasis** is usually limited to the pleura. Invasive thymomas are prone to recurrence, even 10 to 15 years following surgery. The recurrence rates are drastically reduced and the five-year survival rates are drastically increased in patients who receive adjuvant radiation therapy.

Alternative and complementary therapies

Although alternative and complementary therapies are used by many cancer patients, very few controlled studies on the effectiveness of such therapies exist. Mind-body techniques such as prayer, biofeedback, visualization, meditation, and yoga have not shown any effect in reducing cancer but they can reduce stress and lessen some of the side effects of cancer treatments. Gerson, macrobiotic, orthomolecular, and Cancell therapies are ineffective treatments for cancer.

Clinical studies of hydrazine sulfate found that it had no effect on cancer and even worsened the health and well-being of the study subjects. One clinical study of the drug amygdalin (Laetrile) found that it had no effect on cancer. Laetrile can be toxic and has caused deaths. Shark cartilage, although highly touted as an effective cancer treatment, is an improbable therapy that has not been the subject of clinical study. Although the results are mixed, clinical studies suggest that melatonin may increase the survival time and quality of life for cancer patients.

Selenium, in safe doses, may delay the progression of cancer. Laboratory and animal studies suggest that curcumin, the active ingredient of turmeric, has anticancer activity. Maitake mushrooms may boost the immune system, according to laboratory and animal studies. The results of laboratory studies suggest that **mistletoe** has anticancer properties; however, clinical studies have not been conducted.

For more comprehensive information, the reader should consult the book on complementary and alternative medicine published by the American Cancer Society listed in the Resources section.

Coping with cancer treatment

The patient should consult his or her treatment team regarding any side effects or complications of treatment. Many of the side effects of chemotherapy can be relieved by medications. Patients should consult a psychotherapist and/or join a support group to deal with the emotional consequences of cancer and its treatment.

Clinical trials

As of 2009, there were a number of active **clinical trials** studying thymoma. The National Cancer Institute sponsors these studies. One trial was studying the effectiveness and toxicity of **cisplatin** and paclitaxel on thymoma. This study was open to patients with invasive and previously untreated thymoma. Another study was studying the effectiveness and toxicity of octreotide on inoperate thymoma. The National Cancer Institute website has information on these and other studies. Patients should consult with their treatment team to determine if they are candidates for these or any other ongoing studies.

Prevention

Because there are no known risk factors for the development of thymoma there are no preventive measures. However, there may be an association between **thymic cancer** and exposure of the chest to radiation.

Special concerns

Damage to the lungs and/or esophagus caused by radiation therapy to the upper chest is a concern. Biopsy runs the risk of seeding tumor cells to other parts of the body.

See also Thoracotomy.

Resources

BOOKS

Bruss, Katherine, Christina Salter, and Esmeralda Galan, editors. *American Cancer Society's Guide to Complementary and Alternative Cancer Methods.* Atlanta: American Cancer Society, 2000.

Cameron, Robert, Patrick Loehrer, and Charles Thomas. "Neoplasms of the Mediastinum." In *Cancer: Principles and Practice of Oncology*, edited by Vincent T. DeVita, Samuel Hellman, and Steven Rosenberg. Philadelphia: Lippincott Williams & Wilkins, 2001.

PERIODICALS

Giaccone, Giuseppe. "Treatment of Thymoma and Thymic Carcinoma." *Annals of Oncology* 11, Supplement 3 (2000): 245–6.

Muller-Hermelink, H., and A. Marx. "Thymoma." *Current Opinion in Oncology* 12 (September 2000): 426–33.

Thomas, Charles, Cameron Wright, and Patrick Loehrer. "Thymoma: State of the Art." *Journal of Clinical Oncology* 17 (July 1999): 2280–9.

ORGANIZATIONS

American Cancer Society. 1599 Clifton Rd. NE, Atlanta, GA 30329. (800) ACS-2345. http://www.cancer.org.

Cancer Research Institute, National Headquarters. 681 Fifth Ave., New York, NY 10022. (800) 992-2623. http://www.cancerresearch.org.

National Institutes of Health. National Cancer Institute. 9000 Rockville Pike, Bethesda, MD 20982. Cancer Information Service: (800) 4-CANCER. http://cancernet.nci.nih.gov.

Belinda Rowland, Ph.D.

Thyroid cancer

Definition

Thyroid **cancer** is a disease in which the cells of the thyroid gland become abnormal, grow uncontrollably and form a mass of cells called a tumor.

Demographics

Diseases of the thyroid gland affect millions of Americans. The most common diseases of the thyroid are hyperthyroidism (Grave's disease) and hypothyroidism, an overactive or an underactive gland, respectively. Sometimes lumps or masses may develop in the thyroid. Although most (95%) of these lumps or nodules are non-cancerous (benign), all thyroid lumps should be taken seriously.

Thyroid cancer is one of the most treatable forms of cancer with the five-year overall survival rate for all stages and all tumor types at 97%. The American Cancer Society estimates that in 2009, approximately 37,200 new cases of thyroid cancer will be diagnosed in the United States and less than 2,000 individuals will die from the disease.

Women are three times more likely to develop thyroid cancer than men. Unlike many cancers, thyroid cancers are most often diagnosed in younger people, with almost two-thirds of cases diagnosed in individuals between the ages of 20 and 55. Caucasians are affected more often than African Americans.

The incidence of thyroid cancer has increased slightly in recent years although this increase is thought to be primarily related to increased sophistication of detection capabilities. The death rate from thyroid cancer has remained stable for several years.

Description

The thyroid is a hormone-producing, butterfly-shaped gland located in the neck at the base of the throat. It has two lobes, the left and the right. The thyroid uses iodine, a mineral found in some foods, to make several of its hormones. Thyroid hormones regulate essential body processes such as heart rate, blood pressure, body temperature, and metabolism, and affect the nervous system, muscles, and other organs. These hormones play an important role in regulating childhood growth and development.

Types of thyroid cancer

Thyroid cancer is grouped into types based on how cells appear under a microscope. Differentiated thyroid cancers include papillary **carcinoma** (the most common type of thyroid tumor) and follicular carcinoma. Hurthle cell thyroid cancer is a subtype of follicular carcinoma. Other less commonly occurring types of thyroid cancers include medullary thyroid carcinomas, anaplastic thyroid cancers, and thyroid lymphomas. They grow at different rates and can spread to other parts of the body if left untreated. The two most common types of thyroid cancer are papillary carcinoma and follicular carcinoma.

PAPILLARY. The papillary type (60%–80% of all thyroid cancers) is a slow-growing cancer that develops in the hormone-producing cells containing iodine.

FOLLICULAR. The follicular type (30%–50% of thyroid cancers) also develops in the hormone-producing cells.

MEDULLARY. The medullary type (5%–7% of all thyroid cancers) develops in the parafollicular cells

Thyroid cancers

Cancer type	Characteristics	Prognosis
Papillary	60–80% of thyroid cancers Slow-growing cancer in hormone-producing cells	90% of patients will live for 15 years or longer after diagnosis
Follicular	30–50% of thyroid cancers Found in hormone-producing cells	90% of patients will live for 15 years or longer after diagnosis
Medullary	5–7% of thyroid cancers Found in calcitonin-producing cells Difficult to control as it often spreads to other parts of the body	80% of patients will live for at least 10 years after surgery
Anaplastic	2% of thyroid cancers Fastest growing Rapidly spreads to other parts of the body	3–17% of patients will survive for five years

(Table by GGS Creative Resources. Reproduced by permission of Gale, a part of Cengage Learning.)

(known as the C cells) that produce **calcitonin**, a hormone that does not contain iodine.

ANAPLASTIC. The anaplastic type of thyroid cancer (2% of all thyroid cancers), is the fastest growing, most aggressive type.

Risk Factors

Risk factors associated with the development of thyroid cancer include:

- Gender – thyroid cancers are diagnosed in women three times as often as in men.
- Age – most cases of thyroid cancer are diagnosed between the ages of 20 and 55 years.
- Diet – consumption of diets low in iodine have been linked to the development of papillary and follicular thyroid cancers.
- Radiation exposure – radiation exposure, particularly exposure in childhood, places individuals at higher risk for the development of thyroid cancer.
- Heredity – about 20% of cases of medullary thyroid cancer are related to an inherited genetic abnormality; individuals with other inherited diseases such as Gardner syndrome, Cowden disease, and familial adenomatous polyposis (FAP), appear to be at increased risk for the development of certain types of thyroid cancer.

Causes and symptoms

The exact cause of thyroid cancer is not known but as stated above, some risk factors have been identified. Radiation was used in the 1950s and 1960s to treat acne and to reduce swelling in infections of the tonsils, adenoids and lymph nodes. It has been proven that this exposure is a risk factor for thyroid cancer. In some areas of the world, diets are low in iodine. Papillary and follicular cancers occur more frequently in these areas. Iodine deficiency is not a large problem in the United States because iodine is added to table salt and other foods. Approximately 7% of thyroid cancers are caused by the alteration (mutation) of a gene called the RET oncogene, which can be inherited.

Symptoms of thyroid cancer are rare. Many thyroid tumors present as a painless lump in the neck. Some tumors are found during routine health-related checkups. The following are signs and symptoms of thyroid nodules:

- A lump or nodule that can be felt in the neck is the most frequent sign of thyroid cancer.
- The lymph nodes in the neck may be swollen and the voice may become hoarse because the tumor presses on the nerves leading to the voice box.
- Some patients experience a tight or full feeling in the neck and have difficulty breathing or swallowing.

Diagnosis

Examination

A physician will carefully examine the neck and lymph nodes in the area if a thyroid tumor is suspected or if a patient complains of anterior neck pain, swelling, hoarseness, or if a suspicious lump is present.

Tests

Physicians use several tests to confirm the suspicion of thyroid cancer, to identify the size and location of the lump and to determine whether the lump is noncancerous (benign) or cancerous (malignant).

A blood test called the thyroid stimulating hormone (TSH) test checks thyroid function.

The calcitonin test may be ordered to evaluate calcitonin levels in blood. Calcitonin is a hormone produced by the C cells (parafollicular cells) of the thyroid gland. The hormone is produced in excess when the parafollicular cells of the thyroid become cancerous. Results of this test are used to confirm the diagnosis of medullary thyroid. Another blood test, the carcinoembryonic antigen (CEA), test may be done if medullary thyroid cancer is suspected. CEA levels are usually high in patients with this type of thyroid cancer.

Computed tomography (CT) scan or **ultrasonography** (an ultrasound scan) are imaging tests used to produce a picture of the thyroid. A radiologist usually interprets the results of these tests within 24 hours. In ultrasonography, high-frequency sound waves are bounced off the thyroid. The pattern of echoes produced by these waves is converted into a computerized image on a television screen. This test can determine whether the lumps found in the thyroid are benign fluid-filled cysts or solid malignant tumors.

A nuclear medicine radioiodine scan is used to identify abnormal areas in the thyroid. For this test, the patient is given a very small amount of radioactive iodine that can either be swallowed or injected. Since the thyroid is the only gland in the body that absorbs iodine, the radioactive iodine accumulates there. An x-ray image is taken or an instrument called a scanner is used to identify areas in the thyroid that do not absorb iodine normally. These abnormal spots are called cold spots and further tests are performed to check whether the cold spots are benign or malignant tumors. If a significant amount of radioactive iodine is concentrated in the nodule, then it is termed "hot" and is usually benign. A radiologist interprets the results within a day.

An octreotide scan may be ordered to detect the spread of medullary thyroid cancer.

Other tests which may be ordered to assist in the diagnosis of thyroid cancer include **magnetic resonance imaging** (MRI) and **positron emission tomography** (PET) scans.

Procedures

The most accurate diagnostic tool for thyroid cancer is a **biopsy**. In this process, a sample of thyroid tissue is obtained and examined under a microscope by a pathologist. This usually takes a day. The tissue sample can be obtained either by drawing out a sample of tissue through a needle (such as a fine needle aspirate biopsy) or by surgical removal of the nodule (surgical biopsy). A needle biopsy takes a few minutes and can be done by a trained physician, usually a radiologist. The surgical biopsy is done by a surgeon under general anesthesia with the help of an anesthesiologist and takes a few hours. If thyroid cancer is diagnosed, further tests may be done to determine the stage of the disease and help doctors plan appropriate treatment.

Staging

The aggressiveness of each type of thyroid cancer is different. Cancer staging considers the size of the tumor, whether it has grown into surrounding lymph nodes and whether it has spread to distant parts of the body (metastasized). Age and general health status are also taken into account. The **American Joint Commission on Cancer** (AJCC) staging is summarized below for each thyroid cancer type.

PAPILLARY AND FOLLICULAR. In patients younger than 45 years:

- Stage I: Patients without evidence of cancer beyond the thyroid.
- Stage II: Patients with spread of cancer outside the thyroid gland to one or more distant sites.

In patients over 45:

- Stage I: Tumors are smaller than 2 cm (0.3 in).
- Stage II: Tumors are 2–4 cm (0.3–0.6 in) across but have not spread to adjacent lymph nodes or distant sites.
- Stage III: Tumors have spread locally to nearby lymph nodes or are larger than 4 cm (0.6 in) and have grown slightly outside of the thyroid but not into lymph nodes or distant sites.
- Stage IV: Tumors have spread outside the thyroid area (distant metastases).

In the case of Stage IV cancer, the places to which thyroid cancer often metastasizes are the lungs and bone.

MEDULLARY. The stages of medullary thyroid carcinomas for individuals at any age are the same as for papillary or follicular thyroid cancer in people over age 45.

ANAPLASTIC. All cases of anaplastic thyroid cancer are considered Stage IV because this type of cancer is extremely aggressive.

Treatment

Papillary thyroid cancer can be treated successfully. Follicular thyroid cancer also has a good cure rate but may be difficult to control if the cancer invades blood vessels or spreads to nearby structures in the neck. Medullary thyroid cancers are more difficult to control because they often spread to other parts of the body. Anaplastic thyroid cancer is the fastest growing and tends to respond poorly to all treatments.

Like most cancers, cancer of the thyroid is best treated when it is found early by a primary physician. Treatment depends on the type of cancer and its stage. Several treatment modalities are used in the treatment of thyroid cancer including surgical removal of the tumor, external beam **radiation therapy**, thyroid hormone therapy, **chemotherapy**, and radioactive hormone therapy. Using a combination of these therapies typically leads to optimal results.

Surgery

Surgical removal is the usual treatment if the cancer has not spread to distant parts of the body. It is the primary treatment for early stage papillary, follicular, and medullary thyroid cancers. The surgeon may remove the side or lobe of the thyroid where the cancer is found (**lobectomy**) or all of it (total thyroidectomy). If the adjoining lymph nodes are affected, they may also be removed during surgery.

Radiation/radioactive iodine therapy

For papillary and follicular thyroid cancers, radioactive iodine may be used in addition to surgery. In this treatment, the patient is asked to swallow a drink containing radioactive iodine. Because the thyroid cells take up iodine, the radioactive iodine collects in any thyroid tissue remaining in the body and kills the cancer cells. External beam radiation may be used if the radioactive iodine is unsuccessful.

For medullary cancers, radioactive iodine is not used. External beam radiation may be used as a palliative therapy. (A palliative therapy is one intended to make the patient more comfortable, not to cure the cancer.)

Hormone therapy

Removal of the thyroid gland causes levels of thyroid hormones to decrease. The pituitary gland then produces TSH, which normally stimulates the thyroid gland to make thyroid hormone. TSH stimulates thyroid cells to grow, and most likely promotes thyroid cancer growth. Hormone therapy uses hormones after surgery to stop this growth and the formation of new cancerous thyroid cells. To prevent cancerous growth, the natural hormones produced by the thyroid are taken in the form of a pill. This maintains normal hormone levels and inhibits the pituitary gland from making TSH. If the cancer has spread to other parts of the body and surgery is not possible, hormone treatment is aimed at killing or slowing the growth of cancer cells throughout the body.

QUESTIONS TO ASK YOUR DOCTOR

- What type of thyroid cancer do I have?
- Has it spread beyond the thyroid gland?
- Is my thyroid cancer hereditary? Should other members of my family be tested?
- What treatments do you recommend? Do you recommend a clinical trial?
- What are the advantages, disadvantages, and side effects of this treatment?
- How much experience do you have treating thyroid cancer/performing thyroid surgery?

Chemotherapy

For advanced thyroid cancers for which surgery was not an option or that have not responded well to other treatments, chemotherapy may be used. There is no standard chemotherapeutic regimen for advanced papillary, follicular, and anaplastic thyroid cancers. Clinical studies are ongoing for patients with these cancers. Anaplastic thyroid cancer may show an increased local response to the chemotherapeutic agent, **doxorubicin**, which is used as a radiation sensitizer in combination with hyperfractionated radiation therapy. Paclitaxel may provide some palliative benefit. Patients with anaplastic thyroid cancer may be eligible for ongoing **clinical trials**.

Prognosis

As of 2009, the 10 year overall survival rates for individuals with thyroid cancer by type of cancer are:

- Papillary – 93%
- Follicular - 85%
- Medullary – 75%
- Anaplastic/undifferentiated carcinomas – 14%

Prevention

It is not possible to prevent this disease completely because most people with thyroid cancer have no known risk factor. The risk for radiation-related thyroid cancer can be reduced by avoiding radiation to the neck when possible. Inherited cases of medullary thyroid cancer can be prevented. If a family member has had this disease, other family members can be tested and treated early. Carriers of the RET mutation may want to consider a prophylactic thyroidectomy at an early age. The National Cancer Institute recommends that every one or two years, a doctor examine anyone who has received radiation to the head and neck during childhood. The neck and thyroid should be carefully examined for any lumps or enlargement of nearby lymph nodes. Ultrasound may be used to screen for the disease in people at risk for thyroid cancer.

Resources

PERIODICALS

Dackiw, A.P. & Zeiger, M."Extent of Surgery for Differentiated Thyroid Cancer." *Surgical Clinics of North America* 2004, 84(3):817–32.

Davies, L. & Welch, H.G. "Increased Incidence of Thyroid Cancer in the United States, 1973-2002."*JAMA*. 2006, 295:2164–7.

OTHER

Practice Guidelines in Oncology Thyroid Carcinoma v.1.2009. National Comprehensive Cancer Network (NCCN) [cited September 12, 2009]. http://www.nccn.org/ professionals/physician_gls/PDF/thyroid.pdf.

Thyroid Cancer Treatment PDQ. National Cancer Institute (NCI). February 6, 2009 [cited September 12, 2009]. http://www.cancer.gov/cancertopics/pdq/treat ment/thyroid/HealthProfessional/page2.

What is Thyroid Cancer. American Cancer Society (ACS). May 14, 2009 [cited September 12, 2009]. http://www.cancer.org/docroot/CRI/content/CRI_2_4_1X_What_is_thyroid_cancer.43.asp?rnav=cri.

ORGANIZATIONS

American Cancer Society. (800) ACS-2345. http://www.cancer.org.

National Cancer Institute, Cancer Information Service. (800) 4-CANCER (800-422-6237). TTY: (800) 332-8615. http://www.nci.nih.gov/.

Lata Cherath, Ph.D.
Kulbir Rangi, D.O.
Melinda Oberleitner, R.N., D.N.S.

Thyroid nuclear medicine scan

Definition

A thyroid nuclear medicine scan is a diagnostic procedure to evaluate the thyroid gland, which is located in the front of the neck and controls the metabolism of the body. A radioactive substance that concentrates in the thyroid is taken orally or injected into a vein (intravenously), or both. There are three types of radioactive iodine used in these scans. A special camera is used to take an image of the distribution of the radioactive substance in and around the thyroid gland. This is interpreted to evaluate thyroid function and to diagnose abnormalities. Although other imaging methods exist for evaluating thyroid disease, thyroid scanning is the most commonly used and is the most cost-effective.

Purpose

A thyroid scan can help assess the overall structure and function of the thyroid. It can be used to identify benign cancers, to assess nodules, to evaluate masses, to locate the source of a painful gland, to assess gland size, to find differentiated carcinomas, and to identify thyroid tissue. A thyroid scan may be ordered by a physician when the gland becomes abnormally large, especially if the enlargement is greater on one side, or when hard lumps (nodules) are felt. The scan can be helpful in determining whether the enlargement is caused by a diffuse increase in the total amount of thyroid tissue or by a nodule or nodules. The thyroid scan plays a critical role in the diagnosis of **thyroid cancer**.

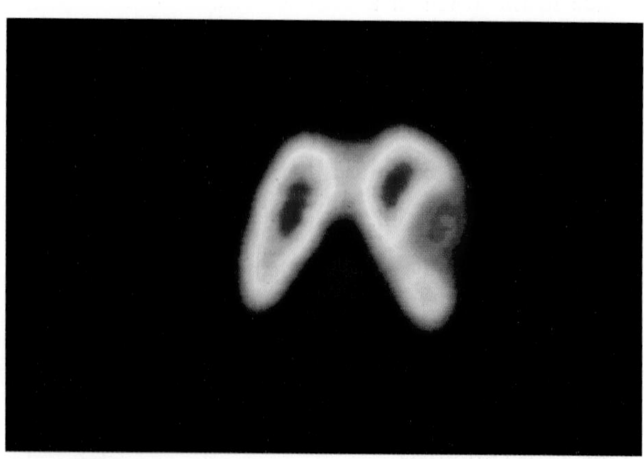

A gamma scan of the human thyroid gland revealing cancer. *(Custom Medical Stock Photo. Reproduced by permission.)*

KEY TERMS

Adenoma—A type of non-cancerous tissue that emanates from glands.

Benign—A type of tissue overgrowth that is not progressive, unlike malignant tissue.

Graves' disease—A condition characterized by bulging eyeballs, among other symptoms, that is synonymous with hyperthyroidism.

Radioisotope—A radioactive or radiation-emitting form of an element.

Radionuclide—A substance that emits radiation as it disintegrates.

When other laboratory studies show an overactive thyroid (hyperthyroidism) or an underactive thyroid (hypothyroidism), a radioactive iodine uptake scan is often used to confirm the diagnosis. A thyroid scan is often performed in conjunction with this scan. Thyroid radionuclide scanning is being considered as a means to screen individuals at risk for thyroid disease following **radiation therapy**.

Precautions

Women who are pregnant should not have this test. Any person with a history of allergy to iodine, such as those with shellfish allergies, should notify the physician before the procedure is performed.

Description

This test is performed in a radiology facility, either in an outpatient x-ray center or a hospital department. Most often, the patient is given the radioactive substance in the form of a tasteless liquid or capsule. It may be injected into a vein (intravenously) in some instances. Generally, the patient lies on an examination table as the scanning is performed. Images will be taken at a specified amount of time after this, depending on the radioisotope used. Most often, scanning is done 24 hours later, if the radioisotope is given orally. If it is given intravenously, the scan is performed approximately 20 minutes later.

For a thyroid scan, the patient is positioned lying down on his or her back, with the head tilted back. The radionuclide scanner, also called a gamma camera, is positioned above the thyroid area as it scans. This takes 30–60 minutes.

The uptake study may be done with the patient sitting upright in a chair or lying down. The procedure is otherwise the same as described for the thyroid scan. It takes approximately 15 minutes. There is no discomfort involved with either study.

A thyroid scan may also be referred to as a thyroid scintiscan. The name of the radioactive substance used may be incorporated and the study called a technetium thyroid scan or an iodine thyroid scan. The radioactive iodine uptake scan may be called by its initials, an RAIU test, or an iodine uptake test.

Preparation

Certain medications can interfere with iodine uptake. These include certain cough medicines, some oral contraceptives, non-steroidal anti-inflammatory drugs, epilepsy drugs, and thyroid medications. The patient is usually instructed to stop taking these medications for a period of time before the test. This period may range from several days up to three to four weeks, depending on the amount of time the medicine takes to clear from the body.

Other **nuclear medicine scans** and x-ray studies using contrast material performed within the past 60 days may affect this test. Therefore, patients should tell their doctors if they have had either of these types of studies before the thyroid scan is begun, to avoid inaccurate results.

Thyroid scan test results can be affected by other conditions, such as kidney failure, **cancer**, cancer **chemotherapy**, hepatitis, cirrhosis of the liver, infections, trauma, poor nutrition, and mental illness.

Some institutions prefer that the patient have nothing to eat or drink after midnight on the day before the radioactive liquid or capsule is to be taken. A normal diet can usually be resumed two hours after the radioisotope is taken. Dentures, jewelry, and other metallic objects must be removed before the scanning is performed. No other physical preparation is needed.

The patient should understand that there is no danger of radiation exposure to themselves or others. Only very small amounts of radioisotope are used. The total amount of radiation absorbed is often less than the dose received from ordinary **x rays**. The scanner or camera does not emit any radiation, but detects and records it from the patient.

Aftercare

No isolation or special precautions are needed after a thyroid scan. The patient should check with his or her physician about restarting any medications that were stopped before the scan.

Risks

There are no risks with this procedure.

Normal results

A normal scan will show a thyroid of normal size, shape, and position. The amount of radionuclide uptake by the thyroid will be normal, according to established laboratory figures. There will be no areas where radionuclide uptake is increased or decreased.

Abnormal results

An area of increased radionuclide uptake may be called a hot nodule or "hot spot." This means that a benign growth is overactive. Despite the name, hot nodules are unlikely to be caused by cancer. Increased radionuclide uptake is indicative of hyperthyroidism and may suggest Graves' disease or an active pituitary **adenoma**.

An area of decreased radionuclide uptake may be called a cold nodule, or "cold spot." This indicates that this area of the thyroid gland is underactive. A variety of conditions, including cysts, hypothyroidism, nonfunctioning benign growths, localized inflammation, or cancer, may produce a cold spot. Single nodules that are not functioning are malignant in about 10–20% of cases. Completely nonfunctioning nodules have a higher probability of being malignant than those that have some degree of function.

A thyroid nuclear medicine scan is rarely sufficient to establish a clear diagnosis. A majority of nonfunctioning nodules are not malignant, but their presence increases the probability of a malignancy. Nodules that are functioning are rarely malignant. Frequently, the information revealed will need to be combined with data from other studies to determine the problem.

Resources

BOOKS

Goroll, Allan H., et al., editors. "Screening for Thyroid Cancer." In *Primary Care Medicine: Office Evaluation and Management of the Adult Patient*. Philadelphia: Lippincott, Williams & Wilkins: 2000.

Siberry, George K., et al., editors. *The Harriet Lane Handbook: A Manual for Pediatric House Officers*. St. Louis: Mosby, 2000.

PERIODICALS

Nusynowitz, M. L. "Thyroid Imaging." *Lippincotts Primary Care Practice* 3 (November–December 1999): 546–55.

Sandhu, A., et al. "Subclinical Thyroid Disease after Radiation Therapy Detected by Radionuclide Scanning." *International Journal of Radiation Oncology, Biology, Physics* 48 (August, 2000): 181–8.

Mark A. Mitchell, M.D.

TNM Staging *see* **Tumor staging**

Topotecan

Definition

Topotecan is a drug used to treat certain types of **cancer**. Topotecan is available under the trade name Hycamtin, and may also be referred to as topotecan hydrochloride or topotecan HCl.

Purpose

Topotecan is an antineoplastic agent used to treat **small cell lung cancer**, and certain cancers of the ovary.

As of late 2003, **clinical trials** are underway in Italy and France to test the effectiveness of topotecan in treating tumors of the brain (glioblastomas) and autonomic nervous system (neuroblastomas). In the French study, topotecan is given together with radiotherapy while the Italian trial uses topotecan as part of combination **chemotherapy**. Early results indicate that the drug may be useful in treating cancers of the nervous system as well as ovarian and small-cell lung cancers.

Description

Topotecan is a synthetic derivative of the naturally occurring compound camptothecin. Camptothecin belongs to a group of chemicals called alkaloids, and is extracted from plants such as *Camptotheca acuminata*. Captothecin was initially investigated as a chemotherapeutic agent due to its anti-cancer activity in laboratory studies. The chemical structure and biological action of topotecan is similar to that of camptothecin and **irinotecan**.

Topotecan inhibits the normal functioning of the enzyme topoisomerase I. The normal role of topoisomerase I is to aid in the replication, recombination, and repair of deoxyribonucleic acid (DNA). Higher levels of topoisomerase I have been found in certain cancer tumors compared to healthy tissue. Inhibiting topoisomerase I causes DNA damage. This damage leads to apoptosis, or programmed cell death.

KEY TERMS

Alkaloid—A nitrogen containing compound occuring in plants.

Anorexia—Loss of appetite and the inability to eat.

Apoptosis—An active process in which a cell dies due to a chemical signal. Programmed cell death.

Topotecan is used in patients whose cancer of the ovary has recurred or progressed after platinum-based treatment such as **cisplatin**. Topotecan is also used to treat relapse of small cell lung cancer that initially responded to other drugs. Increases in survival times have been observed in patients treated with topotecan compared to control populations treated with paclitaxel.

Tumors that are targeted by topotecan sometimes develop resistance to the drug. Although the reasons for this resistance are not fully understood as of late 2003, researchers think that they may be related either to inadequate amounts of drug in the tumor or to alterations in topoisomerase I that make the enzyme resistant to topotecan.

Recommended dosage

Patients should be carefully monitored before and during topotecan treatment for bone marrow function.

Topotecan is administered intravenously over 30 minutes once per day for five consecutive days followed by 16 days of rest. This schedule may be repeated every 21 days. The initial dose of topotecan may be adjusted downward depending on patient tolerance to the toxic side effects of topotecan.

The dose of topotecan may be reduced in patients with kidney dysfunction.

No dose modification is necessary for patients with liver impairment.

No dose modification is necessary for elderly patients.

Precautions

Topotecan should be used only under the supervision of a physician experienced in the use of cancer chemotherapeutic agents. Certain complications will only be possible to manage if the necessary diagnostic and treatment resources are readily available. Topotecan should not be used in patients with bone marrow depression before starting treatment. Skin that comes in contact with topotecan must be washed thoroughly with soap and warm water.

The dose of topotecan may be reduced in patients with moderate kidney dysfunction. Topotecan is not recommended for use in patients with severe kidney dysfunction.

Topotecan should not be administered to pregnant women. Women of child bearing age are advised not to become pregnant during treatment. Women should discontinue nursing prior to taking topotecan.

Side effects

Suppression of bone marrow function is the most serious side effect commonly observed in this treatment and can lead to death. Bone marrow reserves should be monitored by blood cell counts for all patients before and during topotecan treatment. The suppression of bone marrow is not cumulative over time. Additional side effects including **nausea and vomiting**, **anorexia**, **diarrhea**, constipation, headache, and hair loss (**alopecia**) may occur.

Interactions

Suppression of bone marrow is more severe when topotecan is given with platinum drugs. G-CSF (**filgrastim**) may extend the duration of bone marrow suppression. If G-CSF is used, it should not be administered until day six of the 21-day course.

See also Lung cancer, small cell.

Resources

PERIODICALS

Garaventa, A., R. Luksch, S. Biasotti, et al. "A Phase II Study of Topotecan with Vincristine and Doxorubicin in Children with Recurrent/Refractory Neuroblastoma." *Cancer* 98 (December 1, 2003): 2488–2494.

Lesimple, T., M. B. Hassel, D. Gedouin, et al. "Phase I Study of Topotecan in Combination with Concurrent Radiotherapy in Adults with Glioblastoma." *Journal of Neurooncology* 65 (November 2003): 141–148.

Nagourney, R. A., B. L. Sommers, S. M. Harper, et al. "Ex vivo Analysis of Topotecan: Advancing the Application of Laboratory-Based Clinical Therapeutics." *British Journal of Cancer* 89 (November 3, 2003): 1789–1795.

Rasheed, Z. A., and E. H. Rubin. "Mechanisms of Resistance to Topoisomerase I-Targeting Drugs." *Oncogene* 22 (October 20, 2003): 7296–7304.

Rose, P. G. "Chemotherapy for Newly Diagnosed and Relapsed Advanced Ovarian Cancer." *Seminars in Oncology Nursing* 19 (November 2003): 25–35.

ORGANIZATIONS

United States Food and Drug Administration (FDA). 5600 Fishers Lane, Rockville, MD 20857-0001. (888) INFO-FDA (463-6332). http://www.fda.gov.

Marc Scanio
Rebecca J. Frey, PhD

Toremifene

Definition

Toremifene, also known as Fareston, is a synthetic compound similar to estrogen. It mimics the action of estrogen on the bones and uterus, but blocks the effects of estrogen on breast tissue.

Purpose

Toremifene is used as adjuvant hormone therapy immediately after surgery in early stages of **breast cancer** and also to treat advanced metastatic breast **cancer** (stages III and above) in postmenopausal women. Postmenopausal women at high risk of developing breast cancer may take toremifene to reduce risk.

Description

Toremifene is similar to **tamoxifen** in structure and action. Toremifene can be given as sole treatment, but it is often given in combination with other chemotherapeutic drugs.

Toremifene belongs to a family of compounds called **antiestrogens**. Antiestrogens are used in cancer therapy by inhibiting the effects of estrogen on target tissues. Estrogen is a steroid hormone secreted by granulosa cells of a maturing follicle within the female ovary. Depending on the target tissue, estrogen can stimulate the growth of female reproductive organs and breast tissue, play a role in the female menstrual cycle, and protect against bone loss by binding to estrogen receptors on the outside of cells within the target tissue. Antiestrogens act selectively against the effects of estrogen on target cells in a variety of ways, thus they are called selective estrogen receptor modulators (SERMs).

Toremifene selectively inhibits the effects of estrogen on breast tissue, while mimicking the effects of estrogen on bone (by increasing bone mineral density) and uterine tissues. The former makes toremifene an excellent therapeutic agent against breast cancer. Although researchers are unclear of the precise mechanism by which toremifene kills breast cancer cells, it is known to compete with estrogen by binding to estrogen receptors, therefore limiting the effects of estrogen on breast tissue. Toremifene also may be involved in other anti-tumor activities affecting oncogene expression, promotion of apoptosis and growth factor secretion.

In the early 2009, **clinical trials** were underway to test toremifene citrate for treating complications of certain therapies for **prostate cancer** patients. For example, androgen deprivation therapy results in increased bone fractures among prostate cancer patients. Researchers believe that toremifene citrate will help reduce these and other effects.

KEY TERMS

Adjuvant—A treatment added to curative procedures such as surgery to prevent the recurrence of cancer.

Anticoagulant—An agent preventing the coagulation of blood.

Apoptosis—A type of cell death where cells are induced to commit suicide.

Granulosa cells—Cells that form the wall of the ovarian follicle.

Oncogene—A gene whose presence can cause cancer; these genes usually arise through mutation of a normal gene.

Ovarian follicle—Several layers of cells that surround a maturing egg in the ovary.

Thromboembolism—A blood clot that blocks a blood vessel in the cardiovascular system.

Recommended dosage

Toremifene is taken orally, and the recommended dose is usually 40 to 60 milligrams once a day, although larger doses are sometimes prescribed. If a dose is missed, patients should not double the next dosage. Instead, they should return to their regular schedule and contact their doctor.

Precautions

Toremifene is not recommended for use in children. Women who are pregnant or nursing should not use this drug since it has several side effects that, although rare, can be severe. It is known to cause miscarriages and birth defects. Women are encouraged to use birth control while taking toremifene. However, oral contraceptives can negatively alter the effects of toremifene. Therefore, patients should explore other birth control options.

Great care should be exercised when toremifene is used with **warfarin**, an anticoagulant, because toremifene can amplify the effects of warfarin, prolonging bleeding times. The result could possibly be fatal. Patients who are predisposed to the formation of thromboembolisms should use toremifene with caution, because toremifene can increase the risk.

Side effects

Although toremifene is usually well tolerated by patients, there are some side effects. One of the most serious side effects is development of uterine cancer. Less common effects include eye problems such as retinal lesions, macular edema, and corneal changes (most resolve themselves after use is discontinued); neurological problems such as **depression**, dizziness, confusion, and **fatigue**; and genital problems such as vaginal bleeding, vaginal discharge, and endometriosis. Patients also may experience liver problems.

Interactions

Toremifene can interfere with the anticoagulant drug warfarin, resulting in severe consequences and death. If these two drugs are used together, patients will be monitored closely. Oral contraceptives and estrogen supplements can also interfere with the action of toremifene.

See also Raloxifene.

Resources

PERIODICALS

"GTx Starts Phase III Study With Prostate Cancer Drug." *BIOWORLD Today* 219 (November 11, 2003).

Sally C. McFarlane-Parrott
Teresa G. Odle

Tositumomab

Definition

Tositumomab is a mouse monoclonal antibody that directly targets and binds with the CD20 receptor of normal and malignant B-cell lymphocytes. When linked with iodine I-131, Tositumomab creates an effective radioimmunotherapy agent, Iodine I-131 Tositumomab; also known as the BEXXAR(r) therapeutic regimen.

KEY TERMS

Cytopenias—Disorders that cause a severe deficiency in the production of one or more the blood cell types: red blood cells (anemia), white blood cells (neutropenia), and platelets (thrombocytopenia). Cytopenias can be caused by cancer, chemotherapy, and radiation therapy.

Monoclonal antibodies—Monoclonal antibodies recognize and lock onto the proteins found on the surface of cancer cells. They can cause the cancer cells to destroy themselves, as well as directly target the body's immune system against the cancer cells. This form of passive immunotherapy can even be effective for treating patients with weakened immune systems, as the monoclonal antibodies are mass produced outside the body in a laboratory setting.

Myelodysplasia—A group of disorders in which the bone marrow does not function normally and produces insufficient numbers of normal blood cells.

Non-Hodgkin's lymphoma—A disease that causes malignant cancer cells to form in the lymphatic system and is unpredictable in nature and more likely to spread to other sites.

Radioimmunotherapy—A treatment modality, in which cytotoxic radiation is delivered directly to a tumor via binding antibodies. Also known as targeted radiotherapy.

Purpose

As part of the BEXXAR(r) therapeutic regimen, Tositumomab is used in the treatment of patients with CD20 positive, follicular, **non-Hodgkin's lymphoma** (NHL), with or without transformation, whose disease is untreatable with **Rituximab** and has relapsed following **chemotherapy**. Clinical studies of the BEXXAR(r) therapeutic regimen have shown positive overall response rates (approximately 63%) and prolonged response durations (upwards of 25 months).

Description

Tositumomab, a monoclonal antibody, can recognize and target the protein produced by the CD20 receptor commonly found on the surface of normal and malignant B-cell lymphocytes. Once injected into the body, the monoclonal antibody seeks out and binds with the CD20 receptor, much as a key fits into a lock. Once attached to the CD20 receptor, the antibody produces a cytotoxic effect and triggers the body's immune system against the **cancer** cell. This, in turn, exposes the cancer cell, making it more susceptible to radiation. When combined with a radioactive substance, in this case Iodine I-131, the monoclonal antibody allows the ionizing radiation to directly target the cancerous lymphocytes. As lymphomas are particularly vulnerable to radiotherapy, the BEXXAR(r) therapeutic regimen increases the chance of destroying malignant **lymphoma** B-cells.

The Food and Drug Administration (FDA) approved the Corixa Corporation's BEXXAR(r) (Tositumomab and Iodine I-131 Tositumomab) therapeutic regimen for the treatment of NHL in June 2003. Clinical studies based on cumulative clinical experience between 1995 and 2005 showed the benefits of the BEXXAR(r) therapeutic regimen, based on durable responses without evidence of an effect on patient survival.

Recommended dosage

Intended for a single course of treatment, the BEXXAR(r) therapeutic regimen is administered in two discrete stages over a period of one to two weeks. These stages, the dosimetric stage and the therapeutic stage, are conducted over a period of four hospital visits.

Before treatment begins, and for two weeks subsequent to the therapeutic stage, the patient is provided with daily iodine supplements, typically provided in the form of liquid drops or tablets. The supplements protect the patient's thyroid gland from the radioactive I-131 during the treatment.

At the beginning of the dosimetric stage of the BEXXAR(r) treatment, paracetamol and antihistamine drips are administered to counteract possible side effects. The patient is provided with a sequential infusion of Tositumomab, totaling 450 mg, over the next hour. This step of the treatment assures that the infusion of Iodine I-131 Tositumomab will spread evenly throughout the patient's body. Finally, an infusion of 35 mg Tositumomab and 5 mCi Iodine I-131 (Iodine I-131 Tositumomab) is administered for 20 minutes. The patient then undergoes the first of three body scans to determine the levels of radioactivity within the patient's body and where it is located. The patient undergoes a second and third body scan at days two to four and days six to seven, respectively. These scans allow the doctor to determine the appropriate dosage for the therapeutic stage of the treatment. This is a complicated evaluation process, and as such, the BEXXAR(r) treatment is only available to physicians with the required training to make proper assessments.

The therapeutic stage begins on the fourth hospital visit, which typically takes place 7 to 14 days after the dosimetric stage. Once again, the patient is provided with a sequential infusion drip of Tositumomab, totaling 450 mg, over a one-hour period. This is followed by an infusion of Iodine I-131 Tositumomab, consisting of 35mg Tositumomab and a dosage of Iodine I-131 determined by the findings from the dosimetric stage. Additional factors, such as the presence of **thrombocytopenia**, can require the dosage of Iodine I-131 to be reduced.

Precautions

The BEXXAR(r) therapeutic regimen is contraindicated for patients with known hypersensitivity to murine (mouse) proteins and/or intolerance to thyroid-blocking agents. Patients should be screened for human hypersensitivity antibodies (HAMA) to avoid risk of serious reactions, including anaphylaxis. Patients with impaired hepatic or renal function, impaired bone marrow reserves, and/or more than 25% lymphoma marrow involvement should use caution when considering the BEXXAR(r) therapeutic regimen, as safety and efficacy have not as of 2005 been clinically established.

Due to the radioactive components of this treatment, the BEXXAR(r) therapeutic regimen can cause fetal harm and, as such, is contraindicated for pregnant women. Additionally, an effective contraceptive should be used during and for at least a year following therapy to prevent possible birth defects. Patients wishing to have children should speak with their healthcare provider, as Iodine I-131 tositumomab possesses the risk of toxic effects on male and female fertility.

Patients must strictly follow all safety measures associated with radioactivity during and after therapy, as their bodies will remain radioactive during this time. Healthcare providers will inform their patients of specific safety instructions and their duration. Typical precautions include minimizing close contact (within six feet) with family members. Infants, young children, and pregnant women are particularly susceptible and should be strictly avoided. Nursing is strongly contraindicated, as radioiodine is excreted in breast milk and can build up to levels equal to or greater than those found in the mother. Patients should avoid sharing the same bed or using the same hygienic facilities as other people. Finally, prolonged travel (three to four hours) in close proximity to others should be avoided, such as cars, trains, or airplanes. If possible, the patient should remain as far as possible from others during short trips.

Side effects

Clinical studies of the BEXXAR(r) therapeutic regimen have shown prolonged and severe cytopenias to be the most common adverse reactions, occurring in 71% of the patients studied. Thrombocytopenia and **neutropenia** were the primary forms of cytopenia, documented in 63% and 53% of patients undergoing therapy, respectively. **Anemia** also appeared in 27% of the studied patients. These adverse effects also included the consequences commonly associated with cytopenias, such as infections, hemorrhaging, and the requirement of blood growth factors and/or blood support.

Allergic reactions (angiodema and bronchospasm), **pneumonia**, secondary leukemia, solid tumors, and myelodysplasia were also observed. The most frequent non-hematological adverse effects observed in patients included asthenia (weakness), **fever**, **nausea**, gastrointestinal symptoms, chills, and pruritus (intense **itching**). Other known side effects include back pain, constipation, **diarrhea**, dizziness, and headache. The BEXXAR(r) therapeutic regimen is also associated with further risks of infusion-related reactions, delayed-onset hypothyroidism, and HAMA. Health providers should inform patients of these risks before beginning treatment.

Interactions

Although no formal drug interaction studies have been conducted on the BEXXAR(r) therapeutic regimen, patients should avoid certain drugs unless specifically prescribed by their health provider. These drugs include aspirin, ibuprofen, ketoprofen, and naproxen, as these drugs may mask a fever or increase the risk of hemorrhaging. Additionally, anticoagulants and agents interfering with platelet function may increase the risk of bleeding. Tositumomab may decrease the response to and increase the risk of adverse reactions to live-virus **vaccines**. As such, patients undergoing the BEXXAR(r) therapeutic regimen are strongly urged to consult with their health provider before undergoing any form of immunization.

Resources

BOOKS

Lacy, C. F., et al. *Lexi-Comp's Drug Information Handbook* 12th ed. Hudson, OH: Lexi-Comp, 2004.

Souhami, R. L., et al., eds. *Oxford Textbook of Oncology* 2nd ed. New York: Oxford University Press, 2002.

PERIODICALS

Friedberg, J. W., and R. I. Fisher. "Iodine-131 Tositumomab (Bexxar(r)): Radioimmunoconjugate Therapy for Indolent and Transformed B-cell Non-Hodgkin's Lymphoma." *Expert Review of Anticancer Therapy* 4 (February 2004): 18–26.

Kaminski, M. S., et al. " ^{131}I-Tositumomab Therapy as Initial Treatment for Follicullar Lymphoma." *New England Journal of Medicine* 352 (February 2005): 441–49.

Vose, J. M. "Bexxar(r): Novel Radioimmunotherapy for the Treatment of Low-Grade and Transformed Low-Grade Non-Hodgkin's Lymphoma." *The Oncologist* 9 (April 2004): 160–72.

Wahl, R. L. "Tositumomab and ^{131}I Therapy in Non-Hodgkin's Lymphoma." *Journal of Nuclear Medicine* 46 (January 2005): 128S–40S.

OTHER

"Bexxar(r)." U.S. Food and Drug Administration [cited April 14, 2005]. http://www.fda.gov/cder/foi/label/2003/tosicor062703LB.pdf.

"Monoclonal Antibody Therapy: Bexxar(r)." Lymphoma Information Network [cited April 14, 2005]. http://www.lymphomainfo.net/therapy/immunotherapy/bexxar.html.

"Newly Approved Cancer Treatments: Bexxar(r)." National Cancer Institute [cited April 14, 2005]. http://www.cancer.gov/clinicaltrials/developments/newly-approved-treatments/page8.

"Tositumomab." American Cancer Society [cited April 14, 2005]. http://www.cancer.org/docroot/CDG/content/CDG_tositumomab.html.

Jason Fryer

Tracheostomy

A tracheostomy is an artificial airway, which is surgically inserted through the windpipe to allow normal respiration.

The key purpose of a tracheostomy is to provide a patient with an open, functional airway. Normal respiration can become hindered or blocked by an obstruction to the upper respiratory tract; the area between the nose and mouth down through the larynx. When a serious obstruction occurs, normal respiratory techniques, such as oral or nasal intubation, may be inadequate or completely ineffective. Obstructions can come from several sources, including foreign bodies, swollen soft tissue, and injury to the larynx and/or trachea. Furthermore, proper respiration can also be obstructed by the growth of malignant tumors in the mouth, larynx, trachea, nasopharynx (the space above and behind the soft palate), and the nasal cavity and paranasal sinuses.

Proper oxygenation of the lungs may also require the use of a tracheostomy. Malignant pulmonary cancers, such as bronchioloalveolar **carcinoma** and **mesothelioma**, can cause serious respiratory problems, including hypoxia (an insufficient oxygen level in the blood and tissues) or hypercapnia (excess levels of carbon dioxide in the blood due to hypoventilation). A tracheostomy can provide the required oxygen levels via the tracheobronchial tree, also known as the bronchia.

A tracheostomy may also be used to clean and remove secretions that build up in the bronchia and throat due to injury, disease, and tumors. This excess fluid can cause obstructions and/or restrict proper oxygenation. Blood and secretions can be suctioned out through the trachea to relieve breathing problems.

There are no known contraindications for the use of a tracheostomy. However, some surgical modalities, such as removal of malignancies, may be required prior to the tracheotomy procedure.

At the simplest level, a *tracheostomy* is an artificial airway that is inserted into the trachea (windpipe) to bypass the upper airway. The surgical procedure to create this secondary airway is known as a *tracheotomy*. Tracheostomies provide physicians with one of the most effective methods to relieving breathing problems due to obstruction. Indeed, historical evidence reveals that tracheostomies may have been used as far back as 2000 B.C. Since Antonio Brasavola performed the first documented tracheotomy in the sixteenth century, surgeons and doctors have been developing and refining this effective medical procedure.

The most common form of tracheostomy is a hollow tube of plastic, silicon, or metal, also known as a tracheostomy tube or trach. During a tracheotomy, this tube is surgically inserted into the patient's neck just beneath the larynx to provide access to the trachea, thus acting as a secondary airway. The surgical opening through which the tracheostomy is inserted is also known as the stoma. Depending on the underlying cause of obstruction and/or respiratory distress, a tracheostomy may be temporary or permanent in nature. Tracheostomies are far more effective for suctioning purposes and maintaining respiratory function than other artificial airways. There are three key types of tracheotomies: *Elective*, *Awake*, and *Emergent*.

- Elective—The majority of tracheotomy procedures are elective in nature. Most patients will have already been intubated by this point in time and may require more prolonged and/or more effective form of intubation. These procedures are conducted under controlled conditions, usually performed in a hospital's operating room under the supervision of a surgeon and anesthesiologist.
- Awake—Acute respiratory distress may require an "awake" tracheotomy. These procedures are typically conducted under controlled conditions and using local anesthesia. However, the patient remains conscious throughout the procedure, which can be extremely disconcerting for the patient. The operating surgeon must be prepared for difficulties caused the heightened levels of anxiety the patient will undoubtedly exhibit.
- Emergent—Emergent tracheotomies, sometimes crudely referred to as "slash" tracheostomies, generally should not be considered unless the patient is in extremis and intubation is inadvisable. Even in these extreme cases, a cricothyrotomy is more advisable to relieve respiratory distress that a tracheotomy.

There are several variations of the tracheotomy, but follow a basic guideline. Once the patient is anesthetized, either generally or locally, the neck is cleaned and positioned. Surgical incisions expose the tough cartilage rings that form the trachea's outer wall. An incision is made through two of these rings and a tracheostomy tube inserted into the windpipe.

Tracheostomy tubes come in a variety of shapes, sizes, and compositions. Tubes are generally designed to the meet specific medical requirements, and can be either disposable or reusable in nature. The Universal is the most commonly used tracheostomy tube. Also known as the "double-luman" or "double-cannula" tube, the Universal consists of three parts: the outer cannula (with cuff and pilot tube), the inner cannula, and the obturator. Other commonly used tracheostomy tubes include:

- Single cannula (used for patients with long and/or thin necks)
- Fenestrated (allow speech and improve swallow function)
- Tracheostomy Button (used to wean patients before final removal of tracheostomy tubes or in the treatment of sleep apnea)
- Cuffed tube (used commonly when mechanical ventilation is required and prevents aspiration of secretions)
- Cuffless tube (used in long-term management)

If possible, the patient should fully discuss the procedure and other viable opinions with their physician at length before undergoing a tracheostomy. Additionally, cancers of the upper airway and throat may require the use of other surgical procedures beforehand. In these cases, an effective treatment plan incorporating the tracheostomy should be established. Stabilization of precipitating factors may also be required beforehand.

Successful tracheostomies require effective and thorough postoperative care. Patients may require one to three days to breathe normally following the insertion of a tracheostomy tube. The tube may prevent verbal communication for a prolonged period, and other methods of communication should be utilized. All patients with tracheostomy tubes require humidification to prevent further complications associated with inspired gases. Aftercare modalities should strive to accomplish four key goals:

- Maintain the patient's airway
- Maintain tracheal integrity
- Avoid infections
- Avoid tube displacement

Patients and family members should be educated in aftercare modalities and information as soon as possible. Home nursing service may be required for patients. Otherwise, a return to regular home life is encouraged. However, while outdoors, a scarf or similar covering around the throat is indicated.

Directly following the procedure, the trachea will produce excessive secretions due to trauma. In addition to monitoring of these secretions, continual saline irrigation and suctioning will be required. Mucolytic (anti-mucus) agents can be utilized to prevent dangerous obstructions. Assessment of the patient's vital signs should also be maintained, in addition to monitoring for other complications associated with surgery.

Further complications can be encountered at all stages of recovery following a tracheotomy: *immediate*, *early*, and *late*.

Immediate complications can occur directly following the tracheotomy and include:

- Apnea
- Bleeding
- Pneumothorax (accumulation of air or gas in the pleural cavity)
- Pneumomediastinum (escape of air into the pleural tissues)
- Injury to adjacent structures
- Postobstructive pulmonary edema (accumulation of fluid in the lungs)

Early complications typically occur within seven days of the tracheotomy and include:

- Bleeding
- Mucus obstructions
- Inflammation of the trachea
- Inflammation of subcutaneous or connective tissue around the incision
- Tube displacement
- Subcutaneous emphysema (air or gas in subcutaneous tissues)
- Total or partial collapse of the lung

Late complications can occur at any time seven days following the tracheotomy and can include:

- Bleeding
- Tracheomalacia (degeneration of the elastic and connective tissue of the trachea)
- Tracheoesophageal fistula (an abnormal connection between the trachea and the esophagus)
- Tracheocutaneous fistula (an abnormal connection between the trachea and the surface of the neck)
- Granulation and scarring
- Failure to remove the tracheostomy tube

The normal tracheostomy can be used for days, weeks, and even or years with proper treatment. However, tracheostomy tubes should be downsized and removed as quickly as medically viable. Once the tracheostomy is removed, the stoma is sealed and allowed to heal over a period of five to seven days. Typically, a full recovery can be expected within two weeks with little to no scarring.

Several abnormal results of varying seriousness are associated with tracheostomies. However, patients should contact local emergency services if their tracheostomy tube is dislodged and cannot be replaced. Additional concerns include:

- Infection
- Fever
- Chills
- Incision sites problems, such as swelling, increased pain, and excessive bleeding
- Nausea and/or vomiting
- Shortness of breath and/or cough despite suctioning
- Persistent speech difficulties after tracheostomy removal

Resources

BOOKS

Russell, C., and B Matta. *Tracheostomy: A Multiproffessional Handbook*. Cambridge, UK: Cambridge University Press, 2003.

PERIODICALS

Hsu, C.L., K.Y. Chen, C.H. Chang, J.S. Jerng, C.J. Yu, and P.C. Yang. "Timing of Tracheostomy as a determinant of Weaning Success in Critically Ill Patients: A Retrospective Study."9(#1, 2005):R46-R52.

Lewis, C., J Carron, J. Perkins, K. Sie, and C. Feudtner. "Tracheotomy in Pediatric Patients: A National Perspective."129(May2003):523-529.

OTHER

Dixon, S. "Tracheostomy: Postoperative Recovery." http://www.perspectivesinnursing.org/v1n1/Dixon.html.

Morgan, C., and S. Dixon. "Tracheostomy." http://www.emedicine.com/ent/topic356.htm.

"Tracheostomy Home." http://www.tracheostomy.com/.

Jason Fryer

Transfusion therapy

Definition

The process of transferring whole blood or blood components from one person (donor) to another (recipient).

Purpose

Transfusions are given to restore lost or depleted blood components, to improve clotting time, and to improve the ability of the blood to deliver oxygen to the body's tissues. Typical reasons **cancer** patients receive blood transfusions are for **anemia** (low red blood cell count) and for clotting factors or platelets (for example, in certain types of leukemia).

Precautions

For donors, the process of giving blood is very safe. Only sterile equipment is used and there is no chance of catching an **infection** from the equipment. There is a slight chance of infection at the puncture site if the skin is not properly washed before the collection needle is inserted. Some donors feel light-headed upon standing for the first time after donating. Occasionally, a donor will faint. Donors are advised to drink plenty of liquids to replace the fluid lost with the donation of blood. It is important to maintain the fluid volume of the blood so that the blood pressure will remain stable. Strenuous exercise should be avoided for the rest of the day. Most patients have very slight symptoms or no symptoms at all after donating blood. People who have cancer usually are not considered candidates for blood donation.

For recipients, a number of precautions must be taken by the blood bank. The blood given by transfusion must be matched with the recipient's blood type. Incompatible blood types can cause a serious adverse reaction (transfusion reaction). Blood is introduced slowly by gravity flow directly into the veins (intravenous infusion) so that medical personnel can observe the patient for signs of adverse reactions. People who have received many transfusions (such as leukemia patients) can develop an **immune response** to some factors in foreign blood cells. This immune reaction must be checked before giving new blood. Infectious diseases can also be transmitted through donated blood. However, many safeguards are in place in the United States to minimize the risk of transmission of blood-borne pathogens (agents in the blood that cause disease) to recipients.

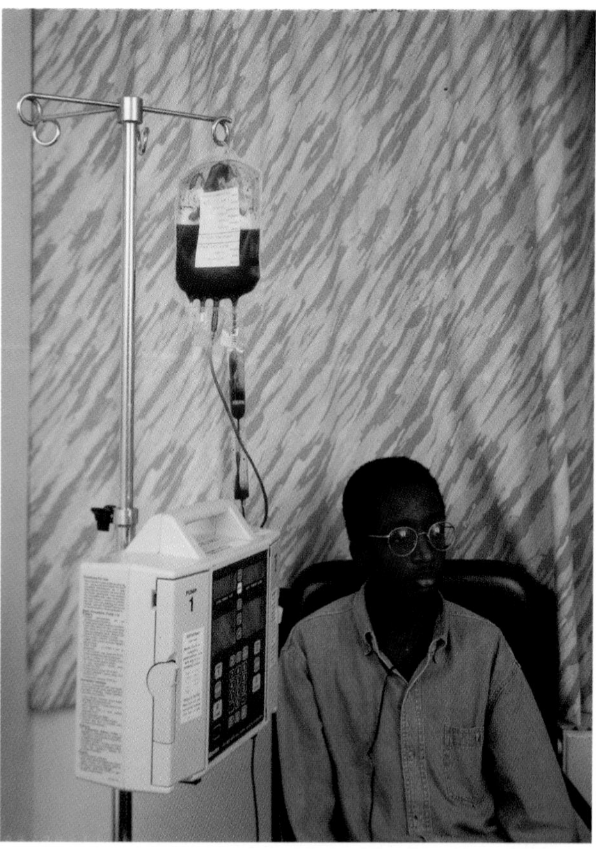

This boy is receiving a transfusion for sickle cell anemia. Cancer patients may receive blood transfusions to treat anemia, or to receive clotting factors or platelets (in certain types of leukemia, for example). *(Custom Medical Stock Photo. Reproduced by permission.)*

Description

WHOLE BLOOD. Either whole blood or blood components can be used for transfusion. Whole blood is used exactly as it was received from the

QUESTIONS TO ASK THE DOCTOR

- Am I a candidate for autologous transfusion?
- Am I a candidate for a directed donation?
- How often will I have blood work done to determine my hemoglobin and hematocrit levels?
- Can I get a stem cell transfusion at this facility if I need one?
- Is a blood transfusion necessary before I have surgery?

KEY TERMS

ABO blood groups—A system in which human blood is classified by whether the red blood cells contain A or B antigens. Type A blood has the A antigen, type B has the B antigen, AB has both, and 0 has neither.

Antibody—A simple protein produced by the body to destroy bacteria, viruses, or other foreign bodies. Production of each antibody is triggered by a specific antigen.

Antigen—A substance that stimulates the immune system to manufacture antibodies (immunoglobulins). The function of antibodies is to fight off intruder cells, such as bacteria or viruses, in the body. Antigens stimulate the blood to fight other blood cells that have the wrong antigens. If a person with blood type A is given a transfusion with blood type B, the A antigens will fight the foreign blood cells as though they were an infection.

Immunoglobulin—An antibody.

Infusion—Introduction of a substance directly into a vein or tissue by gravity flow.

Injection—Forcing a fluid into the body by means of a needle and syringe.

Rh (rhesus) factor—An antigen present in the red blood cells of 85% of humans. A person with Rh factor is Rh positive (Rh+); a person without it is Rh negative (Rh-). The Rh factor was first identified in the blood of a rhesus monkey.

donor. Blood components are parts of whole blood, such as red blood cells (RBCs), plasma, platelets, clotting factors, immunoglobulins, and white blood cells. Whole blood is used only when needed or when components are not available. Most of the time, whole blood is not used because the patient's medical condition can be treated with a blood component. Too much whole blood can fluid-overload a patient's circulatory system. This can create high blood pressure and congestive heart failure (overwork of the heart muscle to pump the extra fluid volume). The use of blood components is more efficient and effective because blood that has been fractionated (processed) into components can be used to treat more than one person.

PLASMA. Plasma is the liquid portion of blood. It contains many useful proteins, especially clotting factors and immunoglobulins. After they are processed, plasma or plasma factors (fractions) are usually frozen. Some plasma fractions are freeze-dried. These fractions include clotting factors I through XIII. Some people have an inherited disorder in which the body produces too little of the plasma clotting factors VIII (hemophilia A) or IX (hemophilia B). Transfusions of these clotting factors help people with hemophilia to stop bleeding. Frozen plasma must be thawed before it is used and freeze-dried plasma must be mixed with liquid (reconstituted). In both cases, these blood fractions are usually small in volume and can be injected by syringe and needle.

RED BLOOD CELLS. Red blood cells are the blood component most frequently used for transfusion. RBCs are the only cells in the body that transport oxygen. A transfusion of RBCs increases the amount of oxygen that can be carried to the tissues of the body. RBCs that have been separated from the liquid plasma (packed RBCs) are given to people who have anemia (low red cell count) or who have lost a lot of blood. There are many causes of anemia. In cancer, anemia is caused by the destruction of red blood cells by disease, by medications such as **chemotherapy**, or by disease in the bone marrow where red blood cells are produced. To determine how serious the anemia is, the physician will do a CBC (complete blood count) to look at the hemoglobin level (the oxygen-carrying capacity of the red blood cells), and a hematocrit (the percentage of RBCs in a given volume of blood).

PLATELETS. Platelets are another component frequently given by transfusion. Platelets are a key factor in blood clotting. The clear fluid that carries blood cells (plasma) also contains blood-clotting factors. The platelets and plasma clotting factors are extracted from donated blood and concentrated for use. These factors are used to treat cancer patients whose bone marrow has been destroyed by disease. Cancer patients may need platelet transfusions when their bone marrow is not producing enough platelets, either because the bone marrow has been damaged by chemotherapy or because it has been replaced by the growth of cancer cells. Dangerous bleeding may occur if the platelet count is too low. However, if there is no evidence of bleeding (no clinical signs of bleeding), platelets may not be given even if the count is low.

IMMUNOGLOBULINS. Immunoglobulins, also called gamma globulin or immune serum, are collected from plasma for use in temporarily boosting the immune capability of a patient. White blood cells (WBCs) are another infection-fighting component of the blood. White blood cells are given by transfusion only rarely. Immunoglobulins are the infection-fighting fraction of blood plasma. This blood fraction is given to people who have difficulty fighting infections, especially people whose immune systems are depressed by diseases, such as HIV/AIDS and cancer. Immmunoglobulins are also used to prevent tetanus after cuts, to treat animal bites when rabies infection is suspected, or to treat severe childhood diseases. Immunoglobulins can also be used to treat idiopathic thrombocytopenic purpura (ITP), a condition characterized by a low platelet count and excessive bruising.

COLONY-STIMULATING FACTORS OR GROWTH FACTORS. Granulocytes are a type of white blood cell that fight infection. Granulocyte transfusion is no longer done because of the **fever** it produces and the potential transmission of infectious diseases through white cells. These infections (CMV or cytomegalovirus) would be particularly dangerous to a cancer patient with a weakened immune system. Chemotherapy patients can develop a low WBC (white cell count). A specific white blood cell called the neutrophil is carefully monitored because it is very important in fighting multiple types of infection. If neutrophil counts are very low, the physician may order special medications that stimulate the production of neutrophils in the bone marrow. These medicines are called colony-stimulating factors or growth factors, and include granulocyte colony-stimulating factor (G-CSF, or **filgrastim**), granulocyte macrophage colony-stimulating factor (GM-CSF, or **sargramostim**), and interleukin-3.

ALTERNATIVES TO BLOOD TRANSFUSION. Researchers have been working to develop a substitute for blood that will avoid the risks associated with blood transfusion. Products are being developed that will perform the functions of red blood cells, such as carrying oxygen through the blood stream, but there is no real substitute for the transfusion of human blood. Two products that are currently available are known as hemoglobin-based oxygen carriers and perfluorochemical compounds. These products can be used on a short term basis to perform the function of blood, but are still considered experimental.

Other types of products that can help patients in need of large volumes of body fluids are volume expanders such as normal saline solution, lactated ringers, or dextran. These are IV (intravenous) solutions that can replace lost fluid volume but not the red blood cells' function of carrying oxygen to the body. Other volume expanders include albumin, a protein solution used to stabilize oncotic pressure (pressure within the veins) and prevent or treat shock. Growth factors, as mentioned earlier, help promote the production of specific white cells needed to fight infections. **Erythropoietin** and **thrombopoietin** are products available to help stimulate the production of red blood cells and platelets. None of these products replace the benefits of blood or blood component transfusions.

New cancer treatments under research

Researchers are looking at the efficacy of using sibling blood components, specifically transfusions of stem cells and T cells, a part of the immune system that can attack and destroy cancer cells. Blood from tissue-matched sibling donors reduces the rejection rate by the patient's body chemistry. This technique is being studied in renal (kidney) tumors, and early results show promise. Researchers are particularly interested in this therapy for renal tumors with **metastasis** (spreading of the cancer to other parts of the body) because this type of cancer does not usually respond to standard cancer therapy protocols. While blood transfusions and bone marrow transplants have been used extensively for cancers of the blood, this is the first time transfusions have been successful in the treatment of solid tumors (such as renal tumors).

Researchers are also looking at the placenta and umbilical cord as a source for blood stem cells for transplant. This method is called cord blood transplantation. It offers an alternative for patients who do not have a sibling donor, or cannot locate a match in the National Marrow Donor Program (NMDP) registry.

Blood donation

Each year in the United States, about 14,000,000 pints of blood are donated. Blood collection is strictly regulated by the Food and Drug Administration (FDA). The FDA has rules for the collection, processing, storage, and transportation of blood and blood products. In addition, the American Red Cross, the American Association of Blood Banks, and most states have specific rules for the collection and processing of blood. The main purpose of regulation is to ensure the quality of blood and to prevent the transmission of infectious diseases through donated blood. Before blood and blood products are used, they are extensively tested for infectious agents, such as hepatitis and HIV/AIDS. Screening prevents blood donation by people who could transmit diseases or by people whose medical condition would place them at risk if they donated blood. Some geographical areas or communities have a high rate of hepatitis or HIV/AIDS. Blood collection in most of these areas has been discontinued.

SPECIAL DONATIONS: AUTOLOGOUS TRANSFUSION. Autologous transfusion is a procedure in which patients donate blood for their own use. Patients who are to undergo surgical procedures for which a blood transfusion might be required may elect to donate a store of blood for the purpose ahead of time. The blood is stored at the hospital for the exclusive use of the patient. This procedure assures that the blood type is an exact match. It also assures that no infection will be transmitted through the blood transfusion. This is most helpful to cancer patients because of the reduction of risk for a transfusion reaction and for infection risks associated with transfusions. As with other forms of specialized blood donations, there is a processing fee for collection and delivering each unit of blood, which may not be reimbursed by **health insurance**.

SPECIAL DONATIONS: DIRECTED DONATION. Directed donors are family or friends of the patient who needs a transfusion. Some people think that family and friends provide a safer source of blood than the general blood supply. Studies do not show that directed donor blood is any safer. Blood that is not used for the identified patient becomes part of the general blood supply.

SPECIAL DONATIONS: APHERESIS. Apheresis is a special procedure in which only the necessary components of a donor's blood are collected. The remaining components are returned to the donor. A special blood-processing instrument is used in apheresis. It separates the blood into components, saves the desired component, and pumps the other components back into the donor. Because donors give only part of their blood, they can donate more frequently. For example, people can give almost ten times as many platelets by apheresis as they could give by donating whole blood.

Preparation

The person receiving a transfusion is made comfortable and vital signs (temperature, blood pressure, pulse and respirations) are monitored closely. The site where the needle will be inserted is carefully washed with a soap-based solution, followed by an iodine-containing antiseptic. The skin is then dried and the transfusion needle inserted into the recipient's vein. During the early stages of a transfusion, the recipient is monitored closely to detect any adverse reactions. If no signs of adverse reaction are evident, the patient is monitored routinely for the duration of the transfusion period. Upon completion of the transfusion, a pressure bandage is placed over the needle-insertion site to prevent bleeding.

Aftercare

Recipients of a blood transfusion have their vital signs monitored during and after the transfusion for signs of adverse reaction. The physician usually orders laboratory tests to check hemoglobin and hematocrit levels, as well as platelet count once the transfusion has ended. This data will help the physician determine if the transfusion of blood or blood products was sufficient.

Risks

Adverse reaction to mismatched blood (transfusion reaction) and transmission of infectious disease are the two major risks of blood transfusion. Transfusion reaction occurs when antibodies in the recipient's blood react to foreign blood cells introduced by the transfusion. The antibodies bind to the foreign cells and destroy them (hemolytic reaction). Transfusion reaction may also cause a hypersensitivity of the immune system that, in turn, may cause tissue damage within the patient's body. The patient may also have an allergic reaction to mismatched blood. The first symptoms of transfusion reaction are a feeling of general discomfort and anxiety. Breathing difficulties, flushing, a sense of pressure in the chest, and back pain may develop. Evidence of a hemolytic reaction can be seen in the urine, which will be colored from the waste of destroyed red blood cells. Severe hemolytic reactions are occasionally fatal. Reactions to mismatches of minor factors are milder. These symptoms include itchiness, dizziness, fever, headache, rash, and swelling. Sometimes, the patient will experience breathing difficulties and muscle spasms. Most adverse reactions from mismatched blood are not life-threatening.

Although transfusions are often necessary, some studies have noted a poorer prognosis if transfusions are done before surgery for **breast cancer**, **colon cancer**, **non-small cell lung cancer**, and sarcomas. A National Institutes of Health (NIH) consensus was that transfusion before surgery should not be given simply to raise the hemoglobin level above 10g/dl. The growth factor erythropoietin may be used more in the future to decrease the need for red blood cell transfusions.

Resources

BOOKS

Berkow, Robert, editor. *Merck Manual of Medical Information.* New York: Pocket Books, 2000.

Dailey, J.F. *Dailey's Notes on Blood.* 4th ed. Arlington, MA: Medical Consulting Group, 2000.

PERIODICALS

Cerhan, James R., R. Wallace, F. Dick, et al. "Blood Transfusions and Risk of Non-Hodgkin's Lymphoma subtypes and Chronic Lymphocytic Leukemia." *Cancer Epidemiology, Biomarkers, and Prevention* 10, no. 4 (2001).

Mullon, J., et al. "Transfusions of Polymerized Bovine Hemoglobin in a Patient With Severe Autoimmune Hemolytic Anemia." *New England Journal of Medicine* 342 (June 1, 2000): 1666–8.

Pysz, Maciej. "Blood Transfusions in Breast Cancer Patients Undergoing Mastectomy: Possible Importance of Timing." *Journal of Surgical Oncology* 75, no. 4 (2000).

Rios, J. A., D. N. Korones, J. M. Heal, et al. "WBC-reduced blood transfusions and clinical outcome in children with acute lymphoid leukemia." *Transfusion* 41, no. 7 (2001).

OTHER

"Blood Product Donation and Transfusion." *ACS Cancer Resource Center* [cited July 17, 2001]. http://www3.cancer.org/cancerinfo.

John T. Lohr
Molly Metzler, R.N.

Transitional care

Definition

According to the National Cancer Institute (NCI), transitional care may refer either to a patient's movement from one level of cancer care to another, or from one place of care to another. Levels of cancer care are defined as active (intended to cure the cancer), supportive (intended to relieve discomfort associated with the symptoms of the cancer or the side effects of treatment), or palliative (intended to manage pain when cure is no longer possible). Places of care are categorized as acute care facilities, subacute care facilities (e.g., rehabilitation centers, nursing homes, and hospices), and home care (usually the patient's or family's house).

KEY TERMS

Biopsychosocial model—A way of evaluating a patient that stresses the importance of considering his or her thinking processes, emotions, and social relationships as well as the physical aspects of his or her disease. The biopsychosocial model was first proposed in 1977 by an American psychiatrist named George Engel.

Hospice—A health care facility for supportive and palliative care of people with a terminal disease.

Description

Transitional care for cancer patients has become a pressing health care issue in the early 2000s. One reason is that health care in the United States and Canada has become increasingly specialized in terms of facilities as well as care givers; in addition, the NCI states that almost 90% of care for cancer patients is now given on an outpatient basis. In an acute care hospital or cancer center, a cancer patient may have a health care team that consists of three or more doctors in various medical and surgical specialties as well as nurses, physical therapists, social workers, nutritionists, and others. As the patient undergoes various forms of cancer therapy, his or her response to treatments as well as financial concerns, family issues, and other considerations may lead to transfer to a subacute care facility or to home care.

Another factor that has led to a new understanding of the importance of transitional care is the growing number of long-term survivors of cancer. Although these people may be able to live at home by themselves or return to work, they still require various types of follow-up to monitor the long-term physical and psychological side effects of the cancer treatment they received.

Because of the growing complexity of cancer treatment and the risk that the patient's care may be fragmented or interrupted by changes in caregivers or facilities, medical professionals and policy makers presently emphasize the importance of integrated or "seamless" care. This concern for continuity is reflected both in the NCI's recommendations about changes in patient care and in its use of the biopsychosocial model of health care. The biopsychosocial model is the medical term for understanding the patient as a human being with thoughts, emotions, spiritual needs, and important relationships with family members and friends as well as physical symptoms related to the

QUESTIONS TO ASK YOUR DOCTOR

- What types of care will I need after I leave the hospital?
- Can I have these services delivered to my home, or must I go to a special facility of some kind?
- Is there someone you would recommend as a transitional care coordinator?
- How much experience do you have in following patients through transitions in their health care?

cancer. The NCI recommends the use of community liaison nurses and social workers as coordinators of patient care in order to relieve the patient or family members of the stress of relaying information from one health care professional to another, and to prevent the patient's care from being interrupted or weakened during transfers from one care facility to another.

The biopsychosocial model is the basis for the comprehensive assessment that precedes planning for transitional care. The patient's health care team will evaluate his or her needs in each of the following areas:

- Physical. This area includes nutritional status, ability to function, smoking history, and future treatment options as well as the current stage of the patient's disease and symptom profile.
- Demographics of the patient and his or her family. This area includes marital status, other family members at home, primary language, cultural background, and educational level.
- Psychological. This part of the assessment covers the patient's (and family members') attitudes toward the cancer, fears and anxieties, habitual coping patterns, history of psychiatric illness, and overall level of family stability.
- Social. This area includes the patient's social support networks, employment history, insurance coverage, availability of transportation, and the patient's knowledge and use of resources in the community.
- Spiritual. This part of the assessment includes the patient's religious beliefs and the level of importance of religion in their life, the extent of their support network in their faith community, and the ways in which their religious beliefs or practices may affect their cancer treatment.
- Legal. This area concerns such matters as the patient's will, estate planning, living will, end-of-life care directives, etc.

This comprehensive assessment should be made at regular intervals during the patient's treatment in order to make any necessary adjustments due to changes in the patient's physical symptoms and level of functioning, family situation, employment, etc.

Special concerns

The NCI notes that some groups of cancer patients are at risk of not receiving adequate treatment planning or transitional care. These patients include low-income and homeless people; members of minority groups living in the inner city; and people living in rural areas.

Treatments

The treatments given during transitional care are highly individualized; they depend on the specific patient's health status, type of cancer, and the types of treatments (surgery, **chemotherapy**, radiotherapy, etc.) that he or she received in the acute care hospital or cancer center. Advances in medical technology, however, have increased the range and variety of treatments that can be delivered by visiting health care professionals in the patient's home. These advances make transitional care at home a possibility for many cancer patients in the early 2000s.

Alternative and complementary therapies

It is usually possible to integrate CAM therapies into transitional care, provided that the patient discusses the specific alternative treatments desired with his or her doctor. Some types of movement or massage therapy may not be suitable immediately following surgery, however, while some herbal preparations or traditional Chinese medicines may interact with the drugs given to treat the cancer itself or to relieve the side effects of treatment.

Patient participation

In addition to consulting with a social worker or other professional coordinator, patients and their families should be actively involved in planning for transitional care. They can gather information about various therapies, care facilities, local support groups, and other resources, and discuss these among themselves as well as with members of the patient's treatment team. The patient and his or her family should not hesitate to ask questions or bring up issues that are not mentioned by the health care team during the patient's evaluation for transitional care. A new interactive resource that may be helpful to many patients in making decisions about treatment is the NexProfiler

Tool for Cancer on the ACS website. The patient chooses a specific type of cancer from a menu, which then allows him or her to locate a detailed analysis of that cancer, statistics about treatment types, and topics for discussion with his or her doctor.

See also Psycho-oncology.

Resources

PERIODICALS

Parks, Susan M., MD, and Karen D. Novielli, MD. "A Practical Guide to Caring for Caregivers." *American Family Physician* 62 (December 15, 2000): 2613–2622.

Sunga, Annette, MD, Margaret M. Eberl, MD, Kevin C. Oeffinger, MD, et al. "Care of Cancer Survivors." *American Family Physician* 71 (February 15, 2005): 699–714.

OTHER

American Cancer Society (ACS), "Finding Support." *Sources of Support*. http://www.cancer.org/docroot/MBC/content/MBC_4_1X_Finding_Support_.asp.

American Cancer Society (ACS), "Making Treatment Decisions." *Treatment Decision Tools*. http://www.cancer.org/docroot/ETO/eto_1_1a.asp?sitearea=ETO.

National Cancer Institute (NCI). *Transitional Care Planning (PDQ®)*, Health Professional version. http://www.cancer.gov/cancertopics/pdq/supportivecare/transitionalcare/HealthProfessional.

ORGANIZATIONS

American Cancer Society (ACS). (800) ACS-2345. http://www.cancer.org.

National Cancer Institute (NCI). Public Inquiries Office, 6116 Executive Boulevard, Room 3036A, Bethesda, MD 20892-8322. (800) 422-6237. http://www.nci.nih. gov.

Rebecca Frey, PhD

Transitional cell carcinoma

Definition

Transitional cell **carcinoma** (TCC) is a type of **cancer** that usually originates in the kidney, bladder, or ureter (the tube that carries urine from the kidney to the bladder). It has also been recently recognized as a subtype of **ovarian cancer**.

Description

A transitional cell is intermediate between the flat squamous cell and the tall columnar cell. It is restricted to the epithelium (cellular lining) of the urinary bladder, ureters (tubes that carry urine from the kidneys to the bladder), and the pelvis of the kidney (that portion of the kidney collecting the urine as it leaves the kidneys and enters the ureters). Transitional cell carcinomas have a wide range in their gross appearance depending on their locations. Some of these carcinomas are flat in appearance, some are papillary (small elevation), and others are in the shape of a node. Under the microscope, however, most of these carcinomas have a papillary-like look. There are three generally recognized grades of transitional cell carcinoma. The grade of the carcinoma is determined by particular characteristics found in the cells of the tumor. Transitional cell carcinoma typically affects the mucosa (the moist tissue layer that lines hollow organs or the cavity of the body) in the areas where it originates.

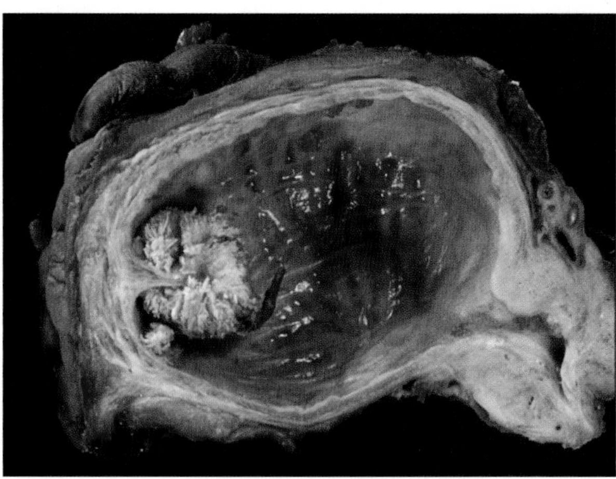

Transitional-cell carcinoma. Seen arising from the dome of the bladder as a fronded cauliflower-like lesion. *(Copyright Biophoto Associates, Science Source/Photo Researchers, Inc. Reproduced by permission.)*

The most common site of transitional cell carcinoma is in the urinary bladder. Transitional cell carcinoma is the form of cancer in about 90% of cancers found in the bladder. The highest grade of transitional cell carcinoma is very likely to spread to other parts of the body. There are two primary ways that transitional cell carcinoma spreads into the surrounding structures. The first is by way of epithelial cells that line the body cavity and many of the passageways that exit the body. The other means of spread is through the lymphatic (network that resembles the circulatory system but transports proteins, salts, water, and other substances) system.

Demographics

Most patients who develop transitional cell carcinoma are older than 40 years of age; the peak age of

KEY TERMS

Analgesic—Drug that relieves pain.

Arylamine—Radical group of the amine chemical family.

Benign—Not progressing or malignant.

Biopsy—Removal of a small piece of living tissue for examination.

Bladder—Muscular and membranous reservoir for urine.

Catheter—Tube that is passed through the body for injecting or removing fluids from body structures.

Chromosomes—Thread in the nucleus of the cell that contains DNA.

Creatinine—End product of creatine metabolism that is found in increased levels in advanced kidney disease.

Immunotherapy—Enhancement of the body's immunity, usually through a biologic agent.

Papilloma—Benign tumor of epithelial tissue.

Tumor—Spontaneous new tissue growth that can be benign or malignant.

Urothelial—Epithelial cells that line the urinary system.

incidence is 60–70 years of age. The male:female ratio for this type of cancer is about 5:2. About 93% of all bladder cancers in North American are of the transitional cell carcinoma type. Only 8% of all renal cancers are of the transitional cell carcinoma type. According to the American Cancer Society (ACS), 70,980 Americans will be diagnosed with **bladder cancer** in 2009 and 14,330 will die from the disease.

Causes and symptoms

The causes and mechanisms of transitional cell carcinoma, like all forms of cancer, are not entirely known or understood. However, researchers have isolated several factors that have been associated with an increased risk for developing this carcinoma.

Cigarette smoking is the strongest risk factor for transitional cell carcinoma. Researchers have found smoking increases the risk for developing this condition by three to seven times. In men with bladder cancer, 50% to 80% have a history of smoking **cigarettes**. Other methods of using tobacco, such as cigar and pipe smoking and chewing tobacco, have been shown to increase the risk of developing this carcinoma but at a reduced rate compared with smoking.

QUESTIONS TO ASK THE DOCTOR

- What type of type of tests are necessary to make an accurate diagnosis?
- Are these tests painful?
- How long will it take to get results?
- If the tests are positive for cancer, what happens then?
- If it is transitional cell carcinoma, is the tumor invasive?
- Has the carcinoma spread to other tissues?
- What stage is the carcinoma?
- What treatment alternatives are there?
- If surgery is necessary, what will the surgery entail?
- What is the recuperation period like after the surgery?
- How long will I be in the hospital?
- If radiation is necessary, what sort of side effects are common?
- If chemotherapy or immunotherapy is necessary, what side effects are common?
- Will chemotherapy cause my hair to fall out?
- Are there any clinical trials that I can participate in?
- What type of surveillance schedule will I be on following the initial surgery and therapy?

Individuals who have undergone long-term exposure to industrial chemicals, such as the class of compounds known as arylamines, are known to have an increased risk of developing transitional cell carcinoma. One of the most dangerous of these chemicals is one known as 2-naphthylamine. Individuals who develop these carcinomas usually do so anywhere from 15 to 40 years following the first exposure to these chemicals. Arsenic is another chemical that has been recently implicated in the development of TCC.

Individuals who have used analgesics for many years, or have used them excessively in the short-term, are at an increased risk for developing transitional cell carcinoma. Many of these patients have suffered at least some damage to the kidneys before developing the carcinoma. Drugs given to patients to treat an earlier cancer, such as the commonly used **cyclophosphamide**, increase the risk of developing transitional cell carcinoma at a later time.

Researchers believe these factors somehow alter genes that are important in the development of transitional cell carcinoma. These changes most often involve the deletions of certain chromosomes but also may result from mutations.

The most common symptom of transitional cell carcinoma is blood in the urine without accompanying pain. There may also be changes in the urge for the patient to urinate and in the frequency of urination. In some cases, urine may be partially obstructed by a tumor in the ureter. Rarely, pain occurs in the pelvic region. Physicians rarely detect a tumorous mass by touch during the first examination.

Diagnosis

There are a variety of ways that can be used to help diagnose transitional cell carcinoma. Many of these involve the use of **imaging studies**. In some cases, traditional **x rays** may be used to image upper urinary tract tumors. One of the things that physicians look for in patients suspected of having transitional cell carcinoma is the abnormal filling of structures in the urinary system. A type of imaging called excretory urography can help detect such flaws in the system. A different imaging method called retrograde urography can help physicians image the process of urinary collection and detect irregularities. **Computed tomography** (CT), more commonly called the CAT scan, is a very useful tool in the imaging of tumors in the upper tract of the urinary system. CT is more sensitive than traditional x rays. In some cases, however, small tumors can be missed using this method.

Ultrasound may also be used to help tell the difference between tumors and normal structures in this region. **Magnetic resonance imaging**, more commonly referred to as MRI, has not been found to have any significant advantage over computed tomography in the diagnosis of transitional cell carcinoma.

Cystoscopy is the examination of the bladder using a cystoscope, an instrument that allows the interior imaging of the ureter and bladder. Cystoscopy is usually mandatory in patients suspected of having transitional cell carcinoma and can be helpful in determining the origin of the bleeding in these patients. Patients who are suspected of having transitional cell carcinoma, or other type of cancer in the upper urinary tract, need to have laboratory analysis of the cells in the suspected mass. This cell analysis tells the physician what type and stage of cell is present.

The easiest but least accurate way to study these cells is to have the patient provide urine samples. Patients who have a low-grade tumor in the upper urinary tract will have normal results in up to 80% of cases when urinalysis is used. However, such urinalysis can be more effective in diagnosis of bladder tumors. Obtaining urine samples from the upper urinary tract using a catheter can provide more accurate analysis of upper urinary tract tumors.

A technique called the brush **biopsy** involves the placing of a tiny brush into a catheter. The catheter is then placed in the ureter and moved into the upper urinary tract where the brush scrapes off cells for later analysis. More modern techniques of imaging and sampling use tiny tubes with attached videocameras called endoscopes. These tubes can be moved into the upper urinary tract to locate bleeding and tumors and can be used to obtain biopsy samples.

Treatment team

The treatment team that treats the patient with suspected and confirmed transitional cell carcinoma usually involves a primary care physician who refers to a specialist, a specialist such as a urologist or nephrologist (kidney specialist), a radiologist who performs the imaging, a pathologist who studies the sampled cells, an oncologist who monitors the overall course of the cancer, and a surgeon who performs the surgical removal of the carcinoma.

Clinical staging, treatments, and prognosis

The International Society of Urological Pathology has developed a classification scheme for grading transitional cell carcinoma. These four grades are urothelial papilloma, urothelial neoplasms of low malignant potential, low-grade urothelial carcinoma, and high-grade carcinoma. Papilloma is usually seen in younger patients and is rare. Neoplasms of low malignant potential are sometimes difficult to differentiate from low-grade urothelial carcinomas. These tumors rarely become invasive to nearby tissue. Low-grade urothelial carcinoma tends to appear in the form of papillomas as well. These tumors can invade nearby tissue but usually do not progress. High-grade carcinomas are flat, papillary, or both. These tumors are larger and are more likely to invade nearby muscle tissue.

The most common means to treat papillary transitional cell carcinoma in the bladder is with surgery. When these tumors are classified as low grade, they can typically be removed completely. Unfortunately, these carcinomas recur 50% to 70% of the time.

Because of this high rate of cancer recurrence, patients with transitional cell carcinoma have to be carefully monitored following surgery with cystoscopy and regular urinalysis.

Other types of therapy called immunologic therapy (immunotherapy) and **chemotherapy** are often used in treating bladder carcinoma. These methods use agents that are directly applied to the bladder. The most commonly used agent in these therapies is called bacillus Calmette-Guérin (BCG). When BCG is placed in the bladder, the body begins an **immune response** that sometimes destroys the tumor. Patients usually receive one treatment per week for six weeks. After this period, a maintenance program involving three-week BCG courses of treatment for up to two years is used. The most common chemotherapy used for transitional cell carcinoma in the past is a combination of the drugs **cisplatin**, adriamycin, **vinblastine**, and **methotrexate**. Newer and less toxic drugs, such as celecoxib, **bortezomib**, ixabepilone, and gallium maltolate are being tested to replace these older agents. A combination regimen of chemotherapy and radiation is being considered as a therapy when the carcinoma invades the muscle surrounding the bladder. The effectiveness of this method has not been studied yet in research studies. **Radiation therapy** alone is not an effective treatment.

Transitional cell carcinoma in the upper urinary tract is also treated with surgical procedures. Affected areas in this region, including the kidney, are sometimes removed. Part or all of the ureter and parts of the bladder are also removed, in some cases.

The noninvasive papilloma rarely recurs once removed. If urothelial neoplasms of low malignant potential recur, they are usually benign tumors. However, in about 3% to 5% of cases, these recurrences are of a higher grade. These carcinomas rarely become invasive, and patients with them have a one-year survival rate of 95% to 98%. Low-grade urothelial carcinomas often show signs of invasion during diagnosis, but are not associated with a high risk for malignancy. High-grade carcinomas have considerable invasiveness into nearby tissue, particularly muscle, and are associated with a very high risk for **metastasis** (movement of cancer cells from one part of the body to another).

Those with superficial, noninvasive, or nonmalignant disease should receive a cystoscopy and a thorough examination every three months for two years followed by a regimen every six months for an additional two years. In those with advanced disease but who did not receive complete bladder removal, a cystoscopy with a thorough examination should be performed every three months for two years, followed by every six months for an additional two years, and then one per year. These patients should also receive a computed tomography (CT) scan of the pelvis and abdomen every six months for two years. Chest x rays, liver function tests, and serum creatinine tests should also be performed on this schedule. Those who had bladder removal should have chest x rays, liver function tests, computed tomography scan of abdomen and pelvis, and serum creatinine tests performed every six months for two years. In addition, an endoscopy of the newly formed bladder structure should be performed.

Coping with cancer treatment

A variety of issues need to be considered when the patient is receiving cancer treatment. One of the most important of these issues is the ability to cope with the emotion of having cancer in the first place. Several techniques, such as relaxation training, meditation, and biofeedback, may be beneficial to the patient in reducing anxiety. Other issues such as missed work and other daily activities need to be planned before the treatment period to reduce emotional stress. The patient needs to consider worst-case scenarios, such as side effects from chemotherapy, when planning these future events. Participation in cancer support groups helps many patients with the stress of the treatment period.

There are physical issues as well during this period. Pain following surgery can be a significant problem. Fortunately, there are many effective pain medications available to handle most pain events. **Nausea** and hair loss (**alopecia**) are two of the more notable effects of chemotherapy. Nausea can be effectively treated with drugs in most cases. Hair loss is only a temporary event, but it often has significant psychological effects that can be somewhat alleviated through social support.

Clinical trials

As of 2009 the National Cancer Institute (NCI) lists 60 **clinical trials** in progress for treating bladder cancer. Several new drugs are being tested, as well as various combinations of drugs, surgery, and BCG therapy. The best way to obtain the most current information is to call the Cancer Information Service at (800) 4-CANCER. The Cancer Information Service is part of CancerNet, a service of the National Cancer Institute. It can also be accessed at: http://cancernet.nci.nih.gov.

Prevention

Cigarette smoking is a major risk factor for the development of transitional cell carcinoma. Cigarette smoking has been associated with 25% to 65% of all cases of bladder cancer. Smokers are two to four times more likely to develop transitional cell carcinoma than nonsmokers. Smoking increases the risk of developing tumors that are at a higher grade, in greater number, and of larger size. Those individuals who have abused analgesics are at an increased risk for developing transitional cell carcinoma. Exposure to the human papillomavirus type 16 also increases the risk of developing transitional cell carcinoma. Petroleum, dye, textile, tire, and rubber workers are at increased risk for developing this carcinoma. Exposure to chemicals, such as 2-naphthylamine, benzidine, 4-amino-biphenyl, nitrosamines, or O-toluidine can also increase the risk of developing transitional cell carcinoma. Eliminating exposure to these substances substantially reduces the risk of developing transitional cell carcinoma.

Resources

BOOKS

Beers, Mark H., MD, and Robert Berkow, MD, editors. "Bladder Cancer." Section 17, Chapter 233 In*The Merck Manual of Diagnosis and Therapy*. Whitehouse Station, NJ: Merck Research Laboratories, 2002.

Beers, Mark H., MD, and Robert Berkow, MD, editors. "Ovarian Cancer." Section 18, Chapter 241 In*The Merck Manual of Diagnosis and Therapy*. Whitehouse Station, NJ: Merck Research Laboratories, 2002.

Ellis, William J. "Malignant Tumors of the Urogenital Tract." *Rakel: Conn's Current Therapy 2000*. Philadelphia: Saunders, 2000.

Ferri, Fred F., et al., editors. "Bladder Cancer." In *Ferri's Clinical Advisor*. St. Louis: Mosby, 2001.

Tierney, Lawrence M., et al., editors. "Cancers of the Ureter and Renal Pelvis." In *Current Medical Diagnosis & Treatment*. New York: Lange, 2001.

PERIODICALS

Bazarbashi, S., et al. "Prospective Phase II Trial of Alternating Intravesical Bacillus Calmette-Guérin (BCG) and Interferon Alpha IIB in the Treatment and Prevention of Superficial Transitional Cell Carcinoma of the Urinary Bladder: Preliminary Results." *Journal of Surgical Oncology* 74 (2000).

Eichhorn, J. N., and R. H. Young. "Transitional Cell Carcinoma of the Ovary: A Morphologic Study of 100 Cases with Emphasis on Differential Diagnosis." *American Journal of Surgical Pathology* 28 (April 2004): 453–463.

Hayashida, Y., K. Nomata, M. Noguchi, et al. "Long-Term Effects of Bacille Calmette-Guérin Perfusion Therapy for Treatment of Transitional Cell Carcinoma in situ of Upper Urinary Tract." *Urology* 63 (June 2004): 1084–1088.

Karagas, M. R., T. D. Tosteson, J. S. Morris, et al. "Incidence of Transitional Cell Carcinoma of the Bladder and Arsenic Exposure in New Hampshire." *Cancer Causes and Control* 15 (June 2004): 465–472.

Konety, Badrinath R., MD, and Georgi Pirtskhalaishvili, MD. "Transitional Cell Carcinoma, Renal." *eMedicine* November 10, 2004. http://www.emedicine. com/med/topic2003.htm.

Maluf, F.C., and D.F. Bajorin. "Chemotherapy Agents in Transitional Cell Carcinoma: the Old and the New." *Seminars in Urologic Oncology* 19 (2001).

OTHER

American Cancer Society (ACS). *Cancer Facts & Figures 2004*. http://www.cancer.org/downloads/STT/CAFF_finalPWSecured.pdf.

American Pain Society. 4700 West Lake Ave., Glenville, IL 60025. (847) 966-5595.

ORGANIZATIONS

American Cancer Society. 1599 Clifton Rd. NE, Atlanta, GA 30329-4251. (800) 227-2345. http://www.cancer.org.

National Cancer Institute. National Institutes of Health. Bethesda, MD 20892. (800) 422-6237. http://www.nci.nih.gov.

Mark Mitchell, M.D.
Rebecca Frey, PhD

Transrectal ultrasound *see* **Endorectal ultrasound**

Transurethral bladder resection

Definition

Transurethral bladder resection is a surgical procedure used to view the inside of the bladder, remove tissue samples, and/or remove tumors. Instruments are passed through a cystoscope (a slender tube with a lens and a light) that has been inserted through the urethra into the bladder.

Purpose

Transurethral resection is the initial form of treatment for bladder cancers. The procedure is performed to remove and examine bladder tissue and/or a tumor. It may also serve to remove lesions, and it may be the only treatment necessary for noninvasive tumors. This

KEY TERMS

Biopsy—The removal and microscopic examination of a small sample of body tissue to see whether cancer cells are present.

Bladder irrigation—To flush or rinse the bladder with a stream of liquid (as in removing a foreign body or medicating).

Bladder tumor marker studies—A test to detect specific substances released by bladder cancer cells into the urine using chemical or immunologic (using antibodies methods).

Bladder washings—A procedure in which bladder washing samples are taken by placing a salt solution into the bladder through a catheter (tube) and then removing the solution for microscopic testing.

Chemotherapy—The treatment of cancer with anti-cancer drugs.

Cystoscopy—A procedure in which a slender tube with a lens and a light is placed into the bladder to view the inside of the bladder and remove tissue samples.

Immunotherapy—A method of treating allergies in which small doses of substances that a person is allergic to are injected under the skin.

Interstitial radiation therapy—The process of placing radioactive sources directly into the tumor. These radioactive sources can be temporary (removed after the proper dose is reached) or permanent.

Intravenous pyelogram—An x ray of the urinary system after injecting a contrast solution that enables the doctor to see images of the kidneys, ureters, and bladder.

Metastatic—A change of position, state, or form; a transfer of a disease-producing agency from the site of disease to another part of the body; a secondary growth of a cancerous tumor.

Noninvasive tumors—Tumors that have not penetrated the muscle wall and/or spread to other parts of the body.

Radiation therapy—The use of high-dose x rays to destroy cancer cells.

Retrograde pyelography—A test in which dye is injected through a catheter placed with a cystoscope into the ureter to make the lining of the bladder, ureters, and kidneys easier to see on x rays.

Ureters—Two thin tubes that carry urine downward from the kidneys to the bladder.

Urethra—The small tube-like structure that allows urine to empty from the bladder.

Urine culture—A test which tests urine samples in the lab to see if bacteria are present.

Urine cytology—The examination of the urine under a microscope to look for cancerous or precancerous cells.

procedure plays both a diagnostic and therapeutic role in the treatment of bladder cancers.

Demographics

Bladder cancer is the sixth most commonly diagnosed malignancy in the United States. According to the American **Cancer** Society, about 70,980 new cases of bladder cancer were projected to be diagnosed in the United States in 2009.

Industrialized countries such as the United States, Canada, France, Denmark, Italy, and Spain have the highest incidence rates for bladder cancer. Rates are lower in England, Scotland, and Eastern Europe. The lowest rates occur in Asia and South America.

Smoking is a major risk factor for bladder cancer; it increases one's risk by two to five times and accounts for approximately 50% of bladder cancers found in men and 30% found in women. If cigarette smokers quit, their risk declines in two to four years. Exposure to a variety of industrial chemicals also increases the risk of developing this disease. **Occupational exposures** may account for approximately 25% of all urinary bladder cancers.

Men have a 1-in-30 chance of developing bladder cancer; women have a 1-in-90 chance of developing bladder cancer. The incidence of bladder cancer in the white population is almost twice that of the black population. For other ethnic and racial groups in the United States, the incidence of bladder cancer falls between that of whites and blacks.

There is a greater incidence of bladder cancer with advancing age. Of newly diagnosed cases in both men and women, approximately 80% occur in people aged 60 years and older.

Description

Cancer begins in the lining layer of the bladder and grows into the bladder wall. Transitional cells line the inside of the bladder. Cancer can begin in these lining cells.

During transurethral bladder resection, a cystoscope is inserted through the urethra into the bladder. A clear solution is infused to maintain visibility and the tumor or tissue to be examined is cut away using an electric current. A **biopsy** is taken of the tumor and muscle fibers in order to evaluate the depth of tissue involvement, while avoiding perforation of the bladder wall. Every attempt is made to remove all visible tumor tissue, along with a small border of healthy tissue. The resected tissue is examined under the microscope for diagnostic purposes. An indwelling catheter may be inserted to ensure adequate drainage of the bladder postoperatively. At this time, interstitial **radiation therapy** may be initiated, if necessary.

Diagnosis/Preparation

If there is reason to suspect a patient may have bladder cancer, the physician will use one or more methods to determine if the disease is actually present. The doctor first takes a complete medical history to check for risk factors and symptoms, and does a physical examination. An examination of the rectum and vagina (in women) may also be performed to determine the size of a bladder tumor and to see if and how far it has spread. If bladder cancer is suspected, the following tests may be performed, including:

- biopsy
- cystoscopy
- urine cytology
- bladder washings
- urine culture
- intravenous pyelogram
- retrograde pyelography
- bladder tumor marker studies

Most of the time, the cancer begins as a superficial tumor in the bladder. Blood in the urine is the usual warning sign. Based on how they look under the microscope, bladder cancers are graded using Roman numerals 0 through IV. In general, the lower the number, the less the cancer has spread. A higher number indicates greater severity of cancer.

Because it is not unusual for people with one bladder tumor to develop additional cancers in other areas of the bladder or elsewhere in the urinary system, the doctor may biopsy several different areas of the bladder lining. If the cancer is suspected to have spread to other organs in the body, further tests will be performed.

Because different types of bladder cancer respond differently to treatment, the treatment for one patient could be different from that of another person with bladder cancer. Doctors determine how deeply the cancer has spread into the layers of the bladder in order to decide on the best treatment.

Aftercare

As with any surgical procedure, blood pressure and pulse will be monitored. Urine is expected to be blood-tinged in the early postoperative period. Continuous bladder irrigation (rinsing) may be used for approximately 24 hours after surgery. Most operative sites should be completely healed in three months. The patient is followed closely for possible recurrence with visual examination, using a special viewing device (cystoscope) at regular intervals. Because bladder cancer has a high rate of recurrence, frequent screenings are recommended. Normally, screenings would be needed every three to six months for the first three years, and every year after that, or as the physician considers necessary. **Cystoscopy** can catch a recurrence before it progresses to invasive cancer, which is difficult to treat.

Risks

All surgery carries some risk due to heart and lung problems or the anesthesia itself, but these risks are generally extremely small. The risk of death from general anesthesia for all types of surgery, for example, is only about one in 1,600. Bleeding and **infection** are other risks of any surgical procedure. If bleeding becomes a complication, bladder irrigation may be required postoperatively, during which time the patient's activity is limited to bed rest. Perforation of the bladder is another risk, in which case the urinary catheter is left in place for four to five days postoperatively. The patient is started on antibiotic therapy preventively. If the bladder is lacerated accompanied by spillage of urine into the abdomen, an abdominal incision may be required.

Normal results

The results of transurethral bladder resection will depend on many factors, including the type of treatment used, the stage of the patient's cancer before surgery, complications during and after surgery, the age and overall health of the patient, as well as the recurrence of the disease at a later date. The chances for survival are improved if the cancer is found and treated early.

WHO PERFORMS THIS PROCEDURE AND WHERE IS IT PERFORMED?

Transurethral bladder resections are usually performed in a hospital by a urologist, a medical doctor who specializes in the diagnosis and treatment of diseases of the urinary systems in men and women and also treats structural problems and tumors or stones in the urinary system. Urologists can prescribe medications and perform surgery. If a transurethral bladder resection is required by a female patient, and there are complicating factors, an urogynecologist may perform the surgery. Urogynecologists treat urinary problems involving the female reproductive system.

Morbidity and mortality rates

After a diagnosis of bladder cancer, up to 95% of patients with superficial tumors survive for at least five years. Patients whose cancer has grown into the lining of the bladder but not into the muscle itself, and is not in any lymph nodes or distant sites, have a five year survival rate as high as 85%. The five-year survival rate may be as high as 55% for patients whose tumors have invaded the bladder muscle, but not spread through the muscle into the surrounding fatty tissue. When the cancer has grown totally through the bladder muscle into the surrounding fatty tissue, and perhaps into nearby tissues such as the prostate, uterus, or vagina, the five-year survival rate is about 38%. For patients whose cancer has spread through the bladder wall to the pelvis or abdominal wall or has spread distantly to lymph nodes or other organs (such as the bones, liver, or lungs), the five-year survival rate is 16%.

The five-year survival rate refers to the percentage of patients who live at least five years after their cancer is found, although many people live much longer. Five-year relative survival rates do not take into account patients who die of other diseases. Every person's situation is unique and the statistics cannot predict exactly what will happen in every case; these numbers provide an overall picture.

Mortality rates are two to three times higher for men than women. Although the incidence of bladder cancer in the white population exceeds those of the black population, African American women die from the disease at a greater rate. This is due to a larger proportion of these cancers being diagnosed and treated at an earlier stage in the white population.

QUESTIONS TO ASK THE DOCTOR

- What benefits can I expect from this operation?
- What are the risks of this operation?
- What are the normal results of this operation?
- What happens if this operation does not go as planned?
- Are there any alternatives to this surgery?
- What is the expected recovery time?

The mortality rates for Hispanic and Asian men and women are only about one-half those for whites and African Americans. Over the past 30 years, the age-adjusted mortality rate has decreased in both races and genders. This may be due to earlier diagnosis, better therapy, or both.

There are over 500,000 bladder cancer survivors in the United States, and approximately 14,330 will die of the disease in 2009.

Alternatives

Surgery, radiation therapy, immunotherapy, and **chemotherapy** are the main types of treatment for cancer of the bladder. One type of treatment or a combination of these treatments may be recommended, based on the stage of the cancer.

After the cancer is found and staged, the cancer care team discusses the treatment options with the patient. In choosing a treatment plan, the most significant factors to consider are the type and stage of the cancer. Other factors to consider include the patient's overall physical health, age, likely side effects of the treatment, and the personal preferences of the patient.

In considering treatment options, a second opinion may provide more information and help the patient feel more confident about the treatment plan chosen.

Alternative methods are defined as unproved or disproved methods, rather than evidence-based or proven methods to prevent, diagnose, and treat cancer. For some cancer patients, conventional treatment is difficult to tolerate and they may decide to seek a less unpleasant alternative. Others are seeking ways to alleviate the side effects of conventional treatment without having to take more drugs. Some do not trust traditional medicine, and feel that with alternative medicine approaches, they are more in control of making decisions about what is happening to their bodies.

A cancer patient should talk to the doctor or nurse before changing the treatment or adding any alternative methods. Some methods can be safely used along with standard medical treatment. Others may interfere with standard treatment or cause serious side effects.

The American Cancer Society (ACS) encourages people with cancer to consider using methods that have been proven effective or those that are currently under study. They encourage people to discuss all treatments they may be considering with their physician and other health care providers. The ACS acknowledges that more research is needed regarding the safety and effectiveness of many alternative methods. Unnecessary delays and interruptions in standard therapies could be detrimental to the success of cancer treatment.

At the same time, the ACS acknowledges that certain complementary methods such as aromatherapy, biofeedback, massage therapy, meditation, tai chi, or yoga may be very helpful when used in conjunction with conventional treatment.

Resources

BOOKS

Hicks, M. *Bladder Cancer*. Cambridge, UK: Cambridge University Press, 2004.

Miller, R. D. *Miller's Anesthesia*, 6th ed. Philadelphia: Elsevier, 2005.

Wein, A. J., et al. *Campbell-Walsh Urology*, 9th ed. Philadelphia: Saunders, 2007.

OTHER

Aetna InteliHealth Inc. *Bladder Cancer*, 2003 [cited April 24, 2003]. http://www.intelihealth.com/IH/ihtIH?t=31066&p=∼br,IHW|~st,24479|~r,WSIHW000|~b,*| (accessed April 12, 2008).

American Cancer Society, Inc. (ACS) *Cancer Reference Information*, 2003 [cited April 24, 2003]. http://www.cancer.org/cancerinfo (accessed April 12, 2008).

ORGANIZATIONS

American Cancer Society. 1599 Clifton Road, N.E., Atlanta, GA 30329-4251. (800) 227-2345. http://www.cancer.org (accessed April 12, 2008).

American Foundation for Urologic Disease. 1128 North Charles St., Baltimore, MD 21201. (410) 468-1800. (800) 242-2383. Fax: (410) 468-1808. E-Mail: admin@afud.org. http://www.afud.org/ (accessed April 12, 2008).

National Cancer Institute Public Inquiries Office. Suite 3036A. 6116 Executive Boulevard, MSC8322. Bethesda, MD 20892-8322. (800) 422-6237. http://www.nci.nih.gov (accessed April 12, 2008).

National Comprehensive Cancer Network. 50 Huntingdon Pike, Suite 200, Rockledge PA 19046. (215) 728-4788. Fax: (215) 728-3877. Email: information@nccn.org. http://www.nccn.org/ (accessed April 12, 2008).

National Institutes of Health (NIH), Department of Health and Human Services. 9000 Rockville Pike. Bethesda, MD 20892.

Kathleen D. Wright, RN

Crystal H. Kaczkowski, MSc

Rosalyn Carson-DeWitt, MD

Transvaginal ultrasound

Definition

A transvaginal ultrasound, also called transvaginal sonogram (TVS), is an ultrasound that uses an internal probe, or transducer, that enters the vaginal cavity. Either a radiology technician or physician performs the test, and a radiologist interprets the results.

Purpose

An internal probe allows for closer access to the structures that need evaluation. With closer access, higher frequency sound waves can be used, which provides a clearer image due to better resolution. It is often used to evaluate suspected **cancer** or abnormal growths in the female reproductive system.

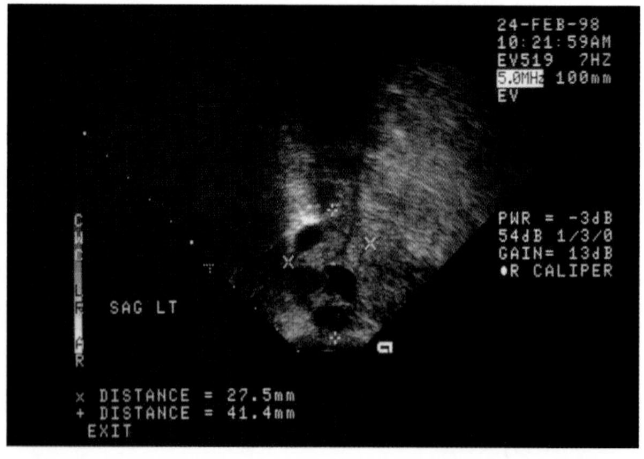

Normal transvaginal ultrasound. The plus marks and x marks show that measurements were taken. Measurements of internal structures, such as ovaries, are often taken to compare one ovary with the other, or to compare this woman's ovaries with other women her age, in order to detect possible abnormal growths. *(Custom Medical Stock Photo. Reproduced by permission.)*

KEY TERMS

False positive—A false positive is a positive finding of a test when, in fact, the true result was negative. This would mean that the test results indicate that a patient had a particular condition or disease when they do not.

Radiologist—A physician with special training in radiology, the study of x rays, magnetic resonance imaging (MRI), ultrasound, and other imaging technology to assist in the diagnosis of a disease or condition.

Precautions

While the transvaginal ultrasound produces a clearer image, it may also create false positive results. This can lead to unnecessary testing to further evaluate the condition, with its accompanying physical and emotional impact.

Description

The transvaginal ultrasound uses a small, wand-like transducer, or probe, which is inserted into the vagina. The probe emits high-frequency sound waves, which are not audible by humans. These sound waves painlessly bounce off the structures in its path. The returning echo wave is picked up by the probe. This information is fed into an attached computer that then creates an image, or sonogram, on a screen. It can differentiate between structures that are solid, such as a tumor, or filled with fluid, such as a cyst. It can be used to measure the thickness of the lining of the uterus, as well as of other organs.

A technique called color flow Doppler imaging may be used to evaluate the blood flow to certain structures. This can be helpful in establishing whether blood flow has been obstructed or enhanced to an organ. It cannot tell if a solid mass is malignant or benign. Other tests, such as a **biopsy**, would be needed to gather that information. It is done on an outpatient basis, is less expensive than imaging tests such as **magnetic resonance imaging** (MRI), and is considered safe, using sound waves rather than radiation to generate an image.

Preparation

Little preparation is needed for the transvaginal ultrasound. A woman will need to undress from the waist down, and lie face-up on the examination surface. Legs may be put in stirrups, or a bolster may be placed under the hips to tilt the pelvic area upwards to facilitate use of the probe, both for insertion as well as for the ultrasound process itself. The test is done with an empty bladder, which is more comfortable than the full bladder required for the abdominal ultrasound. This method may be a preferred choice for women who have difficulty with bladder control. A woman may wish to request that she insert the probe herself, which is similar to the insertion of a tampon. Gel that has been warmed will make insertion more comfortable.

QUESTIONS TO ASK THE DOCTOR

- What are you looking for with this test?
- Who will perform the test? Is that person board-certified?
- Who will read the results? Is that person board-certified?
- Does the facility utilize color flow Doppler imaging?
- When, how, and from whom will I receive the results?
- If the result is positive, how will you evaluate if it was a false positive?
- Will my insurance cover the cost of this test?

Aftercare

Because of the small amount of gel used on the probe for easier insertion, a woman may wish to use a sanitary pad to protect her underpants from any minor leakage after she stands up. After the test a woman will be able to resume her regular scheduled activities.

Risks

The risk involved in using the transvaginal ultrasound is that of obtaining a false positive result, any resulting tests that would be ordered unnecessarily, and their accompanying emotional burden.

Normal results

The normal results of a transvaginal ultrasound are the finding of the normal shape and size of any structure evaluated, with no abnormal thickness, masses or growths of any kind found.

Abnormal results

Abnormal results include the finding of growths, such as masses or cysts, and any unexpected thickness of the structures evaluated. Because of the risk of false positive results, any abnormal findings should be further evaluated and confirmed before undergoing surgery or treatment for the suspected condition. Magnetic resonance imaging (MRI) is often ordered to further evaluate masses. An endometrial biopsy is performed to further evaluate a thickened uterine lining.

Resources

BOOKS

Libov, Charlotte. *Beat Your Risk Factors*. New York: Plume Books, 1999.

Runowicz, Carolyn D., Jeanne A. Petrek, and Ted S. Gansler. *American Cancer Society: Women and Cancer*. New York: Villard Books, 1999.

Teeley, Peter, and Philip Bashe. *The Complete Cancer Survival Guide*. New York: Doubleday, 2000.

PERIODICALS

Rubin, Rita. "Ultrasound Studied as Ovarian Cancer Test." *USA Today* February 8, 2000.

Esther Csapo Rastegari, R.N., B.S.N., Ed.M.

Transverse myelitis

Description

Transverse myelitis (TM) is an inflammation or **infection** of the spinal cord in which the effect of the lesion spans the width of the entire spinal cord at a given level. The spinal cord consists of four regions: the cervical (neck), followed by the thoracic (chest), the lumbar (lower back) and the sacral (lowest back). TM can occur in any of these regions. The disease is uncommon, but not rare, as it occurs in one to five persons per million population in any given year in the United States. It is equally diagnosed in both adults and children. TM may occur by itself or in conjunction with other illnesses such as viral or bacterial infectious diseases, autoimmune diseases such as multiple sclerosis, vascular illnesses such as thrombosis, and **cancer**.

The symptoms of TM depend on the level of spinal cord lesion with sensation usually diminished below the spinal cord level affected. Some patients experience tingling sensations or numbness in the legs with bladder control also being disturbed. The condition is usually diagnosed following **magnetic resonance imaging** (MRI) or **computed tomography** (CT) with "spinal taps" (lumbar punctures) taken for additional analysis. Recovery depends on the general health status of the patient and is usually considered unlikely if no improvement is observed within three months.

Causes

The exact cause of TM is unknown but research results point to autoimmune deficiencies, meaning that the patient's own immune system abnormally attacks the spinal cord, resulting in inflammation and tissue damage.

There is also evidence suggesting that TM occurs as a result of **spinal cord compression** by tumors or as a result of direct spinal cord invasion by infectious agents, especially the human immunodeficiency virus (HIV) and the human T-lymphotropic virus type I (HTLV-1).

TM is also listed among the spinal cord disorders occurring in patients diagnosed with AIDS.

Treatments

There is no specific treatment for transverse myelitis. Treatment of the illness is largely symptomatic, meaning that it depends on the specific symptoms of the patient. The region in which the spinal cord has been infected is critical but a course of intravenous steroids is generally prescribed at the onset of treatment.

Treatment of the bladder function impairment resulting from TM include drugs, external catheters for men, and padding for women, with surgery recommended in certain cases. A common TM side effect is difficulty with stool evacuation and this condition can be treated by diets that include stool softeners and fiber.

As a result of TM, muscle groups below the affected level may become spastic. Treatment of spasticity usually involves prescriptions of drugs such as Baclofen (Lioresal), which stops reflex activity, and Dantrolene sodium (Dantrium), which acts directly on muscle. A new very well-tolerated drug, Tizanidine, has also recently been introduced in the United States. Muscle pain is generally treated with analgesics such as acetaminophen (Tylenol) or ibuprofen (Naprosyn, Aleve, Motrin). Nerve disorders might be treated with anticonvulsant drugs such as **carbamazepine**, **phenytoin**, or **gabapentin** (Tegretol, Dilantin, Neurontin).

Alternative and complementary therapies

Individuals with TM may experience serious difficulty with common tasks such as dressing, bathing and eating. Complementary TM therapies may accordingly include a course of physical therapy so as to help patients recover mobility. This can be achieved with special exercises, canes, walkers and custom-designed braces.

After the acute phase, people with TM start the rehabilitation process. During this period, the focus of care is shifted from designing an effective TM treatment to learning to cope with a serious disease. TM patients must learn to cope with the loss of abilities which healthy people take for granted and this process is necessarily harder if TM is associated with AIDS or another serious autoimmune disease. Resources that may help this required adjustment are psychological assistance from counselors, relatives and friends, and making contact with TM support groups. The Transverse Myelitis Association may also be contacted: 3548 Tahoma Pl. West, Tacoma, WA 98466-2141 (info@myelitis.org; www.myelitis.org); Phone: 253-565-8156.

See also Imaging studies; Lumbar puncture.

Resources

BOOKS

Beers, M.H., and R. Berkow, editors. *The Merck Manual of Diagnosis and Therapy*. 17th ed. Whitehouse Station, NJ: Merck Research Laboratories, 1999.

ORGANIZATIONS

National Institute of Neurological Disorders and Stroke (NINDS), National Institutes of Health. NIH Neurological Institute. P.O. Box 5801, Bethesda, MD 20824. (800) 352-9424. http://www.ninds.nih.gov.

Transverse Myelitis Association. 3548 Tahoma Pl. West, Tacoma, WA 98466-2141. (253) 565-8156. http://www.myelitis.org.

Monique Laberge, Ph.D.

Trastuzumab

Definition

Trastuzumab is a humanized monoclonal antibody produced by recombinant DNA technology that binds specifically to the human epidermal growth factor receptor 2 protein (also known as HER2 or neu or c-erb-2) that is found on the cell surface of some **cancer** tumors, most notably **breast cancer**. The drug is marketed in the United States under the **Herceptin** brand name.

Trastuzumab has been tested in clinical trials for the potential treatment of gastric cancer, and in 2009 positive results were released regarding the increased survival rate of gastric cancer patients receiving trastuzumab alongside standard chemotherapy treatments.

KEY TERMS

Antibody—A protective protein made by the immune system in response to an antigen, also called an immunoglobulin.

Humanization—Fusing the constant and variable framework region of one or more human immunoglobulins with the binding region of an animal immunoglobulin, done to reduce human reaction against the fusion antibody.

IgG—Immunoglobulin type gamma, the most common type found in the blood and tissue fluids.

Interleukins—Cytokines responsible for the activation of B and T cells of the immune system.

Monoclonal—Genetically engineered antibodies specific for one antigen.

Purpose

Trastuzumab is a monoclonal antibody used to treat breast cancers that overexpress the HER2 protein, which occurs in about 25–30% of breast malignancies. By binding the HER2 protein on the tumor cell, the antibody targets it for destruction by the immune system. Based on data gathered in the laboratory, developers believe that trastuzumab triggers cell-mediated means to kill the tumor cells, through the action of natural killer cells and monocytes, two types of white blood cells. As binding of the antibody also slows growth of the tumor, it is theorized that the antibody may also block the interaction of the HER2 protein with a not yet identified growth factor that triggers rapid cell divisions.

Clinical trials have also begun or are soon to begin to test the use of trastuzumab against **osteosarcoma**, as well as endometrial, colorectal, kidney, pancreatic, prostate, ovarian, salivary gland, lung, and bladder cancers, as all of these tumor types can overexpress the HER2 protein on their surface.

Description

Trastuzumab is a genetically engineered monoclonal antibody. In 1998 it was approved by the FDA as a method of slowing growth of breast cancer tumors that overexpress the HER2 protein on the cell surface. Overexpression or overproduction of the HER2 protein is associated with aggressive disease and increased mortality.

Trastuzumab is approved for use either alone, or in combination with paclitaxel, a drug used for chemotherapeutic treatment of breast cancer. In clinical trials treating patients having breast cancer that has spread beyond the breast (metastatic breast cancer), trastuzumab had an overall response rate of 14%, with 2% having a complete response. When used in combination with paclitaxel treatment, the antibody reduced the risk of death by 24%. Higher expression of the HER2 protein on the tumor surface correlates with an increased chance of response to the drug. Additionally, clinical trials using trastuzumab in the TCH **chemotherapy** regime (Taxotere, **cisplatin** or **carboplatin**, and Herceptin) appears to avoid risk of heart problems (cardiotoxicity) seen with the paclitaxel/Herceptin combination.

Other clinical trials have begun testing the use of trastuzumab with other chemotherapy drugs such as **doxorubicin** (an antitumor anitbiotic), **cyclophosphamide** (an alkylating agent that interferes with mitosis and cell division), celecoxib (an aspirin-like drug called a cyclooxygenase-2, or COX-2, inhibitor), **capecitabine** (an antimetabolite that interferes with DNA and RNA growth), and others. Testing the combination of the monoclonal antibody and various cytokines, such as interleukins 2 and 12, is also ongoing. Additionally, doctors are also studying the combination of the antibody with other cancer treatments such as radiation and transplantation with peripheral stem cells.

Most of the trastuzumab sequence is derived from human sequences, while about 10% are from the mouse. The human sequences were derived from the constant domains of human IgG1 (called "constant" because it is essentially the same for all IgG antibodies) and the variable framework regions of a human antibody. These areas do not bind to the epidermal growth factor receptor 2. Using human sequences in this part of the antibody helps to reduce patient **immune response** to the antibody itself and is called humanization. The actual binding site of trastuzumab to the receptor is from a mouse anti-HER2 antibody.

Recommended dosage

Trastuzumab is administered intravenously, at a dose of 4 mg/kg for the initial administration, and 2 mg/kg for weekly maintenance until the disease progresses. The antibody can be given for longer periods to maintain tumor shrinkage.

Precautions

Extreme caution should be exercised when using trastuzumab to treat patients with existent heart problems. Also, patients with lung problems have an increased risk of side effects. Because the drug can pass to the fetus through the placenta and is present in breast milk, the drug should be used during pregnancy and nursing only if clearly indicated.

Side effects

The most severe side effects seen with this drug are heart and lung problems, which tend to occur most often in patients with a history of heart or lung disease. The use of anthracyclines and cyclophospamide in combination with trastuzumab also appears to increase these types of side effects.

The most common side effects with trastuzumab are infusion-associated symptoms, usually consisting of **fever** and chills on first infusion. The symptoms are often mild to moderate in severity and are treated with acetaminophen, diphenhydramine, and/or **meperidine**. Other common side effects include **nausea and vomiting**, and pain (in some cases at tumor sites), which occur less often after the first dose. Lowered red blood cell count (**anemia**), lowered white blood cell count (leukopenia), **diarrhea**, and **infection** occur more often in patients receiving Herceptin plus chemotherapy as compared to chemotherapy alone. The severity of these symptoms usually do not result in discontinuation of therapy with Herceptin.

Other less common side effects are headache, abdominal pain, back pain, flu-like symptoms, sinusitis, rhinitis, pharyngitis, fluid retention (edema), insomnia, dizziness, and **depression**.

Interactions

There have been no formal drug interaction studies done for trastuzumab. However, in clinical trials, this drug has a decreased clearance rate (time of removal from the body) when combined with some chemotherapeutic drugs including paclitaxel.

See also Monoclonal antibodies.

Michelle Johnson, M.S., J.D.

Tretinoin

Definition

Tretinoin, a natural vitamin A metabolite, is an anticancer drug used in the treatment of acute promyelocytic leukemia (APL). Tretinoin is more

KEY TERMS

Leukocyte—White blood cell. Leukocytosis is the medical term for an excess number of white blood cells, and is seen in conditions such as infection and leukemia.

Metabolite—A product of metabolism.

Retinoid—Natural or artificial compound that is similar to vitamin A.

commonly used to treat such skin disorders as acne, warts, hyperpigmentation, and reactions to sunlight.

Purpose

Tretinoin is given to APL patients with the goal of bringing on a remission. The drug is being investigated as a treatment for **skin cancer**, and it is also available in an acne cream commonly called Retin-A.

As of 2004, tretinoin is also being investigated as a possible chemopreventive for **breast cancer**. The drug is thought to slow the spread of tumors and speed up the process of tumor cell self-destruction (apoptosis).

Description

Tretinoin causes abnormal leukemia cells in the blood to mature into normal cells (granulocytes). The exact mechanism of action is not known. In **clinical trials** 72–94% of APL patients experienced a complete remission when taking this drug. Tretinoin can be used to induce remission and to maintain remission.

Recommended dosage

The recommended dosage for adults with APL is 45 milligrams per square meter taken by mouth as two evenly divided doses. The physician will calculate the specific dose for each patient. The drug should be discontinued 30 days after remission or 90 days after treatment begins, whichever comes first.

Precautions

Patients who are hypersensitive to vitamin A or other retinoids should not take this drug. People should avoid tretinoin if they are sensitive to parabens, a preservative used in the drug's capsule. Pregnant or breast-feeding women should not take tretinoin. Women of childbearing age should take a pregnancy test to assure that they are not pregnant prior to starting this drug.

Side effects

Tretinoin has a number of side effects. Patients should discuss the risk of complications with their physician. Some side effects resemble symptoms that are common in APL patients. All side effects should be reported to a patient's doctor.

Side effects that are more commonly reported include headache, **fever**, dry skin and mucous membranes, **bone pain**, rash, **itching**, inflamed lips, sweating, **nausea and vomiting**, abdominal pain, **diarrhea**, constipation, indigestion, bloating, irregular heart beat, visual disturbances, earache, hair loss (**alopecia**), skin changes (including formation of inflammatory growths known as granulomas), vision changes, and bone inflammation.

Hemorrhage is a life-threatening complication. Blood coagulation studies are done while the patient is taking the drug to monitor the risk of hemorrhage. Hepatitis is another life-threatening side effect. Liver function tests can be abnormal in 50–60% of patients taking the drug. Liver function is monitored periodically while a person is taking the drug.

In addition, approximately one-quarter of patients taking tretinoin develop retinoic-acid-APL (RA-APL) syndrome. Symptoms include fever, weight gain, difficulty breathing, and other respiratory disorders. Some patients have cardiac changes and low blood pressure as part of this syndrome. The syndrome can occur two days after treatment begins or three to four weeks later. Symptoms must be reported to the patient's physician immediately so that treatment can begin. In rare cases this syndrome is fatal. Most patients do not need to stop taking tretinoin if the syndrome develops.

Approximately 40% of patients taking tretinoin develop high white blood cell counts (leukocytosis). If the number of white blood cells increases rapidly there is a higher chance of developing life-threatening complications. White blood cell counts are monitored during treatment. As many as 60% of patients taking tretinoin develop increased cholesterol and triglyceride levels. The levels drop when the medication is stopped. Cholesterol and triglyceride levels are monitored while the drug is being taken.

Tretinoin has other side effects that may impact the heart, skin, digestive tract, lungs, central nervous system, and other parts of the body. Patients should report all unusual symptoms to the doctor immediately.

Interactions

Tretinoin interacts with:

- Cimetidine (antipeptic ulcer drug)
- Cyclosporine (immunosuppressant)

- Dilitiazem (heart medication)
- Erythromycin (antibiotic)
- Glucocorticoids (steroids)
- Ketoconazole (antifungal drug)
- Phenobarbital (sedative/hypnotic)
- Pentobarbital (sedative/hypnotic)
- Rifampicin (an antituberculosis drug, also known as rifampin)
- Verapamil (heart medication)

See also Acute myelocytic leukemia; Antineoplastic agents.

Resources

BOOKS

Beers, Mark H., MD, and Robert Berkow, MD, editors. "Acne." In *The Merck Manual of Diagnosis and Therapy*. Whitehouse Station, NJ: Merck Research Laboratories, 2007.

Beers, Mark H., MD, and Robert Berkow, MD, editors. "Warts (Verrucae)." In *The Merck Manual of Diagnosis and Therapy*. Whitehouse Station, NJ: Merck Research Laboratories, 2007.

Wilson, Billie Ann, Margaret T. Shannon, and Carolyn L. Stang. *Nurse's Drug Guide 2003*. Upper Saddle River, NJ: Prentice Hall, 2003.

PERIODICALS

Halder, R. M., and G. M. Richards. "Topical Agents Used in the Management of Hyperpigmentation." *Skin Therapy Letter* 9 (June-July 2004): 1–3.

Kligman, D. E., and Z. D. Draelos. "High-Strength Tretinoin for Rapid Retinization of Photoaged Facial Skin." *Dermatologic Surgery* 30 (June 2004): 864–866.

Simeone, A. M., and A. M. Tari. "How Retinoids Regulate Breast Cancer Cell Proliferation and Apoptosis." *Cellular and Molecular Life Sciences* 61 (June 2004): 1475–1484.

Teknetsis, A., D. Ioannides, G. Vakali, et al. "Pyogenic Granulomas Following Topical Application of Tretinoin." *Journal of the European Academy of Dermatology and Venereology* 18 (May 2004): 337–339.

ORGANIZATIONS

American Society of Health-System Pharmacists (ASHP). 7272 Wisconsin Avenue, Bethesda, MD 20814. (301) 657-3000. www.ashp.org.

United States Food and Drug Administration (FDA). 5600 Fishers Lane, Rockville, MD 20857-0001. (888) INFO-FDA. www.fda.gov.

Rhonda Cloos, R.N.
Rebecca J. Frey, PhD

Trichilemmal carcinoma

Definition

Trichilemmal **carcinoma** is an uncommon malignant tumor of the hair follicle, and is assumed to be the malignant counterpart of the benign trichilemmoma.

Description

Trichilemmal carcinomas most often occur on part of the skin that has been often exposed to the sun, like the face. The tumors look like tan or flesh-colored spots. They can resemble warts and sometimes have a hair in them. Usually, a trichilemmal carcinoma will occur as an isolated lesion.

Trichilemmal carcinomas are thought to be the malignant form of the non-cancerous tumors called trichilemmomas, which are seen in Cowden syndrome. Cowden syndrome is an inherited disorder that predisposes individuals to breast and **thyroid cancer**. The disease is inherited in an autosomal dominant inheritance pattern. With autosomal dominant inheritance, men and women are equally likely to inherit the syndrome. In addition, children of individuals with the disease are at 50% risk of inheriting it. **Genetic testing** is available for Cowden syndrome but, due to the complexity, genetic counseling should be considered before testing. Although they are thought to be related to trichilemmomas, none of the reports of trichilemmal carcinomas have been seen in patients with Cowden syndrome.

It is important to note that trichilemmal carcinoma is not the same as "malignant proliferating trichilemmal tumor," which is usually seen on the scalp and the back of the neck.

Demographics

Trichilemmal carcinomas are most often seen in older people. They occur with equal frequency in both males and females.

Causes and symptoms

The causes of trichilemmal carcinoma are unknown. The only recognizable symptom is the presence of an unusual, tan or flesh-colored spot on the skin.

Diagnosis

Diagnosis of a trichilemmal carcinoma is very important. Because the tumors are so rare, a physician may not immediately recognize its exact diagnosis. A

KEY TERMS

Metastasize—Cancer spreads to remote parts of body.

Pathologic examination—When a physician examines a small section of the tumor under a microscope.

dermatologist will suspect an abnormality on the skin and have it removed. It is only on the pathologic examination (when a physician examines the abnormality under a microscope) that the tumor can be correctly classified.

Treatment team

The treatment of trichilemmal carcinoma will involve a dermatologist (a physician who specializes in diseases of the skin) and a surgeon (a physician who will surgically remove the tumor).

Clinical staging, treatments, and prognosis

Once a trichilemmal carcinoma has been diagnosed, a surgeon must remove it. It is necessary that documented clear margins are obtained, indicating that the entire tumor has been removed. There is a chance that the tumor will recur (return) locally (in the same spot or near the same spot). If this occurs, the recurrent tumor needs to be surgically removed as well. It is very unlikely that a trichilemmal carcinoma will metastasize (spread to other parts of the body), and further treatment with **chemotherapy** is not needed.

Alternative and complementary therapies

Because trichilemmal carcinoma is easily treated with removal, there are no suggested alterative and/or complementary therapies.

Coping with cancer treatment

The surgical procedure to remove a trichilemmal carcinoma is relatively straightforward and low-risk. Most surgeries will be done on an outpatient basis, requiring no stay in the hospital. A small scar on the skin may be left after the tumor is removed.

Clinical trials

No **clinical trials** for trichilemmal carcinoma could be identified.

Prevention

Because the underlying cause of trichilemmal carcinoma is largely unknown, preventive strategies have not been suggested.

Resources

OTHER

Introduction of Skin Diseases. *Handbook of Dermatology and Venereology*. http://www.hkmj.org.hk/skin/skintro.htm.

Kristen Mahoney Shannon, M.S., C.G.C.

Trimethoprim *see* **Antibiotics**

Trimetrexate

Definition

Trimetrexate (Neutrexin) is a drug that was first used to treat bacterial infections, and is now being investigated as a treatment for several different cancers.

Purpose

Trimetrexate is most commonly used to treat **pneumonia** in patients with acquired immunodeficiency syndrome (AIDS). However, it was recently discovered that the drug was able to kill a variety of different **cancer** cells. As a result, trimetrexate is now considered to be an investigational drug for cancer treatment.

Ongoing **clinical trials** are using trimetrexate to treat a number of cancers including advanced colon and rectal cancers, advanced **pancreatic cancer**, and advanced squamous cell cancers of the head and neck. Results from many trials are still preliminary, but trimetrexate appears to be most promising as a treatment for advanced colon and rectal cancers.

Description

Trimetrexate glucoronate works by stopping cells from using **folic acid** (vitamin B9). As a result, cells cannot make essential components they need to survive, and they die. Because trimetrexate is toxic to both cancer cells and healthy cells, it is always used in combination with **leucovorin** (Wellcovorin, citrovorum factor). Leucovorin is a drug that protects healthy cells from the harmful effects of certain types of **chemotherapy**.

KEY TERMS

Leucovorin—A drug used to protect healthy cells from toxic chemotherapy.

Myelosuppression—A condition where the bone marrow makes fewer blood cells and platelets than normal.

Trimetrexate can also enhance the anti-cancer effect of another chemotherapy drug called **fluorouracil** (Adrusil, 5-FU). Fluorouracil is frequently used to treat patients with colon and rectal cancers.

Recommended dosage

In clinical trials, patients with colon and rectal cancers were given trimetrexate, fluorouracil, and leucovorin for eight-week cycles. A cycle consisted of six weeks of treatment followed by two weeks rest with no treatment. Patients received trimetrexate intravenously, with the dose depending on their weight. Twenty-four hours after trimetrexate treatment, patients received intravenous fluorouracil and leucovorin treatment. Some patients also took oral leucovorin every six hours for several days after their intravenous chemotherapy.

Patients with squamous cell cancer of the head and neck received trimetrexate in combination with **cisplatin** (Platinol), leucovorin and fluorouracil in a 21-day cycle. These patients also received surgery or **radiation therapy**. Pancreatic cancer patients received eight-week cycles of trimetrexate, fluorouracil and leucovorin, similar to that given to patients with **colon cancer**.

Precautions

Patients who are given oral leucovorin as part of their chemotherapy must take their medication. Trimetrexate is a toxic drug, and patients who do not take leucovorin may experience severe side effects. Pregnant women should not take trimetrexate because it may harm the fetus. Women who are taking trimetrexate should avoid becoming pregnant. In addition, women should not breast feed while taking this drug. The liver and kidney are used to break down and eliminate trimetrexate from the body. As a result, patients with a history of liver or kidney disease should tell their doctor.

Side effects

Patients taking trimetrexate will have their blood monitored regularly to check for the development of **myelosuppression**. Myelosuppression is a condition where a patient's bone marrow makes fewer blood cells and platelets than normal. As a result of this condition, patients have an increased risk of **infection**, may bleed more, and may experience symptoms of **anemia**. Trimetrexate may also cause damage to the kidneys and the liver. Some patients also experience **nausea and vomiting**, and may develop a rash or inflammation and sores in their mouths. Taking leucovorin with trimetrexate helps to reduce or eliminate the risk of experiencing many of these side effects.

Interactions

Trimetrexate is known to interact with several other drugs. Some antifungal drugs such as ketoconazole (Nizoral) and fluconazole (Diflucan) interfere with the way the body breaks down trimetrexate. The antibiotic erythromycin also has this effect. Patients taking these drugs will be monitored carefully. The toxic effects of trimetrexate can be increased by other drugs. Patients should therefore tell their doctor about any medication they are taking whether it is prescription or over the counter.

Alison McTavish, M.S.

Triple negative breast cancer

Definition

Triple negative **breast cancer** (TNBC) is breast **cancer** in which the cells have neither estrogen nor progesterone receptors nor do they have excess HER2 protein on their surfaces. TNBC is an aggressive form of breast cancer that is more difficult to treat than other types. Also called triple-negative phenotype, the formal name for TNBC is estrogen receptor (ER)-negative, progesterone receptor (PR)-negative, and HER2-negative invasive breast cancer.

Demographics

Breast cancer is the second most commonly diagnosed cancer among women and the second leading cause of cancer death in women. Of the 190,000 new cases of breast cancer diagnosed in the United States each year, 10–20% are TNBC. Only about one-third of breast cancers have cells that lack receptors for both of the female hormones estrogen and progesterone; however only about one in five breast cancers produce excess human epidermal growth factor receptor 2 (HER2).

Whereas most breast cancers are more common in women aged 60 and older, TNBC is more likely to occur before the age of 40 or 50. TNBCs are more common in African American women than in any other racial or ethnic group. This type of breast cancer is also more common in young Hispanic women than among other groups. Asian and non-Hispanic white women are less likely to develop TNBC. The incidence of TNBC among African American women has helped to explain, in part, the longstanding observation that African American women are significantly more likely to die of breast cancer than white American women.

Description

TNBCs are usually invasive ductal carcinomas that originate in the lining of the milk ducts. It is estimated that 65–90% of TNBCs are of a subtype called basal-like, meaning that the cells resemble the basal cells that line the ducts and give rise to mature glandular breast cells. This is a new subtype of breast cancer that has been identified using genetic technologies. TNBCs tend to grow and spread more quickly than other types of breast cancer. Basal-like cancers in general tend to be more aggressive and of a higher grade. Cancer cells are graded on a scale of 1–3, depending on how much their appearance and growth pattern differ from normal healthy breast cells, with grade 3 as the most abnormal. TNBC cells are often grade 3.

Estrogen and progesterone bind to hormone receptors, signaling the cells to grow. About 75% of breast cancers have cells with estrogen receptors and about 65% have cells with both estrogen and progesterone receptors. Hormone therapies such as **tamoxifen** or **aromatase inhibitors** block these receptors, halting the growth of breast cancer cells. About 20–30% of breast cancers have excess HER2. Drugs such as **Herceptin** (**trastuzumab**) target HER2, preventing the cancer cells from growing. These targeted therapies are ineffective against TNBC, making this cancer difficult to treat.

Risk factors

BRCA1 (BReast CAncer) is a gene that encodes a protein that helps to repair damaged DNA. Some inherited forms of breast cancer are associated with specific mutations in the BRCA1 gene and most of these cancers are basal-like triple-negative tumors, especially when the cancer is diagnosed before the age of 50. Women who inherit these BRCA1 gene mutations are at an increased risk for TNBC. However only 5–15% of women with TNBC have a mutated BRCA1 gene. The BRCA genes were originally discovered by studying gene mutations in families with a history of early-onset breast cancer, especially among Ashkenazi Jews; thus, the observation that African American women have a higher risk for TNBC has spurred the search for additional genes that may be involved in TNBC. However many women with TNBC have no family history of breast cancer. Another recent study has suggested that women who breast-feed for six months or longer have a lower risk of TNBC.

Causes and symptoms

The exact cause of TNBC is unknown. Most breast cancers in older women appear to be related to long-term exposure of cells to estrogen. Genetic and environmental factors influence how much estrogen a woman produces, how the estrogen is metabolized, and how many years the breast tissue is exposed to high levels of estrogen. Early-onset menstruation and late-onset menopause increase lifetime exposure and pregnancy and breastfeeding decrease exposure. In addition there are two major pathways for the metabolism of estrogen—one leads to a metabolite that increases the risk of breast cancer and the other leads to a metabolite that may actually reduce the risk. Heredity and diet may influence the pathway that is utilized.

Early-stage breast cancer has few symptoms and the early symptoms of TNBC are the same as for other breast cancers:

- a thickening or lump in the breast or underarm
- a change in the size, shape, contour, or feel of the breast, nipple, or areola—the dark area surrounding the nipple
- a change in the appearance of the breast skin or nipple, such as a puckering or dimpling, ridges or pitting, crustiness or scaliness
- nipple tenderness or discharge
- a nipple that is pulled back or inverted

Diagnosis

Examination

Most breast cancers, including TNBC, are first detected by screening during:

- a self-examination
- an annual clinical breast exam by a healthcare professional

- an annual or biennial screening mammogram or x-rays of the breasts, which can detect cancers that are too small to feel.

Tests

A wide variety of blood and other tests may be performed to diagnose and stage breast cancer. For TNBC the most important tests are for the presence of estrogen and progesterone receptors and excess HER2. Cancer cells removed during a **biopsy** or surgery are tested by **immunohistochemistry** (IHC). The IHC staining test uses specific antibodies that bind to estrogen or progesterone receptors, thereby staining the cells. The test results should indicate the complete absence of both estrogen and progesterone receptors to rule out hormone therapy as a treatment. IHC with specific antibodies that bind HER2 also stain cells and are used to measure the amount of HER2. The IHC test gives a score of 0 to 3+. If the IHC result is 0 or 1+, the cancer is HER2-negative. Test results of 2+ are considered inconclusive and HER2 is re-measured by fluorescent in situ hybridization (FISH), a more sensitive test. Excess HER2 us caused by extra HER2 genes in cancer cells. FISH uses fluorescently labeled pieces of DNA that bind to these genes so that they can be counted under the microscope. There are various other genetic tests that also may be performed on biopsied cancer cells.

Procedures

There are a wide variety of imaging procedures that can be performed to determine the size of the tumor and whether it has spread to the lymph nodes or other parts of the body. These may include:

- diagnostic mammograms
- magnetic resonance imaging (MRI)
- ultrasound
- a ductogram if nipple discharge is present

Staging

Staging of TNBC includes:

- Stage O: cancer cells are within a duct and have not invaded surrounding fatty breast tissue.
- Stages I, II, and III depend on the size of the tumor and whether the cancer has spread to the lymph nodes near the breast and to the chest wall and skin.
- Stage IV: the cancer has spread to other organs or to lymph nodes far from the breast.

Treatment

Traditional

Although TNBC tends to be more aggressive than other types of breast cancer, it is not necessarily treated more aggressively. For example, just because the breast cancer is triple-negative, surgery is not necessarily more likely to be a **mastectomy** than a **lumpectomy**. With stage 1 or stage 2 TNBC, in which the cancer has not spread to the lymph nodes, the tumor tissue is surgically removed, followed by **chemotherapy** and often localized **radiation therapy**. Metastatic TNBC is generally treated with surgery, chemotherapy, and radiation therapy.

Drugs

TNBC often responds better to chemotherapy than hormone receptor-positive breast cancer. Some women with TNBC benefit from so-called neoadjuvant chemotherapy prior to surgery. Sometimes such chemotherapy eradicates all signs of cancer, although surgery is often still performed to ensure the removal of all cancerous tissue. Combination chemotherapy is often used to treat TNBC:

- gemcitabine and carboplatin
- ACT—doxorubicin (Adriamycin), cyclophosphamide (Cytoxan), and paclitaxel (Taxol)
- carboplatin and cisplatin for metastatic TNBC

A new drug for TNBC was in **clinical trials** as of 2009. BSI-201 inhibits a protein called PARP-1 (poly-ADP-ribose polymerase 1) that is involved in DNA repair and cell proliferation. In early clinical trials the drug has shown promise against metastatic TNBC when used in combination with chemotherapy. PARP-1 inhibitors may be particularly useful for treating women whose TNBC is caused by a mutated BRCA1 gene, since without the BRCA1 DNA repair mechanism, these cells rely on PARP for DNA repair. PARP inhibitors are believed to cripple this DNA repair mechanism in tumor cells without harming healthy cells. A second PARP inhibitor called olaparib has also shown promising results.

Avastin, a drug that inhibits a growth-inducing protein called vascular endothelial growth factor (VEGF) has had promising results against metastatic HER2-negative breast cancers. Avastin blocks blood vessel growth to tumors, thereby starving the cancer cells of nutrients.

TNBC tumor cells often have high levels of epidermal growth factor receptor (EGFR), which may help the cells grow. Drugs such as Erbitux (**cetuximab**), which is used to treat some cases of metastatic colorectal cancer, block EGFR and may also be useful against metastatic TNBC.

The anti-leukemia drug **dasatinib** (Sprycel) is in early clinical trials. It targets enzymes called src kinases that transmit growth and survival signals to tumor cells. These enzymes are overproduced in many types of cancer, including some types of TNBC.

Home remedies

Eating a healthy low-fat diet, exercising regularly, and limiting **alcohol consumption** are important for maximizing the effectiveness of breast cancer treatment.

Prognosis

Breast cancers without estrogen and progesterone receptors have a poorer prognosis than cancers that are ER+ and PR+ and basal-like tumors have a poorer prognosis than non-basal cell tumors. TNBC is more likely than other breast cancers to metastasize to other parts of the body. However the majority of women with stage 1 or stage 2 TNBC are cancer-free for many years following treatment and many patients with stage 3 or stage 4 lymph-node-positive TNBC also respond well to chemotherapy.

TNBC is more likely than other breast cancers to recur after treatment. Disease recurrence within five years is about 32% for TNBC compared with only about 15% for other types of breast cancer. The average survival time after recurrence is nine months. However the risk of recurrence is greatest in the first few years after treatment. Studies have indicated that, although TNBC is more likely to recur outside of the breasts, this is true only in the first three years following treatment. After three years the risk of recurrence is similar to that of other breast cancers.

Five-year-survival rates tend to be lower for TNBC than for other breast cancers. A 2007 study of more than 50,000 women with all stages of breast cancer found that 77% with TNBC survived for five years, compared with 93% of women with other types of breast cancer. Another 2007 study of more than 1,500 women found that, although those with TNBC had a higher risk of death within five years of diagnosis compared with women with other types of breast cancer, after five years their risk of death was no greater than that of the other women.

Prevention

Genetic testing is available for identifying BRCA mutations that increase the risk of TNBC. Since early detection is very important for the prognosis of TNBC and other breast cancers, women with a BRCA mutation should use augmented breast cancer surveillance techniques:

- monthly breast self-examinations beginning at age 18
- clinical breast examinations performed by a physician or nurse breast specialist every 6–12 months beginning at age 18
- mammograms every 6–12 months, beginning at age 25–35, or at least five years before the youngest age that breast cancer was diagnosed in a family member

However, mammograms do not detect some breast cancers, especially in younger women such as those who are at risk due to BRCA mutations.

Risk-reducing, prophylactic, or preventive mastectomy—the removal of the breasts and as much at-risk tissue as possible—in healthy women with a BRCA mutation reduces the risk of breast cancer by 90%. However it is not clear whether women undergoing this procedure are at any less risk of dying from breast cancer as compared with women who use careful surveillance methods.

Lifestyle factors that may increase the risk of breast cancer include:

- birth control pills
- obesity
- gaining weight after menopause, especially after natural menopause or age 60
- alcohol consumption, which can shift estrogen metabolism toward the higher-risk pathway, with the effect increasing with the amount of alcohol consumed
- synthetic hormone-replacement therapy after menopause.

QUESTIONS TO ASK YOUR DOCTOR

- Are you sure that my breast cancer is triple-negative?
- What stage is my breast cancer?
- What are my treatment options?
- Should I seek a second or third opinion about the best treatment for my TNBC?
- Are there clinical trials that may be appropriate for me?

Resources

BOOKS

Hirshaut, Yashar, and Peter I. Pressman. *Breast Cancer: The Complete Guide,* 5th ed. New York: Bantam, 2008.

Miller, Kenneth D. *Choices in Breast Cancer Treatment: Medical Specialists and Cancer Survivors Tell You What You Need to Know*. Baltimore: Johns Hopkins University Press, 2008.

Queller, Jessica. *Pretty Is What Changes: Impossible Choices, the Breast Cancer Gene, and How I Defied My Destiny*. New York: Spiegel & Grau, 2008.

PERIODICALS

Bauer, K. R., et al. "Descriptive Analysis of Estrogen Receptor (ER)-Negative, Progesterone Receptor (PR)-Negative, and HER2-Negative Invasive Breast Cancer, the So-Called Triple-Negative Phenotype: A Population-Based Study from the California Cancer Registry." *Cancer* 109, no. 9 (May 1, 2007): 1721-1728.

Cafferky, Monica. "The Hidden Breast Cancer You Need to Know About." *Daily Mirror* (January 17, 2008): 38.

Kõster, Frank, et al. "Triple-Negative Breast Cancers Express Receptors for Growth Hormone-Releasing Hormone (GHRH) and Respond to GHRH Antagonists with Growth Inhibition." *Breast Cancer Research and Treatment* 116, no. 2 (July 2009): 273-279.

Stein, Rob. "Drug-Resistant Breast Cancer Afflicts Blacks; Scientists Look at Genes, Breastfeeding Patterns." *Washington Post* (June 23, 2007): A1.

Viale, Giuseppe, et al. "Invasive Ductal Carcinoma of the Breast with the 'Triple-Negative' Phenotype: Prognostic Implications of EGFR Immunoreactivity." *Breast Cancer Research and Treatment* 116, no. 2 (July 2009): 317-328.

OTHER

"A Breast Cancer Survivor Goes the Distance with her Son." *ACS News*. http://www.cancer.org/docroot/FPS/content/FPS_1_A_Breast_Cancer_Survivor_Goes_the_Distance_with_Her_Son.asp.

Brown, Doris. "Public Health Democracy: U.S. and Global Health Disparities in Breast Cancer." *National Cancer Institute*. http://oia.cancer.gov/pdf/Browne_PublicHealthDemocracyApr2008.pdf.

Lebrasseur, Nicole, and Heather L. Van Epps. "Targeting the Triple Threat." *CureToday*. http://www.curetoday.com/index.cfm/fuseaction/article.show/id/2/article_id/1235.

"Triple-Negative Breast Cancer." *Breastcancer.org* http://www.breastcancer.org/symptoms/diagnosis/trip_neg/.

"What Is Breast Cancer?" *American Cancer Society*. http://www.cancer.org/docroot/CRI/content/CRI_2_4_1X_What_is_breast_cancer_5.asp.

ORGANIZATIONS

American Cancer Society, 1599 Clifton Road NE, Atlanta, GA, 30329-4251, (800) ACS-2345, http://www.cancer.org.

Breakthrough Breast Cancer, Weston House, 246 High Holborn, London, England, WC1V 7EX, 020 7025 2400, 08080 100 200, 020 7025 2401, info@breakthrough.org.uk, http://breakthrough.org.uk/.

Breastcancer.org, 7 East Lancaster Avenue, Third Floor, Ardmore, PA, 19003, http://www.breastcancer.org.

National Cancer Institute, NCI Public Inquiries Office, 6116 Executive Boulevard, Room 3036A, Bethesda, MD, 20006, (800) 4-CANCER, http://www.cancer.gov.

Triple Negative Breast Cancer Foundation, PO Box 204, Norwood, NJ, 07648, (646) 942-0242, (877) 870-TNBC (8622), info@tnbcfoundation.org, http://www.tnbcfoundation.org.

Margaret Alic, PhD

Triptorelin pamoate

Definition

Triptorelin pamoate is a synthetic luteinizing hormone-releasing hormone (LHRH) agonist, which is a substance that reduces the level of sexual hormones in the system.

Purpose

Since its approval by the FDA (Food and Drug Administration) in June of 2000, triptorelin pamoate has been recognized as a successful option in the treatment of long-term **cancer** of the prostate gland. The prostate gland is a solid, chestnut-shaped organ surrounding the male urethra. It produces secretions that become part of seminal fluid. In the case of cancer of the prostate gland, it is advantageous to reduce prostate gland cell activity. One way to do this is to reduce the amount of hormones circulating in the system that will stimulate prostate activity. LHRH-agonists, such as triptorelin, are indicated when either **orchiectomy** (surgical removal of one of both testes) or the administration of the female hormone estrogen is either inadvisable or considered unacceptable by the person suffering from the cancer.

Triptorelin pamoate has been successfully used to alleviate symptoms in cases of such advanced **prostate cancer**, and is now being used and researched as a treatment for:

- all prostate cancers
- ovarian cancer
- *in vitro* fertilization
- endometriosis, or chronic disease of the mucous membrane lining the uterus
- uterine leiomyoma, also called uterine fibroids, a non-cancerous growth on the smooth muscle of the uterine wall

- precocious puberty, a condition in which children of either sex may undergo pubescent changes at an abnormally early age
- fibrocystic breast disease, or the presence of one or more benign tumors in the breast

Description

The human body provides balance in the provision of all chemicals necessary to its function. The pituitary gland and hypothalamus in the brain interact to release substances called gonadotropins, which trigger and regulate the production of estrogen (female) and androgen (male) hormones. Synthetic LHRH medications (similar in chemical makeup to natural LHRH enzymes) reduce the quantity of natural gonadotropins released. This reduces cell activity occurring in organs affected by these hormones, such as the prostate gland, ovaries, testes, uterus, and breasts, therefore slowing the growth of cancerous cells.

Triptorelin is a potent synthetic LHRH medication, effectively reducing gonadotropins if administered to maintain a continuous, therapeutic level in the body. Initially, there is often a temporary surge in circulating amounts of both male and female hormones, but usually within two to four weeks of beginning therapy, there is a marked reduction of these sex hormones. In men, there is a reduction in **testosterone** in the blood stream comparable to the level usually seen in surgically castrated men. Consequently, cells that rely upon these hormones for stimulation become less active. In most cases, the effect of triptorelin pamoate on sexual hormones is reversible once treatment is completed.

Recommended dosage

For advanced prostate cancer, the most common application for triptorelin, the usual dose is 3.75 milligrams (mg) given once per month as a single intramuscular injection. This will normally maintain a therapeutic level. If necessary, this medication may also be given intravenously.

Precautions

In the treatment of prostate cancer, there have been reported flare-ups of the disease at the onset of therapy. Patients with a prostate tumor affecting the spinal cord or urinary flow should use caution, as an increase in tumor activity may initially worsen symptoms. Triptorelin pamoate is capable of causing harm to fetuses if administered to pregnant women. During long-term treatment of endometriosis or uterine fibroids, bone loss has been reported.

Side effects

The following side effects have either been reported or were observed:

- nausea and vomiting
- hot flashes
- vaginal dryness
- impotence
- loss of sex drive
- breakthrough bleeding
- sleep disturbance
- **diarrhea**
- fatigue
- hair loss (**alopecia**)
- mouth sores
- breast tenderness
- weight gain
- pain at injection site
- increases in cholesterol
- headache

Interactions

Because triptorelin pamoate has only had FDA approval since the early 2000s, not all information is known regarding its interactions with other medicines. Currently, no drug interactions have been reported.

Joan Schonbeck, R.N.

Tube enterostomy

Definition

Tube enterostomy, or tube feeding, is a form of enteral or intestinal site feeding that employs a stoma or semi-permanent surgically placed tube to the small intestines.

Purpose

Many patients are unable to take in food by mouth, esophagus, or stomach. A number of conditions can render a person unable to take in nutrition through the normal pathways. Neurological conditions or injuries, injuries to the mouth or throat, obstructions of the stomach, **cancer** or ulcerative conditions of the gastrointestinal tract, and certain surgical procedures can make it impossible for a person to

KEY TERMS

Enteral nutritional support—Nutrition utilizing an intact gastrointestinal tract, but bypassing another organ such as the stomach or esophagus.

Parenteral nutritional support—Intravenous nutrition that bypasses the intestines and its contribution to digestion.

Stoma—A portal fashioned from the side of the abdomen that allows for ingestion into or drainage out of the intestines or urinary tract.

Tube feeding—Feeding or nutrition through a tube placed into the body through the esophagus, nose, stomach, intestines, or via a surgically constructed artificial orifice called a stoma.

receive oral nutrition. Tube feeding is indicated for patients unable to ingest adequate nutrition by mouth, but who may have a cleared passage in the esophagus and stomach, and even partial functioning of the gastrointestinal tract. Enteral nutrition procedures that utilize the gastrointestinal tract are preferred over intravenous feeding or parenteral nutrition because they maintain the function of the intestines, provide for immunity to **infection**, and avoid complications related to intravenous feeding.

Tube enterostomy, a feeding tube placed directly into the intestines or jejunum, is one such enteral procedure. It is used if the need for enteral feeding lasts longer than six weeks, or if it improves the outcomes of drastic surgeries such as removal or resection of the intestines. Recently, it has become an important technique for use in surgery in which a gastroectomy—resection of the intestinal link to the esophagus—occurs. The procedure makes healing easier, and seeks to retain the patient's nutritional status and quality of life after **reconstructive surgery**. Some individuals have a tube enterostomy surgically constructed, and successfully utilize it for a long period of time.

There are a variety of enteral nutritional products, liquid feedings with the nutritional quality of solid food. Patients with normal gastrointestinal function can benefit from these products. Other patients must have nutritional counseling, monitoring, and precise nutritional diets developed by a health care professional.

Demographics

Tube enterostomy provides temporary enteral nutrition to patients with injuries as well as inflammatory, obstructive, and other intestinal, esophageal, and abdominal conditions. Other uses include patients with pediatric abnormalities, and those who have had surgery for cancerous tumors of the gastroesophageal junction (many of these cases are associated with Barrett's epithelium). Intestinal cancers in the United States have declined since the 1950s. However, this endemic form of gastric cancer is one of the most common causes of death from malignant disease, with an estimated 798,000 annual cases worldwide and 21,900 of those in the United States. As gastric cancer has declined, esophageal cancers have increased, requiring surgeries that resect and reconstruct the passage between the esophagus and intestine.

Description

Tube enterostomy refers to placement via a number of surgical approaches:

- laparoscopy
- esophagostomy (open surgery via the esophagus)
- stomach (gastrostomy or PEG)
- upper intestines or jejunum (jejunostomy)

The appropriate method depends on the clinical prognosis, anticipated duration of feeding, risk of aspirating or inhaling gastric contents, and patient preference. Whether through a standard operation or with laparascopic surgical techniques, the surgeon fashions a stoma or opening into the esophagus, stomach or intestines, and inserts a tube from the outside through which nutrition will be introduced. These tubes are made of silicone or polyurethane, and contain weighted tips and insertion features that facilitate placement. The surgery is fairly simple to perform, and most patients have good outcomes with stoma placement.

Diagnosis/Preparation

A number of conditions necessitate tube enterostomy for **nutritional support**. Many are chronic and require a complete medical evaluation including history, physical examination, and extensive imaging tests. Some conditions are critical or acute, and may emerge from injuries or serious inflammatory conditions in which the patient is not systematically prepared for the surgery. In many cases, the patient undergoing this type of surgery has been ill for a period of time. Sometimes the patient is a small child or adult who accidentally swallowed a caustic substance. Some are elderly patients who have obstructive **carcinoma** of the esophagus or stomach.

WHO PERFORMS THE PROCEDURE AND WHERE IS IT PERFORMED?

Gastrointestinal surgeons and surgical oncologists perform this surgery in general hospital settings.

Optimal preparation includes an evaluation of the patient's nutritional status, and his or her potential requirement for blood transfusions and **antibiotics**. Patients who do not have gastrointestinal inflammatory or obstructive conditions are usually required to undergo bowel preparation that flushes the intestines of all material. The bowel preparation reduces the chances of infection.

The patient's acceptance of tube feeding as a substitute for eating is of paramount importance. Health care providers must be sensitive to these problems, and offer early assistance and feedback in the self-care that the tube enterostomy requires.

In preparation for surgery, patients learn that the tube enterostomy will be an artificial orifice placed outside the abdomen through which they will deliver their nutritional support. Patients are taught how to care for the stoma, cleaning and making sure it functions optimally. In addition, patients are prepared for the loss of the function of eating and its place in their lives. They must be made aware that their physical body will be altered, and that this may have social implications and affect their intimate activities.

Aftercare

Tube enterostomy requires monitoring the patient for infection or bleeding, and educating him or her on the proper use of the enterostomy. According to the type of surgery—minimally invasive or open surgery—it may take several days for the patient to resume normal functioning. Fluid intake and urinary output must be monitored to prevent dehydration.

Risks

Tube enterostomies are not considered high risk surgeries. Insertions have been completed in over 90% of attempts. Possible complications include **diarrhea**, skin irritation due to leakage around the stoma, and difficulties with tube placement.

Tube enterostomy is becoming more frequent due to great advances in minimally invasive techniques and new materials used for stoma construction.

QUESTIONS TO ASK THE DOCTOR

- How long will the tube enterostomy remain in place?
- How much assistance will be given in adjusting to the stoma and the special diet?
- If the condition does not improve, what other surgical alternatives are available?
- How long can a person live safely and comfortably with a tube enterostomy?

However, one recent radiograph study of 289 patients who had jejunostomy found that 14% of patients suffered one or more complications, 19% had problems related to the location or function of the tube, and 9% developed thickened small-bowel folds.

Normal results

Recovery without complications is the norm for this surgery. The greatest challenge is educating the patient on proper stoma usage and types of nutritional support that must be used.

Morbidity and mortality rates

Some feeding or tube stomas have the likelihood of complications. A review of 1,000 patients indicated that PEG tube placement has mortality in 0.5%, with major complications (stomal leakage, peritonitis [infection in the abdomen], traumatized tissue of the abdominal wall, and gastric [stomach] hemorrhage) in 1% of cases. Wound infection, leaks, tube movement or migration, and **fever** occurred in 8% of patients. In a review of seven published studies, researchers found that a single intravenous dose of a broad-spectrum antibiotic was very effective in reducing infections with the stoma. Open surgery always carries with it a small percentage of cardiac complications, blood clots, and infections. Many gastric stoma patients have complicated diseases that increase the likelihood of surgical complications.

Alternatives

Oral routes are always the preferred method of providing nutritional intake. Intravenous fluid intake can be used as an eating substitute, but only for a short period of time. It is the preferred alternative when adequate protein and calories cannot be provided by oral or other enteral routes, or when the gastrointestinal system is not functioning.

Resources

BOOKS

Feldman, M.D., Mark. *Sleisenger & Fordtran's Gastrointestinal and Liver Disease*,7th ed. Elsevier, 2002.

Townsend, Courtney M. *Sabiston Textbook of Surgery*, 16th ed. W. B. Saunders Company, 2001.

PERIODICALS

ASPEN Board of Directors and the Clinical Guidelines Task Force. "Guidelines for the Use of Parenteral and Enteral Nutrition in Adult and Pediatric Patients." *Journal of Parenteral Enteral Nutrition* 26, no.1 (Suppl) (January/February 2002).

Chin, A. and N.J. Espat. "Total Gastrectomy: Options for the Restoration of Gastrointestinal Continuity." *The Lancet Oncology* 4, no.5 (May 2003).

Marik, P.E. and G.P. Zaloga. "Early Enteral Nutrition in Acutely Ill Patients: A Systematic Review." *Critical Care Medicine* 29, no.12 (December 2001).

Mentec, H., et.al. "Upper Digestive Intolerance During Enteral Nutrition in Critically Ill Patients: Frequency, Risk Factors, and Complications." *Critical Care Medicine* 29, no.10 (October 2001).

OTHER

Tube Feeding. Patient Handout. MDConsult. www.MDConsult.com.

ORGANIZATIONS

American Society Parenteral and Enteral Nutrition. 8630 Fenton St., Suite 412, Silver Springs, Maryland 20910. (301) 587-6315. Fax: (301) 587-2365. www.clinnutr.org.

United Ostomy Association, Inc. 19772 MacArthur Blvd., Suite 200, Irvine, CA 92612-2405. (800) 826-0826. www.uoa.org.

Nancy McKenzie, Ph.D.

Tumor grading

Definition

Tumor grading is an estimate of the tumor's malignancy and aggressiveness based on how the tumor cells appear under a microscope and the number of malignant characteristics they possess.

Purpose

Tumor grading, together with the stage of the tumor, assists doctors in planning treatment strategies. Although grading is an important part of describing most cancers, it is extremely important in helping to determine the course of treatment for specific cancers such as soft tissue sarcomas, **brain tumors**, lymphomas, and breast and **prostate cancer**. Generally higher grade and higher stage tumors require more drastic therapy than lower grade and stage tumors. Tumor grade and stage also help doctors give an estimation of the prognosis of the patient. Patients with lower grade and stage tumors usually have a more positive prognosis than patients with higher grade and stage tumors. Patients should thoroughly discuss the grade and stage of their tumor with their physician, asking about necessary treatments and prognosis.

KEY TERMS

Anaplastic—Poorly differentiated; immature and abnormal in function.

Benign tumor—A non-cancerous tumor that is incapable of invading surrounding tissue and spreading to other areas of the body.

Differentiated—Description of the similarity of function and appearance of cancer cells when compared to the normal, healthy tissue.

Exfoliative cytology—Evaluating cells that are shed from the body's surface.

Malignant tumor—A tumor that is capable of invading surrounding tissue and spreading to other areas of the body.

Pap smear—Analysis of cells found in vaginal secretions to determine the presence of uterine cancer. Also called a Pap test.

Pathologist—A doctor that examines cells under a microscope to determine the presence of the disease.

Pleomorphic—Irregular shape.

Tumor stage—An objective measurement gauging the cancer's progression.

Description

Before a tumor can be assigned a grade, a sample of tissue must be removed for microscopic evaluation. Tissue samples can be obtained through one of various types of **biopsy** or through exfoliative **cytology** (e.g., Pap smear). A pathologist analyzes various characteristics of the tissue. Some characteristics include the size and shape of the nucleus; the ratio of the volume of the nucleus to the volume of the cytoplasm; the relative number of dividing cells called the mitotic index; the organization of the tissue; the boundary of the tumor;

QUESTIONS TO ASK THE DOCTOR

- What are the microscopic characteristics that this cancer presents?
- What grade is this cancer?
- What courses of treatment do you recommend for this grade of this type of cancer?

and how well-differentiated the cells appear—how close to normal the cells seem in maturity and function.

Benign tumors have normal-looking cells. That is, they have small- and regular-shaped nuclei, small nuclear volume relative to the rest of the cellular volume, a relatively low number of dividing cells, and normal and well-differentiated tissue that has a well-defined tumor boundary. However, malignant tumors generally have all or several of the following characteristics: large and pleomorphic (irregular-shaped) nuclei, large nuclear volume compared to the rest of the cellular volume, a high number of dividing cells, and disorganized and anaplastic (poorly differentiated) tissue that has a poorly defined tumor boundary.

Depending on the number of malignant characteristics present, the **American Joint Commission on Cancer** has recommended that the tumor be given a grade using G0 through G4.

- G1: Well-differentiated (Low-grade and less aggressive)
- G2: Moderately well-differentiated (Intermediate-grade and moderately aggressive)
- G3: Poorly differentiated (High-grade and moderately aggressive)
- G4: Undifferentiated (High-grade and aggressive)

Alternatively, Roman numerals I through IV may be used. Low-grade tumors are assigned lower Roman numerals (e.g., grade I), indicating that the tumor is less aggressive. High-grade tumors are assigned higher Roman numerals (e.g., grade IV), indicating that the tumor is very aggressive, growing and spreading quickly.

- I: Well-differentiated (Low-grade and less aggressive)
- II: Moderately well-differentiated (Intermediate-grade and moderately aggressive)
- III: Poorly differentiated (High-grade and moderately aggressive)
- IV: Undifferentiated (High-grade and aggressive)

There are some cancers that have their own grading convention. For example, the Gleason system is a unique grading system that was developed to describe **adenocarcinoma** of the prostate. Pathologists analyze prostate tissue and give a Gleason score ranging from 2 to 10, subject to the number of malignant characteristics observed. Well-differentiated, less aggressive prostate tumors with only a few malignant characteristics are given lower Gleason numbers, while inadequately differentiated, more aggressive prostate tumors that possess many malignant characteristics are assigned higher Gleason numbers.

See also Tumor staging.

Resources

BOOKS

Bast, Robert C. *Cancer Medicine*. B.C. Decker Inc., 2000.

Sally C. McFarlane-Parrott

Tumor lysis syndrome

Definition

Tumor lysis syndrome is a life-threatening metabolic emergency that complicates the treatment of certain types of tumors (neoplasms).

Demographics

Many factors contribute to the development of tumor lysis syndrome. Most of the research performed to date revolves around high-grade **non-Hodgkin's lymphoma** cases, 40% of which demonstrate laboratory evidence of tumor lysis syndrome. (An estimated 6% demonstrate clinical evidence of the syndrome.) Tumors that carry the highest risk of the development of tumor lysis syndrome are those that are large and bulky, usually greater than eight to ten cm (3-4 in.), and comprised of rapidly dividing cells. In addition, tumors that respond well to treatment are associated with tumor lysis syndrome because treatment results in rupture of a large number of cells.

Most often, the syndrome is associated with blood-based (hematologic) tumors, such as non-Hodgkin's **lymphoma**, particularly **Burkitt's lymphoma**, and acute leukemia. Though less likely because of lower rates of cell division, tumor lysis syndrome can also occur in solid tumors such as **breast cancer**. The Washington Manual of Medical Therapeutics associates the following **cancer** types with tumor lysis syndrome:

KEY TERMS

Dialysis—A medical procedure that uses a special machine to filter waste products from the blood and restore it. It is a life-sustaining procedure in end-stage kidney failure.

Electrolytes—Substances or particles that dissolve into ions, (atoms with a positive or negative charge) such as potassium or sodium, and carry water molecules across cell membranes, regulating electric charge in order to maintain the proper oxygen flow of body fluids.

Metabolic—Pertaining to the physical and chemical process of synthesis and breakdown of substances necessary to sustain life.

Nephrology—The study of the kidneys—their structure and function.

pH—A measure of the alkalinity or acidity of a substance.

- Non-Hodgkin's lymphoma (NHL)
- Acute lymphocytic leukemia (ALL)
- Acute myelocytic leukemia (AML)
- Chronic lymphocytic leukemia (CLL)
- Chronic myelocytic leukemia (CML)
- Breast cancer
- Testicular cancer
- Medulloblastoma
- Merkel cell carcinoma
- Neuroblastoma
- Small cell carcinoma of the lung

Description

Concentrations of intracellular electrolytes, those that are within the cell, differ from extracellular electrolytes, or those that are outside the cell and in the bloodstream. In tumor lysis syndrome, tumor cells lyse, or break apart, releasing their contents into the blood stream. The result is a dangerous alteration in the normal balance of serum electrolytes—potassium, phosphate, and uric acid levels are elevated, while calcium levels are decreased. The changes occur so quickly and can be so dramatic, that immediate death can result.

Causes and symptoms

Usually, tumor lysis syndrome develops after the administration of combination **chemotherapy** regimens, but it may also occur spontaneously or as a result of radiation or corticosteroid therapy. Lactic acid dehydrogenase (LDH) is an enzyme found in cells of body tissues. An increase in the LDH level is considered a marker of bulky disease that correlates with the risk of tumor lysis syndrome.

Patients with underlying kidney (renal) dysfunction and/or decreased urine output are at a higher risk of developing tumor lysis syndrome. Without optimal kidney functioning, waste products that build up cannot be excreted in the urine at a high enough rate. Patients with cancer may be predisposed to conditions that increase the risk of renal failure due to increased uric acid buildup. For example, a patient undergoing chemotherapy may experience **nausea and vomiting**, and may, as a result, be dehydrated, increasing the risk. The same patient may have decreased white blood cell counts, making him or her more susceptible to infections. Many **antibiotics** adversely affect the kidneys, also increasing the risk.

In some cases, the patient does not manifest any symptoms of tumor lysis syndrome. Instead, the electrolyte derangements are noted on blood testing. In other cases, the derangements may be extreme enough to cause overt signs and symptoms, such as:

- Bloody urine
- Flank pain
- High blood pressure
- Decreased urine output
- Lethargy
- Sleepiness
- Muscle cramps and twitching
- Heart arthythmmias
- Fainting
- Nausea
- Vomiting
- Severe diarrhea
- Sudden death
- Confusion
- Seizures
- Coma

Treatments

Treatment is aimed at prevention and supportive care, with the main goals being to prevent renal failure and severe electrolyte imbalances. Patients at risk receive treatment on an inpatient basis to allow for close monitoring by medical personnel. At all times, patients should have reliable intravenous access. Prior to initiating treatment, a patient's hydration status and electrolyte levels are carefully evaluated. If there are abnormalities, a treatment delay may be considered, though this is not always an option.

Laboratory tests are done frequently to monitor levels of calcium, potassium, phosphate, magnesium, and uric acid. A typical hospital protocol may require blood be drawn for these tests every two to six hours over the course of two to three days. Following are prevention and management strategies for each of the major electrolyte imbalances, hyperuricemia, hyperkalenia, hyperphosphatemia, and **hypocalcemia**.

Hyperuricemia is a medical term used to describe an abnormal increase of uric acid levels in the blood that can lead to acute renal failure. There are several methods employed to prevent kidney damage—aggressive hydration being a major focus. Intravenous (IV) hydration is started before treatment and continues throughout to maintain a urine output of 100 to 200 milliliters per hour (ml/hr). Medications called diuretics, such as furosemide or acetazolamide, are given to help increase urine output when necessary.

Urine may be alkalized to prevent uric acid buildup. Alkalization can be accomplished by adding sodium bicarbonate to the patient's IV fluid. For example, the basic maintenance IV fluid may consist of 5% dextrose in 0.25 normal saline, to which sodium bicarbonate, in amounts ranging from 50 to 200 milliequivalents (mEq—the total number of charges of electrolytes in solution), may be added. Urine pH is routinely tested, and the sodium bicarbonate is periodically increased or decreased to maintain a pH level between 7 and 8.

Urine alkalinization is somewhat controversial. If urine is too alkaline, calcium phosphate crystal formation may occur, increasing the likelihood of renal failure. However, it is generally believed that if urine output levels are appropriately maintained, calcium phosphate will be diluted, and the possibility of crystal formation will diminish.

Patients at risk for tumor lysis syndrome may also be given **allopurinol** prophylactically. One dose of 600 milligrams (mg) may be given the day before treatment, followed by 300 mg once a day for the remainder of treatment days. Allopurinol is effective because it inhibits the formation of uric acid. In 2004, a new drug called rasburicase became available in the United States. It prevents the damaging effects of tumor lysis syndrome with fewer side effects.

Hyperkalemia is a medical term used to describe an abnormal increase of potassium levels in the blood that can cause dangerous abnormalities in heart rhythms, heart attack, and muscle weakness. Frequent monitoring with electrocardiography (EKG) is recommended in patients at risk for tumor lysis syndrome so that alterations in the electrical activity of the heart can be caught early. Potassium-rich foods may also be restricted to prevent already elevated levels from increasing. Sometimes, medications such as Kayexalate are administered to help reduce potassium levels.

Hyperphosphatemia is a medical term used to describe an abnormal increase on phosphate levels in the blood that can cause neuromuscular irritability and worsen kidney function. Malignant cells may contain up to four times as much phosphate as non-malignant cells. Patients experiencing acute tumor lysis syndrome may be instructed to reduce their dietary intake of phosphate. In addition, they may be given medications that bind to phosphate, thereby inhibiting its absorption in the intestines.

Hypocalcemia is a medical term used to describe an abnormal decrease in calcium levels in the blood that can cause muscle spasms (tetany), muscle cramps, and seizures. A calcium supplement may be required.

Dialysis is a procedure used to normalize electrolyte imbalances through the diffusion and ultrafiltration of fluid. Potassium, for example, can be separated and filtered from fluid, bringing levels back to a safer range. Hemodialysis is a procedure that removes waste products through the blood. Dialysis can alternatively be performed through the peritoneum, the tissue that lines the abdominal area and surrounds the organs in what is called peritoneal dialysis. Because peritoneal dialysis does not clear phosphate and urate as efficiently, and because it is not feasible in patients with abdominal tumors, hemodialysis is the preferred method. A doctor who specializes in nephrology will generally examine a high-risk patient before cancer treatment begins, to prepare for the possibility of dialysis treatment. In some cases, dialysis is started as a preventive measure, either before or during chemotherapy treatment.

Prognosis

The prognosis of tumor lysis syndrome is good, as long as the problem is identified and treated early in its course. If the process is allowed to continue unchecked, the syndrome can prove life-threatening.

Prevention

Patients who are going to be treated for tumors known to have high rates of tumor lysis syndrome (such as lymphomas and leukemias) should be given medications to prevent the production and/or buildup of uric acid, such as allopurinol or Rasburicase. Patients should be monitored carefully for the advent of electrolyte changes that could suggest that they are at risk for developing full-blown tumor lysis syndrome.

Resources

BOOKS

Abeloff, MD et al. *Clinical Oncology*. 3rd ed. Philadelphia: Elsevier, 2004.

Goldman L, Ausiello D., eds. *Cecil Textbook of Internal Medicine*. 23rd ed. Philadelphia: Saunders, 2008.

Hoffman R. et al.*Hematology: Basic Principles and Practice*. 4th ed. Philadelphia: Elsevier, 2005.

Marx, John A., et al. *Rosen's Emergency Medicine*. 6th ed. St. Louis, MO: Mosby, Inc., 2006.

Tamara Brown, R.N.
Teresa G. Odle

Tumor markers

Definition

Tumor markers are measurable biochemicals that are associated with a malignancy. They are either produced by tumor cells (tumor-derived) or by the body in response to tumor cells (tumor-associated). They are typically substances that are released into the circulation and thus measured in the blood. There are a few exceptions to this, such as tissue-bound receptors that must be measured in a **biopsy** from the solid tumor or proteins that are secreted into the urine.

Purpose

Though tumor markers are rarely specific enough to be used alone to diagnose **cancer**, they do have a number of clinical uses. They can be used to stage cancer, to indicate a prognosis, to monitor treatment, or in follow-up to watch for cancer recurrence. Changes in some tumor markers have been sensitive enough to be used as targets in **clinical trials**. When used for diagnosis, tumor markers are used in conjunction with other clinical parameters such as biopsy and radiological findings. Although there are a multitude of tumor markers, very few of them have found their way into clinical practice because of their lack of specificity. However, some of these non-specific markers have found a place in monitoring cancer treatment rather than in diagnosis.

KEY TERMS

AFP (Alpha-fetoprotein)—A tumor marker associated with liver, testicular, and ovarian cancer.

Beta-HCG (Beta-human chorionic gonadotropin)—A tumor marker associated with testicular cancer and tumors, such as choriocarcinoma and molar pregnancies, that begin in placental cells called trophoblasts.

Biopsy—The process of taking a sample of tumor tissue through a needle.

CA 15-3 (Cancer antigen 15-3)—A tumor marker associated with breast cancer.

CA 19-9 (Cancer antigen 19-9)—A tumor marker associated with pancreatic cancer.

CA 27-29 (Breast carcinoma-associated antigen)—A tumor marker associated with breast cancer.

CA 125 (Cancer antigen 125)—A tumor marker associated with ovarian cancer.

CEA (Carcinoembryonic antigen)—A tumor marker associated with many cancers, especially liver, intestinal, and pancreatic.

Prognosis—The predicted outcome of a disease.

PSA (Prostate specific antigen)—A tumor marker associated with prostate cancer.

Sensitivity—A test's ability to detect all cases of a disease.

Serial measurements—A series of measurements looking for an increase or decrease over time.

Specificity—A test's ability to detect only the disease in question.

Tumor markers—Biochemicals produced by tumor cells or by the body in response to tumor cells. Their levels in the blood help evaluate people for certain kinds of cancer.

Description

As tumor cells grow and multiply, some of their substances can increase and leak into the bloodstream or other fluids. Depending upon the tumor marker, it can be measured in blood, urine, stool, or tissue. Some widely used tumor markers include: AFP, beta-HCG, CA 15-3, CA 19-9, CA 27.29, CA 125, CEA, and PSA. Some tumor markers are associated with many types of cancer; others, with as few as one. Some tumor markers are always elevated in specific cancers; most are less predictable. However, no tumor marker is specific for cancer and most are found in low levels in healthy persons, or can be associated with non-neoplastic diseases as well as cancer. Also, no tumor marker test is free of false negatives or false positives.

Once cancer is diagnosed, tumor marker levels sometimes help to determine the extent of cancer. Higher levels can indicate more advanced cancer and a worse prognosis in some cases. The patient and their physician may use this information to choose between more or less aggressive treatments.

Monitoring cancer treatment is the most common use of tumor markers. As cancer is reduced, levels often decrease. Stable or increasing levels often indicate that the cancer is not responding to treatment. The choice of tumor marker to use for monitoring is important. Only a marker elevated before treatment should be used to monitor a person during or after treatment. Timing of the tests is also important. Each tumor marker has a unique life span in the blood. To monitor a treatment's success, enough time must have passed for the initial marker to be cleared from the blood. Tests done too soon may be falsely elevated because the marker produced by the untreated cancer is still present.

Watching for cancer recurrence after treatment is another reason for tumor marker testing. Periodic testing can sometimes detect a recurrence often months earlier than could an ultrasound, x ray, or physical examination.

Tumor marker tests are performed in a lab using immunological techniques. A sample of blood or other tissue is mixed with a substance containing specific antibodies to each tumor marker. If that tumor marker is present, these very specific antibodies bind to the markers. Some type of label, often a radioactive substance, is then used to measure the amount of bound marker and antibody. From this measurement, the amount of tumor marker is calculated. The results are usually available within a few days.

Conclusions based on tumor marker tests are seldom based on one test result but on a series of test results, called serial measurements. A series of increasing or decreasing values is more significant than a single value.

Tumor marker testing is currently the object of much research and attention. Their use is directed by approval from the Food and Drug Administration (FDA) and guidelines established by organizations such as the American Society of Clinical Oncology and the American Cancer Society. Not all tumor receptor marker tests are widely available nor are they widely accepted.

Oncofetal antigens

There are two common oncofetal antigens, alphafetoprotein (AFP) and carcinoembryonic antigen (CEA). Carcinoembryonic antigen CA 72-4 is a more recently discovered oncofetal antigen just coming into usage. The oncofetal antigens are so named because they are normally produced during embryonic development and decrease soon after birth. Cancer cells tend to dedifferentiate, or revert to a more immature tissue and begin to produce fetal antigens again. Oncofetal antigens are very non-specific and expressed by a wide number of cancer types. However, they are used both to monitor a patient's progress and their response to treatment over time.

ALPHA-FETOPROTEIN (AFP). Elevated AFP typically indicates a primary liver tumor or a germ cell tumor of the ovary or testicle. AFP is a glycoprotein produced in high amounts by fetal tissue and is elevated during pregnancy. It is most widely used as a marker for hepatocellular **carcinoma** and **testicular cancer** but is also associated with **ovarian cancer**. Seventy percent of people with **liver cancer** have increased AFP levels. In China, where liver cancer rates are high, AFP is used as a **screening test** for that disease. AFP levels indicate the extent of cancer, and serial measurements are used to monitor treatment response. Non-cancerous liver conditions such as cirrhosis and hepatitis have moderately increased levels of AFP.

CARCINOEMBRYONIC ANTIGEN (CEA). CEA is a glycoprotein most often associated with colorectal cancer, and used to monitor patients with this type of cancer. Its most popular use is in early detection of relapse in individuals already treated for colorectal cancer. After surgery, serial measurements indicate the surgery's success and are used to detect early signs of recurrence. It has recently been found to be useful when measured during surgery for colorectal cancer to help determine prognosis and who will benefit from adjuvant treatment.

CEA is measured in the blood plasma. It is very non-specific and can be increased in many types of cancer: gastrointestinal, colorectal, ovarian, bladder, cervical, stomach, kidney, lung, pancreatic, liver, prostate, thyroid, **melanoma**, **lymphoma**, and breast. People with noncancerous conditions, such as cirrhosis or peptic disease, or inflammatory intestinal conditions such as colitis or diverticulitis, may also have increased levels. CEA levels can be elevated in elderly patients and in those who smoke.

CANCER ANTIGEN 72-4 (CA 72-4). The more recently identified carcinoembryonic protein is CA 72-4.

Although it is slightly elevated with most carcinomas, it is mostly associated with gastric carcinoma (**stomach cancer**). CA 74-2 is finding a role in the management of patients with gastric carcinoma.

Cancer antigen 15-3 (CA 15-3)

CA 15-3 is produced by cells in the breast and increased levels can be associated with **breast cancer**. Rarely increased in women with early breast cancer, it may be used to detect recurrence of cancer in women following treatment or **mastectomy** and to monitor treatment for women with advanced breast cancer. However, adenocarcinomas of the ovary, lung, colon, and pancreas also express elevated CA 15-3 levels. Non-cancerous conditions sometimes associated with elevated CA 15-3 include benign breast or ovarian disease, endometriosis, pelvic inflammatory disease, and hepatitis. Pregnancy and lactation are also related to high CA 15-3 levels.

Cancer antigen 27-29 (CA 27-29)

CA 27-29, also called breast carcinoma-associated antigen, is used as a marker for breast cancer. Eighty percent of women with breast cancer have an increased CA 27-29 level. This marker may be used with other procedures and tumor marker levels such as CA 15-3 to check for recurrences of cancer in previously treated women. Serial measurements monitor treatment response and identify recurrence.

Levels of CA 27-29 may also be increased in cancers of the colon, stomach, kidney, lung, ovary, pancreas, uterus, and liver. Noncancerous conditions associated with elevated CA 27-29 include first trimester pregnancy, endometriosis, ovarian cysts, non-cancerous breast disease, kidney disease, and liver disease.

HER-2/neu

HER-2/neu is an oncogenic growth factor receptor also known as c-erbB-2. It is measured in the tissue from a biopsy either by immunological assays of the protein or polymerase chain reaction (PCR) to identify the DNA. The presence of HER-2/neu is generally associated with a poorer prognosis for breast cancer. It can also help to determine treatment options, since newer drugs can block this protein and decrease cancer growth. The most widely known of these drugs is **trastuzumab** (brand name **Herceptin**).

Estrogen receptor

Measurement of the estrogen receptor (ER) is used specifically to evaluate breast cancers. It gives an indication of prognosis and responsiveness to therapy. Tissue from a biopsy is used to measure the estrogen receptor. Most breast cancers in post-menopausal women are ER-positive, meaning that they require estrogen to grow. These ER-positive breast cancers are less aggressive than ER-negative breast cancers, which are found generally in pre-menopausal women.

Cancer antigen 125 (CA 125)

Although produced by a number of cell types, CA 125 is primarily produced by ovarian cancer cells. Eighty percent of women with ovarian cancer have increased CA 125 levels. Although the test is not sensitive or specific enough to be used for screening, it contributes to a diagnosis when combined with an ultrasound and pelvic examination. Blood levels of CA 125 are used primarily to monitor the treatment of ovarian cancer. A falling CA 125 level usually indicates that cancer is responding to the treatment. After diagnosis and treatment, serial measurements help detect remaining or recurrent cancer. A negative or normal result, however, does not guarantee the absence of cancer.

Women may have increased CA 125 levels during menstruation and pregnancy. Increased levels are also found in pelvic inflammatory disease, endometriosis, pancreatitis, and liver disease. Elevated levels are also associated with non-ovarian cancers including cancers of the uterus, cervix, pancreas, liver, colon, breast, lung, or digestive tract.

Prostate specific antigen (PSA)

Prostate specific antigen (PSA) levels, along with the **digital rectal examination**, are used to screen for **prostate cancer**. PSA is a protein produced by the prostate gland and can be overproduced in prostate cancer. It is perhaps the best tumor marker in use because of its tissue specificity, meaning that it is produced only by the prostate. Men over the age of 50 years are advised to consider annual screening for prostate cancer. Men at high risk for prostate cancer, such as African Americans or those with a family history of the disease, should begin screening at age 40. Once a diagnosis of prostate cancer is made, PSA levels can help determine the stage of the cancer, monitor the response to treatment, and watch for recurrence.

Measurements of PSA following **prostatectomy** are useful in determining the success of surgery. Any PSA level following surgery would indicate residual prostate tissue, possibly from **metastasis**. PSA levels can also be used to detect a recurrence of prostate cancer. PSA is also increased in benign prostatic hyperplasia (BPH), an enlarged prostate condition common in older men.

PSA can be found in the serum in two states, bound and free. Measuring both PSA levels can provide more specificity to the test and reduce unnecessary biopsies. The percentage of free PSA is greater in BPH than prostate cancer. If the total PSA level is higher than 4.0 nanogram/milliliter (ng/mL) and the free PSA level is less than 25%, a prostate biopsy is indicated.

PSA levels may increase after ejaculation. Men are recommended to abstain from sexual intercourse or masturbation for 48 hours before the test. PSA levels may also increase after prostate manipulation following the digital rectal exam.

Prostatic acid phosphatase (PAP) originally found to be produced by the prostate and thought to be a marker for prostate cancer. It is now found to be elevated with testicular cancer, leukemia, **non-Hodgkin's lymphoma**, and several noncancerous conditions.

Cancer antigen 19-9 (CA 19-9)

CA 19-9 has been identified in patients with digestive tract or intra-abdominal carcinomas such as colorectal cancer, **pancreatic cancer**, stomach cancer, and **bile duct cancer**. In pancreatic cancer, higher levels are associated with more advanced disease. After diagnosis, levels help predict the success of surgery and monitor the course of the cancer. Not all people with pancreatic cancer have increased CA 19-9 levels. This antigen is related to the Lewis blood group and so only patients positive for the Lewis blood group antigen will test positive for CA 19-9. It is also increased in liver and **gastrointestinal cancers** and in noncancerous diseases, including pancreatitis, gallstones, and jaundice.

Human chorionic gonadotropin (hCG)

Human chorionic gonadotropin is normally produced by the placenta during pregnancy. There are two protein subunits that make up HCG, beta and alpha. It is the beta subunit that is increased in women's serum during early pregnancy. It is also the beta subunit that is increased in some malignant tumors. Tumors that secrete beta-hCG are typically **germ cell tumors** such as teratocarcinomas. These are tumors found in the ovaries and testes that contain embryonal tissue. Rarely, these types of tumors are found in the pineal region of the brain where beta-hCG can serve as a marker. Levels of hCG rise with choriocarcinoma and with trophoblastic disease, a rare cancer that develops from an abnormally fertilized egg. **Gestational trophoblastic tumors** also secrete AFP and this test is often used in combination.

HCG is most often used to screen for cancer of the testis or ovary. Serial measurements monitor the progress and treatment of these cancers. This marker can be elevated in individuals who use marijuana.

Squamous cell carcinoma (SCC) Antigen

Squamous cell carcinoma (SCC) antigen was first identified in **cervical cancer**. It is a marker for squamous cell cancers, which can occur in the cervix, head and neck, lung, and skin. Levels of SCC can be used as an aid to stage the carcinoma and to determine the response to treatment.

Bence-Jones protein

Patients with plasmacytomas such as **myeloma** overproduce monoclonal immunoglobulins, also called M proteins. The Bence-Jones protein refers to the immunoglobulin light chain, a portion of these immunoglobulins. The Bence-Jones protein is secreted into the urine where it can be measured. It was the first tumor marker identified.

Neuron-specific enolase (NSE)

NSE is a protein found mainly in neurons and neuroendocrine cells. It is elevated in tumors derived from these tissues, including **neuroblastoma** and **small cell lung cancer**. It can give information about the extent of the disease, the patient's prognosis and the patient's response to treatment. NSE can also be elevated in medullary thyroid cancers, carcinoid tumors, pancreatic endocrine tumors, and melanoma.

Hormone assays

Tumors of the endocrine glands oversecrete their corresponding hormones. By measuring particular hormones, clues can be obtained regarding certain cancers. For instance, breast cancer cells may secrete prolactin and estrogen. Medullary carcinoma can secrete **calcitonin**. Pheochromocytomas secrete catecholamines. Tumors of the pituitary gland may secrete growth hormone or cortisol. Carcinoid tumors secrete serotonin. Some tumors of the pancreas secrete insulin. Serial measurements can also monitor treatment for these tumors.

Enzymes

Several serum enzymes can be measured to help detect metastases in cancer patients. Tumors that metastasize to the liver cause increases in serum alkaline phosphatase, gamma-glutamyltransferase, and transaminases. Although these are not necessarily tumor markers, they indicate liver damage that may be caused by metastatic cancer. Tumors that metastasize to the bone sometimes secrete elevated alkaline phosphatase. Lactate dehydrogenase is an enzyme found throughout the body. Because of this it cannot be used as a marker for cancer. It can, however, be used to monitor the treatment of some types of cancer including germ cell tumors, testicular cancer, **Ewing's sarcoma**, non-Hodgkins lymphoma, and some types of leukemia.

Precautions

There is not a good consensus in the medical community about the value of most tumor markers. Because they lack specificity and accuracy, their use is limited. False positives can cause emotional distress and fear. It is not yet determined if there is a savings of life or money with testing. Currently, much controversy surrounds the issue of mass screening for cancer using tumor markers.

Preparation

Tumor marker tests usually require 5-10 mL of blood. A healthcare worker ties a tourniquet on the patient's upper arm, locates a vein in the inner elbow region, and inserts a needle into that vein. Vacuum action draws the blood through the needle into an attached tube. Collection of the sample takes a few minutes and results are available within a few days.

Some markers, such as those for **bladder cancer**, **multiple myeloma**, and plasmacytomas, are measured in the urine. Typically this requires a 24-hour urine sample, which means that the individual must collect all of his or her urine for 24 hours. This is usually about 1.5 quarts or more. These results are then available within a few days.

Other tumor markers require tissue samples for analysis. These include **receptor analysis** such as estrogen receptor and Her-2/neu. Tissue samples are obtained by biopsy. This is usually done by inserting a needle through the skin and into the tumor. The area is typically numbed prior to the procedure. These results are also available within two to three days.

Aftercare

Discomfort or bruising may occur at the puncture site or the person may feel dizzy or faint. Pressure to the puncture site until the bleeding stops reduces bruising. Warm packs to the puncture site relieve discomfort. There is a rare chance of **infection** occurring especially after biopsy. Any sign of infections should be watched for such as pain and redness.

Normal results

- AFP: 99% of (nonpregnant) people have less than 15 ng/mL; 95% have less than 6 ng/mL. Serum AFP levels higher than 400 micrograms/L are associated with cancer or some other pathology.
- Beta-HCG: in males, less than 2.5 IU/L; in females, less than 5.0 IU/L; in postmenopausal females, less than 9.0 IU/L.
- CA 15-3: less than 40 U/mL.
- CA 19-9: less than 40 U/mL.
- CA 27.29: less than or equal to 38 U/mL.
- CA 125: less than 35 U/L.
- CEA: less than or equal to 5 ng/mL.
- PSA: less than 4 ng/mL; PSA levels increase with age. Age-specific values range from 2.0 micrograms/L at age 40 to 7.2 micrograms/L at age 80. Typically, levels below 4.0 micrograms/L rule out prostate cancer.

Abnormal results

The meaning of an increased tumor marker level depends on the specific marker, the person's medical history, and why the test was done. Knowledge of the patient's history and additional tests and physical examinations are needed to correctly interpret tumor marker test results.

Resources

BOOKS

Eissa, S. *Tumor Markers*. Philadelphia: Lippincott Williams & Wilkins, 1999.

Henry, John B. *Clinical Diagnosis and Management by Laboratory Methods*. 20th ed. Philadelphia: W. B. Saunders Company, 2001.

PERIODICALS

Bast, R. C., P. Ravdin, D. F. Hayes, et al. "2000 Update Recommendations for the Use of Tumor Markers in Breast and Colorectal Cancer." *Journal of Clinical Oncology* 19, no. 6 (2001).

Daugaard, G. "The Clinical Use of Tumor Markers in Germ Cell Cancer." *Journal of Tumor Marker Oncology* 16, no. 1 (2001).

Eriksson, B., K. Oberg, and M. Stridsberg. "Tumor Markers in Neuroendocrine Tumors." *Digestion* 62, no. 1 (2000).

Lindblom, Annika, and Annelie Liljegren. "Tumor Markers in Malignancies." *British Medical Journal* 320 (2000): 424.

Ruckdeschel, John C. "Update in Oncology." *Annals of Internal Medicine* 131 (1999): 760–7.

Salgia, R., D. Harpole, J. E. Herndon, et al. "Role of Serum Tumor Markers CA125 and CEA in Non-small Cell Lung Cancer." *Anticancer Research* 21, no. 2 (2001).

OTHER

National Cancer Institute. "NCI Fact Sheet: Tumor Markers." April 1998. [cited July 17, 2001]. http://www.oncolink.upenn.edu/pdq_html/6/engl/600518.html.

National Cancer Institute. "Screening for Ovarian Cancer." May 1998. June 11, 1998. [cited July 17, 2001]. http://cancernet.nci.nih.gov/clinpdq/screening/Screening_for_ovarian_cancer_Physician.html.

National Cancer Institute. "Screening for Prostate Cancer." May 1998. June 11, 1998. [cited July 17, 2001]. http://cancernet.nci.nih.gov/clinpdq/screening/Screening_for_prostate_cancer_Physician.html.

ORGANIZATIONS

American Cancer Society. 1599 Clifton Rd. NE, Atlanta, GA, 30329. (800) 227-2345. http://www.cancer.org.

American Society of Clinical Oncology. 225 Reinekers Lane, Suite 650, Alexandria, VA 22314. (703) 299-0150. http://www.asco.org.

National Cancer Institute. 9000 Rockville Pike, Building 31, Bethesda, MD 20892. (800) 4-CANCER. http://www.nci.nih.gov.

Nancy J. Nordenson
Cindy L. A. Jones, Ph.D.

Tumor necrosis factor

Definition

Tumor necrosis factor is a protein produced by several of the body's cell types, such as white blood cells, red blood cells, and other cells that line the blood vessels. It promotes the destruction of some types of **cancer** cells.

Description

In the 1970s, researchers took **sarcoma** cells in culture and exposed them to a protein produced by white blood cells. The protein caused necrosis (death) of the sarcoma cells but had little effect on normal cells in the culture. Hence, the protein was called "tumor necrosis factor" (TNF).

TNF is a type of cytokine released by white blood cells. Cytokines are a group of molecules that are released by many different cells to communicate with other cells and regulate the duration of an **immune response**. There are many different kinds of cytokines, each with a different effect on specific target cells.

KEY TERMS

Cachexia—A side effect of cancer therapy characterized by weight loss due to lack of appetite and wasting away due to malnutrition.

Cytokines—Molecules released by cells to regulate the length and intensity of an immune response and to mediate intercellular communication.

Macrophage—A type of white blood cell that produces antibodies and molecules for cell-to-cell immune responses.

Regional perfusion—Forcing a liquid through the blood at the capillary beds at or near a specific site.

Once a cell releases the cytokines, they bind to corresponding receptors located on target cells, thus causing a change to take place within the target cell. Tumor necrosis factor is released by special white blood cells called macrophages. Although researchers are still investigating the exact mechanism by which TNF kills cancer cells, it is clear that TNF binds to receptors located on the surface of cancer cells, causing a change and then death of the cell. This was found to be true in animal models. As a result, researchers thought TNF might enhance the reaction of the human immune system to cancer cells.

In the mid-1980s, TNF became available in recombinant form and was analyzed in clinical human trials. At that time, researchers discovered that TNF administered systemically was toxic to humans' normal tissues at the maximum doses required to kill all of the cancer cells, thus limiting its usefulness. At maximum doses required to kill cancer cells, patients experienced **fever**, loss of appetite (**anorexia**), and cachexia (severe **weight loss**, malnutrition, and wasting away of the body).

However, TNF can be effectively combined with other systemic chemotherapeutic drugs such as **doxorubicin** and **etoposide**. TNF in conjunction with the above drugs enhances DNA breakage in tumor cells, contributing to their death. In addition to administering TNF systemically, TNF (with or without other chemotherapeutic drugs) can be forced through the blood at the capillary beds at or near the site of the tumor. The regional perfusion of TNF allows larger dosages to be administered only in the area requiring the treatment. Therefore, less normal and healthy tissue is disrupted before reaching the maximum tolerable limits. Research performed in 1998 (by Lejeune, et al.) found regional perfusion to be especially successful in the case of **melanomametastasis**, resulting in complete remission of 70% to 80% of patients.

Although TNF is valuable in killing cells in melanoma and sarcoma tumors, it can promote growth of other kinds of cancers. Therefore, the action of TNF is continually under research with the hope of increasing its effectiveness on killing cancer cells, while decreasing the toxic side effects on healthy tissue.

Sally C. McFarlane-Parrott

Tumor staging

Definition

Tumor staging is the process of defining at what point in the natural history of the malignant disease the patient is when the diagnosis is made. The organ and cell type in which the malignancy has developed defines the type of malignancy. For example, **adenocarcinoma** of the lung defines that the **cancer** originated in the mucus-secreting cells lining the airways of the lung. Staging is different than defining the type of cancer; it is the process of defining the degree of advancement of the specific type of malignancy in the patient at the time of presentation (the time when the diagnosis is made). Because there are many different types of malignancy arising from many different organs in body, the specifics of staging systems vary.

Purpose

Staging fulfills an organizational role that is central to treatment of cancer. After the tumor is staged, the treatment team knows to what degree the cancer has evolved in its natural history. This knowledge will provide the information necessary to formulate a plan of treatment and will allow an estimate of the success of that treatment (prognosis). Finally, by establishing uniform criteria for staging, people with the same type of malignancy presenting at the same stage can be treated equivalently. If a new treatment is tested that improves the long-term prognosis then that treatment will become the new standard of care. Thus, staging is vital to the processes of research and scientific reporting.

Prognosis

The first question that most patients want answered when they find they have cancer is "How am I going to do?" They want to know the ultimate outcome—their prognosis. Because of the existing research on the natural history, or progression, of the disease, this information is available on a statistical basis. Staging, then, helps define the patient's prognosis. Intuitively, one would think that those presenting with an earlier stage have a better prognosis. For the most part, that is correct.

Scientific reporting and research

When a patient develops a life-threatening disease such as cancer, the physicians and other members of the treatment team intervene in an effort to improve the prognosis. Treatment regimens are defined as good or bad based on how they influence the prognosis of the disease. Staging allows medical professionals to interpret whether or not their efforts are favorably influencing the natural history of the disease. Once a patient's cancer stage has been established, a baseline exists against which to measure the efficacy of the cancer treatment that follows for that patient.

Staging plays a similar "baseline" role when considering a large group of cancer patients. In order to gauge accurately the effectiveness of any cancer treatment, researchers must know if the patients' conditions really are comparable. If they are, comparisons between treatments are fair. If the patients' conditions vary at the outeset of a study, then comparing the outcomes of different treatments is not useful.

Staging provides that useful, objective standard so that researchers can accurately compare specific treatments in certain stages of particular cancers. Staging allows uniformity in treatment protocol and reporting of the data related to outcome. As new treatment protocols are developed, they can be tested on patients with the same type and stage of cancer and the two groups compared. If there is improvement with a new treatment protocol, that treatment regimen will be adopted as standard. Physicians can use these established best practices to determine treatments for their patients.

Criteria for staging

As it became apparent to medical professionals that staging of malignancies was necessary for accurate assessment of treatment regimens and defining the treatment recommendations themselves, criteria for staging needed to be developed. Initially this was done for individual tumors separately. Because of the need for uniformity, a universal set of criteria was desired. The TNM system of staging has been adopted for the most part for this reason. It has been developed and updated by The American Joint Committee on Cancer (AJCC). Some of the types of malignancy do not fit well into the TNM criteria and others have older systems that are still in use because they are effective and are deeply established in scientific literature.

TNM system

This system of staging is the general format used for staging cancer of all types and is updated and maintained by the AJCC. The "T" stands for tumor size. The "N" stands for spread to lymph nodes, (nodal **metastasis**). The "M" stands for metastasis, (spread of the cancer to sites in the body other than the organ of origin. When the diagnosis of cancer is made, the physical examination along with laboratory testing and **imaging studies** will be performed to define the TNM status of the patient. The TNM status will define stage.

The tumor size, "T" will be assessed by physical examination or various imaging modalities depending on the accessibility of the tumor. The "T" value is generally defined as 1 through 4 on the basis of size and whether or not the tumor is invading structures that surround it. In cancer so early that it is felt to be incapable of spreading, it is assigned a "T" value of 0. The "T" value is, in essence, a description of the tumor in its local place of origin. As time passes and the staging system is updated, the "T" value is being subdivided in certain types of cancer. The subdivisions are indicated by letters "a" through "d" and also have a graduated value system. For example: T1 **breast cancer** is a tumor sized 2 cm or less in greatest dimension. T1a is less than 0.5 cm, T1b is 0.5 to 1.0 cm, and T1c is 1.0 to 2.0 cm.

In many cancers, there seems to be a progression from the place of primary origin, then to the regional lymph nodes, and then throughout the body. Lymph nodes can be thought of as filters that drain tissue fluid coming from a particular organ. If that organ has developed a cancer and some of the cells flow away with the tissue fluid to the lymph node filter that is draining that organ, the cancer may begin to grow there also. Assessment of lymph node involvement thus becomes the next step in staging and defines the "N" value. Since the word metastasis means that the cancer has spread from its point of origin to somewhere else in the body and the lymph nodes are in the region, the "N" value defines presence of regional metastasis. The assessment is performed by physical examination and imaging studies of the region involved. "N" is assigned a value of 0 for no nodes involved, or depending on the anatomic nature of the region, values 1 through 3.

"M" stands for distant metastasis. As mentioned previously, metastasis is the spread of the primary tumor to elsewhere in the body. When that spread or metastasis is outside the region of the primary tumor, the patient has distant metastasis. The "M" value is assessed by physical exam, laboratory studies, and imaging studies. Different cancers have different typical patterns of metastasis. Common areas of metastatic involvement are lung, liver, bone, and brain. The "M" value is assigned either 0 or 1. Another term used to describe the patient who has distant metastasis is that of having systemic disease. In the TNM system virtually all patients with an "M" value of 1 have stage IV disease. The "M" value may also have a subscript defining the organ of metastatic involvement.

After the values for TNM have been determined as accurately as possible, the values are grouped together and a stage value is assigned. The stage value is usually I through IV, (and is written in roman numerals). Each stage may be subdivided if it is useful for treatment recommendations and reporting. In general, stage I implies the tumor is confined to its source of origin and stage IV implies distant metastasis or systemic disease. Because of different anatomical, prognostic, and treatment considerations, the intermediate stages are defined by different tumor sizes, the presence or absence of local invasion of the tumor into surrounding structure, or the number and/or presence of involved lymph nodes. Treatment recommendations and expected outcome are both defined to a large extent by stage. The specific criteria for each stage are contained in the *AJCC Cancer Staging Manual.*

An example of TNM staging follows. This example is the staging criteria for non-small-cell lung cancer.

- Stage 0: A small group of cancerous cells have been found in one location in the lung.
- Stage I: The cancer is only in the lung and has not spread anywhere else.
- Stage II: The cancer has spread to nearby lymph nodes.
- Stage III: The cancer has spread to more distant lymph nodes, and/or other parts of the chest like the diaphragm.
- Stage IV: The cancer has spread to other parts of the body (distant metastasis).

Special staging systems

In the development of staging systems it has been recognized that some malignancies do not fit well into the scheme of the TNM system or that the system in place reflects the same information as the TNM system. Thus there are a few special staging systems in use for specific organs of involvement. The goal is the same for these schema as for TNM—to define the point in the natural history at presentation, to allow establishment of prognosis and treatment recommendations, and to facilitate scientific research and reporting.

COLON CANCER: DUKE'S STAGING. The Duke's staging system is similar to the TNM system when describing colorectal cancer. This was the original staging system for colon and rectal cancers; however, the TNM staging sytem has begun to replace the Duke's system for colon and rectal cancers.

OVARIAN CANCER: FIGO SYSTEM. FIGO stands for the International Federation of Gynecology and Obstetrics. This organization developed staging criteria for the various gynecologic malignancies and the one for cancer of the ovary is still used somewhat though the TNM criteria are gradually replacing the FIGO system. In the FIGO system, **ovarian cancer** is staged I through IV similar to the TNM scheme then each stage is subdivided into A, B, or C, depending on defined criteria.

LYMPHOMA: ANN-ARBOR STAGING. Anatomically, the lymph system and its nodes are found throughout the body. Malignancies involving the lymph system (lymphomas), do not fit the typical TNM scheme well. The Ann Arbor staging criteria are instead utilized to classify this group of malignancies. The goals of the Ann Arbor **lymphoma** staging system are to define the degree of advancement of the disease so that treatment recommendations can be made and prognosis can be estimated, and to facilitate consistent reporting and research.

The Ann Arbor system classifies lymphoma into four stages based on anatomic lymph nodal group involvement. Disease confined to one nodal group or location defines stage I. Disease limited to one side of the diaphragm, (the muscle separating the chest from the abdomen), defines stage II. Stage III patients have disease on both sides of the diaphragm and stage IV patients once again have disseminated disease. Consideration of involvement of the liver, spleen, and bone marrow are also considered in this system. Finally, the stage is subdivided into categories of A and B depending on the presence of symptoms of **itching**, **weight loss**, **fever**, and **night sweats**. Those having symptoms receive the designation "B" and have a worse prognosis.

LEUKEMIA: THE FAB AND RAI/BINET STAGING SYSTEMS. Leukemia is the type of malignancy that begins in the cells of the marrow that produce the cellular components of blood, the progenitor cells. These malignancies are truly systemic from their outset and do not fit any form of the TNM system. Still there is need to categorize the presenting features of the patients with these diseases to help make treatment recommendations, estimate prognosis, and to facilitate scientific research and reporting. The **acute leukemias** are staged by the FAB (French, American, British) system, and **chronic lymphocytic leukemia** is classified by the Rai/Binet system.

LUNG CANCER, SMALL CELL. Unlike other types of lung cancer, the staging of **small cell lung cancer** is relatively simple. This is because approximately 70% of patients already have metastatic disease when they are diagnosed, and small differences in the amount of tumor found in the lungs do not change the prognosis. Small cell lung cancer is usually divided into three stages:

- Limited stage: The cancer is found only in one lung and in lymph nodes close to the lung.
- Extensive stage: The cancer has spread beyond the lungs to other parts of the body.
- Recurrent stage: The cancer has returned following treatment.

Defining the stage

The process of defining stage is quite simple. First, the diagnosis is established by study of the patient and by tissue **biopsy**. Once the cell type and organ of origin are established, the staging criteria are reviewed. The patient will undergo a series of diagnostic tests to define the various parameters of the staging criteria. The results of these tests define the extent of the disease and establish the stage. The known typical natural history of the disease dictates the types of testing done. The tests differ for each type of malignancy.

Special concerns

Clinical vs. pathological stage

The stage of the patient's disease may be categorized into clinical or pathological. As mentioned, the known natural history of the disease and the staging criteria are utilized to define the stage of the patient at the time of presentation. The investigations performed often involve an initial degree of uncertainty when they are based on clinical grounds alone. For example, the physical exam or the imaging of a particular group of lymph nodes may show that they are enlarged but the enlargement may not accurately define whether they are truly involved with cancer. This issue may only be resolved by removing some or all of the suspect enlarged nodes, sometimes by biopsy before treatment or sometimes by the removal of the questionable nodes at the time of definitive treatment. The evaluation under the microscope of the clinically enlarged nodes will define whether they are really involved with cancer or merely enlarged. When staging criteria are based on clinical assessment alone, it is referred to as the clinical stage. Once the results of the microcopic evaluation are known the true stage or pathologic stage may be assigned.

Stage is uniform and accurate

One of the main goals of staging is to facilitate communication so that like patients are compared to like patients. It is imperative that the adopted staging criteria are rigidly adhered to or inaccurate comparisons may be made and the results of research to develop better treatment regimens will be difficult to interpret.

Tumor grade

When the tissue obtained for diagnosis is evaluated under the microscope for cell type, often another index called grade is defined. As the pathologist analyzes the malignant cells, attention will be given to how close to a normal cell the malignant cells appear to be. If they are very similar, the malignant cells are not felt to be too aggressive and a low grade value is assigned. The more atypical the malignant cells appear to be, the more aggressive the tumor is and a higher grade value is assigned. Grade is usually assigned a value of I through IV though more levels can be assigned depending on the particular cancer.

The estimate of grade is just that—an estimation. It is subjective in nature and cannot be determined quantitatively. Though useful in predicting prognosis, the correlation is not exact. Rather, grade is included as only one of the factors influencing prognosis. Grade may be included as part of the actual staging criteria; however, it usually is not part of the scheme.

Tumor boards

A tumor board is a body of specialists in the treatment of cancer that convenes to discuss the aspects of patients presenting with cancer. The AJCC encourages the development of tumor boards throughout the nation to facilitate the use of staging and reporting of cancer statistics from region to region throughout the country. In addition to allowing the collection of vital cancer statistics, local tumor boards create a forum where the clinical aspects of a patient's cancer may be discussed to provide recommendations or to play a role in education.

See also Tumor grading; See individual cancer entries for specific staging information for each cancer.

Resources

BOOKS

Abelhoff, Armitage, Niederhuber, and Lichter. *Clinical Oncology Library*. Philadelphia: Churchill Livingstone 1999.

Richard A. McCartney, M.D.

Tumor suppressor genes *see* **Cancer genetics**

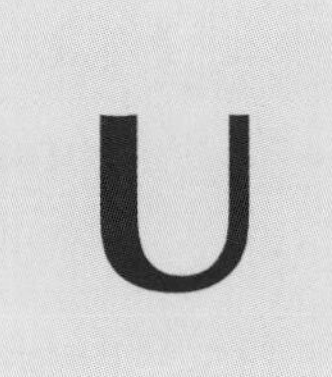

Ultrasonography

Definition

Ultrasonography is the study of internal organs or blood vessels using high-frequency sound waves. The actual test is called an ultrasound scan or sonogram. Duplex ultrasonography uses Doppler technology to study blood cells moving through major veins and arteries. There are several types of ultrasound. Each is used in diagnosing specific parts of the body.

Purpose

An ultrasound is a noninvasive, safe method of examining a patient's eyes, pelvic or abdominal organs, breast, heart, or arteries and veins. It is often used to diagnosis disease, locate the source of pain, or look for stones in the kidney or gallbladder. Ultrasound produces images in real time. Images appear on the screen instantly. It may also be used to guide doctors who are performing a needle **biopsy** to locate a mass. (Needle biopsies are often used to obtain a sample of breast tissue to test for **cancer** cells.) Duplex/Doppler ultrasound aids in diagnosing a blockage in or a malformation of the vessel. Different color flows aid in identifying problem areas in smaller vessels. Endoscopic ultrasound combines a visual endoscopic exam, during which a flexible tube called an endoscope is threaded down the throat, with an ultrasound test. The ultrasound probe is attached to the end of the endoscope. An endoscopic ultrasound is helpful in determining how deeply a tumor has grown into normal tissues or the gastrointestinal tract. During a **transvaginal ultrasound**, the ultrasound probe is inserted into the vagina to obtain better images of the ovaries and uterus. Color flow Doppler imaging, using a transvaginal probe, is being performed to detect abnormal blood flow patterns associated with **ovarian cancer**.

Precautions

Ultrasound is considered safe with no known risks or precautions. The exam uses no radiation. Under normal circumstances the exam is normally painless. However, if the patient has a full bladder, pressure exerted during the exam may feel uncomfortable. An ultrasound conducted in conjunction with an invasive exam carries the same risks as the invasive exam.

Description

The patient will be asked to lie still on an exam table in a darkened room. The darkness helps the technician see images on a screen, which is similar to a computer monitor. Sometimes the patients are positioned so they can watch the screen. The technician will apply a lubricating gel to the skin over the area to be studied. Ultrasound uses high-frequency sound waves to produce an image. A small wand-like device called a transducer produces sound waves that are sent into the body when the device is pressed against the skin. The gel helps transmit the sound waves, which do not travel through the air. Neither the patient nor the technician can hear the sound waves. The technician moves the device across the skin in the area to be studied. The sound waves bounce off the fluids and tissues inside the body. The transducer picks up the return echo and records any changes in the pitch or direction of the sound. The image is immediately visible on the screen. The technician may print a still picture of any significant images for later review by the radiologist.

Preparation

Depending on the type of ultrasound ordered, patients may not need to do anything prior to the test. Other ultrasound studies may require that the patient not eat or drink anything for up to 12 hours prior to the exam, in order to decrease the amount of gas in the bowel. Intestinal gas may interfere in

KEY TERMS

Biopsy—Removal of a tissue sample for examination under a microscope to check for cancer cells.

Endoscopy—Examination of the upper gastrointestinal tract using a thin, flexible instrument called an endoscope.

Radiologist—Doctor who has received special training and is experienced in performing and analyzing ultrasounds and other radiology exams.

QUESTIONS TO ASK THE DOCTOR

- Did you see any abnormalities?
- What future care will I need?

obtaining accurate results. The patient must have a full bladder for some exams and an empty bladder for others.

Aftercare

Remove any gel still left on the skin. No other aftercare is required following an ultrasound.

Risks

Standard, diagnostic ultrasound is considered risk-free. Risks may be associated with invasive tests conducted at the same time, such as an endoscopic ultrasound or an ultrasound-guided needle biopsy.

Normal results

An ultrasound scan is considered normal when the image depicts normally shaped organs or normal blood flow.

Abnormal results

Abnormal echo patterns may represent a condition requiring treatment. Any masses, tumors, enlarged organs or blockages in the blood vessel are considered abnormal. Additional testing may be ordered.

See also Upper gastrointestinal endoscopy.

Resources

BOOKS

Pfenninger, John L. *Procedures for Primary Care Physicians.* 2nd ed. St. Louis: Mosby-Year Book, Inc. 2000.

Rosen, Peter. *Emergency Medicine: Concepts and Clinical Practice.* St. Louis: Mosby-Year Book, Inc. 1999.

Debra Wood, R.N.

Upper gastrointestinal endoscopy

Definition

Upper gastrointestinal endoscopy is a procedure that allows the doctor to visually examine the upper portions of the gastrointestinal tract, using a flexible tool called an endoscope. The endoscope has a light source and projects an image on a video screen. An endoscope may also be used to assist with other diagnostic exams and procedures. For instance, an ultrasound probe can be placed on the end of the endoscope to evaluate how deeply a tumor has penetrated the esophagus or wall of the stomach. An endoscope may be used to assist with placement of a permanent feeding tube or to treat a bleeding ulcer.

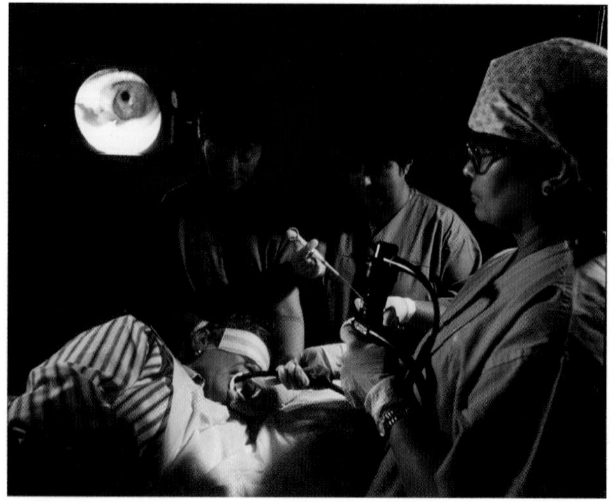

Doctors performing an endoscopy examination of a woman's stomach and taking a biopsy. The endoscope has been inserted through the patient's mouth and fed down her throat. The image obtained by the endoscope is on the screen at upper left. *(Copyright Deep Light Productions, Science Source/ Photo Researchers, Inc. Photo reproduced by permission.)*

KEY TERMS

Biopsy—Removal of a tissue sample for examination under a microscope to check for cancer cells.

Duodenum—The first portion of the small intestine.

Endoscope—A thin, flexible, lighted tube that is passed down the throat and enables the doctor to view the esophagus, stomach lining and duodenum.

Perforation—Puncture or tear.

Staging—Determination of how advanced the cancer is.

Ultrasound—The study of internal organs using high-frequency sound waves.

Purpose

An upper gastrointestinal endoscopy aids in the investigation of the source of pain, difficulty swallowing, bleeding or other symptoms of an upper abdominal problem. During an endoscopy the doctor can obtain samples of tissue for **biopsy**, to check for the presence of **cancer** cells or the bacteria responsible for most stomach ulcers. Various instruments can be passed through the endoscope to treat problems, such as controlling bleeding due to an ulcer. The procedure may be performed on patients who have had stomach surgery to assess for cancer or the return of an ulcer. It may also be used to monitor patients at high risk for upper **gastrointestinal cancers**.

Precautions

Patients with a history of heart and lung disease and those with blood-clotting problems require special precautions. For instance, a patient with artificial heart valves or a history of **infection** of the lining of the heart will need **antibiotics** to prevent infection. Patients with an intestinal perforation, or puncture in the gastrointestinal tract, should not have an upper gastrointestinal endoscopy. Patients must be able to cooperate during the procedure. Those who are not able to cooperate are not good candidates for an endoscopy.

Description

An endoscopy may take place in the physician's office or in a hospital. An intravenous (IV) line will be started in a vein in the arm. Through the IV line, the patient generally receives a sedative and a pain-killer if needed. The medication will help the patient feel relaxed and drowsy. A local anesthetic is usually sprayed into the throat to prevent a gag reflex. Dentures are removed. A mouthpiece will help to keep the mouth open. Patients are positioned onto their sides. The doctor slowly advances the lubricated endoscope down the throat, into the stomach. Air will be passed through the endoscope to make it easier for the doctor to see the lining of the gastrointestinal tract. The endoscope will be repositioned to see different parts of the stomach and the small intestine. The exam usually takes less than an hour. The patient is able to breathe independently during the exam. In some cases a biopsy may be taken. Biopsy forceps or a brush used to secure cells are passed through the endoscope. The tissue sample is taken and then removed through the endoscope.

QUESTIONS TO ASK THE DOCTOR

- Did you see any abnormalities?
- How soon will you know the results of the biopsy (if one was done)?
- When can I resume any medications that were stopped?
- What future care will I need?
- Which problems should prompt me to call you?

Preparation

The doctor should be informed of any allergies as well as all the medications that the patient is currently taking. The doctor may instruct the patient not to take certain medications, like aspirin and anti-inflammatory drugs that interfere with clotting, for a period of time prior to the procedure. The patient should not eat or drink anything for at least eight hours prior to the endoscopy. The doctor should be informed if the patient has had heart valves replaced or a history of an inflammation of the inside lining of the heart, so that appropriate antibiotics can be administered to prevent any chance of infection. Risks and benefits of the procedure will be explained to the patient. The patient will be asked to sign a consent form.

Aftercare

The patient will be monitored for an hour or two after the procedure, while the effects of the medication wear off. Due to the sedative, the patients will need to arrange for someone to drive them home after the procedure.

Patients may feel bloated due to the air that is introduced into the stomach during the procedure, and may have a sore throat for a couple of days. Patient should contact the doctor if they develop difficulty swallowing, chest pain, severe abdominal pain, throat soreness that becomes more severe or rectal bleeding.

Risks

Endoscopy is usually considered safe when performed by a specially trained physician. As with any invasive procedure it is not risk-free. Complications include bleeding and perforation (puncturing a hole in the lining of the gastrointestinal tract). Scopes are cleaned and disinfected between patients so any risk of transmitting infectious disease from one patient to another by the endoscope would be negligible.

Normal results

A pale reddish pink lining with no abnormal-looking masses or ulcerations is considered a normal result.

Abnormal results

Evidence of an ulcer or other lesion would be considered an abnormal result. If the biopsy determines the presence of cancer cells, a diagnosis of cancer is made. The appearance of the lesion, including its size or if there are multiple lesions, often helps with staging and treatment plans. An ultrasound probe attached to the endoscope also may help with staging.

Resources

BOOKS

Fauci, Anthony S. *Harrison's Principles of Internal Medicine.* 14th ed. New York, NY: The McGraw-Hill Companies, 2000.

Pfenninger, John L. *Procedures for Primary Care Physicians.* 2nd ed. St. Louis: Mosby-Year Book, Inc. 2000.

ORGANIZATIONS

American Gastroenterological Association. 7910 Woodmont Ave., Seventh Floor, Bethesda, MD 20814. (301) 654-2055. [cited June 28, 2001]. http:www.gastro.org.

Society of American Gastrointestinal Endoscopic Surgeons (SAGES). 2716 Ocean Park Boulevard, Suite 3000, Santa Monica, CA 90405. (310) 314-2404.[cited June 28, 2001]. http:www.sages.org.

Debra Wood, R.N.

Upper gastrointestinal series *see* **Upper GI series**

Upper GI series

Definition

An upper GI examination is a fluoroscopic examination (a type of x-ray imaging) of the upper gastrointestinal tract, including the esophagus, stomach, and upper small intestine (duodenum).

Purpose

An upper GI series is frequently requested when a patient experiences unexplained symptoms of abdominal pain, difficulty in swallowing (dysphagia), regurgitation, **diarrhea**, or **weight loss**. It is used to help diagnose disorders and diseases of, or related to, the upper gastrointestinal tract, including cases of hiatal hernia, diverticuli, ulcers, tumors, obstruction, **enteritis**, gastroesophageal reflux disease, Crohn's disease, and pulmonary aspiration.

Precautions

Because of the risks of radiation exposure to the fetus, pregnant women are advised to avoid this procedure. Patients with an obstruction or perforation in their bowel should not ingest barium (a radioactive substance used to show contrast in the images) for an upper GI, but may still be able to undergo the procedure if a water-soluble contrast medium is substituted for the barium.

Glucagon, a medication sometimes given prior to an upper GI procedure, may cause **nausea** and dizziness.

Description

An upper GI series takes place in a hospital or clinic setting and is performed by an x-ray technician and a radiologist. A radiologist typically is in attendance to oversee the procedure and view and interpret the fluoroscopic pictures. Before the test begins, the patient is sometimes administered an injection of glucagon, a medication that slows stomach and bowel activity, to allow the radiologist to get a clearer picture of the gastrointestinal tract. In order to further improve the clarity of the upper GI pictures, the patient may be given a cup of baking soda crystals to swallow, which distend the stomach by producing gas.

Once these preparatory steps are complete, the patient stands against an upright x-ray table, and a fluoroscopic screen is placed in front of him. The patient will be asked to drink from a cup of flavored barium sulfate, a thick and chalky-tasting liquid that

QUESTIONS TO ASK THE DOCTOR

- What is the purpose of this examination?
- When will I know the results?
- How will I be notified of the results?
- How will the examination results help to determine the next step in the management of my condition?
- What are the alternatives to this diagnostic exam?

KEY TERMS

Dysphagia—An inability to swallow, or difficulty with swallowing.

Fluoroscopy—Also called radioscopy, this procedure involves the examination of internal body structures using x-rays and projecting images on a fluorescent screen.

Necrosis—Death of cells in a body tissue.

Radiologist—A doctor who specializes in an area of medicine that focuses on the use of radiation to diagnose and treat disease.

allows the radiologist to see the digestive tract, while the radiologist views the esophagus, stomach, and duodenum on the fluoroscopic screen. The patient will be asked to change positions frequently in order to coat the entire surface of the gastrointestinal tract with barium. The technician or radiologist may press on the patient's abdomen in order to spread the barium. The x-ray table will also be moved several times throughout the procedure. The radiologist will ask the patient to hold his breath periodically while exposures are being taken. The entire procedure may take up to 45 minutes.

In some cases, in addition to the standard upper GI series, a doctor may request a detailed intestine, or small bowel, radiography and fluoroscopy series; it is also called a small bowel follow-through (SBFT). Once the preliminary upper GI series is complete, the patient will be escorted to a waiting area while the barium travels down the rest of the small intestinal path. Every 15 to 30 minutes, the patient will return to the x-ray suite for additional **x rays**. Once the barium has traveled down the small bowel tract, the test is complete. This procedure can take anywhere from one to four hours.

Esophageal radiography, also called a barium esophagram or a barium swallow, is a study of the esophagus only, and is usually performed as part of the upper GI series. It is commonly used to diagnose the cause of difficulty in swallowing (dysphagia) and for detecting hiatal hernia. A barium sulfate liquid, and sometimes pieces of food covered in barium or a barium tablet, are given to the patient to drink and eat while a radiologist examines the swallowing mechanism on a fluoroscopic screen. The test takes approximately 30 minutes.

Preparation

Patients must not eat, drink, or smoke for eight hours prior to undergoing an upper GI examination. Longer dietary restrictions may be required, depending on the type and diagnostic purpose of the test. Patients undergoing a small bowel follow-through exam may be asked to take **laxatives** the day prior to the test. Upper GI patients are typically required to wear a hospital gown, or similar attire, and to remove all jewelry, so the camera has an unobstructed view of the abdomen. Patients who are severely ill may not be able to tolerate the procedure.

Aftercare

No special aftercare treatment or regimen is required for an upper GI series. The patient may eat and drink as soon as the test is completed. The barium sulfate may make the patient's stool white for several days, and patients are encouraged to drink plenty of fluids in order to eliminate it from their system.

Risks

Because the upper GI series is an x-ray procedure, it does involve minor exposure to ionizing radiation. Unless the patient is pregnant, or multiple radiological or fluoroscopic studies are required, the small dose of radiation incurred during a single procedure poses little risk. However, multiple studies requiring fluoroscopic exposure that are conducted in a short time period have been known, on rare occasions, to cause skin death (necrosis) in some individuals. This risk can be minimized by careful monitoring and documentation of cumulative radiation doses administered to these patients.

Another risk is barium impaction, which occurs when the patient is unable to completely expel the barium contrast agent before it eventually dries and hardens. The risk of barium impaction is greatest in elderly patients and those with colon obstruction or colon motility disorder.

Normal results

A normal upper GI series will show a healthy, functioning, and unobstructed digestive tract.

Abnormal results

Obstructions or inflammation, including ulcers of the esophagus, stomach, or small intestine, or irregularities in the swallowing mechanism are some of the possible abnormalities that may show up on an upper GI series. Other abnormalities may include polyps, foreign bodies, or congenital anomalies. Upper GI series are helpful in the diagnosis of gastric (stomach) **cancer**.

Resources

BOOKS

Fischbach, F., editor. *A Manual of Laboratory & Diagnostic Tests*. 6th ed. Philadelphia, PA: Lippincott Williams & Wilkins, 1999.

Rosen, P., editor. *Emergency Medicine Concepts and Clinical Practice*. 4th ed. St. Louis, MO: Mosby-Year Book, Inc., 1999.

PERIODICALS

Froehlich, F., and C. Repond, et al. "Is the Diagnostic Yield of Upper GI Endoscopy Improved by the Use of Explicit Panel-based Appropriateness Criteria?" *Gastrointestinal Endoscopy* 52, no. 3 (September 2000): 333–41.

Paula Anne Ford-Martin

Ureterosigmoidoscopy

Definition

Ureterosigmoidoscopy is a surgical procedure that treats urinary **incontinence** by joining the ureters to the lower colon, thereby allowing urine to evacuate through the rectum.

Purpose

The surgery is indicated when there is resection (surgical removal), malformation, or injury to the bladder. The bladder disposes of wastes passed to it from the kidneys, which is the organ that does most of the blood filtering and retention of needed glucose, salts, and minerals.

Wastes from the kidneys drip through the ureters to the bladder, and on to the urethra where they are expelled via urination. Waste from the kidneys is slowed or impaired when the bladder is diseased because of ulcerative, inflammatory, or malignant conditions; is malformed; or has been removed. In these cases, the kidney is unable to get rid of the wastes, resulting in hydronephrosis (distention of the kidneys). Over time, this leads to kidney deterioration. Saving the kidneys by bladder diversion is as important as restoring urinary continence.

The surgical techniques for urinary and fecal diversion fall into two categories: continent diversion and conduit diversion. In continent diversion, an internal reservoir for urine or feces is created, allowing natural evacuation from the body. In urinary and fecal conduit diversion, a section of existing tissue is altered to serve as a passageway to an external reservoir or ostomy. Both continent and conduit diversions reproduce bladder or colon function that was impaired due to surgery, obstruction, or a neurogenically (nerve dysfunction) created condition. Both the continent and conduit diversion methods have been used for years, with advancements in minimally invasive surgical techniques and biochemical improvements in conduit materials and ostomy appliances.

Catheterization was the original solution for urinary incontinence, especially when major organ failure or removal was involved. But catherization was found to have major residual back flow of urine into the kidneys over the long term. With the advent of surgical anatomosis—the grafting of vascularizing tissue for the repair and expansion of organ function—and with the ability to include flap-type valves to prevent back-up into the kidneys, major continent restoring procedures have become routine in urologic surgery. Catherization has been replaced as a permanent remedy for persistent incontinence. Continent surgical procedures developed since the 1980s offer the possibility of safely retaining natural evacuation functions in both colonic (intestinal) and urinary systems.

Quality of life issues associated with urinary diversion are increasingly important to patients and, along with medical requirements, put an optimal threshold on the requirements for the surgical procedure. The bladder substitute or created reservoir must offer the following advantages:

- maintain continence
- maintain sterile urine

- empty completely
- protect the kidneys
- prevent absorption of waste products
- maintain quality of life

Ureterosigmoidoscopy is one of the earliest continent diversions for a resected bladder, bladder abnormalities, and dysfunction. It is one of the more difficult surgeries, and has significant complications. Ureterosigmoidoscopy does have a major benefit; it allows the natural expelling of wastes without the construction of a stoma—an artificial conduit—by using the rectum as a urinary reservoir. When evacuation occurs, the urine is passed along with the fecal matter.

Ureterosigmoidoscopy is a single procedure, but there are additional refinements that allow rectal voiding of urine. A procedure known as the Mainz II pouch has undergone many refinements in attempts to lessen the complications that have traditionally accompanied uretersigmoidoscopy. This surgery is indicated for significant and serious conditions of the urinary tract including:

- Cancer or ulceration of the bladder that necessitates a radical cystectomy or removal of the bladder, primarily occurring in adults, particularly those of advanced age.
- Various congential abnormalities of the bladder in infants, especially eversion of part or all of the bladder. Eversion (or exotrophy) is a malformation of the bladder in which the wall adjacent to the abdomen fails to close. In some children, the bladder plate may be too small to fashion a closure.

Demographics

Bladder cancer affects over 50,000 people annually in the United States. The average age at diagnosis is 68 years. It accounts for approximately 10,000 deaths per year. Bladder **cancer** is the fifth leading cause of cancer deaths among men older than 75 years. Male bladder cancer is three times more prevalent than female bladder cancer.

In the United States, radical **cystectomy** (total removal of the bladder) is the standard treatment for muscle-invading bladder cancer. The operation usually involves removal of the bladder (with oncology staging) and pelvic lymph node, and prostate and seminal conduits with a form of urinary diversion. Uretersigmoscopy is one option that restores continence.

Pediatric ureterosigmoidoscopy is performed primarily for bladder abnormalities occuring at birth. Classic bladder exstrophy occurs in 3.3 per 100,000 births, with a male to female ratio of 3:1 (6:1 in some studies).

KEY TERMS

Bladder exstrophy—One of many bladder and urinary congenital abnormalities. Occurs when the wall of the bladder fails to close in embryonic development and remains exposed to the abdominal wall.

Conduit diversion— A surgical procedure that restores urinary and fecal continence by diverting these functions through a constructed conduit leading to an external waste reservoir (ostomy).

Cystectomy—The surgical resection of part or all of the bladder.

Urinary continent diversion—A surgical procedure that restores urinary continence by diverting urinary function around the bladder and into the intestines, thereby allowing for natural evacuation through the rectum or an implanted artificial sphincter.

Description

The most basic ureterosigmoidoscopy modification is the Mainz II pouch. There is a 2.4 in (6 cm) cut along antimesenteric border of the colon, both on the proximal and distal sides of the rectum/sigmoid colon junction. The ureters are drawn down into the colon. A special flap technique is applied by folding the colon to stop urine from refluxing back to the kidneys. After the colon is closed, the result is a small rectosigmoid reservoir that holds urine without refluxing it back to the upper urinary tract. Some variations of the Mainz II pouch include the construction of a valve, as in the Kock pouch, that confines urine to the distal segment of the colon.

Ureterosigmoidoscopy is typically performed in patients with complex medical problems, often those who have had numerous surgeries. Ureterosigmoidoscopy as a continent diversion technique relies heavily upon an intact and functional rectal sphincter. The treatment of pediatric urinary incontinence due to bladder eversion or other anatomical anomalies is a technical challenge, and is not always the first choice of surgeons. In Europe, early urinary diversion with ureterosigmoidoscopy is used widely for most exstrophy patients. Its main advantage is the possibility for

WHO PERFORMS THE PROCEDURE AND WHERE IS IT PERFORMED?

Uretersigmoidoscopy is usually performed by a urological surgeon with advanced training in urinary continent surgeries, often in consultation with a neonatalist (in newborn patients) or an oncological surgeon. The surgery takes place in a general hospital.

spontaneous emptying by evacuation of urine and stool.

Diagnosis/Preparation

A number of tests are performed as part of the pre-surgery diagnostic workup for bladder conditions such as cancer, ulcerative or inflammatory disease, or pediatric abnormalities. Tests may include:

- cystoscopy (bladder inspection with a laparoscope)
- CT scan
- liver function
- renal function
- rectal sphincter function evaluation (The rectal sphincter will be a critical ingredient in urination after the surgery, and it is important to determine its ability to function. Adult patients are often asked to have an oatmeal enema and sit upright for a period of time to test sphincter function.)

In adult patients, a discussion of continent diversion is conducted early in the diagnostic process. Patients are asked to consider the possibility of a conduit urinary diversion if the ureterosigmoidoscopy proves impossible to complete. Educational sessions on specific conduit alternatives take place prior to surgery. Topics include options for placement of a stoma, and appliances that may be a part of the daily voiding routine after surgery. Many doctors provide a stomal therapist to consult with the patient.

Aftercare

After surgery, patients may remain in the hospital for a few days to undergo blood, renal, and liver tests, and monitoring for **fever** or other surgical complications. In pediatric patients, a cast keeps the legs abducted (apart) and slightly elevated for three weeks. Bladder and kidneys are fully drained via multiple catheters during the first few weeks after surgery. **Antibiotics** are continued after surgery. Permanent follow-up with the urologist is essential for proper monitoring of kidney function.

QUESTIONS TO ASK THE DOCTOR

How many times has the surgeon performed this operation?
Is conduit surgery the best route for protecting renal function?
What is the surgeon's complication rate?

Normal results

Good results have been reported, especially in children; however, ureterosigmoidoscopy offers some severe morbid complications. Post-surgical bladder function and continence rates are very high. However, many newly created reservoirs do not function normally; some deteriorate over time, creating a need for more than one diversion surgery. Many patients have difficulty voiding after surgery. Five-year survival rates for bladder surgery patients are 50–80%, depending on the grade, depth of bladder penetration, and nodal status.

Morbidity and mortality rates

The continence success rate with ureterosigmoidoscopy and its variants is higher than 95% for exstrophy; however, long-term malignancy rates are quite high. **Adenocarcinoma** is the most common of these malignancies, and may be caused by chronic irritation and inflammation of exposed mucosa of the exostrophic bladder. In one series of studies, adenocarcinoma was reported in more than 10% of patients. However, the malignancy is actually higher in untreated patients whose bladders are left exposed for years before surgery.

Upper urinary tract deterioration is a potential complication, caused by reflux of urine back to the kidneys, resulting in febrile infections.

Alternatives

Other options include construction of a full neobladder in certain carefully defined circumstances, and bladder enhancement for congenitally shortened or abnormal bladders. Surgical bladder resection is often followed by continent operations using other parts of the colon, and by various conduit surgeries that utilize an external ostomy appliance.

Resources

BOOKS

"Continent Urinary Diversion." In Walsh, P., *Campbell's Urology,* 8th ed. Elsevier, 2002.

"Pediatric Urology: Continent Urinary Diversion." In Walsh, P., *Campbell's Urology,* 8th ed. Elsevier, 2002.

PERIODICALS

Stehr, M. "Selected Secondary Reconstructive Procedures for Improvement of Urinary Incontinence in Bladder Exstrophy and Neurogenic Bladder Dysfunction in Childhood." *Wiener Medizinische Wochenschr* 150, no.11 (January 1, 2000): 245-8.

Yerkes, B. and H.M. Snyder, H.M. "Exstrophy and Epispadias." *Pediatrics/Urology* 3, no.5 (May 6, 2002). www.author.eMedicine.com.

OTHER

Girgin, C., et. al. "Comparison of Three Types of Continent Urinary Diversions in a Single Center." *Digital Urology Journal.* www.duj.com.

ORGANIZATIONS

American Academy of Pediatrics. 141 Northwest Point Boulevard; Elk Grove Village, IL 60007-1098. (847) 434-4000. Fax: (847) 434-8000. www.aap.org.

National Institutes of Diabetes & Digestive & Kidney Disease. www.niddk.nih.gov/tools/mail.htm.

Nancy McKenzie, Ph.D.

Ureterostomy, cutaneous

Definition

A cutaneous ureterostomy, also called ureterocutaneostomy, is a surgical procedure that detaches one or both ureters from the bladder, and brings them to the surface of the abdomen with the formation of an opening (stoma) to allow passage of urine.

Purpose

The bladder is the membranous pouch that serves as a reservoir for urine. Contraction of the bladder results in urination. A ureterostomy is performed to divert the flow of urine away from the bladder when the bladder is not functioning or has been removed. The following conditions may result in a need for ureterostomy:

- bladder cancer
- spinal cord injury
- malfunction of the bladder
- birth defects, such as spina bifida

Demographics

Bladder disorders afflict millions of people in the United States. According to the American **Cancer** Society (ACS), there were 70,980 new cases of **bladder cancer** in 2009, with approximately 14,330 deaths from the disease.

Description

Urostomy is the generic name for any surgical procedure that diverts the passage of urine by redirecting the ureters (fibromuscular tubes that carry the urine from the kidney to the bladder). There are two basic types of urostomies. The first features the creation of a passage called an "ileal conduit." In this procedure, the ureters are detached from the bladder and joined to a short length of the small intestine (ileum). The other type of urostomy is cutaneous ureterostomy. With this technique, the surgeon detaches the ureters from the bladder and brings one or both to the surface of the abdomen. The hole created in the abdomen is called a stoma, a reddish, moist abdominal protrusion. The stoma is not painful; it has no sensation. Since it has no muscles to regulate urination, urine collects in a bag.

There are four common types of ureterostomies:

- Single ureterostomy. This procedure brings only one ureter to the surface of the abdomen.
- Bilateral ureterostomy. This procedure brings the two ureters to the surface of the abdomen, one on each side.
- Double-barrel ureterostomy. In this approach, both ureters are brought to the same side of the abdominal surface.
- Transuretero ureterostomy (TUU). This procedure brings both ureters to the same side of the abdomen, through the same stoma.

Diagnosis/Preparation

Ureterostomy patients may have the following tests and procedures as part of their diagnostic workup:

- Renal function tests; blood, urea, nitrogen (BUN); and creatinine.
- Blood tests, complete blood count (CBC), and electrolytes.
- Imaging studies of the ureters and renal pelvis. These studies characterize the ureters, and define the surgery required to obtain adequate ureteral length.

The quality, character, and usable length of the ureters is usually assessed using any of the following tests:

- Intravenous pyelogram (IVP). A special diagnostic test that follows the time course of excretion of a contrast dye through the kidneys, ureters, and bladder after it is injected into a vein.
- Retrograde pyelogram (RPG). X-ray study of the kidney, focusing on the urine-collecting region of the kidney and ureters.
- Antegrade nephrostogram.
- CT scan. A special imaging technique that uses a computer to collect multiple x-ray images into a two-dimentional cross-sectional image.
- MRI with intravenous gadolinium. A special technique used to image internal stuctures of the body, particularly the soft tissues. An MRI image is often superior to a routine x-ray image.

The presurgery evaluation also includes an assessment of overall patient stability. The surgery may take from two to six hours, depending on the health of the ureters, and the experience of the surgeon.

Aftercare

After surgery, the condition of the ureters is monitored by IVP testing, repeated postoperatively at six months, one year, and then yearly.

Following ureterostomy, urine needs to be collected in bags. Several designs are available. One popular type features an open bag fitted with an anti-reflux valve, which prevents the urine from flowing back toward the stoma. A urostomy bag connects to a night bag that may be attached to the bed at night. Urostomy bags are available as one- and two-piece bags:

- One-piece bags: The adhesive and the bag are sealed together. The advantage of using a one-piece appliance is that it is easy to apply, and the bag is flexible and soft.
- Two-piece bags: The bag and the adhesive are two separate components. The adhesive does not need to be removed frequently from the skin, and can remain in place for several days while the bag is changed as required.

Risks

The complication rate associated with ureterostomy procedures is less than 5–10%. Risks during surgery include heart problems, pulmonary (lung) complications, development of blood clots (thrombosis), blocking of arteries (embolism), and injury to adjacent structures, such as bowel or vascular entities.

WHO PERFORMS THE PROCEDURE AND WHERE IS IT PERFORMED?

Ureterostomy is performed in a hospital setting by experienced surgeons trained in urology, the branch of medicine concerned with the diagnosis and treatment of diseases of the urinary tract and urogenital system. Specially trained nurses called wound ostomy continence nurses (WOCN) are commonly available for consultation in most major medical centers.

Inadequate ureteral length may also be encountered, leading to ureteral kinking and subsequent obstruction. If plastic tubes need inserting, their malposition can lead to obstruction and eventual breakdown of the opening (anastomosis). Anastomotic leak is the most frequently encountered complication.

Normal results

Normal results for a ureterostomy include the successful diversion of the urine pathway away from the bladder, and a tension-free, watertight opening to the abdomen that prevents urinary leakage.

Morbidity and mortality rates

The outcome and prognosis for ureterostomy patients depends on a number of factors. The highest rates of complications exist for those who have pelvic cancer or a history of **radiation therapy**.

In one study, a French medical team followed 69 patients for a minimum of one year (an average of six years) after TUU was performed. They reported one complication per four patients (6.3%), including a case requiring open drainage, prolonged urinary leakage, and common ureteral death (necrosis). Two complications occurred three and four years after surgery. The National Cancer Institute performed TUU for pelvic malignancy in 10 patients. Mean follow-up was 6.5 years. Complications include common ureteral narrowing (one patient); subsequent kidney removal, or **nephrectomy** (one patient); recurrence of disease with ureteral obstruction (one patient); and disease progression in a case of inflammation of blood vessels, or vasulitis (one patient). One patient died of **sepsis** (**infection** in the bloodstream) due to urine leakage at the anastomosis, one died after a heart attack, and three died from **metastasis** of their primary cancer.

QUESTIONS TO ASK THE DOCTOR

- Why is ureterostomy required?
- What type will be performed?
- How long will it take to recover from the surgery?
- When can normal activities be resumed?
- How many ureterostomies does my surgeon perform each year?
- What are possible complications of the surgery?

Alternatives

There are several alternative surgical procedures available:

- Ileal conduit urostomy, also known as "Bricker's loop." The two ureters that transport urine from the kidneys are detached from the bladder, and then attached so that they will empty through a piece of the ileum. One end of the ileum piece is sealed off and the other end is brought to the surface of the abdomen to form the stoma. It is the most common technique used for urinary diversion.
- Cystostomy. The flow of urine is diverted from the bladder to the abdominal wall. It features placement of a tube through the abdominal wall into the bladder, and is indicated in cases of blockage or stricture of the ureters. It can be temporary or permanent.
- Indiana pouch. A pouch is constructed using the end part of the ileum and the first part of the large intestine (cecum). The remaining ileum is first attached to the large intestine to maintain normal digestive flow. A pouch is then created from the removed cecum, and the attached ileum is brought to the surface of the abdominal wall to create a stoma.
- Percutaneous nephrostomy. A nephrostomy is created when the flow of urine is diverted directly from the kidneys to the abdominal wall. Tubes are placed within the kidney to collect the urine as it is generated, and transport it to the abdominal wall. This procedure is usually temporary; however, it may be permanent for cancer patients.

Resources

BOOKS

Door Mullen, B. & K. A. McGinn. *The Ostomy Book: Living Comfortably With Colostomies, Ileostomies, and Urostomies*. Boulder, CO: Bull Publishing Co., 1992.

Jeter, K. F. *Urostomy Guide*. Irvine, CA: American Urological Association, code 05-006.

PERIODICALS

Cedillo, U., C. Gracida, R. Espinoza, and J. Cancino. "Vesical Augmentation and Continent Ureterostomy in Kidney Transplant Patients." *Transplant Proceedings* 34 (November 2002): 2541-2.

Hiratsuka, Y., T. Ishii, H. Taira, and A. Okadome. "Simple Correction of Ureteral Stomal Stenosis for Cutaneous Ureterostomy." *International Journal of Urology* 10 (March 2003): 180-1.

Purohit, R. S., and P. N. Bretan, Jr. "Successful Long-term Outcome Using Existing Native Cutaneous Ureterostomy for Renal Transplant Drainage." *Journal of Urology* 163 (February 2000): 446-9.

Yoshimura, K., S. Maekawa, K. Ichioka, N. Terada, Y. Matsuta, K. Okubo, and Y. Arai. "Tubeless Cutaneous Ureterostomy: The Toyoda Method Revisited." *Journal of Urology* 165 (March 2001): 785-8.

ORGANIZATIONS

American Urological Association (AUA). 1120 North Charles Street, Baltimore, MD 21201. (410) 727-1100. www.auanet.org.

United Ostomy Association (UOA). 19772 MacArthur Blvd., #200, Irvine, CA 92612-2405. (800) 826-0826. www.uoa.org.

Monique Laberge, Ph.D.

Urethral cancer

Definition

A rare form of **cancer** that can affect both men and women, urethral cancer is a type of cancer that develops in a person's urethra.

Description

The urethra is the tube in a person's body that empties urine from the bladder. In women, the urethra is a very short tube that opens to the outside of the body just above the vagina, whereas in men it is a much longer tube that goes through the prostate gland and penis to the outside of the body.

In both men and women, urethral cancer has a tendency to invade local and adjacent soft tissues. By the time of diagnosis, the majority of tumors are locally advanced, which sometimes results in a poor prognosis despite aggressive treatment. Urethral cancer rarely metastasizes (spreads) to distant locations. In women, the most common sites of tumor invasion

QUESTIONS TO ASK YOUR DOCTOR

- How will having a penectomy affect my survival time?
- When is it safe for me to resume sexual relations?
- Are there any clinical trials I should consider joining?
- How successful is the reconstructive surgery?
- How will the treatment affect my ability to have children?
- How will my ability to urinate be affected if I have an ostomy?

are the vagina and bladder, whereas in men, tumor invasion most commonly occurs in the deep tissues of the perineum, the prostate, and the penile and scrotal skin. Most of the urethral tumors, in both men and women, are the squamous-cell type. The second most common type is transitional-cell **carcinoma**.

Demographics

Because urethral cancer is so rare (approximately 600 cases a year), there is not much data validating the best methods of treatment. Generally speaking, urethral cancer is found more often in women than in men. Although people of many different ages have been diagnosed with urethral cancer, it is usually found in people over the age 50. Urethral cancer is more common in white, than in African Americans; however, African Americans tend to have a worse prognosis after urethral cancer has been diagnosed.

Causes and symptoms

Patients with a history of **bladder cancer** have an increased risk of urethral cancer. Although cigarette smoking and exposure to certain chemicals, such as the ones that used to be used in the rubber industry, can contribute to the development of bladder cancer, the same correlation does not exist with urethral cancer. Certain types of human papillomavirus are suspected as the cause of urethral cancer in some people, although in many cases the cause is unknown.

Often the first symptom of urethral cancer is blood in the urine, although it may be present in such small amounts that it can only be detected in a microscope. Sometimes, however, the urine may be visibly red. There may be pelvic pain and the flow of urine may be obstructed, making it difficult to urinate. A lump may be present on the urethra. In women, tiny growths that bleed may be present at the external opening of the urethra.

Diagnosis

To diagnose urethral cancer, a physician will examine the patient physically for any lumps. A urinalysis may also be done to check for the microscopic presence of blood and to check for **infection**. Patients may need to have a **cystoscopy**, which will allow the physician to see inside the urethra. In adults, the procedure is usually done under local anesthesia, which means that the area around the urethral opening is injected with an anesthetic. The cystoscope, which is a long, flexible tube made of plastic or metal, is inserted through the urethra. The tube has a lens and a fiberoptic light that allows the physician to examine the area through a scope. It may be necessary to take a small sample of the tissue, which is referred to as a **biopsy**. The sample will then be viewed under a microscope to check for any signs of cancer.

Treatment team

The treatment team is comprised of physicians from a variety of medical specialties. For example, a patient diagnosed with urethral cancer may have a treatment team that includes the patient's primary care physician and urologist, as well as a radiologist, oncologist, surgeon, and **pain management** specialist. Women may also seek the advice of their gynecologist. At home caretakers are also part of the treatment team, providing important physical and emotional support to the patient. Physicians and patients that value a holistic approach to fighting cancer may add a variety of other advisors to the treatment team, such as psychologists, pastors, and alternative medicine specialists.

Clinical staging, treatments, and prognosis

After a diagnosis of cancer has been made, patients will need to have more tests to determine if the cancer has spread to other areas of the body. The treatment is gauged depending on the stage of the disease. The stage of urethra cancer is determined by the cancer's location and whether it has metastasized. According to the National Cancer Institute, the following are used to describe the different stages of urethral cancer:

- Anterior urethral cancer: the cancer is located on the urethra near the outside of the body.
- Posterior urethral cancer: the cancer is located on the urethra near the bladder.
- Urethral cancer associated with invasive bladder cancer: the cancer has spread to the urethra because of the presence of bladder cancer.

Surgery, **radiation therapy**, and **chemotherapy** are the conventions treatment options for urethral cancer. According to the National Cancer Institute, the surgeon may remove the cancerous tumor in one of three ways:

- Electrofulguration: electric current is used to kill the cancer cells.
- Laser therapy: a narrow beam of powerful light is used to kill the cancer cells.
- Cystourethrectomy: the urethra and bladder are removed.

Surgical requirements vary depending on the severity of the cancer. The removal of the urethra will require the surgeon to create something called a urinary diversion, meaning another way to urinate will need to be constructed. In some cases, the patient's physician may recommend that men have part of or their entire penis removed, which is called a penectomy. If a penectomy (the total removal of the penis) is done, the patient will need plastic surgery to make a new penis. Lymph nodes in the pelvis may also be removed. In women, surgery to remove the urethra, bladder, and/or vagina may be necessary. Plastic surgery will be necessary to create a new vagina.

When a patient's bladder is removed, the surgeon may use part of the small intestine to create a tube so that the patient can urinate and a mouth-like opening, referred to as a stoma, is made surgically on the outside of the body. This procedure is called an ostomy. The patient then uses glue to connect a bag that is designed especially for the purpose of being connected to the stoma. As a patient urinates, the urine collects in the bag. The patient can then throw the bag away and replace it with a new one. The bag is hidden under the patient's clothing. Ostomy patients can be more prone to infection and some patients with sensitive skin may experience occasional skin irritation due to the glue that holds the bag in place.

It is psychologically difficult for some patients to get used to urinating in a bag. Fears of having "accidents" or "smelling bad" sometimes overwhelm ostomy patients. Support groups and special counseling can be very helpful to patients who are having a difficult time adjusting to their new situation.

Based on the severity and extent of the cancer, radiation and/or chemotherapy treatments may be recommended. The prognosis of urethral cancer depends on a variety of factors, such as the tumor's size and location, as well as the extent of the cancer and the patient's general health. For example, in an article published in the *Journal of Urology*, Drs. Grisby and Corn reported that women who have been diagnosed with posterior urethral cancer that do not have tumors larger than 2 centimeters can be effectively treated with radiation alone, surgery alone, or a combination of the two treatment options. In fact, studies such as the one conducted by Dr. Sailer and colleagues, which was also published in the *Journal of Urology*, have shown that 60% of the women diagnosed with posterior urethral cancer that have tumors smaller than 2 centimeters can expect a five-year survival, whereas only 13% of the women can expect a five-year survival if their tumors exceed 4 centimeters.

Coping with cancer treatment

Patients having difficulty coping with the pain associated with cancer and chemotherapy might find it helpful to be referred to a physician who specializes in pain management or a pain clinic. Physicians specializing in the treatment of pain come from a variety of medical backgrounds, such as anesthesiology, urology, and surgery. Because of the complicated nature of cancer and cancer-related pain, ideally a pain management team should be formed that works with the patient's primary care physician, oncologist, and radiologist to provide comprehensive care to the patient.

But what about the emotional pain that is associated with urethral cancer? Much has been written about coping with the physical side effects of cancer treatment; however, patients with urethral cancer also face emotional challenges associated with their treatment. For example, men and women may be concerned how the treatment will affect their sexual relations. They may have to deal with a variety of psychological issues, such as **body image** versus self-image. Patients may need to be reminded, especially by family members and friends, that they are more than a collection of body parts. Patients having difficulty dealing with the emotional aspects of their cancer may find it useful to see a psychologist. Psychologists can help patients identify a variety of coping mechanisms designed to enable them to deal with what lies ahead.

It is important for cancer patients to understand that they are not alone. Support groups exist to help patients cope not only with the physical aspects of having cancer, but with the psychological ones as well. Patients should be encouraged to talk about their feelings. The positive support (both emotional and otherwise) provided by caregivers can help to improve a patient's quality of life. In addition, support groups on the Internet have made it possible for patients, even those in rural or remote areas, to reach out to one another in ways that allow anonymity.

Resources

PERIODICALS

Grigsby, P. W., Corn, B. W. "Localized urethral tumors in women: indications for conservative versus exenterative therapies." *Journal of Urology* 147 (1992): 1516–1520.

Sailer, S. L., Shipley, W. U., Wang, C. C. "Carcinoma of the female urethra: a review of results with radiation therapy." *Journal of Urology* 140 (1988): 1–5.

OTHER

National Cancer Institute. "Urethral Cancer (PDQ^{R}): Treatment. " 22 Feb. 2005. http://www.cancer.gov/.

United Ostomy Association, Inc. "What is an ostomy?" 3 March 2005. http://www.uoa.org/ostomy_main.htm.

Lee Ann Paradise

Urostomy

Definition

Urostomy is a surgical procedure that creates an opening (stoma) in the abdominal wall through which urine leaves the body.

Purpose

Doctors perform urostomy when a patient has **bladder cancer**, spinal cord injury, specific types of birth defects, or when the bladder is not functioning properly and must be removed.

Precautions

In an individual who is obese or who has folds in the skin or scars in the abdominal wall, an internal collection sac (reservoir) the patient can empty (catheterize) works better than a passage that lets urine flow out of the body into a collection bag (pouch) worn next to the skin under the clothes.

Description

Urostomy is a form of urinary diversion. Surgeons perform this reconstructive procedure when disease, **infection**, injury, or congenital abnormality makes it necessary to remove a patient's bladder and create a new channel (conduit) for urine to leave the body.

KEY TERMS

Bladder neck—The narrowest part of the bladder.

Cystoscopy—Diagnostic procedure that allows the doctor to view the entire bladder wall.

Kidney failure—Inability of the kidneys to excrete waste and maintain a proper chemical balance. Also called renal failure.

Surgeons perform urostomy by separating a short piece of the large or small intestine from the rest of the intestine. They attach the separated intestine to the two thick tubes (ureters) that carry urine from the kidneys to the bladder and connect the ureters to the stoma.

Continent and incontinent diversions

An incontinent ostomy drains continuously into a small pouch fitted over the stoma and worn under the patient's clothes. The patient wears a collection pouch at all times and empties it several times a day.

To perform a continent urinary diversion, the surgeon uses a piece of the patient's intestine to create an internal reservoir to store urine. The patient does not wear an ostomy pouch but empties the reservoir four to six times a day by inserting a drainage tube (catheter) into the stoma.

Types of urostomy

The most common types of urostomy are the ileal conduit, which uses a piece of the small intestine (ileum), and the colonic conduit, which uses a piece of the large intestine (colon). Orthotopic neobladder is a new type of continent diversion that channels urine into the tube that drains urine from the bladder (urethra) and enables the patient to urinate almost normally.

Temporary urostomy does not involve severing the ureters and is most often performed in children.

Doctors consider the likelihood of disease recurring in the pelvis or urethra as well as the patient's gender to determine which type of urostomy is most appropriate. Neobladders are not appropriate for female patients whose **cancer** involves the bladder neck or male patients with problems affecting the right colon or small bowel.

QUESTIONS TO ASK THE DOCTOR

- What type of urostomy will I have?
- Will I have to wear a pouch after the operation?
- Will I be able to take care of myself after the operation?
- Will other people be able to tell that I have had a urostomy?

If bladder cancer has metastasized or cannot be surgically removed, the surgeon may perform a urostomy without removing the patient's bladder.

Preparation

Before undergoing a urostomy, the patient learns where on the abdomen the stoma will be created, what type of collection device (if any) will be worn, and what changes in appearance the operation may cause.

Nurses encourage the patient preparing to undergo an incontinent urostomy to become familiar with the collection device that will be worn after the operation. They may arrange to have someone who has already had the operation (ostomate) reassure the patient preparing for either an incontinent or continent procedure and answer questions about life after the surgery.

Preoperative restrictions

The patient may be told not to eat certain foods before surgery and must fast for eight hours and have a cleansing enema before the operation.

Fluid and **antibiotics** may be given to a patient who is frail.

Aftercare

A patient who has undergone an incontinent diversion wears a collection device that is odor-free, not visible under clothing, disposable or reusable, and available at drug stores or medical supply houses or through the mail.

To prevent urine leakage, infection, skin irritation, and odor, the patient should re-measure the stoma and make any necessary adjustments in the size of the flat sponge-like patch that covers and protects it. This should be done during the first few months after the operation (when shrinkage occurs) or whenever gaining or losing weight. Measuring devices and instructions are included in every box of collection pouches.

Some doctors recommend taking Vitamin C to prevent infection- and odor-causing bacteria from accumulating in the urine. Other recommendations include drinking eight to ten glasses of water a day to reduce the likelihood of kidney infection.

Risks

Because tumors sometimes develop in neobladders, a patient who undergoes this procedure must have a **cystoscopy** within five years.

Normal results

A patient who has had a urostomy can:

- Shower or bathe with or without the collection pouch
- Usually wear the clothes worn before the operation
- Return to work shortly after leaving the hospital (although a doctor's permission is required before doing heavy lifting)
- Enjoy intimate relationships
- Participate in athletic activities, but should avoid strenuous contact sports like football or wrestling

Dietary restrictions are rare.

A woman who has undergone a urostomy should talk with her doctor before becoming pregnant.

Abnormal results

Almost half (40%) of patients who undergo continent diversions and 24.1% of those who undergo ileal or colonic conduits require subsequent surgery to repair leaks or obstructions and correct other surgery-related problems.

A patient who has had a urostomy may also experience:

- kidney damage, infection, or failure
- swelling, shrinkage (stenois), or displacement (prolapse) of the stoma
- infections of the stoma or urinary tract
- fever
- hernia
- **diarrhea**
- urinary problems
- chills
- pain in the leg or abdomen
- blood or pus in the urine

Resources

BOOKS

Kupfer, Barbara, et al. *Yes We Can! Advice on Traveling with an Ostomy and Tips for Everyday Living*. Worcester, MA: Chandler House Press, 2000.

OTHER

"Bladder Cancer: Types of Treatment." *ACS Cancer Resource Center*. [cited July 11, 2000 and July 18, 2001]. http://www3.cancer.org/cancerinfo.

Cherath, Lata. "Bladder Cancer." 1999. [cited May 20, 2001 and July 6, 2001]. http://www.findarticles.com/cf_1/g2601/0002/2601000204/print.html.

Guttman, Cheryl. "Diversion Procedures Require Similar Reintervention." June 1999. [cited July 18, 2001]. http://www.findarticles.com/cf_1/m0VPB/6_27/54852652/print.jhtml.

"Urostomy fact sheet." *United Ostomy Association*. [cited April 15, 2001 and July 18, 2001]. http://www.uoa.org/factsheets/urostomyfs.html.

ORGANIZATIONS

United Ostomy Association, Inc. 19772 MacArthur Blvd., Suite 200, Irvine, CA 92612-2405. (800) 826-0826. http://www.uoa.org.

Maureen Haggerty

Uterine cancer *see* **Endometrial cancer**

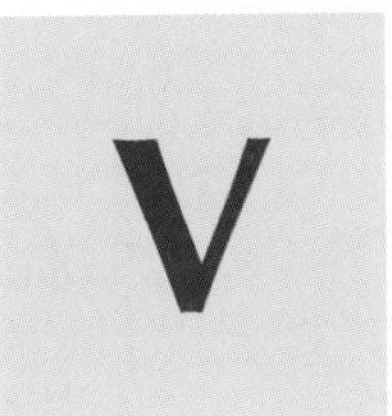

Vaccines

Definition

A **cancer** vaccine is a method of treating the disease involving administration of one or more substances characteristic of the cancer, called antigens, often in combination with factors that boost immune function. This induces the patient's immune system to attack and eliminate the cancerous cells.

Purpose

Unlike traditional vaccines for infectious diseases, at this time cancer vaccines are not given to prevent the initial development of cancer. Instead, cancer vaccines are a method of treating cancer that has already occurred and are given to patients already diagnosed with cancer.

As a cancer treatment method, the ultimate goal of most cancer vaccines is the elimination of tumor or cancerous cells from the body. Other vaccines are given after the use of more traditional treatments, such as **chemotherapy**, radiation, or surgery, with the aim of suppressing the recurrence of the cancer.

Precautions

No vaccine has yet been approved by the Food and Drug Administration (FDA) for the treatment of cancer. Accordingly, vaccines are not standard treatments and other more traditional treatments should be investigated first. Vaccines are available only through participation in **clinical trials**. Each trial has its own criteria that can limit who can participate. However, many cancers have a current trial for one or more types of vaccines. The American Society for Gene Therapy states that as of the early 2000s, vaccines were the most common approach to gene therapy being studied by researchers.

Most vaccine trials test the response of the disease with and without the vaccine or the effect of substances added to the vaccine, called adjuvants. Such trials usually only accept patients who have already tried the standard treatment methods. Others test a standard treatment method with and without the addition of the vaccine. A very few compare the standard treatment to the vaccine.

Looking at cancer vaccines overall, this treatment method has been more successful eliminating very small tumors rather than the getting rid of a large tumor load. So if the size of the tumor is significant, a more realistic goal is to shrink the tumor and reduce its effect on the patient's body, rather than total elimination of the cancer.

The complexity of the human immune system has made it very difficult to develop an effective vaccine. Tumors have strategies to evade detection by the immune system. Most notably, they mimic the outward appearance and antigens of the body's own cells. The immune system's built-in lack of response against "self" allows the tumor to escape notice by the body. Now fully aware of this phenomenon, researchers are working to develop methods of circumventing this problem to develop a highly effective vaccine system.

Description

There are three general types of cancer vaccines: those that use whole tumor cells, those that use only one or more substances derived from the tumors, or those that administer primed cells from the patient's immune system.

Whole cell vaccines

Whole cell vaccines are autologous when they contain only inactivated tumor cells from the patient's own tumors. The cells have been isolated from the tumor and made to grow in the laboratory, a process known as creating a cell line. Allogeneic whole cell

QUESTIONS TO ASK THE DOCTOR

- Have all the standard treatment methods for my cancer been tried?
- Is there a vaccine in clinical trials for my kind of cancer?
- Do I fulfill the requirements necessary for the clinical trial for this vaccine?
- Has this vaccine been tried on human patients before?
- If so, what were the results?

KEY TERMS

Adjuvant—A substance added to a vaccine to increase the immune system's response to the vaccine contents.

Allogeneic—A type of vaccine made up of tumor cells derived from persons other than the patient.

Antigen—A substance characteristic of a tumor that evokes an immune response.

Antigen presenting cell—A cell of the immune system that ingests antigens and exposes them to cells of the immune system in a way that activates the cells to seek out and destroy any other cells displaying that antigen.

Autologous—A type of vaccine made up of tumor cells from the patient's own tumor.

Cytokine—A substance made by cells of the immune system that increases the response to a foreign substance.

Dendritic cell—A special type of antigen-presenting cell that is effective in stimulating T cells.

Epitope—A portion of a protein or other molecule that is the specific target of an immune response.

vaccines are made from inactivated tumor cells isolated from one or more other people. The main advantage to autologous vaccines is the direct relation between the vaccine and the tumor target. However, because of the screening of self antigens away from a body's own immune system, **immune response** to tumor antigens in autologous whole cells vaccines can be low.

Allogeneic vaccines avoid some of the problems of autologous vaccines. First, cell lines do not have to be created for each patient, a labor-intensive process that can have highly variable results. Second, the same vaccine can be given to all patients, making the response to the vaccine more predictable. Third, a use of a pool of tumor cells can increase the possibility of having the full repertoire of the tumor antigens in the vaccine. This helps to overcome the ability of tumor cells to escape notice by the immune system. Finally, by using well-characterized cell lines, it is much easier for the researcher to add genetic modifications that increase the immune system's response to the cells.

Isolated antigen vaccines

There are many kinds of vaccines that deliver only a portion of the tumor cell that will elicit an immune response, called an antigen. Some antigens are unique to a cancer type, some are unique to an individual tumor, and a very few are found in more than one cancer type. For example, vaccines against telomerase and human chorionic gonadotripin (hCG), two proteins produced by many cancers, have been developed, raising hopes for the development of a universal cancer vaccine.

The most common kind of antigen used in cancer vaccines is a protein or a part of a protein. The protein can actually be isolated from the tumor cells, or more commonly, produced in large quantity using genetic engineering techniques. When a part of a protein is used, experimental efforts generally preceded the vaccine production to determine what parts of the protein were often the target of immune responses. Parts of proteins that elicit immune responses are called epitopes.

Antigens do not necessarily have to be proteins. Immune responses are also mounted against the carbohydrate (sugar) molecules present on the surface of the proteins. Tumor proteins can have unusual carbohydrate structures that set them apart from cells from normal tissue. Carbohydrates are also found in abundant numbers on the surface of the tumor cells. Accordingly, researchers have developed cancer vaccines that combine the tumor-characteristic carbohydrates anchored on protein bases. These vaccines are being tested for their ability to reduce the recurrence of **prostate cancer**.

Vaccines can also contain the naked genetic material encoding the protein (either deoxyribose nucleic acid, DNA, or ribose nucleic acid, RNA). After the genetic material gains entry to the cell, the cellular machinery uses it to produce the antigen and an immune response is mounted against it. Animal studies have found that these types of vaccines are very dependent on the particular antigen and the mode of administration of the vaccine. A unique method of delivery used with DNA or RNA vaccines is the coating of tiny gold beads with the genetic material and shooting the beads into the skin.

Genetically engineered viruses can also be used to bring the DNA or RNA into the cell. When used in this way the viruses are called viral vectors. One example of a viral vector currently being used as a cancer vaccine is one based on the adenovirus. When viruses are used as vectors they have been altered to no longer cause disease, but they do retain the ability to infect human cells. Instead of making new viruses, the infected cells make the desired antigen, and the body will respond against it. Viral vectors can also carry the genetic instructions for factors, called cytokines, which boost the immune system's response to the antigen.

Antigen-presenting cell (APC) vaccines

Vaccines can also be made that contain cells from the patient's own immune system, in particular antigen-presenting cells (APCs). These cells play a central role in the development of an immune response against a particular antigen. Specifically, APCs ingest the antigen and present them to the T cells, a type of immune cells responsible for targeting and killing cells seen as foreign to the body. If T cells are exposed to the antigen by an APC, as opposed to seeing the antigen on the cell itself, they are more strongly activated. That is, more T cells that specifically attack that antigen are produced and the immune response against the foreign cell is stronger.

Dendritic cells are a type of APC that is most effective in activating T cells. For this reason, they are often the kind of cells used in APC vaccines. Unfortunately, the number of dendritic cells circulating in the blood at any one time is relatively low. However, new techniques have been developed that allow that small number of dendritic cells to be isolated and then stimulated outside the body to result in a usable number. During stimulation, the dendritic cells are exposed to the tumor antigen, a process known as priming. Thus, when injected into the body, the dendritic cells are primed to recruit large numbers of T cells specific against the tumor antigen.

Cytokines and adjuvants

Because of the ability of tumor cells to escape detection by the immune system, an important component of many cancer vaccines is the addition of biological factors or chemical adjuvants to help boost immune response. One type of adjuvant is a cytokine, a factor normally produced by cells of the immune system to help recruit cells to the site of the foreign cells or help T cells function. Some examples of cytokines used in vaccines are granulocyte/macrophage colony stimulating factor (GM-CSF, or **sargramostim**), the interleukins (especially IL-2), the **interferons** (INFs), and **tumor necrosis factor** alpha (TNF-α).

Adjuvants are chemical additions to vaccines that help boost the response to the contained cells or antigens. Adjuvants are derived from a variety of sources and can be isolated from animals, plants, or are synthetic chemical compounds. Several adjuvants in use with cancer vaccines are keyhole lympocianin (KLH, derived from shell-dwelling sea animals), incomplete Freud's adjuvant (IFA, mineral oil, and an emulsifying agent), and QS-21 (a chemical derived from the soapbark tree).

Administration

The particular administration method and schedule will vary from clinical trial to clinical trial. Administration methods can include intradural (injection within the skin), subcutaneous (injection below the skin), injection into the lymph nodes, or intravenous (injection into the veins). Typically, vaccines are administered as a series of several doses (initial challenge and boosters). Many clinical trials utilize various administration methods and timing strategies in order to try to determine the best means of inducing an antitumor immune response.

Preparation

Before enrolling in a clinical trial, patients should discuss the potential benefits and risks with their doctor. Clinical trials can be located by contacting the research institutes directly or by searching the Internet. A particularly good site for getting information about clinical trials for cancer treatment is run by the National Cancer Institute (http://www.clincialtrials.gov).

Aftercare

One of the most striking advantages of vaccines compared to other cancer treatments is the relatively low incidence of side effects. Particularly if IFN is used as an immunoadjuvant, patients sometimes experience flu-like symptoms. However, other than some soreness at the site of injection, vaccine patients generally have no adverse reactions to this kind of treatment.

Risks

The greatest risk with cancer vaccines is that there will be no immune response and the treatment will be ineffective. Although serious adverse reactions to the antigens, such as the attack of healthy cells, are theoretically possible, these fears have not materialized. Other than some mild adverse reactions, such as **fever** and redness of the skin at the injection site, vaccine treatment appears relatively low-risk in the traditional sense.

Normal results

Based on a review of published clinical trials as of the early 2000s, normal results for this treatment is, unfortunately, little or no effect. Although a response by the immunized patient's T cells against the tumor is often documented by testing, the effect on disease is generally marginal. These results could be at least partially due to the selection process for patients in the trials, who are often suffering from late-stage cancers.

Abnormal results

For each trial, there are a small percentage of patients who have complete, partial, or mixed response to the vaccine. Others show a stabilization of the disease where deterioration of condition would be expected. As traditional treatments were often unsuccessful with these patients, these results are significant. However, the very low rate of success underscores the complexity of the human immune system, the number of variables in the vaccine method, and the amount of research that will need to be done to develop an effective vaccine treatment for this disease.

See also Immunologic therapy; Monoclonal antibodies.

Resources

BOOKS

Restifo, Nicholas, et al. "Therapeutic Cancer Vaccines." In *Cancer Principles & Practice of Oncology*, edited by Vincent DeVita, et al. Philadelphia: Lippincott Williams & Wilkins, 2001, pp. 3195–217.

PERIODICALS

Bocchia, Monica, et al. "Antitumor Vaccination: Where We Stand." *Haematologica* 85 (November 2000): 1172–206.

Monzavi-Karbassi, B., and T. Kieber-Emmons. "Current concepts in cancer vaccine strategies." *Biotechniques* 30 (January 2001): 170.

OTHER

"First Potential Universal Cancer Vaccine Shows Promise In Lab." *ScienceDaily Magazine*. 30 August 2000 [cited April 12, 2001 and June 28, 2001]. http://www.sciencedaily.com/print/2000/08/000830073711.htm.

"Treating Cancer with Vaccine Therapy." *CancerTrials*. July 20, 1999. [cited April 12, 2001 and June 28, 2001]. http://cancertrials.nci.nih.gov/news/features/vaccine/index.html.

Michelle Johnson, M.S., J.D.

Vaginal cancer

Definition

Vaginal **cancer** refers to an abnormal, cancerous growth in the tissues of the birth canal (vagina).

Description

Vaginal cancer is rare and accounts for only 1% to 2% of all **gynecologic cancers**. In the United States, there are approximately 2,000 cases of vaginal cancer diagnosed, and approximately 600 deaths, each year. Vaginal cancer can be either primary or metastatic. Cancer that originates in the vagina is called primary vaginal cancer; if cancer spreads to the vagina from another site, it is called metastatic cancer. Eighty-percent of vaginal cancers are metastatic. Metastatic cancers carry the name of the primary cancer site. For instance, cancer that has spread from the cervix to the vagina would be called "metastatic cervical cancer," not "vaginal cancer."

The vagina is a short tube that extends from the outer female genitalia (vulva) to the opening to the uterus (cervix). It serves to receive the penis during sexual intercourse, as an outlet for shed tissue and blood during menstruation, and as a passageway for a baby during childbirth. Most cancers are located in the upper third of the vagina.

Squamous **carcinoma** is the most common type of vaginal cancer and accounts for 85% of cases. Infrequent types of vaginal cancer include **adenocarcinoma**, **melanoma**, and sarcomas. Adenocarcinoma is usually found in young women (ages 12 to 30 years) while squamous cell cancer (squamous carcinoma) is usually found in older women (ages 60 to 80 years). Although vaginal melanoma can afflict adult women of any age, women are on average in their fifties at the time of diagnosis.

KEY TERMS

Adjuvant therapy—A treatment that is intended to aid the primary treatment. Adjuvant treatments for vaginal cancer are radiation therapy and chemotherapy.

Biopsy—Removal of a small piece of tissue for microscopic examination. This is done under local anesthesia and removed by either using a scalpel or a punch, which removes a small cylindrical portion of tissue.

Colposcope—An instrument used for examination of the vagina and cervix. The instrument includes a light and magnifying lens for better visualization.

Intracavitary radiation—Radiation therapy for vaginal cancer in which a cylindrical container holding a radioactive substance is placed into the vagina for one or two days.

Metastasis—The movement of cancer cells from one area of the body to another. This occurs through the blood vessels or the lymph vessels.

Pelvic exenteration—Surgical removal of the organs of the pelvis, which includes the uterus, vagina, and cervix.

Squamous cells—Scale-like cells that cover some body surfaces and cavities.

Vaginectomy—Surgical removal of the vagina. An artificial vagina can be constructed using grafts of skin or intestinal tissue.

QUESTIONS TO ASK THE DOCTOR

- What type of cancer do I have?
- What stage of cancer do I have?
- What is the five-year survival rate for women with this type and stage of cancer?
- Has the cancer spread?
- What are my treatment options?
- How much tissue will you be removing? Can you remove less tissue and complement my treatment with adjuvant therapy?
- What are the risks and side effects of these treatments?
- What medications can I take to relieve treatment side effects?
- Are there any clinical studies underway that would be appropriate for me?
- What effective alternative or complementary treatments are available for this type of cancer?
- How debilitating is the treatment? Will I be able to continue working?
- Are there any restrictions regarding sexual activity?
- How is a vaginal reconstruction performed?
- How will a vaginal reconstruction affect sexual functioning?
- Are there any local support groups for vaginal cancer patients?
- What is the chance that the cancer will recur?
- Is there anything I can do to prevent recurrence?
- How often will I have follow-up examinations?

Demographics

Vaginal cancer is most common in women who are between the ages of 60 and 80.

Causes and symptoms

Cancer is caused when the normal mechanisms that control cell growth become disturbed, causing cells to grow and divide without stopping. This is usually the result of damage to the genetic material of the cell (deoxyribonucleic acid, or DNA). The cause of vaginal cancer is not known.

Symptoms of vaginal cancer appear when the cancer has become more advanced. Approximately 20% of vaginal cancer cases are asymptomatic (produce no symptoms) and are diagnosed following an abnormal Pap test. Symptoms of vaginal cancer include:

- abnormal vaginal bleeding or discharge
- pain during intercourse
- pain in the pelvic area
- difficult or painful urination
- constipation

Diagnosis

The diagnosis of vaginal cancer is made by physical examination and laboratory analysis of tissue samples. During the physical examination, the physician will place one or two fingers into the vagina and press down on the lower abdomen with his or her free hand to feel (palpate) the reproductive organs and any masses. During a routine speculum examination, the physician will obtain a sample of cervical and vaginal cells (using a swab, brush, or wooden applicator) for laboratory analysis (Pap test).

A special magnifying instrument, called a colposcope, may be used to view the vagina. Additionally, the surface of the vagina may be treated with a dilute solution of acetic acid, which causes some abnormal areas to turn white. Squamous carcinoma and adenocarcinoma usually appear as a growth on the surface of the vagina. Squamous carcinoma may be present as an open sore (ulcer). Adenocarcinoma may lie deeper so that it is not visible and detected only by palpation. Vaginal melanoma appears as a brown or black skin tag (polypoid), growth attached to the vaginal wall by a stem (pedunculated), nipple-like growth (papillary), or fungus-like growth (fungating). Sarcomas often appear as a grape-like mass.

If any area appears abnormal, a tissue sample (**biopsy**) will be taken. The biopsy can be performed in the doctor's office with the use of local anesthetic. A small piece of tissue, which contains the suspect lesion with some surrounding normal skin and the underlying skin layers and connective tissue, will be removed. Small lesions will be removed in their entirety (excisional biopsy). The diagnosis of cancer depends on a microscopic analysis of this tissue by a pathologist.

Chest **x rays** and routine blood work are commonly employed in the diagnosis of any cancer. Endoscopic examination of the bladder (**cystoscopy**) and/or rectum (proctoscopy) may be performed if it is suspected that the cancer has spread to these organs.

Treatment team

The treatment team for vaginal cancer may include a gynecologist, gynecologic oncologist, radiation oncologist, plastic surgeon, gynecologic nurse oncologist, sexual therapist, psychiatrist, psychological counselor, and social worker.

Clinical staging, treatments, and prognosis

Clinical staging

The International Federation of Gynecology and Obstetrics (FIGO) has adopted a clinical staging system for vaginal cancer that is used by most gynecologic oncologists. Vaginal cancer is categorized into five stages (0, I, II, III, and IV) that may be further subdivided (A and B) based on the depth or spread of cancerous tissue. The FIGO stages for vaginal cancer are:

- Stage 0. Cancer is confined to the outermost layer (epithelium) of vaginal cells and is called carcinoma *in situ* or vaginal intraepithelial neoplasia (VAIN).
- Stage I. Cancer is confined to the vagina.
- Stage II. Cancer has spread to the tissues near the vagina.
- Stage III. Cancer has spread to the bones of the pelvis, local lymph nodes, and/or other reproductive organs.
- Stage IV. Cancer has spread to the bladder, rectum, or other parts of the body.

Treatments

The treatment of vaginal cancer varies considerably and depends on the type of cancer, stage of cancer, and the patient's age and overall health. Surgery is the most common treatment for vaginal cancer. **Radiation therapy** and **chemotherapy** are often used as adjuvant therapy to complement the surgical treatment.

SURGERY. The amount of tissue removed depends upon the stage and type of cancer. The local lymph nodes may also be removed (lymphadenectomy). Laser surgery, which destroys the cancerous cells, may be used in the treatment of stage 0 vaginal cancer. With a wide local excision, the cancerous tissue and some surrounding healthy tissue is cut out. Wide local excisions may require skin grafts to repair the vagina.

For more extensive cancer, the vagina may be removed (vaginectomy). Following vaginectomy, skin grafts and plastic surgery are used to create an artificial vagina. Vaginal cancer that has spread to the other reproductive organs would be treated by radical hysterectomy in which the uterus, fallopian tubes, and ovaries are removed. Cancer that has spread beyond the reproductive organs may be treated by pelvic **exenteration**, in which the vagina, cervix, uterus, fallopian tubes, ovaries, and, as necessary, the lower colon, bladder, or rectum are removed.

Surgical complications include urinary tract **infection**, wound infection, temporary nerve injury, fluid accumulation (edema) in the legs, urinary **incontinence**, falling or sinking of the genitals (genital prolapse), and blood clots (thrombi).

RADIATION THERAPY. Radiation therapy may be used as the sole treatment of vaginal cancer or as an adjuvant therapy to aid surgery. Radiation therapy uses high-energy radiation from x rays and gamma rays to kill the cancer cells. Radiation given from a machine that is outside the body is called external radiation therapy. Radiation given internally is called internal radiation therapy or brachytherapy. Sometimes applicators containing radioactive compounds are placed inside the vagina (intracavitary radiation) or directly into the cancerous lesion (interstitial radiation). External and internal radiation may be used in combination to treat vaginal cancer.

The skin in the treated area may become red and dry and may take as long as a year to return to normal. **Fatigue**, upset stomach, **diarrhea**, and **nausea** are also common complaints of women having radiation therapy. Radiation therapy in the pelvic area may cause the vagina to become narrow as scar tissue forms. This phenomenon, known as vaginal stenosis, makes intercourse painful.

CHEMOTHERAPY. Chemotherapy is not very a very successful treatment of vaginal cancer and is generally reserved for patients with advanced disease. Chemotherapy uses **anticancer drugs** to kill the cancer cells. The drugs are usually given by mouth (orally) or intravenously. They enter the bloodstream and can travel to all parts of the body to kill cancer cells. Generally, a combination of drugs is given because it is more effective than a single drug in treating cancer. For vaginal cancer, anticancer drugs may be put into the vagina (intravaginal chemotherapy).

The side effects of chemotherapy are significant and include stomach upset, **vomiting**, appetite loss (**anorexia**), hair loss (**alopecia**), mouth or vaginal sores, fatigue, menstrual cycle changes, and premature menopause. There is also an increased chance of infections.

Prognosis

Survival is related to the stage and type of vaginal cancer. The five-year survival rates for squamous carcinoma and adenocarcinoma of the vagina are: 96%, stage 0; 73%, stage I; 58%, stage II; 36%, stage III; and 36%, stage IV. With a five-year survival rate of less than 20%, melanoma has a poor prognosis. Vaginal cancer most commonly spreads (metastasizes) to the lungs, but may spread to the liver, bone, or other sites.

Alternative and complementary therapies

Although alternative and complementary therapies are used by many cancer patients, very few controlled studies on the effectiveness of such therapies exist. Mind-body techniques such as prayer, biofeedback, visualization, meditation, and yoga have not shown any effect in reducing cancer but can reduce stress and lessen some of the side effects of cancer treatments.

Clinical studies of hydrazine sulfate found that it had no effect on cancer and even worsened the health and well-being of the study subjects. One clinical study of the drug amygdalin (Laetrile) found that it had no effect on cancer. Laetrile can be toxic and has caused death. Shark cartilage, although highly touted as an effective cancer treatment, is an improbable therapy that has not been the subject of clinical study.

The American Cancer Society has found that the "metabolic diets" pose serious risk to the patient. The effectiveness of the macrobiotic, Gerson, and Kelley diets and the Manner metabolic therapy has not been scientifically proven. The Food and Drug Administration (FDA) was unable to substantiate the anticancer claims made about the popular Cancell treatment.

There is no evidence for the effectiveness of most over-the-counter herbal cancer remedies. However, some herbals have shown an anticancer effect. Some studies have shown that polysaccharide krestin (PSK), a substance from the mushroom *Coriolus versicolor*, has some effectiveness against cancer. In a small study, the green alga *Chlorella pyrenoidosa* has been shown to have anticancer activity. In a few small studies, evening primrose oil has shown some benefit in the treatment of cancer. Herbals can have a negative impact on conventional treatment; patients must discuss herbal use with a physician.

For more comprehensive information, the patient should consult the book on complementary and alternative medicine published by the American Cancer Society listed in the Resources section.

Coping with cancer treatment

The patient should consult her treatment team regarding any side effects or complications of treatment. Vaginal stenosis can be prevented and treated by vaginal dilators, gentle douching, and sexual intercourse. A water-soluble lubricant may be used to make sexual intercourse more comfortable. Women with a reconstructed vagina will need to use a water-soluble lubricant during sexual intercourse. Many of the side effects of chemotherapy can be relieved by medications. Women may wish to consult a psychotherapist and/or join a support group to deal with the emotional consequences of cancer and vaginectomy.

Clinical trials

As of 2009, there are no **clinical trials** underway that were specific for vaginal cancer. Women should consult with their treatment team to determine if they are candidates for any ongoing studies.

Prevention

Risk factors for vaginal cancer include:

- Diethylstilbestrol (DES). Young women whose mothers took DES during pregnancy are at a higher risk of developing vaginal cancer, particularly clear cell carcinoma. Between 1945 and 1970, DES was prescribed to pregnant women who were at risk of miscarriage.

- Cervical cancer. Women with a history of cervical cancer have a high risk of developing vaginal cancer.
- Hysterectomy. Up to half of all patients with vaginal cancer have had a hysterectomy. Their vaginal cancer may actually represent an earlier spread from the cervix.
- Chronic irritant vaginitis. Chronic irritation to the vagina, particularly from use of a vaginal pessary, is associated with vaginal cancer. A pessary is an instrument that is placed into the vagina to support the uterus or prevent pregnancy (contraception).
- Vaginal adenosis. This condition, in which cells that resemble those of the uterus are found in the vaginal lining, places a woman at a higher risk of developing vaginal cancer.
- Human papilloma virus (HPV) infection. Infection by this sexually transmitted virus, the cause of genital warts, increases a woman's risk of developing squamous carcinoma.
- Smoking. There appears to be an association between tobacco use and vaginal cancer.

All women, even those who have had a hysterectomy or are past menopause, should get an annual pelvic examination and Pap test. Women who had a hysterectomy because of cancer may benefit from more frequent Pap tests. The earlier that precancerous abnormalities or vaginal cancer are detected, the better the prognosis. Women whose mothers took DES during pregnancy and those with vaginal adenosis should be screened regularly. Women can reduce the risk of contracting HPV by avoiding sexual intercourse with individuals who have had many sexual partners, limiting their number of sexual partners, and delaying first sexual activity until an older age. Avoiding tobacco products may reduce a woman's risk of developing vaginal cancer.

Special concerns

Of special concern to women undergoing treatment of vaginal cancer is the effect surgery and/or radiation therapy will have on sexual functioning. Women of childbearing age may worry about their fertility and whether or not they will be able to bear children. **Depression**, due to the affects of surgery on **body image** and **sexuality**, may occur. Complications, both short term and long term, following extensive surgical treatment of vaginal cancer are not uncommon.

See also Cystoscopy; Fertility issues.

Resources

BOOKS

Bruss, Katherine, Christina Salter, and Esmeralda Galan, editors. *American Cancer Society's Guide to Complementary and Alternative Cancer Methods*. Atlanta: American Cancer Society, 2000.

Eifel, Patricia, Jonathan Berrek, and James Thigpen. "Cancer of the Cervix, Vagina, and Vulva." In *Cancer: Principles & Practice of Oncology*, edited by Vincent T. DeVita, Samuel Hellman, and Steven Rosenberg. Philadelphia: Lippincott Williams & Wilkins, 2001.

Garcia, Agustin, and J. Tate Thigpen. "Tumors of the Vulva and Vagina." In *Textbook of Uncommon Cancer*, edited by D. Raghavan, M. Brecher, D. Johnson, N. Meropol, P. Moots, and J. Thigpen. Chichester, UK: John Wiley & Sons, 1999.

Primack, Aron. "Complementary/Alternative Therapies in the Prevention and Treatment of Cancer." In *Complementary/Alternative Medicine: An Evidence-Based Approach*, edited by John Spencer and Joseph Jacobs. St. Louis: Mosby, 1999.

ORGANIZATIONS

American Cancer Society. 1599 Clifton Rd. NE, Atlanta, GA 30329. (800) ACS-2345. http://www.cancer.org.

Cancer Research Institute. 681 Fifth Ave., New York, NY 10022. (800) 992-2623. http://www.cancerresearch.org.

Gynecologic Cancer Foundation. 401 North Michigan Ave., Chicago, IL 60611. (800) 444-4441 or (312) 644-6610. http://www.wcn.org/gcf.

National Institutes of Health, National Cancer Institute. 9000 Rockville Pike, Bethesda, MD 20982. (800) 4-CANCER. http://cancernet.nci.nih.gov.

Belinda Rowland, Ph.D.

Valacyclovir HCl *see* **Antiviral therapy**

Valrubicin

Definition

Valrubicin (also known as Valstar) is a chemotherapeutic drug that interferes with the metabolism of DNA, thus disrupting the proliferation of cells, including **cancer** cells.

Purpose

Valrubicin is an antineoplastic drug that is used as a treatment for a form of **bladder cancer** called papillary bladder cancer when the bladder cannot be surgically removed due to increased risk of morbidity or mortality. It is also being tested as treatment for several other types of **carcinoma** *in situ*.

KEY TERMS

Carcinoma *in situ*—A malignant tumor in a preinvasive stage.

Instillation—Dropping a liquid into a body part such as the bladder.

Intravesical—Within the bladder.

Urethral—Relating to the urethra, a passageway from the bladder to outside the body.

Description

The Food and Drug Administration approved valrubicin for bladder cancer treatment in 1998. As of the early 2000s, it was being tested in **clinical trials** for both bladder and **ovarian cancer** treatments. It is an anthracycline-like compound that acts by penetrating cells and disrupting the dividing cell cycle by interfering with DNA metabolism. Valrubicin acts by inhibiting nucleoside incorporation into nucleic acids, thus, causing major damage to DNA. Research performed in 1999 indicated that valrubicin entered cells faster than **doxorubicin**, another anthracycline. Research has also shown that complete response is seen in one in five patients.

Recommended dosage

Valrubicin is only available in instillation form and can only be administered under the supervision of a physician. During initial clinical trials patients received doses ranging from 200 milligrams to 900 milligrams each week. The normal dose is 800 milligrams once a week for six weeks. However, dosing may vary from patient to patient. The drug is administered intravesically (directly into the bladder) through a catheter tube that penetrates into the bladder wall. Once delivered to the bladder the solution should be maintained in the bladder for approximately two hours.

During clinical trials for ovarian cancer, valrubicin is administered through the abdomen.

Precautions

There are other bladder problems that may affect the use of valrubicin. Patients with bladder irritation can have an increased risk of unwanted effects. Patients with perforated bladders should not take this medication. Patients with small bladders could have trouble holding all of the medication. Finally, if patients have urinary tract infections, they should use caution when taking this medication.

Valrubicin has not been studied in pregnant women, but it has been studied in pregnant animals. In animals it can cause birth defects. Therefore, women who are pregnant or breast-feeding should not take valrubicin. Additionally, women should not become pregnant while on this medication. Men taking this medication should not engage in procreative activities. Both men and women should use appropriate forms for contraception to avoid causing pregnancy.

There have not been appropriate studies done specifically on children or the elderly to determine the risk of using this medication in these populations. However, this drug is not expected to act differently in the elderly than it does in younger adults.

Side effects

During the six-week course of treatment patients could experience one or more side effects. The most common are loss of bladder control, increased frequency of urination, and blood in the urine. Other less common and rare side effects are bladder pain, pelvic pain, urethral pain, and loss of the sense of taste.

Interactions

As of the early 2000s there were no known drug-drug interactions with valrubicin.

See also Daunorubicin; Taste alteration.

Sally C. McFarlane-Parrott

Vancomycin *see* **Antibiotics**

Vascular access

Definition

Vascular access is the use of flexible tubes (catheters) that remain inserted into blood vessels for weeks or months, and provide a means of infusing **antibiotics**, **chemotherapy**, pain medications, or **nutritional support** into patients, and enable blood samples to be taken from patients.

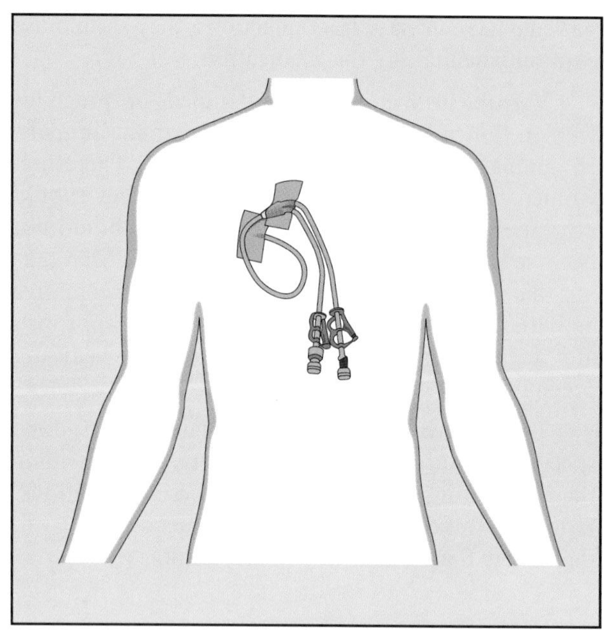

A tunnelled central venous catheter ("Hickman line"). *(Illustration by Argosy. Cengage Learning, Gale.)*

Purpose

Cancer patients may require a variety of treatments over extended periods of time. Many of these treatments are infused directly into the bloodstream (intravenous or IV therapy). For example, a cancer patient may need chemotherapy given through a vein, as well as blood tests requiring frequent samples to be taken from their veins. Indwelling catheters, which stay in place for weeks or months, save the patient the discomfort of undergoing frequent needle sticks (venipuncture), and prevent veins from the trauma of repeated punctures and accidental release of harsh chemical agents into skin and subcutaneous tissues. The catheters are used for continuous, as well as intermittent, treatments and procedures.

Description

The two types of indwelling catheters are external and internal. These devices have been in use since the 1970s.

When deciding which catheter to use, the physician looks at the:

- patient's age and size
- length of time the catheter will be in place
- purpose of the catheter
- patient's previous history with indwelling devices
- condition of the blood vessels

KEY TERMS

Broviac—Long–term external central venous catheter.

Groshong—Long–term external central venous catheter, similar to Broviac or Hickman types, but with a different tip.

Hickman—Long–term external central venous catheter.

Lumen—An external opening in the catheter used for putting fluids in or drawing blood out.

Mediport—A defunct brand of implantable port now used to refer to any implantable port.

Pasport—Long–term implantable port inserted in the arm.

PICC—Long–term silicone or polyurethane catheter inserted into the arm, and threaded into central circulation.

Portacath—Long–term implantable port.

Physicians also consider their own preferences, as well as the treatment team suggestions and any special needs the patient may have.

External catheters are usually made of polyurethane for short–term use, and silicone for long–term use. Long–term devices have an internal cuff surrounding them to prevent catheter movement and **infection**. They have one to three openings, called lumens. One may be used for chemotherapy, a second for nutritional support, and the third for drawing blood samples. The catheters may be inserted into a central vein in the neck or chest, or an arm vein, called a peripheral vein.

External central catheters

External central catheters are divided into the types designed to stay in place for just a week or so, and the long–term devices commonly known as Broviac, Groshong, and Hickman, which can remain in place for months. The short–term devices are placed directly into a vein, while the long–term catheters are tunneled under the skin to the point where they enter a central blood vessel, such as the cephalic, jugular or subclavian vein. Central catheters are inserted using sterile, surgical technique.

External peripheral catheters

A peripherally inserted central catheter, or PICC, is inserted through the arm, and threaded into a central vein. With proper insertion and care, a PICC can remain in place for months. It may be inserted in the patient's room by a specially trained nurse. A PICC

QUESTIONS TO ASK THE DOCTOR

- What type of catheter will I have?
- Why was this particular type chosen?
- Will insertion be an outpatient procedure or require a hospital stay?
- Who will insert the catheter?
- How should I prepare for insertion?
- What are the risks of a complication during insertion?
- Will any special care be needed immediately after it is put into place?
- What treatments will I receive through the catheter?
- What special care does the device require?
- What are the symptoms of a catheter problem?
- Will the catheter cause any physical limitations?
- How long will my catheter be in place?
- How will the catheter be removed?

may limit arm movement, and is usually placed in the patient's least dominant arm. For example, the left arm would be the ideal PICC insertion site for a right–handed person. However, if a procedure such as breast surgery has been performed on one side, the PICC will most likely be inserted into the arm on the other side.

Internal catheters

An internal catheter, such as a Portacath or Pasport, is commonly called an implantable mediport because the catheter connects to a pocket, or reservoir, located under the skin, either in the chest or arm. While the system is entirely internal, the pocket is located near the surface and can be felt through the skin. The range of catheter materials includes plastic and titanium. Over the years, these devices have gotten smaller in size, making them more comfortable for patients. An implantable port is inserted and removed in a surgical or radiology setting using sterile technique. Functionality can be determined by injecting contrast material into the port, a procedure referred to as a port-o-gram. Fluid flow is regulated by a pump located on the outside or implanted internally during a surgical procedure. External pumps are usually portable so patients can move around.

Preparation

External long–term indwelling catheters, such as Hickmans, and internal catheters, such as Portacaths, are inserted in a surgical setting. Patients are positioned with their legs elevated during the procedure and are usually given a local anesthetic to help them relax. Some pediatric patients are given additional anesthesia.

Aftercare

After a long–term external or internal catheter is in place, patients have a chest x ray to assure that it is in the proper position, and that the procedure has occurred without complications.

Special concerns

Catheter Care

Indwelling catheters require frequent care so that they work properly and stay clean. The devices must be cleaned daily and handled carefully. They are flushed with **heparin** or saline, usually every day or every other day, depending on the device. Care techniques vary with the different catheters.

Risks

There are certain complications that may occur during catheter placement. Pneumothorax (air in the pleural cavity) or hemothorax (blood in the pleural cavity) rarely occurs during insertion, and is uncommon after the catheter is in place.

The catheter may leak due to a defect or as a result of being pinched between the collarbone and rib. More commonly, a blockage in the tubing may occur. The first sign of this problem is usually difficulty withdrawing blood, and the blockage can be confirmed with a chest x ray. Flushing will sometimes clear the blockage.

Another problem is that a catheter can move over the course of time. To get a dislodged catheter back into place, patients are sometimes instructed to raise their arms or attempt other maneuvers. If catheter movement recurs, the device will repeatedly malfunction, and may need to be removed.

Another risk over time is that of a vein thrombosis, commonly called a blood clot. The treatment varies for each patient. It may be as simple as changing the arm position or, in more serious cases, may involve removing the catheter. This condition may or may not have symptoms, but is important to diagnose because blood clots that break loose (emboli) can travel around the bloodstream and become potentially fatal.

Infection presents another risk, and may occur on the surface or internally, along the tubing itself. An infection at the surface is usually red, tender to the touch, and may contain discharge. A gram–positive bacteria, such as staphylococcus, is the most common culprit, although other bacteria have been found in these infections. Treatment is determined by the seriousness of the infection, the site of the problem, and the type of catheter involved. A minor infection may clear up with a topical antibiotic applied to the skin. In more severe cases, such as infections along the tubing, in the bloodstream, or in an implantable port, a course of antibiotics will be prescribed.

Resources

BOOKS

Dorland, I., and W. I. Newman, *Dorland's Illustrated Medical Dictionary*. 29th ed. Philadelphia, PA: W. B. Saunders Company, 2000.

Gajewski, James L., and Issam Raad. "Vascular Access Catheters and Devices." In *Cancer Treatment*. 5th ed. Philadelphia, PA: W.B. Saunders, 2001, pp. 225–29.

Libutti, Steven K., and Horne K. McDonald III. "Vascular Access and Specialized Techniques." In *Cancer: Principles & Practice of Oncology*. 6th ed. Philadelphia, PA: Lippincott, Williams & Wilkins, 2001, pp.760–67.

PERIODICALS

Crawford, Marilin, et al. "Peripherally Inserted Central Catheter Program." *Nursing Clinics of North America* 35 (June 2000): 349–59.

Rhonda Cloos, R.N.

Venoocclusive disease *see* **Bone marrow transplantation**

Vinblastine

Definition

Vinblastine is a drug used to treat certain types of **cancer**. Vinblastine is available under the trade names Velban and Velsar, and may also be referred to as vinblastine sulfate. The drug was previously known as vincaleukoblastine or VLB.

Purpose

Vinblastine is an antineoplastic agent used to treat **Hodgkin's disease**, non-Hodgkin's lymphomas, **mycosis fungoides**, cancer of the testis, **Kaposi's sarcoma**, Letterer-Siwe disease, as well as other cancers.

KEY TERMS

Alkaloid—A nitrogen-containing compound occurring in plants.

Microtubles—A tubular structure located in cells that help them to replicate.

Therapeutic index—A ratio of the maximum tolerated dose of a drug divided by the dose used in treatment.

Description

Vinblastine was approved by the Food and Drug Administration (FDA) in 1961.

Vinblastine is a naturally occurring compound that is extracted from periwinkle plants. It belongs to a group of chemicals called alkaloids. The chemical structure and biological action of vinblastine is similar to **vincristine** and **vinorelbine**.

Vinblastine prevents the formation of microtubules in cells. One of the roles of microtubules is to aid in the replication of cells. By disrupting this function, vinblastine inhibits cell replication, including the replication the cancer cells.

Vinblastine is one the most effective treatments for Hodgkin's disease, and is typically used in combination with **doxorubicin**, **bleomycin**, and **dacarbazine**. It is also used to treat non-Hodgkin's lymphomas, mycosis fungoides, and Letterer-Siwe disease. Vinblastine is also used to treat cancer of the testis in combination with other cancer drugs, and Kaposi's **sarcoma** alone or in combination with other drugs. Vinblastine is also used less frequently to treat other types of cancer.

Recommended dosage

Vinblastine is administered by intravenous injection at intervals of at least seven days. Blood tests may be necessary every seven days to ensure that enough white blood cells are present to continue treatment. The initial dose of vinblastine may be adjusted upward or downward depending on patient tolerance to the toxic side effects of treatment. The minimum recommended treatment duration is four to six weeks.

Precautions

Vinblastine must only be administered by individuals experienced in the use of this cancer chemotherapeutic agent. Vinblastine must only be administered intravenously, that is, directly into a vein. Accidental administration of vinblastine into the spinal cord fluid is a medical emergency that may result in death. Vinblastine has a low therapeutic index. It is unlikely there will be therapeutic benefit without toxic side effects. Certain complications can only be managed by a physician experienced in the use of cancer chemotherapeutic agents.

Because vinblastine is administered intravenously, the site of infusion and surrounding tissue should be monitored for signs of inflammation and irritation.

Adverse side effects are more likely in patients with malnutrition or skin ulceration.

Blood tests may be necessary to ensure that the number of white blood cells is adequate for treatment to continue. Vinblastine is not recommended for use in patients with low white blood cell levels. Infections should also be controlled before vinblastine treatment.

Patients should inform their physician if they experience sore throat, **fever**, chills, or sore mouth and any serious medical event.

Vinblastine may cause harm to a fetus when administered to pregnant women. Only in life-threatening situations, should this treatment be used during pregnancy. Women of childbearing age are advised not to become pregnant during treatment. Women should stop nursing before beginning treatment, due to the potential for serious adverse side effects in the nursing infants.

Side effects

The side effects of vinblastine treatment are usually related to the dose of drug and are generally reversible. Toxic side effects are more common in patients with poor liver function. Studies have also shown that patients with advanced **prostate cancer** experienced toxic side effects of **estramustine** phosphage (EMP) plus vinblastine (VBL) and from EMP alone.

A decrease in the number of white blood cells is the principal adverse side effect associated with vinblastine treatment. Blood tests will allow a doctor to determine if there are an adequate number of white blood cells to begin or continue treatment. **Nausea and vomiting** may occur, for which antiemetic agents are usually effective. Shortness of breath is a potentially severe side effect that patients should report to their doctor.

Additional side effects, including loss of appetite (**anorexia**), **diarrhea**, constipation, pain, rectal bleeding, dizziness, hearing impairment, and hair loss (**alopecia**) may occur.

Interactions

Drugs that may alter the metabolism of vinblastine, particularly itraconazole, should be used with caution due to the potential for interactions. Hearing impairment may be enhanced when vinblastine is used with other drugs that affect the ear. These drugs include platinum-containing **antineoplastic agents**, such as **cisplatin**. Seizures have been reported in patients taking vinblastine and **phenytoin**. The doses of vinblastine and phenytoin may need to be adjusted to decrease the chance of this problem.

Marc Scanio

Vincristine

Definition

Vincristine is a drug used to treat certain types of **cancer**. Vincristine is available under the trade names Oncovin, Vincasar, and Vincrex, and may also be referred to as vincristine sulfate, or VCR. The drug was previously known as leurocristine, or LCR.

Purpose

Vincristine is an antineoplastic agent used to treat leukemia, **Hodgkin's disease**, malignant lymphomas, **neuroblastoma**, **rhabdomyosarcoma**, **Wilms' tumor**, as well as other cancers.

Description

Vincristine was approved by the Food and Drug Administration (FDA) in 1984.

Vincristine is a naturally occurring compound that is extracted from periwinkle plants. It belongs to a group of chemicals called alkaloids. The chemical structure and biological action of vincristine is similar to **vinblastine** and **vinorelbine**.

Vincristine prevents the formation of microtubules in cells. One of the roles of microtubules is to aid in the replication of cells. By disrupting this function, vincristine inhibits cell replication, including the replication of the cancer cells.

Vincristine is used in combination with other drugs to treat leukemia. It is also used in combination with other drugs, such as **mechlorethamine**, **procarbazine**, and prednisone, to treat Hodgkin's disease. It is also used in combination to treat non-Hodgkin's

KEY TERMS

Alkaloid—A nitrogen-containing compound occurring in plants.

Microtubles—A tubular structure located in cells that help them to replicate.

Therapeutic index—A ratio of the maximum tolerated dose of a drug divided by the dose used in treatment.

lymphomas, neuroblastoma, rhabdomyosarcoma, and Wilms' tumor. Vincristine is also used less frequently to treat other types of cancer.

Recommended dosage

Vincristine is administered by intravenous injection once per week. The initial dose of vincristine may be adjusted upward or downward depending on patient tolerance to the toxic side effects of treatment.

Precautions

Vincristine must only be administered by individuals experienced in the use of this cancer chemotherapeutic agent. Vincristine must only be administered intravenously—that is, directly into a vein. Accidental administration of vincristine into the spinal cord fluid is a medical emergency that may result in death. Vincristine has a low therapeutic index. It is unlikely there will be therapeutic benefit without toxic side effects. Certain complications can only be managed by a physician experienced in the use of cancer chemotherapeutic agents.

Because vincristine is administered intravenously and is extremely irritating, the site of infusion and surrounding tissue should be monitored for signs of inflammation.

Some experts recommend blood tests to ensure that the number of white blood cells is adequate for treatment to continue. Infections should also be controlled before vincristine treatment starts.

Vincristine is not recommended for use in patients with the demyelinating form of Charcot-Marie-Tooth syndrome.

Vincristine is not recommended for patients receiving **radiation therapy** though a port in the liver.

Vincristine may cause harm to a fetus when administered to pregnant women. Only in life-threatening situations, should this treatment be used during pregnancy. Women of childbearing age are advised not to become pregnant during treatment. Women should stop nursing before beginning treatment, due to the potential for serious adverse side effects in the nursing infants.

Side effects

The side effects of vincristine treatment are usually related to the dose of drug and are generally reversible. Toxic side effects may be more common in patients with poor liver function.

Toxicity of the nervous system is the principal adverse side effect associated with vincristine treatment. This toxicity may cause numbness, pain, especially of the jaw, tingling, and headaches. Lengthy treatment at high doses may cause even more severe toxicity. Constipation is a common side effect. **Laxatives** and enemas are typically used to prevent severe constipation. Shortness of breath is a potentially severe side effect that patients should report to their doctor. Additional side effects, including rash, an increase or decrease in blood pressure, dizziness, **nausea and vomiting**, hearing impairment, and hair loss (**alopecia**) may occur.

Interactions

Drugs that may alter the metabolism of vincristine, particularly itraconazole, should be used with caution due to the potential for interactions. Hearing impairment may be enhanced when vincristine is used with other drugs that affect the ear. These drugs include platinum-containing **antineoplastic agents**, such as **cisplatin**. Seizures have been reported in patients taking vincristine and **phenytoin**. The doses of vincristine and phenytoin may need to be adjusted to decrease the chance of this problem.

Marc Scanio

Vindesine

Definition

Vindesine (desacetyl **vinblastine** amide sulfate) is a synthetic derivative of vinblastine. Vindesine is a **chemotherapy** drug that is given as a treatment for some types of **cancer**. This drug belongs to the group of **anticancer drugs** known as vinca alkaloids. Vindesine is also called vindesine sulfate, desacetylvinblastine

KEY TERMS

Acute lymphocytic leukemia—A rapidly progressing disease where too many immature infection-fighting white blood cells called lymphoblasts are found in the blood and bone marrow. It is also known as ALL or acute lymphoblastic leukemia.

Intravenous (or intravenously)—Into a vein.

Vinblastine—A vinca alkaloid. See definition for vinca alkaloid.

Vinca alkaloid—A group of cytotoxic alkaloids extracted from a flower called Madagascar periwinkle. Cytotoxic chemotherapy kills cells, especially cancer cells. Vinca alkaloids are cell cycle phase specific, and exert their effect during the M phase of cell mitosis and cause metaphase cell arrest and death. These drugs are for antineoplastic therapy (chemotherapy) for cancer treatment. Other vinca alkaloids are: vinblastine, vincristine, vindesine, and vinorelbine.

amide, DAVA, DVA, or VDS, and by its brand name, Eldisine.

Purpose

Vindesine is used primarily to treat **acute lymphocytic leukemia**. Less frequently, it is prescribed for use in **breast cancer**, blast crisis of **chronic myelocytic leukemia**, colorectal cancer, **non-small cell lung cancer**, and renal cell cancer (**kidney cancer**).

Description

Vindesine binds to particular proteins and causes cell arrest or cell death. Metabolized by the liver, vindesine is primarily excreted through the biliary system.

Vindesine is used in other countries around the world such as Britain, South Africa, and several European countries, but it is not approved by the Food and Drug Administration, and is thus not commercially available in the U.S. Eli Lilly discontinued Eldisine in Canada in 1998 to make way for newer, more effective vinca alkaloid drugs.

For acute lymphocytic leukemia (ALL), vindesine is effective in both adult and pediatric populations. As an agent used alone, vindesine has produced response rates ranging from 5% to 63% in several clinical studies. Vindesine has been used in combination therapy using the following drugs: **daunorubicin**, **asparaginase**, prednisone, **cytarabine**, and **etoposide**.

The clinical response rate in children (41%) is better than in adults (26%) for treatment of ALL. Vindesine with combination therapy has shown very high response rates in childhood ALL.

For treatment during the blast crisis of chronic myelocytic (or myelogenous) leukemia, overall response rates of 51% have been reported in adults when vindesine was used alone or in combination therapy with prednisone. Efficacy has not been demonstrated in pediatric groups.

Vindesine may be effective in treating breast cancer. When used alone, one clinical trial reported that vindesine showed an overall response rate of approximately 19% in treating advanced breast cancer.

Vindesine in combination with **cisplatin** is one of the most active treatments for non-small lung cancer, but **vinorelbine** substituted for vindesine has shown higher response rates in treating non-small lung cancer.

Vindesine is not effective for treating acute non-lymphocytic leukemia.

Recommended dosage

There are many dosing schedules that depend on the type of cancer, response to treatment, and other drugs that may be co-prescribed. Dosing guidelines also consider the white blood cell count.

Method of administration: Vindesine is injected intravenously through a fine needle (cannula). Alternatively, it may be given through a central line that is inserted under the skin into a vein near the collarbone.

- Intravenous administration for adults: Each one to two weeks a dose of 2-4 mg/m^2 is given; or each three to four weeks 1.5 mg/m^2/day for five to seven days as a continuous infusion is administered.
- Intravenous administration for children: Once a week with 4 mg/m^2 or twice weekly with 2 mg/m^2.

Precautions

Vindesine may cause fertility problems in men and women. In addition, it may harm the fetus or may damage sperm; therefore, it is not recommended for women to use vindesine during pregnancy or for men to father a child while taking this drug. The physician should be alerted immediately if pregnancy occurs. Due to possible secretion into breast milk, breast-feeding is not recommended.

Other considerations:

- Vindesine is potentially mutagenic or carcinogenic (cancer-causing).

- Vindesine may cause death if injected intrathecally (into the spinal cord). It is for intravenous use only.
- Prior injection sites should be carefully inspected because tissue damage may occur days or weeks after administration.
- Hepatic dysfunction increases the neurotoxic potential of this drug.
- Alert doctors or dentists about vindesine therapy before receiving any treatment.

Side effects

Possible side effects of vindesine therapy:

- Pain or tenderness may occur at the injection site.
- Hair loss (**alopecia**) is common.
- Vindesine can damage the surrounding tissue if it leaks into the tissue around the vein. If vindesine leaks under the skin, a burning or stinging sensation may be felt. Alert the doctor immediately if burning or stinging occurs while the drug is administered or if fluid is leaking from the site where the needle was inserted. Also tell the doctor if the area around the injection site becomes red or swollen at any time.
- Constipation or abdominal cramps; these can be alleviated by drinking plenty of water, eating a high-fiber diet, and light exercise.
- A temporary decrease in white blood cell count and platelets may occur.
- Numbing of the fingers or toes may occur over the course of treatment. It may take several months to return to normal.
- Diarrhea occurs infrequently.
- Mouth sores and ulcers may form.
- Nausea and vomiting rarely occurs.
- Anaphylaxis is rare.
- Jaw pain may be severe, but it is rare.
- Thrombocytopenia (a decrease in the number of platelets in the blood) or thrombocytosis; these conditions are also rare.

Interactions

Vindesine may interact with **mitomycin-C** (brand name Mutamycin), causing acute bronchospasm within minutes or hours following administration. **Phenytoin** (brand name Dilantin) may also interact with vindesine, leading to decreased serum levels of phenytoin.

Other drug interactions may occur with:

- Itraconazole
- Live virus and bacterial vaccines; when taking immune suppressing chemotherapy drugs, live vaccinations should not be given.
- Quinupristin/dalfopristin
- Rotavirus vaccine
- Warfarin

Crystal Heather Kaczkowski, MSc.

Vinorelbine

Definition

Vinorelbine is a drug used to treat certain types of lung **cancer**. Vinorelbine is available under the trade name Navelbine. The drug may also be referred to as vinorelbine tartrate, or didehydrodeoxynorvincaleukoblastine.

Purpose

Vinorelbine is an antineoplastic agent used to treat non-small cell lung **carcinoma**.

More recently, vinorelbine has been used in the palliative treatment of patients with advanced **esophageal cancer** and advanced **breast cancer**. Early reports of its effectiveness are encouraging.

Description

Vinorelbine was approved by the Food and Drug Administration (FDA) in 1994.

Vinorelbine is a semisynthetic derivative of **vinblastine**, a naturally occurring compound that is extracted from periwinkle plants. It belongs to a group of chemicals called vinca alkaloids. The chemical structure and biological action of vinorelbine is similar to vinblastine and **vincristine**.

Vinorelbine prevents the formation of microtubules in cells. One of the roles of microtubules is to aid in the replication of cells. By disrupting this function vinorelbine inhibits cell replication, including the replication the cancer cells.

Vinorelbine is used alone and in combination with **cisplatin** (another anticancer drug) to treat non-small cell lung carcinoma. It has been used in combination with other drugs to treat breast cancer. As of the early 2000s, vinorelbine was under investigation for the treatment for **cervical cancer**.

KEY TERMS

Alkaloid—A nitrogen-containing compound occurring in plants.

Microtubles—A tubular structure located in cells that help them to replicate.

Palliative—Referring to a treatment intended to relieve symptoms rather than cure a disease.

Therapeutic index—A ratio of the maximum tolerated dose of a drug divided by the dose used in treatment.

Recommended dosage

Vinorelbine is administered by intravenous injection (directly into a vein) once per week. The initial dose may be adjusted downward depending on patient tolerance to the toxic side effects of treatment. If toxic effects are severe, vinorelbine treatment may be delayed or discontinued.

Precautions

Vinorelbine must be administered only by individuals experienced in the use of this cancer chemotherapeutic agent. Vinorelbine must only be administered intravenously. Accidental administration of vinorelbine into the spinal cord fluid is a medical emergency that may result in death. Vinorelbine has a low therapeutic index, which means it is unlikely there will be therapeutic benefit without toxic side effects. Certain complications can only be managed by a physician experienced in the use of cancer chemotherapeutic agents.

Because vinorelbine is administered intravenously and is extremely irritating, the site of infusion and surrounding tissue should be monitored for signs of inflammation.

Blood tests are recommended to ensure that bone marrow function and the number of white blood cells is adequate for treatment to continue. Infections should also be controlled before vinorelbine treatment starts. Special caution should be used with patients whose bone marrow reserves have been reduced by previous radiation or **chemotherapy** treatment.

Vinorelbine may cause harm to a fetus when administered to pregnant women. Only in life-threatening situations should this treatment be used during pregnancy. Women of childbearing age are advised not to become pregnant during treatment. Women should stop nursing before beginning treatment due to the potential for serious adverse side effects in the nursing infants.

The safety of vinorelbine in children under 18 years of age has not been established.

Side effects

The side effects of vinorelbine treatment are usually related to the dose of drug and are generally reversible. It is possible that toxic side effects may be more common in patients with poor liver function, and should be used with caution in those patients.

Decreased bone marrow function is the principal adverse side effect. This can reduce the number of white blood cells and increase the chance of infections. Patients should report **fever** or chills to their doctors immediately. Patients should also inform their doctor if they experience abdominal pain, constipation, or an increase in shortness of breath.

Toxicity of the nervous system is another side effect. Shortness of breath is a potentially severe side effect that patients should report to their doctor. Additional side effects, including fever, **anemia**, an increase or decrease in blood pressure, dizziness, **nausea and vomiting**, hearing impairment, and hair loss (**alopecia**) may occur.

Several cases of heart attacks related to vinorelbine have been reported. A group of French researchers estimates that about 1% of patients treated with vinorelbine will develop heart problems; however, vinorelbine does not appear to have a higher rate of these side effects than other drugs in its class.

Interactions

The use of vinorelbine in combination with another anticancer drug, **mitomycin-C**, has caused severe shortness of breath. Patients taking vinorelbine and cisplatin are more likely to experience a decrease in the number of white blood cells. This side effect should be carefully monitored to ensure that the number of white blood cells is adequate for treatment to continue. Patients taking vinorelbine and another anticancer drug, paclitaxel, may be more likely to experience toxicity of the nervous system, and should be carefully monitored for this. Drugs that may alter the metabolism of vinorelbine should be used with caution due to the potential for interactions.

Patients who are treated with vinorelbine during or following radiotherapy may become hypersensitive to radiation treatment.

Resources

BOOKS

Beers, Mark H., MD, and Robert Berkow, MD, editors. "Bronchogenic Carcinoma." In *The Merck Manual of Diagnosis and Therapy*. Whitehouse Station, NJ: Merck Research Laboratories, 2007.

Karch, A. M. *Lippincott's Nursing Drug Guide*. Springhouse, PA: Lippincott Williams & Wilkins, 2003.

PERIODICALS

Garrone, O., E. Principe, M. Occelli, et al. "A Phase II Study of Epirubicin, Vinorelbine and Cisplatin in Advanced Breast Cancer." *Anticancer Drugs* 15 (January 2004): 23–27.

Lapeyre-Mestre, M., N. Gregoire, R. Bugat, and J. L. Montastruc. "Vinorelbine-Related Cardiac Events: A Meta-Analysis of Randomized Clinical Trials." *Fundamental and Clinical Pharmacology* 18 (February 2004): 97–105.

Razis, E., P. Kosmidis, G. Aravantinos, et al. "Second-Line Chemotherapy with 5-fluorouracil and Vinorelbine in Anthracycline and Taxane-Pretreated Patients with Metastatic Breast Cancer." *Cancer Investigation* 22 (January 2004): 10–15.

Richel, D. J., and W. L. Vervenne. "Systemic Treatment of Oesophageal Cancer." *European Journal of Gastroenterology and Hepatology* 16 (March 2004): 249–254.

ORGANIZATIONS

American Society of Health-System Pharmacists (ASHP). 7272 Wisconsin Avenue, Bethesda, MD 20814. (301) 657-3000. www.ashp.org.

United States Food and Drug Administration (FDA). 5600 Fishers Lane, Rockville, MD 20857-0001. (888) INFO-FDA. www.fda.gov.

Marc Scanio
Rebecca J. Frey, PhD

Viruses *see* **AIDS-related cancers; Epstein-Barr virus; Human papilloma virus**

Vitamins

Definition

Vitamins are compounds that are essential in small amounts for proper body function and growth. Vitamins are either fat soluble: A, D, E, and K; or water soluble: vitamin B and C. The B vitamins include vitamins B_1(thiamine), B_2 (riboflavin), and B_6 (pyridoxine), pantothenic acid, niacin, biotin, **folic acid** (folate), and vitamin B_{12} (cobalamin). Vitamins also may be referred to as micronutrients.

KEY TERMS

Antioxidant—A substance that prevents damage caused by free radicals.

Cancer—A term for diseases in which abnormal cells divide without control. Cancer cells can invade nearby tissues and can spread through the bloodstream and lymphatic system to other parts of the body.

Free radicals—Free radicals are highly reactive chemicals that often contain oxygen. They are produced when molecules are split to give products that have unpaired electrons. This process is referred to as oxidation.

Malignant (also malignancy)—Meaning cancerous; a tumor or growth that often destroys surrounding tissue and spreads to other parts of the body.

Oxidative stress—A condition in which antioxidant levels are lower than normal. Antioxidant levels usually are measured in blood plasma.

Description

A guide to the amount an average person needs each day to remain healthy has been determined for each vitamin. In the United States, this guide is called the recommended daily allowance (RDA). Consuming too little of certain vitamins may lead to a nutrient deficiency. Consuming too much of certain vitamins may lead to nutrient toxicity.

Consumption of a wide variety of foods that have adequate vitamins and minerals is the basis of a healthy diet. Good nutrition may assist in the prevention of **cancer** or may help cancer patients to feel better and fight **infection** during treatments. Obtaining nutrients through food remains the best method for obtaining vitamins; however, requirements may be higher because of the tumor or cancer therapy. Therefore, supplements may be necessary.

The following vitamins are important in a healthy diet and also may assist in **cancer prevention**. Their role in maintaining health and the best food sources are listed below.

Vitamin A (retinal, carotene)

- role in growth and repair of body tissues
- important in night vision
- immune function

- Best sources: eggs, dark green and yellow fruits and vegetables, low-fat dairy products, liver

Vitamin B_6 (pyridoxine)

- role in formation of antibodies
- important in carbohydrate and protein metabolism
- red blood cells
- nerve function
- Best sources: lean meat, fish, poultry, whole grains, and potatoes

Folic acid (folate)

- assists in red blood cell formation
- important in protein metabolism
- growth and cell division
- Best sources: green leafy vegetables, poultry, dried beans, fortified cereals, nuts, and oranges

Vitamin C (ascorbic acid)

- resistance to infection
- important in collagen maintenance
- contributes to wound healing
- strengthens blood vessels
- assists in maintaining healthy gums
- Best sources: citrus fruits, tomatoes, melons, broccoli, green and red peppers, and berries

Vitamin E (tocopherol)

- may assist in immune function
- important in preventing oxidation of red blood cells and cell membranes
- Best sources: vegetable oils, wheat germ, nuts, dark green vegetables, beans, and whole grains

Purpose

Specific nutrients have been linked to prevention of several cancers of the colon, breast, prostate, stomach, and other types of tumors. A high intake of fruits and vegetables as well as fiber appears particularly protective, while a diet high in fat has been implicated as a cancer risk.

Vitamins important for cancer prevention

Antioxidant vitamins are believed to protect the body from harmful free radicals that can contribute to diseases such as cancer. Antioxidant vitamins include vitamin A, C, and E. However, doses too high may increase oxidative stress and therefore may increase cancer risk.

A diet rich in fruits and vegetables (containing B_6, folate, and niacin) appears to protect against **stomach cancer** and in particular, intestinal cancer.

One study reported that cruciferous vegetables, especially broccoli, brussel sprouts, cauliflower, and cabbage were associated with a decreased risk of **prostate cancer**. Other foods, such as carrots, beans, and cooked tomatoes, also were associated with a lower risk.

A component of Vitamin E, tocotrienol, has been linked to a decreased risk of **breast cancer** in lab animals. Tocotrienol has been shown to readily kill tumor cells grown in culture. Tocotrienol is not the same type of substance found in generic Vitamin E supplements, but is plentiful in palm oil. Palm oil is difficult to obtain in the Western world, but lower concentrations of tocotrienol are found in rice bran oil and wheat bran oil. In 2004, research showed that the nutrient calcium and vitamin D worked together, not separately, to lower risk of colorectal cancer.

Researchers state that no single nutrient is the answer, but that the effects are cumulative and depend on eating a variety of fruits and vegetables. Because there are many more nutrients available in foods such as fruits and vegetables than in vitamin supplements, food is the best source for acquiring needed vitamins and minerals.

Special concerns

For many years, debate has continued regarding taking vitamin supplements to prevent cancer. In 2004, the U.S. Preventive Services Task Force concluded that the evidence is inadequate to recommend supplementation of vitamins A, C, or E, multivitamins with folic acid, or antioxidant combinations to decrease the risk of cancer. Beta-carotene supplements should not be used in patients with no symptoms because there is no evidence of risk reduction and some evidence that these supplements may cause harm to some patients.

There are concerns regarding antioxidant levels during **chemotherapy** and **radiation therapy**. Researchers report large amounts of Vitamin C are consumed by cancerous tumors during chemotherapy in studies with mice. Vitamin C is an antioxidant that consumes free radicals and is thought to perhaps interfere with the process of killing cancer cells during chemotherapy or radiation therapy. Cancer patients undergoing chemotherapy are advised against taking large amounts of Vitamin C. Another research study also has warned cancer patients about vitamin A and vitamin E during chemotherapy because it has demonstrated a protective effect on cancer cells in mice. These **antioxidants** may protect not only the normal cells from being destroyed, but also may protect dangerous cancer cells from being destroyed during cancer treatment. The researchers suggest an antioxidant-depleted diet may be prudent during cancer therapy.

Smokers are advised not to consume a diet high in beta-carotene (Vitamin A) because research has shown a link to increased lung cancer incidence.

Alternative and complementary therapies

There are a great many claims about particular vitamin and or antioxidants having beneficial health effects. Proper nutrition with an adequate diet is the best way to obtain vitamins, but a supplement may be required when intake is inadequate. It is important to check with a dietitian or doctor before taking nutritional supplements or alternative therapies because they may interfere with cancer medications or treatments.

Resources

BOOKS

Quillin, Patrick, and Noreen Quillin. *Beating Cancer With Nutrition—Revised.* Sun Lakes, AZ: Bookworld Services, 2001.

PERIODICALS

"Calcium and Vitamin D Collaborate to Reduce Cancer Risk." *Health & Medicine Week* January 5, 2004: 190.

Sadovsky, Richard. "Can Vitamins Prevent Cancer and Heart Disease?" *American Family Physician* February 1, 2004: 631.

Singletary, Keith. "Diet, Natural Products and Cancer Chemoprevention." *Journal of Nutrition* 130 (2000): 465–6.

Willett, Walter C. "Diet and Cancer." *The Oncologist* 5, no. 5 (2000): 393–404.

ORGANIZATIONS

The National Cancer Institute (NCI). Public Inquiries Office: Building 31, Room 10A31, 31 Center Dr., MSC 2580, Betheseda, MD 20892-2580 (301) 435-3848, (800) 4-CANCER. http://cancer.gov/publications/, http://cancertrials.nci.nih.gov, http://cancernet.nci.nih.gov.

National Center for Complementary and Alternative Medicine (NCCAM). 31 Center Dr., Room #5B-58, Bethesda, MD 20892-2182. (800) NIH-NCAM, Fax (301) 495-4957. http://nccam.nih.gov.

Crystal Heather Kaczkowski, MSc.
Teresa G. Odle

von Hippel-Lindau disease

Definition

von Hippel-Lindau disease (VHL) is a rare familial **cancer** syndrome. A person with VHL can develop both benign and malignant tumors and cysts in many different organs in the body. Tumors and cysts most commonly develop in the brain and spine, eyes, kidneys, adrenal glands, pancreas, and inner ear.

KEY TERMS

Benign—Not cancerous, not able to spread to new places in the body.

Cyst—A fluid filled sac that can be normal or abnormal.

Hemangioblastoma—A benign tumor caused by the abnormal growth of blood vessels.

Malignant—Cancerous, able to spread to new places in the body.

Mutation—A change in the DNA code.

Tumor—An abnormal growth caused by the uncontrolled growth of cells.

Description

VHL does not have a predictable set of symptoms. VHL affects approximately 1 in 35,000 people, and affects men and women equally. Some families may have different symptoms than other families. Even within a family, there may be people with very mild signs of VHL, and others with more severe medical problems. In one study of a Chinese family with 47 members, 4 were diagnosed as carriers of the VHL gene while 18 others were diagnosed as having VHL itself. Of these 18 patients, 10 had renal cell **carcinoma**, 9 had central nervous system hemangioblastomas, and 7 had multiple pancreatic cysts. The age when symptoms develop can range from infancy to late adulthood, although most people with VHL will have some clinical symptoms by age 65. It is important for a person with VHL to have regular physical examinations to check for signs of VHL in all areas of the body that may be affected.

Tumors in the brain and spine, or central nervous system, are called hemangioblastomas. Hemangioblastomas are benign growths (not cancerous), but they may cause such symptoms as headaches and balance problems if they are growing in tight spaces and pressing on surrounding tissues or nerves. The eye tumors in VHL are called retinal angiomas or retinal hemangioblastomas, and may cause vision problems and blindness if they are not treated. Kidney cysts rarely cause problems, but the kidney tumors can be malignant, and are called renal cell carcinoma. Tumors in the adrenal glands are called pheochromocytomas.

Pheochromocytomas are usually not malignant, but they can cause serious medical problems if untreated. This is because pheochromocytomas secrete hormones that can raise blood pressure to dangerous levels, causing heart attacks or strokes. Benign cysts can be found in the pancreas, and pancreatic islet cell tumors can also occur. These tumors grow very slowly and are rarely malignant. Tumors that grow in the ear are called endolymphatic sac tumors, which can result in hearing loss if untreated. Occasionally men and women with VHL will have infertility problems if cysts are present in certain places in the reproductive organs, such as the epididymis (a duct in the testes)in men or the fallopian tubes in women. A few male patients with VHL develop large testicular masses that can be treated successfully with steroid therapy.

Diagnosis

A clinical diagnosis of VHL can be made in a person with a family history of VHL if he or she has a single retinal angioma, central nervous system hemangioblastoma, or **pheochromocytoma**, or if he or she has renal cell carcinoma. If there is no known family history of VHL, two or more retinal or central nervous system hemangioblastomas must be present, or one retinal or central nervous system hemangioblastoma and one other feature of VHL. Melmon and Rosen published these criteria in 1964, when they first described VHL as a disease with a specific set of features. Because not all people with VHL will meet these diagnostic criteria, VHL may be an under–diagnosed disease. **Genetic testing** can confirm a diagnosis of VHL in a person with clinical symptoms, who may or may not meet the above diagnostic criteria.

Causes

VHL is a genetic disease caused by a mutation of the VHL tumor suppressor gene on chromosome three. It is inherited as an autosomal dominant condition, which means that a person with VHL has a 50% chance of passing it on to each of his or her children. Usually a person with VHL will have a family history of VHL (a parent or sibling who also has VHL), but occasionally he or she is the first person in the family to have VHL. Screening and/or genetic testing of family members can help establish who is at risk for developing VHL. Identification of a person with VHL in a family may result in other family members with more mild symptoms being diagnosed, and subsequently receiving appropriate screening and medical care.

Risks

The United States National Institutes of Health (NIH) has determined risk ranges for a person with VHL to develop certain tumors. Persons with VHL have a 21–72% chance of developing hemangioblastomas of the brain or spinal cord, a 43–60% chance of developing retinal angiomas, a 24–45% chance of developing cysts and tumors of the kidney, an 8–37% chance of developing pancreatic cysts, and an 8–17% chance of developing pancreatic islet cell tumors. It has been proposed that VHL be divided into subtypes depending on the types of tumors present in a family. It is likely that in the future, specific risk figures will be available for the different types of tumors depending on the specific genetic mutation in a family.

Genetic testing

Almost 100% of people with VHL will have an identifiable mutation in the VHL gene. There have been many different mutations found in the VHL gene, but all persons with VHL in the same family will have the same mutation. If a mutation is known in a family, genetic testing can be done on family members who have not had any symptoms of VHL. A person who tests positive for the family mutation is at risk for developing symptoms of VHL and can pass the mutation on to his or her children. A person who tests negative for the family mutation is not at risk for developing symptoms of VHL, and his or her children are not at risk for developing VHL. Screening is needed for people who test positive for a VHL mutation, and people who are found not to have the family mutation can be spared from lifelong screening procedures. Genetic testing can also be used to determine if a pregnant woman is carrying a fetus affected with VHL. Other techniques may become available which allow selection of an unaffected fetus prior to conception. Families work with a physician, geneticist, or genetic counselor familiar with the most up-to-date information on VHL when having genetic testing, in order to understand the risks, benefits, and current technological limitations prior to testing.

Screening and Treatment

Regular screening and monitoring of tumors in people with VHL allows early detection and treatment, before serious complications can occur. A physician familiar with all aspects of VHL can coordinate screening with a variety of specialists, such as an ophthalmologist for eye examinations. Ultrasounds, **computed tomography** scans (CT), and

magnetic resonance imaging (MRI) may be used to screen and detect tumors and cysts. Whether or not treatment is necessary depends on the size of the tumor, where it is growing, what the symptoms are, and if the tumor is benign or malignant. Treatment for benign tumors may include surgery or laser treatments. Cancer in people with VHL is treated just as it would be in someone in the general population with that type of cancer. People with VHL who develop cancer have a better prognosis if the cancer is detected at an earlier stage before it has spread. Urine tests, ultrasound, CT and/or MRI screen for pheochromocytomas. It is especially important to screen for pheochromocytomas prior to surgery, because an undiagnosed pheochromocytoma can cause complications during surgery. Prior to becoming pregnant, a woman should have a full physical examination looking for all signs of VHL, but most importantly pheochromocytomas. It is best for a woman to avoid VHL-related surgery while she is pregnant unless medically necessary. Pregnancy itself does not seem to make VHL worse or make the tumors grow faster, but any tumors that are present should be evaluated, and a plan for surgical removal or monitoring should be in place.

See also Cancer genetics; Familial cancer syndrome; Kidney cancer.

Resources

BOOKS

Beers, Mark H., MD, and Robert Berkow, MD, editors. "Adrenal Disorders." In *The Merck Manual of Diagnosis and Therapy*. Whitehouse Station, NJ: Merck Research Laboratories, 2007.

Beers, Mark H., MD, and Robert Berkow, MD, editors. "Cancer Genetics." In *The Merck Manual of Diagnosis and Therapy*. Whitehouse Station, NJ: Merck Research Laboratories, 2007.

PERIODICALS

Huang, Y. R., J. Zhang, J. D. Wang, and X. D. Fan. "Genetic Study of a Large Chinese Kindred with von Hippel-Lindau Disease." *Chinese Medical Journal* 117 (April 2004): 552–557.

Levy, M., and S. Richard. "Attitudes of von Hippel–Lindau Disease Patients towards Presymptomatic Genetic Diagnosis in Children and Prenatal Diagnosis." *Journal of Medical Genetics* 37 (June 1, 2000): 476–478.

Sgambati, M.T., et al. "Mosaicism in von Hippel–Lindau Disease: Lessons from Kindreds with Germline Mutations Identified in Offspring with Mosaic Parents." *American Journal of Human Genetics* 66 (2000): 84–91.

Vortmeyer, A. O., Q. Yuan, Y. S. Lee, et al. "Developmental Effects of von Hippel-Lindau Gene Deficiency." *Annals of Neurology* 55 (May 2004): 721–728.

Weeks, D. C., M. M. Walther, C. A. Stratakis, et al. "Bilateral Testicular Adrenal Rests after Bilateral Adrenalectomies in a Cushingoid Patient with von Hippel-Lindau Disease." *Urology* 63 (May 2004): 981–982.

OTHER

The VHL Handbook: What You Need to Know about VHL. A Reference Handbook for people with von Hippel–Lindau Disease, their families, and support personnel. Updated 2005. http://www.vhl.org/handbook/index.html.

ORGANIZATIONS

VHL Family Alliance. 171 Clinton Road, Brookline, Massachusetts 02445. (617) 277–5667, (800) 767–4VHL. Email: info@vhl.org. http://www.vhl.org. Dedicated to improving diagnosis, treatment, and quality of life for individuals and families affected by VHL.

Laura L. Stein, M.S., C.G.C.
Rebecca J. Frey, PhD

von Recklinghausen's neurofibromatosis

Definition

Von Recklinghausen's neurofibromatosis is also called von Recklinghausen disease, or simply neurofibromatosis (NF)1. It is an automsomal dominant hereditary disorder. NF is the most common neurological disorder caused by a single gene. Patients develop multiple soft tumors (neurofibromas) and very often skin spots (freckling AND café au lait spots). The tumors occur under the skin and throughout the nervous system. The disease is named for Friedrich Daniel von Recklinghausen (1833–1910), a German pathologist, although cases of it have been described in European medical publications since the sixteenth century.

Description

There are three types of neurofibromatosis, although some researchers have proposed as many as eight categories. The two main types of neurofibromatosis are neurofibromatosis 1 (NF1), which affects about 85% of patients diagnosed with neurofibromatosis, and neurofibromatosis 2 (NF2), which accounts for another 10% of patients. NF1 affects approximately 1 in 2,000 to 1 in 5,000 births worldwide. NF2 affects 1 in 35,000 to 1 in 40,000 births worldwide. Recently, schwannomatosis has been recognized as a rare form of NF. Since NF is the most common neurological disorder, NF is more prevalent than the

KEY TERMS

Audiometry—Testing a person's hearing by exposing ear to sounds in a soundproof room.

Autosomal dominant—Genetic information on a single non-sex chromosome that is expressed with only one copy of a gene. Child of an affected parent has a 50% chance of inheriting an autosomal dominant gene.

Cancer—Abnormal and uncontrolled growth of cells that can invade surrounding tissues and other parts of the body. Although some cancers are treatable, recurrence and death from cancer can occur.

Cataract—Lens of eye loses transparency and becomes cloudy. Cloudiness blocks light rays entering the eye that may lead to blindness.

Chromosome—A structure within the nucleus of every cell, that contains genetic information governing the organism's development. There are 22 non-sex chromosomes and one sex chromosome.

Ependymoma—Tumor that grows from cells that line the cavities of brain ventricles and spinal cord.

Gamma knife—A type of highly focused radiation therapy.

Gene—Piece of information contained on a chromosome. A chromosome is made of many genes.

Magnetic resonance imaging—Magnetic resonance imaging (MRI) measures the response of tissues to magnetic fields to produce detailed pictures of the body, including the brain.

Meningioma—Tumor that grows from the protective brain and spinal cord membrane cells (meninges).

Mutation—A permanent change to the genetic code of an organism. Once established, a mutation can be passed on to offspring.

Neurofibroma—A soft tumor usually located on a nerve.

Radiation therapy—Exposing tumor cells to controlled doses of x-ray irradiation for treatment. Although tumor cells are susceptible to irradiation, surrounding tissues will also be damaged. Radiation therapy alone rarely cures a tumor, but can be useful when used in conjunction with other forms of therapy or when a patient cannot tolerate other forms of therapy.

Schwannoma—Tumor that grows from the cells that line the nerves of the body (Schwann cells).

Tinnitus—Noises in the ear that can include ringing, whistling, or booming.

Tumor—An abnormally multiplying mass of cells. Tumors that invade surrounding tissues and other parts of the body are malignant and considered a cancer. Non-malignant tumors do not invade surrounding tissues and other parts of the body. Malignant and non-malignant tumors can cause severe symptoms and death.

number of people affected by cystic fibrosis, hereditary muscular dystrophy, Huntington's disease, and Tay-Sachs disease combined. In addition to skin and nervous system tumors and skin freckling, NF can lead to disfigurement, blindness, deafness, skeletal abnormalities, loss of limbs, malignancies, and learning disabilities. The degree a person is affected with a form of neurofibromatosis may vary greatly between patients.

Causes and symptoms

A defective gene causes NF1 and NF2. NF1 is due to a defect on chromosome 17q. NF2 results from a defect on chromosome 22. Both neurofibromatosis disorders are inherited in an autosomal dominant fashion. In an autosomal dominant disease, one copy of a defective gene will cause the disease. However, family pattern of NF is only evident for about 50% to 70% of all NF cases. The remaining cases of NF are due to a spontaneous mutation (a change in a person's gene rather than a mutation inherited from a parent). As with an inherited mutated gene, a person with a spontaneously mutated gene has a 50% chance of passing the spontaneously mutated gene to any offspring.

NF1 has a number of possible symptoms:

- Five or more light brown skin spots (café au lait spots, a French term meaning "coffee with milk"). The skin spots measure more than 0.2 inches (5 millimeters) in diameter in patients under the age of puberty or more than 0.6 inches (15 millimeters) in diameter across in adults and children over the age of puberty. Nearly all NF1 patients display café au lait spots.
- Multiple freckles in the armpit or groin area.
- Ninety percent of patients with NF1 have tiny tumors in the iris (colored area of the eye) called Lisch nodules (iris nevi).

QUESTIONS TO ASK THE DOCTOR

- How can I tell if I have neurofibromatosis?
- Which type of neurofibromatosis do I have?
- Will I develop tumors? Will they be cancerous?
- Is my neurofibromatosis genetic?
- What medical tests are important?
- What treatments are available for neurofibromatosis?
- Will I die from neurofibromatosis?

- Two or more neurofibromas distributed over the body. Neurofibromas are soft tumors and are the hallmark of NF1. Neurofibromas occur under the skin, often located along nerves or within the gastrointestinal tract. Neurofibromas are small and rubbery, and the skin overlying them may be somewhat purple in color.
- Skeletal deformities, such as a twisted spine (scoliosis), curved spine (humpback), or bowed legs.
- Tumors along the optic nerve, which cause visual disturbances in about 20% of patients.
- The presence of NF1 in a patient's parent, child, or sibling.

There are very high rates of speech impairment, learning disabilities, and attention deficit disorder in children with NF1. Other complications include the development of a seizure disorder, or the abnormal accumulation of fluid within the brain (hydrocephalus). A number of cancers are more common in patients with NF1. These include a variety of types of malignant **brain tumors**, as well as leukemia, and cancerous tumors of certain muscles (**rhabdomyosarcoma**), the adrenal glands (**pheochromocytoma**), or the kidneys (**Wilms' tumor**). Symptoms are often visible at birth or during infancy, and almost always by the time a child is about 10 years old.

In contrast to patients with NF1, patients with NF2 have few, if any, café au lait spots or tumors under the skin. Patients with NF2 most commonly have tumors (schwannomas) on the eighth cranial nerve (one of 12 pairs of nerves that enter or emerge from the brain), and occasionally on other nerves. The location of the schwann cell derived tumors determines the effect on the body. The characteristic symptoms of NF2 include dysfunction in hearing, ringing in the ears (tinnitus), and body balance. The common characteristic symptoms of NF2 are due to tumors along the acoustic and vestibular branches of the eighth cranial nerve. Tumors that occur on neighboring nervous system structures may cause weakness of the muscles of the face, headache, dizziness, numbness, and weakness in an arm or leg. Cloudy areas on the lens of the eye (called cataracts) frequently develop at an early age. As in NF1, the chance of brain tumors developing is unusually high. Symptoms of NF2 may not begin until after puberty.

Multiple schwannomas on cranial, spinal, and peripheral nerves characterize schwannomatosis. People with schwannomatosis usually have greater problems with pain than with neurological disability. The first symptom of schwannomatosis is usually pain in any part of the body without any source. It can be several years before a tumor is found. About one-third of patients with schwannomatosis have tumors in a single part of the body, such as an arm, leg, or segment of spine. People with schwannomatosis do not develop vestibular tumors or any other kinds of tumors (such as meningiomas, ependymomas, or astrocytomas), do not go deaf, and do not have learning disabilities.

Diagnosis

Diagnosis of a form of neurofibromatosis is based on the symptoms outlined above. Although a visual inspection may be sufficient for inspection of tumors for a clinical diagnosis of neurofibromatosis, **magnetic resonance imaging** (MRI) is the most useful type of imaging study for early diagnosis of tumors while CT scans are better for detecting skeletal abnormalities. Diagnosis of NF1 requires that at least two of the above listed symptoms are present. A slit lamp is used to visualize the presence of any Lisch nodules in a person's eye. A person with a parent, sibling, or child with NF1 is another tool used to diagnose a person with NF1.

NF2 can be diagnosed three different ways and with symptoms different from NF1 symptoms:

- The presence of bilateral cranial eighth nerve tumors.
- A person who has a parent, sibling, or child with NF2 and a unilateral eighth nerve tumor (vestibular schwannoma or acoustic neuroma).
- A person who has a parent, sibling, or child with NF2 and any two of the following: glioma, meningioma, neurofibroma, schwannoma, or an early age cataract.

The presence of multiple schwannomas may be a symptom of NF2 or schwannomatosis. An older person with multiple schwannomas and no hearing loss probably does not have NF2. A high-quality MRI scan should be used to detect any possible vestibular tumors to differentiate between NF2 and schwannomatosis in a younger person with multiple schwannomas or any person with hearing loss and multiple schwannomas.

In prepubertal children a yearly assessment including blood pressure measurement, eye examination, development screening, and neurologic examination is recommended.

Monitoring the progression of neurofibromatosis involves careful testing of vision and hearing (audiometry). X-ray studies of the bones are frequently done to watch for the development of deformities. CT scans and MRI scans are performed to track the development/progression of tumors in the brain and along the nerves. Auditory evoked potentials (the electric response evoked in the cerebral cortex by stimulation of the acoustic nerve) may be helpful to determine involvement of the acoustic nerve, and EEG (electroencephalogram, a record of electrical currents in the brain) may be needed for patients with suspected seizures.

Treatment

There are no cures for any form of neurofibromatosis. To some extent, the symptoms of NF1 and NF2 can be treated individually. Skin tumors can be surgically removed. Some brain tumors, and tumors along the nerves, can be surgically removed, or treated with drugs (**chemotherapy**) or x-ray treatments (**radiation therapy**, including gamma knife therapy). Twisting or curving of the spine and bowed legs may require surgical treatment or the wearing of a special brace.

Prognosis

Prognosis varies depending on the types of tumors which an individual develops. In general, however, patients with neurofibromatosis have a shortened life expectancy; the average age at death is 55–59 years, compared with 70–74 years for the general United States population. As tumors grow, they begin to destroy surrounding nerves and structures. Ultimately, this destruction can result in blindness, deafness, increasingly poor balance, and increasing difficulty with the coordination necessary for walking. Deformities of the bones and spine can also interfere with walking and movement. When cancers develop, prognosis worsens according to the specific type of **cancer**.

Clinical Trials

As of 2009 the National Cancer Institute (NCI) is sponsoring a number of clinical trails regarding neurofibromatosis. One such study is an evaluation of Lapatinib, a drug that may reduce tumor growth in NF2. It is hoped that Lapatinib may prove to be an effective drug treatment for the disorder.

The use of an auditory brainstem implant (ABI) as part of hearing rehabilitation in patients with NF2 has been tested in Europe and the United States.

Prevention

There is no known way to prevent the cases of NF that are due to a spontaneous change in the genes (mutation). Since genetic tests for NF1 and NF2 are available, new cases of inherited NF can be prevented with careful genetic counseling. A person with NF can be made to understand that each of his or her offspring has a 50% chance of also having NF. When a parent has NF, and the specific genetic defect causing the parent's disease has been identified, prenatal tests can be performed on the fetus during pregnancy. Amniocentesis and chorionic villus sampling are two techniques that allow small amounts of the baby's cells to be removed for examination. The tissue can then be examined for the presence of the parent's genetic defect. Some families choose to use this information in order to prepare for the arrival of a child with a serious medical problem. Other families may choose not to continue the pregnancy. **Genetic testing** may also be useful for evaluating individuals with a family history of neurofibromatosis, who do not yet show symptoms.

Resources

BOOKS

Beers, Mark H., MD, and Robert Berkow, MD, editors. "Disorders of the Peripheral Nervous System." In *The Merck Manual of Diagnosis and Therapy*. Whitehouse Station, NJ: Merck Research Laboratories, 2007.

PERIODICALS

Bance, M., and R.T. Ramsden. "Management of Neurofibromatosis Type 2." *Ear Nose & Throat Journal* 78, no. 2 (1999): 91–4.

Evans, D.G. "Neurofibromatosis Type 2: Genetic and Clinical Features." *Ear Nose & Throat Journal* 78, no. 2 (1999): 97–100.

Gillespie, J.E. "Imaging in Neurofibromatosis Type 2: Screening Using Magnetic Resonance Imaging." *Ear Nose & Throat Journal* 78, no. 2 (1999): 102–9.

Huson, S.M. "What Level of Care for the Neurofibromatoses?" *Lancet* 353, no. 9159 (1999): 1114–6.

Khan, Ali Nawaz, MBBS, and Ian Turnbull, MD. "Neurofibromatosis Type 1." *eMedicine* February 10, 2004. http://emedicine.com/radio/topic474.htm.

Laszig, R., et al. "Central Electrical Stimulation of the Auditory Pathway in Neurofibromatosis Type 2." *Ear Nose & Throat Journal* 78, no. 2 (1999): 110–7.

Lynch, H. T., T. G. Shaw, and J. F. Lynch. "Inherited Predisposition to Cancer: A Historical Overview." *American Journal of Medical Genetics, Part C: Seminars in Medical Genetics* 129 (August 15, 2004): 5–22.

Rasmussen, S.A., and J.M. Friedman. "NF1 Gene and Neurofibromatosis." *American Journal of Epidemiology* 151, no. 1 (2000): 33–40.

ORGANIZATIONS

Acoustic Neuroma Association. 600 Peachtree Parkway, Suite 108, Cumming, GA, 30041-6899. (770) 205-8211. http://www.anausa.org.

March of Dimes Birth Defects Foundation. National Office, 1275 Mamaroneck Ave., White Plains, NY 10605. http://www.modimes.org.

Massachusetts General Hospital Neurofibromatosis Clinic. Harvard Medical School, Massachusetts General Hospital, Boston, MA 02114. (617) 724-7856. http://neurosurgery.mgh.harvard.edu/NFclinic.htm.

National Cancer Institute. Information Office, Building 31, Room 10A03, 9000 Rockville Pike, Bethesda, MD, 20892-2580. (800) 4-CANCER. http://cancernet.nci.nih.gov.

National Institute of Child Health and Human Development. Building 31, Room 2A32, MSC 2425, 31 Center Dr., Bethesda, MD, 20892. (800) 370-2943. http://www.nichd.nih.gov.

National Institute of Neurological Disorders and Stroke. Office of Communications and Public Liaison, PO Box 5801, Bethesda, MD, 20824. (800) 352-9424. http://www.ninds.nih.gov. National Organization focused on neurological biomedical research.

The National Neurofibromatosis Foundation, Inc.(NNF). 95 Pine St., 16th Floor, New York, NY 10005. (800) 323-7938. http://www.nf.org.

Neurofibromatosis Association (NFA). 82 London Road, Kingston upon Thames, Surrey KT2 6PX. 0208 547 1636. e-mail: nfa@zetnet.co.uk. http://www.nfa.zetnet.co.uk.

Neurofibromatosis, Inc. 8855 Annapolis Rd., #110, Lanham, MD 20706-2924. (800) 942-6825. http://www.nfinc.org.

Rosalyn S. Carson-DeWitt, M.D.
Laura Ruth, Ph.D.
Rebecca J. Frey, PhD

Vorinostat

Definition

Vorinostat (Zolinza) is a histone deacetylase inhibitor manufactured by Merck & Co., Inc. It is used to treat **cutaneous T-cell lymphoma** that has failed to respond to other drug treatments.

Purpose

Vorinostat is used to treat cutaneous T-cell **lymphoma** (CTCL). CTCL is a rare (about 4 cases per 1,000,000 population) type of non-Hodgkin's lymphoma that affects the skin, most often in individuals ages 40–60 years. Vorinostat is a second-line treatment used in progressive, persistent, or recurrent CTCL after two systemic therapies, one of which must have contained the drug **bexarotene** (Targetrin) have failed.

Description

Vorinostat is sold both in the United States and internationally under the brand name Zolinza. It is a white to light orange water-soluble powder contained in a white hard gelatin capsule. Vorinostat has orphan drug status in both the United States and the European Union. Although approved for the treatment of CTCL in October 2006, as of late 2009, this drug was being tested in **clinical trials** in the United States for use against other cancers, both alone and in combination with other therapies. A list of clinical trials currently enrolling volunteers can be found at: http://www.clinicaltrials.gov.

Vorinostat belongs to a class of drugs called histone deacetylase (HDAC) inhibitors. Histones are proteins around which deoxyribonucleic acid (DNA) is coiled. Too much HDAC activity causes DNA to coil up too tightly. When it is tightly coiled, some of the genes that control cell division and programmed cell death (apoptosis) do not function. This allows abnormal (malignant) T cells to reproduce wildly and uncontrollably. Vorinostat inhibits (slows) HDAC activity so that the DNA becomes less tightly coiled and these genes can function again. Allowing the genes that control cell reproduction and cell death to function slows the spread of the **cancer**.

Recommended dosage

Vorinostat comes only in 100 mg capsules that should be stored at room temperature. The standard dose for all patients is 400 mg by mouth once a day. This can be reduced to 300 mg once a day or 300 mg five days a week if the standard dose causes toxicity. Vorinostat is always taken with food. Capsules should not be opened or crushed.

There are no special dosage recommendations for use of vorinostat in the elderly, those with liver (hepatic) impairment, or those with kidney (renal) impairment, although caution is urged when prescribing for these groups. The safety and effectiveness of this drug

QUESTIONS TO ASK YOUR DOCTOR OR PHARMACIST

- How long will I need to take this drug before you can tell if it helps for me?
- How often do I have to have blood work and other laboratory tests done to check the effect the drug is having?
- Is this drug safe to take with the other drugs that I am currently taking?
- What side effects should I watch for? When should I call the doctor about them?
- Are there any clinical trials of this drug combined with other therapies that might benefit me?

have not been established in children. There is no data on overdosage.

Precautions

Precautions should be taken concerning the following adverse reactions.

- Monitoring should be done for pulmonary embolism and deep vein thrombosis.
- Decrease in the number of blood platelets (thrombocytopenia) may reduce the ability of the blood to clot, and a decrease in the number of red blood cells (anemia) also may occur. Blood count should be monitored regularly. In severe cases, medication may need to be reduced or discontinued.
- Blood glucose (sugar) levels may rise (hyperglycemia). Individuals with diabetes are especially at risk; diet and insulin intake may need to be modified.
- Vomiting and **diarrhea** may be severe enough to require replacement fluids and electrolytes. Blood chemistries should be monitored regularly

Pregnant or breastfeeding

Vorinostat is a pregnancy category D drug. Woman who are pregnant or who might become pregnant should not use vorinostat. It is not known whether the drug is excreted in breast milk. Women taking this drug who are or who want to breast-feed should discuss the risks and benefits with their doctor and err on the side of caution, as there is the potential for this drug to cause serious adverse effects on nursing infants.

Side effects

The most serious side effect in clinical trials was pulmonary embolism in 3.5– 4.7% of patients.

More common but somewhat less serious side effects included:

- loss of appetite
- fatigue
- **nausea and vomiting**
- weight loss
- diarrhea
- fever
- anemia
- distortion or loss of sense of taste (dysguesia)

Interactions

When taken with warfarin-based anticoagulants (blood thinners such as Coumadin), blood clotting time is increased.

When taken with other HDAC inhibitor drugs (e.g. valproic acid), severe gastrointestinal bleeding and severe decrease in platelets may occur.

Resources

OTHER

"Oncolink." Abramson Cancer Center of the University of Pennsylvania. 2009 [October 3, 2009]. http://www.oncolink.upenn.edu.

Pazdur, Richard. FDA Approval for Vorinostat, National Cancer Institute. October 10, 2006 [October 4, 2009]. http://www.cancer.gov/cancertopics/druginfo/fda-vorinostat.

Vorinostat (Zolinza) for Cutaneous T-cell Lymphoma—Second Line. National Institute for Health Research, National Horizon Scanning Centre, University of Birmingham (UK). January 2008 [October 4, 2009]. http://www.haps.bham.ac.uk/publichealth/horizon/outputs/documents/2008/january/Vorinostat.pdf.

What Is Cutaneous T Cell Lymphoma (CTCL)? Cancer Research UK. December 12, 2008 [October 4, 2009]. http://www.cancerhelp.org.uk/help/default.asp?page = 3962.

Zolinza: An Effective Treatment Option for Patients With Advanced CTCL. Merck & Co. 2009 [October 4, 2009]. http://www.zolinza.com/vorinostat/zolinza/hcp/index.jsp.

ORGANIZATIONS

American Cancer Society, 1599 Clifton Rd., NE, Atlanta, GA, 30329, (404) 320-3333, (800) ACS-2345, http://www.cancer.org.

Leukemia & Lymphoma Society, 1311 Mamaroneck Avenue, Suite 310 , White Plains, NY, 10605, (800) 955-4572, http://www.leukemia-lymphoma.org.

National Cancer Institute Public Inquires Office., 6116 Executive Boulevard, Room 3036A, Bethesda, MD, 20892-8322, (800) 4-CANCER. TTY (800) 332-8615, http://www.cancer.gov.

National Organization for Rare Diseases (NORD), P. O. Box 1968, Danbury, CT, 06813-1968, (203) 744-0100, (800)999-NORD (6673), orphan@rarediseases.org, http://www.rarediseases.org.

Tish Davidson, A.M.

Vulvar cancer

Definition

Vulvar **cancer** refers to an abnormal, cancerous growth in the external female genitalia.

Description

Vulvar cancer is a rare disease that occurs mainly in elderly women. The vulva refers to the external female genitalia, which includes the labia, the opening of the vagina, the clitoris, and the space between the vagina and anus (perineum). There are two pairs of labia (a Latin term meaning lips). The labia meet to protect the openings of the vagina and the tube that connects to the bladder (urethra). The outer, most prominent folds of skin are called labia majora, and the smaller, inner skin folds are called labia minora. Vulvar cancer can affect any part of the female genitalia, but usually affects the labia.

Approximately 70% of vulvar cancers involve the labia (usually the labia majora), 15% to 20% involve the clitoris, and 15% to 20% involve the perineum. For approximately 5% of the cases, the cancer is present at more than one location. For approximately 10% of the cases, so much of the vulva is affected by cancer that the original location cannot be determined. Vulvar cancer can spread to nearby structures including the anus, vagina, and urethra.

Most vulvar cancers are squamous cell carcinomas. Squamous cells are the main cell type of the skin. Squamous cell **carcinoma** often begins at the edges of the labia majora or labia minora or the area around the vagina. This type of cancer is usually slow-growing and may begin with a precancerous condition referred to as vulvar intraepithelial neoplasia (VIN), or dysplasia. This means that precancerous cells are present in the surface layer of skin.

Other, less common types of vulvar cancer are **melanoma**, **basal cell carcinoma**, adenocarcinomas, Paget's disease of the vulva, and tumors of the connective tissue under the skin. Melanoma, a cancer that develops from the cells that produce the pigment that determines the skin's color, can occur anywhere on the skin, including the vulva. Melanoma is the second most common type of vulvar cancer, and accounts for 5% to 10% of the cases. Half of all vulvar melanomas involve the labia majora. Basal cell carcinoma, which is the most common type of cancer that occurs on parts of the skin exposed to the sun, very rarely occurs on the vulva. Adenocarcinomas develop from glands, including the glands at the opening of the vagina (Bartholin's glands) that produce a mucus-like lubricating fluid.

Vulvar cancer is most common in women over 50 years of age. The median age at diagnosis is 65 to 70 years old. Additional risk factors for vulvar cancer include having multiple sexual partners, **cervical cancer**, and the presence of chronic vaginal and vulvar inflammations. This type of cancer is often associated with sexually transmitted diseases.

KEY TERMS

Adjuvant therapy—A treatment that is intended to aid primary treatment. Adjuvant treatments for vulvar cancer are radiation therapy and chemotherapy.

Biopsy—Removal of a small piece of tissue for microscopic examination. This is done under local anesthesia and removed by either using a scalpel or a punch, which removes a small cylindrical portion of tissue.

Colposcope—An instrument used for examination of the vagina and cervix. Part of the instrument includes a magnifying lens for better visualization.

Metastasis—The movement of cancer cells from one area of the body to another. This occurs through the blood vessels or the lymph vessels.

Pelvic exenteration—Surgical removal of the organs of the true pelvis, which includes the uterus, vagina, and cervix.

Sentinel lymph node—The first lymph node to receive lymph fluid from a tumor. If the sentinel node is cancer-free, then it is likely that the cancerous cells have not metastasized.

Demographics

Vulvar cancer is most common in women who are between the ages of 65 and 75 years. In the United States there are approximately 3,000 new cases of vulvar cancer diagnosed each year. Vulvar cancer

QUESTIONS TO ASK THE DOCTOR

- What type of cancer do I have?
- What stage of cancer do I have?
- What is the five-year survival rate for women with this type and stage of cancer?
- Has the cancer spread?
- What are my treatment options?
- How much tissue will you be removing? Can you remove less tissue and complement my treatment with adjuvant therapy?
- What are the risks and side effects of these treatments?
- What medications can I take to relieve treatment side effects?
- Are there any clinical studies underway that would be appropriate for me?
- What effective alternative or complementary treatments are available for this type of cancer?
- How debilitating is the treatment? Will I be able to continue working?
- How will the treatment affect my sexuality?
- Are there any restrictions regarding sexual activity?
- How realistic will a vulvar reconstruction look?
- Are there any local support groups for vulvar cancer patients?
- What is the chance that the cancer will recur?
- Is there anything I can do to prevent recurrence?
- How often will I have follow-up examinations?

accounts for only 1% of all cancers in women. Approximately 5% of all **gynecologic cancers** occur on the vulva. For unknown reasons, the incidence of vulvar cancer seems to be rising.

Causes and symptoms

Cancer is caused when the normal mechanisms that control cell growth become disturbed, causing the cells to grow continually without stopping. This is usually the result of damage to the DNA in the cell. Although the cause of vulvar cancer is unknown, studies have identified several risk factors for vulvar cancer. These include:

- Vulvar intraepithelial neoplasia (VIN). This abnormal growth of the surface cells of the vulva can sometimes progress to cancer.
- Infection with human papillomavirus (HPV). This virus is sexually transmitted and can cause genital warts. Although HPV DNA can be detected in most cases of vulvar intraepithelial neoplasia, it is detected in fewer than half of all cases of vulvar cancer. Therefore, the link between HPV infection and vulvar cancer is unclear. As of the early 2000, it is theorized that two classes of vulvar cancer exist: one that is associated with HPV infection and one that is not.
- Herpes simplex virus 2 (HSV2). This sexually transmitted virus is also associated with increased risk for vulvar cancer.
- Cigarette smoking. Smoking in combination with infection by HPV or HSV2 was found to be a particularly strong risk factor for vulvar cancer.
- Infection with human immunodeficiency virus (HIV). This virus, which causes AIDS, decreases the body's immune ability, leaving it vulnerable to a variety of diseases, including vulvar cancer.
- Chronic vulvar inflammation. Long-term irritation and inflammation of the vulva and vagina, which may be caused by poor hygiene, can increase the risk of vulvar cancer.
- Abnormal Pap smears. Women who have had abnormal Pap smears are at an increased risk of developing vulvar cancer.
- Chronic immunosuppression. Women who have had long-term suppression of their immune system caused by disease (such as certain cancers) or medication (such as those taken after organ transplantation) have an increased risk of developing vulvar cancer.

The hallmark symptom of vulvar cancer is **itching** (pruritus), which is experienced by 90% of the women afflicted by this cancer. The cancerous lesion is readily visible. Unfortunately, because of embarrassment or denial, it is not uncommon for women to delay medical assessment of vulvar abnormalities. Any abnormalities should be reported to a gynecologist.

If squamous cell vulvar cancer is present, it may appear as a raised red, pink, or white bump (nodule). It is often accompanied by pain, bleeding, vaginal discharge, and painful urination. Malignant melanoma of the vulva usually appears as a pigmented, ulcerated growth. Other types of vulvar cancer may appear as a distinct mass of tissue, sore and scaly areas, or cauliflower-like growths that look like warts.

Diagnosis

A gynecological examination will be used to observe the suspected area. During this examination, the physician may use a special magnifying instrument called a colposcope to view the area better. Additionally, the area may be treated with a dilute solution of acetic acid, which causes some abnormal areas to turn white, making them easier to see. During this examination, if any area is suspected of being abnormal, a tissue sample (**biopsy**) will be taken. The biopsy can be performed in the doctor's office with the use of local anesthetic. A wedge-shaped piece of tissue, which contains the suspect lesion with some surrounding normal skin and the underlying skin layers and connective tissue, will be removed. Small lesions will be removed in their entirety (excisional biopsy). The diagnosis of cancer depends on a microscopic analysis of this tissue by a pathologist.

The diagnosis for vulvar cancer will determine how advanced the cancer is and how much it has spread. This is determined by the size of the tumor and how deep it has invaded the surrounding tissue and organs, such as the lymph nodes. It will also be determined if the cancer has metastasized, or spread to other organs. Tests used to determine the extent of the cancer include x ray and **computed tomography** scan (CT scan). Endoscopic examination of the bladder (**cystoscopy**) and/or rectum (proctoscopy) may be performed if it is suspected that the cancer has spread to these organs.

Treatment team

The treatment team for vulvar cancer may include a gynecologist, gynecologic oncologist, radiation oncologist, gynecologic nurse oncologist, sexual therapist, psychiatrist, psychological counselor, and social worker.

Clinical staging, treatments, and prognosis

Clinical staging

The International Federation of Gynecology and Obstetrics (FIGO) has adopted a surgical staging system for vulvar cancer. The stage of cancer is determined after surgery. The previous clinical staging system for vulvar cancer is no longer used. Vulvar cancer is categorized into five stages (0, I, II, III, and IV) which may be further subdivided (A and B) based on the depth or spread of cancerous tissue. The FIGO stages for vulvar cancer are:

- Stage 0. Vulvar intraepithelial neoplasia (precancerous cells).
- Stage I. Cancer is confined to the vulva and perineum. The lesion is less than 2 cm (about 0.8 in) in size.
- Stage II. Cancer is confined to the vulva and perineum. The lesion is larger than 2 cm (larger than 0.8 in) in size.
- Stage III. Cancer has spread to the vagina, urethra, anus, and/or the lymph nodes in the groin (inguinofemoral).
- Stage IV. Cancer has spread to the bladder, bowel, pelvic bone, pelvic lymph nodes, and/or other parts of the body.

Treatments

Treatment for vulvar cancer will depend on its stage and the patient's general state of health. Surgery is the mainstay of treatment for most cases of vulvar cancer.

SURGERY. The primary treatment for stage I and stage II vulvar cancer is surgery to remove the cancerous lesion and possibly the inguinofemoral lymph nodes. Removal of the lesion may be done by laser, to burn off a minimal amount of tissue, or by scalpel (local excision), to remove more of the tissue. The choice will depend on the severity of the cancer. If a large area of the vulva is removed, it is called a vulvectomy. Radical vulvectomy removes the entire vulva. A vulvectomy may require skin grafts from other areas of the body to cover the wound and make an artificial vulva. Because of the significant morbidity and the psychosexual consequences of radical vulvectomy, there is a trend toward minimizing the extent of cancer excision. The specific inguinofemoral lymph node that would receive lymph fluid from the cancerous lesion, known as the sentinel node, may be exposed for examination (**lymph node dissection**) or removed (lymphadenectomy), especially in cases in which the cancerous lesion has invaded to a depth of more than 1 mm. Surgery may also be followed by **chemotherapy** and/or **radiation therapy** to kill additional cancer cells.

Surgical treatment of stage III and stage IV vulvar cancer is much more complex. Extensive surgery would be necessary to completely remove the cancerous tissue. Surgery would involve excision of pelvic organs (pelvic **exenteration**), radical vulvectomy, and lymphadenectomy. Because this extensive surgery comes with a substantial risk of complications, it may be possible to treat advanced vulvar cancer with minimal surgery by using radiation therapy and/or chemotherapy as additional treatment (adjuvant therapy).

An intraoperative technique that is used to identify the sentinel node in **breast cancer** and melanoma is being applied to vulvar cancer. This technique, called lymphoscintigraphy, is performed during surgical treatment of vulvar cancer and allows the surgeon to immediately identify the sentinel node. A radioactive compound (technetium 99m sulfur colloid) is injected into the cancerous lesion approximately two hours prior to surgery. This injection causes little discomfort, so local anesthesia is not required. During surgery, a radioactivity detector is used to locate the sentinel node and any other nodes to which cancer has spread. Though still in the experimental stage, vulvar lymphoscintigraphy shows promise in reducing morbidity and hospital length of stay.

The most common complication of vulvectomy is the development of a tumor-like collection of clear liquid (wound seroma). Other surgical complications include urinary tract **infection**, wound infection, temporary nerve injury, fluid accumulation (edema) in the legs, urinary **incontinence**, falling or sinking of the genitals (genital prolapse), and blood clots (thrombus).

RADIATION THERAPY. Radiation therapy uses high-energy radiation from **x rays** and gamma rays to kill the cancer cells. The skin in the treated area may become red and dry and may take as long as a year to return to normal. **Fatigue**, upset stomach, **diarrhea**, and **nausea** are also common complaints of women having radiation therapy. Radiation therapy in the pelvic area may cause the vagina to become narrow as scar tissue forms. This phenomenon, known as vaginal stenosis, makes intercourse painful.

CHEMOTHERAPY. Chemotherapy uses **anticancer drugs** to kill the cancer cells. The drugs are given by mouth (orally) or intravenously. They enter the bloodstream and can travel to all parts of the body to kill cancer cells. Generally, a combination of drugs is given because it is more effective than a single drug in treating cancer. The side effects of chemotherapy are significant and include stomach upset, **vomiting**, appetite loss (**anorexia**), hair loss (**alopecia**), mouth or vaginal sores, fatigue, menstrual cycle changes, and premature menopause. There is also an increased chance of infections.

Prognosis

Factors that are correlated with disease outcome include the diameter and depth of the cancerous lesion, involvement of local lymph nodes, cell type, HPV status, and age of the patient. Vulvar cancers that are HPV positive have a better prognosis than those that are HPV negative. The five-year survival rate is 98% for stage I vulvar cancer and 87% for stage II vulvar cancer. The survival rate drops steadily as the number of affected lymph nodes increases. The survival rate is 75% for patients with one or two, 36% for those with three or four, and 24% for those with five or six involved lymph nodes. The previous statistics were obtained from studies of patients who received surgical treatment only and cannot be used to determine survival rates when adjuvant therapy is employed.

Vulvar cancer can spread locally to encompass the anus, vagina, and urethra. Because of the anatomy of the vulva, it is not uncommon for the cancer to spread to the local lymph nodes. Advanced stages of vulvar cancer can affect the pelvic bone. The lungs are the most common site for vulvar cancer **metastasis**. Metastasis through the blood (hematogenous spread) is uncommon.

Alternative and complementary therapies

Although alternative and complementary therapies are used by many cancer patients, very few controlled studies on the effectiveness of such therapies exist. Mind-body techniques such as prayer, biofeedback, visualization, meditation, and yoga have not shown any effect in reducing cancer but can reduce stress and lessen some of the side effects of cancer treatments. Clinical studies of hydrazine sulfate found that it had no effect on cancer and even worsened the health and well- being of the study subjects. One clinical study of the drug amygdalin (Laetrile) found that it had no effect on cancer. Laetrile can be toxic and has caused death. Shark cartilage, although highly touted as an effective cancer treatment, is an improbable therapy that has not been the subject of clinical study.

The American Cancer Society has found that the "metabolic diets" pose serious risk to the patient. The effectiveness of the macrobiotic, Gerson, and Kelley diets and the Manner metabolic therapy has not been scientifically proven. The FDA was unable to substantiate the anticancer claims made about the popular Cancell treatment.

There is no evidence for the effectiveness of most over-the-counter herbal cancer remedies. However, some herbals have shown an anticancer effect. As shown in clinical studies, Polysaccharide krestin, from the mushroom *Coriolus versicolor*, has significant effectiveness against cancer. In a small study, the green alga *Chlorella pyrenoidosa* has been shown to have anticancer activity. In a few small studies, evening primrose oil has shown some benefit in the treatment of cancer. Patients should discuss the use of any alternative or complementary therapies with their doctor.

For more comprehensive information, the patient should consult the book on complementary and alternative medicine published by the American Cancer Society listed in the Resources section.

Coping with cancer treatment

The patient should consult her treatment team regarding any side effects or complications of treatment. Vaginal stenosis can be prevented and treated by vaginal dilators, gentle douching, and sexual intercourse. A water-soluble lubricant may be used to make sexual intercourse more comfortable. Many of the side effects of chemotherapy can be relieved by medications.

Women should consult a psychotherapist and/or join a support group to deal with the emotional consequences of cancer and vulvectomy.

Clinical trials

There are some active, long-term **clinical trials** for the diagnosis and treatment of vulvar cancer. Two of these trials are sponsored by the National Cancer Institute. One trial (protocol ID# GOG-173) is testing the effectiveness of a **sentinel lymph node mapping** technique which uses a visible dye. The sentinel node is identified and removed. This diagnostic and treatment study is open to patients with invasive squamous cell carcinoma of the vulva. The other trial (protocol ID# GOG-0185) is testing the effectiveness of the chemotherapeutic agent **cisplatin** in combination with radiation therapy. This treatment study is open to patients with stage I, II, or III squamous cell carcinoma of the vulva. Women should consult with their treatment team to determine if they are candidates for these or any other clinical studies.

Prevention

The risk of vulvar cancer can be decreased by avoiding risk factors, most of which involve lifestyle choices. Specifically, to reduce the risk of vulvar cancer, women should not smoke and should refrain from engaging in unsafe sexual behavior. Good hygiene of the genital area to prevent infection and inflammation may also reduce the risk of vulvar cancer.

Because vulvar cancer is highly curable in its early stages, women should consult a physician as soon as a vulvar abnormality is detected. Regular gynecological examinations are necessary to detect precancerous conditions that can be treated before the cancer becomes invasive. Because some vulvar cancer is a type of **skin cancer**, the American Cancer Society also recommends self-examination of the vulva using a mirror. If moles are present in the genital area, women should employ the ABCD rule:

- Asymmetry. A cancerous mole may have two halves of unequal size.
- Border irregularity. A cancerous mole may have ragged or notched edges.
- Color. A cancerous mole may have variations in color.
- Diameter. A cancerous mole may have a diameter wider than 6 mm (1/4 in).

Special concerns

Surgical removal of the cancerous lesion may remove some or all of the vulva. Vulvectomy alters the appearance of the vulva and affects sexual function. **Depression**, due to the effects of surgery on appearance and **sexuality**, may occur. Short-term and long-term complications following extensive surgical treatment of vulvar cancer are not uncommon. Women of child-bearing age should discuss future fertility with their physician.

Resources

BOOKS

Bruss, Katherine, Christina Salter, and Esmeralda Galan, editors. *American Cancer Society's Guide to Complementary and Alternative Cancer Methods*. Atlanta: American Cancer Society, 2000.

Eifel, Patricia, Jonathan Berrek, and James Thigpen. "Cancer of the Cervix, Vagina, and Vulva." In *Cancer: Principles & Practice of Oncology*, edited by Vincent DeVita, Samuel Hellman, and Steven Rosenberg. Philadelphia: Lippincott Williams & Wilkins, 2001.

Garcia, Agustin, and J. Tate Thigpen. "Tumors of the Vulva and Vagina." In *Textbook of Uncommon Cancer*, edited by D. Raghavan, M. Brecher, D. Johnson, N. Meropol, P. Moots, and J. Thigpen. Chichester: John Wiley & Sons, 1999.

Primack, Aron. "Complementary/Alternative Therapies in the Prevention and Treatment of Cancer." In *Complementary/Alternative Medicine: An Evidence- Based Approach*, edited by John Spencer and Joseph Jacobs. St. Louis: Mosby, 1999.

PERIODICALS

Grendys, Edward, and James Fiorica. "Innovations in the Management of Vulvar Carcinoma." *Current Opinion in Obstetrics and Gynecology* 12 (February 2000): 15-20.

OTHER

Cancer Care News. [cited July 3, 2001]. http://www.cancercare.org.

Quackwatch, Questionable Cancer Therapies. [cited July 3, 2001]. http://www.quackwatch.com.

ORGANIZATIONS

American Cancer Society. 1599 Clifton Rd. NE, Atlanta, GA 30329. (800) ACS-2345. http://www.cancer.org.

Cancer Research Institute, National Headquarters. 681 Fifth Ave., New York, NY 10022. (800) 992-2623. http://www.cancerresearch.org.

Gynecologic Cancer Foundation. 401 N. Michigan Ave., Chicago, IL 60611. (800) 444-4441 or (312) 644-6610. http://www.wcn.org/gcf.

National Institutes of Health. National Cancer Institute. 9000 Rockville Pike, Bethesda, MD 20982. (800) 4-CANCER. http://cancernet.nci.nih.gov.

Cindy L. Jones, Ph.D.
Belinda Rowland, Ph.D.

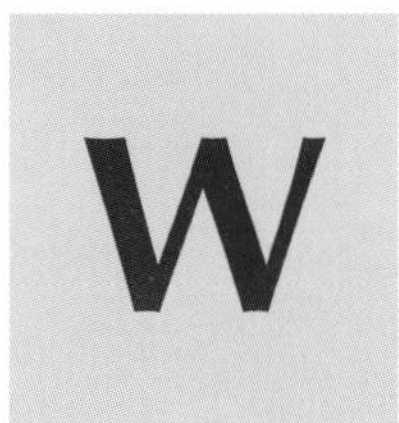

Waldenström's macroglobulinemia

Definition

Waldenström's macroglobulinemia is a rare, chronic **cancer** of the immune system that is characterized by hyperviscosity, or thickening, of the blood.

Description

Waldenström's (Waldenström, Waldenstroem's) macroglobulinemia (WM) is a **lymphoma**, or cancer of the lymphatic system. It was first identified in 1944, by the Swedish physician Jan Gosta Waldenström, in patients who had a thickening of the serum, or liquid part, of the blood. Their blood serum contained a great deal of a very large molecule called a globulin. Thus, the disorder is called macroglobulinemia.

Lymphomas are cancers that originate in tissues of the lymphatic system. All lymphomas other than **Hodgkin's disease**, including WM, are known collectively as non-Hodgkin's lymphomas. There are 13 major types of non-Hodgkin's lymphomas, and others that are very rare. Other names that are sometimes used for WM include: lymphoplasmacytic lymphoma, lymphoplasmacytic leukemia, macroglobulinemia of Waldenström, primary macroglobulinemia, Waldenström's syndrome, Waldenström's purpura, or hyperglobulinemic purpura. Purpura refers to purple spots on the skin, resulting from the frequent bleeding and bruising that can be a symptom of WM.

WM is classified as a low-grade or indolent form of lymphoma because it is a slow-growing cancer that produces fewer symptoms than other types of lymphomas. WM most often affects males over the age of 65. Frequently, this disease produces no symptoms and does not require treatment. It has not been studied as extensively as other types of lymphoma.

The lymphatic system

The lymphatic system is part of the body's immune system, for fighting disease, and part of the blood-producing system. It includes the lymph vessels and nodes, and the spleen, bone marrow, and thymus. The narrow lymphatic vessels carry lymphatic fluid from throughout the body. The lymph nodes are small, pea-shaped organs that filter the lymphatic fluid and trap foreign substances, including viruses, bacteria, and cancer cells. The spleen, in the upper left abdomen, removes old cells and debris from the blood. The bone marrow, the spongy tissue inside the bones, produces new blood cells.

B lymphocytes or B cells are white blood cells that recognize disease-causing organisms. They circulate throughout the body in the blood and lymphatic fluid. Each B lymphocyte recognizes a specific foreign substance, or antigen. When it encounters its specific antigen, the B cell begins to divide and multiply, producing large numbers of identical (monoclonal), mature plasma cells. These plasma cells produce large amounts of antibody that are specific for the antigen. Antibodies are large proteins called immunoglobulins (Igs) that bind to and remove the specific antigen.

A type of Ig, called IgM, is part of the early **immune response**. The IgM molecules form clusters in the bloodstream. When these IgM clusters encounter their specific antigen, usually a bacterium, they cover it so that it can be destroyed by other immune system cells.

Plasma cell neoplasm

WM is a type of plasma cell neoplasm or B-cell lymphoma. These are lymphomas in which certain plasma cells become abnormal, or cancerous, and begin to grow uncontrollably. In WM, the cancerous plasma cells overproduce large amounts of identical (monoclonal) IgM antibody. This IgM also is called M protein, for monoclonal or **myeloma** protein.

KEY TERMS

Anemia—Any condition in which the red blood cell count is below normal.

Antibody—Immunoglobulin produced by immune system cells that recognizes and binds to a specific foreign substance (antigen).

Antigen—Foreign substance that is recognized by a specific antibody.

Autosomal dominant—Genetic trait that is expressed when present on only one of a pair of non-sex-linked chromosomes.

B cell (B lymphocyte)—Type of white blood cell that produces antibodies.

Bence-Jones protein—Light chain of an immunoglobulin that may be overproduced in Waldenström's macroglobulinemia; it is excreted in the urine.

Biopsy—Removal of a small sample of tissue for examination under a microscope; used in the diagnosis of cancer.

Cryoglobulinemia—Condition in which protein in the blood forms particles in the cold, blocking blood vessels and leading to pain and numbness of the extremities.

Hyperviscosity—Thick, viscous blood, caused by the accumulation of large proteins, such as immunoglobulins, in the serum.

Immunoelectrophoresis—Use of an electrical field to separate proteins in a mixture (such as blood or urine), on the basis of the size and electrical charge of the proteins; followed by the detection of an antigen (such as IgM), using a specific antibody.

Immunoglobulin (Ig)—Antibody such as IgM; large protein produced by B cells that recognizes and binds to a specific antigen.

Interferon alpha—Potent immune-defense protein; used as an anti-cancer drug.

Lymphatic system—The vessels, lymph nodes, and organs, including the bone marrow, spleen, and thymus, that produce and carry white blood cells to fight disease.

Lymphoma—Cancer that originates in lymphatic tissue.

M protein—Monoclonal or myeloma protein; IgM that is overproduced in Waldenström's macroglobulinemia and accumulates in the blood and urine.

Monoclonal—Identical cells or proteins; cells (clones) derived from a single, genetically distinct cell, or proteins produced by these cells.

Plasma cell—Type of white blood cell that produces antibodies; derived from an antigen-specific B cell.

Plasmapheresis—Plasma exchange transfusion; the separation of serum from blood cells to treat hyperviscosity of the blood.

Platelet—Cell that is involved in blood clotting.

Stem cell—Undifferentiated cell that retains the ability to develop into any one of numerous cell types.

Macroglobulinemia refers to the accumulation of this M protein in the serum of the blood. This large amount of M protein can cause the blood to thicken, causing hyperviscosity. The malignant plasma cells of some WM patients also produce and secrete partial immunoglobulins called light chains, or Bence-Jones proteins. The malignant plasma cells can invade various tissues, including the bone marrow, lymph nodes, and spleen, causing these tissues to swell.

Demographics

WM accounts for about 1-2% of non-Hodgkin's lymphomas. It is estimated that it may affect about five out of every 100,000 people. It usually affects people over the age of 50, and most often develops after age 65. It is more common in men than in women. In the United States, WM is more common among Caucasians than among African Americans. The disease can run in families.

Causes and symptoms

The cause of WM is not known.

Many individuals with WM have no symptoms of the disease. This is known as asymptomatic macroglobulinemia. When symptoms of WM are present, they may vary greatly from one individual to the next.

Hyperviscosity syndrome

At least 50% of individuals with WM have hyperviscosity syndrome, an increased viscosity or thickening of the blood caused by the accumulation of IgM in the serum. Hyperviscosity can cause a slowing in the circulation through small blood vessels. This condition can lead to a variety of symptoms:

QUESTIONS TO ASK THE DOCTOR

- Why have you diagnosed Waldenström's macroglobulinemia?
- Is my disease likely to progress?
- Do you recommend treatment, and if so, why?
- What are my treatment options?
- What is my prognosis?

- fatigue
- weakness
- rash
- bruising
- nose bleeds
- gastrointestinal bleeding
- weight loss
- night sweats
- increased and recurrent infections
- poor blood circulation in the extremities

Poor blood circulation, or Raynaud's phenomenon, can affect any part of the body, but particularly the fingers, toes, nose, and ears.

Cold weather can cause additional circulatory problems, by further thickening the blood and slowing down circulation. In some cases, the excess blood protein may precipitate out of the blood in the cold, creating particles that can block small blood vessels. This is called cryoglobulinemia. The extremities may turn white, or a patchy red and white. The hands, feet, fingers, toes, ears, and nose may feel cold, numb, or painful.

Hyperviscosity may affect the brain and nervous system, leading to additional symptoms. These symptoms include:

- peripheral neuropathy, caused by changes in the nerves, leading to pain or numbness in the extremities
- dizziness
- headaches
- vision problems or loss of vision
- mental confusion
- poor coordination
- temporary paralysis
- mental changes

Hyperviscosity can clog the tubules that form the filtering system of the kidneys, leading to kidney damage or kidney failure. Existing heart conditions can be aggravated by WM. In extreme cases, WM may result in heart failure. Late-stage WM also may lead to mental changes that can progress to coma.

Anemia

The accumulation of IgM in the blood causes an increase in the volume of the blood plasma. This effectively dilutes out the red blood cells and other blood components. The lowered concentration of red blood cells can lead to **anemia** and cause serious **fatigue**. Likewise, a deficiency in platelets (**thrombocytopenia**), which cause the blood to clot, can result in easy bleeding and bruising. As the cancer progresses, there may be abnormal bleeding from the gums, nose, mouth, and intestinal tract. There may be bluish discoloration of the skin. In the later stages of the disease, leukopenia, a deficiency in white blood cells, also can develop.

Organ involvement

In 5-10% of WM cases, the IgM may be deposited in tissues. Thus, some individuals with WM have enlargement of the lymph nodes, the spleen, and/or the liver.

If Bence-Jones proteins are produced by the malignant plasma cells, they may be deposited in the kidneys. There they can plug up the tiny tubules that form the filtering system of the kidneys. This can lead to kidney damage and kidney failure.

Diagnosis

Since many individuals with WM have no symptoms, the initial diagnosis may result from blood tests that are performed for some other purpose. Blood cell counts may reveal low red blood cell and platelet levels. A physical examination may indicate enlargement of the lymph nodes, spleen, and/or liver. A retinal eye examination with an ophthalmoscope may show retinal veins that are enlarged or bleeding.

Blood and urine tests

Serum **protein electrophoresis** is used to measure proteins in the blood. In this laboratory procedure, serum proteins are separated in an electrical field, based on the size and electrical charge of the proteins. Serum **immunoelectrophoresis** uses a second antibody that reacts with IgM. A spike in the Ig fraction indicates a large amount of identical or monoclonal IgM in individuals with WM.

Normal serum contains 0.7-1.6 gm per deciliter (g/dl) of Ig, with no monoclonal Ig present. At serum IgM concentrations of 3-5 g/dl, symptoms of hyperviscosity often are present. However some individuals remain asymptomatic with IgM levels as high as 9 g/dl.

Urinalysis may indicate protein in the urine. A urine Bence-Jones protein test may indicate the presence of these small, partial Igs.

Bone marrow

Abnormal blood tests usually are followed by a **bone marrow biopsy**. In this procedure, a needle is inserted into a bone and a small amount of marrow is removed. Microscopic examination of the marrow may reveal elevated levels of lymphocytes and plasma cells. However, less than 5% of patients with WM have lytic bone lesions, caused by cancerous plasma cells in the bone marrow that are destroying healthy cells. Bone lesions can be detected with **x rays**.

Treatment team

WM usually is diagnosed and treated by a hematologist/oncologist, a specialist in diseases of the blood. Asymptomatic macroglobulinemia is followed closely by the patient's physician for the development of symptoms.

Clinical staging, treatments, and prognosis

Clinical staging, to define how far a cancer has spread through the body, is the common method for choosing a cancer treatment. However, there is no generally accepted staging system for WM.

There also is no generally accepted course of treatment for WM. Treatment may not be necessary for asymptomatic macroglobulinemia. However, if IgM serum levels are very high, treatment may be initiated even in the absence of symptoms. If symptoms are present, treatment is directed at relieving symptoms and retarding the disease's development. Of major concern is the prevention or alleviation of blood hyperviscosity. Therefore, the initial treatment depends on the viscosity of the blood at diagnosis.

Hyperviscosity

Plasmapheresis, or plasma exchange transfusion, is a procedure for thinning the blood. In this treatment, blood is removed and passed through a cell separator that removes the plasma, containing the IgM, from the red and white blood cells and platelets. The blood cells are transfused back into the patient, along with a plasma substitute or donated plasma. Plasmapheresis relieves many of the acute symptoms of WM. Individuals with WM may be given fluid to counter the effects of hyperviscous blood.

Low blood cell counts

Treatments for low blood cell levels include:

- the drug Procrit to treat anemia
- transfusions with packed red blood cells to treat anemia in later stages of the disease
- antibiotics to treat infections caused by a deficiency in white blood cells
- transfusions with blood platelets

Chemotherapy

Chemotherapy, the use of anti-cancer drugs, helps to slow the abnormal development of plasma cells, but does not cure WM. It can reduce the amount of IgM in the bone marrow. In particular, chemotherapy is used to treat severe hyperviscosity and anemia that are caused by WM.

Chlorambucil (Leukeran), possibly in combination with prednisone, is the typical chemotherapy choice for WM. This treatment is effective in 57% of cases. These drugs are taken by mouth. Prednisone is a corticosteroid that affects many body systems. It has anti-cancer and anti-inflammatory effects and is an immune system suppressant. Other drug combinations that are used to treat WM include **cyclophosphamide** (Cytoxan), **vincristine**, and prednisone, with or without **doxorubicin**. **Fludarabine**, 2-chlorodeoxyadenosine, and **corticosteroids** also may be used.

Side effects of chemotherapy may include:

- Mouth sores
- Nausea and indigestion
- Hair loss (alopecia)
- Increased appetite
- Nervousness
- Insomnia These side effects disappear after the chemotherapy is discontinued.

The long-term management of WM usually is accomplished through a combination of plasmapheresis and chemotherapy.

Alternative and complementary therapies

Biological therapy or immunotherapy, with the potent, immune system protein interferon alpha, is used to relieve the symptoms of WM. Interferon alpha works by boosting the body's immune response. Interferon can cause flu-like symptoms, such as **fever**, chills, and fatigue. It also can cause digestive problems and may affect blood pressure.

The drug **rituximab**, an antibody that is active against antibody-producing cells, is effective in about 30% of individuals with WM. Rituximab is a monoclonal antibody produced in the laboratory. Monoclonal antibody treatment may cause a an allergic reaction in some people.

Prognosis

There is no cure for WM. In general, patients go into partial or complete remission following initial treatments. However the disease is not cured and follow-up treatment may be necessary.

The prognosis for this cancer depends on an individual's age, general health, and genetic (hereditary) makeup. Males, individuals over age 60, and those with severe anemia have the lowest survival rates. The Revised European American Lymphoma (REAL) classification system gives WM a good prognosis following treatment, with an average five-year survival rate of 50-70%. However, many people with WM live much longer, some without developing any symptoms of the disease. About 16-23% of individuals with WM die of unrelated causes.

Clinical trials

Clinical studies for the treatment of WM are ongoing. These studies are focusing on new anticancer drugs, new combinations of drugs for chemotherapy, and new biological therapies to boost the immune system. The drug **thalidomide** is a promising new treatment for WM. Its mode of action is unclear; the drug appears to have various effects on the immune system and may inhibit cancerous plasma cells, both directly and indirectly. If thalidomide is taken during pregnancy, it can cause severe birth defects or death of the fetus.

Biological therapies in clinical trial include **monoclonal antibodies** that contain radioactive substances (radioimmunotherapy), in combination with autologous peripheral blood stem cell rescue or transplantation (PBSCT). With PBSCT, the patient's peripheral blood stem cells (immature bone marrow cells found in the blood) are collected and frozen prior to radioimmunotherapy, which destroys bone marrow cells. A procedure called apheresis is used to collect the stem cells. Following the therapy, the stem cells are reinjected into the individual. The procedure is autologous because it utilizes the individual's own cells. A similar procedure that utilizes chemotherapy with PBSCT also is being tested.

Prevention

There is no known prevention for WM.

Special concerns

WM is a rare disorder and many physicians and even hematologists may not have had experience with it. Furthermore, there is not a clear consensus among professionals as to what constitutes a diagnosis of WM; nor is there a defined course of treatment or accurate prognosis. Thus, it is important that the patient obtain all available information, including seeking second opinions and additional consultations.

See also Bone marrow transplantation; Immunologic therapy; Pheresis; Transfusion therapy.

Resources

OTHER

Complementary and Alternative Therapies for Leukemia, Lymphoma, Hodgkin's Disease and Myeloma. The Leukemia and Lymphoma Society. 27 Mar. 2001. [cited June 28, 2001]. http://www.leukemia-lymphoma.org.

"Macroglobulinemia of Waldenström." *WebMD.* 1999. 14 Apr. 2001. [cited June 28, 2001]. <http://my.webmd.com/content/asset/adam_disease_macroglobulinemia-primary>.

McKusick, Victor A. "Macroglobulinemia, Waldenström; WM." *Online Mendelian Inheritance in Man.* John Hopkins University. 28 Dec. 1999. [cited June 28, 2001]. http://www.ncbi.nlm.nih.gov:80/entrez/dispomim.cgi?id = 153600.

"Multiple Myeloma and Other Plasma Cell Neoplasms." *CancerNet.* National Cancer Institute. Mar. 2001. [cited June 28, 2001]. <http://cancernet.nci.nih.gov>.

"Non-Hodgkin's Lymphoma." *Cancer Resource Center.* American Cancer Society. 20 Dec 1998. [cited June 28, 2001]. <http://www3.cancer.org/cancerinfo/load_cont.asp?ct = 32&st = wi>.

Waldenströms.com. International Waldenström's Macroglobulinemia Foundation.[cited June 28, 2001]. http://www.iwmf.com.

ORGANIZATIONS

Cure for Lymphoma Foundation. 215 Lexington Ave., New York, NY 10016. (212) 213-9595. (800)-CFL-6848. infocfl@cfl.org. http://www.cfl.org/home.html. An advocacy organization; education and support programs, research grants, information on clinical trials for Hodgkin's and non-Hodgkin's lymphomas.

International Waldenström's Macroglobulinemia Foundation. 2300 Bee Ridge Road, Sarasota, FL 34239-6226. (941) 927-IWMF. http://www.iwmf.com. Information, educational programs, support for patients and families, research support.

The Leukemia and Lymphoma Society. 600 Third Ave., New York, NY 10016. (800) 955-4572. (914) 949-5213. http://www.leukemia-lymphoma.org. Information, support, and guidance for patients and health care professionals.

The Lymphoma Research Foundation of America, Inc. 8800 Venice Boulevard, Suite 207, Los Angeles, CA 90034. (310) 204-7040). http://www.lymphoma.org. Research into treatments for lymphoma; educational and emotional support programs for patients and families.

J. Ricker Polsdorfer, M.D.
Margaret Alic, Ph.D.

Warfarin

Definition

Wafarin is a vitamin K antagonist that belongs to the family of drugs called anticoagulants ("blood thinners," although it does not actually thin the blood). The brand name of warfarin in the U.S. is Coumadin.

Purpose

Wafarin is used to decrease the clotting ability of the blood and to help prevent harmful clots from forming in the blood vessels. It is also used for the long-term treatment of thromboembolic disease, a common side effect of **cancer**.

One of the most common hematological complications is disordered coagulation. Approximately 15% of all cancer patients are affected by thromboembolic disease, and it is the second leading cause of death for cancer patients. However, thromboembolic disease may represent only one of many complications in end-stage patients. Thromboembolic disease includes superficial and deep vein thrombosis, pulmonary embolism, thrombosis of venous access devices, arterial thrombosis, and embolism. The cancer itself or cancer treatments may induce coagulation. For example, **tamoxifen**, a drug prescribed to treat **breast cancer**, increases the chance of developing pulmonary embolism or deep vein thrombosis.

Cancer and its treatment can affect all three causes of thromboembolic disease including the alteration of blood flow, damage to the cells in blood vessels (endothelial cells), and enhancing procoagulants (precursors, such as fibrinogen or prothrombin, that mediate coagulation). Cancer can affect blood flow by mechanically affecting blood vessels close to a tumor. In addition, tumors cause angiogenesis, which may create complexes of blood vessels with a disordered appearance and flow (varying in magnitude and direction). **Chemotherapy** or tumors may directly damage endothelial cells. Procoagulants may be secreted into the blood stream by cancer cells or can be increased on the surface of cancer cells.

KEY TERMS

Angiogenesis—The formation of new blood vessels that occurs naturally under certain circumstances, for example, in the healing of a cut.

Anticoagulant—A medication that prevents the formation of new blood clots and keeps existing blood clots from growing larger.

Arterial thrombosis—A condition characterized by a blood clot in an artery.

Blood clot—A clump of blood that forms in or around a vessel as a result of coagulation. The formation of blood clots when the body has been cut is essential because without blood clots to stop the bleeding, a person would bleed to death from a relatively small wound.

Coagulation—The blood's natural tendency to clump and stick.

Embolism—An obstruction in a blood vessel due to a blood clot or other foreign matter that gets stuck while traveling through the bloodstream.

Embolus—A blood clot, gas bubble, piece of tumor tissue, or other foreign matter that moves through the bloodstream from its site of origin to obstruct a blood vessel.

Endothelial cells—The cells lining the inside of blood vessels.

Fibrinolytics—Agents that decompose fibrin, a protein produced in the clotting process.

Pulmonary embolism—A blockage of the pulmonary artery by foreign matter such as a blood clot.

Thromboembolic disease—A condition in which a blood vessel is obstructed by an embolus carried in the bloodstream from the site of formation.

Thrombosis—A condition in which a clot develops in a blood vessel.

Vein thrombosis—A condition characterized by a blood clot in a vein.

Description

Warfarin will not dissolve an existing blood clot, but it may prevent it from getting larger. When warfarin is taken orally, it is absorbed quickly from the gastrointestinal tract. It reaches a maximal plasma concentration in 90 minutes and stays in the bloodstream (i.e. its half-life) 36–42 hours. Warfarin circulates in the bloodstream attached to plasma proteins—in particular, a protein called albumin. The response or effects of a warfarin dose vary from person to person.

Whether anticoagulants like wafarin may also improve cancer survival rates independent of their effect on thromboembolism has been investigated. There is suggestive evidence that warfarin may actually enhance cancer survival rates. Animal studies show that warfarin and other agents such as **heparin**, fibrinolytics, and even antiplatelet agents inhibit tumor growth and **metastasis**.

Recommended dosage

A doctor may prescribe a dosage based on laboratory blood tests that determine a patient's clotting time. This blood test (called prothrombin time) is conducted usually weekly or monthly as suggested by a physician and should always be done at the same time of day. Based on the clotting time, the doctor determines the dose and/or whether the dose should be adjusted. Warfarin is normally prescribed to be taken once a day, and it should be taken at the same time every day.

Precautions

Following certain precautions when taking warfarin may reduce the risk of side effects and improve the effectiveness of the medication. The rate of blood clotting is affected by illness, diet, medication changes, and physical activities. If an individual has other medical problems, this may affect the use of warfarin. Of particular importance are bleeding ulcers, heavy menstrual periods, infections, high blood pressure, and liver or kidney problems. The doctor should be informed of any changes in these conditions so dose alterations can be made, if necessary. If a patient using warfarin is scheduled for surgery or dental work, the doctor or dentist should be informed that the patient is taking this medication. Warfarin should not be prescribed if an allergic reaction has occurred in the past, during pregnancy or while breastfeeding, or if pregnancy is planned. Anyone taking warfarin should exercise extra care not to cut him/herself and not to sustain injuries that can result in bruising or bleeding.

In addition, patients taking warfarin should watch their intake of vitamin K, since too much vitamin K may alter the way in which warfarin works. The amount of foods high in vitamin K (such as broccoli, spinach, and turnip greens) eaten each week should be kept stable. Grapefruit juice should be avoided because it may intensify the effects of this medication. Alcohol should also be avoided while taking warfarin because it interferes with warfarin's effectiveness.

In order to determine a safe and effective dose, regular blood tests to check prothrombin time should be done while taking this medicine. Individuals taking warfarin frequently require dose adjustments.

Side effects

The most common complication of long-term warfarin therapy is bleeding. The intensity of anticoagulant therapy, age, kidney function, and unidentified diseases of the gastrointestinal and genitourinary tracts all directly influence the risk of bleeding. Patients taking warfarin should be aware of the signs and symptoms that may indicate a bleeding problem. These signs and symptoms include:

- bleeding from the gums or nose
- red or black bowel movements
- coughing up blood (hemoptysis)
- heavy bleeding from cuts or wounds that will not stop
- unusually heavy menstrual bleeding
- blood in the urine
- easy bruising or purple spots on the skin
- severe headache

The patient should inform his/her doctor immediately if any of these symptoms is present.

Other side effects that may occur with warfarin treatment include:

- mild stomach cramps
- upset stomach
- hair loss (alopecia)
- poor appetite (anorexia)
- cough or hoarseness
- fever or chills
- skin rash, hive, or itching
- painful or difficult urination

The occurrence of any of these side effects should also be reported to the doctor.

Interactions

Some medications should not be combined. The patient should check with the doctor monitoring the warfarin treatment before taking any new medication, including over-the-counter medication or medication prescribed by another doctor.

Among the medications and dietary supplements that may alter the way warfarin works are:

- other prescription medications
- nonprescription medications such as aspirin or non-steroidal anti-inflammatory drugs (i.e. ibuprofen)
- cough or cold remedies
- herbal products and nutritional supplements
- products containing vitamin K

Studies have shown that Warfarin along with cranberry juice can be big trouble. The volume of the case studies included glasses of cranberry juice daily, not gallons. This drug-food interaction was shown to cause an increased risk of bleeding. This risk prompted the UK's Committee on Safety of Medicines and the Medicines and Healthcare Products Regulatory Agency to warn patients of warfarin to limit consumption of cranberry juice or avoid it altogether. According to Dr. Jacci Bainbrigde of the University of Colorado, Denver, A cranberry juice/warfarin interaction is biologically plausible. Warfarin is metabolized chiefly by cytochrome P-450 in the liver, and the antioxidant flavonoids contained in the juice are known to inhibit the enzyme pathway." However, limited consumption is advised.

See also Low molecular weight heparin.

Crystal Heather Kaczkowski, MSc.

Weight loss

Definition

Weight loss is a reduction in body mass characterized by a loss of adipose tissue (body fat) and skeletal muscle.

Description

Unintentional weight loss is the most common symptom of **cancer** and often a side effect of cancer treatments. A poor response to cancer treatments, reduced quality of life, and shorter survival time may result from substantial weight loss. The body may become weaker and less able to tolerate cancer therapies. As body weight decreases, body functionality declines and may lead to malnutrition, illness, **infection**, and perhaps death.

Most cancer patients in the United States expect to suffer weight loss during treatment for their disease; a study of 938 patients from 17 communities in upstate New York reported in 2004 that weight loss was the fourth most commonly expected side effect of cancer therapy, after **fatigue**, **nausea**, and sleep disturbances.

KEY TERMS

Anorexia—A condition frequently observed in cancer patients characterized by a loss of appetite or desire to eat.

Cachexia—A condition in which the body weight "wastes" away, characterized by a constant loss of weight, muscle, and fat.

Cancer—A group of diseases in which abnormal cells divide without control. Cancer cells can invade nearby tissues and can spread through the bloodstream and lymphatic system to other parts of the body.

Chemotherapy—Chemotherapy kills cancer cells using drugs taken orally or by needle in a vein or muscle. It is referred to as a systemic treatment due to fact that it travels through the bloodstream and kills cancer cells outside the small intestine.

Enteral nutrition—Feedings administered through a nose tube (or surgically placed tubes) for patients with eating difficulties.

Parenteral nutrition—Feeding administered most often by an infusion into a vein. It can be used if the gut is not functioning properly or due to other reasons that prevent normal or enteral feeding.

Protein-calorie malnutrition—A lack of sufficient protein and calories to sustain the body's composition, resulting in weight loss and muscle wasting.

Radiation therapy—Also called radiotherapy; uses high-energy rays to kill cancer cells.

Wasting—When inadequate calories are consumed, it can lead to depletion of body mass. Wasting results in weight loss in tissues such as skeletal muscle and adipose tissue (fat).

Severe malnutrition is typically defined in two ways: functionally (increased risk of morbidity and/or mortality) and by degree of weight loss (greater than 2% per week, 5% per month, 7.5% per 3 months, and 10% per 6 months). Without considering a specific time course, grading is as follows:

- Grade 0 = less than 5.0% weight loss
- Grade 1 = 5.0% to 9.9%
- Grade 2 = 10.0% to 19.9%

- Grade 3 = greater than 20.0%
- Grade 4 (life-threatening) is not specifically defined. Paying attention to weight loss at an early stage is necessary to prevent deterioration of weight, body composition, and performance status.

Causes

There are many reasons for weight loss in cancer patients, including appetite loss because of the effect of cancer treatments (**chemotherapy**, **radiation therapy**, or biological therapy) or psychological factors such as **depression**. Patients may suffer from **anorexia** and lose desire to eat, and thus consume less energy. When inadequate calories are consumed, it can lead to "wasting" of body stores (muscle and adipose tissue). Weight loss may be temporary or may continue at a life-threatening pace.

Weight loss may be also be a consequence of an increased requirement for calories (energy) due to infection, **fever**, or the effects of the tumor or cancer treatments. If infection or fever is present, it is necessary to consider that there is an increased caloric need of approximately 10% to 13% per degree above 98.6°F (37°C). Therefore, energy intake has to be increased to account for this rise in body temperature.

Weight loss may be a result of a common problem in cancer called cachexia. Approximately half of all cancer patients experience cachexia, a wasting syndrome that induces metabolic changes leading to a loss of muscle and fat. It has been proposed that cachexia may be due to the effects of the tumor, but this is debatable considering some patients with very large tumors do not experience cachexia, while others do even though tumors are less than 0.01% of body mass. Cachexia is most common in patients with pancreatic and gastric cancer. Approximately 83% to 87% of these patients experience weight loss. Cachexia is characterized by such symptoms as decreased appetite, fatigue, and poor performance status. It can occur in individuals who consume enough food, but due to disease complications, cannot absorb enough nutrients (i.e. fat malabsorption). Although energy expenditure is sometimes increased, cachexia can occur even with normal energy expenditure. Cachexia is multifactorial in nature and associated with mechanical factors, psychological factors, changes in taste, and cytokines. It should be distinguished from anorexia, in which there is a loss of desire to eat, resulting in weight loss. Cachexia is a serious complication in cancer patients, thought to be responsible for as many as 20% of all deaths from cancer..

Special concerns

In order to allow normal tissue repair following aggressive cancer therapies, patients require adequate calories and macronutrients in the form of protein, carbohydrates, and fat. Inadequate consumption of food and/or poor nutrition may impair the ability of a patient to tolerate a specific therapy. If a low tolerance to therapy necessitates a decrease in dose, the therapy's effectiveness could be compromised. Wound healing may also be impaired with poor nutrition and inadequate energy intake.

Research has demonstrated that men often experience significantly more weight loss than women over the course of the disease and lose weight much faster. On average, survival time for men is shorter than for women. Significant predictors of patient survival are stage of disease, initial weight-loss rate, and gender.

Treatments

Nutritional problems related to side effects should be addressed to ensure adequate nutrition and prevent weight loss. In particular, cancer patients should maintain an adequate intake of calories and protein to prevent protein-calorie malnutrition. The patient's caloric requirements can be calculated by a dietitian or doctor since nutrient requirements vary considerably from patient to patient. Moreover, patient education about nutrition is vitally important; several recent studies have shown that almost half of all cancer patients in the United States receive no nutritional information from health care professionals, including the 18% who experience significant weight loss.

The following dietary tips may help patients to reduce weight loss:

- Eat more when feeling the hungriest.
- Eat foods that are enjoyed the most.
- Eat several small meals and snacks instead of three large meals. A regular meal schedule should be kept so meals are not missed.
- Have ready-to-eat snacks on hand such as cheese and crackers, granola bars, muffins, nuts and seeds, canned puddings, ice cream, yogurt, and hard boiled eggs.
- Eat high-calorie foods and high-protein foods.
- Take a small meal as to enjoy the satisfaction of finishing a meal. Have seconds if still hungry.
- Eat in a pleasant atmosphere with family and friends if desired.
- Make sure to consume at least eight to 10 glasses of water per day to maintain fluid balance.

- Consider commercial liquid meal replacements such as Ensure, Boost, Carnation, and Sustacal.

An appetite stimulant may be given in order to prevent further weight loss such as **megestrol acetate** or **dexamethasone**. In **clinical trials**, both these medications appear to have similar and effective appetite stimulating effects with megestrol acetate having a slightly better toxicity profile. **Fluoxymesterone** has shown inferior efficacy and an unfavorable toxicity profile.

As of 2004, researchers at the Medical College of Virginia are studying a group of compounds known as cannabinoids for the treatment of cachexia and **vomiting** associated with cancer treatment. The best-known natural cannabinoids are derived from marijuana.

Further research is needed in order to devise an effective treatment for the loss of muscle tissue in cachexia. As of 2004, there are no medications, nutritional supplements, or other treatments that are even moderately successful in reversing the wasting of muscle tissue in cachexia.

Alternative and complementary therapies

Depression may affect approximately 15%–25% of cancer patients, particularly if the prognosis for recovery is poor. If anorexia is due to depression, there are antidepressant choices available through a physician. Counseling may be also be sought through a psychologist or psychiatrist to cope with depression.

It is important to check with a dietitian or doctor before taking nutritional supplements or alternative therapies because they may interfere with cancer medications or treatments. St. John's Wort has been used as a herbal remedy for treatment of depression, but it and prescription antidepressants are a dangerous combination that may cause symptoms such as nausea, weakness, and may cause one to become incoherent.

See also Taste alteration.

Resources

BOOKS

Quillin, Patrick, and Noreen Quillin. *Beating Cancer With Nutrition—Revised.* Sun Lakes, AZ: Bookworld Services, 2001.

PERIODICALS

Dahele, M., and K. C. Fearon. "Research Methodology: Cancer Cachexia Syndrome." *Palliative Medicine* 18 (July 2004): 409–417.

Hartmuller, V. W., and S. M. Desmond. "Professional and Patient Perspectives on Nutritional Needs of Patients with Cancer." *Oncology Nursing Forum* 31 (September 17, 2004): 989–996.

Hofman, M., G. R. Morrow, J. A. Roscoe, et al. "Cancer Patients' Expectations of Experiencing Treatment-Related Side Effects: a University of Rochester Cancer Center–Community Clinical Oncology Program Study of 938 Patients from Community Practices." *Cancer* 101 (August 15, 2004): 851–857.

Kant, Ashima, et al. "A Prospective Study of Diet Quality and Mortality in Women." *Journal of the American Medical Association* 283, no. 16 (2000): 2109–15.

Martin, B. R., and J. L. Wiley. "Mechanism of Action of Cannabinoids: How It May Lead to Treatment of Cachexia, Emesis, and Pain." *Journal of Supportive Oncology* 2 (July-August 2004): 305–314.

Muscaritoli, M., M. Bossola, R. Bellantone, and F. R. Fanelli. "Therapy of Muscle Wasting in Cancer: What Is the Future?" *Current Opinion in Clinical Nutrition and Metabolic Care* 7 (July 2004): 459–466.

Tisdale, M. J. "Cancer Cachexia." *Langenbeck's Archives of Surgery* 389 (August 2004): 299–305.

ORGANIZATIONS

American Institute for Cancer Research. 1759 R Street NW, Washington, D.C. 20009. (800) 843-8114 or (202) 328-7744. http://www.aicr.org, e-mail: support@aicr.org.

American Society for Clinical Nutrition. 9650 Rockville Pike, Bethesda, MD 20814-3998. (301) 634-7110. Fax: (301) 634-7350. http://www.ascn.org.

National Cancer Institute (NCI). Public Inquiries Office: Building 31, Room 10A31, 31 Center Dr., MSC 2580, Betheseda, MD 20892-2580 (301) 435-3848, (800) 4-CANCER, <http://cancer.gov/publications/>, <http://cancertrials.nci.nih.gov>, <http://cancernet.nci.nih.gov>.

National Center for Complementary and Alternative Medicine (NCCAM). 31 Center Dr., Room #5B-58, Bethesda, MD 20892-2182. (800) NIH-NCAM, Fax (301) 495-4957. <http://nccam.nih.gov>.

Crystal Heather Kaczkowski, MSc.
Rebecca J. Frey, PhD

Whipple procedure

Definition

A Whipple procedure, or pancreaticoduodenectomy, is a surgical procedure which is most often performed to treat **pancreatic cancer**. The operation may also be performed for **cancer** of the duodenum, cholangiocarcinoma (cancer of the bile duct), cancer of the ampulla (the area where the bile and pancreatic ducts enter the small intestine), and for chronic pancreatitis and benign (noncancerous) tumors involving the pancreatic head.

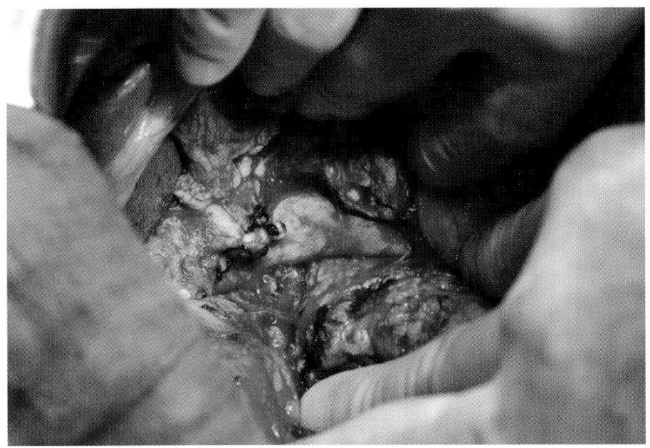

Surgeons performing a Whipple procedure, the removal of the pancreatic head. *(Barry Slaven, MD, PhD/Phototake. Reproduced by permission.)*

During the course of a Whipple procedure, the surgeon removes the head of the pancreas, the majority of the first part of the small intestine (the duodenum), part of the bile duct, and in some cases part of the stomach. Variations on the operation may include removal of the body of the pancreas and/or the entire gall bladder.

Purpose

The Whipple procedure is the most common operation performed for treatment of cancer of the pancreas. The pancreas is an organ located near the liver on the right side of the body. It produces both digestive juices and hormones that are involved in regulation of blood sugar. Pancreatic cancer most often affects what is called the exocrine pancreas, which is the portion of the pancreas involved in producing digestive juices.

Because it initially causes only vague symptoms, pancreatic cancer is often not diagnosed until later stages of the disease. Additionally, it spreads very quickly, so when the disease is often quite widespread by the time it is finally diagnosed. Symptoms of pancreatic cancer can include pain in the upper abdomen, often radiating to the back; jaundice (yellow eyes and skin); decreased appetite; **weight loss**; and **depression**.

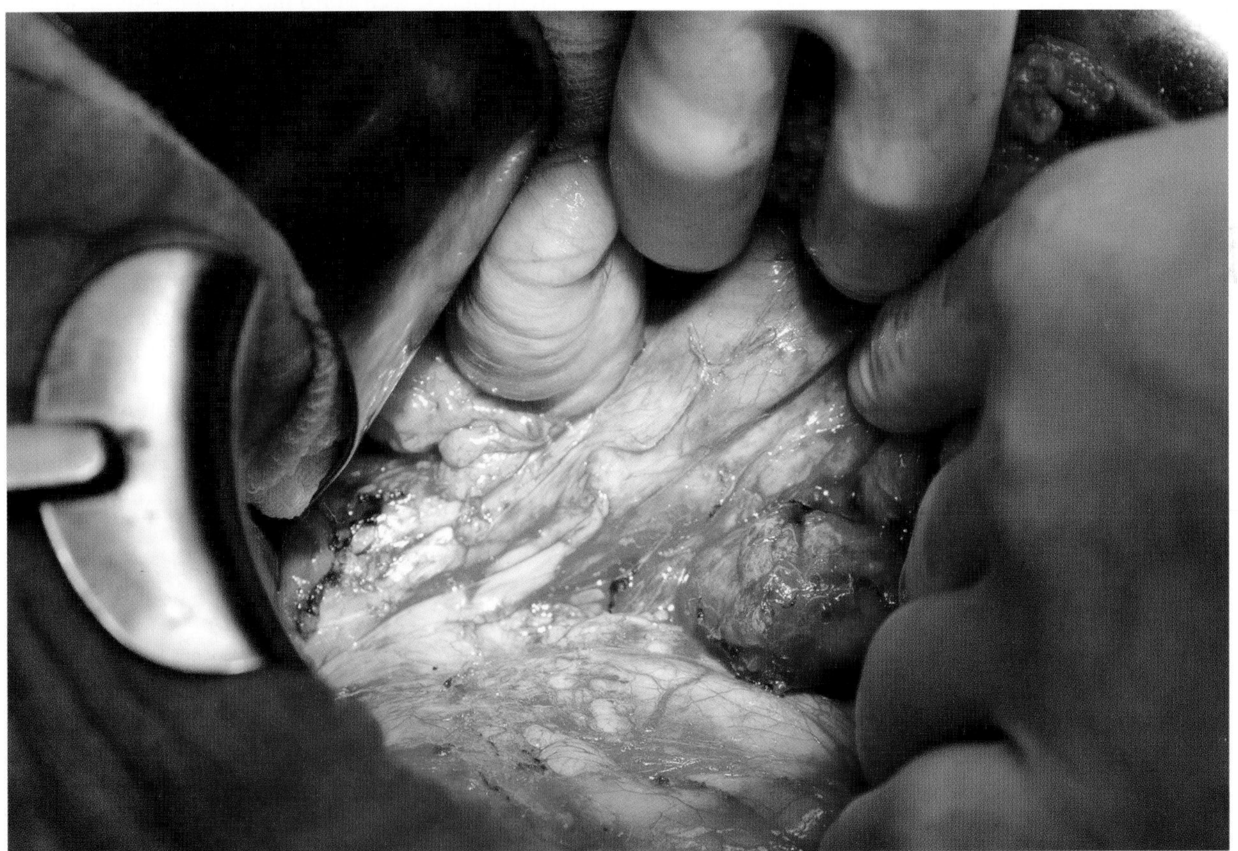

Whipple procedure. *(Barry Slaven, MD, PhD / Phototake. Reproduced by permission.)*

KEY TERMS

Anastomosis—A surgically created joining or opening between two organs or body spaces.

Fistula—An abnormal connection between two organs, or between an organ and the outside of the body.

Jaundice—A yellowish cast to the whites of the eyes and/or the skin, caused by excess bilirubin circulating in the bloodstreatm.

Demographics

The American Cancer Society estimates that approximately 37,680 people will be diagnosed with pancreatic cancer in the United States in 2008. About 34,290 people will die of pancreatic cancer in 2008, making pancreatic cancer the fourth leading cause of cancer death in the United States. Most people who are diagnosed with pancreatic cancer are over age 60. Men and women are about equally at risk. Risk factors for the development of pancreatic cancer include smoking, history of diabetes, family history, and a personal history of chronic pancreatitis. Researchers are still examining the possibility that other factors, such as certain workplace exposures or a high fat diet, may also increase an individual's risk of pancreatic cancer.

Description

A Whipple procedure is a lengthy operation, taking about four to six hours. General anesthesia is required. A classic operation requires a large abdominal incision through which the operation occurs. There are some centers that offer laparoscopic Whipple procedure performed with or without robotic assistance. This minimally invasive method of surgery is performed through four small incisions with the use of a fiberoptic scope and miniaturized surgical instruments.

After the head of the pancreas has been removed during the operation, three important connections (anastamoses) must be performed. The intestine must be connected to the remains of the pancreas, to the bile duct, and to the stomach. These anastamoses must be very carefully achieved, since any leak may allow pancreatic juices to enter the abdomen, risking severe complications.

Diagnosis/Preparation

The patient meets with the operating physician prior to surgery to discuss the details of the surgery and receive instructions on preoperative and postoperative care. Blood tests to evaluate bleeding time and an EKG to evaluate cardiac function may be performed several days prior to the operation. Directly preceding surgery, an intravenous (IV) line is placed to administer fluid and medications, and the patient is given a bowel prep to cleanse the bowel and prepare it for surgery.

Aftercare

Recuperation from Whipple procedure may be slow and difficult. Depending on the type of surgery (traditional open incision or minimally invasive), inpatient stay will range from five to 14 days. Because of the high likeilhood of gastroparesis (slow gastric emptying), patients will remain on intravenous feeding for five or six days following the operation. A nasogastric tube may be required to remove excess stomach acid and juices that accumulate. Advancement of diet through clear liquids, full liquids, soft foods, to regular diet will be slow and the timeframe will depend on the patient's tolerance of each new step. Some patients take as long as 4-6 weeks to have normal stomach emptying return. A feeding tube that delivers a nutritional formula directly into the jejunum may be used if recovery is overly slow.

Risks

Risks associated with the Whipple procedure include excessive bleeding, **infection**, and complications due to general anesthesia. Delayed gastric emptying after eating affects about 19% of patients. Leakage of pancreatic juices into the abdomen is a serious problem, since these digestive juices are strong enough to actually begin to digest the internal organs themselves. This can result in perforations (holes) in the intestine, stomach, or other nearby organs; abnormal communication between organs (fistulas); or necrosis (cell death) within an affected organ. Some patients may develop diabetes following Whipple procedure. Weight loss of 5-10% of original body weight is common after the operation, as is the need to take oral enzyme supplements to aid digestion.

Normal results

Although the recuperative time may be long, most patients return to their usual level of functioning and their usual quality of life after a Whipple procedure. However, the risk for further advancement of pancreatic cancer is very high. Many patients receive **chemotherapy** and radiation for further treatment of the cancer.

WHO PERFORMS THE PROCEDURE AND WHERE IS IT PERFORMED?

A Whipple procedure is performed in a hospital operating room. It is considered one of the most technically difficult operations, and should be performed by a very experienced, skilled surgeon who has successfully performed many of these same procedures. Some of the doctors who perform these operations include general surgeons, surgical gastroenterologists, and surgical oncologists.

QUESTIONS TO ASK THE DOCTOR

- Why is a Whipple procedure being recommended?
- What type of Whipple procedure would work best for me?
- What are the risks and complications associated with the recommended procedure?
- Are any nonsurgical treatment alternatives available?
- How soon after surgery may I resume my normal diet and activities?
- If the Whipple procedure is being done to treat pancreatic cancer, will I require any other treatment?

Morbidity and mortality rates

The Whipple procedure has a high morbidity and mortality rate. It requires the expertise of a surgeon who has performed a large number of these types of procedures. Even when highly skilled surgeons in cancer centers operate, 2-5% of patients die due to surgical complications. When less skilled surgeons perform this procedure, or when it is undertaken at smaller hospitals rather than major medial centers, the death rate from surgical complications may be as high as 15%. The complication rate is very high as well, between 30-50%. Possible complications include leakage from the anastomoses (connections) between organs, infection, bleeding, and slow gastric (stomach) emptying following meals. Risk of death from advancement of the original pancreatic cancer also is quite high, with only about 20% of all Whipple procedure patients surviving for five years after their initial diagnosis. Patients with no lymph node involvement at the time of surgery may have a higher five-year survival rate (about 40%). However, patients who receive chemotherapy but no surgery have only a 5% survival rate at five years.

Resources

BOOKS

Abeloff, M. D., et al. *Clinical Oncology*. 3rd ed. Philadelphia: Elsevier, 2004.

Feldman, M., et al. *Sleisenger & Fordtran's Gastrointestinal and Liver Disease*. 8th ed. St. Louis: Mosby, 2005.

Khatri, V. P., and J. A. Asensio. *Operative Surgery Manual*. 1st ed. Philadelphia: Saunders, 2003.

Townsend, C. M., et al. *Sabiston Textbook of Surgery*. 17th ed. Philadelphia: Saunders, 2004.

Rosalyn Carson-DeWitt, MD

Whole brain radiotherapy

Definition

Whole brain radiotherapy or **radiation therapy** (WBRT) is a type of conventional radiotherapy in which an external radiation source is aimed at the entire brain for treating **cancer**.

Purpose

WBRT is most often used to treat multiple **brain tumors** or metastatic cancer that has spread to the brain. Its purpose is to shrink multiple tumors throughout the brain, both large and small, with one procedure, rather than targeting individual tumors. It also can treat tumors deep in the brain that are inaccessible to surgery. In the past WBRT generally was used only for patients who were expected to live no more than one to two years and for whom no other treatment existed.

WBRT may be:

- the sole form of treatment for brain cancer
- performed in advance of other types of radiotherapy or microsurgery
- performed after surgery to reduce the risk of tumor recurrence

WRBT is most often performed:

- following surgery to treat primitive neuroectodermal tumors (PNETs) in adults and in children over age three

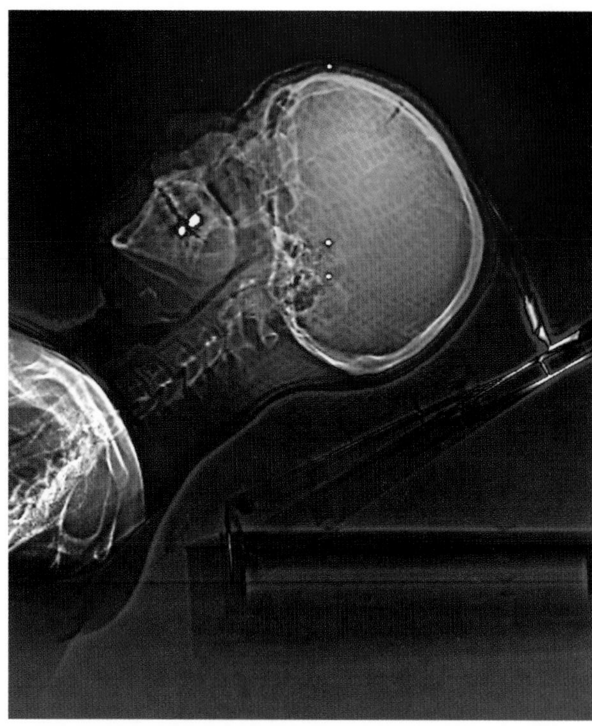

Colored computed tomography (CT) scan of the head of a patient being treated with radiotherapy for brain cancer. *(Zephyr/Photo Researchers, Inc. Reproduced by permission.)*

- following surgery and/or radiosurgery to treat single or multiple metastatic (secondary) tumors that have spread to the brain from other parts of the body
- to prevent metastasized cancer from spreading to the brain
- to treat HIV/AIDS-related primary central nervous system (CNS) lymphoma

Demographics

- Metastatic brain tumors—cancers that have spread to the brain from other parts of the body, most often the lung or breast—are the most common type of brain tumor, with an annual incidence more than four times greater than that of primary tumors that originate in the brain.
- It is estimated that every year more than 150,000 cancer patients will develop symptoms of a metastatic tumor in the brain or spinal cord.
- Medulloblastomas/embryonal/primitive tumors represent just 1% of all primary brain tumors.

Pediatric

Embryonal/primitive neuroectodermal tumors/medulloblastomas are the most common brain tumors in children from birth to age four, with an incidence of 0.92 per 100,000.

Geriatric

The number of elderly patients receiving WBRT for brain metastases is expected to increase in the future.

Precautions

WBRT is the most damaging of all radiation treatments and causes the most severe long-term side effects. It can lead to long-term disability including neurological deterioration and dementia. Furthermore, new brain tumors can begin to develop within a few months of completing WBRT. Therefore this treatment may only benefit patients in the near-short term. WBRT may not be the best option for patients who are expected to live at least 18 months. These patients may have the option of radiosurgery or multi-session stereotactic radiotherapy. These treatments have few or no side effects from damage to healthy brain tissue and, if necessary, can be repeated to treat either the original tumors or new tumors. An increasing amount of research suggests that radiosurgery and stereotactic radiotherapy can be as effective as WBRT without the side effects. A study published in 2009 found that patients suffered more memory and learning difficulties when WBRT was performed in addition to standard stereotactic radiosurgery (SRS). The study was halted early when it was found that patients receiving both SRS and WBRT were 96% more likely to experience declines in function and memory after four months than patients treated with SRS alone.

Pediatric

Children are extremely susceptible to the side effects of WBRT because their brains are still developing. Treatment with radiation is delayed as long as possible, at least until the age of three. PNETs in children under age three may be treated with **chemotherapy** following surgery to reduce or delay the need for WBRT.

Description

WBET delivers an even dose of high-energy **x rays** to the entire brain from two beams of radiation. Unlike radiosurgery or conformal radiotherapy, there is a maximum radiation dose for WBRT. This dose is usually 6,000 gray (Gy). Treatment is divided into daily sessions to allow the healthy tissues surrounding the tumors to repair themselves.

Preparation

WBRT is performed over a period of two to six weeks. Because hair loss is a side effect of WBRT, patients may want to purchase a wig or have a wig made from their own hair before beginning treatment. Corticosteroid treatment is often started at the outset of radiotherapy and continued throughout to help prevent some of the acute side effects.

Aftercare

Acute reactions to WBRT are caused by radiation-induced brain swelling (edema) and intracranial pressure and may include:

- muscle weakness
- headache
- nausea
- vomiting
- speech problems
- double vision

These reactions are temporary and are usually relieved by **corticosteroids** such as **dexamethasone**.

Other neurotoxic side effects of WBRT may include:

- fever
- hair loss (alopecia)
- damage to the skin and scalp (radiation dermatitis)
- hearing loss
- memory loss
- seizures
- lethargy
- fatigue

Some of these effects are transient. However hair loss, dermatitis, and hearing loss can persist for months. **Fatigue** following WBRT can be severe, but usually lessens within a few weeks after completing treatment.

Early-delayed or sub-acute reactions occur a few weeks or months after the completion of WBRT and may include loss of appetite and an increase in pre-existing neurologic symptoms, in addition to lethargy and fatigue. These symptoms usually last about six weeks, but can persist for several months.

Leukoencephalopathy is a type of early-delayed reaction that occurs from irritation to the white matter (mylenated tissue) of the brain from the radiation or from dead tumor cells. The severity of the symptoms depends on the amount of tissue damage. Leukoencephalopathy may be reversible and is usually treated with steroids.

QUESTIONS TO ASK YOUR DOCTOR

- How long will the WBRT take?
- What are the potential side effects of WBRT?
- What are the risks associated with WBRT?
- Are there alternatives to WBRT that may be appropriate for me?
- Should I get a second or third opinion before undergoing WBRT?

Methods for managing acute and early-delayed side effects of WBRT include:

- antiemetics, relaxation, imagery, and/or biofeedback to help control nausea and vomiting
- cutting the hair short before treatment and using satin pillowcases, an infant comb and brush, and only mild shampoo as the hair begins to grow back, and avoiding strong hair products and appliances
- avoiding the sun to protect damaged skin
- eating a balanced diet despite changes in appetite

Late reactions to WBRT are due to changes in the white matter and brain atrophy and tissue death (necrosis) caused by radiation-damaged blood vessels and the buildup of dead tumor cells. Symptoms can occur months to years after therapy is completed. Although symptoms vary from mild to severe, they are permanent and may become progressively worse. Late reactions can include:

- decreased intellectual abilities
- memory impairment
- confusion
- personality changes
- stroke-like symptoms
- general neurological deterioration
- dementia

Severe reactions such as tumor necrosis may require surgery to remove dead tissue.

Risks

WBRT may worsen neurological symptoms such as memory loss and problems with concentration and cognition. Severe radiation-induced dementia following WBRT is estimated to occur in 11% of patients who survive for one year and in up to 50% of those who survive for two years after treatment. Finally, since WBRT targets more healthy tissue than other types of radiotherapy, there is a risk that it will result in the development of new tumors.

Results

New brain tumors can begin to develop within a few months of completing WBRT. However a 2009 study of patients with one to three brain metastases, who were treated with SRS alone or with both SRS and WBRT, found that after one year 73% of the SRS plus WBRT patients were recurrence-free; in contrast, only 27% of the patients treated with SRS alone had no tumor recurrence. However four months after treatment 29% of the SRS plus WBRT patients had died compared with 13% of the SRS-only patients.

Geriatric

Most elderly patients with brain metastases have an unfavorable prognosis. Although WBRT improves symptoms in about 50% of these patients, long-term survivors are at serious risk for neurotoxic effects and dementia.

Resources

PERIODICALS

Aoyama, H., et al. "Stereotactic Radiosurgery Plus Whole-Brain Radiation Therapy vs. Stereotactic Radiosurgery Alone for Treatment of Brain Metastases: A Randomized Controlled Trial." *Journal of the American Medical Association* 295 (2006): 2483-2491.

Fraser, Ginny. "A Life in the Day." *Sunday Times (London)* (January 29, 2006): 86.

"Health Beat." *USA Today* 137, no. 2765 (February 2009): 3.

Nieder, Carsten, et al. "Is Whole-Brain Radiotherapy Effective and Safe in Elderly Patients with Brain Metastases?" *Oncology* 72, no. 5/6 (February 2008): 326-329.

OTHER

"The Essential Guide to Brain Tumors." *National Brain Tumor Society*.http://www.braintumor.org/upload/contents/330/GuideFINAL2007.pdf

"Facts & Statistics, 2009." *American Brain Tumor Association.* http://www.abta.org/siteFiles/SitePages/4E1FE8EDC134B66F0F552257CD4C36F5.pdf

"Help with Side Effects—Radiation Therapy." *American Brain Tumor Association*.http://www.abta.org/index.cfm?contentid = 105

Preidt, Robert. "Focused Radiation Protects Tumor Patients' Brain Function." *HealthDay*.http://www.nlm.nih.gov/medlineplus/news/fullstory_90190.html

"Radiation Injury to the Brain." *International RadioSurgery Association*.http://www.irsa.org/radiation_injury.html

"Radiation Therapy to the Brain." *American Cancer Society.* http://www.cancer.org/docroot/MBC/content/MBC_2_3X_Radiation_Therapy_to_the_Brain.asp?sitearea = MBC

"Understanding Brain Metastasis: A Guide for Patient and Caregiver." *National Brain Tumor Foundation and Lung Cancer Alliance*.http://www.braintumor.org/upload/contents/330/BrainMets%20FINAL.pdf

ORGANIZATIONS

American Brain Tumor Association, 2720 River Road, Des Plaines, IL, 60018, (847) 827-9910, (800) 886-2282, (847) 827-9918, info@abta.org, http://www.abta.org.

American Cancer Society, 1599 Clifton Road NE, Atlanta, GA, 30329-4251, (800) ACS-2345, http://www.cancer.org.

American College of Radiology, 1891 Preston White Drive, Reston, VA, 20191, (703) 648-8900, (800) 227-5463, info@acr.org, http://www.acr.org.

American Society for Radiation Oncology, 8280 Willow Oaks Corporate Drive, Suite 500, Fairfax, VA, 22031, (703) 502-1550, (800) 962-7876, (703) 502-7852, http://www.astro.org.

International RadioSurgery Association, 3002 N. 2nd Street, Harrisburg, PA, 17110, (717) 260-9808, http://www.irsa.org.

National Brain Tumor Society, 124 Watertown Street, Suite 2D, Watertown, MA, 02472, (617) 924-9997, (800) 770-8287, (617) 924-9998, info@braintumor.org, http://www.braintumor.org.

National Cancer Institute, NCI Public Inquiries Office, 6116 Executive Boulevard, Room 3036A, Bethesda, MD, 20006, (800) 4-CANCER, http://www.cancer.gov.

Margaret Alic, PhD

Wilms' tumor

Definition

Wilms' tumor is a cancerous tumor of the kidney that usually occurs in young children. It is named for Max Wilms, a German surgeon (1867–1918) and is also known as a nephroblastoma.

Demographics

Wilms' tumor occurs almost exclusively in young children. The average patient is about three years old, although cases have been reported in infants younger than six months and adults in their early twenties. Females are only slightly more likely than males to develop Wilms' tumors. In the United States, Wilms' tumor occurs in 8.3 individuals per million in white children under the age of 15 years. The rate is higher among African-Americans and lower among Asian-Americans. Wilms' tumors are found more commonly in patients with other types of birth defects. These defects include:

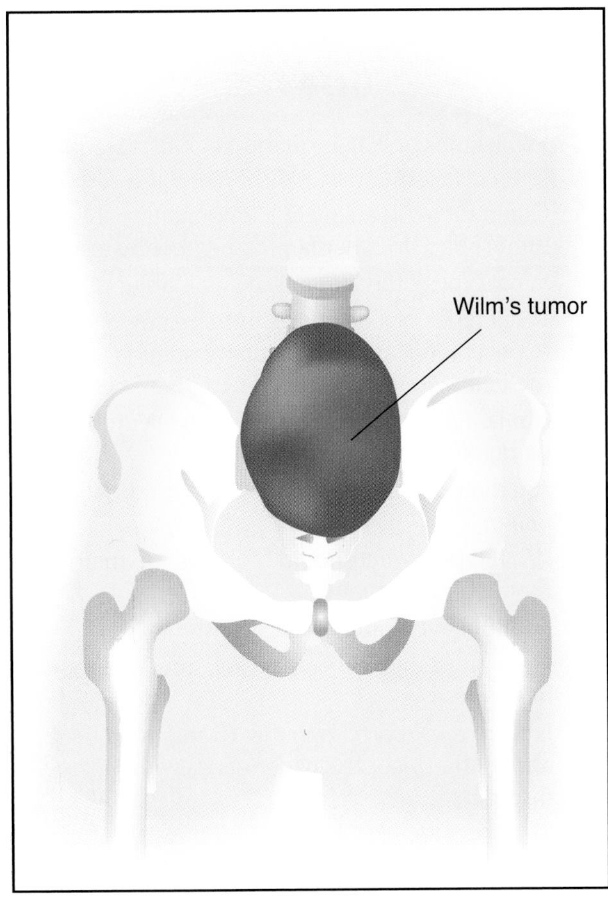

(Illustration by Argosy Publishing. Cengage Learning, Gale.)

- absence of the colored part (the iris) of the eye (aniridia)
- enlargement of one arm, one leg, or half of the face (hemihypertrophy)
- certain birth defects of the urinary system or genitals
- certain genetic syndromes (WAGR syndrome, Denys-Drash syndrome, and Beckwith-Wiedemann syndrome)

Description

When an unborn baby is developing, the kidneys are formed from primitive cells. Over time, these cells become more specialized. The cells mature and organize into the normal kidney structure. Sometimes, clumps of these cells remain in their original, primitive form. If these cells begin to multiply after birth, they may ultimately form a large mass of abnormal cells. This is known as a Wilms' tumor.

Wilms' tumor is a type of malignant tumor. This means that it is made up of cells that are significantly immature and abnormal. These cells are also capable of invading nearby structures within the kidney and traveling out of the kidney into other structures. Malignant cells can even travel through the body to invade other organ systems, most commonly the lungs and brain. These features of Wilms' tumor make it a type of **cancer** that, without treatment, would eventually cause death. However, advances in medicine during the last 20 years have made Wilms' tumor a very treatable form of cancer.

Causes and symptoms

The cause of Wilms' tumor is not completely understood. Because 15% of all patients with this type of tumor have other heritable defects, it seems clear that at least some cases of Wilms' tumor are due to an inherited alteration. A genetic defect known as WT1, the Wilms' tumor suppressor gene, has been identified in some patients on chromosome 11. It appears that the tendency to develop a Wilms' tumor can run in families. In fact, about 1.5% of all children with a Wilms' tumor have family members who have also had a Wilms' tumor. The genetic mechanisms associated with the disease are unusually complex; it is thought as of 2004 that the tumor develops because the defective WT1 gene fails to stop its growth. Other genes that have been linked to Wilms' tumor are located on chromosomes 16q, 7p15, and 17q12.

Some patients with Wilms' tumor experience abdominal pain, **nausea**, **vomiting**, high blood pressure, or blood in the urine. However, the parents of many children with this type of tumor are the first to notice a firm, rounded mass in their child's abdomen. This discovery is often made while bathing or dressing the child and frequently occurs before any other symptoms appear. Rarely, a Wilms' tumor is diagnosed after there has been bleeding into the tumor, resulting in sudden swelling of the abdomen and a low red blood cell count (**anemia**).

About 4–5% of Wilms' tumor cases involve both kidneys during the initial evaluation. The tumor appears on either side equally. When pathologists look at these tumor cells under the microscope, they see great diversity in the types of cells. Some types of cells are associated with a more favorable outcome in the patient than others. In about 15% of cases, physicians find some degree of cancer spread (**metastasis**). The most common sites in the body where metastasis occurs are the liver and lungs.

Researchers have found evidence that certain types of lesions occur before the development of the

Wilms' tumor. These lesions usually appear in the form of stromal, tubule, or blastemal cells.

Diagnosis

Children with Wilms' tumor generally first present to physicians with a swollen abdomen or with an obvious abdominal mass. The physician may also find that the child has **fever**, bloody urine, or abdominal pain. The physician will order a variety of tests before imaging is performed. These tests mostly involve blood analysis in the form of a white blood cell count, complete blood count, platelet count, and serum calcium evaluation. Liver and kidney function testing will also be performed as well as a urinalysis.

Initial diagnosis of Wilms' tumor is made by looking at the tumor using various imaging techniques. Ultrasound and **computed tomography** scans (CT scans) are helpful in diagnosing Wilms' tumor. Intravenous pyelography, where a dye injected into a vein helps show the structures of the kidney, can also be used in diagnosing this type of tumor. Final diagnosis, however, depends on obtaining a tissue sample from the mass (**biopsy**), and examining it under a microscope in order to verify that it has the characteristics of a Wilms' tumor. This biopsy is usually done during surgery to remove or decrease the size of the tumor. Other studies (chest **x rays**, CT scan of the lungs, **bone marrow biopsy**) may also be done in order to see if the tumor has spread to other locations.

QUESTIONS TO ASK YOUR DOCTOR

- What kinds of diagnostic studies will be required to ascertain the type and spread of this tumor?
- Could there be a genetic component to this tumor? Should other family member be tested?
- What types of treatments are available?
- What types of side effects from treatments can I expect? What are your recommendations to help me deal with those side effects?
- Am I eligible for any clinical trials? Would these be helpful to consider?
- Are there any lifestyle changes that I should make?
- What type of diet should I follow? Are there foods I should avoid?
- Should I avoid any medications?
- How often should I be checked after treatment has ended?
- Is there a support group that I can join to hear about other people's experiences with this disorder?

Treatment

In the United States, treatment for Wilms' tumor almost always begins with surgery to remove or decrease the size of the kidney tumor. Except in patients who have tumors in both kidneys, this surgery usually will require complete removal of the affected kidney. During surgery, the surrounding lymph nodes, the area around the kidneys, and the entire abdomen will also be examined. While the tumor can spread to these surrounding areas, it is less likely to do so compared to other types of cancer. In cases where the tumor affects both kidneys, surgeons will try to preserve the kidney with the smaller tumor by removing only a portion of the kidney, if possible. Additional biopsies of these areas may be done to see if the cancer has spread. The next treatment steps depend on whether/where the cancer has spread. Samples of the tumor are also examined under a microscope to determine particular characteristics of the cells making up the tumor.

Information about the tumor cell type and the spread of the tumor is used to decide the best kind of treatment for a particular patient. Treatment is usually a combination of surgery, medications used to kill cancer cells (**chemotherapy**), and x rays or other high-energy rays used to kill cancer cells (**radiation therapy**). These therapies are called adjuvant therapies, and this type of combination therapy has been shown to substantially improve outcome in patients with Wilms' tumor. It has long been known that Wilms' tumors respond to radiation therapy. Likewise, some types of chemotherapy have been found to be effective in treating Wilms' tumor. These effective drugs include **dactinomycin**, **doxorubicin**, **vincristine**, and **cyclophosphamide**. In rare cases, **bone marrow transplantation** may be used.

The National Wilms' Tumor Study Group (NWTSG) has developed a staging system to describe Wilms' tumors. All of the stages assume that surgical removal of the tumor has occurred. Stage I involves "favorable" Wilms' tumor cells and is usually treated successfully with combination chemotherapy involving dactinomycin and vincristine and without abdominal radiation therapy. Stage II tumors involving a favorable histology (cell characteristics) are usually treated with the same therapy as Stage I. Stage III tumors with favorable histology are usually treated with a combination chemotherapy with doxorubicin, dactinomycin, and vincristine along with radiation therapy to the abdomen. Stage IV disease with a favorable histology is generally treated with combination chemotherapy with dactinomycin, doxorubicin, and vincristine. These patients usually receive abdominal radiation therapy and lung radiation therapy if the tumor has spread to the lungs.

In the case of Stage II through IV tumors with unfavorable, or anaplastic, cells, then the previously-mentioned combination chemotherapy is used along with the drug cyclophosphamide. These patients also receive lung radiation therapy if the tumor has spread to the lungs. Another type of tumor cell can be present in Stages I through IV. This cell type is called clear cell **sarcoma** of the kidney. If this type of cell is present, then patients receive combination therapy with vincristine, doxorubicin, and dactinomycin. All of these patients receive abdominal radiation therapy and lung radiation therapy if the tumor has spread to the lungs.

Prognosis

The prognosis for patients with Wilms' tumor is quite good, compared to the prognosis for most types of cancer. One German study reported the overall five-year survival rate to be 89.5%. The patients who have the best prognosis are usually those who have a small-sized tumor, a favorable cell type, are young (especially under two years old), and have an early stage of cancer that has not spread. Modern treatments have been especially effective in the treatment of this cancer. Patients with the favorable type of cell have a long-term survival rate of 93%, whereas those with anaplasia have a long-term survival rate of 43% and those with the sarcoma form have a survival rate of 36%.

Prevention

There are no known ways to prevent a Wilms' tumor, although it is important that children with birth defects associated with Wilms' tumor be carefully monitored.

Resources

BOOKS

Abeloff, MD et al. *Clinical Oncology*. 3rd ed. Philadelphia: Elsevier, 2004.

Behrman, RE et al.*Nelson's Textbook of Pediatrics*.17th ed. Philadelphia: Saunders, 2004.

Brenner, BM et al*Brenner & Rector's The Kidney*. 7th ed. Philadelphia: Saunders, 2004.

Wein, AJ et al. *Campbell-Walsh Urology*. 9th ed. Philadelphia: Saunders, 2007.

PERIODICALS

Boglino, C., A. Inserra, S. Madafferi, et al. "A Single-Institution Wilms' Tumor and Localized Neuroblastoma Series." *Acta Paediatrica Supplementum* 93 (May 2004): 74–77.

Emerson, R. E., T. M. Ulbright, S. Zhang, et al. "Nephroblastoma Arising in a Germ Cell Tumor of Testicular Origin." *American Journal of Surgical Pathology* 28 (May 2004): 687–692.

Glick, R. D., M. J. Hicks, J. G. Nuchtern, et al. "Renal Tumors in Infants Less Than 6 Months of Age." *Journal of Pediatric Surgery* 39 (April 2004): 522–525.

Weirich, A., R. Ludwig, N. Graf, et al. "Survival in Nephroblastoma Treated According to the Trial and Study SIOP-9/GPOH with Respect to Relapse and Morbidity." *Annals of Oncology* 15 (May 2004): 808–820.

OTHER

Online Mendelian Inheritance in Man (OMIM). #194070. "Wilms Tumor 1; WT1." <http://www3.ncbi.nlm.nih.gov/entrez/dispomim.cgi?id = 194070.>

ORGANIZATIONS

American Cancer Society. 1515 Clifton Rd. NE, Atlanta, GA 30329. (800) 227-2345. <http://www.cancer.org.>

March of Dimes Birth Defects Foundation, National Office. 1275 Mamaroneck Ave., White Plains, NY 10605. <http://www.modimes.org.>

National Cancer Institute (National Institutes of Health). 9000 Rockville Pike, Bethesda, MD 20892. (800) 422-6237. <http://www.nci.nih.gov\.>

National Wilms Tumor Study Group (NWTSG). Fred Hutchinson Cancer Research Center, 1100 Fairview Avenue North, P. O. Box 19024, Seattle, WA 98109-1024. (800) 553-4878. Fax: (206) 667-6623. <http://www.nwtsg.org.>

Mark A. Mitchell, M.D.
Rebecca J. Frey, PhD

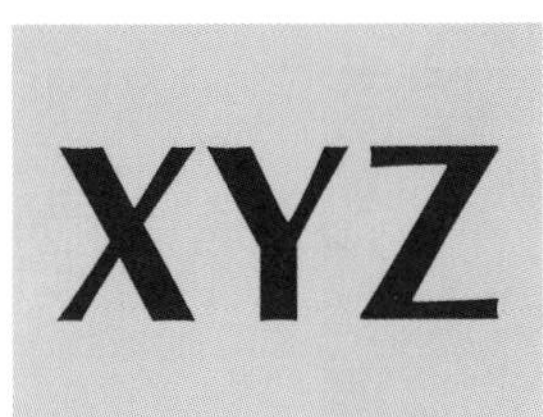

X rays

Definition

X rays are a type of radiation used in imaging and therapy that uses short wavelength energy beams capable of penetrating most substances except heavy metals.

Purpose

Diagnostic x rays are some of the most powerful medical imaging tools available. Other imaging techniques that do not use x rays include **magnetic resonance imaging** (MRI), **ultrasonography**, and radionucleotide imaging. Based on the symptoms presented by the patient, the physician can request specific x rays (such as chest x rays) that help diagnose many types of cancers, including sarcomas, lymphomas, and lung cancers. X rays allow the physician to visualize certain internal body conditions with little or no invasive procedures. Conditions may be visualized on photographic film, or for more complex and detailed information, **computed tomography** (CT scan), fluroscopy, or **angiography** might be used.

Precautions

Before consenting to any x-ray procedure, the patient should consider the impact of existing medical conditions or medications. Sensitivities to contrast dyes may produce allergic reactions. Pregnant women or those who suspect they might be pregnant should consult a physician prior to x-ray treatments to avoid injury to the fetus. Nursing mothers may be required to store enough milk to last for 48 hours following certain procedures. Patient age should always be taken into consideration when choosing the type and intensity of x ray. Patients should be aware that some prescribed **cancer** medications act as radiosensitizers and amplify the effect of x rays. Any patient with a suppressed immune system or diabetes may require special x-ray procedures.

Description

X-ray procedures are administered in a hospital or clinical setting. Most procedures may be conducted on an outpatient basis. The time required for the procedure may vary from a few minutes to more than an hour. There is little or no discomfort associated with diagnostic x rays. The general procedure for diagnostic x rays include:

- proper positioning and shielding of the patient
- administering contrast dyes, if necessary
- administering radiation
- review of the films by a technician to insure proper imaging
- Scheduling a time to review the films with the radiologist. However, if fluoroscopy or angiography is used, the procedure is dynamic (in motion), and the radiologist is present during the x ray administration.
- dismissal of the patient

Preparation

Diagnostic x rays require little preparation. The patient may be required to abstain from food and liquids for a certain period prior to the x ray. For some x rays, enemas may be necessary or a contrast agent may be administered immediately prior to or during the procedure.

Aftercare

For non-invasive diagnostic x-ray procedures, the patient is dismissed immediately after the films have been reviewed, and little or no aftercare is necessary.

Risks

A general rule for x rays suggests that the beneficial effects of x rays far exceed the risks involved. As a result of certified training and strict guideline compliance, risks from technical application are essentially

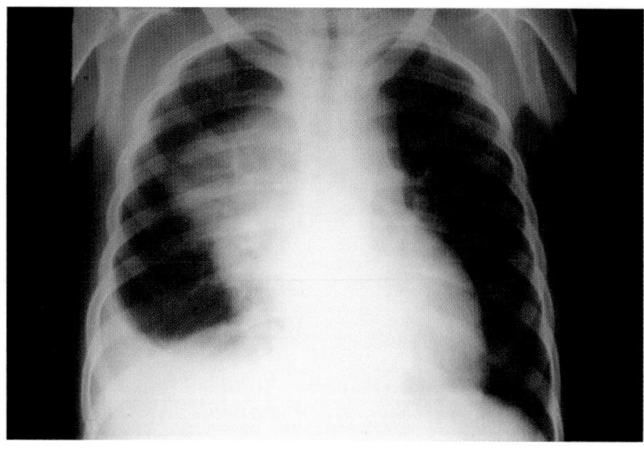

Chest x ray of patient with Hodgkin's disease. *(Custom Medical Stock Photo. Reproduced by permission.)*

nonexistent. However, for any x-ray procedure, radiation exposure is always a concern, and although uncommon, the risk of **infection** during invasive techniques can not be discounted.

Normal results

Diagnostic x rays provide detailed information that the physician can use to determine the best approach to correct or control a medical problem. Normal results would indicate no existing abnormalities.

Abnormal results

Abnormal results would indicate irregularities such as a tumor, an enlarged lymph node, or **pleural effusion**. Although highly unlikely, diagnostic x-ray films can be misread and the wrong diagnosis made.

See also Barium enema; Bone survey; CT-guided biopsy; Imaging studies; Intravenous urography; Lymphangiography; Nephrostomy; Pain management; Percutaneous transhepatic cholangiography; Radiation therapy; Stereotactic needle biopsy; Upper GI series.

KEY TERMS

Angiography—A radiographic technique in which an opaque contrast material is injected into a blood vessel for the purpose of identifying its anatomy on x ray.

Computed tomography (CT)—A special radiographic technique that uses a computer to convert multiple x-ray images into a two dimensional cross-sectional image.

Contrast dye—A radiopaque dye that allows enhancement of the anatomy demonstrable with conventional x ray.

Fluoroscopy—X-ray imaging of moving anatomic structures.

Gene therapy—The delivery of normal genes or genetically altered cells to the site of a tumor.

Interventional radiography—Diagnostic and therapeutic x-ray procedures that are invasive or surgical in nature but do not require the use of general anesthesia.

Pleural effusion—The accumulation of fluid in the pleural space, the region between the outer surface of each lung.

Radiologist—A physician specially trained in the use of x-rays for diagnostic and therapy purposes.

QUESTIONS TO ASK THE DOCTOR

- What type of x-ray procedure is best to diagnosis my condition?
- Will the procedure or treatment hurt?
- How long will it take each time and how many treatments are required?
- What are my chances for a complete recovery?
- Are these procedures covered by insurance?

Resources

BOOKS

Brant, William E., and Clyde A. Helms, editors. *Fundamentals of Diagnostic Radiology*. 2nd ed. Baltimore: Williams & Wilkins, 1999.

PERIODICALS

Henchke, Claudia, et al. "Early Lung Cancer Action Project: Overall Design and Findings from Baseline Screening." *Lancet* 354 (July 1999): 99–105.

OTHER

"CT Screening Detects Majority of Lung Cancer Cases Missed by X ray." *RSNA Meeting*. Dec., 1998. [cited March 29, 2001 and June 28, 2001]. http://www.psl group.com.

Harrison, Pam. *Lung Cancer Detected Earlier with CT Scan than with X ray*. 2000 Reuters Ltd. 29 March 2001. [cited June 28, 2001]. http://www.respiratorycare.medscape.com.

Marchant, Joan. "Pixels Join Cancer Fight." *The Guardian*. Dec. 1999. [cited April 21, 2001 and June 28, 2001]. http://www.guardianunlimited.co.uk.

Jane Taylor-Jones, M.S.

Xerostomia

Description

Xerostomia, also known as dry mouth, is marked by a significant reduction in the secretion of saliva. Signs and symptoms of xerostomia include:

- dryness of the mouth
- cracked lips, cuts, or cracks at the corners of the mouth
- taste changes
- a burning sensation of the tongue
- changes in the surface of the tongue
- difficulty wearing dental appliances (like dentures)
- difficulty swallowing fluids accompanied by an increase in thirst Xerostomia makes the mouth less able to neutralize acid, clean the teeth and gums, and protect itself from **infection**. This can lead to the development of gum disease and cavities.

Saliva is necessary for carrying out the normal functions of the oral cavity, such as taste, speech, and swallowing. Saliva provides calcium and phosphate, minerals that protect the teeth against softening. It also contains substances inhibiting the production of bacteria that cause tooth decay. In addition, saliva buffers the acids produced when leftover food particles are broken down by bacteria.

Xerostomia causes the following mouth changes that can contribute to discomfort for the patient, and an increased risk for oral lesions:

- Saliva becomes thick and is less able to lubricate the mouth.
- Acids in the mouth cannot be neutralized, leading to mineral loss from the teeth.
- There is an increased risk for cavities because the mouth is less able to control bacteria.
- Plaque becomes thicker and heavier because of the patient's difficulty in maintaining good oral hygiene.
- The acid produced after eating or drinking sugary foods leads to further mineral loss from the teeth, causing even more tooth decay.

Causes

Xerostomia in **cancer** patients is primarily caused by the effects of **radiation therapy** on the salivary glands, usually the result of radiation to the head and neck area. These changes may occur rapidly and cannot normally be reversed, especially if the salivary glands themselves are irradiated. Within one week of starting radiation treatment, the production of saliva drops and continues to decrease as treatment continues. The severity of xerostomia is dependent upon the radiation dose and how many salivary glands are irradiated. Typically, the salivary glands inside the upper back cheeks (the parotid glands) are more affected than others. Salivary glands that are not irradiated may become more active as a way of compensating for the loss of saliva from the destroyed glands.

A number of medications can cause xerostomia, including many drugs used in the management of cancer or cancer treatment side effects. Some of these are: atropine, **amitriptyline**, **carbamazepine**, diphenhydramine, **gabapentin**, haloperidol, loperamide, **lorazepam**, **meperidine**, and **scopolamine**, among several others.

Xerostomia may develop in patients with HIV infection, as the virus often damages the salivary glands.

Lastly, xerostomia often accompanies the normal aging process; between 25 and 50% of people over the age of 65 complain of increasing dryness of mouth.

Treatments

A number of **clinical trials** are investigating drugs called radioprotectors, which are given at the time of radiation therapy in an attempt to prevent xerostomia. If xerostomia has already developed, there are a number of measures that may help to both alleviate the symptoms of dry mouth and prevent cavities and gum disease. These measures include:

- cleaning the mouth well at least four times per day (after every meal and at bedtime)
- rinsing the mouth immediately after every meal
- using fluoride toothpaste to brush the teeth
- sipping water frequently
- rinsing the mouth with a salt and baking soda solution four to six times per day (1/2 tsp. salt, 1/2 tsp. baking soda, and 8 oz of water)
- avoiding foods and liquids containing large amounts of sugar
- avoiding mouthwashes containing alcohol
- using moisturizer on the lips
- using saliva substitutes to help relieve discomfort
- using a sialogogue such as pilocarpine (Salagen), which can stimulate saliva secretion from the remaining salivary glands
- applying a prescription-strength fluoride gel daily at bedtime to clean the teeth

Xerostomia usually cannot be reversed when the cause is the destruction of the salivary glands by radiation treatments. It may be reversible if related to a medication. All of the treatment measures serve to increase the level of comfort, decrease the chance for oral lesions, and reduce the occurrence of gum disease and cavities.

Resources

BOOKS

Beers, Mark H., MD, and Robert Berkow, MD, editors. "Dentistry in Medicine." Section 9, Chapter 103 In *The Merck Manual of Diagnosis and Therapy*. Whitehouse Station, NJ: Merck Research Laboratories, 2002.

PERIODICALS

Bruce, S. D. "Radiation-Induced Xerostomia: How Dry Is Your Patient?" *Clinical Journal of Oncology Nursing* 8 (February 2004): 61–67.

Nagler, R. M. "Salivary Glands and the Aging Process: Mechanistic Aspects, Health-Status and Medicinal-Efficacy Monitoring." *Biogerontology* 5 (March 2004): 223–233.

Pinto, A., and S. S. De Rossi. "Salivary Gland Disease in Pediatric HIV Patients: An Update." *Journal of Dentistry for Children (Chicago)* 71 (January-April 2004): 33–37.

Porter, S. R., C. Scully, and A. M. Hegarty. "An Update of the Etiology and Management of Xerostomia." *Oral Surgery, Oral Medicine, Oral Pathology, Oral Radiology, and Endodontics* 97 (January 2004): 28–46.

OTHER

Hodson, D.I., et al. "Symptomatic Treatment of Radiation-induced Xerostomia in Head and Neck Cancer Patients." *Cancer Care Ontario Practice Guideline Initiative*. April 2000. [cited July 18, 2001]. http://hiru.mcmaster.Ca/ccopgi/guidelines/head/cpg5_5f.html.

"Oral Complications of Chemotherapy and Head/Neck Radiation—Supportive Care." *CancerNet PDQ*. [cited July 18, 2001]. http://cancernet.nci.nih.gov.

Deanna Swartout-Corbeil, R.N.
Rebecca J. Frey, PhD

Zoledronate

Definition

Zoledronate, which is also known as zoledronic acid, is a treatment for **hypercalcemia** (high levels of calcium in the blood) caused by tumors. It is sold under the brand name Zometa. New laboratory evidence suggests that, in addition, zoledronate may have direct anticancer effects.

KEY TERMS

Bisphosphonates—A class of drugs that inhibit the action of osteoclasts—the cells that dissolve or break down bone.

Bone metastases—The spread of tumor cells from the primary site of origin to bone. Bone metastases from breast cancer, for example, represent breast cancer cells that have invaded bone. They are not the same as bone cancer cells that originate in bone.

Hypercalcemia of malignancy—Also called tumor-induced hypercalcemia; high levels of calcium in the blood from the dissolving of bone, either directly by cancer cells or indirectly by chemicals released from cancer cells.

Purpose

Tumor-induced hypercalcemia is also known as hypercalcemia of malignancy. Tumor-induced hypercalcemia may be caused by a tumor spreading to and causing breakdown of bone, or by chemicals released from some tumors. The result is high levels of calcium in the blood. High levels of calcium may cause changes in mental status, constipation, and kidney damage.

Zoledronate was approved by the Food and Drug Administration (FDA) in 2002 as a treatment for **multiple myeloma** and bone metastases. Bone metastases may develop if cells from breast, lung, or other cancers are transplanted to bone by the disease process. Bone **metastasis** may cause pain, compression of the nerves of the spine, and bone fractures.

Other drugs in the same class as zoledronate are used to prevent pain or fractures in people with bone metastases. Zoledronate appears to be effective for this use as well, particularly in men being treated for **prostate cancer**. In addition, these drugs (the class of **bisphosphonates**) are being studied to see if they prevent the development of bone metastases in the first place.

Description

Zoledronate is one of a group of medicines known as bisphosphonates. Bisphosphonates prevent bone destruction by inhibiting the action of osteoclasts, cells that break down bone. Zoledronate is one of the most potent bisphosphonates approved for use in the United States.

Recommended dosage

As of 2002 the recommended dosage of zoledronate is 4 mg, given intravenously over a 15-minute period. This short infusion period gives zoledronate an advantage over other drugs in the bisphosphonate class; one study done in Australia found that patients preferred zoledronate to other intravenous bisphosphonates for this reason. The frequency of administration of zoledronate for hypercalcemia depends on the patient's calcium blood level.

Side effects

The most common side effects due to zoledronate that have been reported to date are **fever**, low blood concentration of phosphate, and low blood calcium (not low enough to cause symptoms). Overall, the drug appears to be well tolerated and safe for long-term use in **cancer** patients.

Resources

BOOKS

Wilson, Billie Ann, Margaret T. Shannon, and Carolyn L. Stang. *Nurse's Drug Guide 2003*. Upper Saddle River, NJ: Prentice Hall, 2003.

PERIODICALS

Chern, B., D. Joseph, D. Joshua, et al. "Bisphosphonate Infusions: Patient Preference, Safety and Clinic Use." *Supportive Care in Cancer* 12 (June 2004): 463–466.

Rosen, L. S., D. Gordon, N. S. Tchekmedyian, et al. "Long-Term Efficacy and Safety of Zoledronic Acid in the Treatment of Skeletal Metastases in Patients with Nonsmall Cell Lung Carcinoma and Other Solid Tumors: A Randomized, Phase III, Double-Blind, Placebo-Controlled Trial." *Cancer* 100 (June 15, 2004): 2613–2621.

Saad, F., D. M. Gleason, R. Murray, et al. "Long-Term Efficacy of Zoledronic Acid for the Prevention of Skeletal Complications in Patients with Metastatic Hormone-Refractory Prostate Cancer." *Journal of the National Cancer Institute* 96 (June 2, 2004): 879–882.

ORGANIZATIONS

American Society of Health-System Pharmacists (ASHP). 7272 Wisconsin Avenue, Bethesda, MD 20814. (301) 657-3000. www.ashp.org.

United States Food and Drug Administration (FDA). 5600 Fishers Lane, Rockville, MD 20857-0001. (888) INFO-FDA. www.fda.gov.

Bob Kirsch
Rebecca J. Frey, PhD

Zollinger-Ellison syndrome

Definition

In Zollinger-Ellison syndrome (ZES), a tumor (a gastrinoma) secretes the hormone gastrin, which stimulates the secretion of gastric acid. This leads to the development of ulcers in the stomach and duodenum (the first part of the small intestine).

Description

In normal individuals, the stomach secretes the hormone gastrin after food enters the stomach. Gastrin is carried by the bloodstream to other parts of stomach. The main effect of gastrin is to stimulate the parietal cells of the stomach. Parietal cells are stomach cells that secrete gastric acid to aid in digestion. This acid plays a vital role in the digestion of food. This process is highly regulated so that the stomach produces gastrin in significant amounts only when necessary, as when there is food in the stomach.

The underlying entity of ZES is a tumor called a gastrinoma which secretes gastrin inappropriately. Marked overproduction of gastrin leads to hypersecretion of gastric acid by the parietal cells. The end result is severe ulcers of the stomach and duodenum that are more difficult to treat than common ulcers.

Gastrinomas are generally small tumors located in the pancreas or duodenum. They often occur in multiples in the same patient. More than half of all gastrinomas are malignant, with the potential to spread to nearby lymph nodes and also spread to the liver and other organs by way of **metastasis**. The malignant potential of gastrinoma is ultimately more life-threatening than the associated ulcers.

The ulcers in ZES are frequently located further down the gastrointestinal tract than common ulcers, and they may be multiple.

About 25% of patients with ZES also demonstrate other tumors of the endocrine system in a syndrome called Multiple Endocrine Neoplasia syndrome.

Demographics

ZES occurs slightly more frequently in males than females. The average age of onset is between 30 and 50 years of age. It is difficult to determine the prevalence of ZES, but it is not a common syndrome.

KEY TERMS

Angiography—Radiographic examination of blood vessels after injection with a special dye

Computed tomography—A radiology test by which images of cross-sectional planes of the body are obtained

Duodenum—The first portion of the small intestine in continuity with the stomach

Endoscopy—Examination of the interior of a hollow part of the body by means of a special, lighted instrument

Gastric—Of or relating to the stomach

Gastrin—Hormone normally secreted by the stomach that stimulates secretion of gastric acid

Gastrinoma—Tumor that secretes the hormone gastrin

Magnetic resonance imaging—A radiology test that reconstructs images of the body based on magnetic fields

Malignant—In reference to cancer, having the ability to invade local tissues and spread to distant tissues by metastasis

Metastasis—The spread of tumor cells from one part of the body to another

Parietal cells—Stomach cells that secrete gastric acid to aid in digestion

Scintigraphy—A radiology test that involves injection and detection of radioactive substances to create images of body parts

Ultrasound—A radiology test utilizing high frequency sound waves

Causes and symptoms

The symptoms of ZES are chiefly related to the ulcer disease. The main symptom is abdominal pain, present in the vast majority of patients. Ulcers can also cause **nausea**, **vomiting**, and heartburn. Compared with patients with common ulcers, patients with ZES generally have more severe and persistent symptoms that are more difficult to control. In some cases, the ulcers can bleed or actually perforate completely through the walls of the stomach or duodenum.

Many patients also suffer **diarrhea** in addition to ulcer pain. In fact, diarrhea is the only symptom in a small fraction of patients, and the diarrhea may precede the development of ulcers in the stomach and duodenum.

Diagnosis

A number of clinical circumstances suggest that a patient's ulcer disease may be due to ZES:

- ulcer disease resistant to conventional medical treatment
- recurrent ulcers after surgery intended to cure the ulcer disease
- ulcer disease in the absence of the usual risk factors for ulcers
- ulcers located in abnormal locations in the gastrointestinal tract
- multiple ulcers
- ulcers accompanied by diarrhea
- strong family history of ulcer disease

Diagnosis of ZES must be confirmed by observing abnormally high levels of gastrin in the blood. This is the hallmark of the disease. But it must be mentioned that the gastrinoma of ZES is not the only cause of hypersecretion of gastrin. ZES is distinguished from these other conditions by the presence of appropriate symptoms and high levels of gastrin and gastric acid. In cases where the diagnosis is not clear, several provocative tests can help determine if the patient has ZES. In the intravenous secretin injection test, a standard dose of the hormone secretin is injected intravenously. If the blood levels of gastrin respond by increasing a certain amount, the diagnosis is ZES. Similarly, in the intravenous calcium infusion test, a dose of calcium is injected and gastrin levels are measured. A substantial increase in the gastrin level points to ZES. A newer test measures the response in gastrin level to the ingestion of a standard meal. For example, the standard meal might be one slice of bread, one boiled egg, 200 mL of milk, and 50 gm of cheese.

Treatment team

The surgeon and gastroenterologists are the chief members of the treatment team. Radiologists play a vital role in the localization of the gastrinoma before surgery. Oncologists may be involved after surgery or if surgery is not indicated.

Clinical staging, treatments, and prognosis

The goal of treatment for ZES is the elimination of excess gastrin production, acid hypersecretion, ulcer disease, and malignant potential. This is achieved only by complete surgical removal of all gastrinomas. An attempt at surgical cure is offered to most patients, with the exception of those who already have widespread metastasis to the liver or who are too ill to undergo surgery. It is important to locate the gastrinoma(s) and any possible areas of metastasis before surgery. This can be accomplished with tests such as **computed tomography** (CT), ultrasound, **magnetic resonance imaging** (MRI), **angiography**, scintigraphy, and endoscopy. But as gastrinomas may be small, multiple, and hidden in atypical positions, finding the exact locations of all cancerous tissue can be challenging and sometimes impossible. In that case, surgeons will still proceed and attempt to find the tumor(s) at the time of operation. All identified gastrinoma should be removed if possible, including involved lymph nodes. Metastatic lesions in the liver can sometimes be safely removed, but only when they are isolated to one part of the liver.

Chemotherapy is sometimes able to reduce tumor size, which may relieve some symptoms due to local invasion or massive growth of the tumor. But it has not been shown to consistently prolong survival.

Medical therapy plays a vital role in the treatment of ZES. A group of drugs known as proton pump inhibitors, which includes omeprazole (a drug used to treat common ulcers), is effective in decreasing acid secretion and promoting ulcer healing in patients with ZES. Omeprazole acts by blocking the last biochemical step in acid production. Omeprazole should be prescribed immediately after diagnosis. If surgery is not attempted, or ultimately unsuccessful, omeprazole is also useful for long-term treatment. For reasons that are not fully known, sometimes patients still require omeprazole after successful surgery. Another drug called octreotide is also effective in reducing acid secretion.

The prognosis for ZES depends primarily on whether or not the gastrinoma can be completely removed. If the **cancer** has spread diffusely to the liver, surgical cure is nearly impossible. The gastrinoma tissue is completely removed in about 40% of patients, resulting in reduced acid secretion and resolution of ulcer disease or diarrhea. These patients should expect a normal life expectancy, although they should undergo regular testing thereafter and may also require long-term omeprazole treatment. The prognosis is poor for patients in whom all the gastrinoma cannot be removed.

Clinical trials

In 2001, five **clinical trials** were recruiting patients with Zollinger-Ellison syndrome. These trials were studying various aspects of treatment for the syndrome, including the use of Omeprazole, interferon therapy, and combination chemotherapy. For further information about ongoing clinical trials, patients may consult the National Institutes of Health clinical trials site listed below.

See also Multiple endocrine neoplasia syndromes.

Resources

BOOKS

Thompson, James C., and Courtney M. Townsend, Jr. "Endocrine Pancreas." In *Sabiston Textbook of Surgery*, edited by Courtney Townsend Jr. 16th ed. Philadelphia: W.B. Saunders Company, 2001, pp. 646–61.

PERIODICALS

Norton, J. A., D. L. Fraker, H. R. Alexander, D. J. Venzon, J. L. Doppman, et al. "Surgery to Cure the Zollinger-Ellison Syndrome." *New England Journal of Medicine* 341, no. 9 (August 26, 1999): 635–44.

OTHER

Clinical Trials. [cited July 24, 2001]. <http://clinicaltrials.gov/>.

"Zollinger-Ellison Syndrome." *National Digestive Diseases Information Clearinghouse*. [cited July 24, 2001]. http://www.niddk.nih.gov/health/digest/summary/zolling/zolling.htm.

Kevin O. Hwang, M.D.

Zolpidem

Definition

Zolpidem is a medicine that helps a person get to sleep and stay asleep. The brand name of zolpidem in the U.S. is Ambien.

Purpose

Zolpidem is a sleep medication. It is intended for the short-term treatment of insomnia. Zolpidem may be particularly useful for people who have trouble falling asleep.

Description

Sleep medications are called sedatives or hypnotics. Zolpidem affects brain chemicals, resulting in sleep. It is somewhat similar in its actions on sleep to the group of drugs known as **benzodiazepines**. Zolpidem is only intended for short term use (seven–10 days). Although there is some information published about effectiveness with longer use, some side effects may increase with longer use.

Recommended dosage

The usual dose is 10 mg before bedtime in adults and 5 mg before bedtime in the elderly and in people with liver disease. The onset of effect occurs within about 30 minutes and the effects on sleep last for 6–8 hours.

Precautions

It is suggested that zolpidem not be discontinued abruptly after regular use (that is daily use for even as short a time as one week). Instead, the drug should be gradually tapered. The tapering is recommended to avoid the possibility of a withdrawal syndrome as well as to avoid the possibility of a rebound worsening of insomnia.

Side effects

The most common side effects of zolpidem include drowsiness, dizziness, and headache. Drowsiness, of course, is desirable when it occurs at bedtime. Daytime drowsiness that is left over from the night before would be considered a side effect. Other side effects include **diarrhea**, **nausea and vomiting**, and muscle aches. Rarely, amnesia, confusion, falls, and tremor are seen. Falls probably result from the drowsiness or dizziness. There was also a reported study of a patient sleepwalking when taking Zolpidem along with valproic acid. It is possible that the interactions between the two might have resulted in sleepwalking.

Interactions

Increased effects of zolpidem (eg. more drowsiness, confusion) may be seen with **alcohol consumption** and with other drugs known to cause drowsiness.

Bob Kirsch

APPENDIX I: NCI-DESIGNATED COMPREHENSIVE CANCER CENTERS

Comprehensive Cancer Centers have been designated as such by the National Cancer Institute. They are required to have basic laboratory research in several fields; to be able to transfer research findings into clinical practice; to conduct clinical studies and trials; to research cancer prevention and control; to offer information about cancer to patients, the public, and health care professionals; and to provide community service related to cancer control.

Alabama

UAB Comprehensive Cancer Center
University of Alabama at Birmingham
1802 Sixth Ave. South, NP2555
Birmingham, AL 35294-3300.
Phone: (205) 934-5077
Fax: (205) 975-7428
E-mail: http://www3.ccc.uab.edu/

Arizona

Arizona Cancer Center
University of Arizona
1515 North Campbell Avenue
P.O. Box 245024
Tucson, AZ 85724.
Phone: (520) 626-7685
Fax: (520) 626-6898
E-mail: http://www.azcc.arizona.edu/Default6.htm

California

City of Hope National Medical Center & Beckman Research Institute
1500 E. Duarte Rd.
Duarte, CA 91010-3000.
Phone: (626) 256-HOPE (4673)
Fax: (626) 930-5394
E-mail: http://www.cityofhope.org

Chao Family Comprehensive Cancer Center
University of California at Irvine
101 The City Drive
Building 56, Rt. 81, Room 406
Orange, CA 92868.
Phone: (714) 456-6310
Fax: (714) 456-2240
E-mail: http://www.ucihs.uci.edu/cancer

Jonsson Comprehensive Cancer Center
University of California Los Angeles
Factor Building, Room 8-684
10833 Le Conte Avenue
Los Angeles, CA 90095-1781.
Phone: (310) 825-5268
Fax: (310) 206-5553
E-mail: http://www.cancer.mednet.ucla.edu/

Moores Comprehensive Cancer Center
University of California, San Diego
3855 Health Sciences Drive, Room 2247
La Jolla, CA 92093-0658.
Phone: (858) 822-1222
Fax: (858) 822-1207
E-mail: http://cancer.ucsd.edu

USC/Norris Comprehensive Cancer Center
University of Southern California
1441 Eastlake Avenue, NOR 8302L
Los Angeles, CA 90089-9181.
Phone: (323) 865-0816
Fax: (323) 865-0102
E-mail: http://ccnt.hsc.usc.edu/

UCSF Helen Diller Family Comprehensive Cancer Center
University of California San Francisco
1450 3rd Street
Room HD-371, UCSF Box 0128
San Francisco, CA 94115-0128.
Phone: (415) 502-1710
Fax: (415) 502-1712
E-mail: http://cc.ucsf.edu/

Colorado

University of Colorado Cancer Center
University of Colorado at Denver & Health Sciences Center
P.O. Box 6508, Mail Stop F434
13001 E. 17th Place
Aurora, CO 80045.
Phone: (303) 724-3155
Fax: (303) 724-3162
E-mail: http://www.uccc.info/

Connecticut

Yale Cancer Center
Yale University School of Medicine
333 Cedar Street, Box 208028
New Haven, CT 06520-8028.
Phone: (203) 785-4371
Fax: (203) 785-4116
E-mail: http://www.info.med.yale.edu/ycc/

District of Columbia

Lombardi Comprehensive Cancer Center
Georgetown University
3970 Reservoir Road, NW
Research Bldg., Ste. E501
Washington, DC 20007.
Phone: (202) 687-2110
Fax: (202) 687-6402
E-mail: http://lombardi.georgetown.edu/

Florida

H. Lee Moffitt Cancer Center and Research Institute
University of South Florida
12902 Magnolia Drive, MCC-CEO
Tampa, FL33612-9497.
Phone: (813) 615-4261
Fax: (813) 615-4258
E-mail: http://www.moffitt.usf.edu/

Illinois

Robert H. Lurie Comprehensive Cancer Center
Northwestern University
303 East Superior Street, Ste. 3-125
Chicago, IL 60611.
Phone: (312) 908-5250
Fax: (312) 908-1372
E-mail: http://cancer.northwestern.edu/home/index.cfm

University of Chicago Comprehensive Cancer Center
5841 South Maryland Avenue, MC 2115
Chicago, IL 60637-1470.
Phone: (773) 702-6180
Fax: (773) 702-9311
E-mail: http://www-uccrc.uchicago.edu/

Iowa

Holden Comprehensive Cancer Center
University of Iowa 5970
"Z" JPP
200 Hawkins Drive
Iowa City, IA 52242.
Phone: (319) 353-8620
Fax: (319) 353-8988
E-mail: http://www.uihealthcare.com/depts/cancercenter/

Maryland

The Sidney Kimmel Comprehensive Cancer Center
Johns Hopkins University
401 North Broadway
The Weinberg Building, Suite 1100
Baltimore, MD 21231.
Phone: (410) 955-8822
Fax: (410) 614-6787
E-mail: http://www.hopkinskimmel cancercenter.org/index.cfm

Massachusetts

Dana-Farber/Harvard Cancer Center
Dana-Farber Cancer Institute
44 Binney Street, Room 1628
Boston, MA 02115.
Phone: (617) 632-2100
Toll free: (877) 420-3951
Fax: (617) 632-4452
E-mail: http://www.dfhcc.harvard.edu/pub_index.shtml?bhcp = 1

Michigan

Comprehensive Cancer Center
University of Michigan
6302 Cancer Center
1500 East Medical Center Drive
Ann Arbor, MI 48109-0942.
Phone: (734) 936-1831
Toll free: (800) 865-1125
Fax: (734) 615-3947
E-mail: http://www.cancer.med.umich.edu/

The Barbara Ann Karmanos Cancer Institute
Wayne State University School of Medicine
4100 John R
Detroit, MI 48201.
Toll free: (800) KARMANOS
Fax: (313) 576-8630
E-mail: http://www.karmanos.org

Minnesota

Masonic Cancer Center
University of Minnesota
MMC 806, 420 Delaware Street, S.E.
Minneapolis, MN 55455.
Phone: (612) 624-8484
Toll free: (888) 226-2376
Fax: (612) 626-3069
E-mail: http://www.cancer.umn.edu/

Mayo Clinic Cancer Center
Mayo Clinic Rochester
200 First Street, S.W.
Rochester, MN 55905.
Phone: (507) 266-4997
Fax: (507) 284-1544
E-mail: http://mayoresearch.mayo.edu/mayo/research/cancercenter/

Missouri

Siteman Cancer Center
Washington University School of Medicine
660 South Euclid Avenue, Campus Box 8109
St. Louis, MO 63110.
Phone: (314) 362-8020
Fax: (314) 454-1898
E-mail: http://www.siteman.wustl.edu

New Hampshire

Norris-Cotton Cancer Center
Dartmouth-Hitchcock Medical Center
One Medical Center Drive, Hinman Box 7920
Lebanon, NH 03756-0001.
Phone: (603) 653-9000
Fax: (603) 653-9003
E-mail: http://www.cancer.dartmouth.edu/index.shtml

New Jersey

The Cancer Institute of New Jersey
Robert Wood Johnson University Hospital and Medical School
195 Little Albany Street
New Burnswick, NJ 08903-2681.
Phone: (732) 235-8064
Fax: (732) 235-8094
E-mail: http://www.cinj.org

New York

Herbert Irving Comprehensive Cancer Center
College of Physicians and Surgeons
Columbia University
1130 St. Nicholas Avenue
Room 508
New York, NY 10032.
Phone: (212) 851-5273
Fax: (212) 851-5236
E-mail: http://www.ccc.columbia.edu/

Memorial Sloan-Kettering Cancer Center
1275 York Avenue
New York, NY 10021.
Phone: (212) 639-2000
Toll free: (800) 525-2225
Fax: (212) 717-3299
E-mail: http://www.mskcc.org/mskcc/html/44.cfm

Roswell Park Cancer Institute
Elm and Carlton Streets
Buffalo, NY 14263-0001.
Phone: (716) 845-5772
Fax: (716) 845-8261
E-mail: http://www.roswellpark.org/

North Carolina

Duke Comprehensive Cancer Center
Duke University Medical Center
Box 2714
Durham, NC 27710.
Phone: (919) 684-5613
Fax: (919) 684-5653
E-mail: http://cancer.duke.edu/

UNC Lineberger Comprehensive Cancer Center
University of North Carolina Chapel Hill
102 Mason Farm Road, CB 7295
Chapel Hill, NC 27599-7295.
Phone: (919) 966-3036
Fax: (919) 966-3015
E-mail: http://cancer.med.unc.edu/

Wake Forest Comprehensive Cancer Center
Wake Forest University
Medical Center Blvd.
Winston-Salem, NC 27157-1082.
Phone: (336) 716-7971
Fax: (336) 716-0293
E-mail: http://www1.wfubmc.edu/cancer

Ohio

Case Comprehensive Cancer Center
Case Western Reserve University
11100 Euclid Avenue, Wearn 151
Cleveland, OH 44106-5065.
Phone: (216) 844-8562
Fax: (216) 844-4975
E-mail: http://cancer.case.edu

Comprehensive Cancer Center
Ohio State University
OSU James Cancer Hospital
300 W. 10th Avenue, Ste. 519
Columbus, OH 43210.
Phone: (614) 293-7521
Fax: (614) 293-3132
E-mail: http://www.jamesline.com

Pennsylvania

Abramson Cancer Center
University of Pennsylvania
16th Floor Penn Tower
3400 Spruce Street
Philadelphia,
PA 19104-4283.
Phone: (215) 662-6065
Fax: (215) 349-5325
E-mail: http://www.penncancer.org/

Fox Chase Cancer Center
333 Cottman Avenue
Philadelphia, PA 19111.
Phone: (215) 728-3636
Fax: (215) 728-2571
E-mail: http://www.fccc.edu/

University of Pittsburgh Cancer Institute
UPMC Cancer Pavilion
5150 Centre Avenue,
Suite 500
Pittsburgh, PA 15232.
Phone: (412) 623-3205
Fax: (412) 623-3210
E-mail: http://www.upci.upmc.edu/index

Tennessee

St. Jude Children's Research Hospital
262 Danny Thomas Place
Memphis, TN 38105-3678.
Phone: (901) 595-3982
Fax: (901) 595-3966
E-mail: http://www.stjude.org

Vanderbilt-Ingraham Cancer Center
Vanderbilt University
691 Preston Research Building
Nashville, TN 37232-6838.
Phone: (615) 936-1782
Fax: (615) 936-1790
E-mail: http://www.vicc.org/

Texas

M.D. Anderson Cancer Center
University of Texas 1515
Holcombe Boulevard, Box 91
Houston, TX 77030.
Phone: (713) 792-2121
Fax: (713) 799-2210
E-mail: http://www.mdanderson.org/

Washington

Fred Hutchinson/University of Washington Cancer Consortium
Fred Hutchinson Cancer Research Center
P.O. Box 19024, D1-060
Seattle, WA 98109-1024.
Phone: (206) 667-4305
Fax: (206) 667-5268
E-mail: http://www.fhcrc.org/

Wisconsin

Paul P. Carbone Comprehensive Cancer Center
University of Wisconsin
600 Highland Avenue,
Room K4/610
Madison, WI 53792-0001.
Phone: (608) 263-8610
Fax: (608) 263-8613
E-mail: http://www.cancer.wisc.edu/

APPENDIX II: NATIONAL SUPPORT GROUPS

African American Breast Cancer Alliance (AABCA)
P.O. Box 8981
Minneapolis, MN 55408-0981
Phone: (612) 825-3675
E-mail: aabacainc@yahoo.com
Web site: http://www.geocities.com/aabcainc/
Breast cancer support for patients, families, and communities.

ALCASE - Alliance for Lung Cancer Advocacy, Support, and Education
P.O. Box 849500 West Eighth Street, Suite 240
Vancouver WA 98660
Phone: (800) 298-2436
Fax: (360) 735-1305
E-mail: info@alcase.org
Web site: http://www.alcase.org
Education, regional support group referrals, and Phone Buddies program.

American Brain Tumor Association (ABTA)
2720 River Rd, Suite 146
Des Plaines, IL 60018
Phone: (800) 886-ABTA
Fax: (847) 827-9918
E-mail: info@abta.org
Web site: http://hope.abta.org/site/PageServer
Brain tumor information, support, and resources.

American Cancer Society (ACS)
2200 Century Parkway, Suite 950
Atlanta, GA 30345
Phone: (800) ACS-2345
Fax: (404) 315-9348
Web site: http://www.cancer.org

American Foundation for Urologic Disease (AFUD)
1000 Corporate Boulevard, Suite 410
Linthicum, MD 21090
Phone: (800) 828-7866
Fax: (410) 689-3998
E-mail: admin@afud.org
Web site: http://www.afud.org

American Liver Foundation
75 Maiden Lane, Suite 603
New York, NY 10038
Phone: (800) GO-LIVER
Web site: http://www.liverfoundation.org

American Lung Association (ALA)
61 Broadway, 6th Floor
New York, NY 10006
Phone: (800) LUNGUSA
Fax: (212) 315-8872
E-mail: info@lungusa.org
Web site: http://www.lungusa.org
Promotes research, education, and advocacy for prevention of lung disease.

Association of Cancer Online Resources (ACOR)
Web site: http://www.acor.org
Links.

Association for Research of Childhood Cancer (AROCC)
P.O. Box 251
Buffalo, NY 14225-0251
Phone: (716) 681-4433
E-mail: odonnell@msn.org
Web site: http://www.arocc.org
Provides support to parents of children with cancer.

Brain Tumor Foundation for Children
1835 Savoy Drive, Suite 316
Atlanta, GA 30341
Phone: (770) 458-5554
Fax: (404)458-5467
E-mail: btfc@bellsouth.net
Web site: http://www.btfcgainc.org/index.asp
Brain tumor information, support, and resources for families of children with brain tumors.

The Brain Tumor Society
124 Watertown St., Suite 3-H
Watertown, MA 02472
Toll free: (800) 770-8287
Web site: http://www.tbts.org

Cancer Care, Inc.
275 Seventh Avenue
New York, NY 10001-6708
Phone: (800) 813-4673
Fax: (212) 712-8495
E-mail: info@cancercare.org
Web site: http://www.cancercare.org
Assists patients and families with the emotional, psychological, and financial consequences of cancer. Toll-free counseling hotline, educational pamphlets, newsletter, and referrals.

Cancer Care of New Jersey
141 Dayton Street
Ridgewood, NJ 07450
Phone: (201) 444-6630
E-mail: njinfo@cancercare.org
Web site: http://www.cancercare.org
Provides counseling, information, and financial assistance to patients and families.

Cancer Control Society (CCS)
2043 North Berendo Street
Los Angeles, CA 90027
Phone: (323) 663-7801
Fax: (323) 663-7757
E-mail: cancercontrol@cox.net
Web site: http://www.cancercontrolsociety.com
Educates health professionals and the public about preventing and controlling cancer and other diseases through many various methods.

Cancer Federation (CFI)
P.O. Box 1298
Banning, CA 92220-0009
Toll free: (800) 207-2873
Fax: (909) 849-0156
E-mail: info@cancerfed.org
Web site: http://www.cancerfed.com
Provided education and counseling for patients with cancer and their families.

Cancer Hope Network
Two North Rd., Suite A
Chester, NJ 07930

Phone: (877) HPE-NET
Fax: (908) 879-6518
E-mail: info@cancerhopenetwork.org
Web site: http://www.cancerhopenetwork.org
Matches cancer patients and their families with trained volunteers who have undergone and recovered from a similar cancer experience.

Cancer Information and Counseling Line (CICL)
1600 Pierce Street
Denver, CO 80214
Phone: (800) 525-3777
E-mail: cicl@amc.org
Web site: http://www.amc.org/
A toll-free telephone service for cancer patients, family members, friends, cancer survivors, and the general public. Education, short-term counseling, and referrals.

Cancer Survivors Network
Phone: (877) 333-HOPE
Web site: http://www.acscsn.org
A telephone and Web-based service for cancer survivors, their families, caregivers, and friends.

Cancervive, Inc.
11636 Chayote Street
Los Angeles, CA 90049
Phone: (800) 4-TO-CURE
Fax: (310) 471-4618
E-mail: cancervivr@aol.com
Web site: http://www.cancervive.org
Education, telephone counseling, referrals, and other services.

The Candlelighters Childhood Cancer Foundation
3910 Warner St.P.O. Box 498
Kensington, MD 20895
Phone: (800) 366-2223
Fax: (301) 962-3521
E-mail: info@candlelighters.org
Web site: http://www.candlelighters.org
Education and support for families of children with cancer.

Carcinoid Cancer Foundation (CCF)
333 Mamaroneck Avenue, No. 492
White Plains, NY 10605
Phone: (888) 722-3132
Fax: (914) 683-0183
E-mail: carcinoid@optonline.net
Web site: http://www.carcinoid.org/
Provides information, support, and resources for health care providers and for patients.

Caring and Sharing Cancer Support Group
401 South Freeman Street
Oceanside, CA 92054-4002
Phone: (760) 439-4307
E-mail: oceansidepier@juno.com
Provides support for seniors only. Looks into needs of anyone affected by any form of cancer.

CATS - Survivors Assisting Your Head Injury (CATS SAY-HI!)
P.O. Box 80346
Lansing, MI 48908-0346
Phone: (517) 676-3992
E-mail: catstbi@voyager.net
Web site: http://www.catstbi.org
Peer-led organization that provides support, education, information to survivors, friends, and communities for any head injury including tumors and other diseases and injuries.

Children's Blood Foundation (CBF)
333 East 38th, Room 830
New York, NY 10016
Phone: (212) 297-4336
Fax: (212) 297-4340
E-mail: info@childrensbloodfoundation.org
Web site: http://www.childrensbloodfoundation.org
Provides support to total patient care facility at Cornell Medical Center and sponsors special social events.

Children's Hospice International
901 N. Pitt St., Suite 230
Alexandria, VA 22314
Phone: (703) 684-0330 or
(800) 2-4-CHILD
E-mail: chiorg@aol.com
Web site: http://www.chionline.org
Support network and resource clearinghouse for dying children and their families.

Colon Cancer Alliance
175 Ninth Avenue
New York, NY 10011
Phone: Office: (212) 627-7451
Phone: Toll Free Helpline:
(877) 422-2030
Web site: http://www.ccalliance.org

Colorectal Cancer Network
P.O. Box 182
Kensington, MD 20895-0182
Phone: (301) 879-1500
E-mail: ccnetwork@colorectal-cancer.net
Web site: http://www.colorectal-cancer.net
Support groups, Internet chat room, hospital visitation programs, and a "One on One" service that connects newly diagnosed individuals with long-term survivors.

Corporate Angel Network (CAN)
Westchester County AirportOne
Loop Road
White Plains, NY 10604
Phone: (914) 328-1313
Fax: (914) 328-3938
E-mail: info@corpangelnetwork.org
Web site: http://
www.CorpAngelNetwork.org
Arranges free flights for patients with cancer who must travel to and from recognized treatment centers. All who do not need onboard care are eligible.

Cure for Lymphoma Foundation
215 Lexington Avenue
New York, NY 10016-6023
Phone: (800) CFL-6848
E-mail: info@cfl.org
Web site: http://www.cfl.org
Patient-to-patient telephone network, educational materials, research, and support.

CURE Childhood Cancer Association
200 Westfall Road
Rochester, NY 14620
Phone: (585) 473-0180
Fax: (585) 473-0201
E-mail: curekids@rochester.rr.com
Web site: http://curechildhoodcancer.org
Provides support (financial, educational, and emotional) to families coping with cancer in a child.

Cure Research Foundation
P.O. Box 3782
Westlake Village, CA 91359
Phone: (805) 498-0185
Fax: (805) 498-4868
E-mail: ccf@cancure.org
Web site: http://www.cancure.org
Dedicated to research and treatment in alternative cancer therapies. Also provides information on treatments and counseling services (where funded).

The Cutaneous Lymphoma Network
c/o Department of Dermatology,
University of Cincinnati P.O.
Box 670523
Cincinnati, OH 45267-0523
Phone: (513) 558-6805
Produces a newsletter with articles on this cancer, information on support groups, and opportunities for contact with other mycosis fungoides patients.

Dana-Farber Cancer Institute
44 Binney Street
Boston, MA 02115
Phone: (617) 632-3000

E-mail: dana-farbercontact-us@dfci.harvard.edu
Web site: http://www.dfci.harvard.edu
Dedicated to supporting children and adults with cancer.

Danville Cancer Association
1225 West Main Street
Danville, VA 24541
Phone: (434) 792-3700
Fax: (434) 791-3187
Supports cancer patients with supplies, equipment, transportation, and financial assistance. Also sponsors C.O.P.I.N.G. Cancer Support Group.

EyesOnThePrize.Org
446 S. Anaheim Hills Road, #108
Anaheim Hills, CA 92807
Web site: http://www.eyesontheprize.org
On-line information and emotional support for women with gynecologic cancer.

Federation for Children with Special Needs
1135 Trumont Street
Boston, MA 02120
Phone: (800) 331-0688
Web site: http://www.fcsn.org
Provides information, support, and assistance to parents of children with disabilities, their professional partners, and their communities.

Florida Brain Tumor Association
P.O. Box 770182-0182
Coral Springs, FL 3307-0182
Phone: (954) 755-4307
Fax: (954) 755-3206
E-mail: bt1diva@aol.com
Dedicated to support brain tumor survivors and their families and health care professionals.

Gilda's Club
322 Eighth Avenue
New York, NY 10001
Phone: (888) GILDA-4-U
Fax: (917) 305-0549
E-mail: info@gildasclub.org
Web site: http://www.gildasclub.org
Support groups for children, teens and adults, lectures, workshops, networking groups, special events, and children's programs.

Gyn Cancer Network
c/o Cancer Action Inc.
255 Alexander Street
Rochester, NY 14607
Phone: (716) 423-9700
Fax: (716) 423-9072
Web site: http://www.canceraction.org
Dedicated to supporting women with gynecological cancer.

Gynecologic Cancer Foundation
401 North Michigan Avenue
Chicago, IL 60611
Phone: (800) 444-4441.
(312) 644-6610.
Web site: http://www.wcn.org/gcf
Research, education, and philanthropy for women with gynecologic cancer.

Hairy Cell Leukemia Research Foundation
2345 County Farm Lane
Schaumburg, IL 60194
Phone: (800) 693-6173
Web site: http://www.hairycellleukemia.org/

HOPE Center for Cancer Support
297 Wickenden Street
Providence, RI 02903
Phone: (401) 454-0404
Fax: (401) 454-0411
E-mail: hope@hopecenter.net
Web site: http://www.hopecenter.org

International Myeloma Foundation
12650 Riverside Dr., Suite 206
North Hollywood, CA 91607
Phone: (800) 452-CURE
Fax: (818) 487-7454
E-mail: theimf@myeloma.org
Web site: http://www.myeloma.org
Support and treatment information for myeloma patients and their families.

International Waldenstrom's Macroglobulinemia Foundation
2300 Bee Ridge Road
Sarasota, FL 34239-6226
Phone: (941) 927-IWMF
Web site: http://www.iwmf.com
Information, educational programs, support for patients and families, research support.

The Johns Hopkins Meningioma Society
Johns Hopkins University Harvey
811600 North Wolfe Street
Baltimore, MD 21205-8811
Phone: (410) 614-2886
Web site: http://www.meningioma.org

Kidney Cancer Association
1234 Sherman Ave, Suite 203
Evanston, IL 60202
Phone: (800) 850-9132
Fax: (847) 332-2978
E-mail: office@kidneycancerassociation,org
Web site: http://www.kidneycancerassociation.org
Supports research, offers printed materials about the diagnosis and treatment of kidney cancer, sponsors support groups, and provides physician referral information.

Lance Armstrong Foundation (LAF)
P.O. Box 161150
Austin, TX 78716-1150
Phone: (512) 236-8820
E-mail: livestrong@laf.org
Web site: http://www.laf.org
Serves the public through advocacy, research, and education including LiveStrong (www.livestrong.org) a resource for people dealing with cancer.

Leukemia & Lymphoma Society
1311 Mamaroneck Avenue
White Plains, NY 10605
Phone: (800) 955-4572
Fax: (914) 949-6691
E-mail: infocenter@leukemia-lymphoma.org
Web site: http://www.leukemia-lymphoma.org/hm_lls
Education, free materials, and various support services. Also sponsors research.

Life Raft Group (LRG)
555 Preakness Avenue, Level 2E, Suite 2
Totowa, NJ 07512
Phone: (973) 389-2070
Fax: (973) 389-2073
E-mail: liferaft@liferaftgroup.org
Web site: http://www.liferaftgroup.org
Dedicated to providing support through information, research, and education for patients with Gastrointestinal Stromal Tumor (GIST).

Look Good. . .Feel Better
Phone: (800) 395-LOOK
Web site: http://www.lookgoodfeelbetter.org
For adults and teens undergoing cancer treatment; offers techniques and assistance in improving physical appearance.

The Lymphoma Research Foundation of America, Inc.
8800 Venice Boulevard, Suite 207
Los Angeles, CA 90034
Phone: (800) 500-9976
Fax: (310) 204-7043
E-mail: lrf@lymphoma.org
Web site: http://www.lymphoma.org
Supports research into treatments for lymphoma and provides educational and emotional support programs for patients and families.

Make Today Count (MTC)
1235 East Cherokee Street
Springfield, MO 65804-2203
Phone: (417) 885-2588
Fax: (417) 885-2587
E-mail: czimmerman@sprg.smhs.com;
Provides information, support, and resources to health professionals, patients, families, and friends.

Mothers Supporting Daughters with Breast Cancer (MSDBC)
21710 Bayshore Road
Chestertown, MD 21620
Phone: (410) 778-1982
Fax: (410) 778-1411
E-mail: msdbc@dmv.com
Web site: http://www.mothers daughters.org
Support for mothers of daughters who have been diagnosed with breast cancer.

Multiple Myeloma Research Foundation
51 Locust Avenue, No. 201
New Canaan, CT 06840-4739
Phone: (203) 972-1250
E-mail: themmrf@themmrf.org
Web site: http://www.multiplemyeloma.org
Information for patients and families. Dedicated to raising awareness of the disease and funding research.

The Mycosis Fungoides Foundation
P.O. Box 374
Birmingham, MI 48102-0374
Phone: (248) 644-9014
Web site: http://mffoundation.org

National Alliance of Breast Cancer Organizations
9 East 37th St., 10th floor
New York, NY 10016
Phone: (888) 80-NABCO
Fax: (212) 689-1213

National Association of Prostate Cancer Support Groups
P.O. Box 1253
Lakefield, Ontario
K0L 2H0 Canada
Phone: (866) 810-CPCN
Fax: (705) 652-0663
E-mail: cpcn@nexicom.net
Web site: http://www.cpcn.org

National Bone Marrow Transplant Link
20411 W. 12 Mile Rd., Suite 108
Southfield, MI 48076
Phone: (800) LINK-BMT
(800-546-5268)
Web site: http://www.nbmtlink.org
Web site provides publications about the logistics of bone marrow transplantation, information about the National Bone Marrow Transplant Link, and a peer support program.

National Brain Tumor Foundation (NBTF)
414 13th St., Suite 700
Oakland, CA 94612-2603
Phone: (510) 839-9777 or
(800) 934-CURE
E-mail: nbtf@braintumor.org
Web site: http://www.braintumor.org
Provides patients and their families with information on how to cope with brain tumors. National and regional conferences, printed materials, access to a national network of patient support groups, and answers to patient inquiries.

National Cancer Institute
9000 Rockville Pike, Building 31,
Room 10A16
Bethesda, MD 20892
Phone: (800) 422-6237.
Web site: http://www.nci.nih.gov

National Cervical Cancer Coalition (NCCC)
2625 Alcatraz Avenue, Suite 282
Berkley, CA 94705
Phone: (800) 685-5531. (818) 909-3849
Fax: (818) 780-9-8199
E-mail: info@nccc-online.org
Web site: http://www.nccc-online.org
Information, education, access to screening and treatment, and support services; sponsors the Cervical Cancer Quilt Project.

National Childhood Cancer Foundation (NCCF)
440 E. Huntington Dr., Suite 402 P.O. Box 60012
Arcadia, CA 91066-6012
Phone: (800) 458-6223 or
(626) 447-1674
Fax: (626) 447-6359
E-mail: info@nccf.org
Web site: http://www.curesearch.org/nccfintro.aspx

National Children's Cancer Society (NCCS)
1015 Locust, Suite 600
StreetLouis, MO 63101
Phone: (800) 532-6459
Fax: (314) 241-6949
E-mail: volunteers@children-cancer.com
Web site: http://www.nationalchildren scancersociety.com
Promotes children's health through financial and in-kind assistance, advocacy, support services, education and prevention programs.

National Children's Leukemia Foundation
172 Madison Avenue
New York, NY 10016
Phone: (212) 686-2722 or
(800) GIVE-HOPE
Fax: (212) 686-2750
Web site: http://www.leukemiafoun dation.org
Support network, bone marrow search, patient advocacy, education, and dream fulfillment.

National Coalition for Cancer Survivorship (NCCS)
1010 Wayne Ave., Suite 770
Silver Spring, MD 20910-5600
Phone: (877) 622-7937
Fax: (301) 565-9670
E-mail: info@canceradvocacy.org
Web site: http://www.canceradvocacy.org
A network for cancer support, advocacy, and quality of life issues.

National Comprehensive Cancer Network (NCCN)
500 Old York Road, Suite 250
Jenkintown, PA 19046
Phone: (215) 690-0300
Fax: (215) 690-0280
E-mail: information@nccn.org
Web site: http://www.nccn.org

National Kidney Foundation
30 East 33rd Street
New York, NY 10016.
Phone: (800) 622-9010
Web site: http://www.kidney.org

National Organization for Rare Disorders
100 Route 37 PO Box 8923
New Fairfield, CT 06812
Phone: (203) 746-6518
Web site: http://www.rarediseases.org
The National Organization for Rare Disorders (NORD) is committed to the identification, treatment, and cure of rare disorders through programs of education, advocacy, research, and service. NORD also provides referrals to additional sources of assistance and ongoing support.

National Ovarian Cancer Coalition (NOCC)
500 NE Spanish River Blvd., Suite 8
Boca Raton, FL 33431
Phone: (561) 393-0005 or
(888) OVARIAN
Fax: (561) 393-7275
E-mail: NOCC@ovarian.org
Web site: http://www.ovarian.org

Referral, support, educational materials, and a database of gynecologic oncologists searchable by state.

National Pancreas Foundation
PO Box 935
Wexford, PA 15090-0935
Web site: http://www.pancreasfoundation.org
The National Pancreas Foundation (NPF) was created to initiate and foster the pursuit of medical advancements in pancreatic disease research, as well as to develop a support network for all individuals suffering from pancreatic disorders.

National Retinoblastoma Parents Group
P.O. Box 317
Watertown, MA 02471
Phone: (800) 562-6265
Fax: (617) 972-7444
E-mail: napvi@perkins.pvt.k12.ma.us

Neurofibromatosis (NF)
9320 Annapolis Road, Suite 300
Lanham, MD 20706-3123
Phone: (301) 918-4600
Fax: (301) 918-0009
E-mail: nfinfo@nfinc.org
Web site: http://www.nfinc.org
Provides support for individuals with NF and for their families, health care providers and others.

Nevoid Basal Cell Carcinoma Syndrome Support Network
162 Clover Hill Street
Marlboro, MA 01752
Phone: (800) 815-4447.
E-mail: souldansur@aol.com
Web site: http://bccns.org/nbccs.htm/

Nevus Outreach
1601 Madison Boulevard
Bartlesville, OK 74006
Phone: (918) 331-0595
Web site: http://www.nevus.org/
Discussion groups, chat rooms, message board, and online services for patients with Biant Nevi and Neurocutaneous Melanosis.

OncoChat IRC Channel
Web site: http://www.oncochat.org
Online peer support for cancer survivors, family, and friends.

Pancreatic Cancer Action Network (PanCAN)
P.O. Box 1010
Torrance, CA 90505
Phone: (877) 2-PANCAN
E-mail: information@pancan.org
Web site: http://www.pancan.org
Advocacy, education, support links, and a survivorship forum.

Patient Advocate Foundation
753 Thimble Shoals Blvd, Suite B
Newport News, VA 23606
Phone: (800) 532-5274
Fax: (757) 873-8999
Web site: http://www.patientadvocate.org/
Serves as an active liaison between the patient and their insurer, employer and/or creditors to resolve insurance, job discrimination and/or debt crisis matters relative to their diagnosis through case managers, doctors and attorneys. Seeks to safeguard patients through effective mediation assuring access to care, maintenance of employment and preservation of their financial stability.

R. A. Bloch Cancer Foundation, Inc.
4400 Main Street
Kansas City, MO 64111
Phone: (800) 433-0464
Fax: (816) 931-7486
E-mail: hotline@hrblock.com
Web site: http://www.blochcancer.org
Matches newly diagnosed cancer patients with trained, home-based volunteers who have been treated for the same type of cancer. Offers informational materials, including a multidisciplinary list of institutions that offer second opinions.

Reach to Recovery
c/o American Cancer Society 1599 Clifton Road2454P.O. Box 102454
Atlanta, GA 30368
Phone: (800) ACS-2345
Web site: http://www.cancer.org/eprise/main/docroot/shr/content/shr_2.1_x_reach_to_recovery? sitearea = shr
Trained volunteers provide support and information for patients, families, and loved onew with breast cancer.

Ronald S. Hirshberg Pancreatic Cancer Information and Advocacy Center
375 Homewood Road
Los Angeles, CA 90049.
Phone: (310) 472-6310.
Web site: http://www.pancreatic.org
Provides informative booklets and other educational materials about pancreatic cancer, and offers referrals to support groups and other organizations.

San Francisco AIDS Foundation (SFAF)
995 Market Street, #200
San Francisco, CA 94103
Phone: (415) 487-3000 or (800) 367-AIDS
Fax: (415) 487-3009
Web site: http://www.sfaf.org

Sarcoma Alliance
775 East Blithedale #334
Mill Valley, CA 94941
Phone: (415) 381-7236
E-mail: info@sarcomaalliance.org
Web site: http://www.sarcomaalliance.org

Skin Cancer Foundation
245 Fifth Ave., Suite 1403
New York, NY 10016
Phone: (800) SKIN-490
Fax: (212) 725-5751
E-mail: info@skincancer.org
Web site: http://www.skincancer.org

Spinal Cord Tumor Support
Web site: http://www.spinalcordtumor.homestead.com

STARBRIGHT Foundation
11835 W. Olympic Blvd., Suite 500
Los Angeles, CA 90064
Phone: (310) 479-1212
Fax: (310) 479-1235
E-mail: ford@starbright.org
Web site: http://www.starbright.org
Creates projects and materials that are designed to help seriously ill children and adolescents cope with the psychosocial and medical challenges they face.

Support for People with Oral and Head and Neck Cancer (SPOHNC)
P.O. Box 53
Locust Valley, NY 11560-0053
Phone: (800) 377-0928
Web site: http://www.spohnc.org

United Ostomy Association, Inc.
19772 MacArthur Blvd., Suite 200
Irvine, CA 92612-2405
Phone: (800) 826-0826
E-mail: uoa@deltanet.com
Web site: http://www.uoa.org
Assists ostomy patients through mutual aid and emotional support, provides information to patients and the public, and sends volunteers to visit with new ostomy patients.

US TOO! International, Inc.
5003 Fairview Avenue
Downers Grove, IL 60515
Phone: (800) 80-US-TOO
E-mail: ustoo@ustoo.com
Web site: http://www.ustoo.org
A support group organization for cancer patients.

Vital Options and "The Group Room" Cancer Radio Talk Show
15060 Ventura Blvd., Suite 211
Sherman Oaks, CA 91403

Phone: (800) GRP-ROOM
E-mail: geninfo@vitaloptions.org
Web site: http://www.vitaloptions.org
Vital Options holds a weekly syndicated call-in cancer radio talk show called "The Group Room," a forum for patients, long-term survivors, family members, physicians, and therapists to discuss cancer issues; also simulcast on the Internet.

The Wellness Community
35 E. Seventh St., Suite 412
Cincinnati, OH 45202
Phone: (513) 421-7111 or (888) 793-WELL
E-mail: help@wellness-community.org
Web site: http://www.wellness-community.org
Support groups, stress reduction and cancer education workshops, nutrition guidance, exercise sessions, and social events.

Women's Cancer Resource Center
4604 Chicago Avenue South
Minneapolis, MN 55407
Phone: (877) 892-6742
Fax: (612) 822-4784
E-mail: wcrc@mr.net
Web site: http://www.givingvoice.org
Education, support, special programs, advocacy.

Y-ME National Breast Cancer Organization, Inc. (Now, Breast Cancer Network of Strength)
135 S. LaSalle St., Ste. 2000
Chicago, IL 60603
Phone: (312) 986-8338
Fax: (312) 294-8597
Web site: http://networkofstrength.org
Open-door groups, 24-hour hotline, early detection workshops, and support programs. Numerous local chapter offices located throughout the United States.

APPENDIX III: GOVERNMENT AGENCIES AND RESEARCH GROUPS

Agency for Healthcare Research and Quality
2101 E. Jefferson St., Suite 501
Rockville, MD 20852
Phone: (301) 594-1364
Web site: http://www.ahcpr.gov
Conducts and supports research and provides information for the health care consumer

American Association for Cancer Research
Public Ledger Bldg., Suite 826
150 S. Independence Mall West
Philadelphia, PA 19106-3483
Phone: (215) 440-9300
Fax: (215) 440-9313
Web site: http://www.aacr.org

American Brachytherapy Society (ABS)
12100 Sunset Hills Road, #130
Reston, VA 20190
Phone: (703) 234-4078
Fax: (703) 435-4390
Web site: http://www.americanbrachy therapy.org

American Brain Tumor Association (ABTA)
2720 River Road, Suite 146
Des Plaines, IL 60018
Phone: (847) 827-9910
Fax: (847) 827-9918
E-mail: info@abta.org
Web site: http://hope.abta.org/site/ PageServer

American Cancer Society
2200 Century Parkway, Suite 950
Atlanta, GA 30345
Phone: (800) ACS-2345
Fax: (404) 315-9348
Web site: http://www.cancer.org

American Foundation for Urologic Disease (AFUD)
1000 Coprorate Boulevard, Suite 410
Linthicum, MD 21090
Phone: (410) 689-3990
Fax: (410) 689-3998
E-mail: admin@afud.org
Web site: http://www.afud.org

American Head and Neck Society (AHNS)
c/o Paul A. Levine, Pres.
11300 West Olymic Boulevard, Suite 600
Los Angeles, CA 90064
Phone: (310) 437-0559
Fax: (310) 437-0585
E-mail: pal@virginia.edu
Web site: http://www.headnadneck cancer.org

American Headache Society (AHS)
19 Mantua Road
Mount Royal, NJ 08061
Phone: (856) 423-0043
Fax: (856) 423-0082
E-mail: ahshq@talley.com
Web site: http://www.ahsnet.org

American Institute for Cancer Research
1759 R St. NW
Washington, DC 20009
Phone: (800) 843-8114
Fax: (202) 328-7226
E-mail: aicrweb@aicr.org
Web site: http://www.aicr.org
Charity and research organization that focuses on diet and nutrition as they relate to the prevention and treatment of cancer.

American Lung Association (ALA)
61 Broadway, 6th Floor
New York, NY 10006
Phone: (800) LUNGUSA
Fax: (212) 315-8872
E-mail: info@lungusa.org
Web site: http://www.lungusa.org
Promotes research, education, and advocacy for prevention of lung disease.

American Radium Society (ARS)
53 West Jackson Boulevard, Suite 663
Chicago, IL 60604
Phone: (312) 322-0730
Fax: (312) 322-0732
E-mail: info@americanradium society.org
Web site: http://www.american radiumsociety.org

American Society for Therapeutic Radiology and Oncology (ASTRO)
12500 Fair Lakes Circle, Suite 375
Fairfax, VA 22033-3882
Phone: (703) 502-1550
Fax: (703) 502-7852
E-mail: webmaster@astro.org
Web site: http://www.astro.org

American Society of Breast Disease (ASBD)
P.O. Box 140186
Dallas, TX 75214
Phone: (214) 368-6836
Fax: (214) 368-5719
E-mail: info@asbd.org
Web site: http://www.asbd.org

American Society of Clinical Oncology (ASCO)
1900 Duke Street, Suite 200
Alexandria, VA 22314
Phone: (703) 299-0150
Fax: (703) 2991044
E-mail: asco@asco.org
Web site: http://www.asco.org

American Society of Cytopathology (ASC)
400 West Ninth Street, Suite 201
Wilmington, DE 19801
Phone: (302) 429-8802
Fax: (302) 429-8807
E-mail: asc@cytopathology.org
Web site: http://www.cytopathology. org

American Society of Pediatric Hematology/Oncology (ASPHO)
4700 West Lake Avenue
Glenview, IL 60025-1485

Phone: (847) 375 4716
Fax: (877) 734-9557
E-mail: info@aspho.org
Web site: http://www.aspho.org

American Society of Preventive Oncology (ASPO)
256 WARF Building
610 Walnut Street
Madison, WI 53705
Phone: (608) 263-9515
Fax: (608) 263-4497
E-mail: hasahel@facstaff.wisc.edu
Web site: http://www.aspo.org

Association for Research of Childhood Cancer (AROCC)
P.O. Box 251
Buffalo, NY 14225-0251
Phone: (716) 681-4433
E-mail: odonnell@msn.org
Web site: http://www.arocc.org

Association of American Cancer Institutes (AACI)
200 Lothrop Street
Iroquois Building, #308
Pittsburgh, PA 15213
Phone: (412) 647-2076
Fax: (412) 647-3659
E-mail: mail@aaci-cancer.org
Web site: http://www.aaci-cancer.org

Association of Cancer Executives (ACE)
475 South Frontage Road, Suite 101
Burr Ridge, IL 60527
Phone: (630) 323-1170
Fax: (630) 323-6989
E-mail: info@cancerexecutives.org
Web site: http://www.cancerexecutives.org

Association of Community Cancer Centers(ACCC)
11600 Nebel Street, Suite 201
Rockville, MD 20852
Phone: (301) 984-9496
Fax: (301) 770-1949
Web site: http://www.accc-cancer.org

Breast Cancer Alliance
15 East Putnam Avenue
Box 414
Greenwich, CT 06831-3301
Phone: (203) 861-0014
Fax: (203) 861-1940
E-mail: info@breastcanceralliance.org
Web site: http://www.breastcanceralliance.org

Cancer Treatment Research Foundation
3150 Salt Creek Lane, Suite 118
Arlington Heights,
IL 60005-1090
Phone: (888) 221-CTRF
Web site: http://www.ctrf.org

Cancer Control Society (CCS)
2043 North Berendo Street
Los Angeles, CA 90027
Phone: (323) 663-7801
Fax: (323) 663-7757
E-mail: cancercontrol@cox.net
Web site: http://www.cancercontrolsociety.com

Cancer Federation (CFI)
P.O. Box 1298
Banning, CA 92220-0009
Phone: (909) 849-4325
Fax: (909) 849-0156
E-mail: info@cancerfed.org
Web site: http://www.cancerfed.com

Cancer Research Foundation of America
1600 Duke Street, Suite 500
Alexandria, VA 22314
Phone: (703) 836-4412
Fax: (703) 836-4413
E-mail: info@preventcancer.org
Web site: http://www.preventcancer.org

Carcinoid Cancer Foundation
1751 York Ave.
New York, NY 10128
Phone: (888) 722-3132
Fax: (914) 683-5919
Web site: http://www.carcinoid.org
Research support, news, and education.

Centers for Disease Control and Prevention
1600 Clifton Rd.
Atlanta, GA 30333
Phone: (800) 311-3435
Web site: http://www.cdc.gov
Develops and applies disease control, environmental health, and health promotion and education. Operates the Cancer Control and Prevention program and the Tobacco Information and Prevention Source (TIPS).

Chemotherapy Foundation (CF)
183 Madison Avenue, Room 403
New York, NY 10016
Phone: (212) 213-9292
Fax: (212) 213-3831
E-mail: scox@chemotherapyfoundation.org

Children's Blood Foundation (CBF)
333 East 38th, Room 830
New York, NY 10016
Phone: (212) 297-4336
Fax: (212) 297-4340
E-mail: info@childrensbloodfoundation.org
Web site: http://www.childrensbloodfoundation.org

Children's Leukemia Research Association (NLA)
585 Stewart Avenue, Suite LL18
Garden City, NY 11530
Phone: (516) 222-1944
Fax: (516) 222-0457
E-mail: info@childrensleukemia.org
Web site: http://www.childrensleukemia.org

City of Hope National Medical Center (COH)
1500 East Duarte Road
Duarte, CA 91010
Phone: (626) 359-8111
Fax: (626) 301-8115
E-mail: egoehner@coh.org
Web site: http://www.cityofhope.org

Coleman Foundation
575 West Madison Street, Suite 4605
Chicago, IL 60661
Phone: (312) 902-7120
Fax: (312) 902-7124
E-mail: coleman@colemanfoundation.org
Web site: http://www.colemanfoundation.org

Concern Foundation
8383 Wilshire Boulevard, Suite 337
Beverly Hills, CA 90211
Phone: (310) 724-5333
Fax: (310) 858-1474
E-mail: info@concernfoundation.org
Web site: http://www.concernfoundation.org

Cure Research Foundation
P.O. Box 3782
Westlake Village, CA 91359
Phone: (805) 498-0185
Fax: (805) 498-4868
E-mail: ccf@cancure.org
Web site: http://www.cancure.org
Dedicated to research and treatment in alternative cancer therapies.

CuresNow
1710 North Vermont Avenue,
Suite 102
Los Angeles, CA 90027
Phone: (323) 660-6362
Fax: (310) 244-1480
E-mail: act@curesnow.org
Web site: http://www.curesnow.org
Dedicated to research in regenerative medicine.

Cystic Fibrosis Foundation
6931 Arlington Road
Bethesda, MD 20814
Phone: (301) 951-4422
Fax: (301) 951-6378
E-mail: info@cff.org
Web site: http://www.cff.org

Dedicated to supporting research, professional education, and care centers for patients with cystic fibrosis.

Damon Runyon Cancer Research Foundation
675 3rd Avenue, 25 Floor
New York, NY 10017
Phone: (212) 455-0500
Fax: (212) 455-0509
E-mail: info@drcrf.org
Web site: http://www.cancerresearch fund.org/
Dedicated to advancing cancer research through various monetary awards.

Friends of Cancer Research
3299 K. Street, NW, Suite 100
Washington, DC 20007
Phone: (202) 944-6711
Fax: (202) 333-7840
E-mail: info@focr.org
Web site: http://www.focr.org

Institutos Nacionales de la Salud (National Institutes of Health Hispanic Communications Initiative)
Web site: http://salud.nih.gov
A Spanish-language health information Web site.

International Myeloma Foundation
12650 Riverside Dr., Suite 206
North Hollywood, CA 91607
Phone: (818) 487-7455
Fax: (818) 487-7454
E-mail: theimf@myeloma.org
Web site: http://www.myeloma.org

International Oncology Study Group (IOSG)
4515 Verone
Bellaire, TX 77401
Phone: (713) 432-7229
Promotes clinical therapeutic research.

Kidney Cancer Association
1234 Sherman Ave, Suite 203
Evanston, IL 60202
Phone: (847) 332-1051
Fax: (847) 332-2978
E-mail: office@kidneycancer association,org
Web site: http://www.kidneycancer association.org
Supports research, offers printed materials about the diagnosis and treatment of kidney cancer, sponsors support groups, and provides physician referral information.

Leukemia & Lymphoma Society
1311 Mamaroneck Ave.
White Plains, NY 10605
Phone: (914) 949-5213
Fax: (914) 949-6691
E-mail: infocenter@leukemia-lymphoma.org
Web site: http://www.leukemia-lymphoma.org
Education, free materials, and various support services. Also sponsors research.

Life Raft Group (LRG)
555 Preakness Avenue, Level 2E, Suite 2
Totowa, NJ 07512
Phone: (973) 389-2070
Fax: (973) 389-2073
E-mail: liferaft@liferaftgroup.org
Web site: http://www.liferaftgroup.org
Dedicated to providing support through information, research, and education for patients with Gastrointestinal Stromal Tumor (GIST).

Lymphoma Research Foundation (LRF)
8800 Venice Boulevard, Suite 207
Los Angeles, CA 90034
Phone: (310) 204-7040
Fax: (310) 204-7043
E-mail: lrf@lymphoma.org
Web site: http://www.lymphoma.org

Melanoma Research Foundation (MRF)
24 Old Georgetown Road
Princeton, NJ 08540
Phone: (800) MRF-1290
Fax: (732) 821-5955
E-mail: mrf@melanoma.org
Web site: http://www.melanoma.org

Multiple Myeloma Research Foundation (MMRF)
51 Locust Avenue, #201
New Canaan, CT 06840-4739
Phone: (203) 972-1250
E-mail: themmrf@themmrf.org
Web site: http://www.multiplem yeloma.org

National Association for Proton Therapy
1301 Highland Drive
Silver Spring, MD 20910
Phone: (301) 587-6100
Fax: (301) 913-0372
E-mail: lenarzt@verizon.net
Web site: http://www.proton-therapy.org

National Breast Cancer Coalition (NBCC)
1707 L Street NW, Suite 1060
Washington, DC 20036
Phone: (202) 296-7477
Fax: (202) 265-6854
E-mail: info@natlbcc.org
Web site: http://www.stopbreastcancer.org
Promotes research into the cause, treatments and cures for breast cancer.

National Cancer Center (NCC)
88 Sunnyside Boulevard, Suite 307
Plainview, NY 11803
Phone: (516) 349-0610
Fax: (516) 349-1755
E-mail: info@nationalcancercenter.org
Supports educational programs and cancer research.

National Cancer Institute, National Institutes of Health
31 Center Dr., MSC 2580
Bethesda, MD 20892
Phone: (800) 4-CANCERTTY: (800) 332-8615
Web site: http://www.nci.nih.gov

National Center for Complementary and Alternative Medicine (NCCAM)
P.O. Box 8218
Silver Spring, MD 20907-8218
Phone: (888) 644-6226
Fax: (301) 495-4957
Web site: http://nccam.nih.gov
Conducts research and provides information on the safety and effectiveness of complementary and alternative therapies.

National Coalition for Cancer Research (NCCR)
426 C St. NW
Washington, DC 20004
Phone: (202) 544-1880
Fax: (202) 543-2565
E-mail: md@capitolassociates.com
Web site: http://www.cancercoalition.org
Advocacy group for cancer survivors and researchers—tracks cancer research and monitors legislation and funding.

National Foundation for Cancer Research
4600 W. West Highway, Suite 525
Bethesda, MD 20814
Phone: (800) 321-2873
Fax: (301) 654-5824
E-mail: sdeane@nfcr.org
Web site: http://www.nfcr.org/

National Women's Cancer Research Alliance (NWCRA)
The Entertainment Industry Foundation11132 Ventura Blvd., Suite 401
Studio City, CA 91604
Phone: (888) 87-NWCRA
Fax: (818) 760-7898
Web site: http://www.nwcra.org/

Office of Research on Minority Health
6707 Democracy Blvd., Suite 800
MSC 5465
Bethesda, MD 20892-5465

Phone: (301) 402-1366
Fax: (301) 480-4049
Web site: http://www.ncmhd.nih.gov/

Pediatric Cancer Research Foundation
18 Technology Dr., Suite 147
Irvine, CA 92618
Phone: (949) 727-7483
Fax: (949) 727-9501
E-mail: admin@pcrf-kids.com
Web site: http://www.pcrf.com

The Pediatric Oncology Branch of the National Cancer Institute
Phone: (301)496-4256
Toll free: (877) 624-4878
Web site: http://home.ccr.cancer.gov/oncology/pediatric/.

U.S. Food and Drug Administration
5600 Fishers Lane
Rockville, MD 20857-0001
Phone: (888) INFO-FDA
Web site: http://www.fda.gov/cder/cancer/index.htm
Contains an Oncology Tools section with information on cancer and approved cancer drugs, oncology reference tools, and other resources.

INDEX

In the index, references to individual volumes are listed before colons; numbers following a colon refer to specific page numbers within that particular volume. **Boldface** references indicate main topical essays. Photographs and illustration references are highlighted with an *italicized* page number; and tables are also indicated with the page number followed by a lowercase, italicized *t*.

B

C

D

E

F

G

H

I

J

K

L

M

N

O

P

Q

R

S

T

U

V

W

X

Y

Z